Pharmacopoeia Universalis: Or, a New Universal English Dispensatory. Containing

Robert James

Pharmacopœia Universalis

OR,

A NEW UNIVERSAL

English Dispensatory

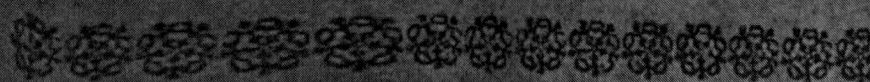

Pharmacopœia Universalis :

OR,

A NEW UNIVERSAL

English Dispensatory

BOOKS *just Published by the same* AUTHOR,

And Printed for J. HODGES at *London-Bridge.*

I. THE Modern Practice of Phyfick, as improved by the celebrated Profeffors *H. Boerhaave* and *F. Hoffman,* Phyfician to the late and prefent Kings of *Pruffia :* Being a Tranflation of the Aphorifms of the former, with the Commentaries of Dr. *Van Swieten,* fo far as was neceffary to explain the Doctrine laid down ; and of fuch Parts of Dr. *Hoffman*'s Works, as fupply the Deficiencies of *Boerhaave,* and render the whole Practice of Phyfick compleat ; wherein the various Difeafes to which the humane Body is fubject, are diftinctly confidered ; whence the Diognoftics and Prognoftics, together with the Method of Cure, are regularly deduced, and the Prefcriptions adapted thereto, from *Boerhaave*'s *Materia Medica,* are added to every Aphorifm. In 2 Vol. 8vo. Price 8 *s.*

II. The Prefages of Life and Death in Difeafes. In Seven Books. In which the whole *Hippocratic* Method of predicting the various Terminations and Events of Difeafes, is in a new and accurate Manner illuftrated and confirm'd, not only by the Sentiments and Opinions of the ancient Phyficians, but alfo by a long Courfe of attentive Obfervation and Experience. By *Profper Alpinus,* Profeffor of Medicine and Philofophy in the Univerfity of *Padua.* Tranflated from the laft *Leyden* Edition, revifed and publifhed by *Gaubius,* at the Requeft of Dr. *Boerhaave.*

Where is likewife to be had, lately Publifhed,

With a Frontifpiece, curioufly engraved, reprefenting an Inftrument neceffary to be ufed in one of the principal Operations,

I. A Phyfical Differtation on Drowning: In which Submerfion, commonly called Drowning, is fhewn to be a long Time confiftent with the Continuance of Life, from a Variety of unexceptionable, tho' furprifing Facts, related by the moft eminent and judicious Authors, and confirm'd by inconteftable Evidence ; which Facts are reconciled and accounted for, from the ftricteft Laws of the Animal Oeconomy. To which is fubjoin'd the proper Meafures for Recovery and Relief; the Obligations we lie under to practife them are clearly fuggefted, and ftrongly enforced ; intended for the Good of Mankind, by reftoring Life to many Perfons who are erroneoufly fuppofed to be irretrievably drowned, Recommended particularly to the Confideration of the Surgeons of the Navy and Army, who have frequent Opportunities of practifing the Methods recommended. With an Appendix, containing fome Methods for the Recovery of thofe who hang themfelves, and of Children fuppofed to be born dead. Price 1 *s.*

II. Obfervations in Surgery: Being a Collection of two Hundred and Forty-three different Cafes, with particular Remarks on each, for the Improvement of young Students. Alfo, the particular Receipts of fuch Remedies, as were ufed by the Author in each Cafe. Vol. I. Containing principally fuch Cafes as relate to the Male Sex. Vol. II. The Method of Practice in difficult Labours, and other Diftempers incident to the Female Sex, are copioufly enlarged. Embellifhed with Copper Plates curioufly engraved, reprefenting thofe Parts where the principal Cafes are particularly concerned. To which is added, a New Chirurgical Dictionary, for the Ufe of young Practitioners and Gentlemen refiding in the Country : Explaining the Terms of Art contained in the Body of the Book : And likewife, all fuch as properly belong to Phyfick and Surgery. Written originally in *French* by *Henry Francis le Dran,* eldeft Surgeon and Demonftrator of Anatomy at the Hofpital *la Charite,* and Mr. *Saviard,* chief Surgeon and Operator in Midwifry, at the *Hofpital Hotel Dieu* in *Paris.* Tranflated by *J. S.* Surgeon.

Pharmacopœia Universalis:

OR,

A NEW UNIVERSAL
English Dispensatory.

CONTAINING

I. An Account of all the Natural and Artificial Implements and Inftruments of Pharmacy, together with the Proceffes and Operations, whereby Changes are induc'd in Natural Bodies for Medicinal Purpofes.

II. Differtations on the various Claffes of Simples ; explaining their Operations and Ufes in Practice.

III. Catalogues of all the Medicinal Simples, wherein their particular Virtues and Ufes are fpecify'd.

IV. The Preparations and Combinations of Drugs ; containing all the Compofitions directed in the *London* and *Edinburgh Pharmacopœias* ; together with others felected from the moft celebrated Writers in Pharmacy and Phyfic.

V. An exact Calculation of the Proportion of each Ingredient in given Quantities of all the Compofitions of any Confequence.

With a Copious INDEX to the Whole.

By R. JAMES, M.D.

LONDON:

Printed for J. HODGES, at the *Looking-Glafs,* over-againft *St. Magnus*'s Church, *London Bridge* ; and J. WOOD under the Piazza of the *Royal Exchange.* 1747.

PREFACE.

MEdicine, like all other Sciences, is, and always must be, subject to Changes; and 'tis impossible it should be otherwise, particularly in the Practice of Physic. For the Discovery of any considerable Simple of great Efficacy, or of any important Virtues in those we were before acquainted with, must necessarily induce considerable Alterations in the Practice of the Art. Thus the Introduction of the Bark, absolutely alter'd the whole Practice of Physicians with Respect to Fevers. And perhaps the greatest Revolution that ever happened in Physic, was brought about by the Discovery of the Virtues of Mercury, a Drug before well known, in the Cure of Distempers. Formerly it was the Custom for the Writers of Dispensatories to embarrass their Compositions, and for Physicians to overload their Prescriptions, with a great Number of superfluous Ingredients; and hence the Efficacy of Medicines was render'd less certain, and the Practice of Physic more precarious. But for the last twenty or thirty Years, Physicians of the first Reputation for Learning, Sense, and Skill in their Profession, seem to have united in their Endeavours, to reduce this Luxuriance within the Bounds of Sense and Science; to prune away the Branches of Physic which bear no Fruit; and to restore the Art to that useful Simplicity which alone is productive of Pleasure and Advantage. And this Spirit of Reformation has induced a very considerable Change in the Modes of Practice, whilst it affords us the agreeable Prospect of having the remaining Superfluities retrench'd.

A new Dispensatory, *therefore, suited to the modern Taste in prescribing, appeared both a useful and necessary Work. And this I have endeavoured to execute in the following Manner:*

First, *I have given a plain and intelligible Account of the grand Implements, by which all the Changes in sublunary Bodies are brought about both by Art and Nature; I mean the Air, Water, Earth, and Fire; particularly so far as they relate to Medicine and Pharmacy.*

Secondly, *I have attempted to give a just Idea of Acids and Alcalis; and of their Influences in the Continuation of Life, the Preservation or Recovery of Health, and the Production of Diseases.*

Thirdly, *I have given some Account of all those Operations, by which Changes are induced in all those Bodies, which are the Subjects of* Pharmacy, *and* Chymistry.

Fourthly, *I have given Dissertations on the various Classes of Medicines, into which Simples are usually divided, in order to explain what is meant by these Divisions, how the Effects ascribed to them are brought about, and how far they may be depended upon, consistent with sound Philosophy, and, what is much better,* Experience.

Fifthly, *I have taken Care to specify the medicinal Virtues and Uses of all the Simples employed in Medicine, from the best Authorities, whether antient or modern. These I have divided into three Classes, that of Vegetables, of Animals, and of Minerals; this Division appearing to me the most commodious. And I have distributed each of them alphabetically, according to the* Latin *Names. The* English *Names are referr'd to from the general Index.*

The last Part consists of Preparations and Compositions; and with Respect to the latter, I think myself under no Necessity of making an Apology to the Public for having been more frugal of them than former Writers; because I am certain that there are

more

more than *sufficient to answer every Occasion ; and besides, a per-*
fect Acquaintance with the Materia Medica, *will enable the Ju-*
dicious to combine Simples, and adapt them to particular Cases
and Constitutions, in such a Manner, as to answer better Pur-
poses than any of the Compositions of the Shops. And I must
farther confess, that I think the unbounded Licentiousness of for-
mer Authors of Dispensatories, *with Respect to the Number of*
Compound Medicines, together with the Encomiums they have be-
stow'd upon each, have greatly prejudic'd true Physic, by inducing
abundant Perplexity, Error, and Confusion ; and after all, the
Physician's Excellence can never depend upon the Multiplicity of
Prescriptions, but upon a judicious Application of a few well-
chosen Remedies.

Tho' the last Attempts of the Colleges of London *and* Edinburgh *have done a great deal towards the Reformation of our*
Dispensatories, *yet I am inclined to believe it would have been*
better if they had proceeded farther, and alter'd, or rather ex-
chang'd their Medicines, whose Composition, notwithstanding
their Antiquity, render them extremely ridiculous ; such I mean, as
in the Quantity commonly given for a Dose, contain the Fraction
of a Grain of some Ingredient, which alone might be taken in
the Quantity of half an Ounce, without any considerable Effect,
or Efficacy, as will appear by the following Table.

In a Book not intended so much to be regularly perus'd, as oc-
casionally consulted, an Index *should seem to be absolutely necessary ;*
I have, therefore, procur'd one, which appears to be more ex-
tensive and useful, than any that have occur'd to me in Books of
this Kind. As it consists of near ten thousand plain References,
the Reader will without Difficulty turn to whatever Subject he
pleases.

In the whole Course of the Work, I have industriously suffer'd
the Names of Bate, Fuller, Quincy, *and even* Salmon, *with the*
rest of the Dispensatory Writers of our Country, to rest in Peace ;
neither disturbing them by Censure, nor perfuming them with In-
cense ; because I apprehend that meer Books of Prescriptions are
of too little Importance to be taken Notice of, much less to be tran-
scrib'd ;

scrib'd; and besides, they tend to promote Quackery, to cover Ignorance, and veil the dirty Craft of the Designing and Ungenerous, without producing any one Advantage as an Equivalent.

But if any one should think otherwise, they are already in the Hands of every male and female Practitioner, and may be consulted without much Embarrasment to their Admirers.

Lastly, I have procur'd an exact Calculation of the Proportion of each Ingredient in given Quantities of all the Compositions of Consequence; which may serve for the Instruction of young Practitioners; and the Reprehension of old ones, who have been accustom'd to give Doses of Medicines, without any (honest) Intention.

As nothing is more uncertain and undetermin'd than the Doses of Simples, and nothing more difficult than to lay down general Rules with Respect to the Quantities adapted to particular Ages, Constitutions, and Distempers, I hope I shall be excus'd for having been less particular upon this Subject than might have been expected. In general, I am afraid 'tis customary to give too small Doses of simple Medicines. This was remarkably the Case of the Bark when it was first known in Europe, of which a few Grains only were exhibited at a Time; and for this Reason it had grown into Disrepute, and had so continu'd, if an Empiric had not learn'd by Experience, that much larger Doses were necessary to effect a Cure. At present, Musk, which may be exhibited to very good Purposes in the Quantity of half a Dram, is only given, generally, in a Dose of four or five Grains; and the same may be said of many others. I should, therefore, recommend it seriously to all Practitioners, as a Thing of the greatest Consequence, to endeavour to determine, by all prudent Means, in what Quantities Simples may be safely exhibited, and with what Effect.

AN

A

CALCULATION

OF THE

Proportion of each Ingredient in given Quantities, of the principal Compositions.

CONFECTIO CARDIACA.

Quant.   *Proportion of the Ingredients.*

Grains

FRESH Rosemary Tops } Juniper Berries }	*each*	$3,4297 = 6,8595$
Lesser Cardamum Seeds, freed from Husks. }	$1,7143$ }	
Zedoary } Saffron }	*each* $1,7143$ }	$5,1430$
Tincture drawn with 7,0001 of } Spirits, and reduced, is }	$5,1430 = 5,1430$	
Compound Powder of Crabs Claws	$4,5714 = 4,5714$	
Cinnamon } Nutmeg }	*each* $0,5714 = 1,1428$	
Cloves	$0,2857 = 0,2857$	
Double refin'd Sugar	$6,8571 = 6,8571$	

Half a Dram.

Grains $30,0025$

            CONFECTI

CONFECTIO PAULINA.

Quant.	Proportion of the Ingredients.		
	Coftus		
	Cinnamon		
	Long Pepper		
	Black Pepper		each ,9375. is in all
Half a Dram.	Strain'd Sterax	}	Grains
	Strain'd Galbanum		7,5
	Strain'd Opium		
	Ruffia Caftor		
	Honey trip. to the whole Species	} is	22,5

Grains 30

DIACASSIA.

Half an Ounce.	Pulp of Caffia	75,7914
	Tamarinds	50,5276
	Calabrian Manna	37,8957
	Syrup of Damafk Rofes	75,7914

240 Grains.

ELECTUARIUM E CASSIA.

Half an Ounce.	Solutive Syrup of Rofes	96,=96,
	Pulp of Caffia frefh extracted	96,=96,
	Manna	32,=32,
	Pulp of Tamarinds	16,=16,

240 Grains.

DIAS

DIASCORDIUM.

Quant.   *Proportion of the Ingredients.*

	Leaves of Water German-der Cinnamon Nutmeg Japan Earth Gum Arabic Olibanum	*each* 1,6326	= 9,7959

One Dram.

Roots of Tormentil Bole Armoniac	*each* 2,4489	= 4,8979
Opium diffolved in a fuffi-cient Quantity of Ca-nary.	*is* 0,3061	= 0,3061
Syrup of dried Rofes boil'd to the Thicknefs of Honey, thrice the Weight of the Powders	*is* 44,9999	= 44,9999

Grains 59,9999

SPECIES E SCORDIO CUM OPIO.

Bole Armoniac	10,0787 &c. [a]
Scordium	5,0393 [a]
Cinnamon	3,7795 &c. [a]
Storax ftrain'd	2,5196 &c. [a]
Roots of Tormentil	2,5196
Biftort	2,5196
Leaves of Cretan Dittany	2,5196
Galbanum ftrain'd	2,5196
Gum Arabic	2,5196
Red Rofes	2,5196
Long Pepper	1,2598 &c.
Ginger	1,2598
Strain'd Opium	,9448 &c. [a]

Two Scruples

Grains 39,9898 = 2 ℈ *feré.*

ELECTUARIUM E SCORDIO.

1 Dram.

Species è Scordio cum Opio	45,
Diacodium	135,

180 *Grains.*

      EELEC.

ELECTUARIUM CARDIACUM.

Quant.	Proportion of the Ingredients.

Conferve of Rofemary.
Red Rofes } each 6,2068 = 12,4137

Orange Peel
Citron Peel, and } each 4,1379 = 12,4137

Thirty Grains. Nutmeg, candied.

Ginger candied 3,1034 = 3,1034
Confection of Kermes 2,0689 = 2,0689
Diftill'd Oil of Cinnamon 10,3448
Syrup of Cloves a fufficient Quantity.

Grains 29,9999

ELECTUARIUM E BACCIS LAURI.

Of the *London* Difpenfatory.

Leaves of Rue dried
Carraway Seeds
Common Parfley Seeds } each 12, = 48,
Half an Ounce. Bay Berries
Sagapenum 6, = 6,
Black Pepper
Ruffia Caftor } each 3, = 6,
Honey clarify'd 180 = 180

240 *Grains*.

ELECTUARIUM E BACCIS LAURI.

Of the *Edinburgh* Difpenfatory.

Conferve of Rue 123,8714
Candied Ginger 61,9352
Bay Berries 30,9676
Half an Ounce. Zedoary 15,4838
Ruffia Caftor
Diftill'd Oil of Fennel } 7,7419
Syrup of Orange Peel, a fufficient
Quantity

Grains 239,9999

ELEC-

ELECTUARIUM LENITIVUM.
Of the *London* Difpenfatory.

fant.   *Proportion of the Ingredients.*

Dried Figs	38,4=38,4
Leaves of Sena	25,6=25,6
Pulp of Tamarinds	
Caffia	each 19,2=57,6
French Prunes	
Coriander Seed	12,8=12,8
Liquorice	9,6= 9,6
Double refin'd Sugar	96,0=96,0

Half an Ounce.

240,0 *Grains.*

ELECTUARIUM LENITIVIUM.
Of the *Edinburgh* Difpenfatory.

Roots of Polypody of the Oak	1,9875= 1,9875
Leaves of Mercury	
Fenugreek Seed	each ,9937= 1,9875
Linfeed	,9937= ,9937
Spring Water	190,8 =190,8
Leaves of Sena	1,9875= 1,9875
Coriander Seeds	0,4968= 0,4968
Honey	23,85 = 23,85
Pulp of Damafk Prunes	11,9250= 11,9250
Pulp of Caffia	5,9625= 5,9625

Half an Ounce.

Grains 239,9905

ELECTARIUM E SCAMMONIO.

Scammony	14,8965
Cloves	7,4482
Ginger	7,4482
Effential Oil of Caraway Seeds	,6205
Honey	59,5860

A Dram and a Half.

Grains 89,999, *&c.*

MITHRI-

MITHRIDATIUM.

Of the *London* Dispensatory.

Quan.   *Proportion of the Ingredients.*

Cinnamon	2,8= 2,8
Myrrh	2,2= 2,2
Agaric	
Spikenard	
Ginger	
Saffron	each 2, =14,
Seeds of Treacle Mustard	
Frankincense	
Chio Turpentine	
Camel's Hay	
Costus	
Indian Leaf	
French Lavender	
Long Pepper	
Seeds of Hartwort	
Juice of the Rape of Cistus	each 1,6=19,2
Strain'd Storax	
Opoponax	
Strain'd Galbanum	
Balsam of Gilead	
Russia Castor	
Poley Mountain	1,4=1,4
Water Germander	1,4=1,4
The Fruit of the Balsam Tree	
White Pepper	each 1,4 is 5,6
Seeds of the Cretan Daucus	
Bdellium strain'd	
Celtic Nard	
Gentian Root	
Leaves of Dittany of Crete	
Red Roses	
Seeds of Macedonian Parsley	each 1, =9,
The lesser Cardamom Seeds freed from Husks	
Sweet Fennel Seeds	
Gum Arabic	
Opium strain'd	

Half an Ounce.

Root

Quant.   *Proportion of the Ingredients.*

	Root of the sweet Flag	
	Root of wild Valerian	each 0,6=2,4
	Aniseed	
	Sagapenum strain'd	
Half an Ounce.	Spignel	
	St. John's Wort	each 0,5=2,
	Juice of Acacia.	
	The Bellies of Scinks	
	Clarified Honey triple the whole Species	each 180,=180

$\mathrm{Z}\,ss.$ 240 Grains.

MITHRIDATIUM DAMOCRATIS.
Of the *Edinburgh* Dispensatory.

	Myrrh	
	Saffron	
	Agaric	
	Ginger	
	Cinnamon	each 1,9191=15,3535
	Spikenard	
	Male Frankincense	
	Seeds of Treacle Mustard	
	Balm of Gilead	
	Camel's Hay	
	Flowers of Arabian Stœchas	
	Costus	
	Galbanum	
	Cyprus Turpentine	
Half an Ounce.	Long Pepper	each 1,5483=20,1249
	Russia Castor	
	Juice of the Rape of Cistus	
	Calamita Storax	
	Opoponax	
	Indian Leaf	
	Cassia Lignea	
	Poley Mountain	
	White Pepper	
	Leaves of Water Germander	
	Seeds of the Cretan Daucus	each 1,3548=10,8384
	Carpobalsamum	
	Trochisci Cypheos	
	Bdellium	

Celticæ

Quant.   *Proportion of the Ingredients.*

Celtic Nard Gum Arabic Seeds of Macedonian Parſley Opium Leſſer Cardamom Seeds Fennel Seeds Gentian Root Red Roſes Dittany of Crete	} *each* 0,9677= 8,7093

Half an Ounce.

Aniſeed Roots of Aſarabacca Sweet Flag Wild Valerian Sagapenum	} *each* 0,5806= 2,9032
Roots of Spignal The true Acacia The Bellies of Scinks Seeds of St. John's Wort	} *each* 0,4838= 1,9352
Clarified Honey, thrice the Weight of the Powders.	} *each* 180, =180,

Grains 239,8648

PILULÆ ÆTHIOPICÆ.

Thirty Grains.

Of pure Quick-ſilver Golden Sulphur of Antimony Roſin of Guaiacum	} *each* 5,=15
Spaniſh Soap	5,= 5
Syrup of Balſam, a ſufficient Quantity.	20 Grains.

PILULÆ COCCIÆ.

Thirty Grains.

Of Succotrine Aloes Coloquintida Scammony	} *each* 8,8888=26,6666
Vitriolated Tartar	2,2222=22,2222
Diſtill'd Oil of Cloves	1,1111= 1,1111
Syrup of Buckthorn, a ſufficient Quantity.	

29,9999

PILULA

PILULÆ EX COLOCYNTHIDE CUM ALOE.

Quant.   *Proportion of the Ingredients.*

Half a Dram.
Socotorine Aloes	11,4285
Scammony	11,4285
Pith of Coloquintida	5,7142
Oil of Cloves	1,4285

                 Grains 29,9999

PILULÆ EX COLOCYNTHIDE SIMPLICIORE.

Half a Dram.
Coloquintida	14,1147
Scammony	14,1147
Oil of Cloves	1,7643

            Grains 29,9938

PILULÆ ECPHRACTICÆ.

Thirty Grains.
Aromatic Pill	13,8461 = 13,8461
Rhubarb	
Extract of Gentian	each 4,6153 = 13,8461
Salt of Iron	
Salt of Wormwood	2,3076 = 2,3076

            Grains 29,9999

PILULÆ ECPHRACTICÆ CHALYBEATÆ.

Thirty Grains.
Of the common Pills	14,4
Gum Ammoniac	
Rosin of Guaiacum	each 4,8 = 9,6
Salt of Steel	6,
Elixir of Propriety, a sufficient Quantity	

            Grains 30.

PILULÆ ECPHRACTICÆ CUM ACULEO.

Quant.	Proportion of the Ingredients.	

Thirty Grains.

Socotorine Aloes		
Extract of black Hellebore	} each 6,8391 = 20,5714
Scammony	
Gum Ammoniac	} each 3,4287 = 6,8574
Rofin of Guaiacum	
Vitriolated Tartar	1,7143 = 1,7143
Diftill'd Oil of Juniper	0,8571 = 0,8571
Syrup of Buckthorn, a fufficient Quantity.	

Grains 30·

PILULÆ E STYRACE.

Eight Grains.

Calamite Storax	1,9047 = 1,9047
Gum Dragant	3,0476 = 3,0476
Olibanum	
Opium	} each 1,5238 = 3,0476
Diacodium, a fufficient Quantity.	

Grains 7,9999·

PILULÆ E STYRACE.

Six Grains.

Strain'd Storax	3,3103
Saffron	1,6551
Strain'd Opium	1,0344

Grains 5,9999·

PIEUL EX DUOBUS.

Thirty Grains.

Coloquintida	} each 12,6312 = 25,2624
Scammony	
Vitriolated Tartar	3,1578 = 3,1578
Diftill'd Oil of Cloves	1,5789 = 1,5789

Grains 29,9999

PILULÆ

PILULÆ FOETIDÆ.

Quant.	Proportion of the Ingredients.	
Thirty Grains.	Affa fœtida	15,
	Ruffia Caftor	10,
	Camphire	5,
	Diftill'd Oil of Hartfhorn, a fufficient Quantity.	
		30 *Grains.*

PILULÆ DE GAMBOGIA.

Thirty Grains.	Socotorine Aloes		
	Extract of Black Hellebore	each 7,0588 = 28,2352	
	Gamboge		
	Calomel		
	Diftill'd Oil of Juniper	1,7647 = 1,7647	
	Syrup of Buckthorn, a fufficient Quantity.		
		Grains 29,9999	

PILULÆ GUMMOSÆ.

Thirty Grains.	Gum Ammoniac	each 6,4864 = 12,9728
	Sagapenum	
	Ruffia Caftor	each 4,8648 = 9,7296
	Myrrh	
	Affa fœtida	each 3,2432 = 6,4864
	Galbanum	
	Diftill'd Oil of Amber	,8108 = ,8108
	Elixir of Propriety, a fufficient Quantity.	
		Grains 29,9999

PILULÆ LAXANTES.

Thirty Grains.	Of pure Quick-filver	12, = 12
	Honey, a fufficient Quantity.	
	Gum Ammoniac	
	Extract of black Hellebore	each 6, = 18
	Rhubarb	
		Grains 30

PILU-

PILULÆ MATHÆI.

Quant.	Proportion of the Ingredients.	
Eight Grains.	Ruffia Caftor	2,2857=2,2857
	Englifh Saffron	
	Opium	each 1,1428=2,2857
	Soap of Tartar	3,4285=3,4285
	Balfam Capivi, a fufficient Quantity.	

Grains 7,9966

PILULÆ MERCURIALES.

Of the *London* Difpenfatory.

Half a Dram.	Quick-filver	16,0714
	Strasburgh Turpentine	6,4285
	Cathartic Extract	4,2857
	Rhubarb in Powder	3,2142

Grains 29,9999

PILULÆ MERCURIALES.

Of the *Edinburgh* Difpenfatory.

Thirty Grains.	Pure Quick-filver	10,
	Honey, a fufficient Quantity.	
	Gum Ammoniac	20,

Grains 30

PILULÆ PACIFICÆ.

Six Grains.	Ruffia Caftor	1,7142=1,7142
	Englifh Saffron	
	Opium	each ,8571=1,7142
	Soap of Tartar	2,5713=2,5713
	Balfam Capivi, a fufficient Quantity.	

Grains 5,9999

PILULÆ

PILULÆ RUDII.

Proportion of the Ingredients.

Eight Grains.	Roots of black Hellebore } Coloquintida }	each 1,0885=	2,1670
	Spring Water	26,0044=	26,0044
	Socotorine Aloes	1,0835=	1,0835
	Scammony	0,5417=	0,5417
	Vitriolated Tartar	0,1354=	3,1354
	Diftill'd Oil of Cloves	0,0677=	0,0677

Grains 29,9999

EXTRACTUM CATHARTICUM,

Of the *London* Difpenfatory.

Thirty Grains.	Socotorine Aloes	2,3376=	2,3376
	Pith of Coloquintida	1,1688=	1,1688
	Scammony } Leffer Cardamum Seeds } huík'd	each 0,7792=	1,5584
	Proof Spirit	24,9344=	24,9344

Grains 29,9999

PILULÆ RUFI.

Of the *London* Difpenfatory.

Thirty Grains.	Socotorine Aloes	15,
	Myrrh	7,5
	Saffron	7,5

Grains 30,0

PILULÆ RUFI.

Of the *Edinburgh* Difpenfatory.

Thirty Grains.	Socotorine Aloes	26,6666
	Myrrh	2,2222
	Saffron	1,1111
	Syrup of Orange Peel, a fufficient Quantity.	

30 Grains,

PILULÆ SAPONACEÆ.

Quant.	Proportion of the Ingredients.	
Ten Grains.	Almond Soap	8,6486
	Strain'd Opium	1,0810
	Essence of Lemon	,1351

Grains 9,8647

PILULÆ SCILLITICÆ.

Thirty Grains.	Spanish Soap	12 = 12
	Gum Ammoniac	
	Woodlice prepar'd } each	6 = 18
	Fresh Squills	
	Balsam Capivi, a sufficient Quantity.	

Grains 30

PILULÆ STOMACHICÆ.

Thirty Grains.	Socotorine Aloes	10,6666 = 10,6666
	Rhubarb	8 = 8
	Gum Ammoniac	4 = 4
	Extract of Gentian } each	2,6666 = 5,3333
	Myrrh	
	Vitriolated Tartar	1,3333 = 1,3333
	Distill'd Oil of Mint	0,6666 = 0,6666
	Syrup of Sena and Rhubarb, a sufficient Quantity.	

Grains 29,9999

PHILONIUM LONDINENSE.

Half a Dram.	White Pepper	
	Ginger } each	2,2222 = 6,6666
	Carraway Seeds	
	Opium strain'd	0,8333 = 0,8333
	Honey clarified, thrice the Quant.	22,4999 = 22,4999

Grains 29,9999

PULVIS ARI COMPOSITUS.

fiat.   *Proportion of the Ingredients.*

Fresh dried Roots of Arum	
Roots of Calamus Aromaticus	$\left.\begin{array}{c} \\ \\ \\ \end{array}\right\}$ *each* 7,8048 = 7,8048
Roots of Pimpinel Saxifrage.	
Crabs Eyes	3,9024 = 7,8048
Cinnamon	1,9512 = 1,9512
Salt of Wormwood	1,4634 = 1,4634
	0,9756 = 0,9756

Twenty Grains.

Grains 19,9999

PULVIS BEZOARDICUS.

Thirty Grains.

Compound Powder of Crab's Claws	$\left.\begin{array}{c} \\ \\ \end{array}\right\}$ 27,6923
Oriental Bezoar	6,5217

29,9999

PULVIS E BOLO COMPOSITUS CUM OPIO.

Half a Dram.

Bole Armoniac	10,6666 &c. ᵃ = $\frac{2}{3}$
Cinnamon	7,1111 &c. ᵃ = $\frac{1}{9}$
Tormentil Root	5,3333 &c. ᵃ = $\frac{5}{7}$
Gum Arabic	5,3333 &c. ᵃ = $\frac{1}{3}$
Long Pepper	,8888 &c. ᵃ = $\frac{8}{9}$ =
Opium	,6669 &c. ᵃ = $\frac{2}{3}$

Grains 29,9999 &c. ᵃ = 30 ½ ʒ

PULVIS E BOLO COMPOSITUS SINE OPIO.

Half a Dram.

Bole Armoniac	10,9999 &c. ᵃ
Cinnamon	7,2727 r.
Tormentil Root	5,4545 r.
Gum Arabic	5,4545 r.
Long Pepper	,9090 r.

Grains 30,0909 &c. ᵃ = ½ ʒ

PULVIS

PULVIS E CHELIS CANCRORUM.
Of the *London* Dispensatory.

Quant.   *Proportion of the Ingredients.*

Thirty Grains.	Tips of Crab's Claws prepar'd	20＝20
	Prepar'd Pearls } each	5＝10
	Red Roses	

                                 30 Grains.

PULVIS E CHELIS CANCRORUM.
Of the *Edinburgh* Dispensatory.

Thirty Grains.	Crabs Eyes } each	5,＝10,
	Red Coral	
	The black Tips of Crab Claws	20,＝20,

            Grains 30

PULVIS E CONTRAYERVA COMPOSITUS.
Of the *London* Dispensatory.

Thirty Grains.	Compound Powder of Crab's Claws }	23,4782
	Contrayerva Root	6,5217

          29,9999

PULVIS E CONTRAYERVA COMPOSITUS.
Of the *Edinburgh* Dispensatory.

Thirty Grains.	Contrayerva	7,0588
	Virginian Snake-root	2,6471
	Cochineal	1,7647
	English Saffron	0,8823
	Bole Armenic	5,2942
	Powder of Crab's Claws	12,3530

       Grains 30

PULVIS

PULVIS DIASENÆ.

Quant.		Proportion of the Ingredients.

Thirty Grains.
Leaves of Sena		
Cream of Tartar	} each 12 = 24
Scammony	
Ginger	} each 3 = 6

Grains 30

PULVIS E SENA COMPOSITUS.

A Scruple.
Leaves of Sena	7,6150, &c. ℈
Cryſtals of Tartar	7,6150, &c. ℈
Scammony	1,9037, &c. ℈
Cloves	,9518, &c. ℈
Cinnamon	,9518, &c. ℈
Ginger	,9518, &c. ℈

Grains 19,9898 = 1 ℈ ferè

PULVIS E MYRRHA COMPOSITUS.

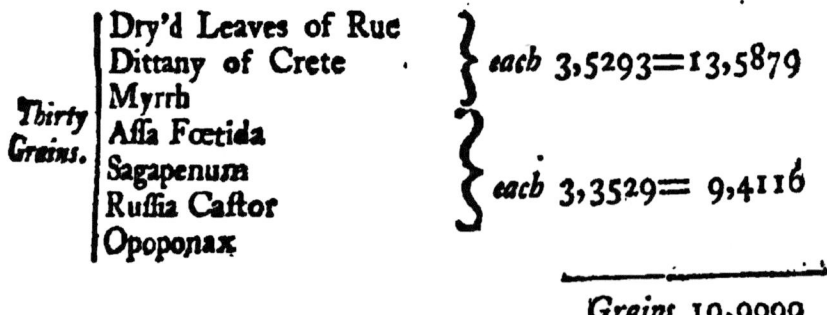

Thirty Grains.
Dry'd Leaves of Rue		
Dittany of Crete	} each 3,5293 = 13,5879
Myrrh	
Aſſa Fœtida	
Sagapenum	} each 3,3529 = 9,4116
Ruſſia Caſtor	
Opoponax	

Grains 19,9999

Pulvis

PULVIS EPILEPTICUS NIGER.

Thirty Grains.	Talus of a Hare calcin'd to Blacknefs Ivory ditto	each 5,2285 = 10,4570
	Roots of Swallow Wort Roots of Piony Roots of Valerian Hartfhorn, calcin'd with- out Fire. Red Coral, prepar'd Elk's Hoof Amber prepar'd Mufcovy Glafs, calcin'd	each 1,5686 = 12,5494
	Shells of Oyfters, prepar'd without Fire.	each 2,0915 = 2,0915
	Herb Carduus Benedictus Seeds of Columbine	each 1,0457 = 2,0915
	Wild Poppies	1,5686 = 1,5686
	Depurated Salt of Amber Salt of Hartfhorn	each 0,3485 = 0,6971
	Oil of Mace Oil of Camomile	each 0,2614 = 0,5229

Grains 29,9780

PULVIS E SCAMMONIO COMPOSITUS.

Eight Grains.	Scammony	4,57142 &c. [a]
	Burnt Hart's-horn	3,42857 &c. [a]

Grains 7,99999 &c. [a] = 8 nea.

PULVIS E SUCCINO COMPOSITUS.

Two Scruples	Prepar'd Amber	10, =
	Gum Arabic	10, =
	Juice of the Rape of Ciftus	5, =
	Balauftines	5, =
	Japan Earth	5, =
	Olibanum	4, =
	Strain'd Opium	1, =

Grains 40, = 2 ℈

THERIACA

THERIACA ANDROMACHI.

Of the *London* Dispensatory.

Quant.	Proportion of the Ingredients.		
	Troches of Squills	1,6	=1,6
	Long Pepper		
	Opium strain'd	each 0,8	=2,4
	Dried Vipers		
	Cinnamon	each 0,5333	=1,0666
	Balsam Gilead		
	Agaric		
	Root of Florentine Orice		
	Water Germander	each 0,4	=2,4
	Red Roses		
	Seeds of Navew		
	Extract of Liquorice		
	Spikenard		
	Saffron		
A Dram.	Amomum	each 0,2666	=1,5999
	Myrrh		
	Costus		
	Camel's Hay		
	Roots of Cinquefoil		
	Rhubarb		
	Ginger		
	Indian Leaf		
	Leaves of Dittany of Crete		
	Horehound		
	Calamint	each 0,2	=?,6
	French Lavender		
	Black Pepper		
	Seeds of Macedonian Parsley		
	Olibanum		
	Chio Turpentine		
	Roots of wild Valerian		

Gentian

Quant.   *Proportion of the Ingredients.*

Gentian Root
Celtic Nard
Spignel
Leaves of Poley Mountain
St. John's Wort
Ground Pine
Tops of creeping Ger-
    mander with the Seed.
The Fruit of Bal. Tree
Aniseed
Sweet Fennel Seed
The lesser Cardamom Seeds
    freed from their Husks.
Seeds of Bishop's Weed
Hartwort
Treacle Mustard
Juice of the Rape of Cis-
    tus
} *each* 0,1333= 1,9999

A
Dram.

Acacia
Gum Arabic
Storax strain'd
Sagapenum strain'd
Lemnian Earth
Green Vitrol calcin'd
} *each* 9,1333= 0,7999

Root of creeping Birth-
    wort
Tops of the lesser Cen-
    taury
Seeds of Carrot of Crete
Opopanax
Galbanum strain'd
Russia Castor
Jew's Pitch
Root of sweet Flag
} *each* 0,0666= 0,5333

Honey clarified, thrice the
    Quantity.
} *is* 44,9999=44,9999

               ———————

Grains 59,9999

THE-

Theriaca Andromachi,

Of the *Edinburgh* Dispensatory.

Proportion of the Ingredients.

Troches of Squills   1,5652＝1,5652

Vipers
The Mass of Hedycroon
Long Pepper   } *each* 0,7826＝3,1304
Opium

Roots of Sclavonian Orice
Red Roses
Leaves of Water Germander
Agaric   } *each* 0,3913＝3,1304
Balsam of Gilead
Juice of Liquorice
Seeds of Navew
Cinnamon

One Dram.

Myrrh
Saffron
Ginger
Rhapontic
Roots of Cinquefoil
Leaves of Calamint
Leaves of Horehound
Leaves of Dittany of Crete   } *each* 0,1656＝2,7384
Flowers of Arabian Stœchas
Camel's Hay
Seeds of Macedonian Parsley
Costus
Cyprus Turpentine
Male Frankincense

White Pepper
Black Pepper
Cassia Lignea   } *each* 0,1956＝0,7824
Spikenard

Polium.

Quant.　　　　　*Proportion of the Ingredients.*

Polium of Crete ⎫
Seeds of the Hartwort of
　　Marseilles
Aniseed
Seeds of Bishop's Weed
Amomum
Lesser Cardamoms
Fennel
Treacle Mustard
Roots of Gentian
Spignel
Wild Valerian
Sweet Flag ⎬ *each* 0,1304 = 3,1304
Leaves of Germandar
Ground Pine
St. John's Wort
True Acacia
Carpobalsamum, or Cubebs
Lemnian Earth
Calcin'd Brass Stone
Calamite Storax
Gum Arabic
Juice of the Rape of Cistus
Celtic Nard
Indian Leaf ⎭

One Dram.

Tops of lesser Centaury ⎫
Seeds of the Carrot of
　　Crete
Roots of small Birthwort
Jews Pitch ⎬ *each* 0,0602 = 0,4816
Galbanum
Opopanax
Sagapenum
Russia Castor ⎭

Of clarified Honey, thrice the ⎫
　　Weight of the Powders, of ⎬ 45, ＝45,
　　Canary a sufficient Quantity. ⎭

—————————————

Grains 59,9598

THE

THERIACA EDINENSIS.

Proportion of the Ingredients.

Virginian Snakeroot		3,6 == 3,6
Wild Valerian	} *each* 2,4 == 4,8
Contrayerva	
Powder of Diambra		1,8 == 1,8
Refine of Guaiacum	} *each* 1,2 == 3,6
Ruffia Caftor	
Myrrh	
Englifh Saffron	} *each* 0,6 == 1,2
Opium	
Honey clarified, a fufficient Quantity.	} 45, == 45,

One Dram.

<hr>

Grains 60,

A

THE
INTRODUCTION.

IT is certain, that simple Remedies were principally employ'd to answer Medicinal Intentions, in the Infancy of Physic, and even after it became considerable under the Cultivation of Æsculapius's Posterity. And I am mvinc'd, that an Ignorance of the History of Diseases and of the real Natures of Simples, concurring with Superstition, and false Theory, have produc'd the copious and frequent Use of compound Medicines, to the great Prejudice of the healing Art; and after all the exaggerated Encomiums of their Inventors and Admirers, the Efficacy of most of them, and even the most celebrated, remains at this Day absolutely undetermin'd and precarious; insomuch, that it is doubted by some whether they are possess'd of any, and by others affirm'd that they have none at all, consider'd as Compounds. It should seem very extraordinary that any one Physician should make Use of any Medicine for six Months only, without being able to arrive at a Certainty as to the Reality of its Virtues, and to such a Degree as to put the Affair beyond dispute. Yet it has happen'd unfortunately, that some Compounds have been us'd for many Centuries, and by a thousand different People, without any uncontroverted Determination with Respect to their Efficacy. Thus the *Venice Treacle* invented by Andromachus under the Reign of *Nero*, and the *Diascordium* of *Fracasto*rius, have been us'd by almost every Physician who has practis'd since their Invention; and notwithstanding this

abundant Experience, 'tis not yet certain, that they answer any medicinal Purpose so well as some one of their simple Ingredients; or that they contribute to the Cure of any one Distemper, better than less complex Remedies; and it even remains a Doubt whether they are best made with or without Honey, a principal Ingredient in the original Prescriptions.

Besides the Inconveniencies arising from this Uncertainty, the Introduction of Compounds into Practice, has been extremely prejudicial to medicinal Knowledge, by depriving Mankind for many Centuries of that Experience, which must long ago have determin'd, to a great Degree of Certainty, the Virtues of Simples; for if these alone had been us'd, their Efficacies must have been long ago ascertain'd beyond all Possibility of Contradiction; whereas at present there is scarcely any one Virtue ascrib'd to any Substance, whether animal, vegetable, or mineral, that has not been, and is not at this Day controverted by some one or other. But as Compositions open a large Field for Sophistications and Frauds, for this, if for no other Reason, their exorbitant Use in Medicine should, in common Prudence, be limited, and more simple and less precarious Medicines, which are not so liable to Adulteration, substituted in their Room. And it is with the greatest Satisfaction I congratulate Mankind on the Prospect of seeing the Grievances I have taken Notice of redress'd, by a Contraction of the Dispensatories, and retrenching superfluous Compositions; and by the united

B   Endeavours

Endeavours of the greateſt Practitioners of the laſt and preſent Age, to
render Phyſic a leſs precarious Science, by eſtabliſhing an accurate Hi-
ſtory of Diſeaſes, and aſcertaining the
Efficacy of Simples, in order to their
Cure. But as even theſe, and particularly ſuch as are produc'd in foreign
Countries, are ſubject to Sophiſticati-
on, Apothecaries ought to make
themſelves acquainted with the Nature
of Drugs, to a great Degree of Accuracy, in order to avoid Impoſition,
and to ſecure to themſelves the Satiſ-
faction of having done their Duty.
They ſhould, farther, uſe no Compoſitions of any Kind, but ſuch as are
made under their own immediate In-
ſpection. And with Reſpect to Chymical Medicines in particular, it
ſhould ſeem not only imprudent, but
diſhoneſt, to place too great Confidence in the Care or Integrity of any
other Perſon; becauſe this Branch of
Buſineſs abounds with infinite Frauds,
in their Conſequences extremely injurious to the Preſcriber, the Diſpenſer,
and the miſerable Patient.

Cuſtom and the Legiſlature, in Imitation of all the civiliz'd Nations of Europe, have very wiſely provided for
the Intereſts and Health of the Subject, by aſſigning to diſtinct Bodies of
People, their different Provinces in
Phyſic; both becauſe each Branch is
ſufficiently extenſive to engroſs the
whole Attention of any one Man;
and becauſe every Diviſion is a Sort of
Check upon another, ſo as to guard
againſt the Effects of Artifice and A-
varice, which might otherwiſe influence theſe as well as all other lucrative
Profeſſions. Thus the Druggiſt is reſtrain'd from providing bad Materials,
by the Knowledge of the Apothecary
who is to purchaſe them. And as an
Encouragement to Induſtry and Integrity, the Apothecary is indulg'd in
ſeveral valuable Privileges and Immu-
nities, which are deny'd to all other
Trades. And beſides this, the univerſal Conſent of Mankind has al-

low'd him very conſiderable Advan
tages in every Thing he vends; an
this with great Juſtice and Prudence
for 'tis certainly the Intereſt of ever
Individual to contribute to the Su
port of the Perſon whoſe Conduct h
ſo great an Influence on Health an
Life, and that in ſuch a Manner, as
place him in a Rank above Tempt
tion to a baſe or diſhoneſt Action. B
leſt this very Indulgence ſhould defe
the End for which it was deſign'
and produce the Inconveniencies
was intended to prevent, it was pr
dently provided, that the Vender
Medicines ſhould not have the Dire
tion of their Uſe; for otherwiſe, t
Conſideration of private Advantag
might influence him to adviſe mo
Remedies, than are abſolutely nece
ſary for a Cure, to the great Prejudi
of the Patient's Fortune and Healt
and Danger of his Life. This Tru
therefore, was repos'd entirely in t
Phyſician, who is ſuppos'd to have t
Advantage of a generous and a learn
ed Education, which is certainly le
ſubject to diſtort the Morals, and bia
them to the Side of Gain, than m
chanical Profeſſions. But in Conſid
ration of human Frailties, he is pr
dently reſtrain'd from vending the R
medies he preſcribes, leſt he ſhoul
alſo, be tempted to deviate from th
Rectitude, which from his Charact
and Situation, the World has Reaſo
to expect he ſhould religiouſly adhe
to.

It is from Conſiderations no le
prudent, that all civiliz'd Nations
the World have divided Surgery fro
Phyſic, and aſſign'd to the Surgeon t
executive Part in all external Diſo
ders, and to the Phyſician the Pr
vince of judging, and directing wh
is proper to be done for the Relief
thoſe who are ſo unfortunate as to fa
under their Care; for by this Mean
the Patient is infinitely better ſecur'
againſt Error and Avarice, than if t
Parts both of Judging and Actin
were truſted to one Individual.

I cannot difmifs this Subject without the Notice of the Chymift, a Weed produc'd within this half Century, in the too rank Soil of Pharmacy for Want of due Cultivation; for if the Apothecaries had, in purfuance of their Duty, taken Care to prepare their own chymical Medicines, this Trade would never have been eftablifh'd as a diftinct Branch; nor would Occafion have been given for the infinite Frauds which are now daily practis'd; becaufe however the Chymift may find his Account in fophifticating his Preparations, which he makes in Quantities fufficient to furnifh perhaps five hundred Shops, no fingle Apothecary could find it anfwer any lucrative Views, to adulterate for the Sake of the trifling Advantage he might expect from the Demands of his own.

But in the prefent Situation of Phyfic, all Manner of Diftinction betwixt the different Provinces, is abfolutely confounded and deftroy'd, and perhaps no one Abufe deferves more the Interpofition of the Legiflature, than thofe introduc'd into Medicine by the Encroachments of the different Branches upon each other. Thus the Chymift compliments his Cuftomers with the Refufe of Drugs; and the Druggift, by Way of Retaliation, furnifhes his with Chymicals equally bad. The Apothecary commences, a moft contemptible Surgeon; the Surgeon on his Part, profeffes Pharmacy with the fame Degree of Knowledge and Succefs; and both in Spight of Education and Reafon, are, by a Kind of Magic, peculiar to themfelves, converted into moft execrable Doctors. Infomuch, that it only remains, that the Phyficians, fhould become very bad Apothecaries; and then we may expect to fee Medicine practifed in Great Britain, much as it is among the Savages of America, tho' I am afraid not fo fafely, nor with equal Succefs.

I would by no means have it underftood, that the private Intereft of the Phyficians, has tempted me to make thefe Obfervations; on the contrary, I folemnly declare, that I now plead as a Member of Society, and out of Regard to the public Welfare. And I am abundantly convinced, that the prefent Confufion among the different Branches of Phyfick, impofes a Tax upon the Public, in Favour of Phyficians, to the annual Amount of a great many thoufand Pounds. Thus if the Druggift, always furnifhed Simples good in their Kind, and the Apothecary difcharg'd his Duty in preparing them, without confiding in Chymifts and wholefale Dealers, more Diftempers would be cured with fewer Attendances. It is farther obfervable, that acute Diftempers in particular, are much more eafily remedied at firft, than after they have made any confiderable Progrefs. Now in thefe Cafes a judicious Phyfician knows the Methods of checking, at leaft nineteen out of twenty, in their Infancy, whilft a fufficient Degree of Strength remains, to co-operate with the Remedies prefcribed; fo that two or three Vifits, are all that can be neceffary. Whereas if the Cafe happens to be conducted, by one, who practices by Habit, and at Random, he generally endeavours to extort Sweats, at the very Beginning, by Cordials and Volatiles; and by this prepofterous Treatment the Difeafe is fo rivetted, and the Conftitution fo injured, as to require fix times the Attendance that would otherwife, have been required. And the Patient has more than common good Fortune, if he efcapes, the fiery Trial, at laft, with Life.

With Refpect to my prefent Undertaking, it may be expected that I give fome Reafons for publifhing a Difpenfatory, after *Quincy*, whom I have reprefented in another Place as an excellent Judge of Pharmacy. In the firft Place then it muft be confider'd, that fince his Time, the Phyficians of *Edinburgh* have publifh'd an excellent Difpenfary, and this Example has been

been followed by our own College. Besides, *Boerbaave*, *Stahl*, *Hoffman*, *Neuman*, and several other Writers, of the first Class, have made many useful Discoveries in the Chymical Pharmacy, to which it appears he was an absolute Stranger. And many Advances have been made, towards a more intimate and certain Acquaintance with the *Materia Medica*, which either escaped his Researches, or came to the Knowledge of the learned World too late to be expected in his Writings.

Secondly, This Author has been much too liberal in his Directions, for the Application of Compounds in particular; and by ascribing to Medicines Virtues, which they in no Degree possess, and bestowing on others Encomiums they by no Means deserve, has misled young Practitioners, and induc'd them to depend too much upon the Efficacy of Prescriptions, and to neglect the more essential Parts of medicinal Knowledge; for whoever should place an implicit Confidence in *Quincy*'s Recommendations, would be inclined to believe no other Book necessary to form a Practitioner; and that no Patient could hereafter die of a Disease, that could be prevailed on to take the Remedies he extols beyond the Bounds of Probability, Reason, and Experience.

Our Author has, farther, done no small Prejudice to true medicinal Knowledge by his great Licentiousness in Philosophizing, and reasoning mechanically, as he calls it, upon Principles either manifestly false, or at best precarious; frequently proposing uncertain Suppositions of his own, or of other Authors, as undoubted Facts, and thus imposing upon the injudicious the Chimæras of a luxuriant Imagination, for physical Truths. *Quincy*, has given a great Number of Prescriptions, from Authors of our own Country, as *Bates*, *Fuller*, and even *Salmon*, which are in the Hands of every Body; and universally known;

but he has taken no manner of Notice of a great Number of celebrated Compositions which occur in foreign Writers, and which it would have been more useful to describe; because theUnderstanding theseAuthors, would thereby have been facilitated; and the Shops would more readily have known what was meant, when these Medicines were taken Notice of in the Prescriptions of foreign Physicians, or our own.

In the Execution, therefore, of the Undertaking, I have endeavoured to preserve the Excellencies of *Quincy*, to avoid his Errors, and to supply his Defects; and how far I have succeeded, must leave to the Judgment of others.

Mean time I must remark, that most of the principal Operations in Chymistry are performed naturally in the open Air, without the Assistance of Art; and that most Bodies, undergo the same Kind of Changes, by the naturalAction of Air, Water, and Fire in a longer Space of Time, as they do in the Laboratories of Chymists in shorter. Thus Hartshorn, for Example, exposed for a long Series of Time to the open Air, undergoes a perfect Distillation; for the Water Oils, and volatile Salts exhale and leave a *Caput Mortuum*, or mere insipid Earth. And the same may be said of all vegetable, and animal Substances. With Respect to Metals, all of them, except Gold, are corroded or dissolved in the Air, and by the very same *Menstruum* which Chymists employ for their Solution, that is, a certain Acid, with which the Air abounds, and which does not much differ from that distilled from Nitre. In order, therefore, to give a perfect Insight into the chymical Part of Pharmacy, I shall first consider the Nature of the Air, as of the greatest Influence and this, both as it affects the human, as well as every sublunary Body. And with the same View I shall enquire into the Nature of Water, Fire, and Earth.

THE NEW
English Dispensatory.

BOOK I.

CHAP. I.
Of AIR.

THE Air in general is that fluid Mass, which every where surrounds the terraqueous Globe. 'Tis call'd the Atmosphere, is so applied to the Surface of our Earth as naturally to touch all the Parts thereof, and is not only the Seat of Winds, Storms and Thunder, but the common Vehicle, or Medium, thro' which, Sounds, Smells, Light are convey'd. The Air in which we continually is impregnated with Corpuscles of all Kinds, insinuates itself the penetrable Interstices of all remains conceal'd in these Interstices, and is again discharg'd from when such Bodies are resolv'd their Elements or constituent This Fluid is absolutely necessary to the Preservation of Life, we draw it in during Inspira-

tion, and force it out in Expiration; so that both Nature and Art seem to use its Influence and Assistance in all their Works; for which Reason it is called the Principle necessary to promote the Generation of Things, and by *Seneca* in *Qu. Nat. L.* 2. *cap.* 4. a necessary Part of the Universe. This is a Description of the Air sufficiently accommodated to the Senses of every one; but if it should be ask'd what this Fluid is, the Philosopher must confess his Ignorance, and be content with describing Air from its most obvious, and best known Properties.

The Air, then, is first to be considered as a fluid Body whose Parts, tho' invisible by means of the finest Microscope are yet continually in Motion. These Parts separately, cannot enter the Pores of many Bodies, thro' which other Liquors readily pass; but the Parts of the Air cannot be excluded from those Places,

into

into which Liquors containing Air can enter. The Parts of this Fluid, have alfo what is call'd a mutual Attraction, and when many of them adhere to each other in a fpherical Form they conftitute what we call a Bubble of Air, and then by a certain Tenacity, greater than in other Liquors, they refift Diffipation, and for that Reafon are with greater Difficulty than any other known Fluids, incorporated with other Liquids. But when thefe Parts are feparated and divided, they forthwith incorporate themfelves with every Body deftitute of Air, and adhere firmly in their Interftices, till a greater Force feperates them, and forces them into Bubbles, either by means of an Air Pump, by boiling over the Fire, by Froft, by fix'd alcaline Salts, by Effervefcence, by chymical Diftillation, Fermentation, Putrefaction, or Combuftion. The Particles of Air difpers'd thro' the minute Interftices of Bodies poffefs a fmaller Space than when being reduc'd to Bubbles, they are feparated or drawn from fuch Bodies. The Quantity of Air contain'd in Bodies bears a Proportion to the Number of their Interftices, and the Particles of the Air by their Tenacity adhere to the very fmootheft and beft polifh'd Surfaces of all Solids, till by Wind, Heat, or a rapid Motion, they are thrown off from them and make Room for the Succeffion of frefh Air. The Air difpers'd thro' the minute Interftices of Bodies, is call'd the internal Air, and does not act like the common Air, fo long as it is divided and not collected together. The external Air is that which furrounds and encompaffes all Objects whatever. We cannot affirm that the Particles of Air are larger than thofe of Water, becaufe thofe of the latter Fluid make their way thro' fome Bodies, thro' which Air cannot pafs; for the Parts of Water, perhaps on Account of their greater Denfity are

better calculated to force a Paffage thro' the Pores of Bodies than thofe of Air.

The fecond Property of the Air is that Refiftance or Oppofition which it makes to Bodies, efpecially fuch as under large Surfaces contain fmall Quantities of Matter, when mov'd thro' it, and this Refiftance is increas'd according to the Augmentation of the Velocity of the moving Bodies, which according to the Principles of Mechanics, is in duplicate Proportion.

The Weight or fpecific Gravity of the Air never remains long the fame, but varies very furprifingly; firft, according to the State of the Weather, fince a Change of its Weight or Gravity is produc'd by Meteors, Rain, Clouds, Hail, Snow, Lightning, Thunder, Winds blowing from various Quarters, Storms, Whirlwinds, Drynefs, and the various Afpects of the Planets. Secondly, according to the Seafon of the Year. Thirdly, according to its different Altitudes, for the inferior Part of the Air is always heavier than the fuperior. In *Europe* it has hitherto been found that the Difference of the greateft and fmalleft Weight of the Air, about the tenth Part of the greateft, and when its Mean or middle Weight is compar'd with the Weight of Water, the former is generally found eight hundred and fifty Times higher than the latter. But the gravitating Force of the whole Atmofphere is generally equal to that of a Column of Water of 32 or 33 Feet high, or that of a Column of *Mercury* 28 or 30 Inches high. Mr. *Homberg* weigh-ed a glafs Globe full of Air, and of 20 Inches Diameter, and found three Ounces, three Drams and heavier than when the Air was exhaufted from it. This Globe or Receiver contain'd two cubical Feet, and ¹⁄₂ of Water fo that a cubical Foot of Air weighs one Ounce and forty eight

eight Grains. *Hales* in his Statics, computes that a cubical Inch of Air, weighs two Sevenths of a Grain. As the Gravity of the Air, is to be determin'd from its Contents, so the following Observations may be taken as so many Axioms. The heavier the Air is, the greater Weight of Mercury it is equal to in the Barometer; hence the Mercury becomes higher in the Tube, but suddenly subsides when the Gravity of the Air is diminish'd. In serene, and especially dry Weather the Air becomes more weighty, and the Water ascends higher, and is more distributed and dispers'd in the Air. But if the Barometer denotes a great Weight of the Air, whilst at the same Time there are thick and fetid Clouds, then the aqueous Parts hang low in the Air, and are almost accompanied with gross oleous and saline Exhalations which cannot at such a Time be accurately and equally mix'd, distributed, and united. Whereas when the Barometer denotes a diminish'd Weight of the Air, in hot and cloudy Weather, then the Water descends to the inferior Parts, but with an equable and very moistening Vapour, tho' it is not as yet rainy Weather.

Upon the Gravity or Weight of the Air also depends its Pressure; hence the greater the Weight of the Air is, the more powerfully it presses Bodies, and the smaller its Weight, the less it presses upon them. The Air also presses Bodies the more, the nearer they are to the Center of the Earth, and the less, the farther they are from it. Bodies lodg'd in the Air are not long press'd by the same Force, so that the Constriction of Bodies, so far as it depends upon the Compression of the Air, varies almost every Moment, only in the same Place, the Difference of Pressure is never greater than one Tenth of the Whole, within which there is a perpetual Vicissitude. Hence in Bodies lodg'd in the Air, there is a Kind of perpetual Oscillation corresponding to the reciprocal Augmentation or Diminution of the Weight of the Air comprehended within the tenth Part of the Whole. Whilst the Air presses, it is also proportionally compressed by all elastic Bodies. But as the heterogeneous Contents of the Air contribute more or less to its Weight, *Boerhaave* suspects that pure Air entirely free from the Admixture of foreign Corpuscules, would perhaps have no Weight at all. On the Force of the pressing Atmosphere it depends that two brazen Hemispheres firmly cohere when the Air is extracted from their Cavities, nor can they be divided unless the Pressure of the incumbent Air is counterballanc'd by the Application of a superior Force. Hence it is that the Sides of a Pair of Bellows cannot be seperated, if all the Holes and Fistures in them are accurately stopt up.

A fourth Property of the Air is its Elasticity: This Quality, among all other known Fluids is at all Times peculiar to the Air alone. In Consequence of this Property, all Air possessing a certain determinate Space from which it cannot make its Escape, is compress'd into a Space smaller in Proportion to the Weight acting upon it, and the more the compressing Weight is diminish'd, the more it spontaneously possesses a larger Space, and at last always returns to its former State when the compressing Force is the same it was before. The smallest Space into which, according to Observation, Air can be compress'd, is sixteen Times less than the Space it naturally occupies; and the greatest Space to which it can spontaneously expand itself is, thirty two Times its natural Space. With respect to this Property of the Air, the following Remarks are to be made: First, Compress'd Air is call'd dense or condensated

Air, whereas that which is expanded is said to be rarified : Secondly, The Density of compress'd Air, bears a Proportion to the compressing Weight : Thirdly, Air when most strongly compress'd neither transfudes thro' Glass nor penetrates the Pores of Mercury : Fourthly, Air is condens'd not only by an Increase of Weight, but more particularly than any other known Body, by Cold. But Air may be condens'd between the Degrees of Heat in boiling Water, and the most intense known Cold, to about one Half of the Whole. It has been affirm'd that Air is capable of Compression, because its Particles do not touch each other, and that if the Particles of Air touch'd each other, it would become as hard as Marble : Fifthly, By Heat, Air is rarified, that is, obtains a Power of expanding itself every where sooner than any other fluid Body, in so much, that there are no known Limits to this Dilatation produc'd by Fire. But the Dilatation is always the same in Degrees of Heat ; so that the action bears a Proportion to the Degrees of the increas'd Heat, and the Compression of the Air before the Rarefaction : Sixthly, The higher or more remote the Air is from the Surface of the Earth, the more rare it always is : Seventhly, The Elasticity of the Air existing in every Portion of it is equivalent to the Weight of the whole Atmosphere, which it can sustain without being any more condens'd than the compressing incumbent Column of Air. The Air by Means of its Elasticity and expansive Faculty repels Objects with a Force equal to that with which they act upon it. Thus *Boerhaave* tells us, " That a small Por- " tion of Air pent up in any Place, " is capable of producing the same " Effects which depend upon a large " Quantity of Air in its natural " State ; for if the common Air is " receiv'd into any Cavity which " may be easily compress'd on all " Sides, it will remain there ; and " from that Place totally remove the " Pressure of the Atmosphere. But " when the Air in such a Cavity is " heated by the Fire, or freed from " external Pressure, it is forthwith so " expanded as to produce Effects equal " to those of the greatest Quantity of " Air. '8thly, The elastic Force is less in Air impregnated with Vapours, than in such as is pure and serene. Ninthly, Air condens'd by Cold produces the same Effects with Air render'd heavier. Hence it is inferr'd that a cold Wind acts more powerfully on the Sails of Ships than such as is warm. Tenthly, Rarified Air possesses the Power of Air render'd more elastic, which Power always increases in a compound Ratio of the augmented Heat, and the former Compressure of the Air. Eleventhly, The Air by its Elasticity produces Effects similar to those of its Gravity, so that its Want of Gravity is compensated by its Elasticity. From this elastic Quality of the Air produc'd by Rarefaction, we can assign a Reason why when the Sun is rising or just appearing above our Horizon we perceive a greater Cold in the Atmosphere than we did the preceeding Night ; for the solar Rays, before they can reach us in such a Quantity as to warm our Atmosphere, have in the superior Region produc'd a Rarefaction of the Air, which by its Elasticity presses and applies more strongly to us the Causes of the Cold before dispers'd thro' our Atmosphere. Thus, also, 'tis said, the Force of Gunpowder exploded from a Gun, depends upon the compress'd Air lodg'd in the Nitre, by the Fire rarified and render'd more elastic. Glass Bubbles, artificial Fountains, and *Aurum Fulminans* are, also, us'd to prove the Elasticity of the Air, produc'd by Rarefaction. The Air Gun also, sufficiently
ently

only evinces the elaſtic Force of the before compreſs'd Air, which is diſcharg'd with a great Noiſe and a Force equal to that of Gunpowder. Various Experiments made on Air-pumps, alſo, evince its Elaſticity: Twelfthly, There is an Elaſticity in the Air contain'd in Liquors, which diſcovers itſelf when the external Air is remov'd, and conſequently the compreſſing Weight no longer acts: Thirteenthly, The Air is continually poſſeſs'd of its Elaſticity which can never be deſtroy'd by any Means whatever. Many learned Gentlemen have indulg'd their Paſſions for Philoſophizing, by endeavouring to account for this Property of the Air, by the Figure of its Parts, and the Action of the ſubtile ætherial Matter thereon. But as I eſteem fabulous and trifling, whatever does not fall under the Cognizance of the Senſes, I ſhall take no farther Notice of theſe uncertain Climæras, always confining myſelf to Facts, confirm'd by Experiments.

Fiſtbly, The Air is to be conſidered as an Aggregate of many and highly heterogeneous Corpuſcules, and as containing in it the moſt minute Particles of all Bodies, which are mix'd with it, fluctuate in it, and are convey'd to it by Way of Exhalations, either in a humid Form as in moiſt Vapours, or a dry one by Way of Powder or Duſt: On this Account ſome divide the Air into different Strata, each of which contains a certain Kind of Corpuſcules, according to the Heighth at which, in Conſequence of their greater or ſmaller Weight, they remain in it. Thus *Mundius* ſays, " The Conſtitu-" tion of the Air generally partakes " of the Nature of the Soil. Thus " in foggy Countries, Iſlands, and " maritime Towns, the Sky is ge-" nerally cloudy, and the Air heavy " and thick; for the Atmoſphere is " full of a Redundance of Moiſture

" lodg'd in its Pores. But the Air " about large and populous Towns, " is render'd opake by Smoke, or " ſome other heterogeneous Particles. But among all the Bodies rais'd from the Earth or reſiding in the Air, the two moſt obſervable are Fire and Water: Fire is always equably diſtributed in it; hence the Air is ſaid to be more or leſs cold; but in ſuch a manner that the Air is the colder the higher it is, and the Increaſe of Cold, other Circumſtances being alike, bears a Proportion to the Degree of Height, for it is colder in open Plains than in Vallies. Thermometers ſufficiently manifeſt the greater Degrees of Heat in the Air. There is always Water in the Air, rais'd from the Waters of our Globe, by the Heat of the Sun, or the Influence of ſubterraneous Fire, by culinary Fires, by Froſt, and eſpecially by Winds: Thus Water may be rais'd to a great Height in the Air, which contains the largeſt Quantities, when it appears ſereue and dry, at which Time it is higheſt, and moſt diſpers'd thro' the aerial Regions. Whereas the Air contains a ſmaller Quantity of Water when it appears moiſt and humid. And in this Reſpect the Air is diſtinguiſh'd into moiſt and dry: This Water in the Air, is the Matter of Dew, Clouds, Rains, Fountains, Rivulets, Rivers, Ice, Hoar-Froſt, Snow, Hail, and perhaps Meteors depending on theſe. This Water alſo, conſtitutes the greateſt Part of the Weight in the Air, but at the ſame Time diminiſhes its Elaſticity. *Bontius* informs us, that the Air of the Iſland of *Java*, in the *Eaſt-Indies*, which might by ſome be thought dry on Account of its Heat, is nevertheleſs incredibly moiſt; for there in the drieſt Seaſon of the Year, Iron, Steel, Braſs and Silver, ſooner contract Ruſt than in the moſt rainy autumnal Seaſons in *Europe*, and that their Cloaths tho' carefully preſerv'd in Cheſts ſoon

become

become mouldy, and would eafily rot if they were not expos'd to the Sun and Wind. The Prefence of Water in the Air is evinc'd by expofing a fix'd alcaline Salt to a free Air apparently dry, by which Means the Salt is diffolv'd, has its Weight augmented, and may be again feparated from the Water by Diftillation. The different Quantities of Water contain'd in the Air at different Times, may be inveftigated by fuch Inftruments as eafily admit the Water into their Pores, by which Means they either fwell and are expanded, are render'd tumid, or retorted, or increafe in Weight. In the Summer when the Air is generally moft dry, it is eafy to perceive that it abounds with humid Corpufcles moving therein, efpecially from that Experiment made by pouring cold Wine or Ale into a Glafs, or fmooth metal Cup, by which Means the exterior Surface of the Cup as far as the Liquor reaches, is bedew'd with aqueous Drops which feem to be nothing but the aqueous Vapours floating in the Air, by the Coldnefs of the Cup condens'd into confpicuous Drops of Water. Other Bodies contain'd in the Atmofphere are the Spirits exhal'd from all Kinds of Vegetables, all Kinds of Oils, Salts, Earths, the Elements of Vegetables, and even their entire Parts, the *Sanctorian* perfpirable Matter of Animals, their Excrements, all the Elements of Animals and their impregnated Eggs, and in the foffile Kingdom, Salts, Sulphurs and Metals. It is fufficiently obvious that thefe Particles are not always and every where the fame in the Air; for the Nature of the Air is various, according as the Winds convey different Corpufcules to it from different Regions through which they pafs, and is alfo vary'd by the Seafons of the Year, Inundations and Earthquakes; and thus Air on Account of the numerous Par-

ticles floating in it, is by fome thoug to be nothing but a Kind of lanu nous Mixture of Earth and Wat impregnated with Effluvia of Kinds.

But the moft remarkable Subfta contain'd in the Air, is the univer Acid, with which Providence has ken Care plentifully to furnifh it many and thofe very important P pofes. The Exiftence of this Aci manifeft by its Effects; for by thi the bafer Metals expos'd to the *A* are corroded. 'Tis this that neu lizes alcaline Salts if long expo to the Air. On this Account Manufacturers of Nitre, prepare B of Earth which they impregnate w Animal and Vegetable alcaline Sa which receive and retain this A in great Plenty; and they rema that it is principally convey'd to th Strata of Earth by the Winds wh blow from any Points betwixt North and Eaft. Now as thefe Wi are generally cold, it fhould fe that there is fome Analogy betw Cold and Acids; and that this A of the Air is the grand Prefervat againft Putrefaction. The *Ete* Winds, frequently mention'd by *E pocrates*, are faid to blow from North-eaft, and to temperate Heat of the Atmofphere. *Pliny* forms us, that the North-eaft Wi blow eight Days before the Dog-S rifes, and that thefe are call'd *P dromi*, and that two Days after Rifing of the Dog-Star, the *Ete* or North-eaft Winds fet in and c tinue for forty Days.

According to *Profper Alpinus*, *Etefian* Winds begin to blow in *gypt*, when the Sun enters Can and blow very conftantly the wh Months of *July* and *Auguft*, as w as almoft all *June*. At the Rifing thefe Winds, which happen nearl the Time when the *Nile* begins increafe, all peftilential Diftemp which were before very commo wl while the contrary Winds blew, are extinguish'd; for, as he says, the southerly Winds which the *Egyptians* call *Campfin*, (as he supposes from *Cambyses*, who with his whole Army was suffocated by the Sand driven upon them by these Winds, as we read in the Life of *Alexander* the Great,) induce a morbid and distemper'd Constitution of the Air. It is but natural to expect that the *Etesian* Winds which are directly contrary to them, should purge the Air and render it wholesome. Besides the Nature of the *Etesian* Winds is opposite to pestilential Constitutions, as much as the southerly Winds are observ'd to promote Putrefaction, agreeable to that of *Galen* in *Lib.* 1. *de Temp.* where he says, "That all "Things are for a long Time pre- "serv'd from Putrefaction by the "North Wind which is cold and "dry by Nature, but are very easily "putrified by southern Blasts." And in many Places he affirms that the former Winds induce an healthy and salubrious State of the Air, as in *Com. in* 3. *Epidem.* "If the *Etesian* Winds, "says he, blow in the Summer, they "prevent many Mischiefs and Dis- "orders, which otherwise would "happen." And speaking of a pestilential Air he says, "If the *Ete- "sian* Winds had blown at this Sea- "son they would have cleans'd the "Constitution of the human Body "from all Distempers." In several other Parts of his Works he assures us that the Summers in which the *Etesian* Winds did not blow, were very sickly. *Hippocrates*, also, when describing a pestilential Summer says, "The Summer was fair and hot, "and the Season was very sultry, "the *Etesian* Winds blowing only "weak and by Intervals."

This Acid I take to be that vivifying Principle in the Air, which is so necessary both to animal and vegetable Life, that neither can subsist

without it. And it is, probably, the grand Instrument of the Destruction, and Dissolution of Bodies; so that it may be consider'd as the Scythe in the Hands of Time, which sooner or later destroys all the Productions of Art and Nature.

Sixthly, The Air is, also, to be consider'd with Respect to Motion or Rest; the Air is said to be at Rest when its contiguous Columns possess an equal Degree of Gravity and Elasticity; for then the Columns of Air press each other equally, and hence arises an Equilibrium and Rest. But when the contiguous Columns of Air are not in a State of Æquilibrium then the most elastic or ponderous Column, presses and acts upon that which is less so: Hence arises that Agitation of the Air which we call Wind. And hence it is that after Showers when our Atmosphere is light, violent Winds generally succeed. As the Matter contain'd in the Air is brought to, or convey'd from different Parts, 'tis obvious that the Qualities of the Air may be greatly varied by the Wind. Hence 'tis evident that Winds may both bring and prevent Rains. The same holds true with Respect to Heat and Cold. And all other Circumstances being alike, another Change produc'd by Winds is to dry Bodies, by removing the Particles of Moisture from them. Thus *Bacon* tells us, "That all Winds "have a greater Power of drying "than the Sun, because the latter "only raises the Vapours, but does "not dissipate them, unless it is ve- "ry hot; whereas Wind both raises "and dissipates them." Hence in the eighth Chapter of *Genesis*, we are told, that after the Deluge, God sent Winds to dry the Face of the Earth. Hence the Reason is obvious, why in Autumn and Spring, Storms and violent Winds are generally more frequent than in Summer or Winter; for in the Autumn and
Spring,

Spring the Vapours in the Atmosphere are more numerous, less dispers'd, and less elevated; for which Reason the Elasticity and Gravity of the Atmosphere are less, according to what has been before observ'd. Hence it yields to the Elasticity and Pressure of the contiguous Column of Air, which rushes impetuously against the heated, rarify'd, and humid Parts of the Atmosphere, in order to restore an Equilibrium. After Winter when the Sun approaches nearer to the Æquator, the Air before condens'd by the Cold is more rarified, and Bodies evaporate more. Hence the Resistance of the Air is less, and by the Pressure of the contiguous Columns, Winds arise, especially such as blow towards the South, where the Rarefaction is already begun, so that at this Season northerly Winds are frequent. These are the principal and most generally assign'd Causes of Winds; but we are, also, to consider the State of the Land or Sea, in which they happen with respect to Vapours and Exhalations, as also the Situation of Mountains, by the Opposition of which the Wind acting upon them is repell'd.

From what has been said we understand the Reason why Winds blowing from cold Quarters, such as the North, render the Atmosphere cold; whilst those coming from a warm Quarter, as the South, render it warm; as also why Winds blowing from moist or dry Countries render the Air moist or dry: And why northerly Winds are cold, dry and generally more impetuous than the Southerly, which are hot and moist. A cold, dry, and condens'd Air, exerts the same Virtues with a ponderous Air, by pressing and propelling that which is adjacent to it, and by that Means inducing serene Weather. On the contrary, a warm and moist Air being rarified, and having its Elasticity weaken'd by the Humidity, cannot long exert its Virtue, but yields to the Pressure and Resistance of the adjacent Air, and by that Means fills the Atmosphere with Moisture and instead of serene, produces cloudy Weather. The other Effects of Winds may be accounted for in like Manner. The Use of Winds is remarkably observ'd in large and populous Cities, where the copious Vapours and Exhalations render the Atmosphere vapid and putrid, unless by the Wideness of the Streets, the Winds have a free Passage thro' them. In Vallies, low situated and shady Places, the Air is, also, frequently noxious, because by the Intervention of Mountains and Woods the salutary Winds are excluded. Calm Seasons, tho' agreeable, are yet often productive of the most fatal Consequences; for during these, the Atmosphere depriv'd of its usual Ventilation, becomes putrid, and by that Means induces the most terrible and malignant Disorders. Hence in most Places on the western Coasts of *Africa,* these Calms are much more dreaded both by Sea and Land, than the most violent Storms. In the Island of St. *Thomas* immediately after the Winter Solstice, the Winds cease for two Months or more; by which Means most of the Inhabitants languish and die, unless grateful Winds blow seasonably to recruit their Spirits. In Ships long becalm'd, so many of the Sailors have died, that hardly a sufficient Number of Men have surviv'd to conduct the Vessels into the nearest Harbours. Unless the Ocean was agitated by Winds, its Water would prove not only fatal to the Fish, but the Air would also become mortal to Land Animals, on Account of the putrid Effluvia rising from it. The Agitation, therefore, of the Atmosphere seems no less necessary than the very Substance itself, to the Support and Preservation of Life, because cafe Winds purge the Air from the Impurities it has contracted, and, by that Ventilation, correct that malignant Quality which it has acquir'd by Reft and Stagnation. But Winds blowing from all Quarters are not equally proper for purging the Air, for in our Hemifphere, the northerly Winds are moft falubrious on Account of the abundant Acid they convey, tho' 'tis better to have any than none of them. Thus *Bacon* tells us, "That all Winds purge the Air "and free it from Putrefaction, fo "that the Years in which Winds "are moft frequent, are for that "very Reafon moft falubrious."

In the free and open Air there is, farther, a particular Virtue abfolutely necessary to the Continuation of the Lives of Animals and Vegetables, for which Reafon it is call'd the latent Support or Food of Life; for in a clofe Air which is not from time to time renew'd, neither Animals nor Vegetables can long protract Life. But this general Propofition admits of fome Limitation; for fome Authors of Candour inform us, that live fhell Fifh of a good Tafte, Toads, Frogs and Serpents, have been found alive pent up in the Midft of Rocks, Stones, and other hard Subftances. But thefe Inftances are fo few, and fo much out of the common Courfe of Nature, befides the Chance of their being falfe, that they fcarcely deferve being taken Notice of as Exceptions to the general Doctrine. There is fomething fo extremely abftrufe in this vivifying Principle in the Air, that the Learned have not yet been able to determine upon what it depends. For my own Part I believe, that a perpetual Supply of the univerfal Acid contain'd in the Air, is indifpenfably neceffary for the Support of Animal and Vegetable Life; and that this Acid is the Ingredient in the Air, which conftitutes the vivifying Principle, fo

much taken Notice of, and fo little underftood.

From the Nature of the Air thus inveftigated from its Properties, Philofophers generally judge concerning the Caufes of thofe Effects produc'd by the Air in the Change of Bodies; for as the Air is always in Motion, 'tis fufficiently obvious that it moves all Bodies, and as it is poffefs'd both of Fluidity and Gravitation, it preffes upon all Bodies, tho' the Preffure is equable on all their Sides. The Air, alfo, keeps Bodies confin'd within certain Limits, for in an Air-pump, when the external Air is evacuated, Fluids rife over the Edges of the Veffels in which they are contain'd; becaufe, fome Portion of the Air has enter'd their Cavities or Interftices. Hence it continually makes an Attrition, Concuffion, and Agitation on the Surfaces of Bodies, determines, applies, and excites their mutual Action upon each other. The Air, therefore, ftrangely mixes Fluids, efpecially the more it is agitated by Heat or Storms; but it does not change the Figures of Bodies, becaufe it preffes every where equably, unlefs when thefe Bodies contain fome Interftices and Cavities free from Air, in which Cafe if they are flexible, it reduces them to a fmaller Bulk. If the Air is at the fame conceiv'd to be elaftic, thefe Effects, will the more infallibly be produc'd. It is, perhaps, from the elaftic Virtue of the Air, which penetrates our Bodies as well as other Subftances, that we are enabled to fuftain the immenfe Weight of the external incumbent Air, which is calculated to be equivalent to 39900 Pound Weight. As the Air contains the Particles of almoft all Kinds of Bodies, fo it will produce the Effects not only of Air as fuch, but alfo of the Subftances contain'd in it. Thus it may be faid to be an univerfal Seminary, rich in all Kinds of Materials, committing to the Earth

thofe

those Elements of Bodies which it first receiv'd from it ; and thus by a Kind of Revolution generating most Sorts of Bodies. And as the Corpuscules contain'd in the Air and perpetually in Motion meet with each other, they may produce the almost infinite Effects depending upon the Combination of their particular Virtues. On this Account in the Schools of experimental Philosophy, the Preceptors generally, with good Reason, begin their Courses with Experiments on the Nature of the Air. And the Teachers of Chymistry can hardly be said to do Justice to their Subject, if they neglect to treat of the Properties of Air, so that *Boerhaave* is unjustly censur'd by some for treating so prolixly of the Air in his Chymistry ; for Air contains not only Water, but also saline, oleous, and other Parts. Hence it surprisingly affects and changes Bodies, promotes many artificial Effects, and by Means of the Corpuscules it contains acts as an universal Menstruum, by mixing, macerating, relaxing, dissolving, drying, corroding, putrifying and fermenting Bodies, according to their Condition, or Disposition to undergo particular Changes ; for it seems sufficiently obvious, that according to the Commixtion, Reaction, and Exhalation of the various Salts in the Air, different Species of Salts may be generated. Thus the *Caput Mortuum* of Vitriol, when long expos'd to the Air, is again impregnated with its acid Salt. Calcin'd Alum, also, soon receives again its aluminous Salt into its Pores, and even exhausted Ores, when expos'd to the open Air, again produce their respective Minerals. Fix'd alcaline Salts, when expos'd to the Air become volatile. Pot ashes when long expos'd to the Air, are in a great Measure converted into a neutral Salt like vitriolated Tartar, or the Arcanum Duplicatum. Dew and Hoar-Frost by their

corrosive Virtue evince their Contents, which are also discover'd by a Chymical Analysis. Thunder and Lightening sufficiently denote the Existence of an inflammable Sulphur in the Air. Vegetables may, also be produc'd in Places where the like Vegetables are not found, because their Seeds are convey'd by the Air to these particular Places. Minute Animals and Insects may also be produc'd in Places where their Parents are not to be found, but whose small impregnated Eggs have been convey'd by the Wind and deposited in other Places. From what has been said the Reason appears obvious, why in some a Ptyalism is induc'd by breathing Air impregnate with Mercury, especially in close Places or Stoves. It is remarkable that Bodies defended from the external Air do not putrify. Thus *I Mort. Lib*. 1. tells us, " That a " Air-pump by extracting the Air " prevents Corruption." This Circumstance seems to add considerable Force to the Opinion that the Air by its Action changes Bodies, by dissolving them, and putrifying such as are subject to Putrefaction. Thus every Body knows that the Putrefaction of such Bodies is prevented by anointing them with oleous and balsamic Substances, so as to prevent the Ingress of the Air, into their Pores. As the Air therefore on Account of its Contents, is vastly different in different Places; so we find that the same Experiments do not answer in all Sorts of Air. The Reason why many Mixtures and Solutions of Bodies do not happen *in Vacuo*, or in high and elevated Places, where the Air is light, is because the Pressure or Motion of the Air, is not sufficiently strong.

Hitherto we have considered the common external Air. With Respect to the internal Air, contained in our Fluids, 'tis certain, that being dispersed

sed and diffused, thro' the Humours of the human Body, it does not produce the Effects of true Air, which it cannot do till it is united in Bubbles, and if this was to happen, it would soon prove mortal. In chymical Distillations, the elastic Force of the Air, which is sometimes so great, as to break the Vessels, is owing to the Extraction and Rarefaction of the latent Air, in the Bodies subjected to this Operation. Bubbles of Air in Effervescencies are excited, whilst the Particles of one Body, entering the Pores of another, expel the Air lodged in them. In the Burning of Bodies, the Fire by destroying the Cohesion of their Parts, expels the Air, which is then united into Bubbles. In the Air Pump, when the external Air is extracted, the internal Air, by its Elasticity, exerts itself, is formed into Bubbles, and produces an Ebullition. Cold expels the Air from Liquors, because the external Air being condensed presses them, and forces from their Pores the Particles of the Air, which are then formed into Bubbles. The Air is discharged from boiling Liquors, by the Fire, which agitates, rarifies, and expels it. Fix'd alcaline Salts, discharge Air from Fluids, because admitting only the solvent Liquid, they exclude the Air lodg'd therein. In Fermentation the Air is excluded, by an Increase of Fire or Heat. In Putrefaction the Air is discharged by an Increase of Heat, disuniting the corporeal Parts of the Bodies, and so seperating their internal Air. The Effects of the *Papinian* Machine, in which, by the Help of Water, hard Bones are resolved, are in a great Measure owing to the Virtues of the Air expanded, pressing, moving, and agitating their internal Structure. The Force with which congealed Water, breaks the Vessels, in which it is contained, is owing to the Cold condensing the

Water, and expelling from its Pores the Air, which is formed into Bubbles, and, makes a Resistance equal to the Pressure it receives. The Air lodged in the Aliments and swallowed with them, being rarified and expanded by the Heat of the Stomach and Intestines, by its Action, assists Digestion, in so far as it consists of a Resolution of solid Food.

The Physician who is careful to preserve Health, and cure Diseases, and who knows that Life cannot be supported, without inspiring the Air; may, from what has been said, understand the Effects of the Air, upon the human Body, and the Necessity of knowing how to direct these Effects prudently, and with Judgment; for he considers that the Air in general, as being possessed of Elasticity and Gravitation, insinuates itself into the patent Cavities of animal Bodies. Hence it is, that when new born Infants first dilate their Thorax, the Lungs, which were before close and compact, are distended, the Ramifications of the *Aspera Arteria* are so dilated, that there is a free Passage of the Air into the Vessels, at the Extremities of these Ramifications; as also of the Blood, thro' the minute Arteries, and Veins, which are interwoven with the Air Vessels, convey the Blood thro' the Lungs, and carry it to the Heart. And such a free Circulation is prevented, when the Lungs are either too much, or too little distended. The Ancients, conscious of the Necessity of Air, for the Support of Life, feigned *Apollo*, meaning the Sun, to be the Inventor of Medicine; *Æsculapius*, that is the Air, to be his Son, and *Hygeia* or Health, to be his Wife, or according to others his Daughter. But it is certain from Experience, that all external Air is prejudicial to Wouxds, which it changes, especially by drying them, preventing a laudable Suppuration, inducing a Putrefaction,

trefaction; and when it is confin'd by Means of a Plaister by infinuating itfelf into the fungous Parts, as the *Membrana adipofa,* and thus producing Emphyfemas; and when rarified and expanded, in the Cavity of the Abdomen, a *Tympanitis.* Thus, alfo, when Wounds of the Cranium are uncovered, the Air mortifies the minute Veffels of the *Pericranium,* and the exterior Lamina of the *Cranium* is exfoliated. All Bones expofed to the Air become gangrenous; for which Reafon the frequent Dreffing of Wounds is difcouraged by fkillful Surgeons. So that in general it holds true; that the Air difpofes to Putrefaction thofe Parts of the human Body to which it ought not to have Accefs; for *Ruyfch* informs us, that the Secundines may remain uncorrupted in the *Uterus* for two Years and longer; provided the Air has no Accefs to them; whereas they forthwith become putrid on the Accefs of this Fluid; hence common external Air, ought to have no Communication with any Parts of the human Body, except the *Epidermis,* the Air Veffels of the Lungs, and the firft Organs of Digeftion.

The Phyfician is, alfo, to confider the Air as fubject to the Influence of two Kinds of Bodies; I mean the heavenly Bodies, and the Exhalations and Vapours arifing from Bodies on the Earth. On the Afpect of the Sun, depend the Seafons of the Year, and Divifion of Difeafes, made according to them into Vernal and Autumnal, thofe of the Summer and the Winter. Hence arofe the aftrological Medicine of the Ancients, according to which they erroneoufly and precepitately, afcribed all Diforders to the Stars. That the human Body is affected, according to the different Nature of Exhalations and Vapours, is obvious, from the Difeafes of thofe who work in Metals, who with the Air infpire

the noxious Qualities communicate to it from the Metal. But the A whether influenced by celeftial terreftrial Bodies, is either prejud cial or beneficial, according to i Heat, Coldnefs, Humidity, Drynef Lightnefs, or Weight.

A too hot and fcorching Air, b drying the Solids, diffipating the mo fluid Parts of the Humours, and thu coagulating what is left in the Body difpofes to inflammatory, and nei vous Diforders. And if the Air be comes fo hot, as the Blood of a foun Perfon is, by the Thermometer, foun to be, 'tis certain from Obfervation that, in fuch an Air, Animals die Hence it is, firft, that by the Summer-Heats, Strength is confiderably impaired, fo that if the intenfe Heat was not temperated by alternate Colds, both Plants and Animals would foon be deftroyed. Secondly, Hence it is that after the Dog-days, Diforders depending on fome Indifpofition of the nervous Syftem often arife. To the Heat alfo of the Air it is owing, that in numerous Affemblies, inclos'd in clofe Rooms, with low Cielings, thofe of weak and delicate Conftitutions, fall into Deliquiums, efpecially in the hotteft Months of the Summer. From what has been faid, we underftand the Reafon of many medicinal Obfervations. Why, for Inftance, an intenfe Heat fuddenly arifing after violent Cold, produces Pleurifies, inflammatory Quinfeys, and fometimes Plagues; becaufe by the Heat, the Blood is deprived of its moft fluid Parts, and whilft the Veffels are dilated by the rarified Liquids, the thick Blood enters Veffels too minute, for its free Circulation. Hence, alfo we underftand, why thofe who remain long in the Sun with their Heads uncover'd, are feized with burning Fevers; as alfo thofe who take long Journies in fultry Weather, as is often experienced by Armies mes which suddenly move their Caps in hot Weather; for on such Occasions, Fevers generally are highly fatal. This is often confirmed by Travellers in *Asia*, where sometimes, almost the whole Caravan die of burning Fevers. Hence, also, we understand why intense Heat long protracted, produces Melancholy; for it is certain, from Observation, that in very hot Countries, vast Numbers of Persons, who in their Youth, were alert, brisk, and lively, after they are forty Years of Age, become hypochondriac, especially if they have used a hot Regimen; because the most fluid Parts of the Blood are dissipated, and the Remainder is consequently inspissated by the Heat. Hence, farther, we understand, why intense Heat succeeding Cold produces a spurious Peripneumony; because the Humours, especially of the pinguious Kind, being rendered stagnant by the Cold, and being resolved, by the succeeding Heat, enter the Mass of Blood by the absorbent Veins, and thus being convey'd into the right Ventricle of the Heart and pulmonary Arteries, produce the Disease.

Too cold and chill an Air, by shortening, condensing, corroborating, and increasing the Action of the solid Fibres upon the Humours, proves hurtful by inducing the Disorders arising from these Circumstances, such as Distillations, and Catarrhs; and a few Degrees of Cold greater than that which produces Ice on Water, congeals the Blood. *Stahl ad Harv. Cap.* 27, tells us, " that a cold Air produces one Effect on the Humours, which it thickens and inspissates, and another on the Solids, which by its Sharpness it stimulates to Contractions. *Hoffman* says, that " too cold an At-

" mosphere compressed by piercing elastic Winds, such as those " blowing from the North, renders " Pains and Spasms more acute, " and generates Coughs, Coryzas, " Hoarseness, Rheumatisms, Catarrhs, and inflammatory Fevers, " especially in Persons, disposed " to these Disorders; we, also, observe that Relapses of intermittent Fevers, and arthritic Paroxysms, are often excited by " northerly Winds. " *Hippocrates* tells us, " that some intensely cold " Bodies, such as Snow and Ice, " rupture the Veins and excite " Coughs." Cold Air to those of a sedentary Life is principally injurious, by generating the Scurvy; and if Persons have before been over-heated, it induces Asthmas, Quinsies, Pleurisies, Peripneumonies, Gouts and Rheumatisms. Cold is, also, highly injurious to the Membranes and Nerves, in the smallest of which it produces Obstructions, which give Rise to Palsies. All the Disorders arising from Cold seem to proceed from a Contraction of the solid Parts, and hence inducing a Change in the Humours on which they act. Hence we observe, that Persons who in Consequence of the State of their Solids, have tender weak Constitutions, and lax or open Pores, are more subject to Diseases rising from Cold than others. *Hoffman* in *Med. Rat.* tells us, " that " the cold Air is principally noxi- " ous to those Parts of the Body, " which have the smallest Afflux " of Blood to them; such as the " nervous and tendinous Parts, the " Abdomen and Intestines, the Head " and Brain, but especially the Feet, " and more particularly the Soles " and Toes, because these Parts " are not only very tendinous and " nervous, but also being at a great " Distance from the Heart, have

C " the

" Blood circulating flowly thro'
" them. " Among the *Spaniards*
who indulge themfelves immoderately in the Ufe of cold Liquors, Tumors in the Glands of
the Fauces are very frequent ; and
from what Authors have obferved
it is fufficiently obvious, that this
Effect may be produced by the
Coldnefs of a Climate, as well as
by cold Liquors ; for it is obfervable that thefe Tumours of the
Neck and Fauces, are more frequent in northerly than in fouth-
erly Countries. The frequent inflammatory Quinfies of Travellers, Couriers, Day-labourers and
Huntfmen, are moft frequently produced by the cold Air, or an ad-
verfe Wind rufhing into the Organs
fubfervient to Deglution and Refpiration. And Quinfies have fometimes happened to whole Armies,
when they have fuddenly remov'd
their Camps and march'd againft
the Wind. *Petrus Bellonius de ad-*
mirabili operum Antiquorum Præ-
ftantia, L. 2. Cap. 10. fpeaks in the
following Manner: " As for thofe
" who in paffing the *Alps* have
" their Fluids fo congealed, that
" they fuddenly drop down dead,
" I affirm that this happens by
" the Infpiration of the cold Air ;
" for the Body by the cold Intem-
" perature of the Air, has its native
" Heat extinguifhed, fo as to be
" congealed and as it were con-
" creted. This is the Caufe why
" Perfons die fo often in paffing
" the *Alps* ; their fudden Death
" is not, therefore, to be afcribed
" to the Snow, but to the cold In-
" temperature of the Air. Ac-
" cidents of this Kind happen not
" only on the Tops of Mountains,
" but alfo in Vallies, Defarts, and
" Forefts, as alfo on the Sea, be-
" caufe the Infpiration of the cold
" Air, by extinguifhing the native
" Heat, puts an End to Life ; but

" the moft effectual Method of p
" venting fuch Misfortunes, is a v
" lent brifk Agitation of the I
" dy."
Too moift an Air, when infpir
conveys too much Water into
Lungs, and is prejudicial to the C
tinuation of Life, by relaxing,
folving, and debilitating. He
proceed the Diforders arifing fr
an *Error Loci* enumerated by *B*
baave in his Inftitutions. If a m
Air is warm at the fame Time, it
poffeffed of a putrefactive Qu:
ty, and is fubject to generate
Plague. In a cloudy moift Air
obferve, that Flefh foon putrifi
and that Oils are colliquated.
late Obfervations we learn, that
Europeans, who firft fettled in fo:
Parts of *America,* were deftroyed
an epidemical Kind of putrid Fev
which foon diffolved their Bodi
but this Misfortune happened pr
cipally to thofe who inhabited ft
Places as abounded with Trees a
Shrubs; for in thefe Woods
Air was exceffively moift, by t
incredible Quantity of tepid V
pours exhaled from the Trees a
Plants ; but after all the Trees a
Woods were burnt, and a f
Air admitted to the Country,
became perfectly falubrious.
moift and cold Air generally exci
intermittent Fevers, as alfo Palfi
Melancholy, and the Gout. Her
it is, that in the Winter, we p
ceive the Cold more intenfe
moift than in dry Weather, tl
in the former, the Thermome
is lower than in the latter. M
fture relaxes the Veffels of the h
man Body, by which Means th
Action upon the Humours is
minifhed, in Confequence of whic
the true Caufe of Heat in t
Body will be foon weakened
whereas in cold dry Weather, t
Veffels having their Elafticity au
mented, act more forcibly on t
H<

Humor, by which Means the Heat of the Body is the longer contained.

Too dry an Air is almost equally injurious, with that which is excessively hot, by drying the Parts of the Body. According, however, to the Observations of *Hippocrates*, dry constitutions of the Air in general are more salubrious and less mortal, than such as are rainy. But in B. 3. *Aph.* 15. and 16. he tells us, that the Diseases which generally happen in rainy Seasons are long continued Fevers, Fluxes, Putrefactions, Anginas, Epilepsies and Palsies; whereas in dry Seasons the Diseases happening are Consumptions, Inflammations of the Eyes, Stranguries and Dysenteries."

An Air which is too heavy, too much compressed, is injurious to Health, by compressing the Vessels and their Contents, and consequently augmenting the Resistance made to the Heart, and by that Means producing a Kind of Suffocation.

Too light or rarified an Air is injurious, because by it the Vessels, being too little compressed, are too much dilated, by which means the Humours rarify, and are driven to improper Places; and by Cause dilating the Lungs, being diminished, the contractile Force of the pulmonary Fibres is increased, and the Lungs themselves are not sufficiently dilated; hence, Respiration is stopped.

The other Causes inducing various Changes and Qualities in the Air, also, alter and affect the human Body, not so much by any Virtue peculiar to the Air itself, as by the Nature of the Corpuscules contained therein, whether these are the Vapours or Exhalations of the Place which it surrounds, or are conveyed to it by Winds from

other Parts. To these Corpuscules we are to refer the acrid, saline, corrosive, and various other Qualities of the Air, as is evinced by the corrosive Nature of Dews. Sometimes a cloudy pinguious and dusky Air lets fall to the Ground, a Kind of Dew in Drops, smelling almost like burnt Milk, and when it is received on a pure marble Floor, it moistens it, as if it had been anointed with Oil. Such an Air when drawn into the Lungs renders them unctuous and inperspirable. Hence arises Accumulations and Congestions of Matter in the Breast. I have already mentioned the Diseases of such as work in Metals, arising from an Air impregnated with the metallic Particles. But Health is principally affected by the excessive Heat, Coldness, Moisture, Dryness, Weight and Levity of the Air, when one of these States suddenly succeeds another; when, for Instance, an intense Heat and Drought succeed an excessive Moisture, or when a severe Cold succeeds an intense Heat. As is observed by *Hippocrates* in *Sect.* 3. *Aph.* 1. and 4. These sudden Changes are the most immediate Causes of epidemical Diseases; for all the People inhabiting the same Place inspire the same Air.

The Motion of the Air is, also, to be considered by a Physician, since Air put into a Commotion, or Wind, exerts its Influences, whether noxious or salutary, more powerfully than Air in a State of Rest. By Wind, Cold is in a particular Manner augmented, and the Vapours penetrate more deeply into the human Body. Hence, we understand the Reason of the three following medicinal Observations. First, that those who being overheated, expose themselves to the Wind, greatly injure their Health. Secondly, that it is a prudent and

laudable

laudable Practice in Countries, where even in the Summer-Time there is a great Inequality in the Air, which is at one Time calm, and immediately after in a violent Commotion, as in *Holland,* and other Places contiguous to the Sea, to wear more and thicker Cloaths, than in other Places, where the Temperature of the Air with reſpect to Heat and Cold is the ſame, but where there is a greater Conſtancy, and fewer Commotions in the Air. Thirdly, As in cloſe Rooms, ſick Perſons of tender and delicate Conſtitutions are greatly injured by the ſmalleſt Cold, ſo we are to take particular Care, that the Air, tho' warm, be not put into any Kind of Commotion near them. Hence, alſo, we underſtand the Method of procuring a requiſite Coolneſs to the Body, by Means of the Air, tho' it is not altered in its Temperature; that is by exciting a Wind or a Motion of the Air by Means of Bellows or Fans, or by a Fire oppoſite to an open Door or Window; for the adjacent Air ruſhes upon that which is rarified by the Fire, by which means a Wind is excited. This End may, alſo, be obtained by cold Water, falling from a Syphon or Pipe perforated with ſmall Holes.

From what has been ſaid the Reaſon is obvious why *Hippocrates in Lib. de Flat.* tells us, " that the " Air is the principal and moſt " conſiderable Agent in all the " Changes and Accidents, which " happen to the human Body. " And why in *Lib. de Humoribus,* he ſays, " ſuch as the Seaſons are, " ſuch will be the Diſeaſes." Thus alſo *Ramazzini in Conſtit. an.* 1691. tells us, " that ſuch as the Air " we inſpire is, ſuch is the Diſ- " poſition of the Blood." Since then, *Hippocrates,* in *Lib. de Flatibus* aſſerts, that nothing contributes

more to Wiſdom and Prudence than a laudable State of the Blood and ſince a good Air has ſuch happy Influence on the Blood, may for that Reaſon, be eſteeme the Source and Origin of Wiſdom It is agreed among Phyſicians, th the ſame Air is not equally prope for all Perſons, whether in a Sta of Sickneſs or Health; for it prodi ces a good or bad Effect accordin to the *Idioſyncraſy,* or peculiar Co ſtitution of the Patient. Thus Perſons of a lax Habit of Body, moiſt Air is more prejudicial tha to ſuch as are of a dry Conſti tion, to whom a dry Air is mo hurtful than to thoſe of a cold ar lax Temperature. A warm Hum dity is beneficial to melanchol Patients; and a dry and ſomewh warm Air is ſerviceable in the Ric ets, according to *Boerhaave.* Son aſthmatic Patients are moſt injur by a dry and thin Air, but li more agreeably in a thick and mo Atmoſphere, ſuch as that of *H laid.* But Patients labouring und a nervous Aſthma, require an eme lient and relaxing Moiſture of t Air, to make the too rigid Fibres the Lungs perform their Function the better. *Hoffman,* ſays, he w " convinced from long and accura " Obſervation, that thoſe who l " bour under the Gout, arthri " Pains, or any other long and vi " lent Diſorder, as alſo under F " vers, and chronical Diſeaſes, " not recover ſo ſoon when t " Mercury is low in the Barom " ter, and a moiſt Intemperature " the Air has prevailed for a lo " Time; but as ſoon as a gra " ful Serenity returns, and the M " cury riſes, there is a remarkal " Change perceived in the Patien " for Tranſpiration and all the " ther neceſſary and critical E " cretions are more expeditiou " carried on, the Appetite is reſt "

" *and* the Sleep becomes founder.
" I *have* often obferved in my Prac-
" *ti*ce, fays he, that all Kinds of
" *Pai*ns, fuch as Cephalagias, Gouts,
" *a*nd Tooth-achs, become more
" acute and intenfe, and in a Pleu-
" rify the Refpiration is rendered
" more difficult and laborious, if
" cold, dry, and elaftic Winds have
" blown for a long Time and a per-
" fect Serenity is obferved. On the
" contrary, Patients labouring under
" a confirmed Phthifis, and intenfe
" Pains, an hectic, or fpitting of
" Blood, live moft agreeably in a
" cloudy, rainy, moift Air, nor are
" their Diforders fo violent as when
" northerly Winds blow." Thus
'tis obvious, that different Airs are
to be recommended according to the
different Nature of Difeafes. Thus
for fuch phthifical Patients, whofe
Diforder arifes from an acefcent
State of the Humours, the beft Air
is that of a Kitchen, which is impregnated with the volatile alcaline
Salt of Fifh and Flefh; whereas fuch
Patients would be palpably injured
by an Air, too much impregnated
with an Acid, fuch as that arifing
from fome Sorts of Wood, when
burnt : Such Patients are not lefs
injured by the acid Smoak of common Coal.

For the great Benefit, therefore, of
Mankind, Methods have been invented of correcting thofe Qualities of the Air, which by their Excefs induce Difeafes. Thus a cold
and moift Air, may be rendered
warm and dry, by Means of Fires
prepared of dry and aromatic Woods;
by the Vapours of hot Aromatics exhaling either fpontaneoufly, or by
Means of Fire; by the Admiffion of
a warm Wind, either natural or artificial. If, on the contrary, the Air
is too hot and dry, it is to be corrected by the Exhalations from cold
Plants immerfed in Water, fuch as
the Sallow, the Poplar, the Rofe-

tree, Elder, and the Mulberry-tree.
If the Water is to be difperfed by
Means of Syringes, let it be mixed
with a Solution of Sal-Ammoniac, in
order to render it more refrigerating.
The *Ægyptians*, according to *Profper Alpinus*, to prevent the Injuries
arifing from the intenfe Heat of the
Air, live in the loweft Appartments
of their Houfes, in the Middle of
which, they have Wells of cold
Water, with which during the whole
Summer they refrigerate the Air of
their Rooms, and near which they
generally fleep in the Night. They
have alfo large Pipes or Tubes, for
receiving the cool Air into their
Houfes. Thefe vaft Pipes, which
are about ten Cubits in Diameter are
carried up to the very Tops of their
Houfes, where they open with a
Mouth refembling that of a Bell,
towards the North, and convey the
cool Air to the loweft Apartments.
This Invention is by *Kircher*, alfo,
applied to other Purpofes, when for
Inftance, the Qualities requifite for
Health are to be procured to the
Air in an Houfe, " Take, fays he,
" a long Tube, which is to be fo
" difpofed, that the larger Orifice be
" fecured without the Room, and the
" reft within it, then gently infert
" into the Tube odoriferous Flowers,
" fuch as Violets, Lillies, Thyme,
" Bafil, and others of a fimilar Na-
" ture, fo that the Wind blowing
" externally, may convey the Odour
" of the Subftances contained in the
" Pipe, into the Chamber." The
Air may be rendered moift and
warm by the Evaporation of hot
Water, as is directed in burning Fevers by *Boerbaave*. An acrimonious
putrifying Air is corrected by burning Nitre or Gun-powder, by the
Steam of Vinegar, or by throwing
Salt on live Coals. Thefe Things
are of great Ufe in a peftilental Air,
againft which the Phyfician in vifit-
ing his Patients ought to guard him-

felf

self by large Spunges, or Handkerchiefs dipt in Vinegar, and applied to his Mouth; that the Air corrected by the Vapour of the Vinegar, may pass thro' these into his Mouth, Stomach, Intestines and Lungs. The Ancients, in order the more effectually to consult the Health of their Miners, used to cloath them in leathern Sacks, and put lax Bladders upon their Faces. At present the Miners, especially those who work at Arsenic, wear glass Masks on their Faces. In all cloudy contaminated Air, 'tis proper to forbear swallowing the Spittle in the open Air; for the acrid noxious Particles of the Air, are by that Means easily conveyed to the Stomach and Intestines. For this Reason 'tis proper to use Tobacco in order to evacuate the infected Spittle. The Advice of Physicians is to be taken, with Respect to the most proper Measures for removing the antecedent Causes of a contaminated Air. Thus, if the Air is infected by stagnant Waters, these are to be conveyed elsewhere by proper Drains, or some other Methods. If the Air is corrupted by unburied Carcasses, Dunghils, or Excrements of any Kind, these are to be buried, burnt, or removed in some other Manner. Noxious Exhalations dispersed thro' the Air, are quickly dissipated by Fire, than which nothing purifies the Air more expeditiously and efficaciously. Thus we are told, that *Hippocrates* removed a Plague from *Greece*, by burning whole Woods. As the Vibration of the Air contributes greatly to its Renovation, so some Authors greatly commend the Ringing of large Bells in the Time of a Plague. Hence Birds, especially Sparrows, Hens, Peacocks, Ducks, and Storks kept tame in Chambers, are thought to purge and ventilate the Air by their flying, or the Agitation of their Wings. *Levinus Lemnius* in *Mir. L. 2. Cap.*

10. tells us, that the frequent Explofions of Cannons and Fire-arms contribute greatly to dissipate Clouds, and contagious Exhalations of the Air. But perhaps the Smoak of kindled Hay, before besprinkled with some Vinegar, may be a more effectual Remedy. In intemperate, unequal and inconstant Weather, it is proper always to be equally cloathed, and to avoid the Inclemency of the Air as much as is possible, by keeping within Doors. With Respect to the Signs of a corrupted, poisonous, or contagious Air, *Mindererus de Peste* tells us, " that we may know such a " State of the Atmosphere, when an " Egg or Apple exposed to the Air " for a Night, becomes highly pu- " trid; or when new Bread, is yet " hot, and erected in the Air " on the Point of a Spear or Pole, " and left for a Night, contracts a " Kind of Putrefaction, becomes " mucid, and requires such a noxi- " ous Quality, that it either cannot be " tasted by Animals, or proves mor- " tal to them when eaten. Such " a Condition of the Air, may also " be known, when the Birds drop " down and die." From what has been said, 'tis sufficiently obvious, that the Air may be possessed either of salutary or noxious Qualities, according to the Natures of those Substances, whose Vapours and Exhalations are mixed therewith. The Health of the Public is, therefore, preserved, by taking care that in populous Places the Air be not polluted by Filth and Nastiness in the Streets, and by making proper Regulations for Soap-boilers, Tanners, Dyers, and Candle-makers. Cleanliness was for this Reason strictly enjoyned the *Jews* in their Camp, as we are told in *Deuteronomy, Cap.* 23. *V.* 12, 13, and 14. And upon this Subject many excellent Treatises have been written. The Reason why a Person who has lived long

ing in the bad Air of a public Hospital, is sometimes indisposed upon his coming out of it, seems to be owing to the Weight of the Air, or the Exhalations therein which he was accustomed to; for according to *Hippocrates* in *Sect.* 2. *Aph.* 50. a Man us'd to an impure Air, cannot bear a better so well.

From what has been said, I think it appears rational to advise the Change of Air, that every Individual may enjoy one suited to his State, Temperament, and Condition.

I have before observed, that an Air close and long pent up, is highly prejudicial to the Continuation of the Lives of Animals; for when long free from all Ventilation, it assumes so pestilential a Quality, as in a Moment to prove mortal to such as rashly expose themselves to it. Thus many by opening Caves and subterraneous Places, which have been long closed, have been forthwith destroyed by the poisonous Air, discharged from them. Hence 'tis obvious, that the Air only by Stagnation, without any foreign Contagion may not only prove useless, but destructive of Life. The Cause of this, *Boerhaave* in his *Instit. Med.* thus gives: "Air, "when not frequently renewed, be"comes mortal, not on Account of its "Heat, Rarefaction, or Density, but "on Account of another more la"tent Cause, which is perhaps the "Destruction of its Elasticity, or of "that Principle which the Alchy"mists call the Aliment of Life." *Vossius* says, that "the vital "and animal Spirit, is not generat"ed of Blood alone, but has also "Air mixed with it, nor could it "subsist, unless it received Nourish"ment from the external Air. But "'tis a childish Error to imagine "that the Air we expire is always "exactly the same with that we in"spire; for a Portion of it remains "within, in order to nourish the

"Spirit, as being a Substance most "similar to it; and the Air that is "expired is no longer pure, but has "reeking Vapours mixed with it." 'Tis certain, that in large Assemblies of People pent up in low close Rooms, such as have weak and delicate Constitutions, fall into Deliquiums, but find Relief in a free and open Air; for it seems probable that when Animals inspire the same Air, which they have not only often expired, but which is also contaminated by the Exhalations perspiring from the Body, such an Air is too light for expanding the Lungs sufficiently, and promoting the Circulation of the Humours. This Doctrine seems to be confirmed, by that Property of Fire, whereby it continues to burn so long as it has the free and open Access of the compressing Atmosphere, but when such an Air is removed, and only the Air expired from the Lungs, is applied to a burning Candle, it is immediately extinguished, but again immediately blown up, by Air collected in the Mouth before it reaches the Lungs. That an Air remaining long without Renovation is contaminated with Exhalations noxious to Health, is sufficiently experienced, also, by those who are frequently near the Beds of sick Persons, especially those labouring under burning Fevers; for those who constantly attend such Patients, have their Eyes and Lips inflamed by that Means. In close Places, such as Prisons, in which many are confined, a highly malignant Species of Scurvy often rages. In public Hospitals, where many lie sick at a Time, Apostems and malignant Ulcers are generally produced by the putredinous Exhalations. Hence appears the Necessity of preventing these Accidents, by the Renovation of the Air. Thus in Prisons, Holes might be made in the Roof or Walls, for removing the old, and bringing new

Air in its ftead. Pure and frefh Air may be admitted to fick Perfons, by opening a Window for a little Time, whilft the Curtains of the Bed are clofed, and then fhutting the former and opening the latter. In the clofeft Places of Ships, where the Air is tainted by the Exhalations of the Men, the Sailors wafh the Floors, and fprinkle them with Vinegar, or pour Vinegar into Iron Veffels heated red hot; but the beft Remedy is certainly the Expulfion of the old, and Introduction of frefh Air.

With Refpect to that Queftion, what Kind of Air, in general, is moft fit for the Prefervation of Health? *Boerhaave* in *Inflit. Med.* fays, " that Air is beft for the Pre-" fervation of Health, which is fe-" rene, heavy, temperately warm, " and dry, which blows from pure " *Mediterranean* Regions, and Ri-" vers; which is agitated by a gen-" tle Wind, free from violent Com-" motions, unconfined, rural and " defecated from faline and oleous " Exhalations;" for a pure ferene and temperate Air preferves the contractile and expenfive Motion of the Solids entire, and communicates a due Tone and Strength to the Fibres; for it neither too much conftricts nor relaxes the Pores and minute Veffels, nor does it refolve and attenuate the Compages of the Fluids, nor induce a Lentor; but rather preferves a due Mixture and Temperature of them. As a pure and temperate Air is of fo great Importance to Health, the Reafon is obvious why elevated Places, efpecially thofe lying expofed to eafterly Winds, and Country Habitations, are fo beneficial to valetudinary Perfons; for high Situations have a thin and pure Air, becaufe they are more frequently expofed to the Wind, and the Impurities of the Air are by that Means diffipated. But no Place is

more proper for living in, than a Plain, or the gentle Declivity of a fmall Hill, where the Soil is barren and gravelly, not fat and bituminous, and confequently lefs fit for the Purpofes of the Hufband-man.

All other Circumftances being alike, we generally perceive ourfelves more cheerful and brifk, when we remove from large and populous Towns, to Country Places, becaufe in the latter we infpire a purer Air, which promotes a free Circulation of the Blood; for it is more ponderous, elaftic, and when infpired, impels the Humours more thro' the Veffels; whereas the Air in Towns being impregnated with Vapours and Exhalations, more light, lefs frequently renewed, and lefs elaftic, is, for thefe Reafons, lefs favourable to the Circulation of the Humours. Hence alfo we underftand the Reafon, why we enjoy not only a freer Refpiration, but alfo a more chearful Temper during the Winter, in a Room heated with a Fire in a Chimney, becaufe then the Vapours and Exhalations are carried up the Chimney, and the Air is conftantly renew'd, than in a Room warmed with a Stove, as is cuftomary in the northern Countries, where the Vapours cannot be difcharged, nor the Air renewed, fo that Refpiration muft be performed in too clofe, vapid and light an Atmofphere. *Voffius* juftly obferves, that every Animal, when the Air is fuited to its Nature, teftifies its Joy either by fome particular Motion, fuch as leaping, running, and flying, or by its Voice; fo great is the Influence of the Air in rendering Life grateful and agreeable. And *Virgil* long ago feems to have been abundantly fenfible of this Influence of the Air, when fpeaking of the Changes of Weather prognofticated by the Behaviour of the brute Creation, he fays:

Non

No equidem credo, quia sic divinitus illis
..., aut rerum fato Prudentia major.
... ibi Tempestas, et Cœli mobilis Humor
...ere Vias, et Jupiter humidus Austris,
... erant quæ rara modo, et quæ densa,
relaxat,
...ntur Species Animorum, et Pectora
Metus
...alios, alios, dum frigora Ventus agebat
...; hinc ille avium Concentus in
Agris,
... læti pecudes, et Ovantes Gutture Corvi.

Those who intend to practise Me-
...ine, ought to remember, that we
...e before evinced that the good
...noxious Qualities of the Air, are
...plied to the human Body in three
...nners ; that is, by Inspiration into
...Lungs ; by its Admixture with
...iments ; and externally upon the
...rface of the Body, and the Vef-
...s distributed upon it ; for a Know-
...ge of these, enables them to direct
...requisite Effects, and remove the
...aries to be apprehended from the
...r. Hence we may, perhaps, con-
...de that the Air produces greater
...anges in the human Body, than
...iments, since the last do not af-
...t us in so many different Ways.
...he Physicians of the methodic Sect,
...o maintained that all Diseases arose
...her from Stricture or Relaxation,
...re more careful in the Choice of
...r for their Patients, than of Meat
...d Drink ; because the Air being
...her hot or cold, may proportiona-

bly relax or constrict the Body. As
another Reason for their Conduct
they also said, that Aliments were
only taken at Intervals, whereas the
Inspiration of the Air was continually necessary.

With respect to the celebrated Question, whether the external, heavy and
elastic Air, during Inspiration, penetrates the pulmonary Vessels, and
mixes with the Blood. *Boerhaave*,
thinks that it does not ; but seems to
be of Opinion, that something passes from the Air-Vesicles in the
Lungs to the Pulmonary Veins.
This *something* I take to be the vital Principle in the Air so often taken Notice of above, and which is
so necessary to the animal Oeconomy, that all Air divested of it by repeated Inspirations, is no longer capable of supporting Life, without a
perpetual fresh Supply. And this,
there is great Reason to believe, is
nothing but the pure ætherial Acid
of the Air ; and 'tis possible, that the
Elasticity of Air may depend entirely
upon it. This however I mention
as a Conjecture, and as a Subject
which highly merits farther Examination.

Thus having considered Air as a
principal Instrument in natural and
artificial Chymistry as well as in e-
very Part of Pharmacy, and as a Non-
natural ; I proceed to Water, another
very important Agent in the Combination and Dissolution of Bodies.

CHAP. II.
Of WATER.

WATER, according to the celebrated *Boerhaave*, is a Liquor highly fluid, inodorous, insipid,
fluid, without colour, and which
in a certain Degree of Cold, is condensed into a brittle, hard and vitre-
ous Substance, commonly called Ice.
Its Weight is to that of Air as 1 to

859. It is heavier than all Wines and Malt Liquors, than the Spirit of Wine, and Oils of Olives, sweet Almonds and Turpentine ; but 'tis almost sixteen times lighter than quick Silver, and considerably lighter than Spirit and Oil of Vitriol, the Spirits of Nitre, Salt, and Sulphur, Aqua-Fortis, Vinegar, distilled Vinegar, the Milks of Cows, Goats and Asses ; Whey, Urine, and Oil of Tartar.

So great is the Fluidity of Water, that by the smallest Heat or Motion, its minutest Parts recede from each other, and 'tis far from being improbable, that in Lakes apparently stagnant, it retains a perpetual, tho' imperceptible Motion on Account of the insensible Undulations of the Air.

The constituent Particles of Water being so small and minute as to escape the Sight, even when assisted by a Microscope, render it capable of penetrating into the invisible Pores and Interstices of many Bodies, into which Air has no Access; and tho' 'tis specifically heavier than Air, yet it may remain in it, and be raised to a considerable Height, just as Earth, which is also heavier than Air, is suspended in it under the Form of Dust. Hence 'tis obvious, that the Water contain'd in the Air will enter these Bodies, into which the Air itself penetrates. The more pure and free from a Mixture of heterogeneous Particles the Water is, the greater Quantity of it will be exhaled, whereas the more Salt it has absorbed the less of it will be evaporated.

Notwithstanding what has been said, there are some Bodies which do not transmit Water thro' their Pores, such as Metals, Flints, hard Stones of all Kinds, Gems, Glass, some Woods of a compact, hard, ponderous and resinous Nature, China Vessels, and well polished Substances. Those Bodies into whose Pores Water cannot enter when cold, also remain impenetrable to it when agitated Fire, and pressed with a great Forc unless the Parts of the Vessel which the Water is contained shou recede from each other, and suff it to pass thro' its Pores. Hen 'tis sufficiently obvious that the hig est Force of Fire cannot divide t Elements of Water into small Parts, but is only capable of exten ing them to a greater Bulk, and agitating them strongly with each ther ; for by the Absence of Fir or rather its Diminution by Col the Particles of Water seem to l contracted, whilst they are concrete into Ice. This Contraction of th Elements of Water cannot be sensibl observed, because the Air expelled b a strict Union of the contracted Ele ments of the Water, begins to forr elastic Bubbles, which more dilat the Ice than it is diminished by th Cold. 'Tis observed by Bricklay ers and Plaisterers, that the colde Water is, the more effectually penetrates Walls ; for Water is mor condensed by Cold than Stones, fo which Reason the Pores of Stone are less contracted by Cold, than the Particles of Water, so that excessively cold Water can pass thro' Pore thro' which warm Water cannot be conveyed. Hence we may infer, that the component Parts of Water are by no Means compressible, but unchangeable in Figure and Bulk, and are probably small Spheres finely polished.

Water contained in the Pores of those Bodies into which it has penetrated, augments their Weight in Proportion to its own. Hence we discover the Frauds of some avaricious Traders who preserve their Goods in a moist Place, or buy them dry in order to sell them in wet Weather. Besides, the Water which insinuates into Bodies, enlarges their Bulk without destroying their Figure. Hence, dry Bodies into which Water insinuates itself, are changed by it. Thus wooden Vessels when

dried

..., have Chinks which admit Water, tho' the same Vessels when moist
no longer suffer any to enter. In
the Night-time when Storms arise,
people often are allarmed at the
cracking of Houses, so much as to
be apprehensive of Thieves on that
Account, whereas this Effect is produced by the moist Air, insinuating itself into the Parts of the Wood,
and forcing them to recede from each
other. The Strings of musical Instruments, prepared of the Intestines
of Animals, are rendered more tense
by the moist Air expanding them:
Water insinuating itself into some Bodies only gently coheres with them,
and is again separated from them,
whereas it is firmly concreted with
them. Hence, wooden Chests, and
the Doors of Houses, which in wet
Weather are firmly shut, in a dry
season open spontaneously, on Account of their Contraction, after the
Expulsion of the Water. On the
contrary, every dry Salt, only by
violent Fire yields Spirits by
Distillation, from which the Water is separated by Rectification,
and sometimes by Means of an
intire Salt. The same holds
true with Respect to Sulphur dissolved into a Spirit. After Water has insinuated itself into other
and Bodies, it adheres so intimately to them, as not to be perceptible,
if at the same Time it constitutes
the of such solid Bodies; as is
shown from dry quick Lime after
the Expulsion of the Moisture in
Calcination. This quick Lime by
the Affusion of Water, is reduced
to a ductile Paste, consisting of
Water, Sand and Lime, which being dried, becomes hard like a
Stone; and yet this Hardness depends
partly on the Water contained therein, but when expelled by the
Fire, the Elements of the Lime
more cohere with each other.
Water, also, concretes with the

most hard and solid vegetable Bodies, as is obvious from the Distillation of *Guaiacum* made by itself.
The hard and driest Parts of Animals, by Distillation, yield a volatile Spirit, which contains a large
Quantity of pure Water. Hence
'tis obvious, that Water enters the
Composition of many Bodies and
proves the strongest Glew or Cement, by which their Parts adhere
to each other. 'Tis also equally
obvious, that the solid Parts of the
human Body, derive their Texture,
from the glutinous and adhesive Quality of Water.

There are Bodies which Water
not only penetrates, but also dissolves, in such a manner as that e-
qual Qualities of such Bodies are
equally distributed thro' all the Parts
of the solvent Water. All Salts
whether in a liquid or solid Form,
are, according to their Natures,
more or less dissolved by Water.
Water in a Commotion always
dissolves a larger Quantity of Salt,
and more expeditiously, than that
which is at Rest, and warm Water
more than that which is cold; so
that the hotter the Water is, the
more Salt it dissolves and retains;
whereas the colder it is the more
of the dissolved Salt it lets fall;
so that during intense Frost, the
Salt is almost entirely expelled from
freezing Water. This is the Reason why Sea-water is not so easily converted into Ice, as fresh Waters; as also why it is more salt
in hot, than in cold Climates. It
seems to be sufficiently certain that
Water, entirely destitute of Heat,
which is the coldest of Ice, can dissolve no Salt. The same Quantity
of Water dissolves one Salt more
quickly than another, and more of
some than of others. 'Tis also observable, that the Water which has
dissolved as much of any given
Salt as it possibly can, so that if
any

any more of the fame Salt is thrown into this *Lixivium*, it remains undiffolved at the Bottom, may yet diffolve a large Quantity of another Salt, when thrown into it, without feparating the Salt which was firft diffolved, from the Water. From fome Salts, when diffolving in Water, arifes Cold, from others Heat, and from others neither Cold nor Heat. Thus Cold is excited by Nitre, Borax, Sea Salt, Vitriol, Verdigreafe, Alum, Rhenifh Tartar, Cream of Tartar, volatile Salt of Urine, and all alcaline volatile Salts. But among all Salts, the greateft Cold is excited by Sal-ammoniac. Heat is produced by common brown Sugar, by Salt of Tartar, Aqua-Fortis, Spirit of Sea Salt and Spirit of Nitre; but the greateft Heat is produced by Oil of Vitriol. Neither Heat nor Cold is produced by diffolving in Water, Oil of Tartar per Deliquium, the recent Urine of a found Perfon, Vinegar, and previoufly putrified human Urine.

Water, alfo, diffolves *Alcohol* of Wine, if ftrongly fhaken with it; but if it be gently poured to the Alcohol, it paffes thro' it, and fubfides to the Bottom, the *Alcohol* fwimming above. But it does not very foon diffolve the Alcohol which after Conquaffation, fluctuates thro' the Water in a Kind of pinguious *Striæ*, tho' it is at laft equally diftributed thro' the whole Water. Now as *Alcohol* is a pure Oil of Vegetables, which by the Efficacy of a due Fermentation is changed into the Nature of Spirits, which deflagrate in Fire, and mix with Water, we know, that Oils themfelves, thus previoufly changed, may be alfo perfectly mixed with Water, tho' this happens the fooner and the more eafily, if they have been before diluted with a fmall Quantity of Water, for com-

mon Spirit of Wine which contains much Water, is more eafily mix'd with Water, than the pureft *Alcohol*. When Water is mix'd with pure *Alcohol* rectified by itfelf, the Mixture produces Heat with an Effervefcence. The fame alfo happens with common Spirit of Wine, tho' in a fmaller Degree; but with alcalizated Spirit of Wine the Heat is lefs, and the Effervefcence none at all. But with Water entirely faturated with diffolved Salts, fuch as Oil of Tartar *per Deliquium*, for Inftance, *Alcohol*, cannot be mix'd by Shaking or Ebullition, for the *Alcohol* always appears uppermoft. But even in this Refpect there is a Difference between Salts; for if the Water be richly impregnated with any Salt which eafily fuffers itfelf to be feparated from the Water, fuch as that of *Epfom*, for Inftance, then the *Alcohol* will be united with the Water pour'd to it, and the Salt difengag'd from the previoufly folvent Water, will be precipitated to the Bottom of the Veffel. If Water is mix'd with *Alcohol* in which a diftill'd Oil is diffolv'd, it forces the Oil from the *Alcohol*. Water alfo feparates any Refin, as alfo Camphire, which has been previoufly diffolv'd in *Alcohol*.

Water alfo diffolves all Soaps compos'd of Oil and alcaline Salts, or all faponaceous Bodies, by which Means a Mixture is produc'd capable of diffolving fome Subftances, which Water alone cannot diffolve; fuch as Oils, oleous Subftances, Refins, refinous Subftances, Gum-Refins, and tenacious Bodies compounded of them. Hence the Power of Water to diffolve Bodies, is much increas'd by the Virtues of Soap. And hence the Method of rendering Oils capable of mixing with Water is fufficiently obvious.

Water alone is capable of diffolving effential Oils, if thefe are before duely mixt with pure *Alcohol*, by

Means

Means of Digestion and repeated Distillations.

Water also diffolves fulphureous Subftances united with thofe of an oilne Nature, as alfo Balfams, Colophonies, and Refins, if they are firft united with alcaline Subftances. Water alfo diffolves the Air itfelf, and receives into its Pores a certain Quantity thereof, which does not act as Air fo long as it remains in thefe Pores. The Air contain'd in Water is fufficiently difcover'd by its Ebullition, when the external Preffure of the Air is remov'd from the Surface of the Water, by Means of an Air-pump. Since, then, Air contains Bodies of all Kinds, hence 'tis obvious that thefe muft alfo with Air be convey'd into the Pores of the Water.

Water is, alfo, capable of diffolving many terreftrial Bodies, if they are firft thoroughly corroded in their proper Acids. Of this Kind, are Oyfterfhels, the Shels and Claws of Crabbs, Shels of Snails, Shels of Fifhes, whether of the Sea or River kind Stones, and ftony Concretions, Horns, Bones, and Hoofs of Animals, Chalk, Pearls, Mother of Pearl, calcin'd Stones and Flints. But as thefe terreftrial Bodies corroded in their Acids become diffolvable in Water, fo on the contrary alcaline Subftances intimately united with Earth, cannot afterwards be diffolv'd in Water, as may be inftanc'd in Glafs; and the highly fubtile and volatile alcaline Salts of Animals intimately united with Earth, conftitute a Mafs which can by no Means be diffolved by Water. But Water is the moft powerful Solvent when rais'd in Vapours by Means of Fire, as is evident from that Species of Calcination which is term'd *Philofophical*.

There are, however, fome Bodies which cannot be diffolv'd by Water, fuch as pure Earth entirely deftitute of foreign Salts, and free from the leaft Admixture of every fulphureous Subftance; as alfo Glafs, Gems, Cryftals, entirely fimple Stones, and feveral other Bodies of a fimilar Nature. To thefe we may add Metals; becaufe the Solutions of Metals faid to be made by Water, feem to be produc'd rather by the Salts contain'd in the Water, than by the Water itfelf. Water, farther, cannot diffolve Oils, Refins, Balfams, Colophonies and Sulphurs, unlefs they are mix'd with fome other Bodies; for which Reafon, Bodies cover'd with thefe Subftances do not admit Water into their Pores. In many Cafes the folvent Force of Water is increas'd, according as its Heat is augmented, and its folvent Power is diminifh'd in Proportion as its Heat is leffen'd. But in other Solutions made with Water, the contrary holds true; for fome Bodies are diffolv'd in tepid, but are indurated in boiling Water, fuch as the White of a new laid Egg, the Serum of the Blood, and fome other Subftances.

Since Water, in Confequence of its folvent Quality, may contain many other Bodies in fuch a Manner as not to appear, but to conftitute in Conjunction with it an aqueous Fluid call'd Water, hence we fee the Abfurdity of thofe who undertake to treat of Water as a pure Fluid perfectly feparated from every other Body; " For, according to the cele- " brated *Hoffman*, there is not to be " found in Nature, any Species of " Water, which does not contain " fomething of a dry and folid Na- " ture; for in every Water, howe- " ver often diftill'd, there is always " fomething dry and folid found in " the Bottom of the Veffel. This " is obvious to the Eye, when the " pureft Water is frozen; for up- " on its being thaw'd, a certain grofs " and earthy Portion fubfides to the " Bottom of the Veffel." Hence 'tis, alfo, farther evident; firft, that the Virtues and Effects of Water often

ten

ten depend upon its Contents. Secondly, that these Virtues are various according to the Substances mix'd with the Water. Thirdly, that one Water differs from another with Respect to the Bodies with which it is mix'd, and that one Water may be said to be purer than another. Fourthly, that it is alter'd or chang'd with Respect to its Fluidity, Smell, Taste and Transparence, by the Bodies which are mix'd with it. And Fifthly, that the Weight of Water is various according to the Bodies contain'd in its Pores; for in Water there are many Substances contain'd, which are lighter than pure and simple Water; this is principally obvious in rain Water and those rais'd in chymical Vessels. There are, however, many more Substances, which are naturally heavier than Water, that mix therewith, insinuate themselves into its Pores, and consequently render it heavier than it would otherwise be.

Since, therefore, Bodies both naturally lighter and heavier than Water may be mix'd therewith, it may seem to be an Error to call that Water purest which we find to be lightest. But 'tis to be observ'd, that in considering natural Water, if we except rain Water, which tho' lighter than other Waters with which the Bowels of the Earth supply us, yet abounds with many heterogeneous Particles, and some mineral Waters impregnated with a large Quantity of etherial Principles, which at the Fountain-head are lighter than common Water, but become heavier when carry'd to a Distance from their Springs, in consequence of the Loss of their spirituous Parts, yet the Goodness of other Waters may be estimated from their Lightness; because, the Water lodg'd in the Bowels of the Earth receives into its Pores, such Bodies as are heavier than the Water itself; whereas Rain

Water, which is rais'd in the Air, admits more light and volatile Bodies; and mineral Waters at their Fountain-head containing an highly subtile Æther, are more rarified, and consequently contain less Matter under the same Bulk. The Weight of Water is therefore to be examin'd in order to know which is most light, and consequently most pure and salubrious. *Sanctorius* orders us to investigate the specific Gravities of different Waters, by weighing some heavy Body in them, because a Body gravitates most in that which is purest and lightest. But the Moderns have invented many more accurate Methods of investigating the Weight or Lightness of Waters, which are now generally known. But 'tis to be observ'd in all statical Experiments, that the different Degrees of Heat vary and change the Weight of the same Water; for in Summer all Water is rarified, and consequently lighter than in Winter, when condens'd. That Water is, also, lightest which boils soonest, whereas that is more heavy which requires a longer Time. And that, also, is the lightest, which cools the soonest.

Besides the Lightness of Water, there are, also, other Tests of its Purity. The most considerable of these is, to dilute a Solution of the purest Silver, made by Aqua Fortis, in the finest Water that can be had; for if the Water to be tried is pour'd into a clear Glass, and some of this Solution dropt into it, without rendering it turbid, opake, or whitish, such a Water may be concluded pure, for nothing can be contain'd in them, except Spirit of Nitre or Aquafortis. Thus, also, if Oil of Tartar *per Deliquium*, well diluted with Water, is drop'd into the Water to be try'd, without inducing any Alteration in the Colour, we are sure nothing is contain'd in it, except an Alcali, for if an Alcali only should be in it, no

Per-

Perturbation or Change of Colour will be produc'd. But nothing discovers the Impurity of Water sooner than a Solution of Sugar of Lead made with the purest Water; for a very few Drops of this soon discovers the heterogeneous Contents, by rendering the Water instantly turbid. The Antients have, also, handed down to us several Signs, by which to judge of the Purity of Waters. Thus 'tis esteem'd good, if it leaves no Stain when thrown upon a brass Vessel; if no Sand or Mud subsides in the Bottom of a Vessel, in which it has been boil'd, when it is pour'd out, after it has been in a State of Rest for some Time; if Pulse boil'd in it are soon reduc'd to Softness; if no Moss nor Rushes grow in or near the Channels where it flows; if it produces in such as drink it no bad Colour, blear'd Eyes, nor Inflammations of the Gums; if it is clear and tasteless; if it readily dissolves Soap, and cleanses Linen from Dirt; if it nourishes good and salubrious Fish, and if it makes good Mortar for the Purposes of Building. To which may be added, if it extracts good Tinctures from Bodies infus'd in it, as from Tea. From what has been said, 'tis sufficiently obvious, that Waters assume different Natures and Qualities, from the Places where they rise, the Soils thro' which they flow, or in which they continue, and the Air to which they are expos'd; and that these different Qualities depend on the heterogeneous Parts with which they are connected.

In order to discuss that important Question, What Species of Water is most useful in common Life? we shall separately consider each of what we commonly call the sweet and simple Waters, beginning with Rain Water.

Rain-Water, then, is a Water distill'd by Nature, for by the Heat of the Air, it is elevated from the Surface of the Earth, to such a considerable Height, as no chymical Distillation can possibly imitate. So that it may truely be said to be the *Lixivium of the Atmosphere*, in which all the various Species of Corpuscules, fluctuating in the Air, are collected. Hence 'tis obvious that there are Variations in rain Water, not only according to the Diversity of the Soils and Climates, but also with Respect to the Seasons of the Year. Thus the vernal Rains are considerably impregnated with mix'd Bodies, which the Cold of the Winter had retain'd in the Earth, but which the Heat of the Spring resolves, disperses thro' the Air, and mixes with the Rain. Hence Spring Rain Water is much fitter than others for some Operations, which in order to render them perfect, require that Force of Water which does not depend upon the Water itself, but upon the Matter which is mix'd with it, as is sufficiently obvious from Fermentations and the Vegetations of Plants; for this Reason it is, that *March* Water is so much celebrated by some. Since, then, Rains vary according to the Constitution of the Air, which is contaminated with more or less foreign Bodies, we may hence judge whether all Rain Waters are good for the Purposes which are excellently answer'd by some.

The most impure Species of Rain Water is that which falls during intensely hot and windy Weather, in populous Cities, and low situated and fetid Places, where the Parts of Animals, Vegetables, and other Bodies are daily and copiously dispers'd thro' the Air, by Reason of the great Multitude of Inhabitants. And the Rain-water will be still worse, if the Air is foggy, and of an ill Smell. Some Rains are observ'd to fall suddenly after violent Claps of Thunder, and these, if collected in clean Vessels, yield a Froth, which seems to contain something like an highly subtile nitrous Salt. Some Rains falling during violent Tempests, have been observ'd to be highly fetid, and in twenty-four Hours to generate Worms in the Cloths they fell upon.

Upon considering all the Waters which fall from the Atmosphere, that of Snow has been found the lightest, and the higher it is carried into the Air, the more it is depurated from its gross Parts in its Descent. If an intense Cold has form'd Water elevated to a great Height, into Flakes of Snow, especially after a Series of serene and dry Weather, and if such a Snow falls upon a barren sandy Soil at a great Distance from Towns and Cities, it will be as pure as it can be made either by Art or Nature; for it will hardly contain either Salt, Air, Oil, or any other Substance. The Water of Snow is unchangeable, may be kept for Years, and is an excellent Remedy for Inflammations of the Eyes. Tho' some are of Opinion that Rain-waters, in Consequence of their Lightness, Purity, and Transparency are of all others the best, especially for medicinal Purposes, yet *Hippocrates* in his Treatise of Air, Water, and Situations, tells us, " That they must be boil'd and puri- " fied, otherwise they have a bad " Smell, and produce Hoarseness in " those who drink them." But he absolutely condemns Snow and Ice-water, tho' some modern Physicians admit the Use of them, when the Snow is pure and not contaminated with earthy Sordes, when the Stomach is overheated, and stands in need of a Cooler, tho' they must not be us'd where there is a scorbutick Cacochymy, or any Disorder of the Viscera. What is said of Snow-water may be, also, applied to that of Hail.

Spring or Fountain-water, it is said, derives its Origin from that of Rain, whilst the aqueous Vapours e- levated from the Earth and dispers'd thro' the Air, striking upon cold and high Mountains, are condens'd into Drops, from a Collection of which flowing down the Sides of these Mountains, Water is produc'd in some subterraneous Cavity, from which it afterwards arises on the Surface of the Earth ; but from the Places thro' which it flows, it acquires a Nature different from that of Rain-water. If it flows thro' Soils which are sandy, and full of pure Flint, it is strain'd, as it were, thro' their Interstices, deposites every Thing of a foreign Nature which adher'd to it, and becomes highly pure. On the contrary, when Spring-water flows thro' Places in which any Matter, which Water can easily dissolve, is contain'd, then it conveys along with it many of the Corpuscules it touches. After this it is of no Importance whether it flows thro' Rocks, Sands, Hills and Mountains, since it will always carry these Corpuscules along with it. Hence 'tis obvious, that nothing can be universally and generally pronounc'd as Truth with Respect to all Spring-water. This is sufficiently confirm'd from a particular Circumstance, which is, that all Spring-water boil'd for some Time, after it remains at rest and becomes cool, deposites more or less Fauces in the Bottom of the Vessel. *Hippocrates,* in his Treatise of Air, Water, and Situations, tells us, " that sound and " healthy Persons may use any " Spring-water without Distinction, " but that such as are sick ought to " drink those which are best suited " to the particular Nature of their " respective Diseases. Those who " are costive ought to use such " Waters as are sweet, light, and " transparent, but those who have a " Solubility of Body and are of " moist and phlegmatic Constituti- " ons, ought to drink Waters which " are crude, hard, and somewhat " saline,

" ſ‥‥, by which Means their Bo-
" ‥‥will be dried, for thoſe Wa-
" ‥‥which are eaſily concoſted and
" ‥‥uated, render the Body ſolu-
" ‥‥, but ſuch as are crude and
" ‥‥rd to be concoſted, render Per-
" ‥‥ coſtive:

River-water has the ſame Origin
‥‥ Spring-water, and only differs
‥ this, that it does not run under
‥ Earth in order to be collected in-
‥ one Receptacle, but flows on its
‥ face in ſmall Rivulets, which
‥ dually concur to the Formation of
‥ge and rapid Rivers, which are
‥ nually expos'd to the Air.
‥ ence whatever is contain'd in the
‥ ir, whatever is convey'd by the
‥ inds, whatever is communicated
‥ om Vegetables and Animals which
‥l into it, and whatever Fiſh and
‥ phibious Animals depoſite in it, is
‥ lected in Rivers, mixed with their
‥ aters, ſubſides to the Bottom, and
‥ y at laſt, by Maceration, be pu-
‥ ied and diſſolv'd. Beſides, as Ri-
‥ rs flow thro' ſo many different
‥ aces, ſuch as Woods, Groves, and
‥ en populous Towns, they muſt in
‥ ſe different Places be of different
‥ alities. Thus River-water will
‥ only receive the Rain as it falls,
‥ d partake of the Nature of the
‥ l thro' which it flows, but will,
‥ ſo, be contaminated by all Kinds
‥ Inſects which fall into it, by A-
‥ mals which live and Plants which
‥ ow in it; for 'tis certain from Ex-
‥ rience that after a Series of hot
‥ d dry Weather, River-water is
‥ ghly unwholſome, on Account of
‥ e many noxious Plants and Herbs
‥ hich in ſuch Weather ſpring up in
‥ . The Water, therefore, of the
‥ me River, is not in every Place
‥ d Seaſon the ſame, but varies in
‥ ferent Places and Seaſons. Hence
‥ me ſurpriſing *Phænomena* have
‥ en obſerv'd of River-water. Thus
‥ the *Philoſophical Tranſactions* we
‥ e told, that ſome River-water

preſerved in Caſks, has emitted
highly fetid Vapours, and ſuch as
were capable of being ſet on a
Flame by a lighted Candle, and
afterwards became inodorous and
ſweet, and in the *Journal des Sca-
vans*. for 1667, we are told, that
if Straw is ſpread on the Banks of
ſome Rivers, a Sort of Froth is collected in it, which depoſites its Humidity, and then concretes into a
tenacious Matter, and by the Force
of Fire acquires the Hardneſs of a
perfeſt Stone.   The River-waters
alſo in the Iſland of *Formoſa* are
highly beneficial in rendering the
Ground fertile, but prove mortal to
ſuch as drink them. But all theſe
and many more ſurprizing Properties of River-waters, are to be a-
ſcribed to their Contents, rather
than to the Waters themſelves, for
if River-waters run for a long Way
upon Sands and pure Flints, they
are not only out of Danger of being
contaminated, but alſo become more
pure, and fit for drinking. 'Tis
commonly ſaid that the Water of
the *Thames* kept in Ships, in hot
Climates ſpontaneouſly ferments and
acquires the Qualities of Spirits of
Wine. But the celebrated Sir
Hans Sloane aſſerts, that this is falſe
and that the *Thames*-water only ferments, and aſſumes a vinous Quality,
in impure and ſordid Veſſels. But
notwithſtanding its Impurities, it is
accounted the beſt Water for the Purpoſes of Sailors.

Well-water, or Pump-water, is properly that which is obtained from a
ſubterraneous Bed of Sand; for by
digging in the Earth, to a certain
Depth, we arrive at pure Sand, out
of which the Water always riſes.
If, therefore, no other Water is
conveyed into the Well, but what
paſſes thro' the Sand, the Water will
be pure and limpid; but if there are
Salts, ſaline or ſaponacious Subſtances
mix'd with the Sand, theſe Bodies

D   diſſolving

diffolving in it, will communicate their Weight, and other Qualities, to the Water ; for which Reafons Well-water is fo rarely to be had good, and always differs according to the Diverfity of Places.

Stagnant, or Pond-waters are fuch as are found in Lakes, Marfhes, and Ditches. Thefe not only retain what they receive from the Bottom or Soil, but are alfo contaminated with other Subftances which fall into them. Hence, by the Heat of the Air efpecially, they become corrupted, putrid, fetid, and turbid. In the hydroftatical Ballances they are, alfo, found to be heavier than pure natural Water, either of Springs, Rivers, or of Rain. Now if we confider that in populous Towns, the ftagnant Waters are filled with the Sordes of Common-Sewers, and all Sort of Filthinefs, we may underftand that fuch Waters may be impregnated with different Qualities, fo that in fome Towns they fhall excellently ferve the Purpofes of Dying, for Inftance ; whereas the ftagnant Waters of another Town, will not anfwer the fame End when employed by the fame Tradefmen ; and the longer fuch Water ftagnates, the more impure it muft become, and the more unfit for all alimentary and culinary Purpofes, and the more offenfive to the Health of the Inhabitants, on Account of the noxious Vapours perpetually exhaling. *Hippocrates* in his Treatife of Air, &c. among other Difadvantages attending ftagnant Waters, tells us, that thofe who ufe them have Diforders of the Spleen, are fubject to be coftive, and have their Faces, Shoulders, and Cavicles, emaciated ; that in the Summer-time ftagnant Waters induce Dyfenteries, Fluxes, and quartan Fevers ; that in Winter, they produce in young Perfons Peripneumonies and Madnefs, where-

as in fuch as are old they bring on burning Fevers.

From what has been faid, 'ti evident that Waters may be im pregnated with an almoft infinit Variety of Qualities, according t the Subftances they receive eithe from the Soil or elfewhere. Hence we are enabled to account fo fome of the wonderful Qualities o Waters, mentioned by Authors fuch as that fome of them indue a ftony Cruft upon Bodies throw into them ; that other Waters drop ping from Rocks are indurate into Stones ; that fome produce In toxication, like Wine ; that fom are hot, and others cold ; and tha fome contribute to the Cure o Difeafes, whilft others foon prov mortal, even by their Exhalations.

We now come to confider th Method of difcovering the Bodie with which Waters are impregnat ed, and the Means of depurating fuch as are impure.

If the Water, then, is of mercurial Nature, a urinous Alcal mix'd with it, caufes a white Precipi tation, but by the Effufion of a fix ed Alcali it becomes red, and witl both thefe mixed, it affumes a dirt Colour. If two Grains of Mercur Sublimate are diffolved in a Quan of Water, this Solution changes th common blue Paper, which is ting ed with Turnfole, to Red, an thereby difcovers its Prefence. I Arfenic or Orpiment is contained i the Water, it becomes black with Solution of Lead, or of *Englifh* o *Dantzic* Vitriol, but affumes a whi Colour, with urinous Salts, and th Water poured upon blue Paper turn it black. But a more infallibl Experiment for this Purpofe is, t evaporate the Water gently, an pour the Refiduum upon a red h Iron Plate, in which Cafe, if tl Water is impregnated with any thefe Subftances, it will render tl

Plat

Pale white, and emit a highly offensive Smell. If Water in its Coat has been impregnated with ammonial Particles, with an Alcali, it turns red, and generates Flowers of a faint red Colour, and fetid Smell. If Water has contracted any ammonious Particles from Silver, a Solution of common Salt produces a white Precipitation. Water impregnated with Copper, is by volatile and urinous Substances changed into a bluish Colour. Chalybeate-waters become black with Galls, and all Astringents, but with a Mixture of Sulphur assumes a blackish Purple Colour; and indeed the best Quality of many hot Springs, seems to consist in Sulphur dissolved by an alcalescent Nitre. Water impregnated with Tin, assumes a dark Purple Colour by a Solution of Gold, whereas those impregnated with Gold assume the same Colour with a Solution of Tin. Sulphureous Waters are known by Sugar of Lead, and a Solution of Silver, which in that Case becomes blackish, but assumes a whitish Colour with other metallic Liquors.

Aluminous-Waters, are not only known by their viscid astringent Taste, but also by their being converted into a viscid Magma, by fixed and volatile Salts of the alcaline Kind. Water impregnated with Lime is frequently to be met with, and becomes cloudy with fixed alcaline Substances, but somewhat more so, with such as are of an urinous Nature; and in the Whiteness of its Colour it resembles Precipitate Mercury. Besides, Silver dissolved in an acid Menstruum renders Water impregnated with Lime turbid and brownish, but with Oil or Spirit of Vitriol it assumes a deep Purple Colour. It becomes greenish with Syrup of Violets, with Turnsole it becomes reddish, not with any Precipitation, but only a Change of Colour.

These are the common Methods of discovering the Contents of Waters.

Some Waters are naturally so impure, as to require Depuration before they are fit to be drank, or employed for culinary Uses. Various Experiments have been thought of, in order to answer this Purpose, but the most natural and easy is, that of permitting them to remain in a State of Rest, till their most gross and sordid Particles subside to the Bottom of the Vessel. When Water is deposited for some Days, or till it becomes fetid, in any temperate or warm Place, in well closed Vessels, but yet so as that there may remain some Communication with the external Air, it will in a little Time become sweet again, and the Water will appear clear, limpid and pure, and a slimy terrestrial Sediment will subside. This Expedient seems to have been discovered by Chance, because those who sail to the *Indies* find that the Water which putrifies and corrupts in the Casks, becomes good and limpid after some Time. The purest Water, under the equinoxial Line, at first becomes mucid and fetid, then of an Ash Colour, then greenish, and last of all assumes an unseemly red Colour; notwithstanding which Changes, it is again spontaneously restored to its natural Colour and State. When Water is strained thro' a linen or woolen Cloth, or thro' pure Sand, the Sordes contained in it remain in the Filtre; for which Reason in Armies they sometimes mix impure and marshy Water with Sand and Chalk, and pour it from one Vessel to another, after which they strain it and permit the grosser Parts to subside, and thus render the Water pure and limpid. Many Inhabitants of *London* depurate the thick and muddy Waters of the River *Thames*,

by

by an Admixture of Sand therewith in their Cisterns, in which the Sordes are deposited whilst the pure Water remains at the Top. What is commonly called the filtrating Stone, is by many used for the Depuration of Water, because its Pores transmit what is pure, but refuse Access to the Sordes. By boiling Water gently in a close Vessel, and permitting it to remain for some Time in a State of Rest, many heterogeneous Bodies subside to the Bottom of the Vessel. The *Egyptians* purify the turbid Waters of the River *Nile*, which is originally unfit to be drank, by Means of a Mass prepared of the Meal of Sweet Almonds, which they rub over the internal Surfaces of their Vessels, by which Means the Water becomes limpid in half an Hour. The *Chinese* depurate their turbid Water and render it drinkable by throwing Alum into it. In the *East-Indies*, turbid and corrupted Water, is corrected and rendered pure by the Admixture of certain Seeds, Beans, or the Nux Vomica. If we may believe the Antients, the Bitterness is removed by throwing the Powder of Coral into it, or by putting a Bag full of bruised Barley into the Vessel in which it is contained. But none of these Methods is sufficient for the Depuration of Water impregnated with Salts : But Distillation is necessary to make the most pure and limpid Part of the Water ascend. The purest Water is obtained from a Distillation of Snow-water.

As for the Preservation of Water, most Species of it cannot be long kept without Corruption, whereas others may be kept for twenty Years in close stopt Bottles. Water in general is best preserved in cold Cellars, and in earthen or glass, rather than in wooden Vessels, because from these last it may

receive into its Pores a Matter which favours Putrefaction. Metallic Vessels are not to be used for this Purpose, lest, if the Water should abound with Salts, it should be impregnated with the Quantity of the Metal by their Means. For the Preservation of Water, nothing more proper, than to drop into a sufficient Quantity of Spirit of Vitriol which resists all Putrefaction, and prevents the Generation of Insects. Another Method of preserving Water is, first to wash the Vessel well into which it is to be put, and then to hold it for some time over the Fume of kindled Sulphur. A small Quantity of Alum put in Water, also, preserves it from Corruption. A small Quantity of distilled Sea Water, all mixed with common Water, preserves it from Putrefaction. But all these Expedients would be entirely useless, if pure Water could always be kept in Vessels in which the Air has no Access ; for according to *Boerhaave*, Water poured into a sound glass Vessel and then hermetically sealed up, that Vessel, so as to admit no external Air, remained for many Years without any sensible Change, so that in so long a Time, it neither concreted, nor generated Earth, nor any other Thing within itself, tho' the Experiment was made in the Air of *Rome*, which is considerably hot.

As for the Uses of Water, they are various; but the most extensive Advantage of Water, depends upon its solvent Quality; for by its Means we seperate the Salts from Bodies, and render such Salts as are dry, active, and fit for medicinal Purposes, by dissolving them in Water. Some Bodies are mixed, others precipitated from each other, and Spirits are diluted and weakened by Means of Water.

1

and hence many extraordinary Effects are produced in the Works both of Art and Nature, as Putrefation, Fermentation, Effervescence, and many others. Thus *Boerhaave* says, " that Water is the " moving Instrument and most universal Vehicle, which dissolves " active Bodies, mixes and applies " them to each other; which tem-" perates the Acrimony of many " Bodies, unites with them, agitates " the whole, and thus becomes the " principal Instrument in all Phy-" fical Changes and Operations." Water is so necessary to apply the Matter of Nutrition to Vegetables, that there can be no Vegetation without it; besides, this Fluid enters the very Composition of Plants. In the fossile Kingdom Water seems to convey the Matter by which all Stones grow, and to be the Cement by which their Parts adhere to each other, just as those of Lime do. Other Fossils so long as they exist in the metallic Veins under the Form of gross, pinguious, and heavy, Juices, resemble a saline unctuous Substance, but may in this State be dissolved in Water, even contain a diluting Water in themselves; for all concreted, saline, vitriolic and metallic Juice, evince the same, since all Experiments shew, that Water acts the most confiderable Part in them, dilutes, moves, changes, augments, and mixes them. The Nutrition of Animals is entirely performed by Water, which is also absolutely necessary to Life, being the most mild and fluid of all the Juices of the Body, and best calculated for penetrating into the most minute Vessels. By an excessive Diminution of this Fluid in the Body, Life immediately ceases, because the Blood and Humours circulate no longer. Nor is there any Liquor known in Nature which can supply the Absence and Defect of Water.

Those who by the gentlest Fire have seperated Water from any of the human Juices, have found, that Water constituted the greatest Part of them, and render'd them fit for passing thro' their respective Vessels. Hence, far the greater Part of the perspirable Matter of *Sanctorius* is Water. Besides, if all the solid Parts of animal Bodies are examined, 'tis found that they owe their Fitness for the Purposes of Life to Water, which being taken away, none of the Conditions requisite to Life remain. For this Reason, the antient Chymists called Water the *Universal Wine,* which was liberally drank by all Animals, Plants, and Fossils; so that in this Sense, we may justly assert Water to be the prolific Principle of which all Things are formed. Health which is the principal Perfection of Life, and the due Exercise of all the Actions subservient to it, are more owing to Water than any Thing. The Growth and Increase of the Body is principally carried on by Water. Many Disorders are brought on, and many removed by Means of Water. Death itself is often to be attributed to an Excess, but much oftner to a Defect of this Liquor, which on various Occasions performs happy and surprising Cures.

Hence 'tis obvious, that the Physician ought to be well acquainted with the Properties of Water, that he may know how to apply it properly to medicinal Uses. As Water is a Menstruum for many Bodies, so we may easily understand its Propriety for culinary and pharmaceutic Purposes. It serves to dilute the Humours of the Body, and preserve them in due Fluidity; and as it is entirely destitute of Taste and Smell, it is highly proper for allaying the Acrimony of the human Juices. Water is, therefore, not only a Vehicle for distributing the nutritive Juice, but is also the best Diluter, when the thick and viscid Fluids are to be divided and attenuated. Water, also, promotes the Concoction of the Aliments, and resolves Obstructions, except those of the oleous and tenacious Kinds, which require Water mixed with saponaceous Substances. It obtunds the Spicula or Asperities of Salts, and consequently checks the excessive oscillatory Motion of the Solids, for which Reason it is justly accounted the most mild, gentle, and anodyne Medicine, excellently calculated for correcting Acrimony, and removing the perternatural Rigidity of the Parts. Water also assists all the Excretions and Secretions, since it proves diuretic, diaphoretic, sudorific or purgative, accordingly as Nature is inclined to one of these Excretions more than another. But it proves injurious when drank to Excess by Persons abounding with aqueous Humours, and by those of phlegmatic or lax Habits, by moistening, softening, and destroying the Tone and Elasticity of the Solids. Hence it may be justly said, that Water judiciously exhibited is an universal Medicine, not only for the Preservation of Health, and Prevention of Diseases, but also for answering the several Intentions of Cure after various Disorders are formed. Water is of singular Use in Medicine on Account of its solvent Quality; for by this Means it is excellently calculated for extracting the medicinal and active Virtues of Bodies, not only in the Solutions of saline and gummatious Substances, but also when used in the Preparations of Infusions and Decoctions. But all these Things are to be understood only of simple fresh Water, the Goodness of which bears a Proportion to its Purity and Lightness. And indeed the Uses of Water are so extensive, in all the Branches of Pharmacy, and Chymistry, that nothing is to be done without it. But since 'tis certain from Experience that an Excess of Water is prejudicial to Health, and that its Effects upon the human Body vary according to the Degrees of its Heat or Coldness, we shall therefore consider cold and hot Water.

Cold-water, then, which is neither heated by the Sun nor Fire, corroborates the Fibres, and increases their Resistance, in Consequence of which it propels the Humours, accelerates their Motion, and preserves Health. But Water so excessively cold as to be near to freezing, too greatly augments the Elasticity of the Parts, injures those of weak nervous Systems, and at last coagulates the Blood. Our Countryman Doctor *Harris* informs us, that cold Water drank in the Morning, alleviates the Heat arising from a Debauch over Night; but he dissuades the Use of it in these Fevers incident to the Inhabitants of the nothern Countries, because it represses the Sweats, augments Coughs and Peripneumonies, and is absolutely prejudicial to the Stomach and Intestines in Persons of cold, weak and phlegmatic Habits. A great many celebrated Physicians have advised the copious Use of cold Water for the Cure of acute and malignant Fevers, provided they are not accompanied with any Disorders of the Lungs and Viscera. *Antonius Michelotti*, a celebrated *Italian* Physician, gives us an Account of a violent Vomiting of Blood cur'd by drinking excessively cold Waters in the Winter-time. Cold Water, both externally and internally used, affords great Relief in many Diseases. Thus in *Ephemerid. Nat. Curiof. Dec.* 1. *An.* 2. *Obf.* 49. we read of a Palsy cured by drinking cold Water. *In Mem. Trev.* we are informed that the Eruption of the Small-

pox

por was promoted only by drinking large Quantities of cold Water. In the *Acta Hafnienfia*, we are inform'd, that the most violent Head-achs were remov'd, by applying a Towel wet with cold Water about the Neck. And in *Eph. Nat. Curiof. Decad 2. An.* 10. *Obf.* 139, we are told, that a bilious Cholic was cur'd by drinking cold Water: In a Weakness of the Stomach, drinking cold Water in the Morning, and two Hours after Meals, is justly recommended as an excellent Remedy, because it not only corroborates the Tone of the Stomach, but also attenuates the Aliments still contain'd in the Inteftines, promotes the Excretion of the Feces, and procures a due Fluidity to the Chyle. Hence the celebrated *Boerhaave* recommends it in a febrile Naufea. But these Things are to be taken under proper Reftrictions; for in tender Bodies which want a due Degree of mufcular Motion, the colder the Water is, and the more of it is exhibited, the more Misfortunes it will produce; for in *Eph. Nat. Curiof. Decad. 3. An.* 2. *Obf.* 166. we are told, that feveral Perfons have become dropfical, and pleuritic, by drinking cold Water on an empty ftomach. Befides, in the laft quoted Work, there is a great Variety of Inftances, in which cold Water has produc'd the moft fatal Effects.

Cold Water fprinkled on the head, recovers Perfons from *Deliriums*, by procuring a contractile force of the Fibres, and confequently promoting the Circulation of the Humours. In the *Memoirs of the Royal Academy of Sciences*, we are told, that by a young Man's immerfing his Feet in cold Water, when he was exceffively hot, he had a Tumor excited of the *Epigaftrium*, and *Hypochondrium*, and an hectic Fever, and an Abfcefs of the Liver produc'd. This happen'd, becaufe

the Fibres of the inferior Parts being contracted, repell'd the Humours to the fuperior Parts, efpecially the *Meanders* of the hepatic Veffels, whence arofe the Tumor, Inflammation, and Abfcefs: With Refpect to the Ufe of cold Water in arthritic Diforders, the Reader may confult the *Eph. Nat. Curiof.* and *Le Clerc's Hiftory of Phyfic.*

Water warm'd to fuch a Degree that an healthy Perfon can bear his Hand in it, is of a far more diffolvent, refolvent, aperient, moiftening, emollient, and relaxing Quantity than cold Water; warm Water according to the celebrated *Hoffman*, when drank in large Quantities, by its elaftic Force enters the Pores, infinuates itfelf every-where, and diffufes a perceptible Heat thro' all the Body; for if the Blood adjacent to the Stomach, is render'd more fluid by its Heat, according to the Laws of the Circulation, the whole Blood muft be render'd more fit for Motion, juft in the fame Manner as the whole Body is warm'd, by applying Heat to its Extremities, the Feet. By this Means, the Spirits being rous'd, perform their Functions the better. Thus by drinking warm Water we are render'd brifk, chearful, and fit for tranfacting Bufinefs. That the *Chinefe* are for the moft Part Strangers to arthritic Diforders, is commonly afcrib'd to the great Quantities of Tea they drink; for warm Water, which is the moft confiderable Ingredient of the Tea, promotes Perfpiration, and carries off the extraneous, and foreign Salts: But thofe who ufe Tea to excefs, do but ill confult their own Health, fince by deftroying the Tone of the Solids, the Circulation of the Humours is fo difturb'd, and the Blood itfelf fo attenuated, as to flow into the lateral Veffels; whence arife Weaknefs of the Vifcera, Anxieties, and other Diforders, caus'd by too

lax

lax a State of the Solids, and the Want of a due Confiftence in the Fluids. *Boerhaave* informs us, that Palfies are produc'd by the conftant and exceffive Ufe of warm Water.

As for boiling Water, 'tis to be obferv'd, that it burns the folid Parts, and could it immediately reach the Blood of a live Perfon, it would inftantly coagulate it,

---

CHAP. III.

Of FIRE.

FIRE is one of the grand Inftruments in natural and artificial Chymiftry; but the Nature thereof is fo extremely abftrufe, as to have perplex'd the greateft Philofophers of all Ages, infomuch, that we are not much the wifer for their Refearches. I will not pretend to affirm, that *Boerhaave* has fucceeded much better than the reft; but as he has contradicted fome popular Opinions, with Refpect to Fire, I fhall take Notice of fome Particulars, and refer the Reader who defires farther Information, to this Author, who in the firft Volume of his Chymiftry has treated very copioufly of Fire.

Tho' 'tis highly difficult, if not abfolutely impoffible, to give a juft and accurate Definition of Fire; yet we may form fuch an Idea of it, as to know, whether it is abfent from, or prefent, in any particular Place, or Body; but at the fame Time, 'tis frequently no eafy Matter, to difcover fuch a Mark of Fire, as will always evince its Prefence, tho' the Quantity of it be ever fo fmall, fince upon Examination it evidently appears, that there is an incredible Quantity of true Fire in thofe Places, where every Perfon not only judges that there is none, but alfo imagines there is really fomething of a different Nature. Thus 'tis certain, from Experience, that

Fire is contain'd in the coldeft Maffes of Ice, tho' none of its Actions and Signs appear, till they are difcover'd by a ftrong Collifion, with fome other hard Subftance.

The manifeft and obvious Signs of Fire, are faid to be: Firft, Heat: Secondly, Light: Thirdly, Colour: Fourthly, Expanfion, or Rarefaction, both of Fluids and Solids: And, Fifthly, the Power of Burning and Melting; together with various other Effects.

Tho' Heat is infeparable from Fire, yet nothing more is meant by it, than a certain Senfation of the Mind, excited by the Application of Fire to the fenfible Parts of the Body.

Tho' Light, is look'd upon as a certain Demonftration of the Prefence of Fire, yet, we know from the Experiments of the celebrated *Hook*, and other natural Philofophers, that it by no Means bears a juft Proportion to the Quantity of Fire contain'd in Bodies; for there may be the ftrongeft Fire, without any vifible Light; and, on the contrary, the moft refulgent Light, without the leaft Degree of fenfible Heat.

As Colour is either Light itfelf, or a various Reflexion of it from opaque Bodies; it is evident, that as Light, fo of Courfe Colour muft be an infufficient Mark of Fire.

A

A great many other suppos'd Effects of Fire are but uncertain, and various Mark of its Presence; but we have one unexceptionable and infallible Mark of the Presence of Fire, which is its expanding Virtue; for upon an accurate Examination of all natural Bodies, whether fluid, or folid, we find none but are expanded by Fire, either of the folar, artificial, or fubterraneous Kind; and this Expanfion bears a Proportion to the Quantity of Fire contain'd in Bodies.

During the moft intenfe Cold, Fire may be produc'd by the Attrition of folid Bodies upon one another, and the ftronger and more rapid the Attrition is, and the harder the Bodies are, the greater Quantity of Fire will be produc'd.

Fire is actually prefent in every Part of Space, tho' we cannot at all Times difcover it, by fearching for it in the common Methods; for the moft accurate Thermometers evince, that there every where actually exifts an Heat, greater than the moft intenfe Degree of Cold, tho' People are fubject to imagine that there is no Heat, or Fire, in the Place where the Fluid of the Thermometer is fallen very low. Befides, Fire not only exifts in every Part of Space, but is alfo equally diffus'd thro' every Body, the moft folid as well as the moft rare, tho' it is not perceptible.

Tho' Fire is of an highly penetrating Nature, yet it cannot infinuate itfelf into what we call the ultimate and impenetrable Elements of Bodies, fince Impenetrability in this Senfe, is infeparable from all Matter whatever.

Fire is produc'd, not only by Attrition, but alfo by Percuffion, and the Vibrations of elaftic Bodies, as is obvious from the Experiments made by Mr. *Boyle*, and other celebrated Philofophers.

Heat, or Fire, may by Means of *Speculums*, be fo collected and concentrated, as to produce very furprizing Effects, fuch as the melting all Kinds of Metals, and even Stones, as is obvious from various Experiments made by fome Moderns.

When Bodies have a greater Heat in them than the ambient Fluids, or adjacent Bodies, the denfer the Fluid is in which they are immers'd, the fooner they will lofe their Heat. Thus Mercury, is a more expeditious Extinguifher of Fire, than either the Air, Water, or any other Fluid.

The larger any particular Body is, if every other Circumftance is alike, the longer it will retain the Heat it has admitted; for the Denfity of the outward Surface, always prevents the quick Egrefs of the Fire, which endeavours to make its Way from the internal Parts. For this Reafon, when Bodies are thoroughly heated, their innermoft Parts require the longeft Time to cool.

Mathematicians have demonftrated, that whilft the corporeal Mafs continues the fame, a Body can never be reduc'd under a fmaller Surface, than when it is form'd into a Sphere; now this Figure is, therefore, the moft tenacious of Heat, both on Account of the Smallnefs of its Surface with Refpect to its Solidity, and the equal Diftribution of all the Parts to the Center, and their equal Recefs from the Surface. But when any Body is divided into Parts, without any other Alteration, then its Surface will be increas'd, tho' its Quantity of Matter continues the fame, and then it will of confequence grow cold fo much the fooner.

What has been faid, affifts us to difcover the Reafons of the Continuance of Heat in other Cafes. It is an old and juft Obfervation, that
Perfons

Perfons of hard, ftrong, and denfe Conftitutions, accuftom'd to Exercife, and full of compact, heavy Fluids, are always found to be hotter and longer in growing cold than others; for fuch Bodies, muft by the ftrong Application of their Solids to their Fluids, condenfe them by this Compreffion, and of Confequence collect more Fire within them, and retain it very tenacioufly. On the contrary, lax, foft, unactive, and weak Perfons, can never communicate fo much Heat to their aqueous Humours; for they always fuffer lefs Attrition, are lefs condens'd, relax'd into larger Surfaces, and confequently, are not fo fit to retain the Heat, when once it is generated. Hence then, we fee what ill Confequences are to be apprehended from both thefe Extremes, and what Kinds of Medicines in particular, are to be exhibited with Succefs. Thus the Ufefulnefs of this Doctrine becomes very extenfive.

Among all the various Bodies of the Univerfe, which have hitherto been examin'd, there is not one which has in itfelf more Heat than another; for *Phofphorus* made of Urine, is as cold as the ambient Water, whilft it is immers'd in it, tho' it foon becomes exceedingly hot and active, when it is expos'd to the Air. That furprizing Spirit of Nitre, call'd the fiery Spirit, and that diftill'd Oil, which the Chymifts obtain from Saffafras, whilft they remain quiet in clofe Veffels, are as cold as the coldeft Ice, tho' when they are mix'd together, they produce the moft terrible Fire. Tho' the Bodies of Animals have a greater Heat in them whilft alive, than inanimate Subftances, yet after Death they are as cold, unlefs there is a Putrefaction begun.

As for the *Pabulum* of Fire, fince Fire itfelf and fome of thofe Bodies in which it is collected, vanifh from our Senfes both together, hence it has become cuftomary to call thofe Bodies, or particular Parts of them, the *Pabulum*, or Aliment of Fire; and thus far it may be allow'd without any Inconvenience. But when Chymifts pretend to call them fo in too ftrict a Senfe, becaufe they look upon them as the Nutriment of real Fire, and imagine them to be chang'd by the Fire, into the very Subftance of elementary Fire, and thus to have their own proper Nature deftroy'd, by affuming that of Fire, then they propofe fomething vaftly different, which ought to be carefully confider'd before it is admitted as true; for tho' the Affertion of it is very eafy, yet the Demonftration of it is exceedingly difficult; and, certainly, whoever runs into this Opinion, muft neceffarily fuppofe, that thofe Bodies which nourifh and fupport Fire, are by this Means conftantly diminifhing; and hence the Quantity of all other Bodies in the Univerfe, muft be continually leffen'd, whilft that of elementary Fire muft be continually encreas'd. Fire, therefore, thus perpetually augmenting, and at the fame Time diminifhing every Thing elfe, would neceffarily have deftroy'd all the Bodies in the Univerfe long ago. But from a Comparifon of the moft early Times with our own, we do not find the fmalleft Indications of any fuch Increafe.

It is concluded, therefore, that when Combuftibles are fet on Fire, no new Fire is generated, nor is any loft when this is extinguifh'd.

Boerhaave has taken a great deal of Pains to prove, that tho' all Bodies whatever are capable of receiving, and retaining Fire, yet it is the Oil only which fupports Flame and is wafted thereby, fo as to be the true *Pabulum*, Food, or Support thereof. And that pure *Alcohol* of Wine, which is an extremely fubtile, and attenuated vegetable Oil, is the only

Thing known that waftes entirely by Fire, fo as to leave no Feces. It does not mean, that either of thefe are actually converted into Fire, or wafted; but that they are diffifed, and entirely chang'd with refpect to their Form, by the Action of Fire. And it appears by his Experiments, that 'tis only a Part of Oils, and even of *Alcohol*, that is the true *Pabulum* of Fire; for it fhould feem, that a great deal of Water, which we know is not inflammable, is feparated from *Alcohol* whilft it burns. Now I think it highly probable, tho' I would only fuggeft this to the Learned, that it may be the Acid, a conftituent Part of all Oils, however it may be difguis'd, that is the Part convertible into Flame, and the real Food of Fire. It will give Light to this Affair, to confider the Nature and Compofition of Gunpowder, and its Effects when Fire is apply'd to it. This, we know, is made of Charcoal, which contains a black and highly inflammable vegetable Oil, and ferves as a Sort of Tinder to kindle the Sulphur, a neceffary Medium betwixt the Coal and the Nitre, which is the third Ingredient, and is known to abound with an Acid, which it receives originally from the Air. When Fire is apply'd to this Compofition, it catches the black Oil of the Coal, which inftantly kindles the Sulphur, and this communicates the Fire to the Nitre, in a Degree fufficient to make it burft out into a lucid Flame.

As, therefore, we find much the fame Ingredients in all Combuftibles, with thofe that enter the Compofition of Gunpowder, I am inclin'd to confider all Flame, as a continu'd Explofion of the Acid included in the Body fubjected to the Action of Fire.

Beerhaave, from his Hiftory of Fire, deduces the following Conclufions:

Firft, That fimple elementary Fire infinuates itfelf into, and rarifies all Bodies in the Univerfe which fall under our Obfervation, whether they are folid, or fluid, or compounded of both.

Secondly, This penetrating and rarifying Quality, is fo peculiar to Fire alone, that it is not common to any other Body we are acquainted with. Neither, do Effervefcences, Fermentations, and particular Rarefactions of Bodies, prove the contrary.

Thirdly, Fire is diftinguifhed by this Property, and is prefent in every Place, as well the folideft *Plenum*, as the moft perfect *Vacuum*.

Fourthly, This Fire is every where diftributed in the moft equable Manner, till there arifes fome Caufe able to collect it thus difpers'd, into one particular Place.

Fifthly, The firft, and perhaps moft confiderable of thefe collecting Caufes, is the Attrition of fome Kinds of Bodies with each other.

Sixthly, Fire is, from its own Nature, mov'd equally every Way, or at leaft is fpontaneoufly expanded in this Manner.

Seventhly, It is, however, poffible, that this Motion, or Expanfion of Fire, may be directed in parallel, or converging Lines, which is a fecond Way of collecting Fire.

Eighthly, The principal Caufe, which compels Fire, of itfelf undetermin'd, into a Parallelifm, is the Sun.

Ninthly, Thefe Rays are made to converge, or are united into a fmall Space call'd a *Focus*, either by Reflexion, or Refraction, which is a third Method of collecting Fire.

Tenthly, The coldeft Steel, violently ftruck againft the coldeft Flint, in the moft intenfely cold Weather, in a Moment produces Fire, which is a fourth Method; fo that Fire does
not

not any Ways depend on the Sun with Refpect to its Matter.

Eleventhly, Fire continues for fome Time in Bodies, and is united to them, whilft the Time of its Continuance is proportionable to the Denfity of the Body with which it is united. But there is no Body as yet not known capable of retaining the Fire always. This is called elementary Fire, but befides this Species of Fire, there is alfo, as fome People imagine, another Sort, which confumes combuftible Bodies, fo as to render them invifible ; which is fuppofed to be fed and fupported, and is falfely believed to convert combuftible Matter into Fire itfelf. This is thought to be produced, when Fire previoufly exifting, is applied in the open Air to a proper *Pabulum*, which is a fifth, and of all others the moft common Method of collecting Fire.

Twelfthly, There is as yet difcovered but one Kind of Matter in the Univerfe which will feed Fire, in fuch a Manner as to be fo entirely confumed by it, fo that nothing fhall be generated but pure fimple Flame, and nothing fhall remain behind when the *Pabulum* is burnt away, and the Flame goes out ; and this Matter is pure *Alcohol*. But other Bodies being mixed with the true *Pabulum* of Fire, and agitated by the Fire along with it, are capable of confiderably increafing its Power.

Thirteenthly, Elementary Fire may be increafed in particular Places to a furprizing Degree, fo that by this Means certain phyfical Effects, not eafily underftood in any other way, may be produced, and reduced to a Kind of natural Hiftory. When this elementary Fire is collected in a particular Place by whatever Caufe, it may there be fupported by the Help of a proper *Pabulum*, which is always either *Alcohol* or Oil, obtained either from the animal, vegetable, or foffil Kingdoms.

Laftly, *Boerhaave* concludes, that Fire is poffeffed of all the Properties of a Body, and that its Corpufcules are highly folid, fmooth, and continually in Motion.

It muft be however carefully obferved :

Firft, That Fire is not an univerfal Solvent, fince it diffolves many Bodies without producing the fame Effects on others, which however are capable of being diffolved by other Means.

Secondly, That Fire is not fo pure a Solvent as to extract from Bodies only thofe Parts which exifted in them before, for at the fame time that it feperates fome Parts, it mixes others together.

Thirdly, That in fome Bodies it produces nothing new, but leaves them without any confiderable Alteration.

Fourthly, That thofe Parts feparated by Fire, however applied, from compound Bodies are not fimple Subftances, but varioufly intermixed and blended with each other.

Fifthly, That Experiments evince, that the Compofition of Bodies is as much affected by the Action of Fire, as their Separation, fince it unites the moft different Bodies fo intimately together, that the new formed Subftance appears perfectly fimple, and is not liable to any Alteration from its Power afterwards.

Sixthly, That the fame Fire applied in different Degrees, will in one Degree compound thofe Bodies, which it will again refolve in another. And,

Seventhly, That the fame Degree of Fire applied to the fame Bodies in different Circumftances, produces

Effects

Effects surprisingly different, especially according to the various Addition of the Air in the Operation.

But as Fire is an Instrument absolutely neceffary for chymical Productions, the laft quoted Author has divided it into fix Degrees.

The firft of thefe is that within the Compafs of which Nature brings about the Work of Vegetation in Plants, fo that it is highly probable that this Degree of Heat is beft fuited to impregnate Oils with the choice Spirit of fome Vegetables, without diffipating the richeft Part of them.

The Second is moft commodioufly eftimated from the higheft to the loweft Degrees of Heat obferved in healthy Perfons. Within the Compafs of this Heat are included the vital Actions of Animals, the Fermentation of Vegetables, and the Putrefaction both of Vegetables and Animals, and the Generation, Breeding, Hatching, Birth, and Nutrition of Animals. This Degree of Heat, Chymifts ufe to prepare their Elixirs, Tinctures, and in many other Procefses which require a gentle Heat.

The Third is from the extreme Degree of the Second, to that in which Water generally begins to boil; and this Degree of Heat ferves for the Diftillation of the Oils, and the medicinal Waters of Vegetables. The fanguineous and ferous Juices of Animals are in boiling Water coagulated into a friable Mafs, whilft all their Solids are deftroyed by it, and reduced to a thick and tenacious Liquid; and hence it is abfolutely deftructive to all Animals.

The fourth is from the extreme Degree of the Third, to that within the Limits of which all Oils, faline Lixiviums, Mercury, and the Oil of Vitriol recede from the Fire, fly upwards, and by this Means diftil. In this Heat Lead and Tin are put in Fufion, and may be mixed with each other. By this, alfo, the Oils, Salts, and faponacious Juices of Vegetables and Animals, are rendered volatile and acrid, and become more or lefs alcacefcent. The folid Parts of them are by this Heat dried, and if they are calcined, they are converted into a very black Coal, are all abfolutely deftroyed, quite altered in their Qualities, and entirely lofe their Virtues. By this Heat too Chymifts fublime fofsil Sulphur, and Sal-ammoniac.

The fifth is from the higheft Degree of the Fourth, to that in which the reft of the Metals are put in Fufion. Glafs, Gold, Silver, Copper and Iron, for a confiderable Time bear this Degree, which deftroys every Thing elfe. In this Heat all other fixed Bodies grow white, the fixed Salts of Vegetables and Fofsils are put in Fufion, are deprived of almoft all their Oils, acquire a greater alcaline Acrimony, and with Sand or Flints are converted into Glafs. In this Heat Lime-ftones are calcined, and other Bodies either vitrify, or become volatile, and are diffipated in the Air.

The fixth and laft Degree comprehends the whole Compafs of catoptrical and dioptrical Fire, which fcarcely any Body is able to refift. By this Gold itfelf fuffers very confiderable Alterations. The ultimate Effect of this Heat on Bodies is their Vitrification. This the Eaftren *Magi* feem to have underftood, when they prophefied that the whole World would at laft be deftroyed by Fire, and that it would then be converted into pellucid Glafs.

It is of the greateft Confequence for the Chymift to know accurately the Methods of raifing and fupporting

porting thefe various Degrees of Fire according as the Intention requires; for on this principally depend all the Operations in Chymiftry.

'Tis to be obferved, that it is far more difficult to preferve a great Degree of Cold for a confiderable Time, than it is to keep up a very great Heat, as is fufficiently obvious from the intenfe Fires requifite in metal and glafs Works. The firft Way of exciting and fupporting a moderate Heat depends upon the Choice of fuch a *Pabulum* as may produce the Strength of Fire requifite for our Purpofe. *Alcohol* of Wine yeilds a Weak and equable Flame, which may be increafed or diminifhed by a greater or fmaller Number of Wicks; when we are therefore refolved upon the Degree of Heat we intend to ufe, we are to light a Lamp with as many Wicks as, by the Thermometer, appear neceffary to excite the Degree defired. Next to *Alcohol* are the light and porous and fpongy Kinds of *Pabulum*, fuch as Rufhes, Straw, dry Leaves, Hair, Shavings of Wood, dried Stalks of Buck-wheat, Chaff, and Bran. Next to thofe are Oils, Tallow, Wax, Camphire, Pitch, Refin, Sulphur, and other Compounds. Next are thick, heavy, hard and compact Woods, and the Coals prepared of them; and laft of all red hot Metals and foffil Coals.

Various Degrees of Fire, the greateft not excepted, may be excited by the Quantity of the combuftible Matter ufed, for if a large Quantity of Fuel is fet on Fire all at once, the Fire thus produced will be proportionably ftronger, the Force of it all being united together.

There is a great Difference in the Heat with Refpect to the Object it acts upon, according to the Diftances at which Bodies are ex-pofed to the Fire, the Heat alw decreafing as they are remo farther off. But the Proportion this Decreafe is not eafily afc tained.

The Degrees of Heat, alfo, pend much on the Agitation, Co cuffion, and Compreffion of the Fi when it is excited by its *Pabula* and included within its aerial Arch for by thefe the Violence of it greatly increafed, and the more the ftronger they are. As we c by no Means procure this Agit tion and Compreffion of Fire mo conveniently and effectually, than blowing the Air forcibly on the Fir fo Bellows are the Inftruments which we direct this Preffure of t Air on the Surface of the Fire, which Means its Parts are agitat with great Violence. Thus if t Wind of feveral large Bellows from different Parts, directed up the Center of the fame Fire, it w act with fo much the more Streng upon the Body placed in that Ce ter, and confequently the Chang induced upon fuch a Body w be fo much the more confider ble.

The Chymifts have many Co trivances for raifing and fupporti the various Degrees of Fire, or He proper for their Operations.

Thus they procure a Sand He as it is called, by placing a Pot Veffel of caft Iron or any ot Subftance that will bear the He upon the Fire. Then this Vel is filled with Sand, and another V fel containing the Matter to be a ed upon, is placed in the Sand. Son times alfo the Filings of Iron, Afhes, are ufed inftead of Iron thefe Purpofes.

The reverberatory Heat is m in a Furnace covered with a Don that by this Means the Heat Flame, which has always a T dency to make its Efcape at

fuper

superior Parts of the Furnace, may be reverberated, or beat back on the Vessel or Body exposed to it.

The naked Fire is, when in distilling their is no intermediate Substance between the distilling Vessel and the Fire, or when it touches the Fire, or receives its Heat without the Intervention of any other Body.

The Lamp Fire is, when any Matter contained in a Glass Vessel is rendered hot by the equable Heat of a lighted Lamp. This Heat is used in order to soften the Necks of small Glass Vessels in order to have them hermetically sealed.

The *Balneum Mariæ* is, when the Vessel containing the Matter to be heated, is placed in a Vessel full of Water, under which a Fire is put, that by this Means the Water becoming hot, may in its Turn heat the Matter contained in the Vessel.

A Vapour Bath is when a Vessel containing any Matter, is heated by the Steam of hot Water.

The Fire of Suppression is, when in order to distil per Descensum, the Fire is laid above the Matter, so that the Moisture forc'd from it by Means of the Heat, is precipitated to the Bottom of the Vessel; or when the Body of a Retort, or other Vessel, is covered over with Fire, this is called a Fire of Suppression.

Insolation is, when any Matter designed either to be put into Fermentation, or dried, is exposed to the Rays of the Sun.

The Heat of Horse-dung, called also the *Horses Belly*, is when a Vessel, containing any Matter either to be digested or distilled, is placed in a large Heap of Horse-dung.

A Heat of the Skins of Grapes collected in large Quantities after the Vintage, may, like the Bath of Horse-dung, serve for Digestions and Distillations.

The Heat of quick Lime moistened, may serve for some Distillations; when, for Instance, after being mixed with Sal-ammoniac, it makes a very subtile Spirit distil from it, without the Assistance of any other Fire.

The Fires of Sand, Filings of Iron, and Ashes, have generally their Degrees from the first to the third, but that of the Filings of Iron has a stronger Heat than the others, because they easily become first hot, and then red; the Fire of Ashes is the most moderate, because they do not retain so great an Heat as the other Substances.

The reverberatory Fire has its Degrees from the first to the fourth, which is that generally raised to the greatest Violence.

A Vessel may receive different Degrees of Heat from a lighted Lamp, by either keeping it at a certain Distance, or gradually advancing it nearer; but when the Vessel is once heated, an equal Heat may be always continued.

The *Balneum Mariæ* and Vapour Bath have also their Degrees; for according as the Water of the Bath is more or less heated, the Distillation is more or less promoted. We may, therefore, call it the first Degree of the *Balneum Mariæ* or Vapour Bath, when the Bath or Vapour are only moderately tepid, as they ought to be when any Matter is put in a Vessel and exposed to them for the Sake of Digestion. Their Heat of the Second Degree is when the Water of the Bath, and Steam of the Water, are so hot that a Person cannot hold his Hand in them, as they ought to be when a gentle Distillation is to be produced. Their third Degree of Heat, is when the Waters of both

both Baths boil, in order to haften the Diftillation.

The Fire of Suppreffion has, alfo, its Degrees; for fometimes warm Afhes are only ufed in order to excite a very mild and gentle Heat, which is the firft Degree. At other times a fmall Quantity of live Coal is mixed with the Afhes, which is the fecond Degree; and at other Times they place upon a thin Bed of Afhes, a large Quantity of live Coals, which is the third Degree of Heat peculiar to this Fire of Suppreffion.

Infolation has, alfo, its Degrees in Proportion to the Heat of the Sun to which Subftances are expofed. The beft Infolation is made in the Months of *July* and *Auguft*, becaufe the Sun has then more Force and Vigour than at other Times.

The Baths of Horfe-dung and grape Skins have alfo their Degrees, according to their Qualities, and the Heat of the Places where they are.

The Heat of quick Lime alfo has its Degrees, for according as we defire it more or lefs ftrong, we expofe it in Powder, a longer or fhorter Time to the open Air.

Another Method of exciting and fupporting a long continued Heat, is by Means of that Furnace which Chymifts call an *Athanor*, which is fo contrived as to keep up a gentle Heat for any Length of Time, by fupplying it every twenty-four, or fometimes every forty-eight Hours, or at longer Intervals, with a proper Quantity of Coals. This Method is very ufeful in Cafes where a long continued Heat is required.

CHAP. IV.

Of EARTH.

BY the Word Earth, Philofophers and Chymifts mean, a fimple, hard, friable foffil Body, which is fixed, but not melted, in the Fire, nor is capable of being diffolved in Water, *Alcobol*, Oil, or Air. What is commonly called Virgin Earth is fo fimple, that it appears as uniform and homogeneous as Metals themfelves. When it is perfectly feparated from every Thing elfe, it is hard and confiftent notwithftanding its exceeding Finenefs. The Matter of Earth is friable, becaufe it always fuffers itfelf to be reduced to a fine Powder, in which Refpect it widely differs from true Metals and Gems. But its greateft Difference

from thefe Subftances confifts in this, that it remains fo fixed and immutable in the moft intenfe Fire, that when it is entirely alone it is impoffible to put it in Fufion.

A moft perfect Earth is procured from Rain Water; for if we catch pure Rain Water, and diftil it carefully, we find at the Bottom of the Veffel a feculent Matter, that when collected, dried, and burned, yields fome Afhes, which being carefully freed from all the Salt it contains, produce a fine pure Subftance called *Virgin Earth*, which if it is throughly feparated from every other Subftance, remains fixed in a Crucible in the ftrongeft Fire, **the** tho' then mix'd with some other Bo-dy may be dissipated into its ulti-me Particles. Of this no other has is necessary, than the burning, of Wood under an high Chimney, in which Case the Smoke fixes a black Soot to the uppermost Parts of the Chimney, which being chy-mically examined by Fire, yields a large Quantity of Earth, which was carried up so high by the Oil and Salt which were mixed with it, and yet this Earth, when purified and se-parated from every Thing else, re-mains fixed in the strongest Fire. Simple Earth, is also obtained by a Distillation of the purest Rain Wa-ter. But even in this Case the Fe-ces produced will contain in them every thing that was together with this Earth floating about in the Air, and at the same time is not volatile enough to ascend, in that Degree of Heat with which the Distillation is performed.

Such a pure and simple Earth may be, also, obtained from the Ashes of burnt Vegetables, for if these are carefully washed with Rain Wa-ter, we may by this Means per-fectly free them from all the fixed Salt which remained in them. And as the Fire had before carried off all the Oil and volatile Salt, the Earth will at last remain in the Water by itself.

By putting any Kind of Vege-table hitherto known into a Re-tort, and raising the Heat from a gentle to the strongest Fire, so that every Thing may come over successively into the Receiver that can be raised by those different Degrees of Heat, the Vegeta-ble will be divided into two di-stinct Parts, one which suffers it-self to be carried up into the Re-ceiver, and another which remains at the Bottom of the Retort and bears the utmost Force of the Fire without ascending, being a fixed

black Coal, the Ashes of which yield an Earth exactly like the for-mer when treated in the same Man-ner. And the volatile Parts which came over into the Receiver, will upon every Rectification, leave some Feces behind, from which a pure virgin Earth may be procured, exactly resembling that which is pro-duced by the Coal.

Hence, therefore, 'tis certain that this Earth may be procured from any Part of Vegetables whatever; and that amongst all the Sorts thus produced, there is not the smallest Difference perceptible by our Sen-ses. Hence too we learn that all this Earth, when absolutely pure, is so fixed in the Fire, that it can bear its utmost Efforts, almost without any Alteration; but that nevertheless when it is mixed with the other volatile Parts of Vegeta-bles, it is, together with them, carried up by the Fire, and is so far volatile. This we see both in the Soot generated by burning them in an open Fire, and the Parts which rise in Distillation in a close Vessel. We also farther ob-serve, that there is not any volα-tile Part of Vegetables which ren-ders Earth more volatile, than Oil; and that among the different Sorts of Oils procurable either by Nature or Art, none carries up more Earth with it in Distillation, than the last thick pitchy Oil, forc-ed out by the ultimate Action of the Fire, and to this it seems owing that these Oils are so very heavy, the large Quantity of Earth which they contain, thus increasing their Weight. Hence, also, arises their great Tenacity, as is obvious from this, that these Oils, when the Earth is separated from them by Distillation, grow immediately very thin, light, and exceedingly volatile.

A pure virgin Earth is, also, ob-tained from fixed alcaline Salts;

E   for

or if we carefully examine that fixed alcaline Salt, which by the Water is washed away from the Earth of burnt Vegetables, we find that by repeated Solutions, Coagulations, and Calcinations, it yields a large Proportion of pure white Earth, exactly similar to that which remains in the Ashes. From this and other chymical Experiments 'tis obvious, First, that the common fixed alcaline Salts obtained from the Ashes of burnt Vegetables, consist in a great Measure of simple elementary Earth, which, whilst they are forming, enters their Composition. Secondly, that this Earth is so concealed and intermixed with these Salts so long as they retain a fixed alcaline Form, that it does not give the least Indication of itself by any Sign, since by Water, or the Moisture of the Air, it is so dissolved, as to be converted into an exceeding simple limpid Liquor. Thirdly, that this Earth of Vegetables can only be subtiliz'd to this Degree by the most violent Action of an open Fire, which, whilst it is thus consuming Vegetables, so intimately, unites this Earth with another alcaline saline Principal, that from both an *Alcali* is generated. Fourthly, hence 'tis certain, that fixed alcaline Salts are not simple Bodies, but compounded of two perfectly distinct Principles, intimately united together. Fifthly, 'tis highly probable that this burning of Vegetables, after it has attenuated the Earth, combines it with that native Salt which was naturally in the Plant. Sixthly, hence we never find in Vegetables any Salt which is naturally fixed, since that which is so, owes its Existence to the Earth with which the Fire has combined it. Seventhly, hence the fixed alcaline Salts obtained from Vegetables, may be again resolved

into a pure simple and imperceptible volatile Salt, and a subtile, pure inactive, and fixed Earth. Eighthly, from this Account of Earth 'tis far more probable that fixed alcaline Salts are generated from Earth and a saline Principle, than that Water, by being intimately united with Earth, should be converted into an Alcali, as some imagine; for tho' all the Methods of Chymistry are used to combine Earth and Water together, yet it has never appeared, that a fixed alcaline Salt has been thence produced, let the Fire be ever so intense. Ninthly, this Earth, therefore, which is always and every where the same, is extracted from Plants in great Quantities, with the Water, Spirits, volatile and fixed Salts, and Oils, when they come under the Management of the Chymist. Hence we are sufficiently certain of the Nature of that Earth which is found in the Class of Vegetables, which as it appears to be every where the same in every Vegetable, constitutes perhaps an immutable Element.

Such an Earth is also to be found in the animal Kingdom; for if Animals after Death are exposed to a warm moist Air they presently putrify, in a Heat less than that of a Man in Health and by this Putrefaction, they are in a short time so much altered, that almost their whole Bodies are resolved into a fetid Matter, which is so volatile, as to be dissipated in the Air, leaving behind it a simple terrestrial and unactive Matter, exceedingly like the Earth obtained from Rain Water, and Vegetables.

The Juices, also, of all Animals by a proper Treatment, yield an Earth of the same Kind; for any of the Humours of every Animal after

for by a due Circulation they have been changed from the crude Condition they had when they were taken into the Body, being chymically treated, yield an incredible Quantity of Water, and a small Quantity of fixed Earth.

This Account of Animals and Vegetables, given with a View to discover the true Nature of Earth, shews us that these two Bodies greatly resemble each other in all their Properties, and in many of them, entirely agree. Hence, therefore, 'tis not surprising that Animals, by Means of their concoctive Faculties, can subsist entirely upon Vegetables, with the simple Addition of Water, and as this appears to be every where the Case, the Bodies of Animals seem in many Respects to be nothing but transmuted Vegetables.

The Union of elementary Earth with all the other Elements of Vegetables, is dissolved by no Action more easily than by that of Putrefaction; for no Vegetables after Putrefaction will, by the Action of Fire, yield a fixed Salt, for the oily and saline Parts recede, and are separated from the Earth, and the Salts are rendered volatile, like those of Animals. The same Effect is produced by the Digestion of Vegetable Food in the Stomachs of Animals, and thus Substances originally of the vegetable Kind, when assimilated to animal Bodies, yield no fixed Salt upon burning. This does not hold true of Fermentation; for tho' this last agitates Vegetables so powerfully, and for so long a Time, yet it is never able to free the elementary Earth from its Salt and Oil, as appears in Tartar, which yields a fixed Salt by Calcination.

Hence we understand the Nature of that elementary Earth, which enters the Composition of Animals and Vegetables, as a true Principle and in both these, this Earth seems to be perfectly of the same Nature, since little or no Difference appears in it. This no where is more evident than in the Cupels which are made as good from the Ashes of Vegetables, as from the pure Earth of Animals, whether procured from any of the Parts of Fishes, Birds, or Beasts. The Earth, then, answers the same Purposes in Animals and Vegetables, since it gives a firm Contexture to their Bodies, and affords a solid Basis for the Rest of the Elements; for these must all be united with this Earth, that by this Means they may be fixed and held together, and thus reduced to the Shape of any particular solid Body. This Earth alone gives all Bodies their proper Form, and when this is separated from them, they either sink into an irregular Mass, or being resolved and disengaged, become volatile, and are dispersed from each other. This Earth by its fixed and tenacious Nature, proves a proper Cement to bind, unite, and properly dispose all the other Parts among themselves, and thus hardens the Body arising from this Conjunction, so that it becomes capable of resisting the Air, Water, Sun, and some Degree of Fire, without any Inconvenience. But then, on the other Hand pure dry elementary Earth requires the Assistance of Water or Oil, as a Kind of Cement to hold together its separate Elements, and thus to form them into one Mass.

If whole Animals are burnt in an open Fire till they are consumed, there then remain no Parts of them but Ashes, which being pounded, exhibit an Earth exceedingly like the former, and free from all Oil or Salt. This cannot be distinguished from the Earth procured from Animals by other Operations, and serves entirely for the same Purposes in every Kind of Experiment.

Elementary

Elementary Earth is, also, obtained from Fossils; for if we take the pure native Salts such as Nitre, Sal-Gemmæ or Sea Salt, dissolve them in clean Water, and digest them in Vessels accurately closed, they will deposite an Earth to the Bottom, which will not be dissolved in the Water. When the Liquor is thus depurated and grown exceedingly clear, let it evaporate in a Place free from Dust, till you observe a Pellicle on its Surface. Then remove it into a cool and quiet Place, and it will Shoot into little saline Glebes, of a particular Figure, which, when dissolved in Water, will also yield a small Quantity of pure Earth; and at last after this Crystallization and Solution has been repeated a great Number of Times, all the Salt will become volatile, be dissipated in the Air, and escape any further Notice of our Senses, leaving the Earth, with which they were firmly united, behind them.

Elementary Earth is, also, obtained from these native Salts by Distillation; for if we reduce any of the above Salts to a Powder, and mix them with three Times the Quantity of dry Clay, Bole, Brick-dust, or pure Earth, and urge the whole with the greatest Degree of Fire, they will by this Means be resolved into a liquid Part, which will be volatile, acid, and corrosive, and a fixed Part, which will remain at the Bottom of the Vessel, among the Earth with which it was mixed. If this fixed Part is depurated by boiling it in Water, letting the Water settle, and afterwards filtrating, and is then reduced to Chrystals, it will yield a Salt pretty much resembling that made use of in the Distillation, except that the Salt from Nitre will be in some Measure alcalescent. And if the Salt thus generated is again dissolved, inspissated, and chrystalized, it will also produce a great

Deal of Earth of the same Nature with that which was procured from the original Salt. The acid Liquor also, thus drawn from the Salt by Distillation, being again distilled in a clean Vessel, will leave some yellow Feces at the Bottom, which when dried, are also found to contain some Earth. These acid Salts are so volatile, when accurately freed from their Earth, as to fly off and be dispersed in Fumes, which can hardly be contained within the Vessels, so that it is not absurd to suppose, that all these acid Salts would not be at Rest in the Air, if it was not on Account of their latent elementary Earth, which being intimately united with them, fix their Volatility and holds them down and that when they are disengaged from their Confinement, they regain their proper Volatility. If for Alum is dissolved, crystallized, and treated in the same Manner as the Salts above mentioned, it also yields a great Quantity of Earth, and this Earth is separated from its Salt these become volatile. By dissolving some Vitriol in Water, and digesting it, we obtain a large Quantity of Earth commonly called *Ochre*.

Elementary Earth is, also, contained from fossil liquid Sulphur and the Substances, produced from them, as *Asphaltus, Bitumens, Naphtha, Petroleum,* and the *Oleum Terræ* for if these are exposed to an open Fire, take Flame, emit black and Fumes, produce Soot and are quite consumed, there is found at the Bottom some Earth, which by being burnt to a Calx, affords a pure Earth exceedingly like that obtained from Animals, Vegetables, and Salts.

If true Sulphur is sublimed into Flowers in a close Vessel, it also leaves some Earth at the Bottom, tho' the Flowers thus obtained scarce yield any in a second Sublimation. But if with the purest Sulphur we mix, over the Fire, an equal Quantity of a pure alcaline lixivial Salt, the Compound arising hence being put into a clean glass Bason, and exposed to the Air in a Place free from Dust, will soon dissolve into a Liquor, to the Bottom of which a great Deal of Earth will subside. And even the Oil itself which produces Sulphur in conjunction with the fossile Earth, contains, and will yeild a pretty large Quantity of Earth.

Tho' some of the Moderns who have treated of the Analysis and Composition of Metals, mention an Earth which will vitrify, as entering their Composition, and which is the Basis of them all, yet this Substance does not at all answer the Characters, and consequently cannot deserve the Name, of Earth ; Mercury, indeed, when brought fresh out of the Mines, and pressed thro' a thick Leather, seems to have some Earth behind it ; and if, when it is thus depurated, we distil it in a clean glass Vessel, it will leave a very small Quantity of Feces but this cannot properly be called Earth, because the genuine Properties of Earth do not appear to be in it. But if we examine all the other Metals with the greatest Accuracy, we find no Earth in them ; for the Calxes of Metals always remain true Metals ; and tho' they are insipid, inodorous, fine, and sometimes capable of being reduced to a Powder, yet by the Addition of some reducing Powders, they may be brought back to their original Form ; whoever, therefore, looks upon these Calxes as true elementary Earth, may with equal Reason suppose that he is able to transmute Earth into Metal whenever he pleases. Besides, calcined Metals may by the Efficacy of Fire alone, or by the

Admixture of some other Substances with them, be converted into true Glass, which cannot be affirmed of pure simple Earth.

From what has been said, we may justly infer, First, That simple elementary Earth concurs as a constituent Principle in the Formation of the particular corporeal Fabric of Animals, Vegetables, and some Fossils of the less simple and durable Kinds. Secondly, That those Bodies which owe their Origin to the very same Earth, must, in this Respect, greatly agree with each other ; nor do they only resemble each other with Respect to their Earth, but also, generally in the great Affinity there is between their other concurring Principles. Thus the Elements of Animals are continually changing into the Matter of Vegetables, whilst on the contrary, the Bodies of Animals are perpetually supported, and nourished, by the Vegetables they take in, and assimilate to their Natures, and which afterwards actually enter their very Make. Thirdly, That Bodies which owe their Origin to the same Earth, are easily transmuted into each other. Fourthly, Iron, which of all the Metals seems to come nearest the Earth of Animals and Vegetables, must be allow'd, also, to come nearest to Animals and Vegetables in Nature, and seems as if it could in some Measure be dissolv'd in them. Hence it yields a noble and safe Remedy for various Diseases of the human Body; whereas the rest of the Metals act with more Violence ; for these, as they have not Earth, but Mercury, for their Basis, seem to remain immutable in all Bodies, and incapable of being digested by our concoctive Faculties. Fifthly, Earth principally furnishes the Chymists with their Instruments and Vessels ; for all Kinds of Glass have a great Quantity of terrestrial Matter uninedted with their fixed alcaline Salts. Sixthly, pure Earth mixed in a proper Quantity with pure fixed Salts, prevents their running into a Mass when they are expofed to a ftrong Fire, which would certainly have been the Cafe had the Earth been away. Seventhly, pure Earth is, alfo of great Service to Chymifts when they want to purify animal or vegetable Salts, from the Oil which tenacioufly adheres to them, and renders them impure, for when thefe are exceeding foul with the empyrcumatic Oil united to them, by the Admixture of pure Earth, they are, in a proper Heat, raifed with an exceeding white Colour, and depofite all their Oil in the bibulous Earth. Eighthly, Earth, when mixed with a great many Subftances, difpofes them to difcharge a flatulent Vapour, which otherwife, upon the Application of Fire, would make them puff up to fuch a Degree, that not being able to bear the Heat neceffary for the Diftillation, they would fwell and rife in the Retort, fo as to run over into the Receiver, and thus confounding every thing together, prevent the defired Effects of the Operation. Thus if for any valuable Purpofes, a Perfon defigns to diftil Honey or Wax, he lofes his Labour if he diftils thofe two Subftances by themfelves. Ninthly, what has been faid of elementary Earth is by no Means to be applied to common Sand, which is falfely taken for true Earth; for pure Sand, upon Examination with a Microfcope,

difcovers itfelf to be an Heap of fmall pellucid and multangular Cryftals, every one of which is of different Size and Figure. Thefe in Conjunction with a fixed *Alcali* will eafily run into Glafs. The wife Author of Nature has difperfed thefe over the Surface of the Earth, that the fructifying Water may be able to infinuate itfelf thro' the Pores of the Ground, which would otherwife very eafily unite and coalefce into one Mafs, and by this Means in a fhort Time acquire a perfect ftony Hardnefs, to the infinite Detriment of Mankind. Neither are we to confound elementary Earth with Bole or medicated Earths, fince thefe are compound Subftances, tho' by the utmoft Action of Fire and Water, they approach nearer to the Nature of true Earth, but in that Cafe they lofe their medicinal Virtues. But leaft of all are we to take for elementary Earth, that Earth on which we tread, and which furnifhes us with the Supplies both of Health and Life; for this our Earth evidently contains pinguious Boles, medicated Earth, barren Sands, Pebbles, Water, Air, Oils, Salts, all the Elements of Animals refolved into their Principles, and all the Principles of diffolved Vegetables blended and confounded together. So that common Earth is fo far from being a pure Element, that it is to be looked upon as a Chaos of all the natural Elements and the various Bodies compounded of them.

CHAP.

CHAP V.
Of ACIDS.

AN Acid is that Body which when applied to the Tongue, or the Nostrils, excites that Taste and Smell which every one calls Acid; so that all those Substances are acid which are capable of exciting the Sensation or Perception of Sourness; these consist of Particles highly rigid, long, subtile, and furnished with the most acute Spicula, by which Means they enter the Pores easily, stimulate the *Papillæ* of the Tongue, and affect the Organs of Taste. Acids are either *Manifest*, and fall under the Notice of the Senses, or *Disguised*, as when they are so sheathed up in oleous or earthy Particles, or so diluted with aqueous Fluids, that they are not perceptible to the Senses, but remain concealed, and disguised. Acids of the first Kind are simple and pure, whereas those of the second comprehend the various Degrees of austere and sweet Acids.

Acids are known from their Origin, Properties and Effects. With Respect to their Origin, they are either spontaneous and native, or factitious, and prepared by Art. The native Acid of the vegetable Kingdom is found almost in all Plants; the austere, crude Acid in the Juice of unripe Fruits, and sometimes in the woody Parts, the Bark and Leaves of Vegetables; whilst an Acid of the sweet Kind, which contains many oleous Parts, is found in some *Fruits* duly concocted and ripen'd by the Heat of the Sun, as in *Cherries*, Strawberries, Apples,

and many others. A simple Acid is, also, found in some ripe Fruits as in Citrons, Oranges, and Lemons. The native Acids of Vegetables, seem to be generated entirely from that Juice, which they draw as Nourishment from the Earth; so that in this Respect, we may perhaps reduce them all to the Nature of Fossils; especially because Plants growing in the Sea, without having their Roots affixed to any earthy Part of its Bottom, consist entirely of alcalescent Parts, and in Distillation yield a volatile oleous Alcali: But as all Plants imbibe the Air at their Surfaces, 'tis possible they may receive a Portion of their Acid by this Means, from the Atmosphere. We have Examples of manifest vegetable Acids in Sorrel and other Plants, from which the Acids may be produced separate, without any Change in the Form of essential Salts, whilst the most liquid acid Juices, being expressed, strained, inspissated, and left at Rest, generate saline Crystals. Which of the latent or occult Acids may be rendered manifest by Art, will afterwards appear, from the factitious Acids, only we shall here observe, that the native Acid of Plants concealed in their expressed and soft Oils, such as that of Olives, for Instance, discover themselves by the solvent Effects they produce on metallic Bodies, not by any Virtue peculiar to these Oils, but by Means of a volatile Acid which adheres to them, and may be expelled by long boiling. That such an Acid is, also, contained in the diftilled Oils of Lavender, Turpentine, and Juniper, is alfo demonftrated by an Experiment of *Hoffman*'s, who by triturating thefe Oils with Salt of Tartar, they produc'd a neutral Salt, compounded of the Acid extracted from them, and the additional Alcali. In the diftilled Waters of many Plants, the Acid, together with the oleous Parts joyned to it, remains concealed fo long as thefe Waters continue limpid to the very Bottom of of the Veffel, in which they are kept; but in the older diftilled Waters, the Acid becomes fenfible to the Tafte, the oleous Parts being then feparated and precipitated to the Bottom, in the Form of a vifcid Matter, in which Cafe thefe Waters are faid to be corrupted by Age.

Very few native foffile Acids are to be found. We indeed frequently meet with Exhalations which refemble a fuffocating fulphureous Acid, and which, alfo, by other Marks difcover the Acidity they contain; but fuch an Acid is very rarely found pure and alone, in the Form of a Liquor. As often, however, which frequently happens, as fuch an Exhalation meets with an hard Body capable of attracting its Acid, this Acid is united to it, is incorporated with it, and becomes fixed. But when this Acid is again extracted from the fixing Body, it fufficiently difcovers itfelf to the Senfes, and fo far as we know, is in every Inftance the fame; for if it meets with pinguious foffil Subftances, it produces various Species of Sulphurs, the Fume of which, when collected, refrigerated, and mixed with moift Air, yields a Spirit or Oil of Sulphur by the Bell. But if we diftil this Acid from a pure glafs Veffel, by expofing it long to the Heat of boiling Water, we obtain a confiderable Quantity of pure Water, which from the Air, in burning the Sul-

phur, had infinuated itfelf into its acid Fume. In this Cafe there will remain at the Bottom of the Veffel a ponderous, thick and burning Acid, which in every Refpect exactly refembles the pureft Oil of Vitriol, except in this alone, that the former contains nothing of a volatile metallic Nature, more or lefs of which is always found in Oil of Vitriol. When this Acid corrodes calcarious Stones, and is concreted with them, it forms various Kinds of Alums, according to the Diverfity of the Materials mixed with it. But all thefe Alums, when previoufly and gently calcined, are by the greateft Force of Fire, raifed into Vapours, and yield a Liquor, which when artificially depurated, is entirely the fame with that obtained from kindled Sulphur. When green native Copperas is, in a gentle Heat, dried to a whitifh Powder, and then urged by the higheft Degree of Fire, it emits white Clouds, which collapfing, yeild a Liquor, which when accurately depurated, is the fame with that obtained from Sulphur and Alum. But blue Vitriol when treated in the fame Manner, yields a Liquor, which is the fame with the former, and cannot be diftinguifh from them, provided it is artificially rectified.

Animals afford no manifeft native Acid; for all animal Juices, left to themfelves, always putrify, and do not become acefcent, whilft all Acids taken along with the Aliments are by a found Body, fubdued and divefted of their Acidity; fo that alcalefcent, putrid, volatile and fetid Salts are rather generated in Animals. Milk, alfo, drawn from the Breafts of a found Woman is never acid, but always of a fweet and mild Tafte. The Urine is, alfo, continualy alcalefcent, even in Perfons who ufe large Quantities of acefcent and acid Food and Liquors. Nor have the Excrements an acid, but rather a putid Smell, unless acefcent or acid Subſtances have been previouſly uſed. Nor is the Blood acid; for ſuppoſing a pure Acid to be, from the Aliments, conveyed with the Chyle to the Blood, it there immediately finds a Principle of an alcaline Nature, with which it engages, and aſſumes a neutral Quality, ſo as to be changed into a tartareous or an ammoniacal Salt. Much leſs are the other Liquors ſecreted from the Blood, ſuch as Bile and Sweat, to be called Acids, ſince they are rather of an alcaleſcent Nature. But if any Acid is found in Animals, it is entirely formed by the Uſe of acid or aceſcent Subſtances and by Reaſon of a Defect of the vital Force in Digeſtion, is depoſited in the *primæ viæ* in the unconcocted Chyle, or in the mammary Veſſels. Hence, in ſome Patients a Sweat manifeſtly of an acid Smell denotes the previous Uſe of Acids, and the languid Force of Nature. Hence if there is any other Acid than this in the ſound Blood, or other Humours of Animals, which have been concocted by the Force of Nature, it is highly latent and involved in oleous Particles, and conſequently cannot act as an Acid.

The factitious or artificial Acids latent in Vegetables, and obtained from them, are: Firſt, A vinous Acid by Fermentation; and this is either a ſimple Acid, or an auſtere Acid, or a ſweetiſh Acid, which are either liquid in the Form of Wine, or ſolid as Tartar. A ſimple Acid is alſo produced by Fermentation, in aceſcent Meals, as is ſufficiently known to Bakers. Secondly, A *fermenting Acid*, when Vegetable Juices are, in the very Act of Fermentation, or in the intermediate State between their native Condition and that which they acquire after the Fermentation is paſt, as is obſervable in recent Muſt, and Ale fermenting in a Bottle. Thirdly, an acetoſe Acid produced, by the ſecond acetoſe Fermentation,

as in Vinegars. Fourthly, an Acid by Diſtillation from ſome Woods diſtilled by themſelves from a Retort, by which Means they yield, firſt, an acidulated Water, and then, by increaſing the Fire, an acid Spirit. The Woods of this Kind, are Guaiacum, the Juniper Tree, the Oak, the Box Tree, the Cedar, and ſome others, which yield a Spirit, acid like Vinegar, oleous, fetid, and empyrenmatic, which when, filtrated thro' Paper, becomes purer by leaving its adherent Oil in the Filtre; but it always remains empyreumatic and pinguious, depoſites an oleous Cruſt on the Sides and Bottom of the Veſſels in which it is kept, and at laſt becomes pure by Rectification in a clean glaſs Veſſel, with a gentle Fire. Theſe acid Spirits are volatile acid Salts diluted with Phlegm, as is obvious from the Smoak produced in burning acid Woods, and the acid Soot generated by it. Of the ſame Nature is that purely acid Spirit obtained by Fire from the native Balſams, as Turpentine and Wax. From all Plants diſtilled with ſimple Water and urged with a great Fire we obtain an Acid, which is the Reaſon why diſtilled Waters prepared by mercenary Diſtillers, who endeavour to obtain too large Quantities, have an ungrateful nauſeous Taſte, and are poſſeſſed of anthelmintic Qualities, in Conſequence of the Corroſion of the Copper of the Still, by the Acidity of the laſt Water. Fifthly, *an Acid by burning* Pieces of Wood, eſpecially ſuch as are green, from the Extremities of which laid upon a large Fire, whilſt the Middles of the Boughs are agitated by the Fire, flows a Liquor like a frothy Water, which is a pure Acid, highly reſembling that which naturally exiſts in moſt Trees, and conſequently is a native Acid. Sixthly, an Acid is obtained from the expreſſed Juices of Plants by cryſtalizing them into

their

their native or essential Salts. But none of these Acids can ever be obtained pure, but are always mixed with other Parts, especially those of the oleous and aqueous Kinds.

Acids obtained from the fossile Kingdom are rarely found in a Solid, but almost always in a liquid Form; among these are the Acid of Sulphur, otherwise called the Oil or Spirit of Sulphur by the Bell; the Acid of Alum expressed by the greatest Force of Fire, and generally called the Oil of Alum; and the Acid of Vitriol, by the greatest Violence of Fire, forced into a Spirit commonly called the Oil of Vitriol. These three Species of Acids duely defecated, seem to differ but little from each other. They are indeed with the greatest Difficulty deprived of all Water, and if they should be totally divested of it, they forthwith attract the Water, from the Air as strongly as fixed alcaline Salts, calcined by the greatest Fire. The other simple fossil and acid Spirts are, the acid Spirits of Nitre and Sea-Salt, which always remain fluid, because the Water cannot be separated from them, since they are so volatile, that by the Degree of Fire requisite to separate the Water, they themselves fly off; *Aqua Fortis* and the *Spirit of Nitre* are much the same, Spirits of Sea-Salt, Fountain-Salt, and Sal-Gemmæ, are esteemed the same; whence 'tis obvious, that there are very few simple fossil Acids. Perhaps the only Instance of a true Acid being obtained in a solid saline Form, is in the Salt of Amber. According to *Homberg,* the acid Spirits of Fossils and Plants, are no more than volatile Salts resolved in a certain Quantity of aqueous Liquor, with which they are carried over in Distillation, but when they are disengaged from this aqueous Liquor, they appear in the Form of concreted or crystalliz'd Salts,

which, when thrown upon live Coals fly off in Smoak, without leaving any Feces.

From the animal Kingdom we obtain an Acid. First, when Milk drawn from an Animal fed with acescent Vegetables, is kept in a warm Place; for in such a State it grows more and more acescent, as is obvious from sour Milk, sour Whey, and Butter-milk. Secondly, we find an Acid in the Spirit of Ants, in these are distilled with their Beds which consist of the Leaves and other Parts of Plants. But this acid Spirit does not derive its Origin from the Ants, but from the Vegetables, since from the Ants distilled alone, we obtain a Spirit, somewhat fetid, but not acid. Thirdly, From distilled Bees we, also, obtain an acid Spirit, which however is not yeilded by the Bodies of the Bees themselves, but by the Wax and Honey they contain and which are vegetable Substances. Fourthly, the small Quantity of Acid which by the most exquisite Torture of the Fire is obtained from Blood is, according to *Homberg,* either the acid Spirit of Sea-Salt mixed with Earth, and procured by the greatest Fire; or if the Blood of an Animal which does not Use such a Salt should yield an Acid without the Addition of any other Substance this Acid must be separated from the pinguious and earthy Principle with which it was intimately united.

The most considerable artificial Acids mention'd by Authors, are Vinegar, Spirit of Nitre, Aqua Fortis, Spirit of Sea Salt, and Oil of Vitriol. But because these Acids can hardly ever be obtain'd pure and free from all adherent Water we shall from the celebrated *Homberg,* lay down the Method of discovering the Quantity of true Acid contain'd in any given Liquor. For this Purpose saturate Salt of Tartar with the acid Liquor, then exhale

O

to evaporate the Phlegm, in which the acid Salt was diffolv'd, which being now retain'd by the faturated and fixd Salt of Tartar, increafes the Weight thereof. And from this Augmentation of Weight, we know the Quantity of true Acid, contain'd in the acid Liquor pour'd upon the Salt of Tartar. Thus according to Homberg's Experiment,

One Ounce of Salt of Tartar abforbed all the Acid from fourteen Ounces of the beft diftilled Vinegar; and hence, after it was dried, it was increafed in Weight three Drams thirty-fix Grains;' the remaining Part of the Vinegar was meer infipid Water. By this Means, then, we difcover the Proportion there is between the Acid, and the Water of the Vinegar.

The fame Quantity of Salt of Tartar abforbed all the Acid from two Ounces five Drams of Spirit of Salt; the Increafe of Weight, when dried, was three Drams, fourteen Grains.

An Ounce of Salt of Tartar abforbed all the Acid from one Ounce, two Drams, thirty-fix Grains of Spirit of Nitre; the Increafe of Weight was three Drams, ten Grains.

The fame Quantity of Salt of Tartar abforbed all the Acid from one Ounce, two Drams, thirty Grains of Aqua Fortis; the increafed Weight was three Drams, fix Grains.

From five Drams of Oil of Vitriol, an Ounce of Salt of Tartar abforbed all the Acid; the increafed Weight in the dried Salt, was three Drams, five Grains.

As thefe are the principal Acids, we may infer, Firft, That in acid Liquors, tho' various with refpect to their Bulk, whilft united with their Water, yet the acid Principle has nearly the fame Weight in all. Thus Vinegar, which is the higheft of all thefe Acids, increafed the Weight of the fame Salt of Tartar, as much as the Oil of Vitriol, which

is the heavieft and ftrongeft. The fame too is true with refpect to the other Acids, the Difference between the greateft and leaft Increafe of Weight, being no more than thirty-one Grains, and only in the Vinegar, and this becaufe the *Tartarus Regeneratus,* that is, the compound Salts formed by the Union of the Salt of Tartar and Acid of the Vinegar, is not dried without a vaft deal of Difficulty.

Secondly, Acids feem to differ principally as to the Quantity of Water they are diluted with, fince the pure Acid when it is attracted, difcovers always the fame Weight. If fourteen Ounces, therefore, of the ftrongeft Vinegar could by any Contrivance be reduced to five Drams, by feparating the Water from it only, and collecting the Acid into a fmaller Compafs without altering it; it is poffible, that Vinegar thus reduced in Bulk, would be as ftrong as Oil of Vitriol. It is however certain, that it would be then capable of faturating the fame Quantity of alcaline Salt.

Thirdly, We have perceived, how great a Part of thefe acid Liquors, is Water.

Fourthly, It is probable, that if thefe acid Salts could be obtained pure without Water at all, they would then appear in a folid Form. This, however, has never yet been acomplifhed: Very intenfe Cold has come neareft it of any Thing, but not quite compleated it. Hence alfo, we may conceive what furprifing Effects *alcaline Menftruums* may produce, when they act upon Subftances that have any latent Acid in them, or upon thofe that are actually confolidated, and held together by an Acid; and hence, when this Acid is abforbed, they fall again into their conftituent Elements.

The common Properties, or Effects, by which Acids are known,

are

are thefe. Firft, Acids once generated, are fcarcely alter'd in the the Fire, even tho' long continued ; for by an Obfervation of *Homberg,* Aqua Fortis, Aqua Regia, Spirit of Nitre, Spirit of Salt, and Oil of Vitriol, digefted for four Years in Glaffes hermetically feal'd, by Means of the equable Heat of an *Athanor,* retain'd the fame folvent Power ; only the diftill'd Vinegar became almoft infipid, and acquir'd an aromatic Smell. The Spirit of Salt began to corrode the Glafs in which it was contain'd ; and a great Part of the Oil of Vitriol which was next the Fire, was form'd into Cryftals as it cool'd. Secondly, The Strength of Acids is as their Weight, on Account of their true Acid mixed with the Water, fo that the heavieft Acids are accounted the ftrongeft. Thus foffil Acids are heavier, and confequently ftronger, than thefe of the vegetable Kind. Hence one Acid exerts the Power of an Alcali with refpect to another, fince the ftronger is receiv'd by the weaker, as it were by an alcaline Salt ; but the Acid of Vitriol is of all others the ftrongeft. Thirdly, All Acids may be diluted with common Water, and confequently fo weakened, that the moft corrofive acid Poifons may be converted into the moft falutary Medicines. Fourthly, Acids may be united with inflammable Spirits, as the Spirit of Nitre with *Alcohol,* which upon Mixture excite a great Heat, emit red Fumes, and produce a terrible Effervefcence. Foffil Acids united with Spirit of Wine, by Digeftion, or Diftillation, are weaken'd and dulcified ; an Inftance of which we have in the Shop Preparations, commonly call'd, the *Spiritus Nitri Dulcis,* and, the *Spiritus Salis Marini Dulcis.* Fifthly, Acids may be alfo united with Oils. Thus Spirit of Nitre, may be mix'd with fome di-

ftill'd Oils, during which a great Heat, and fometimes a lucid Flame are excited. But when Acids are united with oleous Liquors, they always produce a Subftance of a bituminous, pitchy, or fulphureous Nature. Sixthly, Acids pour'd upon the Flowers of Mallows, the Syrups of Violets and Rofes, but efpecially upon a Solution of Heliotropium, or upon blew Paper, immediately turn them of a Colour more or lefs red, according to the Quantity and Quality of the Acid. Seventhly, Acids mix'd with an oleous Principle, quickly produce a Liquor of a redifh Colour. Eighthly, All fluid Acids added to earthy alcaline Subftances, call'd Abforbents, and to alcaline Salts, whether of the fix'd, or volatile Kind, produce an Effervefcence with them, diffolve them, and in Conjunction with them form a neutral Subftance. Ninthly, Acids added to Solutions, made by *Alcalies,* frequently caufe a Precipitation. Tenthly, Acids produce an Effervefcence with Metals, and other Minerals ; all Acids, however, do not equally affect all Metals and Minerals, but fome act more ftrongly with fome, and others more faintly. Eleventhly, Acids diffolve the folid Parts of Animals, as Horns, Hoofs, and Bones. Twelfthly, Acids coagulate Milk, and the Whites of Eggs. Thirteenthly, Strong foffil Acids put a Stop to Fermentations. Fourteenthly, Strong Acids applied to the folid Parts of live Animals corrode them, and induce a yellow Spot, but when applied to nervous Parts, excite convulfive Motions. Fifteenthly, Acids refift Putrefaction, and when applied to putrefcent Subftances, as the Flefh of Animals, preferve them from Corruption. Sixteenthly, Different Acids taken into the human Body, excite a certain Stimulus in the Solids, with Forces and Effects peculiar to themfelves.

felves. Laftly, Acids are more flowly congeal'd than fimple Water, and require a greater Cold for that Purpofe.

As for the Ufe of Acids in Medicine, 'tis certain, that there is a great Difference betwixt the Strength of vegetable and foffil Acids. Hence thefe laft, are for the moft Part only employ'd for external Ufe by Surgeons, when they want corrofive and cauftic Medicines; but cannot be exhibited internally, till they are diluted with aqueous Liquors, or dulcified with Spirits of Wine. And as vegetable Acids are of various Kinds, and different Virtues, fo nothing concerning their Ufe in Medicine, can be advanced, which is equally applicable to them all. However, that we may be enabled to form as juft an Opinion of their Effects, as poffible; we fhall obferve, that fome are afraid of Acids, on Account of their corrofive and diffolving Quality, whilft others are apprehenfive of their Strength and coagulating Virtue. Both are in the right, if their Opinions are underftood, with a due Reftriction. As all foffil Acids are of a corrofive Quality, we fhall fay no more of them, but confine ourfelves to vegetable Acids, which, as they are weaker than the former, may confequently be more eafily fubdu'd, by the digeftive Powers. But 'tis carefully to be obferv'd, that vegetable Acids, obtain'd from the very fame Plant, often produce widely different Effects; for, we muft accurately diftinguifh between aftringent, and refolvent Acids; thus there is a refolvent Acid in ripe Summer Fruits, which when eaten copioufly, prove purgative; whereas, before they are ripe, they contain an aftringent Acid, which produces Coftivenefs, and all the Difeafes arifing from a Conftriction of the capillary Veffels, and a Coagulation of the Fluids, of which Kind, is a particular Species of Itch, to which the poorer Sort of People are fubject, on Account of their eating four and unripe Fruit. Among vegetable Acids, therefore, we find that the *Omphacium*, or Juice of unripe Grapes, is aftringent, whilft that of fuch as are ripe, fo refolves the Humours, as to induce fatal Diarrhæas, and Choleras. This Juice of ripe Grapes, when fermented, produces Wine, which when recent, is ftill more refolvent, and at the fame Time hot and productive of Commotions; but old Wine is not refolvent, tho' it becomes more hot. Of Wine, is prepar'd Vinegar, which is ftill more refolvent. But as the moderate tho' daily Ufe of Vinegar, cannot be prejudicial to Health, when fubdued, and chang'd by the concoctive Powers; fo the immoderate Ufe of it produces thofe Diforders which arife from a predominant Acid, and which are either produc'd by the too copious Ingeftion of acid Subftances, or by the languid Condition of the concoctive and digeftive Powers. The celebrated *Helmont*, juftly informs us, " That " in any other Part than the Sto- " mach, all Acidity is preter-natu- " ral, and unfriendly; for that in " the Inteftines it produces Gripes; " in the urinary Paffages, a Stran- " guary; in Ulcers, a Corrofion of " the Parts; in the Skin, the Itch; " and in the Joints, the Gout.--The " Truth of this Affertion, fubjoins the " Author, is evinced from this, that " recent Urine difcharged without " any Pain, produces great uneafinefs " in the urinary Paffage, when " mixed with a few Drops of tar- " tifh Wine, and injected with a " Syringe." Diforders, alfo, frequently happen in the Stomach, from a redundant Acid, as is obvious from the Heat, Uneafinefs, pungent Pains, difficult Concoctions,

acid

acid Eructations and Vomitings with which it is afflicted. When, therefore, 'tis certain that an Acid predominates in the Body, we may, from what has been said, discover what Medicines are to be opposed to it; that is, aqueous Diluents, mitigating and obtunding Substances, mild oleous Medicines, Alterants, earthy Absorbents, and saline alcaline Substances.

If in sedentary Persons the Humours are disposed to Acidity, the Disorder is more properly removed by due Exercise, than by the Exhibition of alcaline Salts, by which the Humours are no less resolved, than the Fibres corroded and abraded. For Persons afflicted with acid Eructations, the Antients ordered Vociferation. It is absurd to assert that all Disorders have a peccant Acid for their primary and fundamental Cause, since different Acids produce different Effects, and since the animal Functions, when too vigorous, spontaneously dispose to Diseases arising not from Acidity, but from Alcalescence and Putrefaction. Besides, 'tis certain from Experience, that Acids not only prevent, but also cure many Diseases; for when the Body is over-heated; and the Motion of the Blood preternaturally accelerated, Acids are so far from being injurious, that they excellently allay the Heat and Thirst, excite a keen Appetite, and procure a laudable Digestion. Acids, also, resist Putrefaction, and change the alcalescent Salts of the Body, into those of a neutral, mild Kind, which greatly contribute to the Preservation of Health. Hence nothing is more efficacious for guarding against the Contagion of malignant Diseases, than Acids, of which Wine Vinegar and Lemon Juice are the most considerable for this Purpose. Acids frequently prove beneficial to dropsical Patients, both on Account of their stimulating Quality, and because they change the putrid Salts into those of a compound neutral Nature, which excellently resist Putrefaction. Mild and grateful Acids, such as ripe Summer Fruits, are proper in Apostems of the Lungs, or Empyemas. As Acids moderately used contribute to Health, so when taken to Excess, they are highly injurious; but in a particular Manner both Meats and Drinks of an acid Kind, are prejudicial to those who have weak Stomacks, in which the Juices easily turn acescent, are long retained, and do not pass duely off by Stool. Among Persons of this Kind are Children, old Persons, those exhausted by previous Diseases, or Grief, but especially hypocondriac, and gouty Patients, hysteric Women, and Persons labouring under Disorders of the Head, or Spasms. All these are greatly injured by ripe Fruits, which contain a large Quantity of Acid, and which by Fermentation, are changed into acid Juices. Some by taking a small Quantity of any Acid, such as rhenish Wine, immediately perceive an Uneasiness in their whole Bodies; and 'tis remarkable, that some Persons who have Issues, soon after the the Use of Acids, perceive a Pain and Itching in these Parts. Acids are always prejudicial to the Bones, so that in spreading and malignant Ulcers 'tis an absurd Practice to apply Acids, in order to prevent a Caries of the Bones. 'Tis customary with some to Use highly acrid Acids in order to beautify the Teeth, which by this Means are soon rendered dull, torpid, and so loose that they drop out.

CHAP.

CHAP VI.

Of ALCALIES.

THE Name of *Alcali* was originally given to the Salts of Vegetables procured by burning them, from *Kali* a Word well known in the East and in *Egypt*, which fignifies a certain Herb replete with Salt, which grows about the Sea Shore, and the Banks of the *Nile*, and also those of the celebrated River *Belus* in *Syria*, as *Pliny* affures us from the Testimony of antient Authors. This Plant, if burnt when it arrives to its full Growth produces Afhes, remarkable for their falt and acrid Tafte, an Evidence of its abounding with Salt. When thefe Afhes are boiled in Water, they yield a ftrong acid falt Lixivium or Lye confifting of the Salt communicated by them to the Water which being properly feparated, there remains a greyifh Part, which will neither diffolve in Water, nor burn in the Fire, but is perfectly infipid, and of the Nature of Earth. If this Lixivium or Lye is evaporated to a Drynefs in an Iron Veffel, a white folid Mafs, of a moft acrid cauftic Tafte and perfectly foluble in Water, is left behind. This Salt only is properly an *Alcali*; but becaufe other Bodies produce much the fame Appearances upon being mixed with Acids, all Subftances that raife an Effervefcence with Acids have been called *Alcaline*; as the volatile Salts of Animals, thofe procured from fome acrid Vegetables, and thofe arifing from putrified Vegetables, in Diftillation. And not only alcaline, fixed, and volatile Salts, but also fome other Bodies produce almoft the fame Ef-

fects with Acids. Hence we generally refer to the Number of Alcalies, Firft, fuch Subftances as are purely of an earthy Nature, fuch as Lime, Marble, and the feald Earths. Secondly, ftony Concretions formed in the Bodies of Animals, fuch as the Stone in the human Bladder, Bezoar Stones, and Crabs Eyes. Thirdly, teftaceous Subftances, fuch as Pearls, Oyfter Shels, the Bone of the Cuttle Fifh, the Claws and Eyes of Crabs. Fourthly, thofe Parts of Animals, which in Procefs of Time have affumed a Stony hardnefs, or are changed into Earth. Fifthly, all Plants of a ftony Nature, or Sea Lithophytes, as Coral, all which Subftances are called Abforbents, or earthy Alcalies. Sixthly, to the Clafs of *Alcalies* alfo belong metallic Subftances. But this Property of uniting and producing an Effervefcence with Acids, is not the peculiar Characteriftic of alcaline Subftances alone; for all diftilled Oils produce an Effervefcence with Acids, which is fometimes fo ftrong as to excite a Flame, which never happens in the Admixture of Alcalies with Acids. Thefe Oils, alfo, after the Effervefcence, yield a Subftance concreted of themfelves and the Acids; but by this very Circumftance they are diftinguifhed from Alcalies, becaufe, like, thefe they do not produce a faline Subftance capable of being diffolved in Water; but only a refinous or bituminous Matter.

With Refpect to genuine *Alcalies*, as all our phyfical Knowledge of
Things

Things depends upon the Discoveries which our Senses make in natural Bodies, hence all their Characteristics must be taken only from such sensible Signs thus discovered. Nor are we able to distinguish Bodies in any other Manner. The following Characters, therefore, of an *Alcali*, may be laid down as genuine, and sufficient for the Purposes both of the Chymist, the Philosopher, and Physician.

First, A fixed *alcaline Salt*, is produced from a vegetable Substance.

Secondly, It is only prepared from a Vegetable by the Action of Fire, which converts it into Ashes.

Thirdly, When it is thus prepar'd, it will remain a considerable Time in the Fire, thus demonstrating its Fixity.

Fourthly, In a moist Air, it perfectly dissolves, and deposites some Fœces, being impatient of a continued Dryness, if any Part of the Air has Access to it.

Fifthly, It impresses an acrimonious Taste upon the Tongue, somewhat caustic, and it excites a Taste of Urine, on which Account these Salts have, though not very properly, been call'd *urinous Salts.* For the Taste of this Salt does not resemble that of Urine, at the first Application. But when this has been in the Mouth some Time, and by its Stimulation caused a Discharge of the Saliva, then the neutral animal Salts which are in the Saliva, deposite all their Acid on the fixed *Alcali*, and thus becomes volatile and *alcaline*, and then impress upon the Tongue a disagreeable urinous Taste, of which this is the true Origin.

Sixthly, This Salt, when it is perfectly pure and without Mixture, has not the least Smell, being extremely fixed, even in the Fire. But as it attracts every Acid, if it meets with any Body, which contains a volatile *alcaline Salt*, fixed by an Acid, and

therefore without any Smell, it then immediately absorbs the Acid, and the *Alcali* being by this Means disengaged, and rendered volatile, affects the Organs with an *alcaline* Smell, which is falsly ascribed to the fixed Salt. This appears evidently upon mixing a fixed *alcaline Salt* with warm fresh Urine, upon which the Liquor that was inodorous before, instantly emits a disagreeable *alcaline* Smell.

Seventhly, Another Property of this Salt is, that when mixed with any Acid whatever, it immediately produces an Ebullition and Effervescence; and afterwards is so intimately united with it into one Mass, that if the Saturation is compleat, the Compound discovers no Sign either of an *Alcali*, or an Acid; but there is always by this Means produced a Salt of another Nature, which is usually called *neutral.*

Eighthly, If a pure fixed *Alcali* is mixed with the Juice of the Turnsole, Roses, or Violets, it presently changes their natural Colour, which is a Kind of Purple, into a Green.

Ninthly, When this *alcaline Salt* is applied for some Time to a human Body that is warm, and consequently exhales some Moisture, it excites an acute Inflammation, attended with all its Symptoms, which soon becomes a grey, hard, dead, and often black Escar; it is therefore capable of producing a true Sphacelus, or Mortification.

Tenthly, All these Salts have the Faculty of deterging and cleansing, which is not the Case with respect to those call'd *neutral.* These, then, are the Marks by which fixed *alcaline Salts* may be known and distinguished from all others; and by these we shall be able to avoid Confusion.

Such *alcaline* fixed Salts may be procured from any crude, fresh Vegetables burnt to Ashes, and treated in the Manner above-mentioned. But few Plants by this Management, yield a very small Quantity. Such as these, which, when crude, have a pungent Smell, which strikes the Nose, and makes the Eyes water; for almost all the Salt of these Plants being volatile, is dissipated by the Heat of the Fire. Garlic, the bulbous rooting Roots, Onions, Scurvy-Grass, Lady's-Smock, Rockets, Hedge-Mustard, Cresses, Radishes, Rapes, Squills, Leeks, Mustard, and the like, are of this Class, in which Nature has so far perfected their *alcaline Salts*, as to render them volatile, as in Animals.

These lixivious acrid Salts, have been known to the Antients in almost all Ages of which we have any Account. *Aristotle* tells us, that the Ashes of burnt Reeds and Bulrushes, boil'd in Water, yield a plentiful Salt. And *Varro*, informs us, that some People about the *Rhine*, having neither Fossil, nor Sea-Salt, instead of those made Use of a salt Coal, which they prepared from some Sorts of Wood, burnt: From which it is plain, that they knew a Method of preparing these Salts, not unlike that of *Tachenius*, so as to make them less acrid, and to come nearer to the Nature of the native *neutral* Salt. Hence *Pliny* asserts, that Ashes have the Quality of Salt, but are milder. And that the burnt Fœces of Wine have the Virtues of Nitre (the antient Nitre) And in another Place, he speaks of the Nitre produced from burnt Oak, which, he says, yields but a small Quantity, *L.* 31. *C.* 10. We farther learn from *Pliny*, that Ashes were in his Time used medicinally, and the Lixivium made of them drank as a Remedy. All these Authorities, to which more might be added, sufficiently evince, that the Discovery of *Alcalies* is not so modern as some imagine.

No native Salts have yet been discovered, with which the preceding Characteristics agree, *alcaline Salts* being procured from vegetable Substances only, by the Action of the Fire. But since the first Calcination of Vegetables that ever happened in the World, these Salts have been produced. Hence therefore, in all Ages and Places where this has happen'd, there must have been a prodigious Quantity of this Salt generated, which always is at last, together with the Ashes, returned to the Earth. In the Revolution, therefore, of such a Number of Years, the whole Earth must have been converted into this Salt, provided it was immutable. But this is not the Case, for these Salts, when committed to the Earth, render it indeed fruitful, but then they change their *alcaline* Nature, and, imbibing the Acid of the Air, become *neutral* Salts, and act as such.

It is farther remarkable, that no Plant which ever grows upon the Surface of the Earth, if it was suffered to become dry, carious and rotten, would ever yield a single Grain of a fixed *Alcali*; but on the contrary, they are always either dissipated into such minute volatile Particles, as escape the Notice of our Senses, or leave behind them a Substance, which upon Examination appears to be simple Earth. This Experiment, therefore, confirmed universally in all Ages, evidently demonstrates, that Nature never produces a fixed *alcaline Salt*, either in the Solids, or Fluids of Vegetables.

Hence it is certain, that fixed *alcaline Salts* have their specific Nature imparted to them by Fire, and not by any natural vegetable Operation. But this is still farther evinced by the following Experiment, which never fails to succeed in the same Manner: Take any Vegetable, which, if burnt, would yield a large Quantity of a fixed *alcaline Salt*, let them be reduced to Putrefaction by Art, so

that

that their whole Subftance fhall be perfectly putrified, they will then be rendered exceedingly fœtid, and a great Part of them volatile, and, if they are burnt in an open Fire, will not yield the leaft Portion of a fixed Salt, but what remains will be a perfectly infipid Earth : If therefore we view this Experiment in a juft Light, we muft be of Opinion, that fixed alcaline Salts are as much the Creature of Fire, as Glafs, which no Body ever fufpected to be a vegetable Production, tho' vegetable alcaline Salts enter its Compofition, and are neceffary to its Exiftence.

It muft, alfo, be remarked, that thefe alcaline Salts are capable of being refolved into a confiderable Part that is faline, hard, bitter, and almoft vitrefcent; into a fimple Earth; and into an alcaline Salt, that is ftronger and more pure : And thus we may obferve, that thefe alcaline Salts are no fimple Bodies, but that they are compounded of different Parts united together; and that the Conjunction of their Principles into one Mafs, which has the Appearance of being homogeneous, is effected by the Strength of the Fire. Hence it will follow, that Nature never acts by fixed alcaline Salts, as by her proper Inftruments, unlefs when they are received firft prepared by the Fire. And that even then, when fhe makes Ufe of them, thus prepared, in bringing about her Purpofes, fhe only operates by them, as they are compounded of the three above-mentioned Principles ; to which, however, as a fourth Part, there ftill feems to remain a Portion of Oil, as many Arguments evince.

Hence it appears, that as thefe fixed alcaline Salts are rendered more and more fimple by a Separation of their conftituent Parts, the Salt that thus arifes will be continually different ; for that which remains after a Separation of fome of its Principles, will always be of another, and more fimple Nature, and confequently will have a different Power of acting Thus in Pot-afh, which yields the beft Alcali, a confiderable Part of it is a bitter, hard, pellucid Salt which does not very readily diffolve in Water. If this is carefully feparated from the reft, a purer Alcali i obtained, fitter than the former, before this Separation, for many Operations that are performed by Alcalies.

It is farther to be obferved, that thefe alcaline Salts may be greatly altered by the cafual Admixture of fome other Body, whilft the Vegetables are burning, which being alfo of a fixed Nature, may be united with them, and remain in the Afhes; fuppofe, for Inftance, that Nitre fhould happen to be among them; then this being fixed with the other vegetable Salt, would produce an Alcali to which, if Oil of Vitriol was added it would emit a fœtid Fume, that would in Smell refemble Spirit of Nitre, which never is the Cafe, if the Alcali is pure. The fame is true with refpect to Sea-Salt, and many others. And laftly, We muft take Notice, that the very Burning of Vegetables, as it is performed in different Manner, will produce different Salts; for it is a known Truth, that if the fame Vegetable burnt in a ftrong brifk Fire, it will yield a Salt different from what produced by burning it in a flow fmothering Fire.

Amongft alcaline Salts, the moft common is, that which is ufually called Pot-Afh. This is imported great Quantities from Courlan Ruffia, Poland, and other Parts the North, where it is prepared from the Wood of green Firs, Pin Oaks, and others of the like Natu of which they make large Piles proper Trenches, and burn them they are reduced to Afhes. Thefe are immediately fifted, and were by the Antients called *Lix*, by the Moderns *Cineres Clavellati*, a Name taken from the *Clavi, Kiln*, into which the Wood is def, to make it burn the more readily. Thefe Afhes are then diffolv'd in boiling Water, and when the Liquor, which contains the Salt, is departed by fubfiding, it is poured off clear, and makes a Lixivium. This is immediately put into large Copper Veffels, and is there boiled for the Space of three Days and Nights, till at laft a Salt is left, which takes the Name of *Pot-Afh*, from the Pots the Lixivium is boiled in. This Salt whilft it is hot and dry, muft be put up in Cafks, made of dry Wood, and which is not impregnated with Oil of any Kind; and by this Means it may be preferved dry; otherwife, if it is expofed to the Air, efpecially one that is moift, it will run into a pinguious *alcaline Fluid*, exactly like Oil of Tartar *per Deliquium*.

By the Manner in which thefe fixed alcaline Salts are produced, one would not fufpect them to contain any confiderable Quantity of Earth, and yet upon Examination, we find they yield a great deal, even after they have been rendered as pure as it is poffible to make them.

The Properties of fixed *alcaline Salts*, are as follows:

They attract Water very powerfully, and at a great Diftance, and from every known Body in which it abides. This is plain to the Eye, for when fuch an *Alcali* is taken out of a ftrong Fire, if it is fuffered to remain in a very hot Air, clofe by the Fire, where Water can by no other Art be difcovered, it will even there grow moift, and diffolve: And it is then put into a clean, dry, Veffel, and dried over the Fire, the Vapour that exhales, is re-

ceived, and condenfed in an Alembic, it will yield again the pure Water which the *Alcali* had attracted. Other Salts, if moift before, would have been deprived of their Water in the very fame Degree of Heat, and the fame Place where the dry *Alcali* attracted Moifture. Thefe *alcaline Salts*, therefore, are true Magnets to Water; by this they are diffolved, and are ftrongly united with it; and hence, when they are once diffolved in Water, a Heat equal to that of boiling Water will not perfectly dry them again.

But to come to a more accurate Knowledge of this Attraction of Water by *alcaline Salts*, *Boerhaave* took a large glafs Bottle, very clean, and dry, and hot, as if it had juft been taken out of the Glafs-houfe-Oven. Into this he put fome pure Salt of Tartar, very hot and dry alfo, and reduced to Powder, in the Manner above defcribed. He then immediately ftopped the Mouth of the Bottle with a dry Cork, and tied over it a Hog's Bladder foftened with Oil, and made very fupple: The Effect of this Experiment was, that the Salt which adhered to the Sides of the Glafs, was grown moift with the Water contained in that fmall Quantity of Air included in the glafs Bottle, tho' the Air was extremely hot and dry, at the Time that the Bottle was clofed.

It has not yet been determined with any Degree of Certainty, whether fixed *alcaline Salts* repel Air, or attract it fo ftrongly, as not to part with it again readily. Experiments that have been made with this View leave the Thing dubious. It is very certain that Oil of *alcaline Salts per Deliquium*, examined by the Air-Pump, gives not the leaft Indications of containing Air, fince none is feparated from it, when the Preffure of the Atmofphere is taken away, even tho' the Oil is made very

hot

hot in Order to expel the Air. On the contrary, it is equally certain, that when *alcaline Oils per Deliquium*, are mixed with Oil of Vitriol, from which the Air has been extracted by the Air-Pump, a surprising Quantity of elastic Air is produced, or, as it is called, generated. Upon considering these Circumstances, it appears most probable that fixed *alcaline Salts* actually attract Air, and unite it with themselves so strongly, that it is not to be dislodged, till the Texture of the Salt is destroyed by the Effervescence upon mixing it with an Acid.

These pure, acrid, fixed, *alcaline Salts*, if they are mixed with the purest *Alcohol*, when they come very hot out of the Fire, attract it, and unite with it; but if there is the least Mixture of Water, either in the Salts or the *Alcohol*, then the Salts repel the *Alcohol*, nor can they be united by any Art whatever. In this Manner, therefore, pure, fixed *alcaline Salts* divide strong Spirit of Wine into two Parts that, are not afterwards miscible with each other, that is, into a Water saturated with the *alcaline Salt*, and into a pure *Alcohol*, which swims at the Top. And thus, again, plainly appears the reciprocal Attraction betwixt Water and fixed *alcaline Salts*: Take a Pint of the purest *Alcohol*, mix with it a small Quantity of Water, and then a dry *alcaline Salt*, and the *Alcali*, will in an Instant draw into it that little Portion of Water, and will appear in the Form of a thick Oil, about the Sides; and, at the same Time, the Combination of the *Alcohol* and Water will be utterly prevented.

These *alcaline Salts* act also upon vinous Spirits in another Manner; for, as every Spirit drawn by Fire, from Wine of any Sort, has always a volatile Acid intermixed with it, the Acid being greedily attracted by the *alcaline Salts*, the Spirit by this Means becomes much more pure, when freed from the Acid which adhered to it, and consequently will be very different, both in its Nature and Virtues, from what it was before this Operation. And the *Alcali* itself will also, at the same Time, be entirely altered, and become a Salt compounded of an Acid and an *Alcali*, insomuch that, if it is perfectly saturated in this Manner, a Salt perfectly *neutral* will be produced.

These Observations direct us to a Method of prepaing a pure *Alcohol*, without Distillation, or any Assistance from Fire; for add a sufficient Quantity of *Pot-Ash* to common Spirit of Wine, and stir them about till they are thoroughly mixed together, the Water will be attracted by the *alcaline Salt*, and the *Alcohol* will swim at the Top, which, by a gentle Decantation, will come off good at the first Time. If any Doubt remains, whether it is quite pure, or not, put some more *Pot-Ash* into the *Alcohol* thus prepared, and by stirring them about, and then pouring the Liquor off, as before, it may be rendered so. In this Operation, however, the Spirit of Wine always discovers an Oil, which before appeared neither in the Spirit of Wine, nor the *alcaline Salt*, but is generated when they are thus mixed together.

Another Property of *alcaline Salt* is, to unite intimately with distilled vegetable Oils: For if the most acrid, pure, dry, *alcaline Salt*, is thrown very hot into a distilled Oil, it attracts the Oil greedily, with a considerable hissing Noise, and unites it so with its own Substance, that there is immediately formed a Kind of Soap; and the Oil is more firmly united to the *alcaline Salt*, and the Soap is rendered more perfect, if the Mixture is set in a subterraneous Place; for by this Means both of them

them become femi-volatile, and form a Mafs diffolvable in Water, which is endued with excellent medicinal Virtue. This is the *Ens parvum fapientum*, the *Sapo Helmontianus*, the fil-volatile *Tartari* of *Starkey*, and the Corrector of *Matthews*. It was formerly in great Reputation, firft in *England*, and afterwards all over *Europe*; for it powerfully refolves almoft every Kind of vifcid Concretion that is generated from the Humours of the human Body: Hence it invades and attenuates the tenacious Concretions that obftruct the Veffels, and at the fame Time it gently ftimulates the Veffels themfelves; and thus, by acting both upon the Solids and Fluids, it promotes the Secretions by Sweat and Urine, and by thefe Evacuations carries off the Caufe of many chronical Diftempers. This foap alfo entirely alters the Nature of many Simples, when digefted with them; and hence, depriving fome of their Virulence, imparts to them Virtues very different from what they naturally poffeffed. The Chymifts, however, as is ufual with them, have been too lavifh in the praife of this Medicine, which they have extolled as an univerfal Remedy. But it muft be obferved, that this Combination of a fixed *alcaline Salt* and diftilled Oil, can never be wrought about, if the leaft Portion of Water adheres either to the Salt, or Oil; and for this Reafon, it is neceffary, the Salt fhould be hot when mixed with the Oil. It will even hinder the Succefs of the Operation, if a fmall Portion of the *alcaline Salt* ftands above the Oil in the Veffel, and thus, by being expofed to the Air, grows ever fo little moift.

Fixed *alcaline Salts*, are eafily united, alfo, with the expreffed Oils of Vegetables, or Animals, as is daily feen in their Combination, into artificial Soap, by the Affiftance of quick Lime, Water, and Fire.

But *alcaline Salts* remarkably attract all Kind of Acids whatever, whether animal, vegetable, or mineral, and that whether dry or moift, pure or diluted. And this Force, with which *Alcalies* thus attract Acids, is incomparably greater than that with which they attract Water: For in this Action, by which they unite thefe Acids with themfelves, they violently expel the Air that refides both in the Salt and Acid, whence arife fuch Numbers of Air-bubbles, which fuddenly appear, and burft. This Union alfo makes them repel even Water, and when they are thus faturated, they will eafily fuffer themfelves to be dried, or deprived of their Water, which before, when they were feparated, they retained moft tenacioufly. Pure Oil of Vitriol, for Inftance, when it is alone, can fcarcely by any Art be utterly deprived of its Water; Oil of Tartar not without a great deal of Difficulty: And yet, when you mix them together, the Water is expelled in fuch a Manner, that a Salt almoft dry appears in the Veffel under it. The fame is true, alfo, of other Acids, when they are combined with an *Alcali*. This Power however, by which *Alcalies* attract Acids, is limited to certain Bounds; hence there appears a great Diverfity among them, though this, indeed, feems more owing to a Difference in the Acids, than in the *Alcalies*. Upon this Subject, the illuftrious *Homberg*, has communicated to the World many ufeful Obfervations, fome of which are mention'd in the Article of Acids.

When an Affufion of an Acid to an *Alcali*, is performed gradually and cautioufly in warm Liquors, and in a large Veffel, if at the fame Time the Veffel is fhaken after every Inftillation of the Acid, the Mixture at laft arrives to fuch a Temperament, that it will admit of no farther Ebul-lition,

lition, and this is called, the *Point of Saturation.* If Acids are after added, no more Agitation will be excited, than there is upon mixing Water with Water: And the Compound thus produced, is neither *alcaline* nor acid, but *neutral,* formed by the Union of both. Hence Acids have been called, Males, and *Alcalines,* Females, and the Compound of them both Hermaphrodites. The *Alcali,* the Vacuum; the Acid, the Implent. The *Alcali* the Chaos, and the Acid the impregnating Spirit.

The violent Ebullition and Effervescence, that appear upon the Mixture of an *Alcali* and an Acid, whilst the Air and Water are forcibly expelled, may possibly arise, because these Bodies impetuously drive out whatever lies betwixt them, when they rush strongly into mutual Contact; and if so, the Ebullition and Effervescence do not arise from any Disagreement, but from an Association of Principles. Hence the following Queries will naturally arise: First, Whether Acids abound plentifully with Air, whilst *Alcalines* contain none at all? So far is certain, that the strongest *Alcali,* taken out of the Fire, and so probably deprived of all its Air, will, if it is thrown into an acid Liquor, produce a prodigious Effervescence, and a great Quantity of Air will be generated. Hence may we not arrive at the true Reason, why Acids, when they are predominant in animal Bodies, are productive of so much Flatulency? Do not *neutral* Salts, produced from a Combination of *Alcalies* and Acids, lose the greatest Part of their Air; and are they not, for this Reason, found to be very little flatulent in the human Body? Are not acid, or at least acefent Bodies, the only Substances which are disposed to ferment, because of the latent Air they contain? And is not this latent Air,

the Source of that prodigious Quantity of Air, which is generated by Fermentation? Does Fermentation therefore, naturally tend to the Generation of Acids, whilst an intense Fire produces *Alcalies?*

From what has been said, it appears, that amongst natural Causes, by which Motion is excited in the Universe, we reckon *Alcalies* and Acids, at the Time when these are mixed together, which Motion ceases, as soon as ever this Combination is compleated.

The Motion thus excited, seems of considerable Importance in Vegetation, or rather in preparing the Earth. People concerned in Husbandry are sensible, that frequent ploughing or digging the Earth, mellows it, as they call it, and renders it fertile; or, to speak more philosophically, disunites the Parts of the Earth, which otherwise cohere together, and form large Glebes, and reduces them into small Particles, better suited to the subsequent Solution they are to undergo, in Order to the Production of a Plant. Now when the Earth is once furnished with an *alcaline Salt,* and that is immediately united with the earthy Particles, which soon happens, because these Salts, attracting the Water floating in the Atmosphere run into an *Oil per Deliquium,* and sink into the Ground the same Salts attract, also, the Acid of the Air, till they are saturated, and both together rendered *neutral* Whilst, therefore, this Neutralization is effecting, an Effervescence is made leisurely, and by Degrees, as the *alcaline Salt* imbibes the Acid Hence Motion is excited in the Part of the Soil which were impregnated with the *Alcali,* and by this Motion the Particles of the Earth are separated from each other, more effectually than either by ploughing or digging. This Separation is an excellent Preparation for a future Solution

tion, and indeed is one Step towards it, since the Solution of a Body is only the reducing it into Particles fine enough to float in the Menstruum that dissolves it, and small enough to be transparent, and consequently not visible.

There can be no doubt, but that in the Action of these *Alcaline* Menstrua upon Acids, the Water is expelled out of them, as well as the Air, when they thus unite together, for tho' they are perfectly fluid, when they are mixed, yet they harden in the very Act of Combination into little saline Globules, and appear in the Water in the Form of pellucid Crystals, the watery Liquid being driven out, and swimming at the Top. And when the Saturation is complete, the Water may be separated pure, and without any saline Taste, and then the Remainder is easily dried into the Form of a white, farinaceous, opake Powder, and that too by a gentle Heat, whereas the Parent *Alcali* and Acid, by whose Combination they are produced, either cannot be dried at all, or not without the greatest Difficulty.

It is farther remarkable, with Respect to these compound Salts thus prepared, that it is extremely difficult to separate again the Alcali from the Acid, so as to procure either of them pure, by the Assistance of Fire only. Sal-Ammoniac, for instance, made by a Combination of an Alcaline Spirit and Spirit of Sea Salt, may be sublimed by exposing it to a sufficient Degree of Fire; but it will not be thus possible to separate it into the saline Principles of which it was compounded. The same is true with regard to *Tartarus vitriolatus, Sal-marinus regeneratus, Nitrum Refusitatum, Tartarus regeneratus,* and others. There are, however, some Methods discovered, by which this Resolution of compound Salts, into

their constituent *Alcaline,* and acid saline Particles, may be accomplished, and the Knowledge of those will make us acquainted with some of the most secret Mysteries of Chymistry. In Order, therefore to arrive at the Knowledge of these, it is necessary to examine some farther Properties of Alcalies.

Alcalies, therefore, though they attract all known Acids, at the same time it is remarkable, that they attract some, much more powerfully than others. This Assertion is abundantly confirmed by Experiments. Thus, if upon an *Alcali* perfectly saturated with Vinegar, or upon *Tartarus regeneratus,* Spirit of Salt or Nitre, or Sulphur, or Vitriol is poured, then the latent *Alcali* will attract that Acid, and repel from it the Acid of the Vinegar with which it was before saturated; and, hence a Liquor, nearly of the same Nature with the Spirit of Vinegar, may be afterwards drawn from this Compound with a moderate Heat, there remaining a considerable fixed, regenerated, nitrous Salt, at the Bottom of the Vessel: Again, if Spirit of Nitre is poured upon an *Alcali,* saturated with Spirit of Salt, an Aqua regia will arise in Distillation; and a nitrous Salt will be left at the Bottom; but much changed from its former Nature. On the contrary, if Spirit of Salt is poured upon an *Alcali,* saturated with Spirit of Nitre, the Mixture will in Distillation also yield an Aqua regia, and the Salt that remains will be of a nitrous Nature, and somewhat inflammable; however of a Nature very different, both from Sea Salt, and Nitre. In both these Cases, as there is no considerable Difference betwixt the Acid of Nitre, and that of the Salt, with respect to their Strength, each of these Acids, in some Degree, dislodges, and expels the other, by which Means they rise mixed together

her, and both of them alſo remain united with the Alcali in the Reſidum.

Pour Oil of Vitriol upon an *Alcali,* ſaturated with Spirit of Nitre; a pure Spirit of Nitre is immediately expelled, and the Acid of the Vitriol unites with the alcaline Part of the Nitre, and forms a Salt at the Bottom, ſomewhat of the Nature of *Tartarus vitriolatus,* though different from it in ſome of its Properties; it has, however, ſcarcely any Thing in common with Nitre. And, laſtly, if Oil of Vitriol is poured upon factitious, or natural Sea-Salt, a very volatile Acid, fuming Spirit of Sea-Salt, will inſtantly ariſe, endowed with almoſt all the known Virtues of Spirit of Salt, except that it fumes more, is more volatile, and its Vapour is noxious and ſuffocating, till it is corrected by repeated Dephrations. All theſe Experiments, therefore, certainly prove that thoſe Acids which are naturally diluted with a leſs Quantity of Water, have a greater Power of uniting themſelves with *Alcalies,* than thoſe, which are naturally diluted with a greater. And this Rule, ſo far as has yet appeared by Experiments, may be laid down as general, that the ſtronger Acid always expels from the *Alcali* that which is weaker, and which is the leaſt powerfully attracted by the *Alcali.* And then the ſtronger Acid always unites with that *Alcali* from which the weaker was expelled, and takes Poſſeſſion of the Place in which that reſided.

Again, the Salt thus generated, loſing the Diſpoſition it had acquired from the firſt and weaker Acid, which is now removed, puts on very nearly the Nature of that Salt, from which the laſt and ſtronger Acid, which is now united with the alcaline Part, was drawn. It muſt however be confeſſed, that there is always ſome remarkable Difference betwixt the Salts thus generated, and

the native Salts from which thoſe ſtronger Acids were procured. Thus, for Inſtance, the *Sal Mirabilis Glauberi* which is prepared by a Diſtillation of Sea-Salt, with the beſt Oil of Vitriol, is of a very different Nature from that *Tartarus vitriolatus,* which is obtained by a Saturation of Oil of Tartar with Oil of Vitriol. This is alſo true, with reſpect to other compound Salts. Thus the Salt which is procured by diſtilling *Glauber's* Spirit of Nitre, is entirely Different from the *Sal Mirabilis* of the ſame Author, though both theſe are ſuppoſed to be produced from the ſame Acid, and the ſame *Alcali.* This Rule therefore, which has been laid down by the moſt eminent Chymiſts, *that* Acids *always convert* Alcalies *into their Nature in ſuch a Manner, that from theſe Compounds, may be conſtantly regenerated thoſe Salts, which before yielded thoſe Acids,* is too general, and muſt be underſtood with ſome Reſtriction.

It is farther remarkabe, that when theſe ſtronger Acids thus poured upon compound Salts, expel thence the weaker Acids which were united with them before, and join with the remaining Alcalies, this new Combination is effected without any conſiderable Efferveſcence or Conflict: For the firſt and weaker *Acid* quits the *Alcali,* and the laſt and ſtronger takes its Place, without any great Ebullition, notwithſtanding there ariſes ſuch a prodigious Emotion, when a pure *Alcali* is mixed with a pure *Acid.* Nor does it appear that any Air is generated by this Union, though in the other Caſe it was expelled in ſo large a Quantity. It is probable, therefore, that the Efferveſcence which was excited in the firſt Saturation of the *Alcali,* had expelled all the Air, ſo that now the new Acid does nothing more than enter into the ſaturated *Alcali* thus deprived of its Air, and remains there, without either expelling or attracting any Air; and it

ſeems

forms a farther Confirmation of this, that if the Acid which is expelled by a stronger Acid, is mixed with another *Alcali*, it will with it raise a violent Effervescence, so that a great Heat, Noise, and Generation of Air will be produced, whilst in the compound Salt, there was very little of any such Appearances.

With Respect to the Effects of fixed Alcaline Salts, considered as Medicines, it must be remarked, that they soon destroy all the Acid in the Body, for there it meets but with a small Quantity, and that too, a mild vegetable Acid only residing in the Primæ Viæ, that is in the Stomach and Intestines.

If they meet with an Acid there, they Cause an Effervescence, generate Wind, and cause Eructations, stimulate by their Activity, and are converted, together with the Acid, into a neutral Salt, which then becomes harmless, penetrating, aperient, diaphoretic, diuretic, and antiseptic, and productive of new Effects by Virtue of their Neutralization, which are sometimes attributed to the *Alcaline Salts*, because subsequent to their Exhibition.

By Means of this Effervescence they stimulate the Nerves, move the Spirits, and incline both to Motions different from what they had before ; hence they often cure the Spasms of hypochondriacal Men, and hysterical Women, and the Distempers depending on them, an Instance of which we see in the celebrated Anti-Emetic of *Riverius*, consisting of an *Alcaline Salt* mixed with the Juice of Lemons, which if drank in the Act of Effervescence, cures the Cholera Morbus, and stops obstinate Vomitings, which resist all other Methods.

They attenuate and resolve whatever is coagulated by an Acid, and hence when Milk is curdled in the Stomach they have very good Effects, if prudently administered ; they are also capable of resolving other tenacious Concretions.

They attenuate glutinous, oily, and fat Concretions, and render them more easily mixable with Water, and hence become Detergents. Fullers, Laundresses, and Diers are sensible of this Property in a Lye of these Salts, and therefore they use them to remove viscid greasy Concretions from Cloths ; if moderately used, therefore, they free the Chylopoietic Organs from all glutinous Impurities.

They resolve Coagulations of the Bile, Lymph, Blood, and Serum, when admitted into the internal Parts of the Body, and there agitated by the vital Powers.

By their acrid Stimulus they put in Motion Bodies that were before unactive, and hence they provoke Urine, Sweat, and Perspiration ; and for this Reason are numbred amongst Diuretics, Diaphoretics, and Sudorfics ; the Intestines also they stimulate to a Discharge of their Contents.

In Diseases, therefore, attended with unactive mucous Viscidities ; where an Acidity prevails in the Stomach and Intestines from acescent Aliment, where there is Load of acescent austere Crudities manifest by the Coagulations it produces, where a watery Serum, or fat tenacious Concretions abound, or where Distempers have been generated by these Causes, as the Dropsy, Jaundice, Leucophlegmatia, Gout, Rheumatism, and Scurvy, in these Cases, this Salt is of great Use, if prudently given, that is, well diluted, in small Doses, and those are administred at a proper Time, and properly repeated. That Species of Gout which is caused by an abundant Acid, scarcely admits of a more successful Method of Cure, than that which may be performed by a con-

tinued

tinued Use of these Salts, taken in small Doses. But it does not follow from their Effects in this Case that they are to be extolled as universal Remedies for the Gout; for they will do a great Deal of Prejudice to a gouty Patient, whose Bile is exalted into an acrid Alcalescence, and whose Humours tend spontaneously to an alcaline Putrefaction.

These Salts are also of considerable Use to the Surgeons; for as Caustics they are employed to raise Escars, in order to make Issues; and by a temperate Lixivum of these, sordid, putrid Ulcers are successfully mundified; Parts that are corrupted by a Gangrene, if scarified almost to the Quick, and then fomented with a Lixivium of these Salts, contract into a Cruft, and then admit of a Separation from the living Part, and by these Means the Mortification is prevented from spreading farther, and a Cure is happily effected. They extirpate Warts, also, and eat away small Cancers with Safety, and if sufficiently diluted, they will effectually take away Discolorations or Spots of the Skin.

It is, however, necessary to remark, that the Use of these Salts is highly pernicious in every Disease, where the native animal Salts begin to degenerate into an acrid, alcalescent, putrid, volatile Nature; or where the natural Oils of our Bodies are disposed to turn acrid, fetid, putrid, rancid and volatile, which is manifested by a disagreeable Smell, peculiar to this Kind of Putrefaction, and a Redness of the Urine. But these Salts are particularly destructive, when the Bile is thus degenerated into an acrid *Alcaline* Nature, and when the Humours of the Patient are too much dissolved, fluid, and putrid; hence in the Plague they are almost an immediate Poison; and this pernicious Quality is even communicated to the Soap in which they are an Ingredient. Hence, therefore, in Inflammations, Suppurations, Gangrenes, a Sphacelus, continued, putrid Fevers, and Diseases arising from too great a Velocity of the Blood, the internal Use of these Salts must be absolutely forbid.

CHAP. VII.

Of MENSTRUUMS.

THE old Chymists in some of their Solutions, used a moderate Fire, for a philosophical Month, that is forty Days; and hence their Solvents were called Menstrual Solvents, and at last *Menstrua*, and hence arose this Term now applied to all Dissolvents.

It is customary to divide Menstruums into Solid and Fluid. Thus Metals, and Semi-metals, dry Salts, hard fossil sulphureous Bodies, and

what the Refiners call Cements, which consist of Salts, Sulphurs, and powdered Brick, are accounted solid Menstruums.

In order to constitute a Menstruum, properly so called, it is necessary that the Solvent together with the Solvent, should be so united, as to become one homogeneous Fluid. Hence it appears that solid Menstruums cannot act as such, till they are reduced by Fusion to Fluidity.

The

The first Class of fluid Menstruums, consists of Water, and aqueous Liquors. But Water, in the Form of Ice, is a Solid, which dissolves into a Liquor, upon being mixed with dry, or fluid Salts, of the fixed and volatile alcaline Kind, with fixed, or volatile acid Salts, compound Salts, and the fermented Spirits of Vegetables, and this even, in the highest Degree of Cold. As a fluid Menstruum, it begins to act in the Degree next below that of freezing. In many Solutions, where Water is the Menstruum, the dissolving Power increases, and diminishes, with the Degree of Heat. Thus Water, thirty-three Degrees hot, dissolves a certain Proportion of Sea-Salt, which prevents the Water, from turning to Ice, by the same Degree of Cold, which would freeze Water, without any Salt dissolved in it; and this probably happens, by the Interposition of the Salt, by which, the Surfaces of the Particles of the Water, are hindred from coming into mutual Contact. But when the Cold is increased, far beyond the Degree, which freezes pure Water, then the Salt Water begins to contact, and the Salt to be collected at the Bottom, of the Vessel, in little Crystals. And as the Cold gradually increases, this Water gradually deposites more Salt, till at last, being nearly deprived of all its Salt, it is changed into Ice, and when this is thawed, all the deposited Salt, will be again taken up by the Water. On the other Hand, if Water thirty-three Degrees hot, has dissolved as much Salt, as it could in that Degree, and be afterwards gradually heated farther, to the Degree of boiling, and upon the Increase of every Degree, a little more Salt be added, this additional Salt, will be dissolved every Time, till the Liquor boils, after which it will dissolve no more, tho' boiled never so long.

Hence 'tis obvious, First, That the Parts of the Salt, and Water, are not here changed, but so conjoyned, that the Water now touches the Parts of the Salts, as the Particles of the Salt, or Water, before touched each other, so that this Species of Solution, is no more than a simple Permixtion. Secondly, that the Increase of Heat, increases the Power of Permixtion, so long as the Water, can receive any higher Degree of Heat. Thirdly, that aqueous Menstruums, saturated with Salt, grow turbid in the Cold, and deposite saline Crystals; but when heated, become transparent again, and dissolve the Salt they had deposited. Fourthly, That boiling Water, saturated with Salt, is heavier than common Water; whence Brine in a boiling State, is found hotter than pure boiling Water, and requires a greater Heat to boil it. Fifthly, that the solvent Power of Water, does not depend upon the Water alone, but requires the Assistance of Fire, to render the Solution perfect.

These Discoveries, applied to the animal Juices, especially those of the human Body, are of the last Importance; for Water is the principal, and most copious of all the Fluids, contained in an healthy human Body. So that in this the other Principles of the animal Fluids, are dissolved, mixed, combined, and preserved fluid. As Water, then, is so liable to Changes, by Heat and Cold, the human Juices, must of Consequence, be proportionably altered. Thus how greatly is Blood drawn from the Veins, changed by Cold, from what it was in the Body; and the Urine of an healthy Person, soon deposites a Sediment, which is again taken up, by warming the containing Vessels. So that it is highly probable, that the solvent Power of Water, almost always increases in Pro-

Proportion to the Heat, applied in boiling it, tho' at the fame Time, there are various Experiments which evince, that the folvent Power of Water upon fome Bodies, decreafes as the Degrees of Heat increafe. Thus Balls made of Flower, and Water, are refolved in the cold or tepid, but hardened in boiling Water; the Serum of the Blood, and the Whites of Eggs, alfo, coagulate in boiling Water. But certain Bodies, are always diffolved by Water, in all its Degrees of Heat. Of this Kind are, Firft, all the known neutral Salts. Secondly, all the known pure, volatile, alcaline Salts, obtained from Animals or Vegetables, by Putrefaction or Diftillation. Thirdly, all fixed alcaline Salts, obtained from Vegetables by Calcination. Fourthly, all Kinds of Acids, naturally found in Vegetables, and in all the acid Salts; all Kinds of native, foffil, acid Salts, with all the vegetable acid Juices, which afford a Spirit or Vinegar, by Fermentation; the Acids obtained from Woods by Diftillation, diftilled Vinegar, Oil of Sulphur by the Bell, Oil of Vitriol, Spirit of Alum, Spirit of Nitre, and Spirit of Sea-Salt. Fifthly, artificial compound Salts, by the Combination of Acids, and Alcalies, fo as to render them neutral, all which eafily diffolve in Water; but Tartar of Vitriol, with the greateft Difficulty. Sixthly, Salts of the Borax kind, which are alfo with Difficulty diffolved by Water. Seventhly, the native Salts of Plants, which are artificially procured, and which eafily diffolve, and run fpontaneoufly in the Air. Eighthly, the vegetable Salts called Tartar, which require twenty times their own Quantity of Water, to diffolve them by boiling.

Water, as a Menftruum, diffolves all thofe Bodies called *Saline,* and which contain fome of the above-mentioned Salts, as a principal Part in their Compofition. Such are, Firft, The native Soaps of Vegetables, as all the ripe Juices of Summer Fruits, being a Mixture of Water, Oil, Spirit, and Salt. Secondly, Certain concreted Juices perfected in particular Parts of Plants: As the Pulp of *Caffia,* Manna, Sugar, and Gums; which are Soaps containing a copious Oil mixed with Salt. Thirdly, The more fluid Juices of Vegetables circulating through the Veffels, and whole Structure of the Plant. Fourthly, All known animal Juices except Fat; though none more eafily than Bile. Fifthly, All the Soaps made of expreffed vegetable Oils, and fixed vegetable *Alcalies,* mix'd by Means of boiling Water with the fiery Part of quick Lime, and by Boiling reduc'd to an hard Mafs. Sixthly, Vitriols, efpecially of the acid Kind, are diffolv'd in Water, whilft they retain their true tranfparent Form; but when the Water is exhal'd by a gentle Heat, fo as to render the Cryftals opake, the metallic Parts are thereby lefs difpos'd to diffolve in Water; and if highly dry'd, will not diffolve at all. Hence Water diffolves Metals, only on Account of the Acid adhering to the Surfaces of their Particles, and therefore quits the Metals fo diffolv'd, as foon as the Acid is remov'd. Thus Metals diffolv'd in Acids, and largely diluted with Water, become potable, fo as to be receiv'd into the Body, mix'with the Fluids, act upon the Solids, and produce confiderable Effects; though this Power lafts no longer than they remain diffolv'd; and their Solution depending principally on the Acid, that being remov'd, the Metal is no longer potable, but turns to a Calx. What is faid of the Action of an Acid with refpect to Water, alfo holds true, of thofe Metals which are diffolv'd by *alcaline Salts:* This however

however, does not hold true of all Metals; for tho' Butter of Antimony is highly acid, yet instead of being diluted with Water, it immediately upon the Effusion thereof, lets fall the Antimony into a white Calx, which being fus'd by a strong Fire, affords a fine Regulus of Antimony, incapable of being dissolv'd in Water.

If pure earthy Bodies be first dissolv'd in Acids, they may afterwards be perfectly diluted with Water, so as to escape the Cognizance of the Senses, and leave the Whole of the Liquor limpid, so that 'tis unsafe to infer that a Liquor is free from Earth, because it appears pellucid.

Alcalies intimately united with Earth, as in Glass, cannot be afterwards diluted with Water, so great is the Difference between the Solution of Earth with one Kind of Salt and another. Sulphurs are not of themselves dissolv'd in Water, but when intimately mixed with *Alcalies*, they readily unite with it; whence we may easily understand the medicinal Virtues of sulphureous medicinal Waters. Volatile-alcaline Salts, also, dissolve Sulphurs, and render them miscible with Water, so that Water by the Assistance of *Alcalies*, becomes an excellent Solvent for Sulphurs.

Tho' Bodies of a glutinous, viscid, or hard Substance, remain untouch'd by Water, yet these may be render'd perfectly soluble in it, by being intimately united with fix'd or volatile *Alcalies*: Thus Soap, Honey, Sugar, and the Yolks of Eggs, being mix'd with these tenacious Bodies, render them commodiously dissolvable in Water, which by this Means generally acquires a detergent Quality. Oils, Balsams, Gums, and the like, are also to be mix'd with Water by this Treatment. Hail collected in the Summer-time after Thunder, consequent upon a Series of a hot Weather, when kept in clean Vessels, has a different Effect from all other Water, perhaps on Account of its being purer, carried higher into the Atmosphere, and frozen before it fell to the Ground. Next to this in Purity, is Snow-water, collected in a cold Winter in a still Air, and in high sandy desart Places. Dew being a Mixture of aqueous, spirituous, saline, and unctuous Vapours, and of all Sorts of dry Exhalations, differs greatly from all other aqueous Menstruums, so that its Effects can hardly be determin'd, or brought under one Class: Hence many have imagined, that the Matter of the universal Salt was contain'd in it, and that a saline Substance, which they call the congeal'd Spirit of the Universe, might be extracted from it. It is to be observ'd, that the Water floating in the Air, may often act as a Menstruum, and the Action be falsly ascrib'd to the Influence of the Air.

Oil consider'd as a Menstruum, is a Juice either fluid, or capable of being rendered so by a small Degree of Heat. It is of an unctuous Nature, inflammable, and immiscible with Water. *Alcohol* is excluded from the Class of Oils, by its being easily mix'd with Water, whilst in other Properties, it has a perfect Resemblance to them.

The dissolving Power of Oils is not exerted, unless they are in a fluid Form; and as some of them freeze sooner than Water, their dissolving Power is less durable with respect to Cold, than that of Water; but those which remain fluid in all the Degrees of natural Cold, constantly retain their dissolving Power; whence it appears difficult to fix a common Point of Heat, at which the dissolving Power of Oils begins, though it may be nearly estimated in any one Species of Oil, after it has been once accurately observed. But it is　*surprising,* furprifing, that tho' Linfeed Oil remains fluid in the keeneft Froft, yet it is then no hotter than Ice, or any other congealed Oil.

When Oil is gradually heated, it does not boil, like Water, with two hundred and twelve Degrees of Heat, but grows conftantly hotter without boiling, till the Heat rifes to fix hundred Degrees; whence we fee why boiling Oil is fo much hotter, and more fcalding than boiling Water: But the moft fubtile Oils boil the fooneft, whereas others bear a great deal more Fire before they boil. Hence 'tis very difficult to determine the diffolving Power of Oils; becaufe in Linfeed Oil, for Inftance, this Power begins with the greateft Degree of natural Cold; whence it increafes to that Degree of Heat, which is capable of melting Lead.

As Oil receives almoft thrice as much Fire as Water, we may hence, eafily underftand, why the diffolving Power of Oils, which in Menftruums depends upon Fire, muft be greater than that of Water; for 'tis obvious from many Experiments, that the Power of Heat in Linfeed Oil is, to that of Water, as ten to three; and as many Oils infpiffated by Boiling, may thus receive much more Fire, fo the Scale of the Power of Heat, may be ftill farther extended in fuch Oils.

Some Metals may be intimately diffolv'd in particular Oils, by Boiling; and by this Means various ufeful Difcoveries have been made, both for mechanical and medicinal Purpofes. But in order accurately to explain the diffolving Power of Oils, 'tis to be confidered, that every expreffed crude Vegetable Oil, conftantly contains Water, as is obvious by boiling expreffed Oil of Almonds in chymical Glaffes, for by this Means, an aqueous Vapour is raifed, and condenfing in the Neck of the Veffel, forms vifible Drops, which falling back upon the boiling Oil, occafion great Commotion, and crackling, which may in fome Degree affect the Manner of Solution. Hence after this Water is difcharged by boiling, the Property of Oil, as a Menftruum, is changed.

Befides this Water, Oils contain a fubtile latent Salt, fuppofed to be very penetrating, which is generally acid, and volatile, as in fome of them is obvious from the Smell. Thefe Salts appear in the Form of acid Spirits, collecting themfelves like Water, and feparating from the Oil, fo as not to be again eafily mixed with it; tho' 'tis not eafy, perfectly to free the Oil from its acid Spirit, which rifes in the whole Diftillation, but in the greateft Quantity at firft.

We ought, therefore, carefully to examine, whether the diffolving Power of Oils, does not depend on the Water and Acid they contain, otherwife we may fall into egregious Errors; for in Painting, Colours which have been diffolved, in boil'd Oil, unite and fink in better, dry quicker, and remain more beautiful, than when mixed up with crude Oil. Thus alfo the particular Power, which the fofteft Oils are fuppofed to have, in diffolving Metals in a gentle Heat, feems principally to proceed from the latent Acid, and not from the oleous Part; fince when Olive Oil is mixed with very fine Filings of Iron, Copper, or Lead, and long digefted together, a Part of the Metal is taken up by the Oil, fo as to give it a new Colour, and other Properties. Hence the Power of Oil, fimply confidered, has been carried too far, as a Solvent; for this Power does not remain in them, after they have been boiled, and are deprived of their latent Acid, which by Experiments, *Hoffman*, has fhewn shewn to be contained in distilled Oil.

Oils obtained by Distillation, with or without Water, by the Retort, mostly leave Earth behind them, upon being redistilled to Dryness in dry Vessels, and gradually become more subtile, less adhesive, more fluid, and trasparent, and when redistilled fourteen Times or more, they each time become different Oils, and different Menstruums, so as at last to become penetrating, anodyne Medicines, highly beneficial in many obstinate Disorders. Whence *Helmont* the Elder imagined that the Oil of human Blood, several Times distilled with Spirit of Salt, till no Fæces were left behind, would prove a diaphoretic Medicine, capable of dissolving, like a *Menstruum*, all preternatural Obstructions, and Coagulations in the human Body. *Hoffman,* also, assures us, that he has prepared Oils in this Manner, and greatly extols their medicinal Virtues.

All Oils have a certain subtile, volatile Substance, adhering to them, and separable from them, which is called their *presiding Spirit*, which is a movable, odorous, high tasted Substance, and the genuine Cause of great Effects; this innate Spirit, when confined in Oils, communicates to them a singular efficacious Virtue, to be found no where else. But it is from many Oils spontaneously exhaled, by a gentle Heat, mixes with the Air, and when entirely evaporated, leaves them insipid, and inactive, so as to be hardly distinguishable from each other. So that the dissolving Power of Oils seems principally to depend upon this Circumstance, that they are disposed to receive into themselves, a great Deal of Fire, which they apply to other Bodies.

Most Oils are capable of being mixed and incorporated; First, with other Oils, tho' some of them not easily, as in the Distillation of Turpentine and Amber, where the Oils raised by different Degrees of Fire, are different in Weight, Consistence, Colour, and Situation, so as not readily to unite with each other. Secondly, True resinous Bodies melt and dissolve in Oils. Thirdly, So do many of those Gums, which have a Mixture of Rosin. Fourthly, So, likewise, do condens'd Oils or Balsams. Fifthly, So do Sulphurs, natural and artificial, liquid or solid, tho' conceal'd in other Bodies. Thus Antimony, finely powder'd, or sublim'd into Flowers, when boil'd with Oil, soon yields a red Balsam of Antimony, dissolv'd by the Oil, which leaves the metallic Parts untouch'd; and the same holds true of the other Semi-metals abounding with Sulphur.

As for spirituous Menstruums, properly so call'd, Chymists assert, that *Alcohol* cannot be united with a pure fix'd *Alcali,* because this Effect may be prevented by the least aqueous Moisture, either in the Salt, or in the *Alcohol.* But if pure *Alcohol* is applied to perfectly dry Salt of Tartar, a rich Tincture is immediately extracted, and a true Combination made. Hence we ought to be highly inquisitive about the Nature of this Liquor, which is the most considerable of spirituous Menstruums.

Perfectly pure *Alcohol* dissolves, First, Water, and all aqueous Liquors. Secondly, Consequently Wines of all Kinds. Thirdly, it dissolves all spirituous fermenting Acids, such as Vinegars. Fourthly, All pure Oils. Fifthly, All true vegetable Resins. Sixthly, Most of the gummy Resins. Seventhly, Pure volatile alcaline Salts. Eighthly, Perfectly dry and fixed Alcaline Salts. Ninthly, Most of the Soaps. Tenthly, Sulphurs, first opened and dissolv'd by an Alcali. But it does not touch compound or native Salts, as Sal-ammoniac, Sea-falt, and Nitre ; nor pure Earth, pure Sulphur, Mercury, Metals, Semi-Metals, nor Stones, whether of the common, or of a more pretious Kind.

As for alcaline and acid fpirituous Menftruums, Chymifts, under oleous and fpirituous Menftruums, have ranged thefe two Kinds, which might rather be term'd faline or compound. This happens, becaufe the Menftruums ufually appear under an unctuous Form, and are, generally, not only volatile, but, alfo, liquid and fubtile. Whence fome Acids, and Alcalies, have been called Spirits, on account of this fubtile, volatile, and unctuous Appearance, tho' they greatly differ from each other, not only in Kind, as to Acid and Alcali, but alfo Acid from Acid, and Alcaline from Alcaline Spirit. We muft, therefore, neceffarily divide the faline fpirituous Menftruums into thofe of the acid and alcaline Kinds ; whilft we divide the alcaline Spirits into fimple and compound. The fimpleft of thefe confift of Water, and an extremely fubtile, volatile, alcaline Salt, both together appearing in the Form of a thin, pellucid, and fomewhat unctuous Liquor, as the pure alcaline Spirit of Sal-ammoniac. And to this Clafs belong the numerous alcaline Salts, obtain'd both from Animals and Vegetables, after they are deprived of the Oil which adheres to them. The more compound Kind generally confift of Water, the volatile Salt now mentioned, and a fetid Oil, into which three Parts they may be feparated, and are therefore a Kind of volatile alcaline Soap, diluted with a Portion of Water juft fufficient to diffolve it. The Acid and commonly volatile Liquors, by the Chymifts call'd Spirits, when examined, prove to be acid Salts, diffolved in pure Water ; fo that we may properly call them, faline Menftruums.

As for the fimple, faline Menftrnums, 'tis certain that various Salts have great Energy in the Diffolution of Bodies. But as the ultimate Particles of Salt are fo minute, that they cannot be diftinctly viewed, by the Affiftance of the beft Glaffes, and fo volatile, that they can hardly be confined in Veffels, fo they muft be reduced to Clufters, by Means of fome Cement, the moft confiderable Parts of which are Water and Earth, before we can arrive at any great Certainty with Refpect to their chymical Action.

We muft alfo confider the principal Difference of Salts, arifing from the different faline Principles of which they are compofed, and tho' thefe Principles are known feparately, yet doubtlefs they have a certain peculiar Virtue refpectively. A fecond Difference arifes from the other Principle, which, uniting with the Saline, conftitutes the Salt. We therefore divide all Kinds of Salt into fuch as differ, either with Refpect, to their faline Principle, their connecting Principle, or both. With Refpect to the firft Divifion, we diftinguifh Salts and faline Menftruum into the following Claffes. Firft fixed Alcalies. Secondly, volatile Alcalies. Thirdly, native vegetable Acids. Fourthly, fermenting vegetable Acids. Fifthly, fermented vegetable Acids. Sixthly, vegetable Acids obtained upon burning. Seventhly, vegetable Acids procured by Diftillation. Eighthly, native foffil Salts. Ninthly, foffil Salts obtained by Burning. Tenthly, Foffil Acid procured by Diftillation. Eleventhly, neutral Salts, as Borax, Nitre foffil Salt, Sea-Salt, Sal-Gemmæ and Sal-Ammoniac. Twelfthly, other Salts compounded of thefe fimple ones. Each of which fhould be examined in order, to find out their peculiar Properties whereby we may come to a true Knowledge of their

fo far as regards the Diſſolution of Bodies.

As for fixed alcaline Menſtruums, 'tis certain that not only theſe, but alſo volatile Alcalies have a ſolvent Power, Firſt, upon animal, vegetable and mineral Subſtances ſo far as thoſe contain Oils, Balſams, Gums, Reſins, or gummy Reſins, or conſiſt of unctuous Matter; as alſo upon Sulphurs, whether pure, compounded, or joined, with other Materials, all which theſe Alcalies excellently open, attenuate, reſolve, and diſpoſe to mix intimately with Water, Alcohol, and Oils. Secondly, Theſe Alcalies alſo act as a Solvent, upon thoſe Bodies whoſe component Parts are held together by an acid Cement, which being thus attracted by the Alcali, the component Parts thus ſeparate or fall aſunder. Thirdly, after certain Bodies have been diſſolved by an acid Menſtruum, pure Alcalies, often exert a new Force, ſo as to diſſolve ſuch Bodies better than if applied to them before they were thus diſſolved by the Acid. Hence, Alchymiſts, in order to obtain, the Mercuries of Metals, direct the Metals, to be firſt calcined by Acids, and afterwards treated with Alcalies.

But there is a Difference, in the Manner, in which fixed, and volatile Alcalies act; for volatile Alcalies act and are agitated ſpontaneouſly, or by a ſmall Degree of Heat, whereas thoſe of the fixed Kind, require a much ſtronger Aſſiſtance, from the Fire, in order to their acting; volatile Alcalies, fly off the Moment they are heated, and therefore do not exert, their ſolvent Power, when applied to hot Bodies, whereas fixed Alcalies, ſooner enter the Bodies they diſſolve when aſſiſted by Heat, and remain conſtantly applied to every fixed Subject they act upon. But when volatile Alcalies, are purpoſely kept cloſe

to a Subſtance to be diſſolved, a moderate Heat increaſes, and quickens their diſſolving Power, as we obſerve, for Inſtance, upon applying the volatile Salt of Urine to the warm Skin, and covering the Salt, with an adheſive Plaiſter; for thus there ſoon ariſes Heat, Pain, and Inflammation, followed by an Ulcer, and a black Eſchar.

As to acid Menſtruums, the Acids, can hardly be obtained pure, but blended with other Bodies, ſo that 'tis exceedingly difficult, to treat of their proper Action; yet we know the Virtues of ſome of them, by their Effects upon certain Bodies; ſince the freſh Juices of Oranges, Citrons, and Lemons, diſſolve Lead, Tin, Copper, and Iron, and pretty ſtrongly calcines them, as well as foſſil Acids.

There are in Vegetables, certain Acids, of an oleous and balſamic Quality; for if the Woods of Guaiacum, Juniper, Oak, and a great many others, are reduced to dry Shavings, and carefully diſtilled in a Retort, they yield a limpid, rediſh Liquor, which is very acid, eſpecially, if depurated by Filtration, and permitted to ſtand quiet; and the ſolvent Power of this Menſtruum is perfectly ſingular, ſince, in the human Body, it produces wonderful Effects, by attenuating, preſerving, ſtimulating, and reſiſting Putrefaction, and carrying off the peccant Matter, by Sweat and Urine. If in theſe Menſtruums, therefore, the medicated Virtues of Plants are diſſolved, the Solutions become exceedingly efficacious, as they act by their highly ſubtile, penetrating Acid, and exalt the Qualities of the Bodies diſſolved in them. All theſe vegetable Acids, are capable of diſſolving many animal, vegetable, foſſil, and metalline Subſtances; for by Digeſtion and Coction, they diſſolve Horns, Hoofs, Bones, and the Fleſh of

G   Animals.

Animals. The Shells of Fishes and other Animals, they corrode into a pellucid Liquor, but do not dissolve Mercury, Silver, nor Gold.

Some fossil Acids, readily dissolve Iron, Copper, somewhat slower, Silver, with a good Deal of Difficulty, and Mercury, not at all, except placed in an intense Degree of Heat.

Neutral Salts are also found, in many Cases to be Menstruums; for Sal-ammoniac, which easily dissolves in Water, and runs *per Deliquium* in a moist Air, thus makes an extremely pungent, penetrating Liquor, capable of dissolving, grofs, gelatinous, pituitous, and gummy Concretions, in the Bodies of Animals, being not only admirably, attenuating, resolving, and inciding, but also diuretic, sudorific, stimulating to the salival Glands, and at the same Time, greatly preventive of Putrefaction. This Solution, of Sal-ammoniac boiled, or digested with gummy, or resinous Vegetables, resolves them intimately, and disposes them to be dissolved, in aqueous or spiritous Menstruums. Filings of Iron, boiled in it, are excellently dissolved, and converted into an admirable, aperient, and invigorating Medicine. When digested with Filings of Copper, it produces a beautiful blew Liquor, a few Drops of which, taken upon an empty Stomach, often prove good against Worms, and epileptic Fits.

The pure dry Salt, sublim'd into Flowers, well ground, mixed with Fossils, and sublimed together in close Vessels, produces very extraordinary Effects, as a Menstruum; for which Reason the Alchymists have called it the *White Eagle*, or the *Philosophical Pestle*. If sulphureous Bodies, Metals, or Semi-metals, are thus treated, they are attenuated, opened, volatilized, and perfectly changed, whence most excellent Medicines are prepared in this Manner, and hardly so well in any other.

Tho' Sea-Salt, Sal-gemmæ, and Fountain-Salt, differ in their Origins, yet they easily dissolve in Water, and run *per Deliquium* in a moist Air, so as to make a Brine, or an excellent Menstruum, producing nearly the same Effects, as the Brine of Sal-ammoniac.

Common Nitre, is easily turned to a fixed Alcali, and a volatile Acid. It also appears of a particular Nature, when applied to Bodies as a Menstruum, in which Case its Operations are sometimes so intricate, as to be hardly explicable. When exposed to the Fire in a pure and dry State, it flows with certain Bodies like Water, and thence surprisingly promotes their melting, tho' otherwise of difficult Fusion, and thus attenuates, divides, and intermixes their Parts, even whilst it acts upon them in no other Respect, for which Reason, it is used as a Flux for Metals.

If the Matter, thus mixed with the Nitre, contains any Thing oleous, unctuous, or sulphureous, this suddenly deflagrates with the Nitre in the Fire, raises a violent Flame, and greatly increases the Heat; whence the Application of the Nitre being stronger, it greatly divides, fuses, changes, and separates the Bodies, in a different Manner from what is otherwise known; the Nitre, at the same Time, losing its own Nature, and becoming a Kind of *Sal Polychrestum*, which has a dissolving Power, different from that of Nitre. Whence the Action of Nitre upon Bodies, is of one Sort, before it deflagrates them, of another during the Deflagration, and of a third, after the Deflagration is over.

When

When Nitre is melted along with a vegetable Coal, its Parts are so strongly agitated, as to produce a similar Agitation in the Bodies to be dissolved ; at the same Time emitting particular active Fumes, capable of dissolving and penetrating many Bodies in the Fire. But when the Nitre is thus changed to a fixed Alcali, it does not flow, unless the Fire be violent, and then according to its penetrating, and particular Nature, it begins to act as a fixed alcaline Menstruum, and thus acquires and exerts a new dissolving Power.

If the Bodies to be dissolved, by Fusion with Nitre, contain Earth, Stone, Alum, Vitriol, Bole, or any other similar Substance, the Nitre is immediately changed into a strong Acid, volatile Salt, or Spirit of Nitre, which being agitated by a violent Fire, penetrates, dissolves, and changes the Subject, acting with one of its Parts like *Aqua Fortis,* while the other Part, remaining at the Bottom, acts by a very different dissolving Power.

From what has been said, we may easily conceive, that various Combinations of Salts, may produce many new Kinds of Saline Menstruums, of singular, and uncommon dissolving Powers. So that 'tis easy to confute the Error of the modern Chymists, who make *Alcalies* and *Acids,* the Principles of all Things, and assert that their Virtues are destroyed, by mixing them together. On the contrary, 'tis certain, that the pure *Alcali* of Tartar, mixed with the volatile Acid of Vinegar, forms a neutral Salt of a much greater Virtue, than the separate Acid, or Alcali. When a pure volatile Alcali, is exactly saturated with strong Spirit of Vinegar, we have a limpid, slightly saline, volatile and compound Liquor, able to pass thro' almost all Bodies, so as to dissolve them, without any considera-

ble visible Conflict. Whence, some have greatly extolled this Liquor, in curing Disorders of the Eyes and Ears, arising from Concretions. What has likewise been accounted, a great and successful Secret, for resolving cold and glandulous Swellings, is to foment them, with a Mixture of putrified Urine, and Vinegar, the Part being first rub'd, and the Liquor applied warm.

When pure volatile alcaline Salts are mixed with vitriol or aluminous Waters, or their unctuous Sediments, a particular Kind of ammoniacal Salts, are produced, which may be called a Semi - volatile, vitriolated Tartar, and highly deserve, to be regarded by Chymists, on Account of their remarkable dissolving Property, and by Physicians, on Account of their aperient, attenuating, resolving, and stimulating Virtues.

Some Menstruums arise from the Combination of fixed Alcalies, with fossil Acids, obtained by Fire. Thus when a pure fixed Alcali is perfectly saturated, with the Acid of Sea-Salt, Sea-Salt seems to be regenerated. When saturated with the Acid of Nitre, it reproduces Nitre, and with the Acid of Oil of Sulphur, or Vitriol, it constantly produces vitriolated Tartar. Hence it appears how many, and what surprising Actions of Menstruums, arise from the mixing of certain Bodies together, and applying them to the Fire, and without an exact Knowledge of all these Particulars, we can never have an adequate Comprehension of the chymical History of *Menstruums.*

Menstruums, are also obtained, by uniting pure simple Salts, with other Salts. Thus, if a pure Alcali be added to the Brine of Sea-Salt, an earthy Matter is precipitated, and the Salt obtained by Crystallization from the clear Liquor, will be a purer Sea-Salt. The same fixed Alcali added to the Brine of Ni-

milky

tre, changes the Liquor thick, and milky, and precipitates an earthy Matter, whereby the Nitre obtained from this Solution, becomes extremely pure. Numberle§s §urprizing In§tances of this Kind, in the Hi§tory of Men§truums, may be under§tood, from the§e Principles; only 'tis to be ob§erved, that in whatever manner Salts are combined with Salts, new §aline Produ¢tions and Men§truums will ari§e; whence the Art of Chymi§try may be perpetually improved, and new Phenomena produced, which not only afford Plea§ure to the Mind, but al§o increa§e our Knowledge of the natural Properties of Bodies, and often lead to great and unexpe¢ted Di§coveries, for the various Purpo§es of Life.

New Men§truums, of particular Virtues, may be infinitely made, by variou§ly combining different Men§truums together, by bringing each Men§truum to its greate§t Purity, and reducing §ome of them, to their mo§t minute Particles; for upon the§e three Particulars, depend the Skill of the Chymi§t. But in order to §hew, that by compounding one Men§truum with another, new and excellent Salts may be procured, let it be ob§erved, that regenerated Tartar, properly prepared, may be intimately united with pure *Alcohol,* and thus produce a vegetable Men§truum, compo§ed of the clo§e Union of the mo§t §ubtile vegetable Particles, an Alcali, an Acid, and a Sulphur. Whence the Effe¢t of §uch a Liquor is extreamly great, both as a Medicine, and a Men§truum. From what has been §aid we may infer,

That it is not certain, whether any Men§truum has a Power of di§§olving any Subje¢t, without the A§§i§tance of Fire, §ince no Experiment could ever be made in a Place de§titute of all Fire, and as mo§t of the known Men§truums a¢t the better when a§§i§ted by a certain Degree of Fire.

That Men§truums can §carcely a¢t as §uch, unle§s they are reduced to a fluid Form, or at lea§t approach to it, as they generally do by Means of Fire, Air, Water, and Trituration, which four Cau§es u§ually excite the latent Powers of Men§truums.

That the Acrimony of a Men§truum, which excites Pain, corrodes and con§umes the Parts of the human Body, is no Proof that §uch a Men§truum is §uited to di§§olve other Bodies. Thus the Oil of Vitriol, Spirit of Nitre, Spirit of Salt, and *Aqua Regia,* readily con§ume the Fle§h, yet they do not di§§olve Wax and Sulphur, tho' the§e two may be ea§ily di§§olved in human Bodies.

That many Bodies incapable of Di§§olution in certain Men§truums, may be fitted for a Di§§olution in them, by being previou§ly di§§olved in another Men§truum. Thus if common Sulphur is boiled ever §o long in Alcohol, it is no more di§§olved than a Stone in Water; but if it is fir§t melted with Salt of Tartar, it is §oon di§§olved by cold *Alcohol.*

That certain Men§truums di§§olve §uch Bodies, as before Trial they were thought little §uited to, and this holds true both of the Solvent and Solvend. Thus the vi§cid and tenacious Body of native Turpentine is §o penetrating in the Body, as §oon to give a Violet Smell to the Urine, change its Colour, and warm the Per§on who takes it. It al§o di§§olves Oils and Re§ins with a gentle Heat, and even gummy Re§ins, which can hardly be di§§olved otherwi§e.

The Yolk of an Egg would hardly be §u§pe¢ted of any §olvent Power, from its mo§t perceptible and obvious Properties, yet by being ground with any of the Oils, Gums, Rms or Balfams, it diffolves them better than any other Menftruum, deftroys their Tenacity, renders them mifcible with aqueous and fpirituous Liquors, and fit to enter the circulating Fluids of Animals. The White of an Egg, boiled to Hardnefs, and diftilled in *Balneo Mariæ*, affords a limpid aqueous Liquor, of no confiderable Smell or Tafte, and of no faline Acid, or alcaline Nature; yet what a confiderable Power it may have upon Metals, appears from *Paracelfus*, and *Helmont*, who judged it the moft proper Thing, in preparing their medicated Mercury; and if the White of an Egg after boiling, be fuffered to run *per Deliquium*, it runs to a Kind of pure Water, which diffolves the hard, tough Subftance of Myrrh, better than any other Menftruum.

That Acidity, Acrimony, or a faline Property, in any Menftruum, can never affure us, that fuch a Menftruum will diffolve a given Body, till we find by particular Experience, that a Solution enfues, upon putting the Bodies together. Thus if any known Acid, whether ftrong or weak, be put to common Sulphur, and affifted by Heat, it will not diffolve the Sulphur. Thus Spirit of Nitre, which diffolves other Metals, does not touch Gold, fo that we cannot fay that Acids, Alcalies, or Salts, are univerfally Solvents, but only with Refpect, to their determinate, definite Subjects, to which Nature has fitted and limited them.

That a cautious Phyfician, upon finding a Body diffolved, will not thence infer, that an Acid, an Alcali, or a neutral Salt, was the Caufe of the Solution, unlefs other Circumftances, determine which of them it is; for fuppofe a Perfon,

fure that Gold was diffolved, into its leaft Particles, and that there was no other known Salt, which would diffolve Gold, befides Sea-Salt, or the Preparations of it, yet he could not juftly infer, that in this Cafe the Sea-Salt is the only Solvent; for pure Quick-filver, alfo, diffolves Gold, tho' Quick-filver, be as far from an Acid, Alcaline, or acrimonious faline Nature, as any known Subftance in the World.

That there is no general, or abfolute diffolving, or corrofive Acrimony, this being always relative, and holding only true, of the Solvent, and Solvend, and not of the Solvent with refpect to all other Bodies. If upon feeing the corrofive Virtue of *Aqua Fortis* in a thoufand Inftances, we fhould conclude that it would diffolve all other foft and tender Subftances, we might foon correct our Error, by obferving that it will not diffolve foft Wax, or brittle Sulphur.

That we ought not to infer, that becaufe a Menftruum proves innocent to the human Body, it will not therefore diffolve other Bodies; for Oil of Olives, may be fafely taken into the Stomach, tho' it readily diffolves Sulphur, and Wax, which Acids will not touch; fo that tho' the Cancer, and the Stone have hitherto proved incurable, yet we ought not to defpair of finding Remedies for them, and particularly of finding a Method of diffolving the Stone without injuring the Bladder, fince it by no Means follows that the Bladder fhould be corroded, by the fame Remedy which diffolves the Stone.

That moft Menftruums, at the Time they diffolve, and change the Subject, are alfo changed by it, the Action being reciprocal, and tho' Water, Alcohol, and Mercury, receive but little Alteration, yet

they

they are gradually chang'd in the Operation.

That it is an Error to suppose, that the purer any Menstruums are made, the more purely and perfectly they always dissolve, because their solvent Power is often diminish'd, in Proportion to their Purification. Thus Lead is the more difficultly dissolv'd in *Aqua Fortis,* the more strong the *Aqua Fortis* is made, and the more easily when the Menstruum is diluted with a due Proportion of Water. And

That there is nothing more' re-

markable in the Doctrine of Menstruums, than the Production of new Powers by their Action, which before existed not either in the Solvent or Solvend; but depend entirely upon the Union of both after the Solution is perform'd. Thus an Infant may safely swallow a few Grains of Quick Silver, or a very few Drops of the Spirit of Salt, but if those are so united as to form corrosive Sublimate, three or four Grains of this last will prove a violent Poison.

CHAP. VIII.

Of CALCINATION.

CALCINATION, by some called, Chymical Corrosion, is that Operation in Chymistry, which produces a Destruction of the former Connection and Cohesion of all the Particles of Bodies, together with a Change of Colour, Smell, Taste, and other Qualities of a like Nature, depending upon the entire Texture of the whole Body; so that the Bodies subjected to this Operation, are reduc'd to a Powder, or into small Portions, or at least become friable; for which Reason, Calcination is, also, called, a chymical Pulverisation. Thus by *Etmuller*, Calcination is defin'd, "A " Corrosion and Dissolution of com- " pact Bodies, into their minutest " Parts, by which Metals and Mi- " nerals are reduc'd to a Calx, and " Vegetables to Ashes, or at least, " whereby the Body, whatever it " is, becomes friable."

Calcination receives different Names, according to the various

Manners in which it is perform'd; and the Effects resulting from these several Methods, are no less various, than the several Names, the Methods themselves have received. In that Method, which by Way of Eminence we commonly call *Calcination,* the combustible Parts of the Bodies are consum'd, by being expos'd either to the common Fire, or to that of the Sun, while such Parts as elude the Action of the Heat, are left behind, and this may be properly call'd *Calcination by actual Fire.* Of this Kind' are not only the *Calcinations* of metallic and other mineral Substances, but also the Incineration observable in the Deflagration of Vegetables, for preparing lixivial Salts, and in the Calcination of some Animals, as Crabs, Moles, and others of a like Nature. *Calcination,* is call'd *Ustion,* when applied to Harts-horn, Alum, and Brass; and these Substances themselves, are distinguish'd

by

by the Epithet, *Burnt*. This Operation, is, also, call'd, *Toasting*, when applied to Rhubarb, and some other Substances: When Bodies are mixed, and reduc'd to a Powder, by the Reflexion of Flame or Heat from the Sides and Top of a Furnace, *Calcination* is, in this Case, call'd *Reverberation*, and when common Salt is calcin'd, *Decrepitation* is the Term which Custom has made expressive of the Thing.

Another Species of *Calcination*, is perform'd by the Addition of proper Menstruums, either with, or without the Assistance of Fire, and this is properly call'd *Corrosion*, or *Calcination by potential Fire*. Of this Kind are, First, The immersive and vaporose Calcinations, or Corrosions of Bodies; when, for Instance, the Body to be calcin'd, is either immers'd in its proper Menstruum, as Copper in Spirit of Nitre, and Lead in Vinegar; or when the Body is suspended in a close Vessel in such a Manner, that the Steams arising from the Menstruum may act upon it; as when Iron is suspended over *Aqua Fortis*, in Order to be calcin'd into Crocus of Mars; or when Copper and Lead are suspended over Vinegar, in Order to be converted into Verdigrease, and Ceruss. Of this Kind, in a particular Manner is, that Species of Calcination, call'd *Philosophical Calcination*, or *Calcination without Fire*; when some Parts of Animals, as Bones, Horns, and Hoofs, are, in the Distillation of Waters, suspended in the Head of the Still, that being penetrated by the ascending Vapour, they may become more porous and friable. But in the Shops, Bones are sometimes not philosophically calcin'd in an Alembic, but boil'd in Water till they are render'd soft and friable by the Hand; then after they are cleans'd, and the black exterior Scurf taken off, they are dried, and reduced to a Powder. The *Cornu Cervi philosophicum*, the human Cranium, the Tooth of the Boar, and that of the Sea-horse, are sometimes thus prepar'd. 2dly, To the *Calcination by potential Fire*, belongs that, by *Illinition*, when neither the Steam of the Menstruum, nor Immersion in it are us'd, but the Body to be calcin'd, is only anointed with it, as when Oil or Spirit of Vitriol, or of Sulphur, are laid upon a Plate of Iron, in Order to produce a Corrosion. Thirdly, To the same Kind of Calcination belongs *Amalgamation*. Fourthly, *Fumigation*. Fifthly, *Detonation*. Sixthly, *Granulation*, which is also call'd, *fusory Calcination*. Seventhly, *Cementation*, or *Stratification*. Eighthly, *Extinction*, or *extinctory Calcination*, as when ignited Crystal is extinguished in common Water, and then reduc'd to a Powder. That Species of *Calcination*, which is perform'd by Fire alone, or by Means of a dry Menstruum, is call'd *dry Calcination*; whereas, that which is perform'd by Means of a liquid Menstruum, is call'd, a *moist or humid Calcination*. *Bohnius*, calls that Species of *Calcination* perform'd by Fire with the Addition of a Menstruum, *mixed Calcination*. The Calcinations of Minerals perform'd by the Air, or rather in the Air, do not constitute a particular Class, but are to be rank'd among those perform'd by a liquid Menstruum; because such a Menstruum, capable of calcining metallic Bodies is lodg'd in the Air; whilst, for Instance, the saline corrosive Particles with which it is impregnated, being dissolv'd by its humid Parts, and applied to the metallic Body, corrode it; or whilst the Humidity of the Air itself, penetrates the saline Parts of the mineral Body, dissolves, and puts them into such a Commotion, that

they

they corrode, and, as it were, calcine the Body in which they reside.

From what has been said, 'tis sufficiently obvious, not only what a *Calx* is, but, also, that the several Species of *Calxes* must vary,

First, According to the Substances or Bodies, from which they are obtain'd.

Secondly, According to the Nature of the particular Menstruum us'd in the Preparation. And

Thirdly, According to the greater or smaller Degree of Fire applied ; or according to the greater or smaller Quantities of humid inflam-
: ble Parts expell'd; or according
a Parts of the Bodies, are more
o1 divided by the Calcination,

'1 is also obvious, that all Calcinations of Bodies are perform'd by taking away the aqueous, oleous, and combustible Substances, connecting the Parts with each other, or by interposing some foreign and heterogeneous Substance, which destroys the Connection and Cohesion of the Parts. From what has been said, we may also conceive, how in some calcin'd Bodies, something is lost, that is, those Parts which can either be destroy'd or exhal'd by the Fire; and how in some others there is an Addition made, by Means of the Menstruums, of which they retain some Parts in the Calcination, and consequently have their Weight increas'd. Hence we may, also, comprehend how some *Calxes* by the Expulsion of that Part of the Menstruum which they retain, may be restor'd to their original Form, and how some others may be so, by a Restitution of what they lost in the Calcination. Of the former Kind, are the Calxes of Metals produced by corrosive Menstruums ; and of the latter Sort are metallic Calxes produc'd by Fire alone. 'Tis an Observation of no small Importance in Medicine, that as Substances calcin'd by Menstruums, or what we call potential Fire, retain something of the Menstruum employ'd, by which a Change is induced on their Natures, which are to be judg'd of by the respective Menstruums us'd , so, also, Substances calcin'd by actual Fire, undergo a certain Change, and assume an acrid, heating, and drying Nature, which they before were destitute of. Thus Shells when calcin'd become Lime, and have very different Effects in Medicine, from the same Substances reduc'd to Powder by Trituration.

CHAP. IX.

Of CLARIFICATION.

THE Apothecaries are said to clarify any thick and turbid Liquors, the express'd Juices of Vegetables, for Instance, Decoctions, or Syrups, when they render them more transparent, pure, and free from Feces. There are many Ways of doing this, as by setting the Liquor in a cool Place, and suffering it to settle for some Time, that the earthy and feculent Parts may gradually and spontaneously subside to the Bottom : This is by Chymists call'd *Clarificatio per Subsidentiam*, or *Clarificatio per Residentiam*. Liquors are, also, clarified by Filtration or Colation, by which Method the grosser Parts remain in
the

the Filtre, whilſt the finer and more ſubtle paſs thro' it. Fermentation is, alſo, another Method of clarifying Liquors, ſince by the fermentative Motion, the groſſer Parts are carried to the Bottom. Another Method of Clarification is by the Affuſion of other Liquors, according to the Nature of the Liquid to be clarified, by which Means being render'd turbid, and a Precipitation produc'd, it becomes more clear and pure.

Another Method of clarifying Liquors, is to beat them, with the Whites of Eggs, to a Froth, and then to boil them; for by this Means the groſs Parts, which render the Liquor turbid and foul, will riſe to the Top, together with the Egg, in the Form of a Scum, which may be taken off with a Spoon, or ſeparated from it by ſtraining.

This Method renders a Medicine more ſightly and neat, but in no Degree augments its Virtues, and in many Caſes impairs them; as wherever they depend upon a mucilaginous and viſcid Texture, which, by Clarification, is in a great Meaſure deſtroy'd. Thus *Quincy* remarks, that the Clarification of the Decoction for the Syrup of Marſh Mallows, abſolutely ſpoils the Medicine, by deſtroying that mucilaginous Contexture, upon which its Virtues depend; and that to clarify a Decoction of Poppies for the *Diacodium*, is to take from it, the principal Part of the Efficacy, expected to be communicated to it from the Poppy, for the like Reaſons.

CHAP. X.

Of CORRECTION.

THE Word *Correction* in Pharmacy has ſeveral Ideas affixed to it; thus draſtic Medicines, or ſuch as operate with Violence, are ſaid to be corrected, when in their Compoſition, ſome Ingredient, is added, which proves a Kind of Check or Ballance to their violent Operation, or prevents the Misfortunes which they generally bring on without ſuch a correcting Ingredient. Thus, for Inſtance, ſome Carminatives, ſuch as the Seeds of Fennel or Aniſe, are added to Senna Leaves, which, when exhibited alone, generally produce Flatulences and Gripes.

Correctors have a Reference either to the noxious Quality, the Viſcidity and Toughneſs, the Coldneſs, the narcotic Nature, the emetic Virtue, or the violent Operation of the Medicines to which they are added. 'Tis therefore, ſufficiently obvious, that Correctors muſt conſiſt of ſuch Parts as are of an oppoſite Nature to thoſe which prevail in the Subſtances to be corrected. Thus, for Inſtance, Alcalies are corrected by Acids, Acids by Alcalies, and Subſtances of any given Nature by thoſe of directly oppoſite Qualities. The univerſal Correctors of ſuch Medicines as operate too violently, are, Firſt, Water, which dilutes Acrimony; and Secondly, mild and balſamic Oils, which obtund and ſheath up the ſtimulating and irritating Spicula of any Medicine. To this Species of Correction,

Correction, also, belongs such a Preparation of Medicines, as weakens or impairs their violent and drastic Operation; when, for Instance, the Root of Arum is rendered milder, and less violent in its Operation, by being dried, or macerated in some proper Liquor: But Corrections are sometimes boasted of in Consequence of an Ignorance of the Nature of Medicines, to which Correctors are added; when, for Example, Opium is thought to be corrected by Castor, and an Addition of other heating and aromatic Substances, because the Antients imagin'd, that Opium prov'd prejudicial by its excessive Coldness. Thus, also, some Corrections are made, which rather deserve the Name of *Castrations*, as, when the Seeds of Coriander or Cumin, are macerated in Vinegar. According to *Helmont*, some boil Scammony in acid Liquors, in Order to correct, or render it more mild in its Operations: But every one, who is in the least vers'd in medicinal Affairs, knows, that when Scammony is expos'd to the acid Steam of Sulphur, it is entirely divested of its Properties, and recedes from the Nature of Scammony in Proportion to the Quantity of the Acid it has imbib'd. With Respect, therefore, to such Corrections, we may affirm, that they are made without any Knowledge of Qualities, Parts, and mutual Relations of the Correctors, and Substances to be corrected. It is surprising, that some Substances should by Correction, have their Qualities and medi-

cinal Virtues directly inverted an revers'd, which happens to Asara bacca upon being boil'd.

Medicines which operate in a slow and languid Manner, are, also, said to be corrected, when they are so prepar'd, as either to accelerate, o augment their Operation; as whe Salts are mix'd with evacuating Me dicines of a gummy and viscou Nature, that by this Means bein more resolv'd or attenuated, the may operate more powerfully Thus with this very Intention, Sal of Tartar, or Sal Prolychrestum are added to Infusions of Senna, an Ingredients added with this View are call'd *Adjuvantia*, assisting Medicines. But when more drasti Substances of the same Virtues are added, in order to augment the O peration of the Composition, these additional Ingredients are call'c *Acuentia*, or sharpening Medicines

Nauseous and ungrateful Medi cines are said to be corrected, whe they are prepared in such a Mannei as to become more acceptable and agreeable to the Palate. But as the Sense of Taste is not the same in al Mankind, the Corrections of thi Sort must necessarily vary accordin to the peculiar Taste of different Pa tients. Medicines intended fo Children, are generally corrected o rendered agreeable, by an Additio of Sugar. In like Manner Substan ces of an ungrateful and disagreea ble Smell, are to be corrected by a Addition of fragrant Ingredients of an agreeable Smell.

C H A P.

CHAP. XI.

Of CRYSTALLIZATION.

CRYSTALLIZATION is that particular Operation, by which folid Parts, which in any Fluid highly attenuated, extended, or engag'd, are reduc'd to a Body which is dry, hard, compact, diaphanous, or at leaft femi-diaphanous, and either foliaceous, or of a geometrical Figure, fuch as tetrahedral, prifmatical, or conical. The Cryftallization of Salts and like Subftances, is perform'd, in a Liquor which is generally aqueous, and contains a Salt diffolv'd in it, is depurated, and inflpifated by a flow and continued evaporation, till a Pellicle appears on its Surface, which may be called the Beginning of Cryftallization: the Evaporation is generally thought to be completed, when a drop of the Solution pour'd upon the Nail of the Finger, or any cold Substance, is forthwith concreted into a Salt. The Evaporation may be perform'd either by the Fire, or the Heat of the Sun, in which laft manner, Sea-Salt is better cryftal-lized than any other. This Evaporation muft be made in large mouth'd Veffels, the beft of which are glafs, and the next to thofe are earthen ware well bak'd, and fuch as will not fuffer the Salts to pafs thro' their Pores. But mettal Veffels are corroded by the Salts, and fubject to be fpoil'd by Ruft. The infpiffated Liquor is to be depofited in fome cool Place, and kept in Veffels of Glafs, Wood, or Earth, with confiderably large Mouths, that the cryftalliz'd Matter may be the more commodioufly taken out. Some Time after, the latent Particles of Salt difpers'd thro' the Liquor, are approximated, brought together, and at the Sides of the Veffel form faline Cryftals, which are greater or fmaller according to the Quantity of the Solution. In either Cafe all the Cryftals are not equally large, but are endowed with the Figure peculiar to each Salt, fingle, beautifully fhining, and the more elegant and large, the more flowly the Evaporation has been made. But the whole faline Subftance is not found form'd into Cryftals, but there is a large Number of irregular Concretions, efpecially in that Bafe, in which the larger Cryftals are planted, and which feems to be, as it were, the Matrix, from which thefe Cryftals arife. Nor is all the diffolved Salt, which was in the Liquor, form'd into Cryftals, but a Quantity of it remains fufficient to faturate the Fluid; hence when the Cryftals form'd are taken out, there is a Neceffity for a new Evaporation, and the Liquor muft be lodged in a cool Place, in Order to obtain more Cryftals; and thefe Meafures are to be repeated, till no more Cryftals can poffibly be form'd. But fince, for the Purpofes of Cryftallization, fome Quantity of Fluid is always required, the Salt cannot poffibly be totally extracted from the Liquor by Cryftallization, but Exficcation becomes neceffary for drawing off the Remainder. Sometimes, in Order to obtain the more elegant Cryftals, Twigs are put into the Veffel, or

Threads

Threads are stretched in it as proper Supports, to which they may adhere, as is usual in collecting the Cryſtals of Alum, Copper, and Sugar. The collected Cryſtals are in the Shops dried on coarſe Paper, by the Heat of the Sun. Theſe, however carefully they may be freed from the Humidity adhering to their Surfaces, ſcarce afford ſo genuine a Salt, but that it contains ſome Mixture of Earth and Water. This ſupplies the Place of a Glue or Calx, for uniting, as it were, the ſaline Cryſtals, for the Union is diſſolv'd when the Water is expell'd, or by Calcination, as we may obſerve in decrepited Sea-Salt, Alum, and Vitriol calcined. Some Salts undergo a better and more perfect Cryſtallization, when, to their Solution, a calcarious Earth is added, as is proved by *Geoffroy* in the Subſtance of Borax, thoſe Salts to which an Oil adheres, are unfit for Cryſtallization, and proportionally more ſo according to its Quantity, becauſe the Oil interpoſed between the ſmall Portions of Matter, by its Tenacity prevents the Union of the ſimilar Particles, and if in ſome Meaſure, they ſhould happen to unite, yet they never acquire a due Degree of Solidity, but are forthwith melted down, on the Acceſs or Contact of a moiſt Air. Hence the Salters of Herrings take Care, that in Boiling no Fat be mix'd with the Salt Water; and ſkilful Chymiſts, when they ſuſpect an Admixture of oleous and pinguious Parts, after a proper Evaporation pour Spirit of Wine upon it, which diſſolves the oleous Parts, receives them, as it were, into its Boſom, and ſo ſeparates them from the ſaline, by which Means they facilitate the Concretion of the Cryſtals. This Obſervation is of ſingular Uſe to Phyſicians, with Reſpect to the Formation of Stones in the human Body, and points out the moſt effec-

tual Remedies, by which their Coi cretion may be prevented. Hem we learn, that Salts, diveſted of a pinguious Parts, are moſt eaſil cryſtallized. The white Colour the ſaline Cryſtals is ſomewhat dark ned by the adhering Oil; this Co lour is alſo variegated by metallin Particles, almoſt infinitely divide and combined with their ſolvei Salt, as appears in the blueiſh V triol of Copper, and the green V triol of Iron, which conſiſts of Metal, which is kept diſſolved t an acid Salt, and a little pure Wate

The Uſe of ſaline Cryſtallizatioi is.

Firſt, To ſeparate Salts, in a di Form, from their ſolvent Liquor.

Secondly, To depurate Salts; f the Water, leaving the Sordes, re tains the Salts; for which Reaſoi the better theſe are depurated, th more elegant Cryſtals they yield i Cryſtallization.

The Ætiology of theſe Cryſtall zations is obvious, if we conſide that in order to their Production there is requiſite too ſmall a Quar tity of Water, to keep them di ſolved; Secondly, the Reſt of th particular Liquor, in which the di ſolved Salt is lodged; and thirdl Cold, for when the ſolvent Mer ſtruum begins to prove defectiv a ſlender Pellicle is form'd on th Surface of the ſaline Parts, whic can no longer be kept in a State c Solution by the Liquor. Then thi Pellicle becomes gradually thicke till at laſt becoming ſpecifically hea vier than the reſt of the Solution it is broken into different Parts, ſub ſides, and forms itſelf into differep Molecules, or Cryſtals, of differen Bulks, which could not be produc ed, unleſs the Liquor was in a Stat of Reſt, becauſe then the Principl of Solution, which is Motion, prov ing defective, nothing hinders th Approach of the ſaline Parts to eacl othe ther, for as the Want or Defect of Humidity, hangs the Parts nearer to each other, it conſequently lays a Foundation for their Union. Thus the Diminution of Motion renders the Fluid unfit for ſeparating the Parts, when they happen to adhere. But when Liquors are compreſſed by the cold Air, many of the Particles lying off from the ſolvent Liquor, the contained ſaline Parts, are by the Conſtriction, more and more expelled, and thrown out from the Pores of the fluid Maſs, and the more intenſe the Cold is, the larger Cryſtals are formed, but theſe are continually mov'd upon the Acceſſion of Heat. Hence it happens, that in a warm Air, very ſmall Cryſtals are generally formed. Cryſtallization is therefore performed, when a ſufficient Quantity of Moiſture, Motion, and Heat, which are the Cauſes of Solution, prove defective. Cryſtallization indeed of Salts happen, when their highly ſaturated, and warm Solutions are left to themſelves, in which manner volatile Salts, ſuch as that of Harts-horn, Vipers, and Silk, and others obtained from the animal Kingdom, are cryſtallized. But theſe are very near to a State of Cryſtallization for the Evaporation is performed with the Deſign, that the Solution which remains after the Diminution of the Liquor may become more ſaturated. But even in an highly ſaturated Solution, a very ſmall Quantity of Cryſtals are formed without a previous Evaporation. 'Tis therefore obvious that Evaporation, that is a Diminution of the ſolvent Liquor, is abſolutely neceſſary to the Cryſtallization of any Salt. Hence, alſo, it is obvious, why in a Receiver from which the Air is extracted, as alſo in a cloſe ſtopt Veſſel, Cryſtals are not formed; becauſe in theſe Caſes, a very ſmall Evaporation or none at all is made. We muſt carefully conſider, that the Cryſtals of Salts, peculiar to each Species, are not obtained by every Kind of Concretion, for when the Solution of any Salt ſufficiently warm is ſuddenly cooled, when for Inſtance the Veſſel containing it, is put into cold Water, the diſſolved Salt lodged in the Liquor, is precipitated to the Bottom, in the Form of a Powder, for then the Solution is, with a Kind of Impetus, condenſed, and forced too precipitately to depoſite its Salts; nor does the Salt acquire its peculiar Figure by a ſudden and continued Evaporation on the Fire, till the whole Liquor is totally exhaled, or at leaſt rendered thicker than it ought to be, for the Heat exciting a preternatural Commotion in all the Parts, hinders the ſaline Parts from receeding from each other, but being forced to run, in all Directions, with a tumultuous Confuſion, and being prepoſterouſly mixed, they are formed into leſs elegant Cryſtals. As therefore a precipitate Refrigeration ſo alſo an intenſe Heat hinders Cryſtallization, the beſt Evaporation is made without boiling, and the Place fitteſt for Refrigeration, is that which is of the ſame Temperature with Cellars about the Months of *June* and *July*. But there are ſome Salts, which are more commodiouſly cryſtallized in pretty warm Air, ſuch as rich and acid Alcaline Salts; and for the Cryſtallization of Sugar in the Pans, a pretty briſk Heat is neceſſary, perhaps becauſe Salts of this kind require little Moiſture for their Solution, and retain it cloſely, which muſt be afterwards leſſened by Evaporation, and a Continuation of the Heat, for it muſt be obſerved that the Salts which require a large Quantity of Water to keep them diſſolved, are firſt formed into Cryſtals; on the contrary they more eaſily and quickly and with the ſmaller Quantity of Water Salts are diſſolved, the more firmly

ly

ly they feem to retain the Water they receive. Salt of Tartar, for Inftance, which of all Salts requires the fmalleft Quantity of Water, for its Solution. Hence if different Salts are diffolved in the fame Water, fome of them will be formed into Concretions fooner than others, and each of them will be diftinguifhed by the particular Figure of its Cryftals. Thus for Inftance, the Cryftals of common Salt are quadrilateral Pyramids, with a fquare Bafe; thofe of Sugar are oblong, and have rectangular Bafes; the Hexagonal Cryftals arifing in Alum, have alfo hexagonal Bafes; the Cryftals of Vitriols, for the moft Part refemble Ificles varioufly interwoven, and Polygons interpofed, or lying between them, Sal-ammoniac elegantly refembles the Branches of a Tree; and Salt of Hartfhorn, Arrows placed in a Quiver; in the Sal Mirabilis Glauberi, which is made of common Salt and Vitriol, the Figures of both Salts are exhibited; Nitre is formed into prifmatical Columns, not unlike Faggots of Wood, and between thefe are fome Figures, fometimes Rhombaidal, and fometimes pentagonal, which feem to approach pretty near to common Salt. In the Salt of Tin, fmall Lines like Pins, fo run out in every Direction from the Center, as to from a Star, fuch as that obferved in the martial Regulus of Antimony. 'Tis furprifing that the Cryftals of the fame Salt, fhould be perpetually formed in the fame Figure, *Willis*, in order to account for this Phenomenon affirms, that the Author of Nature granted fuch particular Modes of Figuration to Salts, as well as other natural Concretions according to the Prepollence of the Spirit or Salt, and their Commixture with the other Principles; but this is no more than a formal and explicit Declaration, that we are ignorant of the phyfical Caufe of this furprizing Appearance. *M chenbrock* alfo denies, that this hitherto been accounted for by : one, any more than this other P nomenon, Why green Vitriol, Alum, diffolved and mixed w Water, returns to their own C ftals, and do not become a th Salt, of a different Kind. If it fho be afked, why fometimes the Wei of Salt ufed in the Solution, is minifhed in the concreted and dr Cryftals, we anfwer with *Gulielm* that the Salt is fo eafily diffolved the Water, that the aqueous Exh lation, efpecially when rifing large Quantities from the Wat may contain fome of the diffolv Particles of the Salt, efpecially they are very minute and fine, li thofe fent up by Water, when i State of violent Ebullition, a Evaporation. As much Salt, the fore, as is carried off by the Exh lation, fo much muft be wanti or defective in the concreted Cr ftals. Some who are fond of redu ing Phenomena to a certain Caul in order to explain faline Cryfti lizations, think the Principle of A traction, beft calculated and adapt to explain faline Cryftallization they affirm that the Parts the Salt, diffolved in a lar Quantity of Water, are more a tracted by the Particles of the W ter, than by each other, and r main feparate from each other for confiderable time; but after a lar Quantity of the Water is expelle in Vapours, and a fmall Pellicu of Salts begins to be formed on th Surface, fince the faline Parts a brought nearer to each other, an almoft into a mutual Contact, an as the Fore of Attraction is greate during the Contact, this Pellicul more ftrongly attracts the Salt fror the fubjacent Water, than an equa Quantity of Solution which confif partly of Water, and partly of Salt When this Pellicule becomes fpeci ficall)

ly heavier by Inspissation, it is
then into Parts, subsides, and by
using the saline Parts to itself,
this Crystals, which they say,
not form'd into Concretions, so
long as the Solution is warm, be-
it so long as the Motion excited
Heat remains, the Whole of
it Motion which ought to be
duced by the attractive Force is
der'd and destroy'd; but since
the Figures of the most simple Parts
remain invariably the same, 'tis ne-
ssary the Form of the Bodies into
which they are concreted, should al-
be the same. And because on one
side of the same saline Particle, the
attractive Force is greater than on
the other, the Concretion always
happens on those which attracts most
powerfully: Hence it may be demonstrated, that the Figures of the
minute constituent Particles, is different from that of the Crystal itself. From what has been said, 'tis
sufficiently obvious, that Crystallization may be called a Species of Coagulation, and that it is a surprising
geometrical Operation of Nature,
in which she exhibits herself to the
Eye of the Spectator, not in a false
and varnish'd, but in her genuine
and real Dress.

CHAP. XII.

Of DETONATION.

DETONATION may be look'd
upon as a Kind of Calcina-
on, perform'd in the Fire, by
leans of Nitre, and other sulphu-
ous Substances. Thus, for In-
ance, the Detonation of Antimo-
y is made with Nitre, in the Pre-
aration of diaphoretic Antimony,
Ceruss of Antimony, and the *Crocus
Metallorum.* A Detonation, also,
happens when Tin is mix'd with
Nitre or Sulphur, since on that Oc-
asion the sulphureous Part of the
Tin is kindled and deflagrated by
the Nitre. The same happens with
Copper, and a similar Detonation is
observ'd in the Preparation of fix'd
Nitre, or the *Sal Polychrestus,* when
the Charcoal is added to the Nitre
in Fusion.

If metallic or mineral Substances
are subjected to such a Detonation,
Calxes or Crocuses are produced; because in Consequence of the acid
and nitrous Particles intimately in-
terspers'd in their Pores, they are
converted into a solid white Powder,
which, by the Addition of a sulphureous *Alcali,* is easily restor'd to
its original Form, whether of a
Metal or a Mineral. By a repeated
Ignition and Extinction in Water,
solid Bodies, especially Stones,
Flints, Crystals, and Corals, are
converted into a quick Lime, or a
calciform Powder; because the Fire,
which by its violent Motion enters
their Pores, attempts a certain Rarefaction, whilst, at the same Time,
the aqueous Fluid, by its more impetuous Motion, produces a Divul-
sion of their most minute Parts.

CHAP. XIII.

Of DIGESTION.

SOLUTION is that Operation, by which the Cement which holds together the Particles of a solid confistent Body, is fo deftroy'd or alter'd by a proper Menftruum, as to permit the Particles thereof, to be fo minutely divided, as to unite intimately with the Solvent, and be equably and invifibly fufpended therein. In Order to bring this about, Heat is always neceffary; but fometimes the Heat of the Atmofphere being not fufficient, the Solvent and Solvend included in a proper Veffel, are expos'd for a Time to a due Degree of Fire, which is generally very gentle, in Order to promote the Solution. And this is call'd Digeftion. This is the common Acceptation of the Term; but in general it imports the Application of a gentle continu'd Heat, to any Body included in a Veffel, that is intended to be acted upon, tho' not with a View to Solution; as when two or more Liquors are expos'd in this Manner to a Heat, in Order to unite them the more intimately. In this Operation, for whatever Purpofes defign'd, the Fire rarifies and agitates the Air, Water, and whatever elfe is contain'd both in the Solvend and Solvent, and makes the conftituent Particles of the Body to be diffolv'd, recede from each other, by which Means the Menftruum has a more eafy Ingrefs into the Pores, where by its Rarefaction, and increas'd Activity, it produces greater Effects, than it could do in a lefs Degree of Heat.

To this Article, *Circulation* may be refer'd, which is perform'd in a particular Species of glafs Veffel call'd a *Circulatory*, in which the contain'd Liquor, when put over the Fire, performs certain Gyrations, and circulates by afcending and defcending, in fuch a Manner, that the more volatile Part of the Liquor rais'd by the Fire, not finding a Paffage, may always fall back; Pelican conftitutes fuch a Veffel. But in the Room of thefe, we may fubftitute Phials with long Necks, hermetically feal'd; or a Cucurbit with a blind Alembic plac'd upon it; or a Cucurbit or glafs Bottle with a fufficiently long Neck is fo difpos'd, that having firft put in the Materials, another lieffer Phial, whofe Neck may enter it, is placed upon it. Then the Joynings are to be carefully luted after the Veffels and Materials are become fufficiently warm for carrying on the Procefs; for then the Air being heated and expanding itfelf goes out of the Veffels, the Joynings of which being afterward luted, the Fire may fafely be rais'd and continu'd at Pleafure. But in this Procefs it generally happens that the Liquor falling cold on the warm Bottom of the Glafs, cracks it; for which Reafon, we muft proceed cautioufly in raifing the Fire Hence 'tis obvious, that what we commonly call Circulation, is no more than a certain Species of Digeftion, and that to circulate a Liquor is to put it in Digeftion, that its more volatile Parts may be continually rais'd and fall back, and
thus

this paſſing as it were in a Circle, may become finer and more atteneated. According to *Sennertus*, Circulation is only us'd for thoſe Liquors, which are already depurated, or freed from their Feces, or at laſt whoſe higheſt Degree of Subtilization is required. Thus the rectified Spirit of Wine is, by Circulation, ſaid to be transform'd into what we call the Quinteſſence. According to *Barnerus*, Circulation is principally inſtituted for two Reaſons, the firſt of which is, that the Spirits and Liquors to be joyn'd, being driven backwards and forwards, may be the more effectually incorporated. The Second is, That any ſubſtance to be diſengag'd from its Feces, or the Liquor in which it

is contain'd, may be the ſooner and more effectually ſeparated from it. Since, then, Circulation is no more than a Species of Digeſtion, 'tis obvious, as *Hoffman* obſerves, that the Subjects of this Operation, may be either Liquids alone, or Solids mix'd with Liquids, either for the Purpoſes of Clarification, Depuration, Exaltation, or Maturation; and ſometimes to obtain the Volatilization of fix'd Subſtances, or the Fixation of ſuch as are volatile: But the Veſſels muſt be very cloſely joyn'd, or hermetically ſeal'd, and a proper Time allow'd for the ſeveral different Intentions of the Operator. That this Proceſs may be ſupplied by repeated Diſtillations, is ſufficiently obvious.

CHAP. XIV.

Of DISTILLATION.

DISTILLATION may be juſtly defin'd, a cloſe Evaporation; for Evaporation in an open Veſſel, is exactly the ſame as Diſtillation in a cloſe Veſſel.

Every Diſtillation ſuppoſes Air and Heat, ſo that an Half, or a third of the Veſſel in which the latter to be diſtill'd is plac'd, muſt neceſſarily be left empty.

The Air, rarified by the Heat, receives into its Pores the Fluid which is ſtrongly agitated by the Heat, and its own inteſtine Motion, ſo that the Air aſcending, raiſes along with it the moſt minute Particles of the Fluid, which being condens'd form a Liquor or Fluid.

There are Examples of Diſtillation perform'd without the Application of Fire; when, for Inſtance, highly rectified Spirit of Nitre is

pour'd upon highly rectified Spirit of Wine, an intenſe Heat is produced, and the Spirit of Nitre is rais'd in Vapours.

All Bodies incapable of Evaporation, or which do not emit Exhalations capable of being eaſily influenc'd by the warm aerial Fluid, are improper Subjects for Diſtillation. Of this Sort are Sugars, all Kinds of Earths, neutral Salts, Stones, and Bones. Neither can thoſe Bodies be diſtill'd, which when agitated by Heat, diffuſe no Smell; whereas thoſe Subſtances which, when triturated or agitated, emit a Smell, may be diſtill'd; and the more penetrating the Smell is, the greater Quantity they yield, in Diſtillation, of an aqueous Fluid.

The more ſubtile Fluids are, the more eaſily they are diſtill'd: where-

H

as the more thick and heavy they are, they are rais'd with the greater Difficulty, and require the more Fire. Among all the Parts fit for rising, the phlogistic inflammable Spirits, and the volatile Salts rise first, whether by themselves or combined with ethérial Oils; and after these the aqueous Phlegm ascends. But Acids cannot be distilled without a greater Heat.

When Spirit of Wine is distilled, the Spirit first rises, and then the Phlegm; but when Vinegar, or any other acid Liquor, is distilled, the Phlegm is first discharged, and then an acid Spirit.

Among Acids, the most easily distilled are, the acid Spirit of Ants, then Spirit of Nitre, Spirit of Salt, Spirit of Vitriol, and Oil of Vitriol, which two last ought not to be distilled by an Alembic, but by a Retort.

Express'd Oils do not admit of Distillation with Water by the Worm; but ætherial, aromatic, and subtile Oils, are commodiously distilled in this Manner, but require a greater Degree of Heat.

Distillation is either moist or dry. Moist, when the Body to be distilled, is put into a fluid or spirituous Liquor; or when it is distilled alone, if it is a Fluid. But dry Distillation is, when the Body distilled is solid and dry; when, for Instance, Hartshorn, Amber, Ivory, Tartar, and Soot are distilled. Distillations, also, differ with Respect to the Degrees of Heat, and some are performed in Horses Dung, the *Balneum Mariæ*, or Vapour-Bath; whilst others are accomplished by Means of Sand, Salt, Ashes, or the Filings of Iron.

That Distillation is most violent, which is performed in a naked Fire, in such a Manner as that the Fire acts immediately upon the Vessel, in which the Substance to be distilled, is contained; as in the Distillation of Spirits from Salts. There are, also, Differences in Distillation with Respect to the Vessels, some of which are high, as Cucurbits, whether of Glass or Stone; and others low, as Retorts, and some others, either of Glass or Stone.

Those Substances whose Particles are subtile and easily evaporated, require but a gentle Heat; and may be distilled in tall Vessels. But such Substances as consist of more fixed Parts, and such as are not easily and speedily evaporated, require a greater Heat, and lower Vessels.

As various Bodies are subjected to this Operation with different Views, Chymists have contrived a great many Machines, to answer their Purposes. The first of these is the cold Still, as it is called, which consists of an Iron Grate, a few Inches above which, a Plate is fix'd, for the Reception of the Vegetable to be distill'd, which is cover'd with a large conical Pewter Head, furnish'd with a long Tube or Beak, that opens into the Head. When any fresh Vegetable is laid upon the Plate abovemention'd, and a very gentle Heat is excited in the Grate immediately below it, the Water together with the Spirit, or that volatile Substance, which imparts the distinguishing Smell and Taste to the Plant, evaporate, are collected in the Head, condens'd into Drops, and thence convey'd by the Beak to a Receiver, fix'd to the other End thereof. Mean Time the Plant loses all its Verdure, and Succulency, and the greatest Part of the Smell, and becomes shrivel'd dry, and lighter than before.

Another Way of distilling, is by the *Alembic*, the whole Apparatus of which consists of a *Body*, or Vessel to contain the Ingredients to be distill'd, which is usually of Copper; to this a Head is exactly fitted, which opens into a long spiral Tube, call'd the

the Worm, which passes thro' a Tub, that is to be fill'd with Water, and comes out at the lower Part of the Side thereof, in Order to be join'd to a Receiver. When the Body is fill'd about two Thirds with the Vegetables to be distilled, and as much Water as will cover them, the Head is to be fitted exactly to the Receiver, and luted, so that no Vapour may pass thro' the Juncture. Then the Materials are to be digested for some Time, in a moderate Heat, which is to be afterwards rais'd gradually till they boil, upon which the volatile Parts arise in Vapour, and condense in the Head, and Worm, by which last they are convey'd to the Receiver, in the Form of Water, impregnated with the Spirits and Oils of the Plants employ'd in the Operation. The same Apparatus serves for the Distillation of vinous Spirits from fermented vegetable Juices, and of spirituous Waters.

Chymists, also, perform many Distillations by the Retort, which is a glass Vessel with a long Neck, bended in such a Manner, as to form nearly a right Angle with the Body of the Retort. In this, the Materials subjected to Distillation, are included, and the volatile Parts are forc'd by the Fire into the Neck, which conveys them into the Receiver, fix'd and luted to the End thereof, where they are condens'd into the Form of a Liquor. The Retort and Receiver generally now supply the Place of the glass Body, and Head, or Alembic, formerly much in Use for the same Purposes.

But for such Substances as require a very intense Heat to make them rise, the most commodious Method of Distillation, is by the *Reverberatory*. For this Purpose, the Materials are included in an earthern Vessel shap'd much like a Bottle, and made so as to endure a very great Fire, call'd a *Long-Neck*; this is fix'd in the Wall of the Furnace, in such a Manner, that the Body is within Side, expos'd to the naked Fire, whilst the Neck coming thro' the Wall, is joyn'd with a Receiver on the other. But as all these Instruments are better understood in an Hour, by examining a Laboratory, than by all the Descriptions that can be given, I should advise those who desire a farther Knowledge of them, to learn it by inspecting them, and seeing the Operations perform'd by them.

CHAP. XV.

Of Effervescence *and* Ebullition.

EFFERVESCENCE, or Ebullition, is said to happen, when the most intense Motion is made, by Liquids mix'd with each other, or by Solids mix'd with Liquids, accompanied with a copious Elevation of Bubbles, an Eructation of Vapours, and Smoke, and a more or less intense Heat.

The Cause of an Effervescence is the impetuous Discharge of the aereo-ætherial Fluid from the Pores of Bodies, whether Liquid or Solid; by which quick Motion, and Discharge of the ætheral Fluid, the Turgescence of the Liquor, the Heat and the Bubbles are produc'd.

Every

Every Fluid does not produce an Effervescence with every other Fluid, nor every Liquid with a Solid, but only these Bodies produce an Effervescence with each other, whose Parts are disposed to enter the Pores of each other, that by this Means, the Æthereal Fluid lodged in them, may be expell'd copiously, and violently.

Every manifest Acid produces an Effervescence with Alcalies, whether saline, earthy, volatile, or fixed. The Effervescence between an acid, and alcaline Substance lasts but for a short Time, and the Tastes of both are abolished, and so contemperated as to form a neutral Substance of a saline Taste.

• All concentrated acid Spirits, totally freed from their aqueous Parts, such as Oil of Vitriol, Spirit of Nitre, and Spirit of Salt, produce an Effervescence with the most subtile, etherial Oils, such as those of Turpentine, Cloves, Sassafras-Wood, and a Heat is generally excited.

The more sulphureous, concentrated acid Spirits are, such as concentrated Spirit of Nitre, the greater Heat they produce, and even take Flame, when joined with heavy etherial Oils.

Acid Spirits concentrated with highly rectified Spirit of Wine, which is only an Oil, by Fermentation resolved in to aqueous Parts, excite the quickest Ebullition; unconcentrated Acids do not act on sulphureous etherial Substances, but leave them untouched.

The Bodies of Metals and Minerals, with proper Acids, or such as have an Ingress into their Pores, in the very Act of Solution produce an Effervescence. Thus Gold produces an Effervescence with *Aqua Regia*, and Silver, Mercury, Copper, and Iron with *Aqua Fortis*, which Effervescence lasts till the particular Body is dissolved.

Every Effervescence does not depend upon Acids and Alcalies; for common Water poured upon highly calcined terreo-saline Bodies, such as Shells, Coral, burnt Stones, and Salt of Tartar, produces a violent Effervescence, because the Water, by its Weight, enters the Pores of the calcined Substances from which it forces the aereo-etherial Particles with a violent Force.

Recent and highly concentrated Oil of Vitriol, by an Addition of common Water, or of Ice, becomes hot, with a violent Effervescence; because the Oil of Vitriol is a concentrated acid Salt, which on Account of the great Quantity of ætherial Particles interpersed with the Acid, remains in a State of Fluidity. Then the Water takes Possession of its Pores, and expels this subtile etherial Matter with Violence.

It is false to assert that an Acid produces an Effervescence with another, as Butter of Antimony, for Instance, with Spirit of Nitre, or Aqua Fortis. It is certain indeed that a violent Effervescence arises from their Admixture, but this does not proceed from the Acids mixed with each other, but from this, that the Acids mixed with each other constitute a Menstruum which acts upon the *Mercurius vitæ* lodg'd in the Pores of the Butter of Antimony.

All Effervescences are not accompanied with Heat, for some are entirely without it. Thus Chalk produces a considerable Effervescence without any Heat, with the Spirits of Nitre, Sal-ammoniac, Vitriol and Salt. This Effervescence may be stopt by an Affusion of highly rectified Spirit of Wine, which in a Moment acts upon the Acid, and unite with it, so as to render it milder.

CHAP

CHAP. XVI.
Of EXTRACTION.

EXTRACTION, in Pharmacy, is the Separation of the pure, and medicinal Part of a Body, from the impure and unactive, by means of a Menftruum which is capable of diffolving the Parts required, and leaving the reft untouched; and when the folvent Menftruum is feparated from the diffolved Body, by Diftillation, or Evaporation, the remainder is called *An Extract*. All Medicines, whofe Virtues confift in Parts that are very volatile, are improper for this Operation, becaufe fuch Parts evaporate in a Heat fufficient for performing it. All the Judgment required in this Procefs, confifts in adapting the Menftruum to the Parts intended to be procured, and regulating the Degrees and Continuance of Heat neceffary for the Solution, and fubfequent Evaporation.

CHAP XVII.
Of FERMENTATION.

BOERHAAVE very juftly diftinguifhes Fermentation, from Effervefcence and Putrefaction, and limits the Term *Fermentation*, to that inteftine Motion in vegetable Fluids, which tends to the Production of an inflammable vinous Liquor, mifcible with Water, and intoxicating; or an Acid uninflammable Liquor called Vinegar. That which produces a vinous Liquor he calls the firft Fermentation; that which generates Vinegar the fecond. He remarks, that all Vegetables are not difpofed to Fermentation, for fuch as abound with a native alcaline Salt, or are eafily changed into it, will not ferment, but are inclined to Putrefaction, as Onions, and Turnips; and that tho' all Fermentables will undergo Putrefaction, yet all Putrefcibles are not capable of Fermentation.

This great Author divides fermentable Vegetables into different Claffes. The firft of thefe comprehends all thofe Seeds of Vegetables, which when ripe and dry, are reducible by Trituration to a fine Powder called Meal, and not to an oily Pafte; and among thefe he reckons Seeds, which tho' they abound with a pinguious Oil, may be fo changed by Art, as to be converted into a Meal of a lefs unctuous Nature. Under this Clafs are contained; firft the Seeds of culmiferous, graminifolious, fpicated Plants, called Corn; the Seeds of all thofe of the Cucumber kind, of Buck-Wheat, Flax, Lettice, and many others of the fame Nature.

H 3   Secondly,

Secondly, The Seeds of almoft all the leguminous, podded Plants with a papilionaceous, or any other Sort of Flower.

Thirdly, Nuts not too oily, as Almonds, Filberts, Chefnuts, Wallnuts, and others of a like Kind; but when thefe abound with Oil, fome Management is neceffary in order to deprive them of Part of it, and this is beft done by fuffering them to begin to fhoot, and then fcorching them.

In order to difpofe thefe to ferment, it is neceffary to fteep them when in their utmoft Perfettition, dry and entire, in Water, till they are fwelled, and have imbibed all the Water they can. Then they are to be taken out, and laid in Heaps in an open airy Place, upon which a gentle Heat will be excited in the Mafs, and the Seeds will begin to germinate, but the Germination muft not be fuffered to proceed too far, but muft be ftopped by fpreading the Seeds abroad, that they may be ventilated, cooled and dried. Then they are to be dried in a Kiln. By this Means the Vifcidity is deftroyed, and the Body of the Seeds is fo attenuated, as readily to permit the greateft Part thereof to be diffolved in Water. They are then ground, and afterwards infufed in a due Proportion of Water.

The fecond Clafs includes all the pulpous Fruits, whofe Juice when ripe, is of an acid Sweet, and which do not incline to a fetid alcaline Putrefattion. Thefe require only to be trod, preffed, or pounded, that their Juices may be feparated from them.

But if their Subftance be too hard, they may boiled in Water, and then reduced to a Pulp. Or if they are dry they may be rafped, and then pounded with Water to a Pulp.

The third Clafs comprehends all the Parts of all fucculent Herbs, as their Leaves, Flowers, Roots, and Stalks, which are fpontaneoufly inclined to grow acid, rather than putrid. Thefe are fufficiently prepared by being beat into a Pulp, whilft they are frefh and juicy, adding a fmall Quantity of Water, to render the Mafs of a thinner Confiftence.

The fourth Clafs contains all the frefh vegetable Juices expreffed from the Fruits and Herbs of the fecond and third Claffes. All the Management here required is to bring them to a due Confiftence, by boiling them fufficiently, in a wide fhallow Veffel, if too thin; and by adding Water to them if too thick.

Thofe vegetable Juices, which are infpiffated into a faponaceous Kind of Subftance, in the Form of a faline and puinguious Coagulum conftitute the fifth Clafs. Among thefe are Manna, Honey, Caffia, Sugar, and feveral others. Thefe only require Dilution with Water, in order to difpofe them to ferment.

In all the Vegetables comprehended under thefe Claffes, fome certain phyfical Conditions are required, in order to render them the fitter for Fermentation. Thus they muft firft arrive at the utmoft Perfection intended by Nature; for when they are harfh, crude, and watery, they are lefs difpofed to ferment. They muft, alfo, be but moderately oily, becaufe very oily Subftances, inftead of fermenting, grow rancid; and thofe without any Oil, are unfit for Fermentation. They muft not be too rough or aftringent; and it is abfolutely neceffary, that they fhould be diffolvable in Water.

Many of the vegetable Subftances mentioned above, fpontaneoufly ferment, and frequently too much, fo as to require a Check; but others ferment more fluggifhly, fo as to require the Addition of fomething to accelerate the Fermentation; and the Things

Things which anfwer this End are called *Ferments*. Thefe are principally: Firft, The frefh Juices of Summer Fruits, which are fo much difpofed to Fermentation, that 'tis not eafy to reftrain them from it.

Secondly, Frefh Yeaft, Barm, or Flowers of Malt Liquors, or Wine, which work up to the Top, during the Action of Fermentation; for thefe are very active, and greatly promote Fermentation, when mixed with other fermentable Liquors.

Thirdly, The fame Yeaft afterwards grown more ponderous, and funk to the Bottom of the fermenting Liquor. This is very active, but not fo much fo as before.

Fourthly, Caffia, Manna, Honey, Sugar, and the like infpiffated Juices.

Fifthly, The acid, mealy, fermented Leaven of the Bakers; this is made by kneading frefh, fweet, wheaten Meal, with Water into a foft Dough of a moderate Denfity, which is to be fet afide in a warm Place, flightly covered; and then in an Hour it will begin to fwell, open on all Sides, rife in Bladders, lofe its Smell, Tafte, and Tenacity, and become acid.

Sixthly, The Refiduums of former fermented Liquors, which adhere to the Sides of the Cafks, for thefe Cafks remarkably promote the Fermentation of frefh Liquors put into them.

Seventhly, The Whites of Eggs, tho' not fermentable, yet by Accident become Helps to Fermentation, when they are beaten up and mixed with Liquors, fo diluted, and thin, that they fuffer the Air and Spirits, too readily to difcharge themfelves, and do not retain them long enough to change their fermentable into a fermented State. In this Cafe the Whites of Eggs infpiffate the Fluid, and enable it to retain fufficiently the Air and Spirits.

Eighthly, Alcalies by Accident, likewife affift Fermentation, when prudently mixed with vegetable Liquors too acid for Fermentation. And Acids do the fame, when added to Fluids, which are hindred from fermenting, by any Tendency to *Pu*trefcence. Thefe are not Ferments themfelves, but remove the Impediments to Fermentation. Good Tartar, however, may in fome Refpects be efteemed a Ferment.

Ninthly, fome auftere Bodies, as Quinces, unripe Medlars, rough Cherries, and fuch like Subftances, when added to Liquors too thin, weak, and watery to retain their volatile Spirits, have accidentally affifted Fermentation.

The Preparations of the firft Clafs reduced to Malt, fcarcely require the Affiftance of Ferments, but are difpofed fpontaneoufly to ferment fufficiently, and fometimes too much. In Winter, however, an Addition of fome Ferment, and of an artifical Heat is neceffary to excite a proper Degree of Motion. An Ounce of Yeaft, or Honey, or Sugar, is fufficient for twenty Pints of Liquor, or double that Quantity of Baker's Leaven, provided the Liquors are kept in a very warm Place.

Thofe of the fecond Clafs feldom require any Addition, unlefs the Weather is very cold; and then a little Yeaft may be added to it, if the Fermentation proceeds too flowly.

Thofe of the third Clafs, in the Summer, and warm Weather efpecially, readily ferment fpontaneoufly; in cold Weather, if the Fermentation is checked, it may be promoted by the Additon of a little Sugar or Honey.

Thofe of the fourth Clafs fpontaneoufly ferment too violently, if the Weather is warm, and efpecially if the

Seafon has been favourable to their Maturation.

Thofe of the fifth Clafs require no additional Ferment, but rather ferve as Ferments to other Subftances that require it.

When Fermentables have been duly prepar'd, and diluted with Water, they are to be put into an oaken Cafk well feafon'd with a Liquor of the fame Kind, fermented in it before. Then let it ftand in a Heat, betwixt fixty and feventy Degrees on *Fahrenheit*'s Thermometer, and let the Bung-hole be left open, that the Air may have free Ingrefs and Egrefs; or it may be flightly cover'd with a Flannel, to prevent Duft and Infects from falling in; and upon this the Fermentation commences, and regularly proceeds.

Boerhaave, in Order to obferve the Phænomena in Fermentation, took a large Glafs Cucurbit, and plac'd it upright in a wooden Box, in fuch a Manner, as to be able to fupport an equal Heat, by fupplying the Bottom of the Box with Fire; then he fill'd three Fourths of the Cucurbit, with a crude fermentable Matter, properly prepar'd for Fermentation, and remark'd the following Appearances:

Firft, then, the Mafs which in the Beginning was at reft, and took up a certain Space in the Veffel, began infenfibly to fwell, and rarify, to be elevated and conceive an intenfe Motion thro' all its Parts, which difcovers itfelf by the ftrange Gyration of the Liquor, upwards, downwards and fide-ways, nor ceafes, tho' the Force changes every Moment. In the mean Time, Bubbles appear to be generated in every Part of the Mafs, which, with a ftrong Tendency, endeavour to afcend, fometimes burfting as they rife, or elfe at the Surface, with an hiffing Noife. Hence the whole Matter, but efpecially the Surface, becomes frothy;

and with a Noife like that of Ebullition, emits an acrid Spirit, which affects the Noftrils with its Acrimony, is fomewhat acid, wonderfully elaftic, incoercible, burfting by its immenfe Force almoft all Veffels in which it is confin'd. Hence *Helmont*, in Order to diftinguifh it by a particular Name, call'd it *Gas Sylveftris.*

Secondly, Whilft Things proceed in this Manner, the thicker Part of the fermentable Mafs, begins to be feparated from the thinner, and is thrown up to the Top, where it is collected in a thick, fpongy Cruft, which accurately covers the Liquor underneath, and confines, and repels its more active Parts; fo, that they cannot eafily exhale, before they have perform'd their proper Office. On this Occafion, it is highly entertaining, to obferve the violent and conftant Agitation, thro' all the moft minute Parts of the Liquid, which lies under the incumbent tenacious Cruft. Nor is it, perhaps, poffible to conceive a greater Attrition, than that arifing from the rapid Agitation of thofe Corpufcules among each other. Hence, the Cruft being elevated, and feparated by the repeated Explofions, a Vapour burfts out thro' the Clefts, with a confiderable Noife, upon which, the Cruft falling down, prefently clofes again, and confines as before, the active Principles, fo, that they cannot too eafily exhale, and be diffipated. The Formation, and Continuance of this Cruft, tend above all Things to bring about a perfect Fermentation.

Thirdly, 'Tis alfo to be obferv'd, that, whereas all the thick Part of the fermentable Matter, was at firft, carried up, and collected at the Top, there are now fome Parts at the Bottom of the Cruft, which growing lefs rare, and being no longer fupported by the Bubbles, which render'd them light, begin to defcend thro' the liquid Part, are agitated

upwards

upwards and downwards, form Bubbles about them, by whose Assistance they rise, then by their Explosion sink again, and when this has happen'd alternately, for a considerable Time, at last subside to the Bottom, and remain at rest. Then other Globules act the same Part; and, when this has proceeded for some Time, it often happens, that the whole upper Crust becomes heavier and less rare, on Account of the Explosion of the Spirits, sinks down at once, and soon after rises again almost entire, and with such a Force, as is hardly credible. When the whole Crust is perfectly dissipated, and sunk to the Bottom, the Fermentation ceases, tho' the same Degree of Heat is still continu'd; a clear, thin, light Liquor swims at the Top, and the Feces subside to the Bottom.

Hence in every true Fermentation, the fermentable Matter is, at first, of an unequal Consistence, but afterwards separated into two Parts, the more liquid which is undermost, and the more solid Crust, which covers it. This Crust, so long as it keeps the upper Place, is called the *Flowers* of the fermentable Liquor or *Yeast*, and is the most convenient and serviceable of all Ferments. But in the second Stage of Fermentation, it is separated into three Parts, the *Flowers* at Top, the *Liquid* in the Middle, and a third Part, which begins to fall, and be collected at the Bottom, under the Title of the *Feces*, which, are the thicker and heavier Part, now quite exhausted of that Principle which caused the Fermentation. And lastly, in the third Stage, it is again divided into two Parts, the Upper, which is clear, fine, and thin, and call'd *Wine*; and the Lower, which is thick, and lies at the Bottom, named the *Lees*, or Mother of Wine.

But there is nothing more surprising, and more carefully to be observ'd, in this Affair of Fermentation, than that prodigious *Spiritus Sylvestris*, or incoercible Spirit, which rushes out with such a Force when the Fermentation is at the Height, nor is there any known Poison that is so subtile, swift, and fatal; for if a large Vessel full of the best fermented Must in the Height of Fermentation, should discharge this Spirit thro' a small Vent-hole in the upper Part, and the strongest Man should but once draw this Vapour into his Nostrils, he would drop down dead that very Moment; or if he drew it in but a little, he would be taken with an Apoplexy; if still less, he would be depriv'd of his Understanding, and be a meer Idiot the rest of his Life, or else become Paralytic; and hence, the like Misfortunes happen to those who are imprudently busy in close Wine-Vaults, where the Wines are fermenting in the Time of Vintage. For this Reason, those Places ought to be purified by Fires, and aired by setting the Windows open. From Sugar dissolv'd in Water, and its Froth first fermented, we have an Account of a Spirit produced, which being drawn into the Lungs in a small Quantity, in an Instant stopped all Respiration, exciting an intolerable Asthma.

Let Physicians, then, consider the Force of Liquor drank in the very Act of Fermentation, and how violent that Spirit may be, which in Summer is generated in the human Body, from a too free Use of Summer Fruits when very ripe, if by a convulsive Constriction of the Stomach, they are prevented from passing any farther, and by being kept in a warm Place, acquire and exert an extreme Elasticity and Acrimony. Hence in *Alcohol*, there still remains a great deal of this Poison, and therefore,

therefore, if the Vapour of it be taken into the Nofe, in a great Quantity, and for a long Time, it caufes the greateft Degree of Drunkennefs, or a flight Apoplexy. If it be ufed too freely internally, it affects the Brain and Nerves particularly, and their Functions. In Chymiftry, we are ftill at a Lofs, from whence this Spirit arifes; we know, indeed, it is the Production of an actual and prefent Fermentation, nor do we know that fuch a one is generated in any other Way; but we cannot conceive, how it caufes Death without any Difeafe, or how it affects the Cerebrum, Cerebellum, or Nerves, without Matter, or without any vifible Alteration, either in the Solids, or Fluids.

As foon as the Fermentation is over, it is proper to clofe the Veffel, and let the fermented Liquor reft awhile upon its Lees, for it will ftill confume much of them, and affimilate them to itfelf, and fo be ftronger, more fpirituous, and much fitter for Diftillation.

The Time neceffary for compleating a perfect Fermentation, can fcarce be determined exactly, as depending upon the Place where the Veffel ftands, the Seafon of the Year, the Heat, and Wind it is expofed to, and the Nature of the fermentable Matter itfelf. In *Africa*, the Liquor of the Palm Tree paffes thro' this Operation, in the Space of a few Hours: In *Afia*, too, the Bufinefs is very foon over; but, in the northern Countries, it proceeds but very flowly. The hot Summer Seafon quickens, the Winter checks it. The South Wind promotes, the North Wind retards it. The expreffed Juice of Grapes and Sugar ferment fuddenly and violently, other Fermentables more flowly. It is eafy, however, to know when a perfect Fermentation is at an End,

which is, when all the Phænome mentioned, have appear'd in t Order defcribed, and at laft ce fpontaneoufly; and then the Ve muft be immediately ftopped, and t fermented Liquor kept upon its Le for otherwife, the Spirit generat by the Fermentation, would in ﹤ fhort Time exhale, and leave the Li quor vapid, and good for nothing whereas, if the Liquor is kept qui in a Veffel well ftopped, it grow gradually finer, more fubtle, an fuller of Spirit. Thus the frefh ex preffed Juice of Grapes may, b boiling, be infpiffated without loofin any of its Virtues; but after Fermen tation, if it be only expofed to th cold Air, it is foon exhaufted of al its Spirits.

The Circumftances neceffary to ﹤ fuccefsful Fermentation, are princi pally thefe:

Firft, It is requifite that the fer menting Liquor fhould remain a reft, that the Cruft which forms itfel at the Top, may keep entire, for t be continually ftirring, and mixing i with the Liquor underneath, prevent a perfect Fermentation.

Secondly, There muft be a fre Ingrefs and Egrefs of the commo Air, which muft, alfo, be intimatel mixed with the fermentable Matter by treading, kneading, or preffing ﹔ otherwife the Fermentation will no proceed.

Thirdly, A Degree of Heat, be tween Forty, and at moft Eighty.

Fourthly, The Spring and Au tumn in particular, are faid to favou this Operation; and when thofe Ve getables are in Flower, from which the Wine was made, 'tis faid, th Fermentation is fubject to be reviv'd Hence the Wine of Grapes is re puted to grow foul, and eafily fer ment again, when the Vine is in Bloffom.

The Checks to Fermentation, by
which

which it is either impeded after it is begun, or entirely stopped, are as follow:

The acid Vapour of burning Sulphur long included, and in a considerable Quantity, with the Air which is in the Cask, above the fermenting Liquor; for if a Vessel first thoroughly penetrated, and replete with this Vapour, receives the fermenting Liquor, and the upper empty Part be afterwards filled with the same Vapour, and carefully stopt, you will prevent any farther Fermentation, which, after some Time, may be reviv'd by proper Means, and restrain'd by the same Fumes. The same Effect follows, from mixing a large Quantity of a strong Acid with the fermenting Matter. The Acids of Alum, Nitre, Salt, Sulphur, and Vitriol, prevent Fermentation, but at the same Time spoil the Liquors.

Alcaline Salts, also, if they are mixed in great Quantities with fermenting Liquors, excite for the present, a very considerable Effervescence; but that soon ceasing, leaves the Liquor incapable of farther Agitation, its Nature being so utterly destroy'd, that it can scarcely be afterwards rais'd to a Fermentation, but rather tends to Putrefaction. Hence it appears, that Alcalies are a greater Obstacle to Fermentation than Acids, the former destroying or suffocating all the Acid. Wherefore,

All Bodies entirely absorbent of Acids, if mixed with fermenting Liquors in a proper Quantity, after a short Struggle and Effervescence, put a Stop to this Operation. Chalk, Crabbs Eyes, Coral, Pearls, Oystershells, Iron, Lead, and Tin, have the same Effect.

Stopping the Vessel so closely, that nothing can pass in or out, provided the Vessel be so strong, as not to burst by the Force of the included Liquor, also, stops Fermentation. This is evident, by new Ale put into very strong Bottles, where the Admission of Air converts the Fermentation, so long suffocated and prevented, into the most violent Effervescence, and discovers a prodigious collected Force. The same Thing happens also in Casks, for there is a constant Struggle and Renitency between the fermenting Body and its containing Vessel.

A great Degree of Cold destroys all Fermentation, for under thirty-six Degrees of Heat, it will hardly make any Progress. Nor is too much Heat a less Obstacle to it, which if it exceeds ninety Degrees, rather dissipates the active Principles of Fermentables, than assists and quickens them. Hence an Exhalation under a greater Degree of Heat, inspissates Fluids to a Degree of Density, unfit for Fermentation. Boiling has a much quicker Effect, so that the richest Juice of Grapes, which can hardly be kept from fermenting, will by quick Boiling loose all its Disposition to ferment, and be converted into a Mass that will rest for Years without Alteration.

The Separation of the elastic Air, by Means of the Air Pump, stops Fermentation, for during the Absence of the Air, the fermentative Motion entirely ceases.

Lastly, An extraordinary Condensation of the same Air, with the fermentable Matter, absolutely prevents both the Beginning and Progress of Fermentation.

Having taken a distinct View of the first Fermentation of vegetable Juices, by which a vinous Liquor is produc'd, that is intoxicating, and yields an inflammable Liquor by Distillation, let us now consider the second Fermentation, by which an acid Liquor is generated, call'd Vinegar, that extinguishes Fire, and is so far from inebriating, that it is a Preservative against, and a Remedy for, Drunkenness.

The Ferments by which an acetose

tofe Fermentation is moft fuccefsfully promoted, are particularly thefe.

Firft, The acid Feces, or Lees of an acidifh Wine, call'd the Mother of Wine. —

Secondly, Feces of Vinegar collected in old Cafks, efpecially fuch as are well faturated with very ftrong Vinegar.

Thirdly, Tartar of an acid Wine, reduc'd to Powder.

Fourthly, Vinegar itfelf, firft well prepared, and brought to its greateft Degree of Acidity.

Fifthly, Old wooden Cafks, which have been for a long Time full of the ftrongeft Vinegar, and hence are thoroughly penetrated with its fharp Acid.

Sixthly, The frequent ftirring up of the Lees in its own Wine.

Seventhly, The Stalks, Twigs, and Skins of Cherries, Currants, and Grapes, the Tendrels of Vines, and the like Parts of other acid, auftere Vegetables.

Eighthly, The acid Rye leaven of the Bakers.

Ninthly, A Compofition of all the Preceeding mix'd together, efpecially if there are fome very warm Aromatics added to the Acids, for then the ftrongeft Vinegars are produced.

Glauber, long ago, gave the whole Hiftory of the Generation of Vinegar with great Accuracy, an Account of which was afterwards publifh'd in the *Philofophical Tranfactions.* The Purport of which, is as follows :

Two large oaken Veffels are prepar'd, in the Shape of common Cafks; in each of thefe, at about the Diftance of a Foot from the Bottom, as they ftand upright, a wicker Grate is fix'd; upon thefe Grates is a moderate thick Stratum of frefh, green Tendrels of Vines, and over thefe fuch fuch a Quantity of the Pedicles of Grapes, from which the Grapes have been ftripped, as is fuf-

ficient to fill the Veffel to within a Foot of the Top. When thefe two Veffels are thus prepar'd, the Wine, of which the Vinegar is to be made, is pour'd into both of them, but in fuch a Manner, that one of them is filled quite full, the other half-full, and then every Day alternately, the Veffel which was half-full, is filled out of the other, fo that neither remains full above twenty-four Hours ; after proceeding in this Manner for two or three Days, a Fermentation arifes in the Wine, with a fenfible Heat in the half-fill'd Veffel, and this increafes gradually every Day. Mean Time the Motion and Heat are almoft fuffocated in the Cafk which is quite full, fo as nearly to ceafe in the Space of the twenty-four Hours, during which it remains full. Thus Fermentation and Heat are alternately excited and fuffocated in the two oaken Veffels.

In this Manner the Operation is continued, till the Heat is extinguifhed, and there appears no more Motion, in the half-filled Veffel; and this is a Sign that the acetofe Fermentation is compleated ; the Vinegar, therefore, muft be then put up in Cafks well ftopped.

The hotter the Room is where thefe Veffels, in which Vinegar is prepared, are placed, the fooner it will be made ; in *France* it is compleated in Summer in about fifteen Days ; but in cold Weather, and a cold Place, the Operation is more flow ; but whenever the Seafon, or the Workhoufe, is very hot, it is often neceffary, to fill the half-filled Veffel, out of that which is full, every twelve Hours ; for otherwife there arifes fuch a Heat and Fermentation in the Veffel half-full, that the volatile Spirits of the Wine, not being yet fufficiently fixed, are diffipated by the Heat, and fly off before they can be properly entangled, and converted into the acid Spirit of Vinegar:

Vinegar; and hence the Liquor tho' it would be four, would, at the fame time, be vapid, and in no Refpect ftrong generous Vinegar. For this Reafon, alfo, the Veffel which is half-full, is always accurately clofed with a Cover of Oak, that the foaming Ebullition of the fermenting Liquor may be reftrained and checked, and thus the repelled Spirits, may act longer and more forcibly, upon the auftere Subftances underneath, and by the Reaction of them, be better fecured from Diffipation. But the full Veffel is not covered, but left quite open, that the Air may have free Accefs to the Liquor defigned to be changed. This is the fecond Fermentation, which tends to the Production of Vinegar, and there terminates. Vinegar is erroneoufly by fome efteemed a Liquor, produced after the Evaporation of the inflammable Spirits generated by the firft Fermentation; for this would be vapid, and nothing like Vinegar. On the contrary, the more generous, and the more replete with Spirits Wine is, which is ufed for this Purpofe, the better will the Vinegar be, and the weaker the Wine is, the lefs acid is the Vinegar prepared from it. For this Reafon the ftrongeft Malt Liquors, if they are treated in the fame Manner, yield an exceeding good Vinegar, as do the richeft *Spanifh* Wines. In this Operation it, is particularly remarkable, that this Converfion of Wine into Vinegar, is not brought about without the Generation of a confiderable Heat, during the Fermentation. Whereas Muft fermenting in the Time of Vintage fcarcely generates any Heat: And Malt Liquor, notwithftanding the violent Motion which is excited whilft it works, does not grow warm; is Heat therefore always required for the Generation of an Acid? It is certain that Corn, and Milk, and Food prepar-

ed from thefe do not grow acid, without a Heat either of the Seafon, of artificial Fire, or that of the Body. And we find that a violent Fire converts Nitre, Sulphur, and Salt, which are . t, acid, into Spirits extreamly acid. Hence, perhaps, upon Reflection, we fhall find Reafon to believe, that almoft every Change that is brought about in Nature, requires a certain Degree of Heat.

In this Operation, another Circumftance occurs, which deferves our Confideration, which is, that whilft Wine is thus converted into Vinegar, this clear thin Liquor depofites an incredible Quantity of thick, pinguious, oily, and as it were foapy Feces, which hang about the Sides of the Veffel, the Vine-tendrels, and the Pedicles of the Grapes. Whence fhould this arife? In the Wine, there is not the leaft Sign of any fuch Thing, and in the auftere Tendrels and Pedicles, one would expect to find nothing like a pinguious oily Subftance; and it is in this Manner formed from the Wine, for if it is wafhed off, it will be generated again, infomuch that it is neceffary once a Year, to clear away all this grofs unctuous Matter, otherwife when the Wine was put into the Veffels, it would not be chang'd into a thin fharp Vinegar, but to a thick corrupted pinguious Liquor, fit for no Ufe whatever.

But Care muft be taken to clear the Pedicles, and Twigs from this pinguious Matter, which adheres to them by a fudden Affufion of Water upon them, which muft be fuffered to run thro' them, left, if it fhould remain, it fhould deprive them of their acid Ferment, with which they are now impregnated. After this the Grates, Sides and Bottoms of the Veffels in which the Vinegar is made, are cleared with the fame Caution, and as foon as ever the pinguious Impurities are removed, the
Grates,

Grates, Twigs, and Stalks, are disposed of as before, and are then again fit for making Vinegar, till, by a long Use, the same oily Crust will be formed again, which evidently demonstrates, that the Wine actually throws out an Oil, whilst it is changed from its own proper Nature, to that of Vinegar. At the same time too, the acetific Ferment, remains in the Vessels, Grates and Stalks, and hence when these Vessels have been used a considerable Time, they acquire very strongly, the Power of converting Wine into Vinegar, and with the Grates and Stalks, &c. become as it were spungy Reservoirs of Vinegar.

It is farther to be remembered, that as *Alcohol*, prepared from very strong old Malt Liquor, can scarcely be distinguished from that drawn from the richest Wine, so here the same Malt Liquor, treated in the Manner explained, may be converted into Vinegar, as good, pure, and fit for any Use as can be made from the best Wine; nor is it easy to find any Difference betwixt them, except what is owing to the Bitters put into Malt Liquor, to make it keep, which give it a Colour and Taste, different from what it would have had, if prepared from Corn alone; in other respects they are entirely the same.

The Effect, therefore, of this second Fermentation, when compleated, is the Production of good Vinegar. In order now to understand this the better, let us consider what Vinegar is. Vinegar is an acid, penetrating, subpinguious, volatile, vegetable Liquor, produced from Wine by a second Fermentation; the first Part of this which rises in Distillation, is truly acid, and by no Means inflammable, but extinguishes Fire and Flame, like Water; and by these remarkable Properties, Wine is distinguished from Vinegar.

The Promoters of this second Fermentation are:

First, A sufficient Degree of Heat.

Secondly, The free Access, and even Admixture of the Air.

Thirdly, Motion, Conquassation, and frequent stirring the Liquor in the open Air.

Fourthly, The Addition of some very warm Aromatic during the Fermentation. The Impediments to this Fermentation are all those Things which retard the first Fermentation, except that stirring the Liquor about here is of Service, whereas in the other it does Harm.

Upon reflecting on the Appearances in both the Fermentations necessary to the Generation of Vinegar, I think there is reason to believe that the Acid of Vinegar, is not a new Production, but that it rather lay concealed, and enveloped in the Oil of the vegetable Juice, till disengaged from it by two Fermentations, which are nothing more than continued Efforts of the extreamly elastic Acid, assisted by a proper Degree of Heat, to disunite itself from the vegetable Oil, which disguises it, and detains it, thereby preventing it from flying off, and mixing with the Air, of which perhaps, it was originally a Denizon, and from whence it may be entertaining to trace it, till it disentangles itself from the vegetable Juices, and exhaling, leaves the remaining Fluid tasteless, and vapid, being only Water, with a small Portion of mucilaginous and unactive Oil.

There is an Acid perpetually floating in the Air. This Acid is so strongly attracted by alcaline Salts of all Kinds, that in Time they become so saturated therewith, as to be entirely neutral. Now alcaline Salts are the great Promoters of Fertility, insomuch that, unless the Earth is sufficiently saturated with them, no Vegetable of any Kind will grow in it.

it, because these Salts are necessary to the Formation of a saponaceous, neutral Menstruum, capable of dissolving Earth; otherwise Earth, which is incapable of Solution by Water alone, could not enter the Pores of the Roots, and contribute to the Formation of the solid Parts of Plants.

If we examine all the Substances in Nature, that are used to promote Fertility, we shall find they contain an alcaline Salt. Thus all the Parts or Excrements of Animals, contain an alcaline Salt; and the same Kind of Salt is found in all Vegetables that have undergone Putrefaction. Thus Lime, also, contains an extremely volatile and penetrating alcaline Salt, of singular Efficacy in fertilizing barren Lands. Amongst Limes may be reckoned a Kind of *Sal Terræ*, to be discovered by its Effects in all Countries: For Earth, by the continual Action of the Sun upon it during Summer, is in some Measure calcined, and furnished with a Salt of the Nature of Lime, Hence the Advantages of a Summer Fallow, as the Farmers call it, which is only exposing the naked Earth to the Influence of the Sun. Hence, also, the great Fertility of Meadows from Inundations; for the Waters having in their Passage taken up and dissolved large Quantities of this *Sal Terræ*, deposite them upon the Lands they overflow.

But this is no where so remarkable as in *Ægypt*, whose prodigious Fertility seems to depend entirely upon this Kind of alcaline Salt; for the Water of the *Nile* being gathered in the parched Mountains of *Æthiopia*, collects in its Passage this Salt, which it afterwards deposites on the Soil of *Ægypt*.

This Kind of Salt is, perhaps, that which the Inhabitants in all Ages have collected in great Quantities, under the Name of *Natron*, which is not unlike the *Cineres Clavellati*, and may be used for the same Purposes. When these alcaline Salts are committed to the Earth, and consequently exposed to the Air, they attract the Acid floating therein, till they are saturated therewith, and become neutral. At the same Time they attract the Moisture, and with it the volatile Oil of Animals and Vegetables floating in the Air. These, then, mixed with the Oil of the Earth, being digested by the Heat of the Sun, form a penetrating, neutral Soap; which, when diluted by the Rains, becomes a Menstruum capable of dissolving Earth, or reducing it to Particles fine enough to enter the Pores of the Roots of Plants.

I call this a Soap, because it has all the Ingredients of Soap in its Composition, and answers the same End; that is, it dissolves Concretions of Earth, or, in other Words, Dirt. And I believe every Body has observed the Earth to foam and lather upon a hasty Shower of Rain. The Ingredients of Soap, are an alcaline Salt, and Oil. Now, all Oils contain an Acid, and this Acid neutralizes the alcaline Salt, as it mixes with it in the Formation of the Soap. It is, perhaps, on Account of this Acid, that Oils flame, for Acids, tho' not readily inflammable, yet flame with the utmost Violence, and greatest Degree of Explosion, when once set on Fire, and I do not recollect any Body in Nature that will flame, that has not an Acid in it. Turpentines, which are vegetable Oils, and contain a great Quantity of Acid, are remarkable for the Violence of the Flame they emit.

From this *Sapo Terræ*, or Soap of the Earth, is made that neutral Salt which we call Nitre, perhaps the greatest Dissolvent in Nature, and for that Reason a Medicine of the greatest Impor-

Importance in the Practice of Phyfic. It muft be obferved here, for the better underftanding and Confirmation of what I am going to fay, that the Acid of the Air, which enters the Compofition of common Nitre, is not loft or deftroyed, but only difguifed and concealed under the Mask of the alcaline Salt, and Oil, with which it is united, and from which it may again be feparated, as it actually is in making Spirit of Nitre.

This faponaceous Menftruum, then, together with the diffolved Earth, is conveyed into the Pores of the Roots of Plants, where a Part of the Earth and Salt is employed in the Formation of the Solids, and a Part of the Oil ferves as a Cement for joining the Particles of Earth together, which otherwife would not cohere, but fall from each other like the Afhes of Vegetables, which are nothing but Earth and Salts, deprived of their cementing Oil, by Fire. Mean time the Juices, deprived of Part of their Earth, Salt, and Oil, are fomewhat acid; that is, the Acid in fome Degree difengaged from the enveloping Oil, neutralizing Salts, and auftere Earth, has Liberty to act and affect the Organs of Tafte. But as the Plant approaches to Maturity, lefs of the Oil and Earth received by the Root is employed in Accretion. They mix, therefore, with the Juices, and contribute by Degrees to their Neutralization, which is farther promoted by the Heat of the Sun, which digefts them together, and mixes with them itfelf; for Heat is a Body, as has been proved by many Experiments; and according to its different Degrees, has the Power of neutralizing Acids, or expelling them from the Subftances to which they adhered; but I do not know that it has been proved by any Experiment, that it can utterly deftroy them.

It muft, alfo, be remembered that Vegetables imbibe the Air, and no Doubt the Acid thereof. And indeed this Kind of Refpiration is not lefs neceffary to Vegetables, than to Animals; for without an open Intercourfe with the Air, no Plant can live, but very foon withers away and dies. If we farther confider, that this Sort of Refpiration is performed by Means of the Leaves, and that in moft Plants the Leaves by Degrees decay and wither, as the Fruit approaches to Maturity, we may perhaps, find Reafon to believe, that the Jucies of Vegetables receive an additional Acid by Refpiration, which ceafes by Degrees, when the Acid is no longer of Ufe, and when the Neutralization of the Juices is neceffary to the Maturation of the Fruits.

And this will be farther confirmed by moft of thefe Vegetables, that produce a Fruit very acid, when full ripe, as the Lemon, Orange, Citron, and others of the fame Kind, which do not loofe their Leaves as the Fruit ripens. Upon the different Combinations of the acid, alcaline, Salts, Oils, Water, and Fire, depend the different Taftes of Vegetables. Hence, alfo, fome Plants are falutary and medicinal, whilft others are deleterious and fatal, to Animals that eat them. How far the Acid may be concerned in rendering them poifonous, I cannot determine; but it is well known that Acids, when naked, are the greateft Poifons known in Nature; tho', when properly combined with Things of a different Nature, they are not only falutary, but endued with excellent medicinal Virtues.

The Example of the Vine may ferve for an Illuftration of what I have advanced, whofe Juices in the Spring are much inclinable to Acidity, whilft the folid Parts, that is the Tendrels and Branches, increafe

fur

surprisingly fast. The Juices of the Fruit, that is, the Grape, are also very acid, till arrived at their full Growth, and neutralized by the Accession of oily and alcaline Particles, and the Admixture of Heat or Fire, a great deal of which last is necessary to bring them to Maturity.

When these Juices are neutralized, that is full ripe, they are sweet, or in other Words, the Acid is enveloped in Oil, and a Portion of Earth and Salts, and mixed with Particles of Fire; for an Acid thus modified seems necessary to the Formation of a sweet Taste, as is evident in Sugar and Honey.

Thus Must and Wort are sweet, which put in a proper Vessel, and set in a sufficient Degree of Heat, begin to ferment; that is, the Acid which is extreamly elastic, begins to expand and disengage itself from the inveloping Oil. Mean time a Part of the Acid flies off with so prodigious a Force that no Vessel is strong enough to confine it. This is what *Helmont* called the *Gas Sylvestris*, or incoercible Spirit, which is the most sudden and deleterious Poison known in Nature, and to a Portion of this remaining in the fermented Liquors, the intoxicating Faculty of such Liquors is indisputably owing.

This *Gas Sylvestris* I call Acid, because it has an acid Smell, and because its expansive Force is greater than that of any known Body in Nature, scarcely excepting the Acid of Nitre, to which it seems nearly related.

Mean time the more gross Particles of the Oil are separated and rise to the Top of the fermenting Liquor in a Froth, where they condense by Degrees and become at last heavier than the Liquor, when they sink to the Bottom, and remain there under the Name of Lees, or Mother of Wine. When this

Fermentation is compleated, the Liquor changes its sweet Taste, for one somewhat inclined to Acidity, and the finer and lighter Parts of the Liquor, separated from the heavier by Distillation, will take Fire and flame, and therefore must be an Oil attenuated by Fermentation, and containing an Acid.

During the second Fermentation, the more gross Particles which entered the Composition of the Oil, and inveloped the Acid, are separated from the Fluid, and deposited on the Sides and Bottom of the containing Vessels; and then the naked Acid is at Liberty to act, and affect the Organs of Taste with that Sensation which we call Sour; but if the second Fermentation is carried on a little too far, the Acid making its Escape, mixes with the Air, from whence it came, and leaves the remaining Liquor a tasteless vapid Mass.

What *Galen* observes with regard to Vinegar makes very much for what I have advanced; this Author tells us, that Vinegar in its penetrating Quality resembles the *Northern Air*. Now *Hoffman* informs us, that those who are concerned in the making Nitre observe, that the northern and easterly Winds favour the Production of Nitre, that is, bring the Acid which fixes on the Earth impregnated with alcaline Salts, and render it nitrous.

'Tis probable a Portion of this Acid, which, uniting with the grosser Particles of the Oil, fixes to the Sides and Bottoms of Casks, and forms Tartar. Hence that incoercible Spirit or Gas, which rises from Tartar in Distillation, that either perspires thro' the Lute, or bursts the Vessel.

If it should be mentioned as an Objection to what I have said, that the Spirit of Wine is lighter than

Water, and rifes firft in Diftillation, but that the Acid of Vinegar is more fixed and rifes after the Water, it would not much embarrafs the Affair; for when the Particles of the Acid are divided minutely, and kept from joining by the Tenacity of the Oil, they muft neceffarily be affected by a lefs Degree of Heat, than when their Gravity is increafed by their Union, which happens as foon as they are in fome Meafure releafed from their Confinement; and then their Cohefion muft be confiderable, for Acids are of all Fluids the moft ponderous and confequently very folid.

CHAP. XVIII.
Of FILTRATION.

FILTRATION is the paffing any Fluid thro' a Strainer, or Filtre, in order to feparate from it any grofs Particles it contains, and render it limpid. To filtrate Fluids of any Kind, Chymifts and Apothecaries fold a Piece of bibulous or coarfe Paper, in fuch a Manner as to fit a Funnel, the fmall End of which they place in the Mouth of the Veffel intended for the Reception of the filtrated Liquor. Then they pour the Liquor into the Paper, permitting it to drop gradually thro' it, and taking Care not to put in too much at a Time, for fear of burfting the Paper. Filtration may be, alfo, performed by Means of a conical, woolen or linen Bag, commonly called *Hippocrates's Sleeve*. But we muft be directed in our Choice of one or other of thefe, by the particular Nature of the Fluid to be filtrated.

CHAP. XIX.
Of the Fixity *and* Solidity *of* BODIES.

FIXITY is oppofed to Volatility, and Solidity to Fluidity; for as thofe Subftances are called volatile, which eafily and with a gentle Heat fly off in the Air, fo fixed Subftances are fuch as remain in the ftrongeft Fire or are difficultly diffipated by Heat.

Thofe Bodies are called fluid, which confift of fine fubtile Parts, agitated with a rapid inteftine Motion, and having a large Quantity of etherial Matter intermixed with them.

Firm and folid Bodies are fuch as confift of larger and groffer Parts fo connected with each other, not to move feparately, but in common Mafs. Bodies are fixed in different Degrees and Refpects; Firft, Thofe which are diftilled with Difficulty, as the Oils of Vitriol:

Sa

Salt. Secondly, Those which remain fixed in the Fire, without any considerable Decrease, as the Calxes of Lead and Tin, Cerufs of Antimony, the Anti-hecticum Poterii, fixed Salts, Earths and Stones. Thirdly, Glasses are faid to be of all other Substances the most fixed, since they sustain the highest Degree of Fire, and lose nothing of their Substance. Hence, the most penetrating folar Fire either diffipates or vitrifies all Substance except Glafs, which alone can remain in it.

It is obfervable that some Bodies naturally volatile, acquire the greatest Degree of Fixity by an Admixture of other particular Substances. Thus Sulphur, which when kindled and retained in the Fire, totally flies off, by an Addition of fixed vegetable Salts, becomes capable of sustaining the Fire, as we fee in the Liver of Sulphur. Sulphur also mixed with Silver, Iron or Copper, and melted over the the Fire, obstinately adheres to thefe Metals, and cannot be separated from them by any Force of Fire. The most volatile Spirit of Sulphur faturated with fixed Salt of Tartar, conftitutes a Salt, which remains highly fixed in the Fire.

Thus, also, Spirit of Vitriol, or of Sulphur, frequently abftracted from Quick-filver, produces a Coagulum which is not easily diffipated by the Fire, and is called coagulated Mercury.

Sulphur, Sal-ammoniac, and Mercury, are highly moveable Substances, and eafily fly off in the Air; but when duely mixed with each other and fublimed, they leave a reddifh brown Mafs, which refifts the most intenfe Fire, is incapable of being fublimed farther, and is called fixed Cinnabar.

Spirit of Salt eafily flies off into the Air, but when mixed with quick Lime, it is fo fixed as to fuftain the most violent Fufion; for by this Means it is transformed into a fixed Sal-ammoniac.

Spirit of Salt mixed with Chalk, and diftilled with it, ftill remains in the Chalk, and produces a fixed cauftic Salt of the alcaline Kind. Tho' Spirit of Nitre is highly volatile, yet when mixed with any fixed alcaline Salt, it is fixed and becomes a regenerated Nitre, which when diffolved in Vinegar, is not diffipated in the Air by the most intenfe Heat.

It is furprifing, that Coals prepared of Vegetables, if treated with the highest Degree of Fire, in a clofe Veffel, cannot be burnt to Afhes, nor a certain earthy Subftance be feparated from them; whereas if the Air has free Accefs to them, their earthy Portion is foon diffipated and flies off. Lead is by a violent Fire eafily refolved into Smoke, but by the Addition of Flints it is converted into a yellow Glafs, called the Glafs of Lead, which remains fixed in the Fire, and contributes much to facilitate the Fufion of Metals and Minerals.

Antimony, together with its Sulphur and Regulus, as alfo Mercury, when calcined with Earths, burnt Harts-horn, or other Afhes of Animals, fixed Salts, or quick Lime, have fome of their Parts fo fixed as to elude the Force of the greatest Fire. The Fixity of Bodies principally depends on fuch a peculiar Connection, Implication, and Adhefion of their conftituent Corpufcules, that the Motion of the Fire and Air may no longer have any Influence upon them. The Fixity of Bodies, alfo, depends upon the Diffipation of the fluid etherial Matter; for the more of a volatile Matter Subftances contain, the more volatile they are.

CHAP. XX.

Of Fluidity *and* Solidity.

ALL Bodies are either folid or fluid, or compounded of thefe two. The principal Fluids are Air, Water, and the fubtile Æther, with which laft we are very little acquainted. The univerfal Solid is the Earth, but every Fluid is not moift, as Mercury and Air; tho' all Moifture is properly fluid.

Fluid Bodies are not continuous, but contiguous, and confift of fmall moveable Particles actually feparated; fome of which may be moved out of a Place, whilft the others remain in their former Situation.

To conftitute a Fluid it is requifite; Firft, That the Particles be highly minute, and divided from each other. Secondly, That they be of a globular Figure, and have a fmooth Surface; and, Thirdly, That they all have an equal moving Force, whereby they tend downwards if the Fluids are homogeneous; fo that Fluids are always difpofed parallel to the Horizon, and conftitute a Kind of natural Ballance.

The Properties of Fluids are, that they may be compreffed and dilated. Delatation is no more than a Rarefaction, and an Enlargement of the Pores, or an Expanfion of the Fluid to a larger Space. The finer and more thin a Fluid is, the lefs it is capable of Rarefaction or Expanfion, according to *Stbal.* Compreffion is an Anguftation of the Pores, and Reduction of the Parts to a fmaller Space. And, in Compreffion, the highly fubtile Matter is expreffed from the Pores, but in Rarefaction it enters them. All Fluids may, therefore, be either condenfed or fubtilized, by the different Admixture of a fubtile Matter.

Tho' the Parts of Fluids have perpetually a Kind of *Nifus* towards the Center of the Earth, and are confequently poffefs'd of a gravitative Motion, yet every Part is alfo conveyed round its own Center or Axis, which is that Motion, which in a great Meafure conftitutes the Nature of Fluidity, and the greater the Admixture of the ætherial Matter is, and the more fubtile the fluid Particles are, the greater are the inteftine Motion, and Fluidity.

The Parts of Fluids yield in different Directions to any external Impulfe. They have, alfo, an elaftic Motion, by which they reftore themfelves to their former State, when the compreffing Force is removed.

Solid and hard Bodies are fuch as confift of grofs Parts, not actually divided, but cohering with each other by their Ramifications. Whence if one Part is removed from its Place, all the others are moved at the fame Time.

But Hardnefs does not confift in this, that the hard Particles remain at reft by each other, as *Des Cartes* imagined; for the Particles of Sand remain at reft by each other, tho' they do not conftitute one continued hard Body. But what is principally requifite to Hardnefs is, that the Particles fhould not be regular and fmooth, but fo furprifingly angular and ramified, that they on Account of a Sort of concatenated Structure, cannot be divided without Difficulty.

Fluid

Fluid Bodies are more active than those of the solid Kind, which are of a more passive Nature. Fluids, as they are disposed to an intestine Motion, and fit for undergoing all Kinds of Motion, induce Changes in Solids, and become most apt to alter their Texture, as is obvious in Air, Fire, and Water. When the Parts of Fluids are agitated round their own Axis or Center, they easily divide Solids into their most minute Parts, which becoming specifically lighter than the Fluid itself, are received into its Pores, and constitute one seemingly homogeneous liquor. The Solution, or Fluidity, of solid Bodies is obtained by Fluids, when their Parts are in an intestine Motion, and at the same Time, by their Gravity and Elasticity penetrate into the most minute Interstices of the Solids, from which they expel the ætherial Fluid, divide the Parts from each other, and at last receive them into their Pores. Hence in every Solution Bubbles rise, and Heat often produced.

The smaller Parts a Body is divided into, the more its Surface is enlarged; whence the smaller the Particles of Bodies are, the more easily they ascend, and are detained in the Pores of Fluids, on account of their greater Surface.

A certain Proportion between the Solvent and Solvend is always requisite. Thus one Ounce of Camhire requires at least two Ounces of a Menstruum. Thus, also, a certain Quantity of *Aqua-Fortis* only dissolves a certain Portion of Silver; and a certain Quantity of Water, a certain Portion of Salts.

When in a Fluid there is every where an equal Pressure and Resistance, and when this Fluid is every where equally acted on by another heterogeneous Fluid, it easily acquires a round Figure, as is observed of Mercury.

The Hardness or Solidity of Bodies, arises from the Dissipation of the Fluid, or the Expulsion of the ætherial Matter from their Pores. Hence a Reason may be easily assigned, why, when Salts are dissolved in Water, and the Humidity dissipated by Heat, they again acquire a solid Form.

As Heat rarifies the Pores, so Cold renders Bodies more firm and hard, by constricting their Pores, as is observable in Water converted into Ice. Oils, especially of the expressed Kind, and such as abound with volatile Salts, as the Oils of Anise, Mint, and Caraway, as also all aqueous Liquors, easily acquire a solid Form in a cold Air. Hence the Reason is obvious, why the Precipitations of Salt, or of resinous Substances, from their Menstruums, are most easily performed in the Cold; and why Gums, such as Opium, Bdellium, and Aloes are easily reduced to a Powder in Winter, but with Difficulty in Summer. Rigid, acid, and angular Parts, easily induce a Coagulum in thick Fluids; thus the White of an Egg is coagulated by Alum; Milk and Blood by the acid Spirit of Salt, and by a Solution of Sublimate, because Fluidity consists in the spherical Figure of the Parts, and their Division by an intestine Motion: But rigid, angular Particles being unfit for Motion and heavy, not only stop this intestine Motion, but join themselves with oleous and mucilaginous Substances, whence happens a Precipitation of the thick from the liquid Parts, and consequently a Coagulation.

The intestine Motion in thick Fluids is augmented by Conquassation; or by the Addition of fixed or volatile Alcalies, or of aqueous Liquors, they become more fluid. Thus the Blood becomes the more fluid and frothy, the more it is shaken.

I 3   CHAP.

CHAP. XXI.

Of FUSION *and* LIQUIFACTION.

FUSION is the Reduction of folid Bodies into a State of Fluidity, by Means of Fire.

Solid Bodies whofe Parts cohere, are at reft, and, as it were, interwoven with each other, become fluid, by Means of an igneous Motion, which is the moft rapid, and violent Agitation of the highly moveable, etherial Matter, procuring an inteftine Motion to the folid Parts, in which the very Nature of Fluidity confifts. But when thefe igneous Particles fly off, or when the igneous Motion ceafes, the inteftine Motion of fluid Bodies, and confequently their Fluidity, is deftroy'd, fo that they acquire their former Solidity.

As Cold renders Bodies firm and confiftent, by hindering their inteftine Motion, and making their Parts approach to the Center, fo Heat or Fire, by relaxing their Pores, producing an inteftine Motion of their Parts, and propelling them from the Center to the Circumference, procures the Fluidity or Liquifaction of Bodies Among folid Bodies fome are more, and fome lefs difpos'd to become fluid; for fuch Subftances as confift only of a fimple and unactive Earth, deftitute of all Salt, Sulphur, and aqueous Principles, are either fus'd with Difficulty, or abfolutely incapable of fuch a Change. But the more any Subftance contains of a faline, fulphureous, or mercurial Earth, the more eafily they are fus'd and liquified. All Stones calcin'd by the higheft Degree of Fire, fo as to be reduc'd to a Calx, as quick Lime, calein'd Coral, calcin'd Shells, calcin'd Flints, Emeralds, and Jacynths, cannot be rendered fluid by the moft violent Degree of Fire, even that of the folar Kind collected by Glaffes not excepted.

The folid Parts of Animals, fuch as Bones and Shells of Eggs reduc'd to a Calx, can be fus'd by no Degree of Fire, except that of the folar concentrated Kind, obtain'd by a large convex Glafs, which with Difficulty produces the defign'd Effect.

All the Species of Talc, Amianthufes, Mufcovy Glafs, Clays, Boles, and fandy Earths, becaufe they have in their Compofition a fubtile, faline and etherial Principle, may be fus'd or vitrified, but only by a folar, or moft intenfe Degree of Fire.

Among Metals, thofe fus'd with the greateft Difficulty are: Firft, Iron: Secondly, Copper: Thirdly, Gold: Fourthly, Silver: Fifthly, Lead: And Sixthly, Tin.

Calcin'd metallic Subftances, as alfo, metallic Ores abounding with a fulphureous Acid, are not fus'd without great Difficulty; but they fly off by the Application of the moft intenfe folar Heat.

The Fufion of folid Bodies is furprifingly promoted by the Addition of Salts, or Sulphurs; for which Reafon, all Earths, Stones and Calxes, may be vitrified by Means of alcaline or neutral Salts.

Some Metals not to be fus'd without Difficulty, fuch as Iron, Gold,

and

and Copper, are eafily melted by the Addition of alcaline Salts, or fuch as contain a fulphureous vegetable Earth, as Salt of Tartar, Pot-Afh, and the black Flux Powder.

Iron Ores are fus'd by the Addition of quick Lime, and Charcoal, which is of great Efficacy both in the Calcination, and Fufion of metallic Ores, becaufe it abforbs the acid, fulphureous, and vitriolic Particles, which prevent their Fufion or Fluidity.

All metallic and mineral Subftances, that have been fubjected to the Action of acid, or fulphureous Spirits, are not without Difficulty reduc'd to Metals; but when Charcoal and Nitre are added, the defired Effect is fpeedily produced, becaufe the alcaline Earth of the Coal abforbs the fulphureous Acid, which is at the fame Time kindled by the Nitre, and with it carried off into the Air.

'Tis fomewhat curious, that mineral Sulphur difpofes fome Metals, not render'd fluid without Difficulty, to an eafy Fufion; and in procuring to others eafily fus'd, a great Refiftance to the Influence of the Fire. Thus Sulphur added to Silver, or Iron, confiderably promotes their Fufion; for an ignited Bar of Iron melts into Drops, upon the Application of mineral Sulphur to it; whereas Sulphur mix'd with Lead or Tin, fo deftroys their Difpofition to Fluidity, that the moft intenfe Fire is requifite to their Fufion.

All metallic Ores which contain a large Quantity of Sulphur, ought to be previoufly calcin'd in a gentle Fire, before their Fufion is attempted; for by this Means, their Fufion is render'd much more eafy than it would otherwife have been.

Pinguious Subftances united with alcaline Salts, and all Sorts of Soaps, difpofe Metals, metallic Ores, and Calxes to an eafy Fufion; partly becaufe they unite with the Sulphur, and partly becaufe they confume and temperate the arfenical, rigid Acids, which hinder Fluidity. Fufory Fires differ in this, Firft, That the folar Fire fufes in a fhort Time, whereas a Coal Fire requires a longer Time. And Secondly, becaufe by the folar Fire, all Metals reduc'd to Calxes, Minerals, or earthy Subftances, which have a Sulphur, or a Salt intimately mix'd with them, are, after Liquifaction, render'd volatile, and carried off into the Air, which by no Means happens with a Coal Fire.

C H A P. XXII.

Of I N C O R P O R A T I O N.

INCORPORATION confifts in the Mixture of certain Subftances that will not fpontaneoufly unite together. The Incorporation of Metals, and dry fufible Subftances, is brought about by Fufion, and fometimes by Amalgamation. Liquids are fometimes incorporated by Agitation, Digeftion, or Circulation; Liquids and Solids, by Solution. But what is ufually meant by this Term is, the Union of two Liquids, of themfelves incapable of Mixture, by Means of a third Subftance added to them. Thus Syrups and Oils will not fpontaneoufly unite;

nite; but if a due Portion of Sugar, Salt, or any Thing else capable of destroying their Viscidity, be first rubb'd with the Syrup, and the Oil be then gradually dropp'd into the Syrup, they will then unite, and form a Substance which is call'd an *Eclegma*, or *Linctus*, of a thicker Consistence, than either the Oil or Syrup separately. Thus, also, Balsams and Turpentines, which alone will not mix with an aqueous Liquor, are brought to unite with it, if the Balsam or Turpentine, is previously mix'd with the Yolk of an Egg. Tho' I am far from thinking, that this Treatment, in either Instance, imparts any additional Virtue to the Medicine. Other Methods of Incorporation are taken Notice of under the Article of Menstruums.

CHAP. XXIII.

Of PRECIPITATION.

PRECIPITATION is a Dejection of the Particles of a solid Body, from the Pores of a fluid, so as to make them subside to the Bottom. That which causes the Precipitation, is call'd, the *Precipitant*; whereas, that which falls to the Bottom, is call'd the *Precipitate*, or *Magistery*.

There are various Causes of this Dejection, from the Pores of a Fluid. The first of these Causes is, that the Menstruum in which a solid Body is dissolv'd, more readily lays hold of the Precipitant, than the dissolv'd Body; so that whilst the Solvent endeavours to dissolve the Precipitant, the Particles lodg'd in the Pores of the Menstruum must necessarily be precipitated thence, because two Bodies cannot possibly exist in the same Place, at the same Time. Thus common Salt, or a Solution thereof, precipitates Silver, Mercury, or Iron, dissolv'd in Aqua Fortis, or Spirit of Vitriol. And, indeed, whatever is dissolv'd in Spirit of Vitriol, may be precipitated by the Addition of common Salt. Iron precipitates Copper from Spirit of Nitre, or from any acid Menstruum, because Acids more readily dissolve Iron than Copper.

Silver dissolv'd in Spirit of Nitre, or Aqua Fortis, is precipitated by the Addition of Copper, because the Spirit of Nitre more readily dissolves Copper, than Silver, which must, for that Reason, necessarily be precipitated. Mercury dissolv'd in Aqua Fortis, is precipitated by Zinc, or Bismuth; because, the Bismuth is much more easily dissolv'd in the Aqua Fortis than the Mercury.

All Metals dissolv'd in acid, corrosive Menstruums, are precipitated by the Addition of alcaline Bodies, and alcaline Salts, because Acids quickly unite with alcaline Substances.

Another Cause of Precipitation is, when the solvent Liquor intimately mixes with the added precipitating Liquor, so as to produce a Third, which is no longer fit to retain the Body before dissolv'd in its Pores. Thus all resinous and sulphureous Substances, distill'd Oils, and resinous Gums, dissolv'd in rectified Spirit of Wine, are precipitated by the

the Affusion of common Water, by which Means the Mixture becomes not only turbid, but also whitish, if the Refin is pure: By this Means Refins are prepar'd, whilst the Spirit of Wine extracts the refinous Parts, which afterwards being precipitated, coalesce and constitute refins. Thus the Refins of Storax, Aloes Wood, Ladanum, Guaiacum, Jalap, and Scammony, are generally prepar'd in the Shops.

The Reason of this Precipitation is, because the best rectified Spirit of Wine, intimately and quickly mixes itself with the aqueous Particles, which are very congruous to its Pores, so that the refinous Parts lodg'd in the Pores of the rectified Spirit of Wine, are precipitated thence.

An Example of this Kind of Precipitation, we have in the Precipitation of Milk, Blood, and the gelatinous and glutinous Parts of Animals, by Means of highly rectified Spirit of Wine, because the rectified Spirit of Wine readily unites with the Water, which is, also, generally the Vehicle of the Spirit, so that the gross and solid Parts lodg'd in the Pores of the Fluid, must necessarily be precipitated to the Bottom, where uniting, they often form a firm and solid Mass.

Volatile Salts dissolv'd in Phlegm to the Point of Saturation, or all volatile urinous Spirits prepar'd with Water, and well saturated, are precipitated by the Addition of highly rectified Spirit of Wine.

Another Example of this Species of Precipitation is, when Spirit of Nitre, or *Aqua Fortis*, are pour'd upon Butter of Antimony; for the Spirit of Salt in the Butter of Antimony, intimately unites with the Spirit of Nitre. Hence a Precipitation, and some Time after a violent Effervescence is produc'd; because from these Spirits is generated

an *Aqua Regia*, which violently dissolves the antimonial Part. Thus, also, Silver dissolv'd in Spirit of Nitre, is precipitated by the Addition of Spirit of Salt; and Silver dissolv'd in *Aqua Fortis*; is precipitated by Spirit of Vitriol; for these Spirits mix with each other, and afterwards produce an incongruous *Menstruum* for Silver.

A third Cause of Precipitation is, when the *Precipitant* imparts an additional Weight to the Corpuscules dissolv'd in the Menstruum, so that they can be no longer sustain'd in the Fluid. Thus the Solutions of Galls, Essences of Aloes Wood, Tormentil, Peruvian Bark, Japan Earth, and Infusions of Orange and Pomegranate Peel, precipitate Solutions of Vitriol, and all Tinctures of Iron, in which they produce an inky Colour. All aqueous Gums, as Gum Tragacanth, Gum Arabic, and Cherry Tree Gum, are precipitated by Acids, because Acids joyn'd to the gummy Parts, coagulate the Particles, and thus produce a Precipitation.

All Acids precipitate Milk, Blood, Serum, and Emulsions of various Kinds; because the Particles of Acids joyn'd with the oleous Parts of these Substances, not only increase their Weight, but also procure a closer and stronger Union between them; whence arise a Coagulation and Precipitation.

All astringent Liquids, consisting of an Acid, and an earthy Principle, for the same Reason coagulate Milk, Serum, and Blood. On this depends the Operation of Styptics, and such Medicines as stop violent Hæmorrhages. A Solution of Alum precipitates almost all vegetable Juices; by which Means, the Magisteries of Herbs are obtained; when, for Instance, this Solution of Alum is pour'd upon their Juices; for the heavy and earthy Particles of the

the Alum, adhering to the alcaline and gummy Parts of the Vegetables, render them heavier; in Consequence of which they subside, and quit the Pores of the Menstruum.

Ising-glass dissolv'd in Water, clarifies turbid Wine, and the same Effect is produc'd by Litharge. The Reason is, that when the sulphureous and earthy Particles lodg'd in the Pores of the Wine, and preventing its Clearness, intimately unite with the gummy Parts of the Ising-glass, they have their Weight by this Means increas'd, and fall to the Bottom.

Spanish Wine may be clarified and rendered pellucid, by an Addition of Milk; for when the spirituous Particles mix with the aqueous Parts of the Milk, the caseous and earthy Parts fall to the Bottom, and carry with them the thick and viscid Parts of the Wine.

Sugar dissolv'd in Water precipitates Ink, because a Solution of Sugar, as being heavy, tends to the Bottom, and carries with it the Chalybeate and earthy Particles lodg'd in the Ink.

The heaviest Mercury added to Solutions of Metals, precipitates those Metals, because the metallic Particles amalgamate themselves with the Mercury, and are with it carried to the Bottom.

A fourth Cause of Precipitation is, the Narrowness of the Pores of the Menstruum, for it is sufficiently known, that Cold precipitates dissolv'd Substances; because the cold Air operates partly by diminishing the Pores of the Fluid, partly by preventing the Motion of Fluidity, and partly by moving the Particles from the Circumference to the Center, by which Means the dissolved Corpuscules are united and subside. This is the Reason why various Kinds of Salts dissolved in Water to a sufficient Degree of Satura-

tion, when exposed to the cold Air, are precipitated and crystallized, whilst the plain Filaments of the Salts are firmly joined together, and constitute a firm crystalliform Substance.

It is remarkable, that various Tinctures, Solutions, and Essences, as the Tinctures of Sulphur, *Zwelfer*'s Tincture of Mars, a Solution of the Vitriol of Mars, and the Essences of Myrrh, and Gum-ammoniac, are rendered turbid, and precipitated in the Winter Time, or when the Weather is very cold.

All alcaline Substances, together with all Metals and Minerals, dissolved in an acid Menstruum, are precipitated by alcaline Salts; as for Instance, by Oil of *Tartar per Deliquium*, a Solution of Pot-ash, Lime-Water, the Liquor of fixed Nitre, and by all the fixed Salts of Vegetables; for the *Alcali* unites with the Acid, and both together become a neutral Salt.

All Substances dissolved in acid Menstruums are precipitated by volatile urinous Salts and Spirits, as the Spirit of Sal-ammoniac, and the volatile Salts of Harts-horn, or of Urine.

A Solution of Mercury precipitated with Oil of *Tartar per Deliquium*, yields a reddish Magistery, or *Turpeth Mineral*. But when it is precipitated with Spirit of *Sal-ammoniac*, a Magistery as white as Milk is produced.

Hence 'tis obvious, that volatile Salts added to precipitated Substances induce a different Quality and Alteration, than when they are precipitated by fixed Salts.

All Kinds of Sulphurs, together with resinous and oleous Bodies, dissolved in alcaline Menstruums, whether volatile or fixed, are precipitated by all Kinds of Acids, as Vinegar, Solution of Tartar, the Spirits of Salt, Vitriol, and Alum.

Sul-

Sulphureous Bodies diſſolved in lixivial Menſtruums, are precipitated by thoſe neutral Salts, in which an Acid predominates; by the Solution, for Inſtance, of Nitre, Lead, Coal, Sal-ammoniac, and Vitriol, but not by common Salt, vitriolated Tartar, and the Arcanum duplicatum; becauſe in theſe the Acid is firſtly united with the Alcali, but more looſely in the other earthy Bodies.

Alcaline or metallic Subſtances precipitated, are called Magiſteries, eſpecially if they are of a whitiſh Colour. But it is to be obſerved, that Magiſteries are always heavier than the Bodies themſelves before the Solution, which ſufficiently evinces, that the Menſtruum and *Precipitant* intimately add ſome Particles to the Subſtances precipitated; for which reaſon Magiſteries are not ſo much eſteemed in Medicine, as the Subſtances themſelves, prepared, and reduced to a Powder.

All alcaline Subſtances and fixed Salts, without Solution diſſolve mineral Sulphur, and by this Means precipitate the Metal detained by it.

On this depends the Method of obtaining the *Regulus* from Antimony, of ſeparating Metals from their Ores, of reducing Calxes and Magiſteries to their former Subſtances, and of reviving Mercury coagulated under various Forms.

All the Calxes of Minerals prepared with an Acid, or with Fire, may be reduced to the former Metals by Means of Nitre and Charcoal, or fixed Nitre. In this Manner *Mercurius Vitæ*, diaphoretic Antimony, Ceruſs of Antimony, the Anti-hecticum Poterii, the Magiſtery of Lead, Minium, the Flowers of Antimony, and the Magiſtery of Biſmuth, are reduced to their original metallic Bodies.

The mercurial reguline Part of Antimony is precipitated either by fixed alcaline Salts of all Kinds, which unite with and detain the Sulphur, or by metallic Bodies of an alcaline Nature, ſuch as Iron or Copper.

All metallic Ores containing Sulphur, when treated in a dry Manner with Charcoal, Nitre, fixed and eſpecially oleous Salts, precipitate the Metal contained in them.

CHAP. XXIV.

Of PUTREFACTION.

PUTREFACTION is an inteſtine Motion of mixed Subſtances, intimately deſtroying the Craſis and Union of the Parts which conſtitute ſuch a Mixture. Hence it changes the Texture, and together with it, the Colour, Smell, Taſte, and all the Qualities. The Subjects of Putrefaction are Animals, and all their Parts, as alſo Vegetables.

All thoſe Subſtances which conſiſt of heterogeneousParticles, a large Quantity of ſulphureous, ſubtile Earth, but a ſmall Portion of Acid, ſuch as the Bodies of Animals, are highly diſpoſed to Putrefaction. But no homogeneous Bodies, ſuch as diſtilled and expreſſed Oils, inflammable Spirits, Metals, Minerals, reſinous Subſtances, Acids, and earthy Bodies,

dies, are fubject to Putrefaction.

Moifture and Heat, grealy promote Putrefaction. Hence, all Bodies which putrify, whether of the animal or vegetable Kind, muft be moift, fince by this. Means the heterogeneous Parts are diffolved, and the more expeditioufly fubjected to the Motion of the ethereal Fluid. Hence animal and vegetable Subftances, when fo dried as to be totally deprived of their Moifture, are no longer fubject to Putrefaction.

A moift and temperate Heat is highly neceffary to Putrefaction, becaufe it affifts the inteftine Motion, and confequently the Putrefaction of the mixed Body. Hence the more intenfe the Cold is, the more effectually it prevents Putrefaction, by refifting the inteftine Motion of the Parts of Bodies, and conftricting and condenfing their Pores more effectually. The free Accefs of the Air is abfolutely neceffary to Putrefaction, for which Reafon Bodies do not putrify *in Vacuo,* or in Places from which the Air is fecluded.

All fpirituous Subftances deprived of their Phlegm, as, alfo, diftilled Oils, and liquified Refins, furprifingly prevent the Corruption and Putrefaction of Bodies. Firft, Becaufe they render them hard, by imbibing and carrying off the Moifture they contain. Secondly, Becaufe they prevent the Accefs of the Air into their Pores; and Thirdly, Becaufe as being homogeneous Bodies, they are not themfelves difpofed to Putrefaction.

Lixiviums impregnated with Salts, efpecially of the neutral Kind, preferve Bodies from Putrefaction, partly by rendering their Texture more firm and folid, and partly becaufe they are abfolutely unfit for undergoing Putrefaction themfelves.

A Body already in a State of Putrefaction, eafily produces the fame Condition in another before free from it; becaufe the former having an inteftine Motion excited in its Parts, readily communicates the fame to the latter; which however muft be fufficiently difpofed to fuch an inteftine Motion.

Every putredinous Fermentation yields a volatile Salt, tho' of the fetid Kind. Hence all putrified Infects and Animals, in Diftillation yield a volatile Salt, which is highly fetid. Worms and other Species of Animalcules are, alfo, frequently generated from Putrefaction; becaufe the inteftine Motion in the putrifying Matter, by producing a fimilar one in the Ova or Eggs, gives Rife to the Production of thefe Animals.

CHAP. XXV.
Of SUBLIMATION.

SUBLIMATION may be call'd a dry Diftillation, perform'd in a clofe Veffel, with a violent Degree of Heat, by which fome Bodies divided into extremely fubtile Parts, are elevated in the Form of Flowers, without having their Texture deftroy'd. The principal Subftances among Vegetables, fubjected to this Procefs, are Camphire and Benzoin;

kmein; among Animals, their volatile Salts. Sal Ammoniac not only flies very easily itself, but also carries along with it many other Bodies, which when alone are fix'd, and incapable of being sublim'd; and hence by the Chymists it is call'd *the Eagle*. Sulphur and many sulphureous Minerals, are capable of Sublimation themselves, and render many other Bodies, which alone will not sublime, volatile. Hence the great Art of separating Metals from their Ores consists in destroying the mineral Sulphur contain'd in them, which carries away the metallic Particles, when subjected to a sufficient Degree of Fire, instead of fusing them.

Sublimation is frequently perform'd in Glass Vessels of various Sorts; as in a Body fitted with a blind Head, that is, one without an Orifice or Beak on the Side, that the Matter in the Body may be confin'd and collected in the Head; or in a common Matrass, or a Florence Flask; or in Vessels made on Purpose, call'd *Subliming Vessels*. Sometimes earthen Vessels are employ'd. But *Stahl* recommends as the most commodious two very large Crucibles, the one inverted up-

on the other and closely luted together. The lowermost is expos'd to a naked Fire, and the Uppermost receives the sublim'd Matter. This Method is very convenient, when a great Heat is requir'd.

Sometimes Aludels are made Use of. Many of these are generally employ'd at the same Time in the following Manner: The Matter to be sublim'd is put into a Body, or Pot, the superior Part of which is fitted into a Hole on the lower Part of an Aludel, and the superior Part of the Aludel is received into the inferior Part of the next Aludel, and so on, till as many Aludels are set one upon another, as the Process requires; to the superior Part of the uppermost Aludel, a Head or Alembic is fix'd, to receive the Matter which sublimes. So that there is a continu'd Tube form'd by the Aludels, from the Pot which contains the Matter to be sublim'd, to the Head or Alembic which receives it, in the Manner that a continued Channel is form'd by a Number of Elm Pipes. The Use of Aludels seems to be, to remove the Matter sublim'd in the Head, to a Distance from the Fire.

CHAP. XXVI.

Of SULPHUR *and* INFLAMMABILITY.

SULPHUR is a mix'd Body consisting of acid, aqueous, and gross earthy Parts, and a subtile etherial Earth, which is highly dispos'd to take Flame; and that an Acid enters the sulphureous inflammable Substance, is sufficiently obvious from many Experiments; for

every mineral Sulphur, whether dug pure, or adhering to Portions of Ore, when kindled emits an acid Spirit, which is the Reason why Sulphurs are absorb'd and dissolv'd by Alcalies, whether moist or dry, because the Acid intimately unites with the Alcali. Among Vegetables,

bles, all Woods, Refins, and Gums, which are inflammable, when diftill'd, yield an acid Spirit.

The diftill'd Oils have not a predominant and difengag'd Acid, yet that they retain fome Degree of Acidity in their Receffes, is fufficiently certain, fince when mix'd with an alcaline Salt, and expos'd to a long protracted Digeftion, they are converted into a volatile Salt, whilft the alcaline Salt affumes the Nature of a neutral Salt, or of a vitriolated Tartar.

All expref's'd Oils and Fats, when diftill'd with alcaline Subftances, become highly penetrating, as is obvious from diftill'd human Fat, the *Oleum Philofophorum,* and the Oil of Soap; becaufe the acid Water and groffer Earth remain in the alcaline Body, whilft the more fubtile, etherial, faline and fulphureous Parts are difengag'd and exalted. That highly rectified Spirit of Wine, which is nothing but an Oil fubtiliz'd, and refolv'd in Phlegm by Fermentation, contains an Acid, is fufficiently obvious, becaufe it reduces volatile Salts to Cryftals, which are never produc'd without an Acid. Befides, highly rectified Spirit of Wine generally corrodes Lead and Tin into a white and fweetifh Calx. And that every Thing which affords an inflammable Spirit is generated from an Acid, is fufficiently obvious from unripe Grapes, Apples, and other Fruits.

That a mineral Acid enters the Compofition of Sulphur is fufficiently certain from its artificial Regeneration; for when Oil of Vitriol is mix'd with Oil of Turpentine, and diftill'd in a Retort, a Subftance exactly refembling mineral Sulphur, in its Effects, Colour and Smell, is fublim'd into the Neck of the Retort: Or, which is ftill plainer, when the Spirit of Sulphur, or the

acid Spirit of Vitriol concentrate in a fix'd Salt, is mix'd with an fulphureous Vegetable, or even ani mal Earth, fuch as Coals or Soot a perfect Liver of Sulphur is pro duc'd, which when diffolv'd, an precipitated by the Acid of Wine conftitutes a Milk of Sulphur which is nothing but a perfect an inflammable Sulphur.

The pinguious Earth of Animal impregnated with the univerfal Acid and pinguious Salts, as Pot-Afh impregnated with the aerial Salt conftitute Nitre, which is an in flammable Salt, if a fulphureou Earth is added to it, that this Earth by faturating the fuperfluous Acid may produce an inflammable Sub ftance.

A true mineral Sulphur is pro duc'd from Antimony diffolv'd i diluted *Aqua Regia;* for the ful phureous Earth in the Antimony upon the Approach of the Acid, i transform'd into a true inflammable Sulphur.

That Water is, alfo, an Ingre dient in Sulphur is fufficiently ob vious, from Fats, expref's'd Oils, an rectified Spirit of Wine; for the Water refifts the Conception o Flame, which it rather extinguifhes and if it is mix'd in a due Propor tion with an etherial phlogiftic Earth, and a fubtile acid Salt, i proves the Occafion why the Flame is not foon diffipated, bu lafts the longer. Thus we fee di ftill'd Oils, which contain a fmal Quantity of Water, are very foon diffipated by Flame. But in recti fied Spirit of Wine the Flame laft longer, becaufe in it there is hardly a thirtieth Part of the diftill'd fubtile Oil, whilft all the other Parts ar aqueous. Befides, expref's'd Oil and Fats, which contain a large Quantity of Water, fuftain the Flame longer than if they were di ftill'd and depriv'd of their Phlegm

I

It is, alfo, certain from Experience, that Oils burn longer by an Addition of Water.

That an earthy Principle is, alfo, found in the Compofition of Sulphurs, is certain from their Soot; for all Oils and Fats emit an oleous, black, and earthy Soot; which, alfo, holds true of the finer diftill'd etherial and fpirituous Oils.

Camphire, according to Mr. *Boyle*, is by Flame almoft all converted into a black, inodorous, and infipid Soot. It is obfervable farther, that a great deal of Earth may be extracted from exprefs'd and diftill'd Oils, when by mixing them with Spirit of Nitre, or Oil of Vitriol, a Refin is form'd, which, when deflagrated, or rather diftill'd, leaves a copious Earth in the Retort.

It is, alfo, remarkable, that the etherial Oils of Amber and Juniper, when diftill'd by themfelves, always leave a certain vifcid earthy Magma, whilft the fine fpirituous Oils fly off. The more thin and fubtile this Earth is, the more volatile, hot, and fit for conceiving Flame are the Oils; and the grofler the Earth is, the more fix'd the Oils are, tho' they do not take Fire fo foon, but retain it longer. This Earth is of an alcaline Nature, which is the Reafon why Oils, whether exprefs'd or diftill'd, as, alfo, highly rectified phlogiftic Spirits, produce a confiderable Effervefcence, and an intenfe Heat, with acid, fuming and concentrated Spirits, fuch as concentrated Spirit of Nitre, and fuming Spirit of Salt. This is, alfo, the Reafon why highly rectified Spirit of Wine generally mitigates and corrects the Acidity of mineral Spirits, as is obvious in the Preparation of fweet Spirit of Nitre, of Salt, or of Vitriol.

CHAP. XXVII.

Of TRITURATION *and* LEVIGATION.

THESE are the two moft fimple Operations in Pharmacy, and are principally employ'd in reducing hard confiftent Subftances to the Form of a Powder. I fhould chufe to fix the Term *Trituration* to the Operation which is perform'd in a Mortar; and that of Levigation, to that which is executed by rubbing or grinding on a Porphyry, or Marble. And in this Senfe, I think, the Terms are generally us'd.

Mortars are generally made of Wood, Marble, Iron, Brafs, Lead, or Glafs; but they muft not be ufed indifcriminately, fince acid and corrofive Subftance, corrode Metals, and if pounded or triturated in metal Mortars are impregnated with the Qualities of the particular Metals, in Confequence of which they can never anfwer the Purpofes for which they were primarily intended; and hard Subftances were away a Part of all Kinds of Mortars, fo that their Qualities muft be in fome Meafure altered by this Means.

It is alfo to be obferved, according to *Quincy*, that in powdering every Preparation, the whole Ingredient, or Ingredients, with all their Parts to be ufed, fhould pafs thro' the Sieve, and be equally mixed before any is ufed, fince thro' a Neglect

glect of this Kind, several Medicines will in different Parts have different Efficacies, according as the most efficacious Parts, being more or less friable, pass the Sieve first, or remain behind; both which Circumstances will render particular Parts of the Medicine either too strong or too weak. Besides, in preparing Medicines of different Textures and Cohesions, some of the Ingredients pass the Sieve much sooner than others; so that there is an absolute Necessity of mixing them carefully after the whole is passed. Thus in powdering Jalap, Ipceacuanha, and other Substances, whose Virtues lie in their most resinous Parts, these being most brittle, break in the Mortar, and pass the Sieve first, in Consequence of which the Patients who use the first, are over-dosed, whilst those who use the last,

which is only the fibrous and woody Parts, are miserably disappointed in their Expectations.

Those Medicines, also, whose Efficacy consists in the peculiar Shape and Points of their component Part are considerably altered by Trituration; for the finer they are powdered the less powerfully they operate Thus Calomel may be rendered much gentler, and consequently capable of being exhibited in far larger Doses, when it is thoroughly triturated in a Glass Mortar; for the continual Trituration has the same Effect upon it as repeated Sublimation, by breaking the saline Spicula till the Medicine becomes almost plain Mercury. But in resinous Substances, especially those of the purgative Kind, this Observation is reversed.

CHAP. XXVIII.

Of VOLATILIZATION.

THOSE Substances are said to be volatile, the Mobility of whose Parts renders them capable of being easily moved upwards, and dissipated in the Air. These Bodies consist of the most subtile, slender, highly divided, and fluid Particles; and as Æther and Air are the most moveable and pure of all Fluids, 'tis hence obvious, that volatile Substances must admit into their Mixture a large Quantity of etherial and aerial Particles. But there are volatile Bodies, which consist partly of an etherial or sulphureous Earth, partly of a saline etherial Earth, and partly of a subtile mineral Earth.

Among those of the sulphureous Kind are; First, Inflammable Spi-

rits, which are nothing but etheri Oils, resolved or subtilized by a fermentative and intestine Motion.

Secondly, Etherial distilled Oil from Aromatic Roots, Seeds, an Resins; the Oils of Cloves, Amber, Juniper, Turpentine, Cinnamon; or the native Oils, as Petroleum.

Thirdly, Empyreumatic Oils extracted by a dry Fire; such as the fetid Oil of Tartar, Oil of Hartshorn, Oil of fossil Coals, and Oil any Wood

The Sulphur of Mineral is highly volatile, so that by a gentle Fire it is raised in a close Vessel, and generally carries along with it considerably heavy, metallic Parts. Saline vol tile Subftances are of two Kinds, either urinous, or acid; the urinous are of all others the moft volatile, and are produced from the animal Kingdom.

The beft of the acid Volatiles are the Spirit of Sulphur, or the volatile Spirit of Vitriol; prepared in the open Fire, in fuch a Manner as that the Air may have Accefs to it. This Spirit in its Volatility, almoft furpaffes the urinous Salts, and flies off by the moft gentle Fire.

Next to thefe are the Spirit of diftilled Vinegar, prepared with the Cryftals of Verdigreafe, efpecially when concentrated by Sugar of Lead; the fuming Spirit of Nitre; and the fuming Spirit of Salt, which can hardly be retained in Glaffes; as alfo Spirit of Nitre, and the volatile acid Spirit of Ants.

Among Minerals confifting of a volatile mercurial Earth, are Arfenic, Quick-filver, Bifmuth, Cobalt, Antimony, and efpecially its Regulus. There are, alfo, various volatile Compofitions. Thus Refins and bituminous Bodies are prepared of acid Subftances and diftilled Oils. Of volatile urinous Salts, and acid Spirits of Salt is prepared a Sal-Ammoniac, which when added to fixed Subftances, Earths, and Metals, renders them volatile. Of Sal-ammoniac and Nitre is prepared a volatile acid Spirit, or fuming *Aqua Regia*.

Of Oil of Vitriol and common Salt is prepared the fuming Spirit of Salt. Of Oil of Vitriol and Nitre is obtained the fuming Spirit of Nitre; and of fublimate Mercury and Tin, is prepared the fuming Spirit of Salt.

The moft fixed Metals may be rendered volatile, by the Addition of volatile Subftances, as is obvious in *Aurum fulminans*, the whole of which flies off when it takes Flame. Thus, alfo, the *Luna Cornua*, which is nothing but a Magiftery of Silver prepared with Spirit of Salt, or with common Salt, flies off in the Fire; as does alfo the *Saturnus Cornuus*, or a Magiftery of Sugar of Lead precipitated with Spirit of Salt. Silver diffolved in Spirit of Nitre, if highly rectified Spirit of Wine is poured upon the infpiffated Solution, is totally evaporated and flies off when Fire is applied to it. The fuming Spirit of Salt drawn off from Gold, Iron, or Copper, carries fome of the metallic Particles along with it. Regulus of Antimony diffolved in concentrated Spirit of Salt, afcends in Diftillation, as we obferved in Butter of Antimony.

By Means of common Sulphur, Metals, and efpecially Silver, fly off in the Air; and mineral Sulphurs may be rendered totally volatile, by Means of volatile urinous Salt.

C H A P. XXIX.

Of L U T E S.

BY the Name of Lute or Luting, Chymifts underftand a fixed, tenacious, ductile Subftance which proves folid with drying,

and, being applied to the Junctures of Veffels, clofes them in fuch a Manner, as to prevent the Air from either getting in or out; but thefe

K

Lutings

Lutings are of principal Use, in confining the Particles rais'd by the Fire in Distillation, so as to prevent their escaping out of the Vessel; and hence it appears, that different Lutings are required, according to the Difference of the Subjects to be distilled.

Boerhaave's Directions for Luting are thus:

" When the Subject is meerly aqueous, Linseed Meal ground to a fine Powder, and well mix'd, or work'd up into a stiff Paste with the White of an Egg, makes a proper Luting; for being applied to the Junctures of distilling Vessels, it grows hard with Heat; and if it happens to crack, it is easily repair'd by a fresh Application, which soon grows solid. But a Paste made of the same Meal well work'd up with cold Water, very well answers the End in the Distillation of all fermented inflammable Spirits, and all volatile alcaline Salts. This Paste will not answer in the Distillation of mild Acids, or acetous Liquors, which soften and dissolve it, so as to let the Fumes escape: In these Cases, therefore, a Bladder steeped in Water till it grows slimy, makes an excellent Luting, by being applied and press'd wet upon the Junctures of the distilling Vessels.

A Luting that acquires a stony Hardness, is necessary in the Distillation of fossile Acids, as those of Vitriol, Sea-Salt, and the like, which is call'd the Philosophical Luting, and may be prepared from the Calx of Copperas, and quick Lime, by boiling the Caput Mortuum of Vitriol, in several Parcels of Water, till it be thus thoroughly wash'd from its saline Parts; then drying the Powder, and preserving it in a close Vessel. This Powder is to be rubb'd with an equal Quantity of strong quick Lime, and wrought into a Paste with the White of Eggs, first

beat thin; and this Luting is immediately to be applied to the Junctures of the Vessels, the Vessels being first a little heated. If it be not applied quick, it presently dries to a stony Hardness, so as to be untractable; but, when properly us'd, it confines all the saline Spirits, like Glass itself. Or, a Luting for the same Purpose may be prepar'd without much Trouble, in this Manner: Beat pure Sand and Potters Clay together, in such Proportion, with Water, till the Matter no longer sticks to the Fingers; then add one fourth Part of common Lime, so as to make the Paste sufficiently strong; and the drier this is applied, the better for the Purpose, provided it be left ductile; for thus it hardens into an excellent Cement, and the Cracks, if any should happen, are easily stopt up with the same.

It is a great Inconvenience in the stronger Distillations with a naked Fire, that, when the Vessels are violently heated, they are subject to crack, and fly to Pieces, upon opening the Door of the Furnace, and letting in the cold Air, or throwing in fresh Fuel; and it is highly proper here to defend the Vessels by a Coating from this sudden Impulse of Cold; and this is frequently necessary, also, when the Operation is perform'd in glass Vessels, and a Sand Heat, if the Fire be so strong as to indanger the Melting of Glass. The best Luting, for this Purpose, is made, by beating fat Potters Earth and powder'd Sand, with Water, into a well wrought Paste, which will not stick to the Fingers, adding thereto a little common Lime at the last, and beating them well together. Then the Vessel to be coated, being warm'd and expos'd to the Vapor of hot Water, that its whole Surface may become dewy, let this Cement be spread all over it equally with the Hand; afterwards sprinkle the Suface of the Coating with hot and dry Sand, and set the Vessel in a cool Place, that the Coating may dry slowly, taking Care to fill up the Cracks in the same Manner, if any should happen in the drying. If thus the Coating should be thoroughly dried, the Vessel will sustain the Action of a violent Fire unhurt.

There is another Kind of Cement, made Use of by some Chymists of London, to answer the same End, consisting of sifted Wood Ashes beat up to due Consistence with the White of Eggs and a little Gum Water. The same Service may be had in a more excellent Manner, as well for crack'd Glasses as broken China, or the like, from what the Painters call drying Oil, or a Mixture of Linseed Oil and Ceruss, made by Insolation or Decoction, into a perfectly white Balsam, and afterwards ground upon a Marble with fresh Ceruse, till the Whole is perfectly fine, and become of the Consistence of an Unguent. This dries slowly, but is very effectual.

The End of the First BOOK.

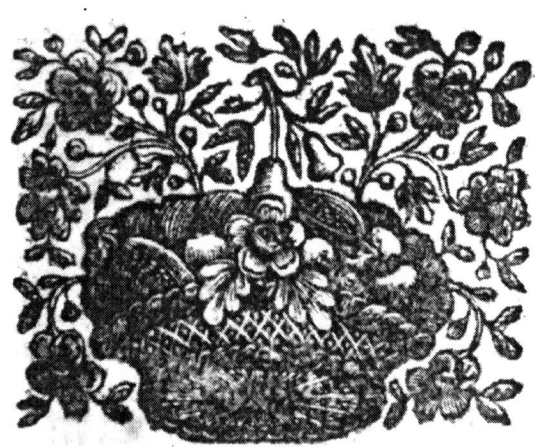

THE NEW
Englijh Difpenfatory.

***

BOOK II.

Of the Operation *of* MEDICINES.

SINCE almoſt the whole Duty of a Phyſician conſiſts in ſeaſonably adminiſtring ſuch Things as are proper to preſerve or reſtore Health, and are effectual to relieve the Sufferings of his Patient, and at the ſame Time in artfully avoiding whatever may be unwholeſome, or prejudicial, it is plain, that nothing is ſo neceſſary to accompliſh theſe Purpoſes to a deſirable Degree of Perfection, as a diſtinct and accurate Knowledge of the Inſtruments by which Health is preſerv'd or reſtor'd: Now this Knowledge ſuppoſes not only an Acquaintance with their Efficacy and Vertues, but, alſo, with their Elements and Manner of Operation; by which Means a Phyſician may be enabled to judge, by ſolid Reaſon, what are the Things, in all the *Materia Medica* which are ſerviceable, or prejudicial, in this or that Diſtemper, to this, or that peculiar Perſon, at ſuch or ſuch a Seaſon, with a due Regard to all other Circumſtances. That he may rightly conduct himſelf in theſe Affairs, and be ready furniſh'd with proper Means to anſwer all Emergencies, nothing ſeems fitter, and more conducive to the Purpoſe, than an artful and compendious Diſtribution of all the *Materia Medica* under certain Heads, according to their Principles, their Way of Operation; and the Effects, which under ſuch and ſuch Conditions, they are adapted to produce.

Medicines may be diſpos'd under their general Heads in a proper and compendious Way, if we conſider, that whatever is ſubſervient to the Ends of Medicine, is directed in its Manner of acting towards the Removal of the Cauſes of Diſeaſes. But in every Diſeaſe there is a Depravation, either in the Motion, or

in

in the Matter which is moved, or even difpofed to move: And fince Motion is exceffive or defective, either in the Whole, or fome Part of it, and Matter is in the Fault either upon Account of its Quantity or Quality, all Remedies, muft, in general, be concerned in the Regulation of depraved Matter or Motion. To Matter vitiated in Quality, we appropriate *Alteratives*; to Matter offending in Quantity, *Evacuants*; if, on the other Hand, Motion is defective, or impair'd, or if the Parts have loft their proper Tone, reftorative and corroborative Medicines are to be us'd; and if the Motion is too intenfe and accelerated, or the Parts wrack'd with Spafms, then and in that Cafe, fedative and compofing Medicines are, of all others, moft efficacioufly adminifter'd.

These are the few general Claffes of Medicines, to which all the Stores, with which indulgent Nature has enrich'd the Art of Phyfic, may be reduced; for by this Means, and by the Affiftance of thefe Helps, all the feveral Intentions of the medicinal Art, may be exactly and effectually anfwer'd. So that *Hippocrates* has given a Definition of Phyfic, which is at once beautiful, and truly mechanical, when he fays that it is, " No more than an Addition and " Subftraction feafonably made; a " Subftraction of thofe Things " which exceed; and an Addition of " thofe Things which are defective. " He who beft can do thefe two " Things, is defervedly efteemed " the beft Phyfician; and the lefs a " Man is qualified for carrying on " thefe two Defigns, the more ig- " norant he is of the true and ge- " nuine Principles of Phyfic." *De Flatibus, Lib.* 3.

Then as to what relates to the Influence and Operation of Medicines, they act directly and immediately, either upon the fluid, or the folid Parts of the Body; fo that the alterative and evacuating Medicines are appropriated to the Fluids, and thofe of a corroborative and compofing Quality to the Solids. But as liquid as well as folid Bodies are of different Qualities, fo they produce their refpective Effects in different Ways; for fome Medicines by their immediate Action, affect the moft fubtle, and eafily moveable Fluid which is lodg'd in the Brain and Nerves, and is the chief Inftrument of Motion and Senfation, either by augmenting its Quantity, or accelerating its Motion: Such as analeptic, cordial, and fragrant Medicines; or by quelling, and becalming its more violent Motions, fuch as anti-hyfteric and anodyne Medicines, Opiates and Fœtids, which even when exhibited in very inconfiderable Dofes, produce very fudden, and almoft inftantaneous Effects. Other Medicines operate immediately upon the Blood and Juices themfelves, fuch as thofe of the diluting, incraffating and attenuating Kinds; and, alfo, fuch as are endowed with an abforbent Quality, or are calculated for fubduing any corrofive or fulphureous Acrimony.

Thofe Medicines which induce a Change upon the Solids, produce their immediate Effects upon the more nervous Parts, as the Stomach and Inteftines, which are endowed with a moft exquifite Senfation. To this Clafs belong all the medicinal Preparations of Minerals, which produce their Effects when given in fmall Dofes, refolve themfelves into Particles of an incredibly fmall Size, without loofing their Texture and Vertues, enter the minuteft Receffes of the nervous Parts, and are with fome Difficulty wafh'd away: Such as, among Emetics, *Emetic Tartar*; among falivating Medicines, *White Precipitate*; among Sulphurs, the *Sulphur of Antimony*; to which volatile Salts may be added; Other Sub-

*ftances

stances strongly stimulate the nervous Parts, by that subtle cauſtic Salt with which they abound; such as among Poiſons, *Arſenic*; among Purgatives, *white* and *black Hellebore*, *Gamboge*, *Reſin* of *Jalap*, and some more of the same Kind, together with all Inſects, eſpecially *Cantharides*. 'Tis nevertheleſs to be obſerv'd, that of Medicines of this Kind, some affect particular nervous Parts more than others; for Inſtance, mercurial Preparations affect the Glands, the Lymphatic Ducts, and the Fauces; Emetic Preparations of Antimony affect the biliary Ducts; Preparations of Colcynth, the nervous Coat of the Inteſtines; Hellebore of Æſophagus, Larynx, and Aſperia Arteria; Cantharides and other Inſects, the nervous, urinary, and ſeminal Ducts; and in fine, oily volatile Salts, and Sudorifics prepared of the volatile Salts of Animals, affect the Coats of the arterial Veſſels. Some others of thoſe Medicines that are appropriated to the Solids, inſinuate their Virtues more effectually into the muſcular and fibrous, than into the nervous and membraneous Parts; among the Number of which are all thoſe Corroboratives which abound with a ſulphureous, or with a mild Aſtringent, fix'd, and earthly Principles.

The whole Body of Medicines in general, is with Reaſon diſtinguiſh'd in this Manner, and in this Manner are we to form our Ideas of their reſpective Methods of acting, and Manner of operating. But as the Art of Phyſic, in Order to become rational, muſt be built upon moſt evident Cauſes, all obſcure ones being rejected, as *Celſus* ſays, not only by the Phyſician, but alſo from the Art of Phyſic itſelf, ſo that particular Branch of Phyſic which diſplays the Vertues of Medicines, and accounts for their Methods of Operation, is to be drawn, not from obſcure and too remote Cauſes, nor from the atomical and geometrical Principles of the Magnitude and Figure of the Parts, which are in reality incomprehenſible; but from Cauſes that are evident, immediate, comprehenſible, ſubjected to our Senſes, and made known by Experience.

CHAP. I.

Of EMETICS.

AMONGST the ſeveral Medicines of the evacuating Kind, *Emetics*, or ſuch as excite Vomiting, are none of the leaſt conſiderable. Theſe are either mild and gentle, or of a more ſtrong and draſtic Nature. Among the former, we may juſtly reckon common Water render'd tepid, with the Addition of a little Salt and Honey, or expreſs'd Oil or Fat; or a Decoction of the Seeds or Root of Horſe Radiſh, or the Seeds of Dill with Water, or the Waters of warm mineral Springs drank in large Quantities at a Time.

Among thoſe of the more violent and draſtic Kind, the vegetable Kingdom ſupplies us with the following. The Leaves and Root of Aſarabacca, white Hellebore, the Juice of the middle Bark of the Elder Tree, Gamboge, Ipecacuanha, and all the draſtic Purgatives exhibited in too large Quantities. Among

Metals

Metals and Minerals, all Preparations of Copper, such as white *Cyprian* Vitriol, the *Gilla* of *Paracelsus*, and *Angelus Sala*, prepared of the *Caput Mortuum* of the Oil of Golfar Vitriol, which partakes of the Nature of Copper; the Cryftals of Verdigreafe, as, also, such Subftances as receive their Emetic Qualities from the reguline Part of Antimony they contain, such as Emetic Tartar, Glafs of Antimony, and the Preparations thereof, the *Mercurius Vitæ*, efpecially when prepared of the rectified Butter of Antimony by Precipitation with common Water, or Oil of *Tartar per Deliquium*; the Golden Sulphur of Antimony, and many others. The milder Emetics, and such as are pretty much of a diuretic Nature, were much ufed by *Galen*, and the Ancients, as they are fafe, and generally by their Quantity, ftimulate the Stomach to vomit, efpecially when it is weak, and difpofed to throw up its Contents, which may be difcover'd by a Naufea, Eructations, Bitternefs of the Mouth, and the uneafy State of the Patient. But thefe do not act beyond the Limits of the Stomach, from which they very advantageoufly evacuate crude, phlegmatic and bilious Humours, produced by improper Aliments, or a bad Digeftion.

The more ftrong and draftic Emetics, when exhibited in a fmall Dofe, by their fiery, cauftic, faline-fulphureous Acrimony, act not only on the nervous Coat of the Stomach and Inteftines, by fpafmodically contracting them, but if exhibited in a fomewhat larger Dofe, they penetrate beyond the Stomach into the highly nervous biliary Ducts, into the Glands of the Inteftines, Myfentery and Pancreas, as also into the Liver, and expel their contain'd Humours from thefe Parts; fometimes, also,

they affect the whole nervous Syftem, and prove highly injurious to the Conftitution.

The Ancients as an Emetic of the moft draftic Kind, us'd white Hellebore, as *Celfus*, in his 13th *Chapter* of his *Second Book*, informs us, in Epilepfies, Madnefs, and other terrible Diforders, when not accompanied with a Fever; but he juftly advifes, that the Body fhould be duly moiften'd, before this Medicine is ufed; but in our Days as we have more fafe Emetics, we juftly abftain from this draftic Medicine, and make Choice of fuch of the abovementioned, as are more friendly to Nature and the nervous Syftem, and may be exhibited with lefs Danger: Among which we may juftly give the Preference to that *American* Root Ipecacuanha, half a Dram or more of which may be exhibited for a Dofe: This Root befides its faline, fubtile, and acrid Principle, also, contains one of a balfamic and corroborating Quality, and has this particular Advantage attending it, that it foon produces its Effects, for which Reafon it is very properly us'd where Delays may be attended with bad Confequences. And becaufe in vomiting the periftaltic Motion of the Stomach, and by Confent that of the Inteftines, is inverted, if the Vomiting is very intenfe in a Diarrhæa or Dyfentery, the Flux is by that Means checked and ftopt for fome Time. Thus *Celfus* juftly affirms, that Vomits ftop Fluxes, and render the Body foluble when coftive. The moft commodious Succedaneum for Ipecacuanha is Afarabacca, the Root and Leaves of which are poffefs'd not only of a fubtile, acrid, volatile and cauftic Principle, which in boiling exhales, but, also, of a corroborating and balfamic Quality, and afford fingular Relief in inveterate Fevers of the

Tertian

Tertian and Quartan Kind, as, alfo, in Dropfies, and the Jaundice. Among antimonial Preparations, we give the Preference to emetic Tartar, prepared of the *Crocus Metallorum*, and not of Glafs of Antimony, which is as ftrong again. Three or four Grains of this Tartar, either alone, or in a fmaller Dofe with Ipecacuanha, prove an excellent Vomit. And if the Intention is to purge, at one and the fame Time, two or three Grains of Emetic Tartar may be added to a Decoction of Manna; and in a pituitous Afthma, this End is fometimes very commodioufly anfwer'd, by two or three Ounces of Oxymel of Squills; but as for the Emetic Preparations of Copper, which by their conftructive Quality long exagitate the nervous Coats of the Stomach, and other Parts, as, alfo, the reguline Powders of Antimony, the Glafs of Antimony, and the *Mercurius Vitæ*, whofe Effects cannot be depended on, fince they act either too ftrongly or too weakly, according to the State and Difpofition of the Humours in the Stomach, we ought carefully to abftain from their Ufe, and may be very well without them in the *Materia Medica*.

Draftic Emetics are fometimes not only ufeful, but abfolutely neceffary, for expelling Poifons, efpecially of the Narcotic Kind, as, alfo, the infectious Particles, which exhale from Patients labouring under contagious Diforders, which defcending to the Stomach, there mix with the Juices, and unlefs foon carried off, are convey'd into the Mafs of Blood. In like Manner, draftic Emetics are neceffary for evacuating the corrupted and peccant Humours arifing from the Commixture of heterogeneous Aliments, the Bile, and fermenting falival Humours, which ftagnating in the Stomach and Inteftines, efpecially the *Duodenum*, become corrupted by their Continuance there, and frequently give Rife to Fevers of the flow, the Quotidian, and Quartan Kind, as, alfo, to chronical Coughs, to violent Diforders of the Head, Melancholy, a Hemicrania, and fometimes to an Epilepfy, or Apoplexy.

In Difeafes arifing from thick Bile, form'd, as it were, into a vifcid Coagulum, and obftructing the biliary Ducts, fuch as the black and yellow Jaundice, a Cachexy, and fome others, Emetics are fometimes ufed with Succefs, when other Medicines prove ineffectual; fince they attenuate the bilious Sordes, which give Rife to thefe Diforders.

In Anafarcas, Leucophlegmatias, Ædematous Swellings of the Parts, and a curable Afcites, Emetics exhibited in a pretty large Dofe, frequently carry off by Stool, but rarely by Vomit, the aqueous Serum from the Liver, and the Ducts and Glands of the Inteftines, Myfentery, and Pancreas.

In all feverifh Paroxyfms, Inflammations of the Stomach, or Cafes where it is affected with Spafms, as for Inftance, in Cordialgias, violent Anger, hyfteric and hypochondriac Spafms, and where there is a Difpofition to Spitting of Blood, or an immoderate Difcharge either by the Menfes, or hæmorrhoidal Veins, as, alfo, in all Difeafes arifing from a Congeftion of Humours to the Head, fuch as Apoplexies, Palfies, Vertigoes, violent Head-achs, a Lofs of Hearing, or Sight, Vomits are never to be ufed; nor are they to be exhibited to plethoric Patients, till the Plethora is remov'd by Bleeding; nor to thofe whofe Inteftines are ftuff'd with Feces, till they are previoufly evacuated, and purged off.

'Tis proper, in order to make Emetics work more eafily, to exhibit them always in a liquid Form, or in a fufficient Quantity of fome moiftening,

ning, relaxing, and pinguious Vehicle; for Vomiting not only requires a powerful Conftriction of the Pylorus, and Bottom of the Stomach, but alfo a Relaxation of the fuperior Orifice of the *Æfophagus.*

During the Operation of Emetics, and after it is over, the Patient is carefully to guard againft Cold, to abftain from cold Liquors, from the fallies of Paffion, from hot and ftimulating Medicines, from acrid and falt Aliments, and rather to ufe fuch as are of a demulcent Nature, afford laudable Juices, and are of eafy Digeftion. It is of fingular Ufe to drink a few Ounces of Affes Milk,

if it can be had, about four Hours after the Operation of the Vomit is over.

It is laid down as a perpetual Rule, by the beft practical Authors, that, in acute Cafes, Bleeding fhould always precede the Exhibition of an Emetic.

Common Salt is given to check the too violent Operation of Emetics, which it does by inclining them to pafs off by Stool. Violent Vomitings, are, alfo, ftopp'd, by copious Draughts of warm diluting Fluids; by mild Oils, by Opiates, Aromatics, grateful Acids, and corroborating Medicines, either taken internally, or applied externally to the Region of the Stomach.

CHAP. II.
Of CATHARTICS.

AMONG the feveral Species of Evacuants, none are of greater Importance than thofe which iminate and difcharge the recrementious and peccant Matter contained in the Body, by Stool; the Medicines of this Kind are either mild and gentle, or ftrong and draftic. Thofe which fafely, mildly, and without any injury to the Stomach, and nervous fyftem, render the Body foluble, are called *Lenitive*, or *Laxative* Medicines, or *Eccoprotics.* Thofe which evacuate the Contents of the Inteftines, in a more efficacious and forcible Manner, come under the Denomination of *Purgatives.* Of the former Kind the principal are, among vegetable Subftances, Manna, Rhubarb, Caffia, Agaric, Tamarinds, Sena Leaves, Aloes, Buckorn Berries, Raifins, Polypody, Peach Flowers, thofe of the *Egyptian* Thorn, as alfo the Flowers and Seeds of Violets. Among Salts, common Salt, Borax, and Nitre; as

alfo thofe obtained from medicinal Springs, fuch as thofe of *Epfom,* and many others. Among Subftances fupplied by the animal Kingdom, Milk, efpecially that of Affes, and Whey. Among chymical Preparations, the Terra foliate Tartari, vitriolated Tartar, Cream of Tartar, a Salt prepared of Alum and Salt of Tartar, the effential Salt of Wood Sorrel, the Magnefia, Sal Polychreftum, Aurum fulminans, Mercurius dulcis, Flowers of Benjamin, as alfo many compound Medicines. Thefe gentle Laxitives, without greatly difturbing or weakening the periftaltic Motion of the Stomach and Inteftines, not only evacuate the Feces, but when exhibited in pretty large Dofes, copioufly difcharge the Serum from the Glands of the Inteftines. Nor, like the more draftic Purgatives, do they operate by an acrid, fubtile, and cauftic Salt, which proves noxious to the nervous Parts, but, by an innocent and harmlefs

Kind

Kind of Subftance, which, however, is of a fine faline, and ftimulating Nature, and which evaporates, and is loft by long boiling, as is obvious from Manna, Rhubarb, Aloes, and Sena Leaves, which for this very Reafon, are more properly infufed than prepared by Decoction. But thefe Laxatives act either by a certain faline and ftimulating but mild Principle, as Manna, Caffia, Raifins, and Polypody; or by a certain fubtile, fulphureous, bitterifh, and earthy Salt, as Aloes, and Rhubarb; or by an acid Salt, which vellicates the Fibres, as Tamarinds, Cream of Tartar, and Salt of Wood Sorrel; or they act by Means of a neutral Salt, as Nitre, Borax, Sal Gemmæ, the Arcanum duplicatum, vitriolated Tartar, Salts obtained from medicinal Waters, and the effential Salts of Herbs; or they operate by Means of a certain calcarious and bitterifh Salt, as the Salts of fome mineral Waters; or, laftly, they act by Means of a calcarious Earth, as the Magnefia, which being diffolved by the Acid of the Primæ Viæ, is converted into a neutral, acrid, and ftimulating Salt.

Thefe highly fafe laxative Medicines, which are of fingular and uncommon Ufe in the Cure of many Diforders, and for that Reafon by fome diftinguifhed by the Epithet *Benedicta,* were little known to the Ancients, in whofe Works we find not the leaft Mention of Aloes, Rhubarb, Tamarinds, Sena Leaves, and Agaric, but only of Caffia and Polypody, among the gentler Purgatives. *Diofcorides* was the firft who wrote any Thing concerning Rhubarb and Aloes, and from him *Pliny* and *Galen* took what they delivered concerning thefe Medicines: But Tamarinds, and Sena Leaves, were firft known to the *Arabian* and *Egyptian* Phyficians. But tho' all Laxatives agree in this, that they render the Body foluble, without Danger, Violence or Commotion, yet in Practice, they ought neceffarily to be diftinguifhed according to the Differences of Difeafes, and the various Conftitutions of Patients. Manna, for Inftance, Caffia, Raifins and Polypody are exhibited with fingular Advantage in Diforders of the Breaft, fuch as a Cough, a Spitting of Blood, a Pleurify and a Phthifis; as alfo in thofe Difeafes which arife from a faline, acrid and fcorbutic Serum, fuch as Gouts, Rheumatifms, Itches and purple Eruptions. In thefe Cafes, the abovementioned Medicines are preferable to others, becaufe they not only difcharge the internal Fæces, but, at the fame time, allay, and correct the faline Acrimony of the Fluids. Gentle Acids, fuch as Tamarinds, Cream of Tartar, Salt of Wood Sorrel, as alfo the effential Salts obtained from nitrous Herbs, Sal Polychreftum, and antimoniated Nitre, are highly proper in hot Climates, and in the Summer-time, for Patients of choleric Habits; as, alfo, in Diforders arifing from too large a Quantity of Bile, and thofe attended with a perternatural Heat, in continued, double, and Summer teritans, as, alfo, in a burning Fever, attended with an infatiable Thirft. In thefe Cafes the Medicines now mentioned are preferable to others, not only on Account of their evacuating Quality, but, alfo becaufe they check the inteftine Motion of the fulphureous Parts of the Blood, and correct the exorbitant Acrimony of the Bile. In Diforders arifing from a Defect of Bile, and the Want of a balfamic Sulphur in the Blood, fuch as Cachexies, and almoft all chronical Diforders, which are attended with an Infpiffation of the Juices, and an Infraction of the Vifcera, bitter Laxatives, fuch as Preparations of Rhubarb and of Aloes duly corrected, are juftly preferable to all other Medicines; but in

Diforde

orders arising from tough and vis-
id Humours lodged in the *Primæ*
iæ, and producing Loss of Appe-
te, Distentions of the Hypochon-
ria, Eructations and Flatulencies,
l neutral Salts, whether chymical-
prepared, or the native Salts of me-
dial Springs, exhibited in a pretty
ge Dose, and with a sufficient
uantity of some proper Liquor,
der the Body *soluble*, and dis-
arge the thick and viscid Recrement. When an Acid, as it gene-
ly happens in hypochondriac and
melancholic Patients, as also those
bearing under quartan Fevers, a-
bounds in the Habit, and eludes the
force of the most acrid Purgatives,
this Case, besides Preparations of
uma, the Magnesia is singularly
beneficial, which, as it is entirely
solved by Spirit of Vitriol, and
les into a neutral Salt of a bitte-
Taste, and purgative Quality, so
assumes the same Virtue and Na-
re, when it meets with an Acid in
Stomach. But, on the contrary,
in a dissolvent Liquor is not found
the Body, it operates little or
e, and proves more injurious than
eficial.

Aurum fulminans and Mercurius
is, are, indeed, generally classed
mong the Laxatives, but their Use
ot altogether safe ; for when Au-
fulminans is thoroughly edulco-
d, its Operation is very languid,
absolutely none at all. On the
rary when it is richly impregna-
with Salino-Nitrous Spiculæ, it
ed renders the Body soluble, be-
e, in Consequence of its Gra-
, it strongly adheres to the Coats
he Stomach, and Intestines ; but
elicate Patients, it excites violent
pes, Flatulencies and other terri-
Symptoms ; besides, it proves
ly prejudicial, where there is a
e Quantity of Acido-corrosive Hu-
rs, or caustic Bile lodged in the
mach or Duodenum. Many, in
r to heighten the purgative Qua-

lity of Aurum fulminans, mix neutral Salts with it, such as the Arcanum duplicatum, or vitriolated Tartar. Nor is it to be denied, that
half a Dram of either of these Salts
triturated with two Grains of Aurum fulminans, acquires a mettal-
line Taste, and, by stimulating the
Intestines, eliminates their Contents ;
but this Effect is rarely produced by
it without Gripes. But we are a-
bove all Things to take Care, that
Mercurius Dulcis, be not triturated
along with Salts, especially those of
an alcaline Nature, or Sal ammoniac, since by this Method of preparing, its corrosive Quality is reviv'd,
by which it acts upon the glandular
and nervous Systems, and often excites a troublesome Salivation.

All the Salts above enumerated,
especially those of the neutral and bitterish kind, when half an Ounce or an
Ounce of them is exhibited for a
Dose, in a sufficient Quantity of
some proper Liquor, are possessed
of a singular Virtue in rendering the
Body soluble, without any Commotion of the Blood, or Loss of the
Appetite and Strength. And they
may be at once more safely and efficaciously used, than the drastic Purgatives obtained from the vegetable
Kingdom, especially in Diseases and
Constitutions, where a large Quantity of thick and viscid Humours
are lodged in the *Primæ Viæ*,
or in the Vessels. Hot and cold mineral Springs, generally called *Acidulæ*, and which are singularly efficacious, both for the Preservation
and Cure of chronical and obstinate
Disorders, derive their aperient, detersive, and purgative Qualities, from
the aqueous, but much more from
the saline Principle they contain.

Among Flowers of a laxative Quality, the most considerable are those
of the *Egyptian* Thorn, Peaches,
Violets, and Roses ; but they ought
to be recent, and be only infused,
but not prepared by Way of Decoction.

coction. Thefe are moft advantageoufly exhibited with fweet Whey, or Affes Milk, efpecially in the Spring; and the Patient, efpecially when delicate and tender, ought every Morning, for fome Weeks, to drink about half a Pint of fuch a medicated Draught, in order to purify his Blood; for both Whey and Affes Milk are poffeffed of a certain laxative Quality, as *Celfus Lib.* 2. *Cap.* 12. thus informs us, " There are " (fays he) certain Difeafes, in which " purging by Milk is highly proper. " And a little after he fubjoins.; " The Ancients, after adding a little " Salt to the Milk of Affes, Cows, " or Goats, boiled it, and remov- " ing the coagulated Parts, ordered " their Patients, in certain Cafes, to " drink the remaining Whey. "

Laxative Preparations of Aloes, either heptic or fuccotrine, are Medicines of uncommon Efficacy, if the Aloes is, by a proper Method, previoufly freed from its prejudical, fulphureous and volatile Principle, and from its Refin, which firmly adheres to the Coats of the Inteftines. But even after thefe Precautions, the Dofe muft be fmall, and mixt up with bitter Extracts, and mild balfamic Ingredients. Pills made upon this Model, may be advantageoufly prefcribed, not only with Intention to render the Body gently foluble, but alfo in order to reftore and corroborate the Tone of the Inteftines, which, being weakened in many Difeafes, is ftill more impaired by the Ufe of draftic Purgatives. And tho' thefe Pills produce but faint and almoft infenfible Effects in Patients of robuft Conftitutions, and fuch as abound with Blood, yet their Operation is more fpeedy and confiderable in Perfons naturally delicate, or fuch as are weakened by the Shock of a Diftemper; as alfo in Child-bed Women, or thofe whofe monthly Evacuations are irregular or obftruc-

ted. For Patients whofe Digeftion is weak, when recovering from any Diforder, they are alfo highly proper, for correcting and evacuating crude Juices; as alfo for hypochondriac Perfons, whofe Stomachs continually throw up acid Crudities. On the contrary, Preparations of Aloe exhibited in large Dofes, and without proper Correctors, throw the Blood into violent Commotions; fo which Reafon plethoric Patients, thofe of delicate Conftitutions, and fuch a are fubject to Evacuations of Blood ought entirely to obftain from them becaufe, when prepofteroufly exhibited, they are attended with this particular Difadvantage, that they excite very painful blind Hæmorrhoides and drive the Blood to the Region of the Loins, and the Parts contained in the Pelvis.

But the Contents of the Inteftine are evacuated in a far more efficacious and powerful Manner, by what we call ftrong *Purgatives.* Of this Clafs the moft confiderable are, the Roots of black and white Mechoacan, of Jalap, of black and white Hellebore, common Flower de Luce Bryony, and Efula, the Herbs, Soldanella, Gratiola, purging Flax, Coloquintida, purging Nuts, the Seed of the Cataputia, Turbith, the middle Bark of Elder, Gamboge, wild Cucumber, and Scammony, together with the Shop Preparations of thofe.

The Principle by which thofe draftic Medicines operate, is of a highly virulent Nature, and the fine cauftic and inflammatory Salt, which in a very fmall Dofe attacks the nervous Membranes, not only of the Stomach and of the Inteftines, but alfo of the whole Body, in the fame Manner Poifon does, act with Violence on thefe Membranes, and generally excite fpafmodic Conftrictions and Uneafinefs of the Præcordia Cardialgias, and Gripes, accompanied with frequent Stools, Hiccup

Inflammations of the Stomach and Intestines, Coldness of the Extremities, and sometimes Convulsions; for that the Salt contained in these Purgatives, is highly subtile and active, and diffuses its Virtue thro' the whole Mass of Humours, is sufficiently obvious from this, that the Child is purged by the Milk of the Nurse who has taken such a Purgative. And sometimes by the external Application only of Purgatives, violent formidable Fluxes have been brought on. Thus *Heurnius* in *Comment. in Hippocrat.* informs us, that the Antients purged themselves by washing their Feet in a Decoction of white Hellebore. *Walæus de Meth. Med.* informs us, that a Piece of Hellebore, used for cleansing an Issue, excited a Vomiting, and proved purgative. And an Ointment in which Coloquintida is an Ingredient, laid upon the Navel, purges not only Children, but also Adults. But the caustic and Inflammatory Nature of strong Cathartics, is sufficiently obvious from this, that, when externally applied, they burn the Skin, and excite Blisters like a Vesicatory. The Juice of the Esula consumes Warts, and the Essence extracted from the drastic Purgatives, such as Jalap, Mechoacan, and Scammony, when swallowed, burns and corrodes the Fauces, and Æsophagus, and excites hot Pustules and Aphthæ. And certainly the virulent and poisonous Quality of drastic Purgatives is sufficiently evinced by the Experiments of *Wepfer*, who in his *Inst. de Cicuta aquatica* informs us, that he gave various Purgatives in a certain Quantity to Whelps, immediately after which, Vomitings, Convulsions, and at last Death ensued. Upon dissecting these Animals, the Stomach and small Intestines were found inflamed, and marked with red Spots, as if they had taken Arsenic: and what deserves our Attention is,

that according to the express Words of the Author, the same Phenomena are exhibited, and the same Effects produced, by the Resin of Jalap, so much used in our Days.

Since, therefore, the Operation of the more acrid and drastic Cathartics is so violent, dangerous, and sometimes fatal, the prudent, rational, and cautious Physician ought seldom to prescribe them. 'Tis sufficiently confirmed by Experience, that in all Ages greater Havock, or more terrible Consequences, have not been produd by any Medicine, than by drastic Purgatives preposterously and unskilfully exhibited. None of the Shop Preparations so quickly and powerfully impair the Strength, change the Pulse, injure the Stomach, or prejudice and disturb the natural Strength thereof, and the Intestines, as acrid and drastic Purgatives. *Hoffman* takes Notice of several Patients who by a frequent and repeated Use of these, have brought on themselves Dropsies, hypochondriac Disorders, Inflammations of the Stomach, accompanied with Fevers which have proved mortal, Dysenteries, a Cholera Morbus, and sometimes a Palsy of the right or left Side. The Antients, indeed, to whom the mild Laxatives, and the Use of the Salts were in a great Measure unknown, frequently prescribed these drastic Purgatives; and *Hippocrates* himself purged his Patients principally with Elaterium, and Hellebore; but if we carefully look into their Works, we find that they did not exhibit these drastic Purgatives, except in Cases where the Danger of the Patient rendered them necessary, and even then they made their Patients drink Milk before and after the Exhibition of the Elaterium, to the Virtues of which they attributed a great deal; and they corrected the Hellebore with an Admixture of Mulsum, Oil, or Milk. Besides, they

they did not promiscuously use these Medicines, but accurately distinguished in what Cases they were proper, and in what not. And *Hippocrates* expresly forbids the Use of them in all Fevers, and inflammatory Disorders. Besides, that the bad Consequences produced by drastic Purgatives were not unknown to the most skilful of the ancient Physicians, is sufficiently obvious from the Precepts and Maxims every where occuring in their Works. This is asserted in express Words, in the 37th *Aphorism* of the *Second Section*, where we are told, " That " those who are in a State of perfect " Health, are speedily reduced to a " deplorable Condition, by being " purg'd." And in the 16th *Aphorism* of the *Fourth Section, Hippocrates* confirms this Truth. *Heurnius,* in his Attempt to demonstrate the Truth of this *Aphorism,* adds, " I " have seen sound and healthy Per- " sons, to whom a simple Purgative " Apozem of Fumitory and Sena " Leaves, rashly exhibited, has pro- " ved fatal." *Celsus,* also, in *Lib.* I. *Cap.* 3. informs us, That as Purgatives are sometimes necessary, so when frequently used, they prove dangerous; and in the 12th *Chapter* of his *Second Book,* he has these Words, " Purgatives generally injure the " Stomach, weaken the Patient, and " are never properly prescribed, ex- " cept in Disorders unaccompanied " with a Fever." *Dioscorides, Lib.* 4. *Cap.* 178. declares himself of the same Sentiments, and affirms, that Purgatives are highly prejudicial and unfriendly to the Stomach. But *Campegus* in a particular Book, has treated of the poisonous and hurtful Quality of Purgatives, in a more full and circumstantial Manner than any who went before him. *Helmont,* also, and his Followers, as also *Bontekoe,* did not scruple to call Purgatives mortal Poisons. *Montanus, Crato,* and *Selenander,* Men well ac-

quainted with the healing Art, were much afraid of prescribing them, but frequently used Pills of bitter Extracts, Gums, and Aloes. But the drastic Purgatives, are in a particular Manner hurtful and injurious to Patients of weak Constitutions, Children, and old Persons, to those who are recovering from a Disease, whose Stomachs are weak, or whose nervous System are subject to disorderly Motions. Nor is there any Medicine more prejudicial to Men of choleric and delicate Constitutions, after the uneasy Shocks of Grief and Sorrow, than drastic Purgatives, by the Use of which several Patients have been taken off, in Consequence of an Inflammation of the Stomach and a subsequent Cholera. Those who are subject to hæmorrhoidal Colics, and hypochondriac and hysteric Spasms, ought, also, carefully to abstain from drastic Purgatives, unless they are in Love with Pain, and fond of Misery. This Species of Medicine is, also, highly prejudicial to Children especially when struggling with the Pangs of a difficult Dentition.

But however terrible the Consequences to be apprehended from the Use of Purgatives are, yet as Poison carefully and circumspectly exhibited becomes a Medicine, as is obvious from Mercurials, and antimonial Emetics, so there are, also, some tho' very few Cases, where strong and drastic Cathartics are properly prescrib'd: In an *Anasarca,* for Instance, especially when it does not arise from an Induration, or a scirrhous State of the Viscera and Glands but from a sudden Stagnation of Water, in Consequence of a Suppression of the menstrual or hæmorrhoidal Discharges, or from too great Voracity in or after a Disease. *Frederic Hoffman* says, he has seen a few Ounces of the Juice of common Flower de Luce, as also Gamboge Elaterium, and Extract of *Esula,* successfully

sfully exhibited with Half a Pint of Milk. The Dose may, also, be several times repeated, as the State of the Patient shall require; for by this Means, a surprising Quantity of Water is not only discharged by the Anus, but also in Women sometimes from the Uterus; and these drastic Purges are sometimes evacuated only a small Quantity of Excrements, but excited a very copious and salutary Discharge of Urine; for hydropic Patients, in Consequence of the relaxed and torpid State of the intestinal Fibres, are the better able to bear these Purgatives, and these Fibres require a strong and powerful Stimulus, to excite and rouse them to their proper excretory Motion. These acrid and drastic Purgatives may, also, be properly prescribed in paralytic Resolutions of the Limbs, lethargic Disorders, and also where the languid State of the Patient requires an efficacious Medicine; as also in Madness, agreeable to which *Celsus* in the twelfth Chapter of his second Book informs us, that " black Hellebore is properly exhibited to those who abound with black Bile, who are melancholy mad, or whose Nerves are, in any Part of the Body, become paralytic." The above noted *Hoffman* affirms, that he has had from Experience, that violent

Pains of the Os Ischium and Os Coccygis, which now and then affect the Thighs, have been relieved by drastic Purgatives, which by procuring seven or eight brisk Stools, have removed the Load of bilious and ill concocted Juices, which was the Cause of the Disorder.

Men of robust Constitutions, who live in the more northerly Climates, and use Aliments which are coarse and hard of Digestion, may, if Necessity requires it, have the drastic Purgatives exhibited to them; but the Dose must be very small, either in Powder in Conjunction with Salts, such as Cream of Tartar, or vitriolated Tartar, with an Addition of a few Grains of a diaphoretic Antimony. Or let the Extract of black Hellebore, Scammony, Resin of Jalap, or other Substances of the like Nature, be reduced into the Form of Pills, together with such Things as allay and correct their virulent Quality; such as Cinnabar, Vitriol of Mars, Saffron, Castor, Salt of Amber, Amber, and Myrrh. 'Tis however always to be remember'd, that where a strong Evacuation is required, 'tis far more proper to excite it by an increased Dose of the more gentle Purgatives, than to force it by those which are highly acrid and virulent.

CHAP. III.
Of ALTERATIVES.

ALTERATIVES are principally employ'd in correcting Matter that is faulty as to Quality; and because the Matter to be corrected in Diseases may be faulty in divers Respects, so it is plain that

there must be various Species of Alteratives adapted to the various Defects of the offending Matter. For Instance, if the Juices of a human Body, which in their natural State are benign, mild, and balsamic;

should

should either acquire a *Salino-acid* and corrosive Quality, or assume a hot, subtile, sulphureous Intemperature, or become thick, viscid, and tenacious, or over acid and corrosive, in such an Instance Alteratives of different Kinds should be administer'd: that is, Absorbents for imbibing and blunting the Acid ; temperating Medicines for dissolving and attenuating the thick and viscid Juices ; and in fine, Demulcents for sheathing and mitigating the burning and corrosive Acrimony.

In the first Kind of Alteratives are included Absorbents, the principal of which are of marine Substances, as the Mother of Pearl, Cockle-shells, Oyster-shells, all the Species of Coral, red, and white, and the Bones of the Cuttle Fish; of Animals the Bones and Horns whether subjected to Boiling and softened by Evaporation, or burnt in an open Fire, the Teeth, the Claws and Eyes of Crabs, the Jaws of Fishes, the animal and fossile Unicorn; of subterraneous Substances, the *Lapis Specularis*, Chalk, prepar'd Crystal, Osteocolla, all Stones calcin'd and burn'd, and various Kinds of Boles, Clays, and sealed Earths ; of Metals, the Filings of Steel; of Chymical Preparations, all Salts prepar'd by Incineration, Cineres Clavellati, Salt of Tartar, fixed Nitre, the urinous Spirit of Sal Ammoniac, volatile Sal Ammoniac, the Magnesia Alba, Tincture of Salt of Tartar, and of Antimony.

'Tis the Nature and Property of all these Absorbents, that they speedily incorporate with any Acid that falls in their Way, imbibe it, blunt, and destroy its corrosive Quality, and are along with it changed into a third, neutral, and inoffensive Body. This Effect is plain from the Example of extremely corrosive *Spiritus Nitri Fumans*; from Oil of Vitriol, sublimate Mercury, Aqua Regia,

Aqua Fortis, and other highly caustic Liquors, which, by the Addition of the Filings of Iron, the Mixture of an alcaline Salt, and an earthly absorbent Substance, loose the Whole of their acid and corroding Quali ties ; but altho' all saline and earthly Alcalies agree in this, that they subdue an Acid, and change it into a third Substance, yet there is this Difference between them, that alcaline and lixivious Salts are quickly and totally dissolv'd in the Body, not only by an acid, but likewise by any aqueous Fluid ; whereas earthly Substances are not without Difficulty entirely dissolved, as is plain in Coral Filings of Steel, and quick Lime which are never thoroughly dissolv'd by an Acid, especially of the vegetable Kind, but always remain Kind of fix'd earthly Substance; and which is still more, alcaline Salts, besides their absorbent Quality, after they have in a Manner embraced the Acid, acquire a new and additional medicinal Vertue, which is that of attenuating and colliquating the viscid, slimy, and tenacious Juices they are, likewise, gently stimulating, and either open the Belly, or promote a Discharge by Urine, or even by Perspiration ; and are, besides, attended with this Advantage that they quickly pass thro' the excretory Ducts. But many other alcaline Substances instead of being calculated to quicken and forward the Secretions, rather prove astringent by their Effects, which is usually the Case with Filings of Steel, Corals, Boles, and sealed Earths.

Since, then, as earthly Alcalies are not dissolv'd but by an Acid, we ought to be cautious in exhibiting them in Disorders where the first Organs of Digestion, the Scene where Absorbents produce their principal Effects, are loaded with a Collection of crude and viscid Juices, lest they should adhere to them undissolve bled, and so oppress the Stomach, destroy the Appetite, and Digestion, and render the Belly more costive, as is sometimes happen'd in Fevers of the burning, bilious, and hectic Kind, which were attended with a Decay of the peristaltic Motion, or of the nutritory or retentive Force of the Stomach.

On the other Hand, because these Absorbents so readily destroy and consume the Acid, and because Acidity is what principally infringes and interfers with the Efficacy of Cathartics and Emetics, they are very usefully, where there is any just Suspicion of the Redundance of an Acid, prescribed before Vomiting and Purging, by Way of Digestive. 'Tho' all earthly Substances absorb and blunt an Acid, yet upon Account of their different Natures and Textures, it sometimes happens, that they produce very different Effects, and such as are often contrary to the Intention of the Prescriber; 'tis therefore necessary we should be very cautious in our Choice of such as we design to use: When for Instance, a Physician desires, besides an absorbent Quality, corroborative and astringent Virtue, marine Substances are chiefly proper for answering his Intention, such as Coral, Oyster-shells, the Shells of Eggs, and the various Species of Earths, or Marls, especially such as are call'd sealed Earths. If he desires a gentler Astringent, Mother of Pearl, and Shells best answer his Intention; and if a Flux of the seminal Matter is to be restrain'd, the Bones of the Cuttle Fish are peculiarly proper for that Purpose. When by Absorbents a laxative Effect is, at the same Time, to be produc'd, the Magnesia Alba duly prepared of a Lixivium of Nitre, is to be administ'd, which being entirely dissolv'd by an Acid, is chang'd into a bitter Salt, of a middle Nature, which occasions a speedy Discharge of the Excrements; for this Reason 'tis of singular Efficacy in hypochondriacal Cases, and when the first Organs of Digestion abound with acid Juices; or when the Belly is costive. When the Effects of diuretic Medicines are to be produced by Absorbents, the Claws and Eyes of Crabs, Shells, or Coral calcin'd, and Osteocolla, are in that Case most efficacious. For procuring a free and plentiful Perspiration in any Disease, the Bones of Animals burned and philosophically prepared, are of all other Medicines the best calculated, and most effectual; and, in fine, for resolving the stagnating and condensed Humours, and the Blood itself when coagulated, nothing is more proper then a Medicine, which consists of the Eyes of Crabs dissolved in Vinegar.

Tho' absorbent Medicines are very simple, and generally speaking very easily prepared, yet their Virtues and Efficacies are almost superior to those of all others, nor can they be sufficiently commended; for none of all the Tribe of Alteratives are endowed with such a Power of speedily subduing the bad Qualities of noxious Juices; nor are any of them so safe and innocent as Absorbents, where not used to Excess. Add to this, that the Body is very subject to be affected by an Acid, especially in those whose Bile is deficient, such as Women, and old Men, those who lead a sedentary Life, or drink freely of Liquors abounding with an Acid; and in many Disorders, especially those of the melancholic and hypochondriacal Kind, the Quantity of Acid in the Body is scarcely credible: But Acids by their coagulating Quality, are hurtful to the human Constitution, obstruct the Circulation of the vital Juices, and lay too sure a Foundation for very terrible Disorders, especially of the chronical Kind. 'Tis therefore evident, that

L   Absorbents

Absorbents are endowed with singular Virtues, and accommodated to a great Number of Diseases; but they were very sparingly used by the Ancients, and only brought into Credit by *Helmont* and *Tachenius*, and their two Followers in *Holland, Sylvius* and *Bontekoe*, who assigned an Acid as the Cause of many Diseases, and prescribed *Absorbents* for their Cure.

The second Class of Alteratives comprehends those Medicines which are of a lenient and temperating Quality, such as check the hot intestine Motion of the sulphureous Particles of the Blood, and qualify, subdue, and cool the scorching hot and bilious Humours in the Intestines themselves. Of Vegetables, the principal of this Kind are, the Root and Herb of Sorrel, Wood-Sorrel, Citrons, Oranges, China Oranges, Pomegranates, Strawberries, Barberries, Cherries, and the Juices of them prepared, and likewise Syrups and Water distilled from these; add to these the four greater cold Seeds, and Decoctions of Oats, Whey, Butter-Bilk, the Juice of Craw Fish, a Decoction of Tortoises, thin Decoctions of the Shavings of Harts-horn, and Vipers Grass, with or without Barley, Jellies of Harts-horn, and Water distilled from the Shavings of Harts-horn. Of the mineral Tribe, well purified Nitre is the best and most efficacious, and becomes still better if restored from *Aqua Fortis*, to its former State, by the Addition of Salt of Tartar. Of chymical Preparations, the essential Salt of Wood Sorrel, Cream of Tartar, Phlegm of Vitriol, Tinctures of Roses, Daisy Flowers, and Violets, prepared with Spirit of Vitriol, are good temperating Medicines.

Temperating Medicines act in three several Manners, for they either by their acid Salts bind up the volatile sulphureous Particles, and by fixing and coagulating them, lessen in some Measure their Intestine and gyratory Motions; or they operate by an expansive and aerio-lastic Quality, such as that which is inherent to Nitre, which consisting of an acid and alcaline Salt, contains great Store of sulphureous Particles, and also, of a subtile aerio-etherial Fluid, by Means of which it dispels the hot Matter whilst in a gyratory Motion, and forces it, as it were, from the Center to the Circumference; by its neutral Salt attenuates, dissolves, and separates the viscid Matter, which is the Matrix of Heat, and Sulphur, and at the same Time by its subtile Acid, retards the accelerated Motion of the sulphureous Parts; or, in the last Place, they restore, the Moisture consumed by the Heat, by diluting and dissolving the sulphureous Parts, and at the same time lessens the too great Elasticity of the Vessels, upon which the Heat in a great Measure depends, as is observable in the Use of Watery Liquors, Whey, Decoctions of Hartshorn, and of Oats.

These temperating and qualifing Medicines are of great Use in Physic, wherever a preternatural Heat is to be extinguished, and therefore cannot be wanted in Fevers of all Kinds, Inflammations, Spasms and grievous Pains, which almost always are occasioned by too great a Commotion of the Blood. But nitrous Preparations are deservedly to be preferred to Acids, for Nitre is not only cooling, but Antispasmodic, and relaxes the Rigidity of the Parts; it, in like Manner, promotes the Discharge by Urine, and Stool; besides, as those cooling and acid Fluids condense and coagulate, and as Nitre rather colloquates, rarifies, and attenuates thick and viscid Humours, so when sprinkled either in Powder, or dissolved in Water, upon black coagulated Blood, it renders it more florid:

iii. For this Reason, Nitre is not only preferable to Acids in Inflammations, and even in inflammatory fevers, which arise from a black coagulated pent up Blood, but is likewise a noble and efficacious Preservative against Inflammations; because it effectually fuses and dissolves the viscid Serum, which is easily to be observed in the Blood of those who are subject to Inflammations.

In chronical Fevers, such as those of the flow and hectic Kind, which for the most Part owe their Origin to a Defect or Putrefaction in some of the Viscera, and when a Cough or Spitting of Blood is joined with them, or when the Lungs themselves are faulty, not Acids but nitrous and diluting Remedies, especially such as are taken from the animal Kingdom are to be used, such as, Whey, the Decoction and Jelly of Harts horn. When, also, a feverish Heat accompanies Diarrhœas, Dysenteries, or a Cholera Morbus, cooling Acids are to be abstained from, and diluting, gelatinous, and mucilaginous Medicines, and temperating and absorbing Powders, with the Addition of a Grain or two of Nitre, are to be used.

In the third Class of Alteratives, are comprehended inciding and attenuating Medicines, among which may be reckoned, the Roots of white Burnet, Dragons, Sweet Flag, Asabacca, wild Radish, Elecampane, Succory, Florentine Orris, Salomons seal, Swallow Wort, the Herbs Leopards Bane, Brook Lime, Scurvy Grass, Water Cresses, and Indian Cresses, Dittander, Rosa Solis, Fumitory, Buck Bean, the lesser Centaury, Hyssop, Germander, Cher-Carduus Benedictus, lesser Houseleek, the several Species of Garlick, Leeks, and Onions, Guaiacum Wood, its Bark, the Spices, Pepper, and Ginger, the Seeds of Mustard, Scurvy Grass, and Water Cresses, the

Gums Amoniacum, Galbanum, Sagapenum, Opopanax, Myrrh, Benzoin; of chymical Preparations, Mercurius Dulcis, Æthiops mineral, Flowers of Sulphur, fixed alcaline Salts of Vegeteables reduced to Ashes, especially Salt of Tartar, and of Wormwood; also neutral Salts, as Sal-ammoniac, Sal-polychrestum, Epsom Salt, vitriolated Tartar, Terra foliata Tartari, Arcanum Duplicatum, a Solution of Crabs Eyes, of Nitre and Sal-ammoniac; Volatiles, as volatile Sal-ammoniac, urinous Spirit of Sal-ammoniac, and Oxymel of Squills, acrid Tincture of Acrimony, Essence of Gum-ammoniac, and of Indian Pepper, Resin of Guaiacum; Syrup of Tobacco, of Hedge Mustard, Fæcula of Arum; and medicinal Waters, also, which besides their diluting and opening Virtue, are possessed of an attenuating and inciting Quality; as also, Infusions in the Form of Tea, which by their great Store of an aqueous Element, exert their Virtues, disjoin the coalescent Globules; and lastly, sweet Whey, which on Account of the sweet and subtile Salt it contains, is detersive, and opens the excretory Ducts.

Of these, some act upon the fluid, and others upon the solid Parts of the Body; those which affect the Fluids by immediate Contact, are very few in Number, and those either consist of aqueous Diluters, which are very efficacious for fusing the glutinous and viscid Juices, or of alcaline fixed and volatile Salts, and nitrous Salts, which when mixed, especially in an liquid Form, with thick and coagulated Blood and Humours, liquify and attenuate them in such a Manner, as even to be perceptible to the Eye. All the rest operate upon the Solids by augmenting their Tone, their Strength, and contractile Force, and by adding to the elastic Powers of the Vessels,

sels,

fels, by which Means they ftrongly prefs and agitate the contained Juices, accelerate their progreffive and inteftine Motions, and forcibly and frequently propelling them thro' the capillary Veffels, divide and disjoin the vifcid Juices into fmall Globules, upon which Fluidity depends. This Action upon the Solids, is in fome Medicines perform'd by a fix'd acrid Salt, as in the Roots of Arum, white Burnet, Afarabacca, Florentine Orris, Solomons Seal, the Herbs German Leopards Bane, Ditander, Rofa Solis, Pepper, and Ginger, which are indeed of an acrid Smell, but being diftilled with Water by an Alembic, neither yield a volatile acrid Oil, nor a Water of an acrid Tafte, which is a fufficient Proof, that they are of a fix'd Nature. Other Medicines, again, produce their Effects by an acrid, fubtile, and volatile Salt, fuch as wild Radifh, Elecampane, Water Creffes, Scurvy Grafs, Muftard, and all Kinds of Onions, Garlick, and Leeks. Some act by their ftimulating neutral Salts, of which Kind are thofe Salts whofe Acrimony and irritating Quality, are not only difcoverable by their Tafte, but by their Effects, for which Reafon when exhibited in large Dofes, they open the Belly and prove diuretic. Others produce their Effects by an acrid Salt, which contains many fulphureous Particles, as is obvious in Gum Ammoniac, Sagapenum, Opopanax, Guaiacum, and its Refin, which befides their acrid Salt, contain an Oil, which upon Diftillation they yield in Abundance. Laftly, Some Medicines perform their Work, by a penetrating, fubtile, and metallic Salt, as Mercury, and efpecially Mercurius Dulcis, and Æthiops Mineral.

The Virtues of attenuating and inciding Medicines are fo extenfive, that, on Account of the great Variety of their Effects, they are ufu-

ally ranged under different Denominations; for when tenacious vifcid Humours not only ftagnate in the Cavities of the Veffels, but ftuff up and obftruct the fmall Tubes of the Inteftines and Emunctions, thefe Medicines, by their inciding and attenuating Quality, difengage the impacted Humours, remove the Obftructions, and may, for that Reafon, be called Aperients, fince they produce the fame Effect; they alfo deferve the Name of Anti-Scorbutics, and Purifiers of the Blood; for fince the Purity and good State of the animal Juices, depend upon the due Secretion add Excretion of fuperfluous and recrementitious Matter, and fince Secretion and Excretion cannot be carried on, if the fmall Canals of the Glands and Emunctories are block'd up by vifcid and tenacious Humours, 'tis therefore plain, that thofe Medicines which are endowed with a Power of inciding vifcid Juices, and removing Obftructions, muft not only be Purifiers of the Blood, but alfo Prefervatives againft the Scurvy, in which the Juices are of a bad Quality, and loaded with various heterogeneous, vifcid, falt, fulphureous, and fharp Particles. Now fince attenuating Medicines produce fo different Effects, the Phyfician ought to know, what particular Attenuants are beft adapted to particular given Cafes.

In Diforders of the Stomach, and firft Organs of Digeftion, for inciding and attenuating vifcid Humours, the following Medicines are excellently calculated: The Root of Arum, of white Burnet, and of Calamus Aromaticus, Pepper, Ginger, purified Sal Ammoniac, vitriolated Tartar, Arcanum Duplicatum, Salt of Wormwood, Spirit of Salt, fimple or dulcified; and if crude and ill concocted Juices are to be evacuated by Way of Excrement, the neutral Salts are preferable, efpecially specially the Sal Polychreſtum, and the Epſom Salts taken in large Doſes, and drank in a ſufficient Quantity of ſome aqueous Vehicle.

In Diſorders of the Breaſt, when viſcid Humours are to be attenuated and thrown up by Spitting, the moſt effectual are the Roots of Elecampane, and of the Florentine Iris, Roſa Solis, Hyſſop, Germander, Maidenhair, Gum Ammoniac, Myrrh, Benzoin, Sulphur, Balſam of Peru, Terra foliata Tartari, Oxymel of Squills, Solution of Crabs Eyes in diſtill'd Vinegar, and Syrup of Hedge Muſtard.

When the Blood is tainted with any thick tenacious Impurity, and by that Means the Embuctories are clogged and the Humours polluted by a ſalt, ſulphureous, and ſcorbutic Dyſcraſy, the Medicines chiefly in Uſe in that Caſe are, the wild Radiſh Root, Garden Scurvy Graſs, Water Creſſes, Indian Creſſes, Dittander, Brook Lime, the leſſer Centaury, Marſh Trefoil, Carduus Benedictus, Fumitory, the Smaller Houſe Leek, Muſtard, Gum Ammoniac, Sagapenum, Myrrh, the Liquor of fix'd Nitre, Oil of Tartar *per Deliquium*, the Solution of Nitre, Tincture of Antimony, the Eſſences of the Woods, Spirit of Sal Ammoniac, Salt of Wormwood with Lemon Juice, and ſome Sorts of medicinal Waters.

When grumous Blood occaſioned by Contuſions, Blows, or Suffuſions, is to be diſſolved and fus'd, the Medicines moſt to be commended in this Caſe is, Solomon's Seal, German Leopard's Bane, Chervil, Vinegar neutraliz'd with Crabs Eyes, Terra foliata Tartari, and antimoniated Nitre.

In Diſeaſes where the Lymph is become thick, eſpecially from a venereal Taint, the principal and moſt efficacious are, Guaiacum, Sopewort, *Mercurius dulcis*, and Æthiops Mineral, which if prudently uſed, is of uncommon Efficacy, for colliquating and reſolving the viſcid Humours lodged in the Glands and Liver.

I come now to the fourth and laſt Claſs of Alteratives, which comprehends the emollient and ſoftning Medicines, of which the chief are, Roots of Marſh Mallows, of white Lillies, of Liquorice, and of Vipers Graſs, the five emollient Herbs, Lettice, Bears Breech, Pellitory of the Wall, the Flowers of Elder, of Mellilot, of Mallows, of Mullein, of Yarrow, of Camomile, of white Lillies, of Borrage, of the wild Poppy, of the Lime Tree, of the Egyptian Thorn, of Violets, and moſt of all Saffron; the Seeds of Flax, of Fenugreek, of Aniſe, of Quinces, of Flea Bane, of white Poppies, the four greater and leſſer cold Seeds, ſweet Almonds, Figs, Pine Nuts, Piſtaches, Cherry Tree Gum, Gum Arabic, Gum Tragacanth, Shavings and Jelly of Hartshorn, human Greaſe, that of a Dog, of a Capon, the Marrow of their Bones, the Fat about their Omentum, Bones, and Myſentery; the native Oils of Animals, freſh Butter, Cream, Milk, Cryſtals of Milk, Sperma Ceti, Honey, the Yolk of an Egg, and its White dried and reduced to Powder. Of prepared Medicines, Oil of ſweet Almonds, Linſeed Oil, Rape Oil, Oil of the Male Balſam Tree, Decoctions of Harts-horn, and Vipers Graſs, mix'd with the Juice of Citrons, the common Ptiſan, ſweet Whey, *Fernelius*'s Syrup of Marſh Mallows, Ointment of Marſh Mallows, ſimple Diachylon Plaſter, that of Melitot, and that of Frogs Spawn.

The Virtues of theſe Medicines is twofold; the one appropriated to the Solids, the other to the Fluids, in the Solids they relax, ſoften, and render moveable the hard, ſtiff, and tenſe Fibres, and at the ſame Time

enlarge

enlarge and dilate the Channels of the small contracted Vessels ; but in the Fluids they, by their viscid Mucilage, bind up, involve, and as it were, inclose in a Sheath the piercing Points of the sharp corroding Salts, and by that Means prove excellent lenitive Medicines, and when externally applied, they convert into a laudable *Pus,* any Collection of extravassed Humour, which cannot be resolved, or taken into the refluent Mass by the lymphatic Vessels ; so that having by their moderate Warmth, dissipated the most subtile Part of the extravasted Humour, the remaining viscous Matter is happily disposed to maturate, the Pores being now gently closed up, left too much Moisture should be exhaled, and the nutritious Juice, of which Pus chiefly consists, being excited to flow more plentifully thro' the small relaxed Tubes.

These lenitive Medicines are of incredible Efficacy, if any one has the Misfortune to take a caustic Poison, and scarce can more powerful Antidotes than these be used, for checking and subduing the Virulence of vegetable and animal Poisons, especially if Abundance of Milk, and oily Liquors, are used as their Vehicles ; because these not only sheath up and blunt the sharp Points of the Poison, but, also, relax the Membranes contracted and render'd subject to Spasms, by the violent Shocks of the Poison ; and by these Means they always promote the Evacuation of Poisons, either by Vomit, or by Stool.

In long and violent Distempers, especially such as arise from an Acrimony of Humours, and which prey upon the Nerves, Infusions, and Decoctions of these emollient Medicines are of singular Advantage ; thus Convulsions, attended with Madness, scorbutic Contractions of the Joints, and intolerable

Gripes of the Belly, are often cur'd by Decoctions of Piony Roots, Marsh-Mallows, Pellitory of the Wall, Bears Breech, Flowers of Mullein, of white Lillies, of Elder, of Borage, of Camomile, and wild Poppy, and by Figs and Fennel Seed, prepared with Water, or Whey ; but, they are to be us'd in large Quantities, and for a long Time, with the Addition now and then of a Spoonful or two of Oil of sweet Almonds, sometimes bathing in fresh Water with Milk.

Fresh Fat and Grease of Animals, especially the Marrow of Bones, which abounds with a very subtile Oil, are us'd internally with Success, in a sharp scorbutic Disposition of the Humours.

In a Dryness of the Parts, and when the Joints can scarce move without making a Noise, and in arthritic Pains, these emollient Medicines produce wonderful Effects, but these fat Substances are to be used when the Stomach is empty, and not in large, but frequent Doses, drinking some suitable warm Draught after them.

In Exulcerations of the Kidnies, and Discharges of bloody Urine, which sometimes happen in the Small Pox, on Account of the Acrimony of the Humours, Cherry Tree Gum, or even Tragacanth, or the dried White of an Egg dissolv'd in Whey, are of singular Use : But in Disorders of the Breast, for blunting the Acrimony, which is the Cause of the Cough, and disposing the Matter for Expectoration, the following Medicines are excellently calculated : Decoction of Oats, Sperma Ceti, Liquorice, the Oil of sweet Almonds, Saffron, Figs, Syrup of Violets, and Flowers of Poppy, and Elder.

In continual hectic Heats, and if the sweet Juices, by a continued slow Fever, acquire a saltish alcaline Acrimony, cimony, Cream and new Butter, on account of their demulcent Qualties, are found to produce excellent Effects.

In a Cholera Morbus, also, in a Dysentery, a Scurvy, or scorbutic Decay, a Consumption, and in general, where-ever the Acrimony of the Humours gives Rise to the Disease, gelatinous Decoctions of Flesh, of Bones, and especially of Harts-horn, Calves Feet, and Sheeps Feet, are of singular Efficacy and Advantage, as well used internally by Way of Drink, as injected by Way of Clyster.

When the Intestines are violently contracted, and the Excrements pent up by Flatulencies, emollient demulcent Medicines, such as Oil of sweet Almonds, Whey, Decoctions of Oats, and Hartshorn, produce very great Effects; but should rather be injected by Way of Clyster, than taken by the Mouth.

Emollient Flowers and Herbs, if boil'd with a small Quantity of Saffron, inclosed in a Bladder, and externally applied over the internal Part affected, procure almost incredible Ease and Relief, as may be experienc'd in a Pleurify, an Inflammation of the Liver, a Cholic, or when the Anus suffers by the blind Hæmorrhoids.

When any extravassed and impacted Humour, is to be converted into Pus, no Applications can be more properly us'd than Liniments and Cataplasms, made of emollient Fats and Milk; but especially of the Flowers and Leaves of white Lillies, Saffron, Figs, roasted Onions, Bean Meal, Yolks of Eggs, and Honey; but these are not to be us'd, when the Matter is contain'd in hardened and scirrhous Parts, where it cannot be converted into Pus, unless we are inclin'd to bring on a fatal Putrefaction.

Mucilages made of the Seeds of Quinces, and Flea Bane, with Rose Water, or Frogs Spawn Water, often afford immediate Relief, in excoriated and exulcerated Parts, attended with Heat and Pain, such as the ulcerated Aphthæ in the Mouth, blind and painful Hæmorrhoids, a Tenesmus, Gonorrhæas, or a corroding Fluor Albus.

CHAP. IV.
Of ANODYNES.

SOPORIFICS, if they are of a potent Nature, take the Name of *Narcotics* or *Stupefactives*, and are such Kind of Remedies, as by their subtile, noxious, deleterious Exhalations, diminish, or quite destroy, the Sense and Motion of the solid Parts. Among *Soporifics*, the most eminent are those which are usually prepared for medicinal Uses, of the whole Poppy, as *Opium*, which by the Antients was called *Lacryma Papaveris*, the Tear of the Poppy, and *Meconium*, which is the Extract of the Poppy made by Boiling. In the Class of Stupefactives, which are of a violent Nature, are all such Remedies as are prepared of the Mandragoras, Hyoscyamus, Stramonium, and Datura. Stupefactives and Soporifics are, not without good Reason, reckon'd amongst Poisons, since they exert their noxious Influence in a

short

short Space of Time, when taken in a small Quantity and a Quantity a little larger than ordinary, proves mortal ; besides, their principal Operation is on the noblest Parts of the Body, which are the Origins of Sense and Motion, and, moreover, they act by Means of an Element quite opposite to Nature, a noisome sulphureous Vapour, by which they diminish to a considerable Degree, or quite destroy, the Sense and Motion of the motive Fibres.

The Operation of stupefactive Poisons is directly opposite to that of Caustics, these latter with their highly acrimonious, and penetrating Salts, excite preternatural and violent Motions ; the other by their sulphureous Vapour, retard or stop those Motions and Sensations, which principally belong to the nervous Membranes, and by that Means render the Circulation of the Blood more languid, and the Excretions slower and more imperfect.

The Life of the human Body, and the Integrity of its Functions, consists in the due Tone of the Solids, and the free and equable Motion of the Fluids : The first depends on their moderate and equable Systole and Diastole, or their Contraction and Dilatation ; the other in a proper Temperament, Quantity, and Ventilation of the Blood. Whatever, therefore, in a speedy and effectual Manner destroys that due Tone of the Solids, and disturbs the equable Motion of the Fluids, is naturally qualified to subvert all the Functions of the animated Body, and if it works such an Effect in a violent Manner, it may be justly called Poison ; and when Soporifics and Narcotics in too great a Measure diminish the Motion, and injure the Tone of the solid Parts, or render the Circulation of the Blood more languid and imperfect, they are highly destructive to Nature.

We are assured by undoubted Experience, that the Effects of Opiats and Narcotics, especially when taken in an immoderate Quantity, are a weak, low, and small Pulse, a Straitness, and Difficulty of Breathing, a soporous Indisposition, and Heaviness of the Head, a Dullness of the Senses, and oftentimes a Deliriousness, attended with a Diminution of Appetite, Costiveness, a Defect in Digestion, and a remarkable Decay of Strength. All these Symptoms proceed from no other Cause, than a too flow Progress or Stagnation of the Blood and Fluids ; for since the Motion of the Fluids depends only on the Tone, Strength, and systolic and diastolic Motions of the solid Parts, it plainly appears, that the animal Spirit, that Fluid of the Brain, which directs and regulates the Motion of all the other Fluids, is primarily and preternaturally affected by these Remedies.

The Elements by which Narcotics operate, are of an highly volatile, and penetrating Nature, since they so deeply insinuate themselves, like a Vapour, into the Pores of the Membranes and Nerves, and by contaminating that most pure and moveable Fluid, deprive, by little and little, the Solids of their Tone and Motion.

That the Elements by which Narcotics exert their Force are extremely volatile and penetrating, may be proved by several Arguments : First, Their Virulence is almost entirely destroyed by long and vehement Boiling. Secondly, If they are applied in Ointment or Epithems to the Head, or other nervous Parts, as the Soles of the Feet, the Palms of the Hands, or only received by Way of Smell, they induce a Sleepiness. *Dioscorides* affirms Opium to be soporiferous by Smell alone. And *Plutarch* in his *Symposiacs* relates, that the Vapours proceeding

ceeding from the Poppy have, for
Want of due Caution, proved fatal
to those who have gathered the
Juice. And Thirdly, It is found by
manifold Chymical Experiments,
that there are no better *Correctives*
of their Virulence then *Acids*, such
as the Juice of Quinces or Citrons,
Wine Vinegar, or Spirit of Vitriol,
which have a great Influence in
fixing the volatile Sulphur; and Opi-
m is well known to lose its Virtue by being roasted on an heated
Plate. All *Narcotics* and *Hypnotics*
exhale a strong and malignant Kind
of Vapour, as we are assured by the
Smell, which is a manifest Indication of an ungrateful Sulphur contained in them.

Narcotics act on the nervous
Membranes of the Stomach and Intestines, principally by Means of a
vaporous and fetid Sulphur. For as
the Stomach and Intestines first and
immediately feel the Force and Efficacy of Remedies, they are so much
more liable to suffer from the Influence of Medicines, which are of a
stronger and more penetrating Nature than ordinary. *Opium* or any
other Narcotic, after it is taken,
and begins to be dissolved by the
internal Heat and Moisture, diffuses
its noxious Vapours, which being
received into the Pores of the nervous Membranes, the Fluid on
which their Tone and Motion depends, loses its Nature: Hence the
Sensation, and, also, the peristaltic
Motion of the Intestines become
more languid; for if a strong Smell,
as in the Case of Hysterics, are received up the Nostrils, such, for
Instance, as proceeds from burnt
Feathers, or Asa Fœtida, has so
sudden an Effect in composing the
turbulent and disorderly Motions in
the nervous and membraneous System, and if, on the contrary, a fragrant Vapour has the Force of immediately disturbing the whole Frame

of the Muscles by violent Spasms,
why may not the foul and noisome
Exhalations of *Narcotics*, by contaminating a Fluid of consummate
Activity, as well injure or put a
Stop to its Motion? But those
Things which act on the Nerves,
are most speedy in their Effects, because their Influence is immediately
diffused over the whole nervous System. An Opiate as soon as taken,
or before it is out of the Stomach,
very soon causes an Inclination to
Sleep, and Relief from Pain in distant Parts; and Opiates, most of
all, exert their Influence on the
Nerves, by Virtue of which, those
wracking Pains which are incident
to the Intestines, are remitted in a
Moment, being succeeded by a
Nausea, Loathing of Food, and, if
there be sufficient Strength, by Vomiting.

Narcotics have, also, a considerable
Influence on the Membranes of the
Brain, where, by gently diminishing the Spring and Systole of the
Arteries, which are furnish'd with
very thin Membranes, they cause a
Stagnation of the Blood therein, with
Distensions of the Vessels of the Head;
by which Means they induce a Torpor, Drowsiness, Deliriousness, with
frightful and troublesome Dreams.

There is nothing in the Nature of
Things that will render a wise and
intelligent Person a Fool, and stupid,
so soon as a *Narcotic*. That the
Datura has such an Effect is well
known, and that the *Solanum Furio-
sum*, and its Berries, will suddenly
render a Man of Sense a Maniac, is
confirm'd by many Observations in
*Matthiolus Comment. in Dioscorid.
Wierius de Præstigio, Mercurialis
de Venenis*, and *Lobelius* in *Adversa-
riis Stirpium*. To these we may
add the following Observation of
Frederic Hoffman: A certain Person
labouring under an Hæmoptoe, having, thro' Want of Care, taken too
large

large a Dose of a Medicine containing a good Quantity of the Seeds of Henbane, was deprived of all Sense and Memory, and continued waking for some Days. And something like this happen'd from Pills of Houndstongue given in too large a Dose to repress Vomiting. Even an external Application of Henbane may procure Madness, as *Platerus* assures us on the Testimony of *Rondeletius*; and the pernicious Effects of these Kind of Remedies were not unknown to the Ancients. Hence *Cælius Aurelianus, Lib.* I. *Cap.* 4. says, " They soon become delirious, " who take the *Papaver, Mandra-* " *goras,* or *Hyoscyamus* inwardly; " but their Pulse at such Time is " very slow." and *Helmont, Lib.* I. *de Lithiaf,* says very justly of Opium, " That they are guilty of a " very great Error, who endeavour " to cure a Mania with Opiates, " since every Opiate is mad in it- " self." And in another Place, " Narcotics will hardly procure " Sleep to mad Persons, tho' given " in a quadruple Dose, but will in- " crease the Madness " To this Purport also is, *Obf.* 78. *Dec.* 11. M. *Naturæ Curioforum,* of a Person labouring under a Dysentery, who was made delirious with a Clyster of a Pint of a Decoction of Hyoscyamus, and continued in that State for six Weeks.

Narcotics or stupefactive Remedies, were always very much suspected by the wisest Physicians amongst the Ancients in the Cure of Diseases, on Account of their deliterious Quality. For a Proof hereof, we shall give a few Testimonies selected from innumerable others. *Galen* was very fearful of exhibiting Opium, and *Lib.* III. *de Medicam. Composit. Cap.* 10. he says, " That " living Bodies suffer something " like Mortification, from the Use " of every Remedy composed of

" *Opium, Hyoscyamus,* and *Mandra-* " *goras.*" And *Celfus, Lib.* III. *Cap.* 18. pronounces, " That if Sleep " must be procured by Medicines, " Moderation is necessary in exhi- " biting them, left we should never " be able to rouse the Person from " the Sleep into which we have " cast him." And *Lib.* V. *Cap.* 25. he says, " To use Anodynes " without urgent Necessity, is a " wrong Step, for they are a vio- " lent Kind of Medicine, and in- " jurious to the Stomach." But the Effects are worse which *Scribonius Largus Compof.* 106. *Cap.* 48. enumerates. " Opium, says he " taken, induces Heaviness of the " Head, Refrigeration and Livid " ness of the Limbs, and cold " Sweats, besides a Difficulty o " Respiration, Stupidity, and Loss " of Reason." *Trallian, Lib.* III. *Cap.* 5. writes, that a certain Person by the sole Use of Opium, had lost his Voice and Senses in such a Manner, that he could never afterward be recovered. Nor must we omit *Ætius,* who very well describes the pernicious Effects of Opiates in the following Manner: " Opiates, says he " never cure the Disease them " selves, on which the Pains at " tend, but by inducing a Stupor " and Dullness of Sensation on the " Parts, procure a Kind of Rest to " the Pains, " and in another Place, to the same Purpose, he says, that " They cause, indeed " an immediate Cessation of the " Pain, but protract the Cause " thereof, and in a little Time af " terwards induce Faintings and " Death, or long and incurable " Disorders." And to speak the Truth, so sudden and pernicious have been the Effects which Physicians of all Ages have recorded from the Use of Narcotics, that they are by no Means to pass unregarded, but to be esteem'd as

E

Evidence of some very active and keen Principle, which has Power to hurt; for which Reason Physicians ought to be careful and circumspect in the Use of these Kinds of Remedies.

Tho' much Mischief and Danger may attend the Effects of Narcotics, so that they may be esteemed not far removed from the Nature of Poisons, Physicians, however, both ancient and modern, have at all times experienced great Benefit from hypnotic Anodynes, especially in violent Pains and Fluxes; for what greater Benefit can we receive, than to be delivered from intolerable Pains? Besides such is the Nature of Pain, that if it be of any long Continuance, it either weakens the Powers of the Mind and Body, to such a Degree, as to render a Disease, otherwise favourable, evidently mortal, or else brings Death itself. Whoever, therefore, shall be so happy as to know how to remove these Pains, and avert so great Dangers, most certainly confers an extraordinary Benefit, and administers, I had almost said, divine Consolation to the miserable Patient; and therefore if we consult the most antient Compositions, of which *Scribonius Largus* has principally made a Collection, or *Celsus*, we shall find many Descriptions against Pains and Fluxes, of which Opium is commonly the Basis. Thus the Theriaca Andromachi, Mithridate, and Philonium, with an infinite Number of modern Preparations, enough to fill a Volume with their bare Titles, are but Corrections of Opium, and Compositions which have for their Basis Opium, celebrated by some as an universal Remedy; and some endeavour to extract a Panacea from it. It were indeed heartily to be wished, that some eminent Physicians had not been so profuse in their Encomiums on this Remedy, since it has been so freely, and with

Impunity, abused to the Destruction of Mankind, especially in our Times, on which Subject, *Stbal de Imposturis. Opii* deserves to be consulted. I cannot avoid taking the Opportunity here to remark, that there is a Custom too prevalent in our Times, when we would repress an Hœmorrhage, or alleviate a Pain, of exhibiting Pills of Hounds-tongue, which having a Mixture of Opium, and the Seeds of Henbane, and often leaving behind them an extraordinary Stupor of the Head, ought to be used with the greatest Caution, and never but when milder Remedies will not answer the Intention, nor then, if the Body be very weak.

In Disorders of the Stomach and Intestines, all Things which induce a Stupor, are very cautiously, or never at all, to be exhibited; because no Kind of Medicine is so pernicious, and injurious to the Tone and Motion of the nervous Parts.

To preserve Health, and prevent Diseases, nothing is so effectual, as to maintain the Tone, Strength, and Motion of what they call the *Primæ Viæ*, or first Passages; because the most salutary Excretion which is performed by Stool, and discharges the Sordes, which are the Recrements remaining after Digestion, or are collected from all Parts of the Body, depend chiefly thereon. Where this Evacuation is surpressed, or else performed after a slow and remiss Manner, a Deluge of vicious Humors is soon collected, and becomes the Cause as well as Fomentor of Diseases. Now there is nothing which so effectually diminishes the peristaltic Motion of the Intestines, and surpresses the intestinal Excretion, as *Sedatives* and *Anodynes*, the Truth of which is attested by Experience: For as all Remedies, so especially those which are of a violent Quality, exert their Efficacy

ficacy first and principally upon the Stomach and Intestines.

It is very dangerous to administer Opiates and Anodynes, where the Stomach and Intestines are inclining to an Inflammation and Sphacelus, or where an extraordinary Impurity disposes them to Corruption.

That a firm Rest and Stagnation of the Blood in the Vessels, which are productive of an Inflammation, will end in a sphacelous Putrefaction, unless seasonably discussed, is not to be questioned. Whenever, therefore, these Parts, I mean the Stomach and Intestines, labour under violent Pains and Spasms, and the Body is infirm or impure, an Inflammation is justly to be apprehended. 'Tis, therefore, the Business of every prudent Physician, in a Dysentery, an iliac Passion, a spasmodic Cholic, and a violent Cardialgia, diligently to confider, not only the Strength of the Patient, but also the various Stages of the Distemper, and the Disposition of the Humours, before he exhibits Medicines of a sedate Quality; otherwise instead of affording seasonable Relief, he procures the Death of the Patient. Thus some of the best Authors inform us, that mortal Symptoms have forthwith been produced by Opiates taken internally, or injected by Way of Clyster. Instances of this Kind occur, in *Thonnerus* in *Observat. Lib. 3. Cap. 5. Waldschmidius* in *Dissert. de Noxa Opiat. Tillingius de Opio. Sennertus Lib. 6, Praxeos. P. 3. Cap. 1.* and *Marcellus Donatus* in *Hist. Med. Mirabil.*

Since Medicines of the sedative and stupifying Quality, so effectually destroy, and impair the Strength of the Intestines, hence it is obvious, that nothing has a more effectual Tendency both to produce and cherish hypochondriac Disorders, than a frequent Use of such Medicines. That the hypochondriac Disorder arises from continual Inflations and Spasms of the Stomach and Intestines, which are of a nervous Nature, and that it is the Effect of the Suppression of the Discharge by Stool, and the large Congestion of peccant Humours arising from that Circumstance, are Things so certain, that they cannot be doubted of. Since, therefore, Medicines of this Kind, by producing Costiveness, weaken the Strength and Force of the Intestines, hence nothing can be more prejudicial in this Disorder, and it is frequently observed, that the immoderate Use of Opiates and Astringents in checking Diarrhœas, Dysenteries, and intermittent Fevers, has produced a violent hypochondriac Disorder, or in Women *Hysterics*, which generally afflicted the Patient during the remaining Part of Life: And if a Physician, by the frequent Use of Anodynes, checks the Pain, and other Symptoms accompanying the Disorder, he by that Means alleviates them for a Time, but lays a Foundation for their recurring with greater Violence.

Sedative Medicines, especially those of the somniferous and stupifying Kind, are, also, injurious to the Head, and increase the Disorders incident to it; because by rendering the Motion and Pulsation of the carotid Arteries, which consist of tender Coats, more languid, they occasion a slow Circulation of the Blood through the Head. Hence the Stagnations of Blood there produced, generate formidable Disorders. In order to keep the Head free from Diseases, it is of the last Importance to preserve the Tone of the Membranes of the Brain, and the due Circulation of its Blood thro' its Vessels. Now nothing is more injurious to the nervous Coats of the Brain, than all Vapours, fetid, and strong smelling Substances, by their Means, since their Strength and Tone is diminished, the systolic and diastolic Force of the small Arteries impaired, and consequently the Circulation of the Blood thro' the Head render'd slower : and this slow Circulation is succeeded by a Secretion of the serous Humour, which lays a Foundation for the most considerable Disorders of the Head, such as Palsy, an Abolition of Memory, an Aphony, Difficulty of Hearing, lethargic Disorders, Hemiplegies, and fixed Pains ; or in Consequence of the too great Distention of the Vessels of the Brain, by the infracted Blood, Melancholy, which is frequently accompanied with a palpable Depravation of the Fancy, an imaginary Appearance of Spectres, horrible Dreams, and a Madness which easily degenerates into Fury. These vapourous and stupifying Medicines have an uncommon Tendency not only to generate, but also to support and cherish these Disorders ; and by the incautious Use of them, it has been frequently observ'd, that wild Disorders of the Head have been converted into Misfortunes of a more terrible Kind ; an Head-ach, for Instance, has been transformed into a Lethargy ; an Hemicrania into Stupidity ; a Palsy into an Apoplexy ; a Vertigo into an Epilepsy ; and a Difficulty of Hearing into a confirmed Deafness.

Anodynes and Opiates are so friendly to the Membranes of the Brain and Intestines, by diminishing their Tone and Strength, Children and old Persons ought in a particular Manner to abstain from the Use of them ; first, because they retard the Discharge by Stool ; and secondly, because they weaken the nervous System and Membranes, two Circumstances highly prejudicial, because the Disorders

principally incident to these Ages, arise either from Costiveness, or a Weakness of the Brain and Nerves.

'Tis certain from Experience, that by a liberal Use of Anodynes, Children contract a Dullness of Genius and Memory, which lasts for a considerable Time ; for a violent Injury done to the tender Structure of their Brain, is not easily repaired. For this Reason *Stalpart Vander Wiel Cent*. 1. *Obs*. 42. justly orders, " That Women and Nurses, should " not, when the Children commit- " ted to their Care are first affect- " ed with Pain and Uneasiness, " forthwith exhibit Anodynes ; since " tho' they do not generally by " that Means destroy them, they " yet often weaken their Brain and " Nerves to such a Degree, as to " induce violent Tremors, Palsies, " and Stupidity. " Of the same Opinion is Dr. *Willis* who in *Pharm. Rat. P*. 1. informs us, that by Medicines of this Kind, he knew some seized with Slowness of Genius and Stupidity, and others with Dotage.

Anodynes and Opiates are highly injurious to Persons naturally weak, to those whose Strength is impaired by Age or Diseases, to those whose Pulse is languid, whose vital Motions are defective, or whose Fluids have a Tendency to Corruption. It ought to be a constant Rule to Practice, never to exhibit strong Sedatives, where the Strength is small, and the Pulse, which is always lessened by Opiates, already weak ; Opiates and Anodynes are scarcely ever useful when the Viscera are infracted, and their Tone destroy'd, as in chronical Disorders. Nor are such Medicines to be exhibited, in Cases where the Blood and Humours are highly impure, as in cacochymic and scrobutic Habits, in which the immoderate Use of Opiates, in Order to remove Pains and Spasms, proves mortal, because it
quickly

quickly induces a Sphacelus. When violent Pains have greatly diminished the Strength, or a profuse Sweat been excited, these Medicines should be sparingly used, lest a Palsy, or some other nervous Disorder, should be induced. For this Reason, 'tis far more expedient to use Opiates and Anodynes in the Beginning of Diseases, when the Strength is entire, than when it is exhausted by the long continued Shock of the Disorder.

As the two principal Indications for stopping Pain are, its Violence, and the Hardness and Strength of the Pulse, so when these happen, an Hypnotic may be used, especially when the Pain proceeds from an external Cause, such as Worms, the Stone, the Eruption of a Tooth, the Puncture of a Tendon or Nerve, a Division of the Nails by some sharp Instrument, or the thrusting a Nail

deep into the Sole of the Foot which not only frequently induces a terrible Train of Symptoms, but also sometimes proves mortal.

As in all Cases mild and safe Medicines are preferable to those of a more dangerous and drastic Nature so in mitigating Pain, we are never to have recourse to strong Anodynes provided those of a mild and gentle Kind prove sufficient. Among these Hoffman recommends anodyne Sulphur prepared from Vitriol, *Spiritus Nitri dulcis* duly prepared ; among vegetable Substances, Saffron and Nutmeg, of fragrant Substances Musk and Amber ; and of Shop Preparations the Oils of Chamomile and Yarrow. To this Class also belongs Opium depurated with Rain Water, and corrected by a due Addition of Analeptics, Purgatives, or Alexipharmics.

CHAP. V.

Of DIURETICS.

THOSE Medicines which eliminate the salt Serum, impregnated with gross, terrestrial, and recrementitious Parts, by the urinary Passages, are called *Diuretics* ; the Medicines of this Kind are, by *Celsus*, in the thirty-first Chapter of his second Book, characterized and enumerated as follows: " Every fra-" grant Vegetable which is cul-" tivated in Gardens, provokes a " Discharge of Urine ; such as " Smallage, Rue, Dill, Basil, Mint, " Hyssop, Anise, Coriander, Gar-" den Cresses, Rocket, Fennel, A-" sparagus, Capers, Catmint, Thyme, " Savory, Nipple-wort Parsnip, " Skiret, and Onions. " But of

the Vegetable kind, *Hoffman* recommends as Diuretics, the Root of Parsley, Celeri, Asparagus, Grass Liquorice, Madder, Parsnip, Crowfoot, Pareira-brava, Acmella, the the Herbs Parsley, Ground Ivy Horse Tail, Chervil, common Nettle, all Leeks, and all the Species of Garlick, the Flowers of Butcher Broom, and blew Bottles, the Seed of Carrot, Parsley, Celeri, Fennel Groomwell, common Nettle, Violets, the four greater cold Seeds, the Seeds of Clubmoss, Winter Cherries, Doghips, Juniper Berries, Strawberries, the Wood of the Juniper Tree, Sassafras and its Bark. Among Resins and Balsams, Mastich Amber

Amber, the *Balsam of Mecha*, and the Balsam of Capivi. In the animal Kingdom, Catharides, Millepedes, May Worms, Scorpions, Toads, EarthWorms, Cochineal, and Whey. To the Class of Diuretics, also, belong all alcaline Salts prepared by Incineration, as also the Salt of Amber, the *Arcanum Duplicatum*, a Solution of Crabbs Eyes and Nitre. The compound Medicines belonging to this Class are, the Tincture of Tartar, and acrid Tincture of Antimony, the *Terra foliata Tartari*, soluble Tartar, the Spirit of Turpentine, Mastick and Amber, Balsam of Sulphur with Oil of Turpentine, Balsam of Juniper, Oil of Juniper, the *Syrupus Dialthææ*, the *Trochisci Alkekengi*, and many others.

As the Discharge of the Urine may be impaired and rendered difficult from several Causes, such as, first, a Defect of due Moisture in the Blood; or secondly thick and tenacious Juices, obstructing the small urinary Ducts of the Kidnies; thirdly, a violent spasmodic Constriction of the Renal Ducts; or fourthly their perternatural Relaxation and Weakness, so also the Medicines calculated for restoring a due Discharge of the Urine, must be adapted to the Removal of those several Causes. Thus, for Instance, some substances, by conveying a due Degree of Fluidity to the inspissated Blood, augment the Discharge of Urine, of which Kind are all aqueous diluting Medicines, liberal Draughts of Spring Water, whether cold or warm, especially if Herbs of a diuretic Quality are infused in them. This Intention is likewise answered by Tea and Coffee, as also by mineral Waters, either hot or cold, as they not only dilute the Blood, but by their alcaline Quality dissolve the viscid and tenacious Humours, and remove

the Obstructions of the Kidneys. The same Effect is produced by Whey, which is possessed of an aqueous, abstergent, and gently stimulating Principle, as also of a sweet nitrous Salt. Other Substances dissolve the tough viscid Humours which obstruct and block up the secretory Ducts of the Kidneys, and by that Means render them fit for performing their Functions; of this Kind are all fixed Salts, and the Lixiviums prepared from them, as also Tincture of Tartar, and the acrid Tincture of Antimony, the *Terra foliata Tartari*, the *Tartarus tartarisatus*, the *Arcanum duplicatum*, a Solution of Crabbs Eyes, and the *Magnesia Alba*, which, with the Acid of the *Primæ Viæ*, is converted into an aperient Salt; as also the Tincture of Quick-lime, Mother of Pearl, and Coral prepared with Lemon Juice, as also the Salts obtained by Exhalation from mineral Waters. Other Substances sooth and alleviate the spasmodic Constrictions of the Emunctories of the Kidneys, which obstruct and prevent the due Discharge of the Urine. The most considerable and efficacious of this Kind are Nitre, the four greater cold Seeds, and Emulsions prepared from them, the Seeds of the white Poppy, of Carrot, and of Club-moss, as also Winter Cherries and Troches prepared of them: The same Intention is answered by the anodyne mineral Liquor, which is both a safe and efficacious Medicine, as also by Saffron and its Essence, the Juice of Grass in Consequence of its nitrous Salt, a Decoction of the Roots of Grass, and Asparagus, the Oil of sweet Almonds, which is a Liquor of a highly demulcent Quality. Other Substances by their oleous, subtile, and balsamic Principle, corroborate and strengthen the Kidneys, such as Mastich, Amber, the *Balsamum de Mecha*, the Balsam of Capivi, Turpentine, the Wood and

and Berries of the Juniper Tree, Saffafras, Parfley, Fennel, Anife, Crow-foot, Celeri, and the Oils, Effences, Spirits, Decoctions and Infufions of them; other Medicines corroborate the Kidneys by their ftrengthning fixed, terreftrial, and fulphureous Principle. Of this Kind are Dog-hips, Rob of Juniper, and dried Strawberries, Pareira brava, Ground Ivy, the Bark of the Root of the Egyptian Thorn, Horfe-tail, Pauls Betony, and Chervil. Laftly, other Medicines powerfully ftimulate the renal Ducts, when they are fo far weakened, as to have their Functions either impaired, or totally deftroyed: Of this Kind are almoft all Infects, efpecially Catharides, Millepedes, Spiders, Scorpions, and dried Toads; and in the vegetable Kingdom, all the Species of Leeks, and Garlick.

Since there is fo great a difference between diuretic Medicines, with refpect to the Principles and Manner of Operation, their Ufe muft of Courfe be different, and they muft be judicioufly adapted to the particular Nature of different Cafes; for if to plethoric Patients labouring under the Stone, we fhould before Venefection and the Diminution of the Quantity of Blood, exhibit hot Subftances impregnated with a fubtile balfamic Oil, fuch as Preparations of Turpentine, and Juniper, or the Balfams of *Mecha, Capivi*, or *Peru*, or acrid Subftances, or fuch infects as abound with a cauftic Salt, Garlick, Onions, or Leeks, we fhould certainly injure the Patient, bring on an Inflammation of the Kidneys, and promote the Generation of Stones. On the contrary, in moift, lefs delicate, and more robuft Patiens, who live upon coarfe Food, as alfo in Difeafes arifing from a Redundance of impure Serum, a Fluor Albus, a Gonorrhæa, a Difpofition to an Ana-

farca, and Leucophlegmatia, thefe draftic Medicines are of fingular Ufe and Service.

Still greater Misfortunes are produced by acrid and ftimulating Subftances, in Cafes where in Confequence of Spafmodic or nephritic Pains, a Difcharge of the Urine is fuppreffed. Diforders of this Nature are far more fafely and efficacioufly removed, by fuch Medicines as alleviate Pain, and relax Strictures; fuch as Winter Cherries, the Seeds of Carrot, Club-mofs, white Poppy, and Gromwell, as alfo Emulfions of the four greater cold Seeds, the *Trochifci Alkekengi* with Opium, antimoniated Nitre depurated, the Water of the Leaves of Meadow fweet, of the Lime Tree, and of the *Egyptian Thorn*, Oil of fweet Almonds, fweet Spirit of Nitre, the Anodyne mineral Liquor, Whey; and externally, emollient Baths and Fomentations, the Virtues of all which are fo great, that by alleviating the wracking Spafms, they not only reftore the free Difcharge of the Urine, but alfo facilitate the Progrefs of the Stone thro' the Ureters, and promote its Expulfion.

In Diforders arifing from a Redundance of Salt and tartareous Serum, which is generally the Caufe of arthritic and rheumatic Pains, this peccant Humour is carried of by gentle Diuretics, tho' not of the hot Kind, left by their Means the Spiculæ of the Salt fhould be put into a brifker Motion, and the Parts in which they are lodged be more violently racked. The gentle Diuretics, by which this Intention is moft effectually anfwered, are, the Roots of Sarfaparilla, Pareira brava, Saffafras, and China-Root; as alfo thofe of Liquorice, Afparagus, Madder, Succory, Fennel, Parfley, and Grafs, together with the Wood of the Juniper Tree, and the Preparations of thefe boiled in Broth made

made with Flesh, or in Water. To this Class, also, belong Whey, and more especially the temperate mineral Waters, and warm Springs.

But in Cases where peccant, viscid and tenacious Humours are lodged in the urinary Bladder, and especially when the Intention is to expel the first Rudiments of a Stone, more acrid and powerful Medicines become necessary. This Intention is answered by Garlick, exhibited with Spirit of Juniper, as, also, by the Powder of Millepedes, May Worms, Essence of Cantharides, Tincture of Cantharides, Tincture of Antimony, and Infusions of Quick-Lime; which may also be cautiously exhibited in a virulent Gonorrhæa, when a viscid and tenacious Matter lodged in the Prostratæ, the Neck of the Bladder, or the Urethra, is to be carried off by Urine.

But the more safe and efficacious Medicines for procuring a free Discharge of Urine are, all Kinds not only of alcaline fixed Salts, but also of those called neutral, for they not only dissolve the tough and viscid Juices, which obstruct the urinary Ducts, but also by a gentle Stimulus promote their Discharge. This Intention is excellently answered by Solutions of the Salt of Tartar, Pot-ash, and fixed Nitre, as also the *Tartarus vitriolatus*, Salt of Wormwood, *Arcanum duplicatum*, a Solution of Crabbs Eyes, soluble Tartar, the *Terra foliata Tartari*, antimoniated Nitre, and *Sal Polychrestum*.

These Medicines not only contribute to restore a due and natural Discharge of the Urine, but also produce some other excellent Effects in the Cure of Diseases; for as many of them are possessed of an aperient and inciding Quality, as others of them are corroborative, balsamic, and restore the Tone of the Parts, and others are of an anodyne Nature, so they prove highly efficacious in those chronical Disorders, which arise from an Obstruction of the Glands of the Viscera, and Emunctories, or from a Impurity of the Juices, or a Redundance of saline, acrid, and tartarous Serum; and certainly, if Relief is to be expected from any Medicines in Dropsies, Ædematous Swellings, stony Concretions, the Gout, and arthritic Pains, we are to look for it from the prudent Use of Diuretics: But we are to be aware of all hot, acrid, and caustic Diuretics, and use those which are of a milder Nature, and fit for common Use, such as small *Moselle* Wine, the mild mineral Waters, and such Ales and Decoctions as are gently diuretic.

M   C H A P.

CHAP. VI.

Of ALEXIPHARMICS.

AN Alexipharmic seems originally to have signified a Remedy
to expel, or prevent the ill Effects
of Poisons taken internally, and this
is *Galen*'s Explanation. But since
some among the Moderns have con-
jured up a chimerical Poison, in order to inflame, or otherwise affect
the imaginary animal Spirits in a-
cute Distempers, Alexipharmics have
been understood to mean Remedies
adapted to expel this Poison by the
cutaneous Pores, in the Form of
Sweat. Hence it appears, that Alexi-
phamics mean just the same as Sudorifics. I am persuaded that few
Theories have ever been introduced
into Medicine, so as to be much depended upon, without very ill Effects upon Practice, but that which
paved the Way for Alexipharmics,
has exerted extraordinary Heroisms,
and made uncommon Havock a-
mongst Mankind.

Hippocrates in his Treatise *de Ratione Victus in Acutis*, has the following Passage : *Whoever in the Beginning of an inflammatory Disease attempts the Cure by Cathartics, does not
in the least diminish the Tension and
Inflammation of the Part affected, for
the Distemper in this State of Crudity,
will not yield to such Medicines ; on
the contrary, this Method of Treatment liquefies and wastes the found
Parts, which would otherwise resist
the Distemper, and when the Body is
in this Manner weakened, the Disease
gets Ground, till at last it becomes incurable.*

Tho' this is said with a great Deal
of Justness and Propriety, I am persuaded it may with stronger Reason
be applied to Sudorifics, that is, to
Alexipharmics, which frequently do
a great Deal of Mischief, and indeed there is nothing in which the
lower Class of Practitioners in Physic make more Errors, than in the
Use of *Alexipharmics*, which I have
frequently known exhibited to young
People, of plethoric Habits, in the
very Beginning of Fevers, and even
without previous Evacuations.

About the Year 1723, 1724, and
1725, a Fever appeared with uncommon Virulence, and was more universal than any I have ever known ;
and by this, great Numbers of working People perished, in so much,
that in many Countries scarce e-
nough were left to gather in the
Fruits of the Earth ; and this Sort
of Fever continued many Years after. In this Disorder it was remarkable, that a warm Regimen or hot
Medicines, seldom or never failed to
render the Fever continual, and keep
it so, bringing on Deliriums, and all
Symptoms of Malignity ; whereas
a cool Regimen, with Evacuations
by bleeding, and purging with Caution, and an entire Abstinence from
hot Medicines, almost always brought
the Fever to a regular Intermission,
and then the Bark effectually took it
off. As I had an Oportunity of
seeing a great Number of Patients
under this Fever, I was abundantly
convinced, that more died of *Alexipharmics*, than of the Distemper.

But that I may not appear singular with Respect to this Sort of Medicine, I shall give the Opinion of
the

the illuftrious *Hoffman* upon this Subject, who having juft before mentioned Cathartics goes on thus.

There is another Sett of Evacuants which carry off the more fubtile Parts of the morbific Matter, by the Pores of the Skin, in a plentiful, offenfive, gentle and more imperceptible Manner. The Remedies moft conducive to this are Sudorifics, by whofe Operation a fenfible Moifture is perfpired through the cutaneous Glands. Of the vegetable Kind the moft efficacious for this Purpofe, are the Roots of a very acrid, penetrating, oily Tafte, as thofe of *Angelica*, the different Species of Mafter-wort, Butter Burr, Elecampane, Lovage, Swallow-wort, Valerian, Contrayerva, *Virginia* Snake-root, Woods of Guaiacum and Saffafrafs, with their Barks. In the mineral Kingdom, crude Antimony, Regulus Antimonii Medicinalis, volatile Tincture of Sulphur prepared with Quick-lime, Sal ammoniac and Sulphur, corrected and fixed Sulphur of Antimony, and alfo the Mixtura Simplex: Likewife, *Venice* Treacle, its Effence, Spirit and Water, all Spirits, and volatile Salts prepared from the Parts of Animals, particularly Harts-horn, Ivory, and Earth-worms, Spirit of Silk, Soot, the Effences of the Woods, and the diftilled fetid Oils, as fetid Oil of Harts-horn diffolved in Spirit of Wine.

Thefe nobler Medicines of the Sudorific Kind, owe the Virtue of their Operation to the Power they poffefs of increafing the fyftaltic Motion of the Heart, and the Elafticity of the Arteries, as to the Number and Force of their Vibrations, by which Means a greater Velocity being added to the Circulation, they protrude the perfpirable Matter thro' the outward and porous Subftance of the Skin. This they perform either by a fubtile, acrid, hot Oil, as the

Roots above-mentioned, which are called *Alexipharmics*, or by a volatile empyreumatic Salt of an igneous Nature; fuch as are all the Spirits, volatile Salts, and Oils from Animals; or by an acrid refinous Salt, more or lefs fixed, as the Root of white Burnet, Guaiacum, and its Bark, Contrayerva, *Virginia* Snake-root: Or laftly they act, and that very powerfully, by Means of a very fine mineral Salt and Sulphur, by which they roufe the nervous Fibres to a violent Motion, and for this purpofe a very fmall Dofe is fufficient. Thus a fingle Grain of diaphoretic Mercury, or two or three Grains of fixed Sulphur of Antimony, will raife a Sweat over every Part of the Body; a Decoction of the Woods, as alfo *Regulus Antimonii Medicinalis*, have the fame Effect.

Thefe ftrong Sudorifics, tho' given in a larger Quantity, will by no Means raife a Sweat, unlefs the porous Subftance of the Skin be fufficiently open and lax, or unlefs the Blood be enough diluted. Wherefore if any one, in the Cure of a Difeafe, thinks fweating required, it will be neceffary for him to give the above-mentioned Sudorifics, with a fufficient Quantity of fome Liquid to dilute the Blood, for Example, a weak Tea, or a Decoction of Barley; and that the Pores of the Skin may obtain a due Relaxation, the Perfon to be fweated fhould be put in a warm Bed, or hot Stove, or into a Bath, efpecially a vapour Bath, that a plentiful Sweat may be excited.

Thefe very active Sudorifics rarely find a Place in Medicine, and are not to be adminiftered but with fingular Caution. For a Sweat never arifes in a healthful and natural State, unlefs the Blood is put into an extraordinary Motion; nor when this happens is it a Sign of Health, like infenfible Perfpiration, the Matter of which is void of Acrimony, watery, of Kin to the nutritious Juices, and almoſt without either Taſte or Smell, and differs very much from Sweat, which is of a ſalt Taſte, a fetid Smell, and approaches the Nature of Urine. Beſides, theſe Sudorifics excite a great Commotion and notable Orgaſm; for they act not with Moderation but Rapidity; whence it comes to paſs, that in Bodies full of Blood, or contaminated Serum, by impelling the Fluids with too much Violence to the ſmall narrow Veſſels, they bring on dangerous and acute Symptoms, occaſioned by the Inflammation, and Redundance of Humours. But they are moſt injurious where the *Primæ Viæ* are obſtructed by a Load of vicious Humours, where the Body is coſtive, and when they are adminiſtered immediately after a violent Fit of Anger. By this pernicious Practice, arthritic and rheumatic Pains, ſlow and hectic Fevers, which have proved of long Continuance, and been attended with eminent Danger, have been excited.

In all acute Caſes, as inflammatory and ſcarlet Fevers, *Sudorifics* are to be entirely baniſhed, or at leaſt to be adminiſtered very ſeldom, and that with great Caution, for the promiſcuous Uſe of *Alexipharmics*, as the Cuſtom too generally prevails, only ſerve to increaſe Heat, Anxiety, and the Violence of the Symptoms. Theſe Remedies are called *Alexipharmics*, as are alſo all thoſe of the Theriacal Kind, from a Virtue attributed to them of reſiſting Poiſons, and malignant Humours, for which Reaſon they are highly extolled by Phyſicians in the Plague, and other contagious Diſtempers; but the Truth is, they are much more powerful for the Prevention, than Cure of theſe Diſeaſes, eſpecially when an epidemical and malignant Diſtemper owes its Birth to an

over wet, foggy, cloudy Seaſon, which has been long deſtitute of the Eaſt and North Winds; or to a Deluge or Inundation of Waters. But in this Caſe it will be much better and ſafer to give them in Wine Vinegar diluted with Water, or to infuſe the ſudorific Roots in Vinegar, which by this Means being impregnated with their *alexipharmic* Virtue, two or three Spoonfuls may be drank in any convenient aqueous Vehicle.

But ſweating is very ſervicable in thoſe Diſtempers which proceed from an external Cold, and obſtructed Perſpiration, as in Catarrhs, Rheumatiſms, Fluxes, Stoppages of the Head, Coughs, and glandular Tumors; alſo, when Danger is apprehended from a Perſon's having drank a large Quantity of cold Liquor, when very hot, or in a Sweat. But then they ſhould be adminiſtered in the Beginning of theſe Diſorders. Nor is a Sudorific of leſs Service in the Beginning of any infectious Diſtemper, taken immediately after a mild Emetic. But perhaps Camphire is the beſt of Alexipharmics.

Likewiſe in thoſe Diſeaſes which have their Seat in the porous and fibrous Subſtance of the Skin, and conſiſt of an acrid viſcid Matter, which deſtroys and deforms its Texture, as an inveterate Itch, the Ring-worm, Leproſy, and venereal Puſtules, and Ulcers, a plentiful Sweat may be excited to great Advantage with proper Remedies. The ſame may be alſo practiſed in arthritic and rheumatic Pains in any Part of the Body; for by this Means the acrid, viſcid, and ſtagnating Serum, which adheres to the nervous Membranes, is thrown off and diſcharged. For the ſame Reaſon in all thoſe Diſeaſes which are called *Cold,* as in Dropſies of every Kind, the cold Scurvy, Pox, ſettled Gout, Sciatica, Palſy, and thoſe of the ſame

Na-

Nature, Sudorifics are of great Efficacy, becaufe they promote and reftore the Elafticity and contractile Power of the Heart and Veffels, which in Diforders of this Kind are very much depreffed, and increafe the Circulation of the Blood, for the better Separation of the morbid Matter. But this Courfe muft be perfifted in for fome time.

Sudorifics always operate beft, when taken with a fufficient Quantity of fome warm Liquid. *Celfus* in the fixth Chapter of his third Book commends warm Water for this Purpofe, his Words are thefe. " When " you perceive the Sweat approaching " you fhould give warm Water to " drink, which hath a moft health- " ful Effect, if it excites a Sweat " over the whole Body." It is notorious that this is procured in the moft plentiful Manner by a Decoction of the Woods, whofe Ufe in venereal Cafes, and other cold Diftempers, cannot be enough commended. Several Country People have been happily cured of intermitting Fevers, and tertian and quartan Agues, by taking a few Hours before the Fit a Vomit, and immediately after it, a Sudorific of Rob of Elder, Salt of Tartar, and a few Corns of Pepper, mixed together in a Spoonful or two of Brandy.

Diaphoretics are inferior in their Power of acting to Sudorifics, but much fuperior to them in their healthful Qualities, as they gently increafe and promote Perfpiration. Of thefe the chief in the vegetable Kingdom are, the Roots of *China*, Sarfaparilla, the *Carline* Thiftle, and Gentian ; of Herbs the holy Thiftle entire, its Seeds, and all the Preparations from it, whether Effences, Waters, Extracts, or Salts, Water Germander, the Elder and Dwarf Elder with its Flowers, Rob and Water; alfo Fumitory, Scabions,

Saffron, the Flowers of Marygold, and Opium. In the animal Kingdom, all Bones, Horns, and Teeth of Animals, whether rafp'd or burnt to Afhes, and chymically prepared, efpecially thofe belonging to the Stag, the Stones, Shells, and Claws of Crabs. Of Earths, all feal'd Earths, and different Kinds of Marle. Of Salts, the Salts of Plants procured by burning, and Nitre. Of precious and exotic Stones, the *Petra di Porco*, the Eaftern and Weftern Bezoar-Stone. Of Minerals and chymical Breparations, the Flower and Milk of Sulphur, Cinnabar, Native, Common, and that of Antimony, Diaphoretic Antimony, Cerufs of Antimony, Magiftery of Antimony, the Bezoardic-Mineral, and *Poterius*'s Antihectic. Of Compounds Goa-ftone, which is compounded of oriental Bezoar, Tragacanth, and Ambergreafe, *Sennertus*'s Bezoardic-powder, the *English* and *Pannonian* Red-powder, the Mineral anodyne Liquor, Wine-vinegar, or diftilled Vinegar with Elder-flowers or Crabs-eyes infufed in it.

The Operation of Diaphoretics is manifold and various ; for either they act in a privative Manner, by abforbing and changing the Acid in the *Primæ Viæ*, which carried into the Blood depreffes its Spirituofity, Fluidity, and inteftine Motion ; of which Kind are all the Earths of an alcaline Nature : Or by imbibing the fuperfluous Moifture, and bracing the relaxed Fibres, as the feal'd Earths, Boles and Marles, alfo Bones and Horns, both thofe burnt and thofe chymically prepared, and the Unicorns Stone : Or by relaxing and mollifying, in Difeafes of the Skin, its contracted Superficies, by their mild, anodyne and vaporous Sulphur, as the different Species of Elder, efpecially the Flowers, Saffron and its Extracts, the Flowers of Red

Poppy, or Corn Rofe, the Anodyne Mineral Liquor, the Emulfions of Poppy Seed, corrected Opiates: Or by compofing and quieting the too violent inteftine Motion of the Blood, as the Remedies of the nitrous Kind, corrected by being joined with the more fixed Diaphoretics; as alfoSpirit of Nitre dulcified, Emulfions of the Four greater cold Seeds, and the milder Acids, as Juice of Lemons, and Vinegar: Or laftly in a pofitive Manner, by gently ftimulating the Fibres and languid Veffels, of which Sorts are, the holy Thiftle, Water Germander, Fumitory, China, Sarfaparilla, the leffer Centaury, Seabious, Carline Thiftle, and Gentian.

Now as the Evacuation of the finer Parts of the morbific Matter, thro' the Pores of the Skin, by infenfible Tranfpiration, is of all others the moft healthful, and as the Obftruction thereof is the Occafion of many Maladies, fo the Ufe of Diaphoretics, which promote this cutaneous Excretion, is certainly very great, univerfal, and almoft infallible, in almoft all Difeafes, even thofe which from their prefent Symptoms, we are not thoroughly acquainted with; fo that a Phyfician can by no Means be without them; for an increafed Circulation of the Blood, and an enlarged Perfpiration, are the grand Mediums and Inftrument of Nature, by which the morbific Matter in any Difeafe is corrected, digefted, refolved, and at laft thrown off; and thus the Diftemper is cured without Danger. Particularly in all acute Difeafes, as Fevers and Inflammations of all Kinds, thefe alone given in fome convenient Vehicle, in fmall Dofes, and continued for fome time, anfwer every Intention of Cure, and are in Truth the beft Difcutients, and Purifiers of the Mafs of Blood.

Becaufe exceffive Heats, efpecially in Summer, and in choleric and bilious Conftitutions, as alfo in choleric and bilious Fevers, dries too much, confumes Moifture, and hinders Perfpiration, acidulated and nitrous Remedies, and particularly Crabs Eyes with Nitre, given in a Julep of Diaphoretic Waters, and Syrup of Lemon Juice, by moderating the too great Heat, and procuring a plentiful Diaphofis, give great Relief to the Patient.

When, thro' the Violence of any Diforder, the Skin is dry, and without Moifture, and its Pores become narrow and contracted, it is always beft to join fome mild Anodynes and Antifpafmodics to the Diaphoretics; and in this Cafe the Anodyne Mineral Liquor mix'd in the Quantity of three Parts with one Part of the *Spiritus Bezoardicus Buffii,* is of admirable Virtue, as are alfo fixed, diaphoretic Powders with a little Nitre and Cinnabar, and a fmall Quantity of an Opiate.

In acute Difeafes and Fevers, where but little Acid is lodged in the *Primæ Viæ,* it will be fafer and of more Service, to give the fixed and earthy Diaphoretics in a fmall Quantity, and well mixed with Syrup of Citron Juice, or Wine Vinegar, which will not coagulate, but often refolves and throws off the ftagnating Blood, efpecially if joned with Diaphoretics.

Thus *Hoffman* very juftly diftinguifhes between Sudorifics or Alexipharmics, and Diaphoretics; fince the former are fuch Medicines a excite a violent Heat and Motion and a confiderable Orgafm in the Body, which tend to extort profufe Sweats, and do a great deal of Violence to Nature, which is by this Means deprived of a large Quantity of the more fluid Parts of the Blood that might otherwife be highly beneficial in preferving the whole Mafs in a due State of Fluidity, in promoting the Diffolution of the ftagnant and obftructing Humours, and affifting affifing the Expulfion of the morbific Matter from the Limits of the Circulation; whereas Diaphoretics are Medicines endued with a gently ftimulating and perhaps refolvent Quality, by which they affift Nature in carrying on her own falutary Purpofes, without any Tendency to do her any Violence, or divert her from the Method fhe has begun to purfue.

In order to account for the fudden Effects of fome Alexipharmics in raifing a Sweat, before they can well be fuppofed to enter the Mafs of Blood, we muft obferve, that Alexipharmics confift of highly penetrating and ftimulating Particles, fo that when thefe act upon the nervous Coats of the Stomach, the Stimulus thereby produced, derives a greater Fluid (if any fuch there be) into thefe Nerves, and all the correfpondent nervous Ramifications diftributed from the fame Trunk. Now the Stomach receives a great many Nerves from the defcending Trunks of the Par-vagum, and fome Branches immediately from the Plexus Cardiacus, formed by the fame Par-vagum, and fituated a little above the Heart, from which Plexus the Heart is alfo furnifhed with Nerves; whatever therefore ftimulates the Nerves of the Stomach, muft alfo proportionably affect thofe of the Heart, the Confequence of which is, that the Force and Frequency of the Contractions of the Heart, muft be increafed, and of Courfe the general Heat of the Fluids circulating by Means of fuch Contractions, augmented, becaufe the Motion and Friction is greater than before. The Blood thus circulating with greater Velocity, muft be impelled more frequently with greater Force towards the Surface of the Body, by which Means an increafed Evacuation by the cutaneous Pores is procured. Tho' I am far from being abfolutely certain that what we commonly call the nervous Fluid or animal Spirits, have a real Exiftence in Nature, yet, let the immediate Vehicles of Senfation and Motion be what they will, what is above advanced with Refpect to the Stimulus of the Nerves, is by Experience found to hold true.

CHAP. VII.
Of CARDIACS.

CARDIACS are properly fuch Medicines, as preferve or increafe the Strength of the Heart, and by that Means the vital Forces, tho' they do not immediately act upon the Heart, nor are particularly appropriated to the Corroboration of that Part. This Effect they perform either by replenifhing the exhaufted Veffels with good Humours, or exciting Motion where it was deficient. Nutritives therefore or Repletives duly chofen with refpect to particular Conftitutions, belong to this Clafs, as well as Aftringents, Corroboratives, and Stimulants, which are ufually accounted the only Cardiacs. In this Senfe we are to underftand the Definition given by *Harvey* of a Cardiac, which he fays is fomething that is endow'd with a Vertue of fpeedily recollecting the fcatter'd and broken Spirits, and recruiting them with plentiful Supplies

plies

plies, and of corroborating the flaccid Fibres of the Heart.

Hence it appears, that *Cardiacs*, are principally deftined to the Removal of fome Weaknefs, and that any thing may be called a *Cardiac*, which removes the Obftacles to Circulation. Wherefore *Valcarengus* was very juft in his Notion when he fays, that " A *Cardiac* is whatever " deftroys, or at leaft blunts the " Force of the morbific Caufe, re- " ftores the loft Tone of the Solids, " and gives due Motion to the " Fluids, and by that Means pro- " cures a juft Equilibrium, which is " the only and lafting Principle of " all the Motions in our Body." Generally what promotes Motion is alfo a Caufe of the Heart's acquiring a greater Strength for Action.

But fince Weaknefs does not only arife from a Defect of good Humours, and a flaccid Indifpofition of the Veffels, but often times from a Redundance of Humours, a thick and ftagnating Blood, with an Obftruction of the Veffels form too great a Rigidnefs, Contraction, or Compreffion, it follows that what we call debilitating, refrigerating, relaxing, refolvent, and evacuating Medicines, belong to the Clafs of *Cardiacs*, in as much as they remove a prefent Weaknefs of the Body, by acting immediately and directly in Oppofition to the Caufe of that Weaknefs. *Riverius* juftly obferves, that as the Heart may be debilitated fometimes by a hot, and fometimes by a cold Intemperature, fome Cardiac Medicines muft of Courfe be of a hot, and others of a cold Nature. *Lind ftolpe* in his Treatife *de Venenis*, fays, that " the Vulgar, indeed, " are of Opinion, that there are " fome Medicines that immediately " cotroborate and exhilerate the " Heart, but I have as yet found " out none of this Kind, for all

" Subftances which corroborate the " Heart; or occafion its ftrong and " frequent Contraction, are the moft " violent Poifons, and of a Quality " the moft unfriendly to the Conftitu- " tion; of this are all acrid, mettalic, " acid, and alcaline Poifons, and the " putrefactive Poifons of Animals " for by large Dofes of thefe Sub- " ftances, the Motion of the Heart " is increafed, and the Ruin of the " Conftitution promoted at the fame " Time. And as the Difeafes arife " from different Caufes, fo whatever " Medicine is contrary to a Difeafe, " may be faid to be poffeffed of a " Cardiac or Cordial Quality, not " becaufe it corroborates the Heart, " but becaufe it proves grateful and " agreeable to the whole Habit. " Thus in putrid Fevers, and fuch " as arife from a predominant Alca- " li, all acid; metallic, and vegetable " Subftances, are Cordials. On the " contrary, in Diforders arifing from " a predominant Acid, we are to " have recourfe to alcaline Subftan- " ces, as the moft proper Cordials; " in Difeafes produced by Rage and " Wrath, we muft enjoin Calmnefs " and Compofure of Temper; in " Grief and Sorrow, Joy and Chear- " fulnefs; and in every Diforder, what " feems moft directly oppofite to it."

Volatile and diffolvent Cardiacs which ftimulate the Fibres, raife the drooping Spirits, and over-heat the Body, univerfally and indifcriminately exhibited to Patients of all Conftitutions, are by no Means to be approved of. 'Tis become however, almoft univerfally cuftomary, to ufe inflammable Spirits, and balfamic and aromatic Medicines, in order to raife the Spirits, when funk and render'd languid, by whatever Caufe. It muft, indeed, be confefs'd that fuch Subftances roufe the Spirits, and procure a momentary Eafe to the Patient; but when unfeafonably or exceffively ufed, they ex-

cite

ate too violent Commotions in the Juices, and diſſipate thoſe which are noſt fluid, by which Means thoſe which are too thick, and unfit for Circulation, are left behind in the Body. Hence ariſes Dryneſs and Rigidity of the ſolid Parts, and a Weakneſs ariſing from Obſtructions, and if, in Caſes of this Nature, the Uſe of theſe Cordial Medicines is repeated or perſiſted in, theſe Diſorders are augmented and increaſed. In a word, the Man who fooliſhly attempts to reſtore his Strength, or raiſe his Spirits, by this Method, has the Fate of him, who by blowing Fire, renders it indeed briſker, but at the ſame Time leſs durable, than it would otherwiſe have been. *Paulus Valcarengus*, in his *Medicina Rationalis*, endeavours to ſhew, that what proves a Cordial to one Patient, may prove a Poiſon to another. The Origin and fatal Conſequences of this wretched Cuſtom, are by Dr. *Cheyne* in his Eſſay of Health and long Life, excellently deſcribed in the following Manner, when ſpeaking of the idle Habits of ſome Ladies drinking Cordials, " A ' Fit of the Cholic, or of the Va- ' pours, a Family Misfortune, a ca- ' ſual Diſappointment ; the Death ' of a Child, of a Friend, with the ' Aſſiſtance of the Nurſe, the Mid- ' wife, and the next Neighbour, ' often give Riſe, and become the ' weighty Cauſes of ſo fatal an Ef- ' fect. A little Lowneſs requires ' Drops, which readily paſs down ' under the Notion of Phyſic. ' Drops beget Drams, and Drams ' beget more Drams, till they be- ' come without Weight, and with- ' out Meaſure ; ſo that at laſt the ' miſerable Creature ſuffers a true ' Martyrdom, between its natural ' Modeſty, the great Neceſſity of ' concealing its Cravings, and the ' ſtill greater one of getting them ' ſatisfied ſomeway. Higher and ' more ſevere Fits of Hyſterics,

" Tremors, and Convulſions, begot " by theſe, bring forth farther Ne- " ceſſity upon Neceſſity of Drops, " Drams, and Gills, till at laſt a Kind " of Dropſy, Nervous Convulſions, " Nervous Atrophy, or a Colli- " quative Diarrhæa, if not a Fever, " or a Frenzy ſet the poor Soul free."

Give me leave to remark, that Dr. *Cheyne* might have added as a frequent Cauſe of the horrid Cu- ſtom of drinking Drams, to theſe above mentioned, the habitual U- ſage of any warm diluting Fluids, ſuch as Tea, which in Conſequence of their Warmth, relax the digeſtive Organs, whence Flatulencies, Low- neſs of Spirits, and a Neceſſity for Drops, or ſomething elſe, in order to raiſe the ſinking Spirits.

There are, however, ſome Caſes, in which Cardiac Medicines of this Kind may be properly exhibited. In Palpitations of the Heart, for Inſtance, and Syncopes, when theſe Diſorders ariſe from a cold and aque- ous, or an inert and mucous State of the Juices ; in which Caſes the diſtil- led cohobated Waters, and the di- ſtilled eſſential Oils of Baum and Le- mon-peel, are principally proper.

Etmuller informs us, that the Cephalico-cardiac Medicine commu- nicated by *Elizabeth* Queen of *Eng- land*, to the Emperor *Rudolphus* the Second, conſiſted of Amber, Muſk, and Civet, diſſolved in the Spirit of Roſes. According to the celebrated *Hoffman* in his *Medicina Rationalis*, " We are not to imagine, that a " true and permanent Reſtoration of " Strength is to be procured by ſuch " Medicines, as communicate Moti- " on to the Spirits, and ſolid Parts, " ſince in various Diſorders, eſpe- " cially Fevers and Convulſions, the " moving Force of the Heart, Arte- " ries, and Membranes, is ſuffi- " ciently great, and yet the natu- " ral Strength is languid and im- " pair'd ; ſo that the true and ge- " nuine

" nuine Perfection of the natural
" Strength, for the moft Part de-
" pends upon proper Aliments, and
" Liquors converted into laudable
" Juices and Blood; of which is af-
" terwards generated, that highly
" fubtile Fluid which is feparated in
" the Brain, convey'd thro' the
" Nerves to the Mufcles and mufcu-
" lar Coats, and which imparts
" Strength and Vigour to the Body,
" and all its Parts. The beft Ana-
" leptics are, therefore, thofe nutri-
" tive Subftances which are poffefs'd
" of the moft falutary Qualities; of
" this Kind are Jelly, Broths of
" Fifhes, Capons, Bones, and their
" Marrow, prepared by boiling in
" Water, in a clofe Veffel, with an
" Addition of a little Wine, a few
" Slices of Lemon, a little Salt,
" Powder of Mace and Cloves. Of
" this Kind is alfo the Broth prepar-
" ed of coarfe Bread, Water, Wine,
" and Eggs. To this Clafs alfo be-
" long Chocolate with or without
" Milk, Affes Milk, Water diftilled
" from coarfe Bread, and Lemon-
" peel; Wine, efpecially old gene-
" rous *Rhenifh* Wine, and genuine
" *Hungarian* Wine. But thefe Nu-
" tritive and Alimentary Medicines
" are moft proper for recruiting and
" reftoring the Strength, tho' not im-
" mediately under the Difeafe itfelf,
" nor when the whole Mafs of Blood
" and Humours is highly impure;
" but in the Decline of the Difeafe,
" and in Cafes where the Strength
" has been exhaufted and impair'd
" by the Shocks of a previous Difor-
" der, the Sallies of exorbitant Paffi-
" ons, exceffive Watchings, Labour
" and Fatigue of Body and Mind,
" or profufe Hæmorrhages, and e-
" ven in thefe Cafes, a cautious and
" prudent Moderation is to be ufed;
" becaufe thefe Subftances very
" quickly pafs into the Mafs of
" Blood, and augment its Quantity."
With refpect to the Ufe of Cor-

dials in hot Diforders, fuch as continued Fevers, the incomparable
Sydenham delivers his Sentiments
thus, " Cordials, as I have experi-
" enced, when exhibited too foon,
" do Mifchief; and unlefs Bleeding
" has preceeded, may derive the
" crude Matter of the Diftemper up-
" on the Membranes of the Brain,
" or upon the Pleura; for this Rea-
" fon I never exhibit them, when
" either no Blood, or but a little, has
" been previoufly taken away, or
" when no other confiderable Eva-
" cuation has been made, or the Pa-
" tient has not paffed the Meridian
" of Life; for whilft the Blood re-
" mains rich enough of itfelf, it
" fhould not be render'd richer, to the
" endangering the Patient; nor does
" it require to be raifed and exalted,
" fo long as no remarkable Evacua-
" tions have diminifh'd its natural
" Heat. Patients of this Kind have
" Cordials ftored up within themfelves
" which render thofe of the external or
" adventitious Kind either fuperflu-
" ous or prejudicial. In Cafes of this
" Nature, therefore, I either prefcribe
" no Cordials at all, or thofe of the
" weakeft Kind. But if the Patient
" fhould be greatly weaken'd, and
" difpirited by copious Evacuations,
" or if he fhould be in the Decline of
" Life, I generally admit of Cor-
" dials, even in the Beginning of a
" Fever; and on the twelfth Day of
" the Diforder, when the Crifis is
" juft approaching, I think a freer
" Ufe of the hotter Remedies allow-
" able, and they may be exhibited
" fooner, provided there is no Dan-
" ger of the febrile Matter falling
" upon the principal Parts; for at
" this Time, the more the Blood is
" heated, the more the Bufinefs of
" Concoction is promoted." And
a little after he fubjoins, " In this
" Diftemper I ufe the milder Cor-
" dials at the Beginning, when the
" Exæftuation is moft violent, and
"   " gradually

"gradually proceed to the hotter, "according as the Fever, or the De- "grees of Ebullition require, al- "ways remembring, where Vene- "section has been freely used, or "when the Patient is advanced in ".Years, to administer those of a "stronger Kind , than when no "Blood has been previously taken "away, or when the Patient is in the "Vigour of Life. The milder Cor- "dials, are such as are made of the "distilled Waters of Borage, Le- "mons, Strawberries, and the com- "pound Scordium Water, with a "Mixture of the Syrup of Baum, "Cloves, or Juice of Lemons. But "the stronger are *Gascoign*'s Powder, "Bezoar, Confection of Hyacinth, "Venice Treacle, and others of a like "Nature."

All the modern Dispensatories are so full of Cardiaca or Cordials, both of the dry and liquid Kind, that these alone would take up a Volume, was I to specify them all, and that to very little Purpose, because they are generally very insignificant and tri- fling Medicines. The best Cardiacs are those Remedies which remove the Disorders of which Lowness of Spirits is the Consequence ; and next to these is Wine, which exhi- bited in proper Quantities, and more or less diluted, as Circumstances re- quire, will generally answer better Purposes than the more pompous Cordials, whilst it is less capable of doing Mischief.

I shall conclude this Article with the Opinions of *Harvey* and *Vallisneri* with respect to the cardiac Powders of the Shops. The former of these affirms, that there is more of a real cordial Quality, in a Spoonful of good Broth, or a few Drops of Brandy, than in a whole Ounce of those officinal Powders, distinguish- ed by the pompous Epithet of Cor- dials.

Vallisneri, in his *Opere Fisico Me- diche T.* 3. informs us, that those are mistaken who imagine, that ear- thy Substances, such as *Armenian* Bole, seal'd Earth, *Samian* Earth, Pearls, and Bezoar are, in malig- nant and pestilential Fevers, proper- ly exhibited with an Intention to resist the Putrefaction, which is generated by an Excess of Heat and Moisture, since this Putrefaction arises purely from Obstructions, and must be great in Porportion to them; and since by earthy, cold, and dry Sub- stances, Obstructions, and consequent- ly the Putrefaction arising from them are augmented.

CHAP. VIII.

Of CEPHALICS.

UNDER the Denomination of Cephalics, are comprehended all those Medicines, which have a peculiar Relation to the Brain ; so that cephalic Remedies in general, are such as promote the Secretion and Distribution of the Spirits. This Intention is answered by all such Substances as procure a free Circulation of the Humours through the Vessels of the Brain : Hence Ce- phalics are different, according to the Diversity of Causes which may hap- pen to obstruct or hinder the Circu- lation of the Humours in the Brain. If the Cause, is of the cold and mucous Kind, the Cephalics to be prescribed, must be of an heating, stimuftimulating, fragrant, and aromatic Quality, ; if on the contrary, the Diforder arifes from an Excefs of Heat in the Body, the Cephalics to be exhibited muft be of a cooling and refrigerating Nature. Thus Correctors, univerfal Evacuants, and other Medicines deferve to be dignified with the Epithet, *Cephalic*, when they have a Tendency to weaken or remove the Caufe, which produces any particular Diforder of the Head; fince, therefore, different Diforders of the Head, draw their Origins from oppofite Caufes, thofe muft certainly be in a palpable Error, who only give the Title of Cephalics, to heating and volatile Subftances, which have often been found to prove prejudicial in Diforders of the Head. The various cephalic Remedies are, therefr ., to be taken from the general Titles or Claffes of Medicines oppofite to the morbific Caufe. Cephalic Medicines are either internal, when for Inftance, they are exhibited by the Mouth, in Order to produce their Effects by the general Circulation of the Fluids; or by Way of Clifters, which often produce the moft happy Confequences, by making a Revulfion from the fuperior, and more noble Parts; or they are fuch as are applied externally to the Head, to which Clafs belong Errhines, proper Liquors for wafhing the Head, medicated Caps, and other Remedies commonly called *Topics,* the Materials of which are, alfo, ufed againft the Diforders of other Parts of the Body. With refpect to cephalic Topics in general, we muft obferve, that the Head is lefs capable of bearing moift than dry Applications, becaufe the former, by diftending or relaxing the Veffels, produce Congeftions of Humours, which prove hurtful and prejudicial to the Brain. Nor do moift Preparations applied to the Head ever anfwer any valuable

Purpofe, except in thofe Cafes alone, where the Diforder arifes from an Excefs of Heat and Drynefs, or from an inflammatory Difpofition in the Head; for in this Cafe, agreeably to the antiphlogiftic Method, moiftening Fomentations, and Epithems, applied to the Head, Neck, and Throat, generally produce happy Effects, fince by thefe Means, the Water infinuating itfelf into the Pores of thofe Parts, renders them more pervious, fo that the Blood paffes more freely thro' them, and confequently preffes lefs forcibly upon the Brain; Decoctions, then, of the Flowers of Marfh-mallows, Mullein, and other Emollients, or moderaely warm Oxymel, or Water and Elder Vinegar, are proper, for Inftance, in Deliriums, according to *Boerhaave Aph.* 702. in Comas, *Aph.* 706. in obftinate Watchings, *Aph.* 709. in a Phrenitis, *Aph.* 781. in an inflammatory Quinfey, *Aph.* 809, and in a Hydrophobia, *Aph.* 1143. *N.* 5. In Wounds of the Head and Pericranium, we muft not according to *Hoffman* ufe oleous or pinguious Subftances and Ointments, becaufe, by obftructing the Pores, they bring on violent Inflammations. But in their room, we muft fubftitute either dry Subftances, fuch as the Powders of *Florentine* Orris, Maftich, and Amber; or Honey, with an Admixture of a fmall Quantity of *Peruvian* Balfam. In other Diforders of the Head, fuch as Pains arifing from a cold Caufe, medicated Bags ftuffed with heating Ingredients, fuch as Sage, Marjoram, Frankincenfe and Salt, are generally ufed with Succefs. The Patient's Head is alfo to be wafhed with a Lixivium, in which Ingredients of a heating Quality have been boiled, fince they are highly proper for attenuating the obftructing Matter, and corroborating the Brain.

Sennertus in his *Inftitutiones Medicinæ* informs us, " that tho' Liquors

" for

for wafhing the Head, are by fome abfolutely condemned and rejected, yet they are not altogether ufelefs, fince they open the Pores of the Skin, that the Fumes, pent up in the fmall obftructed Veffels, may be exhaled; but they muft not be ufed, when the Patient labours immediately under a Catarrh, or a Head-ach; for they are more properly and with greater Succefs applied, in the Intervals of thefe Diforders. As for the Method of ufing them, the Head muft be wafhed either in the Morning, or an Hour before Supper; and when it is fufficiently wafhed, it muft be dried with moderately warm linen Cloths. Wafhing of the Feet is, alfo, proper, not only with a View to remove the fordid Matter collected about them, but alfo to derive the Humours from the Head." *Campegius* his *Campus Elyfius Galliæ* gives the following Cautions with refpect to the ufe of heating medicated Bags. " Let them (fays he) be applied after a confiderable, but gentle Evacuation, and at the Height, or in the Decline, but not in the Beginning or Increafe of the Difeafe, nor before a gentle Evacuation is made, leſt by their hot and attracting Influences, they fhould draw the Humours to the Head, and by that Means do more harm than good."

Cheyne tells us, that the greateft Advantages accrue to the Eyes, Ears, and whole Head, from fhaving t frequently, and bathing it daily in old Water, mixed with a few Drops of Lavender or *Hungary* Water. The Benefits, fays he, arifing from his Method, abftracted from the Pleafure it affords, are only known and relifhed, by fuch as have experienced them. To rub the Head after it is fhaved, proves an inftantaneous Cure for a Cephalalgia, a ftuf-

fing of the Head, and a Weaknefs of the Eyes, arifing from a languid and relaxed State of the nervous Fibres. And as by every frefh Evacuation of the Humours, their Quantity is not only leffened, but alfo their recrementitious Parts derived thither, fo the more frequently the Head is fhaved, the larger Quantity of Humours is difcharged; fo that the frequent Shaving of the Head and Beard is like a perpetual Fontenel, or Veficatory. From frequently wafhing the Skin of the Head with Soap and Water, and then fhaving it, arifes another confiderable Advantage, which is the cleanfing the Mouths of the cutaneous Pores, from the Scurf and Scales, which block them up; by which Means a free Difcharge is procured to the perfpirable Matter, which, when retained, proves highly prejudicial to the Head and Brain. Then by plunging the Head in cold Water, and carefully wafhing it, the Scales of the Cuticula are clofely braced up, and hindered from gaping, in an unfeemly Manner, fo that too large a Quantity of the perfpirable Matter fhould be difcharged, and that they may the better refiſt the Influence of the external Cold; by which Means Perfons of an infirm State of Health, fuffer very confiderably; for which Reafon all valetudinary Perfons fhould fhave every Day, or at leaſt as often as they conveniently can, and then wafh their Heads with cold Water. *Celfus*, in the fourth Chapter of his firſt Book, gives the following Directions, with Refpect to the Management of the Head. " The Perfon (fays he) who has a " weak Head, provided his Digefti- " on is good, ought gently to rub " it with his Hands in the Morn- " ing, never if poffible to keep it " covered, nor to fhave it clofe to " the Skin. It is proper he fhould " avoid the Influence of the Moon, " efpecially

" especially before her Conjunction
" with the Sun ; he muft alfo take
" care not to go abroad immedi-
" ately after Meals. If he has Hair
" he muft daily comb it, and walk
" much, but neither in the Houfe
" nor in the Sun. He muft alfo in
" a particular manner avoid the Heat
" of the Sun after Meals, or the
" Ufe of Wine ; he muft rather a-
" noint than bath, and when he
" does it, it muft never be before a
" violent Fire, where there is an
" Eruption of Flame, but fome-
" times before a gentle Fire where
" the Coals are alive and clear. But
" if he intends to ufe a Bagnio, he
" muft firft fweat a little, covered
" with Cloths in the *Tepidarium,*
" where he muft, alfo, be anointed,
" thence be muft go to the fweating
" Room. When he has fweated, he
" muft not go into the bathing Cif-
" tern, but pour large Quantities of
" Water, firft moderately warm,
" and then cold upon his Head, and
" whole Body, but he muft pour it
" longer on his Head than upon
" the other Parts ; then he muft
" rub his Head for fome Time,
" and at laft of all wipe himfelf
" and anoint. *Nothing is fo benefi-*
" *cal to the Head as cold Water.*
" He therefore who has an infirm
" Head ought, during the Summer,
" daily to plunge it in a pretty
" large Veffel of Water ; and tho'
" he fhould anoint without bath-
" ing, or cannot endure the Influ-
" ence of the cold over his whole
" Body, yet he ought always to
" pour cold Water on his Head.
" When he has not an Inclination
" to have the Water touch any o-
" ther Parts of his Body, he muft
" bend his Head downwards, that
" it may not reach his Neck, and
" that the Eyes and other Parts of
" the Face may partake of the com-
" mon Benefit, he is every now and
" then to apply it to thefe Parts

" with his Hands, as it runs down ;
" he muft neceffarily ufe a fpare Di-
" et, and fuch as is of eafy Digefti-
" on, and if his Head is prejudiced
" by Fafting, he may, alfo, eat in
" the Middle of the Day ; but if he
" fuftains no Injury by Fafting, it
" is more advifeable to eat only once
" a Day. For his ordinary Drink,
" 'tis more expedient he fhould ufe
" mild diluted Wine, than Water ;
" it is alfo proper that when his
" Head begins to ach violently, he
" fhould have a Place proper for his
" Repofe to betake himfelf to ;
" Wine or Water ufed continually
" by themfelves, are not proper for
" him ; fince they only prove Medi-
" cinal when ufed alternately ; he
" muft neither write, read nor dif-
" pute after Supper : But of all o-
" ther Circumftances, Vomiting is
" moft prejudicial to one in his
" State." From what has been faid
we fee, that there are two principal
Claffes of Cephalics, and thefe are
the Medicines of the refrigerating or
cooling, or of the warming and heating Kind ; for fince, as *Riverius* juftly
obferves, the Brain is fometimes attack'd with cold, and fometimes with
hot Diforders, the Medicines calculated for its Relief muft, alfo, be of two
Kinds, in order to remove the fevera
Indifpofitions to which it is fubject
" Heating Medicines (fays the laf
" quoted Author) not only heat an
" dry the Brain, but alfo incide an
" attenuate the Phlegm, contain'd i
" it ; whereas thofe of a refrigeratin
" Quality, partly correct the hot In
" temperature of the Brain, and part
" ly infpiffate the acid faline Phlegm
" and other ferous Humours, whic
" produce violent Defluxions." T
thefe two Claffes of refrigeratin
and heating Medicines we may r
fer what *Hoffman* in his *Annotat.* a
Poter. propofes in the followin
manner. " Two Kind of Medicin
" are principally proper in Diforde
" (

of the Head, which arise from an irregular and desultory Motion of the Spirits; or from Obstructions of the Nerves and Vessels of the Brain. Of the former Kind are Anodynes, which, by their grateful Exhalations stop the tumultuous and disorderly Motions of the Spirits, such as the Flowers of the Cowslip, of the Lime, of Piony, of the *Egyptian* Thorn, of Elder, of Roses, of Violets, of the wild Poppy, and of Lillies of the Valley, as also odoriferous and scented Substances, such as Musk, Castor, Amber, and Saffron. To the latter Class belong such Substances, as contain a subtile oleous Salt, of which Kind are all oleous Substances, and volatile Spirits obtain'd from Animals; as also Marjoram, Rue, Lavender, Valerian, Aloes Wood, Garden and wild Rosemary, Cardamoms, Cubebs, Mother of Thyme, Basil, Amber, Ambergrease, and Peruvian Balsam, all which boil'd with Water or Wine, or infused in any proper Menstruum, prove excellent Medicines for Disorders of the Head."

But such Substances as relax the too much constricted Vessels (in consequence of which Constriction, a brisker Motion of the Humours, and greater Heat in the Body are procured) retard the accelerated Motion of all the Humours. As to what we call cephalic Specifics, which by a peculiar Virtue act upon the Head, and remove its Disorders, without influencing any other Parts of the Body, and are consequently indiscriminately proper in all Indispositions of the Head, from whatever Cause they may arise, we must in this Affair be cautious in passing our Judgment, since some maintain, that there are really such Medicines, whilst others deny the Fact, and engage the opposite Party with Experience, the most conclusive of all Arguments. *Wedelius* in his *Centuriæ Exercitationum Medicarum Cent.* 1. *Dec.* 7. informs us, that Hyssop was the cephalic Specific of *Hippocrates*, as appears from his Book *de Morbo Sacro*, compared with what he has said concerning Hyssop. But this Plant can only be proper in one Species of Epilepsy; when, for Instance, it is produced by a Redundance of Phlegm, concerning which Species *Hippocrates* treats in that work. In this Case, indeed, heating and drying Medicines are proper: Hyssop is a Plant of this Kind, and *Wedelius* himself informs us, that it abounds with a volatile oleous Salt. *Hippocrates*, also, in his Work *de Diæta Lib.* 2. informs us, that Hyssop is hot, and evacuates Phlegm.

CHAP. IX.

Of BALSAMICS.

THE very word *Balsam* seems, in all Ages, to have had an Idea of Excellence and Efficacy affixed to it, above any other Branch of the *Materia Medica*; for the ancient Physicians, by this Word, meant any Species of Medicine, which powerfully recommended itself by a grateful and delicious Fragrance, and whose Use, both internal and external, was of singular Efficacy in preventing Putrefaction, and resisting fifting Corruption. *Balfams,* 'tis true, were originally ufed, for embalming and preferving the dead Bodies of thofe, who had fignalized themfelves by great and heroick Deeds, or endeared themfelves to Mankind by the Practice of the focial Virtues. And when the thinking and fagacious Part of Mankind obferved, that the Bodies of the Dead, were, by Means of *Balfams,* enabled to defy the Attacks of Corruption, for an immenfe Series of Years, they began to imagine, that their Virtues might extend to the Living, protract Life, and corroborate what they called the *Calidum Innatum* in the Blood. But however unintelligibly they may have talked upon this Subject, yet it is certain, that the Notion was juft and well grounded, fince we are taught by Experience, that amongft the vaft Variety aud infinite Store of Medicines, with which the Mineral, Animal, and Vegetable Kingdoms fupply Mankind, none are more powerful, none more efficacious, than thofe which come under the Denomination of *Balfams,* and *Balfamics.* But as all *Balfams* are not alike efficacious, nor equally adapted to medicinal Ufes, I fhall only confider thofe *Balfamics* which feem beft calculated to anfwer the Intentions of Medicine, whether Prefervative or Curative : I fhall farther fpecify the Principles by which they operate, enumerate their feveral Virtues, and give Directions with regard to their Ufes. Mean time, it may not be improper to enquire into the Origin of the word *Balfam,* and afcertain the precife and determinate Idea, which ought to be affix'd to it.

Since, then, the Inhabitants of *Paleftine* and the Coafts of *Phœnicia,* and perhaps their Neighbours the *Arabians* and *Egyptians,* were, according to the beft Accounts, the firft who ufed *Balfams,* common Senfe

directs us to the Genius of the or ental Languages for the Origin of th Name. Whether then it is a fimpl Word, which is moft probable, an moft confonant with the Genius of th *Eaftern* Language, and derived fror *Bofem,* a Word peculiar to the *Hi brews,* for expreffing the moft fra grant and delicious Subftances, and i which other Nations have probabl inferted an additional Letter, as i many other inftances they did ; o whether, with others, we maintai that it is compounded of *Baal Sche men,* which fignifies, the chief o Prince of Oils and Spices, yet ftill i amounts to the fame Thing, finc by the Import of the Word in botl Cafes, it is plain, that only the bel Spices, Oils and Refins, and fuch a excell'd all others in their Virtue: the Fragrancy of their Smell, an the Sweetnefs of their Tafte, wer called *Balfams* ; and the Idea whicl the word *Balfam* or *Balfamic,* fhoulc now convey, is that of a Medicine poffeffed of a fulphureous, refinous and oleous Principle, which at th fame Time muft be fragrant anc friendly to Nature, and by Means o which it operates. Two things muft therefore, concur to characterize anc conftitute a *Balfam* : the Firft is that the greater Part of its Subftance ought to be inflammable, that is either of an oleous, or refinous Na ture. The fecond Circumftance ne ceffary to conftitute a *Balfam* is, thai its Subftance be of a grateful Smell and pungent Tafte, that it may give Proof of its Efficacy, and of the Smallnefs and Minutenefs of its Parts. So that according to this Doctrine, all Sulphurs, and refinous Subftances, as alfo all inflammable Oils, tho' of the Confiftence of a *Balfam,* are yet to be excluded from the Clafs of genuine *Balfamics,* if they want the Fragrancy of Scent, and Delicioufnefs of Tafte, which are requifite to conftitute a Balfam. Thus Naphtha, or Roch Oil,

Oil, Jews Pitch, Refin of the Pine, the Oils of Turpentine, and Fir, ought by no means to be rank'd among the Clafs of *Balfamics,* tho' they are inflammable penetrating Subftances, excellent for the Purpofes of embalming, and promife very falutary Effects, both when ufed internally and externally. Yet becaufe they abound in a too ftrong acrid, and penetrating Sulphur, which is not altogether friendly and agreeable to Nature, they are therefore lefs fit for reftoring loft Vigour, and recruiting impair'd Strength. Nor are Subftances whofe fole Property is Fragrancy of Smell, fuch as Civet, Mufk, and the fragrant Flowers of Jeffamine, Oranges, or the Hyacinthus Tuberofus, to be properly efteem'd *Balfamics*; becaufe Fragrancy alone, which is owing to a fine and eafily exhalted Sulphur, is not fufficient to conftitute a *Balfam*; but 'tis neceffary, that this fragrant Principle be blended and incorporated with a fubtile acrid Oil, and an inflammable Refin. •

'Tis, therefore, juftly to be doubted, whether a true and genuine *Balfam* is to be found in the animal Kingdom. Mean time the vegetable Kingdom is richly ftored with Medicines of this Clafs, of which the moft ancient, and that which firft bore the Name of *Balfam* by way of Excellence, is the *Opobalfam* of the *Arabians,* and *Egyptians.*

This *Balfam* was alway had in fo great Efteem by the Antients, that they made it an Ingredient in their moft noble Antidotes, which were fold for double their Weight in Silver, according to *Theophraftus, Pliny,* and *Diofcorides.* This is eafily accounted for, fince the *Balfam-tree* being very fmall, and not able to afford a great Quantity of *Opobalfamum,* its Price muft of courfe run high. This, alfo, was the Reafon why the *Opobalfamum* of the An-

cients, according to *Lobelius in Animadverfionibus,* was often vitiated with Cyprus Turpentine, or the Oil of the Maftich-tree. Since, then, the *Balfam* of *Meccha,* of all others the fineft, is without doubt the True *Opobalfamum* of the *Egyptians,* true exactly refembles it in all its Qualities, its Ufe in Phyfic is to be highly recommended; and of this, diffolved and prepared with a fpirituous Menftruum, very efficacious and elegant Medicines may be made for internal Ufe.

The *Balfam* of *Tolu* is the next in Value, as a Medicine, and is frequently us'd as a *Succedaneum* to the true *Opobalfamum.*

The next is that which is brought from *Peru,* and is called *Peruvian,* and *Indian Balfam.* It is poffeffed of very fingular and efficacious Qualities, as is fufficiently obvious from its fragrant Smell, and aromatic Tafte. It was at firft only ufed as an external Medicine; but in Procefs of Time, fome Phyficians and Chymifts began to ufe it internally, fometimes mixing it with Pills, at other times diffolving it in highly rectified Spirit of Wine, and on other Occafions incorporating it with Sugar, or any other Ingredients they thought moft likely to anfwer their Intention.

The next is the *Balfam* of *Capivi* or *Copaiba,* which has of late Years acquir'd an uncommon Reputation, and not undefervedly.

Having taken Notice of the liquid *Balfams,* with which Nature has fo bountifully fupplied us, I fhall confider thofe which are of a more dry and folid Nature, fuch as the refinous fragrant Gums, impregnated with an agreeable Oil: Of thefe the principal are, Benzoin, pure Storax Calamita, Ladanum, Myrrh, and Maftich. Thefe are produced by making an Incifion in the Bark of the *Balfam bearing Trees,* which are always

N　　　　　　　　　　　green,

green, in the hotteſt Seaſon. From theſe Trees a tenacious Liquor drops. which becomes, gradually more ſo-lid, as its humid Parts are exhal'd by the Heat of the Sun ; for which Reaſon theſe reſinous Gums are juſt-ly called dry *Balſams,* becauſe in all Points they agree with *Balſams.* For their whole Subſtance is inflammable, they have a frequent Smell, are of a penetrating Taſte, they are diſſolved, tho' not totally, in highly rectified Spirits of Wine, and yield an Oil when ſubjected to Diſtillation.

Having mention'd the *Balſamic* Gums and Reſins, it remains that I direct my View to thoſe Woods which are impregnated with a balſa-mic Principle ; among theſe the firſt Place has been univerſally aſſigned to Aloes Wood, otherwiſe called *Xylo-aloes,* the whole of which is reſinous, of an aromatic and bitter Taſte, and of a fragrant grateful Smell, 'eſpeci-ally when reduced to Powder.

The *Lignum Rhodium* deſerves to be conſider'd. Its Root is reſinous, and of an aromatic Taſte, and a fra-grant roſy Smell ; it grows in the *Canary Iſlands,* and, when ſubjected to Diſtillation, yields a very fragrant Oil, the Uſe of which is highly ex-tolled.

The next in order is the Yellow-Sanders, which abounds with a fra-grant Reſin : This is plain, from the Spirit of Wine drawn off this Wood, which ſmells almoſt like Am-ber ; and if the Tincture is made with rectified Spirit of Wine, and the Spirit is drawn off by a gentle Heat, a moſt fragrant oily Liquor remains, of the Conſiſtence of *Peruvian Bal-ſam.* A Decoction of this Wood is highly to be valued on Account of its penetrating Reſin.

Of the *Balſamic* Barks the prin-cipal are, the Bark of the Saſſafras Wood, *Peruvian* Bark, Winters Bark, that of Caſcarilla, and the true Coſtus. They are endow'd with a reſinous, *Balſamic,* and ſubaſtrin-gent Principle, which is not only diſcovered from their penetrating Taſte and Smell, but, alſo, from the highly penetrating Oil, which theſe Barks yield, upon being diſtil-led with Water.

In the Northern Countries the Ju-niper-tree is truly of the *Balſamic* Kind ; for not only its Wood and Leaves, but particularly its Berries, abound with a ſubtile penetrating Oil, which they yield in great Quan-tities, when ſubjected to Diſtillation by the Worm. And this Oil, when pure and unadulterated, is an excel-lent Strengthner of the Nerves, and powerfully promotes a Diſcharge of the Urine, as moſt other *Balſams* do. There is alſo a Decoction prepared of the Wood itſelf, which is of ſingular Uſe in the Cure of the Scurvy.

But beſides theſe Simples already mentioned, of a fragrant Smell, and penetrating Taſte, with which Na-ture has bountifully furniſh'd us, Oils alſo of the ſame Qualities ought to be reckoned among *Balſamics* or *Balſams* ; for ſubtile etherial Oils, are certainly liquid Reſins, or *Bal-ſams* : For the principal Element which is the Source of the fragrant Smell, the penetrating Taſte, and healing Quality, by which all *Bal-ſams,* whether liquid or ſolid, act, is no other than a ſubtile, volatile Oil, which being taken away, the Subſtance in which it was lodged be-comes effete and uſeleſs.

For this Reaſon it may be aſſerted for Truth, that all thoſe Aromatics, which in Diſtillation yield a fragrant and penetrating Oil, ſuch as Cinna-mon, Cloves, Nutmegs, Mace, Car-damoms, Cubebs, Lemon and O-range peels, are juſtly to be rank'd among the principal of the *Balſamics.* For this very Reaſon, *Valerius Cor-dus* in his Diſpenſatory, orders Oil of Cloves to be uſed as a *Succedaneum*

to

to the *Opobalsamum*, in all the Antidotes in which it is ordered for an Ingredient. " There are not, says " he, in our Days, *Opobalsamum*, " *Carpobalsamum*, and *Xylobalsamum* " to be found, which come up to the " true Descriptions given us of them; " but as we are taught by Experi- " ence, that the distill'd Oils of Cin- " namon and Cloves, of which the " Ancients were ignorant, are equal " in their Virtues to the *true Bal- " sam*, for this Reason we have, in " our *Theriaca*, substituted the Oil of " Cloves instead of the *Opobalsa- " mum*. It would not be improper " to substitute instead of *Carpobalsa- " mum*, Cubebs or Cloves, or Car- " damoms and Aloes Wood, instead " of the *Xylobalsamum*."

These aromatic Oils, then, are subtile spirituous *Balsams*, of so uncommon Virtues and Efficacy, that the other oriental *Balsams* can scarcely be expected to come up to them; for these produce their Effects only by a subtile Oil; neither is it difficult to reduce these very penetrating and liquid Oils, either to the Consistence of a *Balsam*, or to the Form of a Resin, provided a concentrated acid Spirit, such as the Oil of Vitriol, be duly mixed with them.

In our own Country there are also spirituous *Balsams* of this Kind, which both on Account of their Virtues and Fragrancy, render it a dubious Point, whether they are not of equal Value with the oriental *Balsams*, and aromatic Oils; and these *Balsams* produced in our own Country are Oils distilled from aromatic Herbs, of a fragrant Smell, and penetrating Taste.

The principal Herbs of this Kind are Rosemary, Lavender, common Spike, Marjoram, common and *Turkish* Baum, Basil, Mother of Thyme, *Roman* Chamomile, and all the Species of Mint, Water-Mint, Cost-mary, Field and Mountain Calamint, curl'd Mint, that Origanum commonly called the wild Marjoram. These Herbs when duly distilled, yield very fragrant and efficacious Oils; but as these Oils are rarely to be met with pure in the Shops, but are adulterated in their Distillation with Turpentine, it happens that they do not discover the Efficacy of which the genuine Sorts are possessed, in corroborating the Tone of the Nerves, and of the other solid Parts. They are most conveniently used when dissolved and reduced to Essences; and *Quercetan* in the End of his *Pharmacopoeia Restituta*, has these remarkable Words concerning them. " In " *Germany* an Expedient is lately " found for reducing the penetrating " Oils into some pure and grateful " Essences, which preserves the Co- " lours, Smells and Tastes of the " peculiar Oils, without any other " Mixture, than the *Celestial Manna* " well purified, which extracts the " Virtue of these Oils, and by its " Admixture proves an excellent " Corrector to them." There is no doubt but the Menstruum so highly commended by this Author, is highly rectified Spirit of Wine, prepared according to Art for a thorough Dissolution of their Oils.

From what has been said, I think it plainly appears, that the vegetable Kingdom supplies us with the noblest and most efficacious *Balsams*, which, when skillfully used, are of singular Service in curing Diseases, and preserving Life and Health. Neither is it to be forgot, that the *Balsamic* Plants and Trees, produced by the bountiful Parent of the human Race, for their Comfort and Preservation, are distinguish'd, as it were, by an external Mark or Characteristic, expressive of their latent and inherent Efficacy against Corruption, and consequently of their *Balsamic* Nature: And this Characteristic is, that almost all of them flourifh perpetually, and are what we call *Ever-greens.* We are, alfo, on this Occafion to enquire, whether Heaven, who in all her Meafures confults the Intereft of Mankind, has not conceal'd *Balfams,* for the Prefervation of the human Species, under the Earth, and in the Bottom of the Sea; if we then diligently enquire into the Nature of the Bodies lodged there, we fhall find two dry *Balfams* hid under the Earth, and diffufed thro' the Seas, which feem to vie with the other *Balfams* procured from the vegetable Kingdom. Thefe are *Ambergreafe,* which in the Eaftern Countries. is very fine, and had in great Efteem; and the Amber produced in the Northern Climates. Both of them furnifh us with *Balfamic* Medicines, which produce very inftantaneous, and fpeedy Effects.

Thefe, then, are the natural *Balfams* known to us, which are certainly fine Prefervatives of Life and Health; and from which a fkillful Phyfician may, by a judicious Mixture of other Subftances, prepare the beft and moft efficacious Medicines.

Befides, thefe *Balfamic* Species were with Succefs join'd by the Ancients to laxative and purgative Medicines, for they thought, that the violent Strength of Purgatives was unfriendly to Nature, and ftood in need of a Corrector, in order to ftrengthen and corroborate.

The *balfamic* Species are, alfo, excellent Correctors to Medicines of a ftupefying and narcotic Quality. For this Reafon we find, that the Antients always mixed them with Opiates; becaufe they imagined, that by their Means the cold Qualities of Opium, and other Narcotics, were deftroyed; and that the Spirits when laid afleep by them, were roufed and rendered active; and undoubtedly the *Pil de Cynogloffo* could

not be fo fafely ufed, unlefs the Roots of the Hounds-tongue, and the Seeds of white Hen-bane, and the Extract of Opium, were mixed with Olibanum, and Refin of Storax. Nor would the *Pil de Styrace* be fo effectual in diffolving acrid Humours in Coughs, and Catarrhs, unlefs they had at the fame time in their Compofition, Olibanum, Refin of Storax, and Myrrh. The *Laudanum* of *Sydenham,* which is much ufed, not only in *England,* but in other Countries of *Europe,* is not a little corrected by the Addition of thefe aromatic Subftances, Cinnamon, Nutmegs, Cloves and *Spanifh* Wine. The *Elixir Psoprietatis* invented by *Paracelfus,* and the *Pil Ruffi* and *Pil Avicennæ,* prepared of the fame Species, have retained their Reputation for a great while, becaufe by the Addition of Myrrh, which is of a *balfamic* Nature; and Saffron, the cathartic Violence of the Aloes is much corrected and fubdued.

Balfamics are, therefore, very properly mixed with evacuating Medicines, not only in order to correct their draftic Qualities, but alfo to affift Nature in performing the feveral Excretions, and to preferve the Strength which Evacuants generally impair. For this Reafon, they are very properly combined with Emetics; as alfo with Sudorifics. 'Tis fufficiently known to every Practitioner, how efficacious balfamic Medicines are in curing the Diforders of the Glands, and removing thofe Difeafes which arife from their too great Laxity, a Defluxion of Humours upon them, or too copious a Difcharge of their Contents. Balfamics are, alfo, excellent Pectorals, becaufe they remove Obftructions of the Lungs, promote Expectoration, and furprifingly corroborate the pulmonary Veficles. Medcines of the balfamic Kind afford confiderable Relief

Relief, in Pains arising from the Stone in the Kidneys, or Bladder. Besides, when the Menses are either defective or too copious, or when too frequent Abortions, or Sterility on some other Account, destroy the Prospect of a hopeful Progeny, no Medicines are better calculated than Balsamics, for corroborating the relaxed Tone of the Uterus, that Nature may be thus rendered able to subdue and eliminate what is noxious, and by that Means provide a proper Receptacle for cherishing and perfecting the Foetus.

The celebrated *Frederic Hoffman* asserts, that balsamic Medicines are truly universal, and of extensive Use in Physic, and that their Virtues are as great as those of any other Class of Medicines whatever, since they are suited to all Constitutions, easily incorporated with all other Remedies, and exquisitely calculated for subduing and removing almost all Diseases. Balsamics have this peculiar to themselves beyond other Medicines, that they are friendly to the human Constitution, and conspire as it were, and contract an Affinity with it. Of this we may easily be convinced, by observing how speedily Strength impaired by chronical Disorders, old Age, or any other Accident, is restored by the timely and seasonable Use of Balsamics. For this Reason no Medicines are so effectual in Faintings from whatever Cause, as *Balsamics*; and in a Word, they wonderfully recruit, restore, and preserve that which is the original Source of Life, and imparts Strength, Pulsation, and Tone to the Heart, Arteries, and Nerves, whether we call it Principle, Spirit, Soul, or Nature; for they seem to be transformed into the Nature and Genius of that noble and wonderful Substance, which is the Director and Source of Motion in all our Mem-

bers; for, in a *Syncope* they so suddenly restore Motion to the oppressed Heart, purely by their Smell, that we cannot enough admir'd their Efficacy; for such is the Nature of all Substances which abound with a penetrating and fragrant Oil, that when used either internally or externally, they singularly cherish and preserve the Strength of our Constitutions. On the contrary, every Thing that is putrid and fetid, and the Reverse of Fragrant, is highly prejudicial to Strength, and the vital Motions which it soon oppresses and destroys; for every Degree of Putrefaction is highly prejudicial to Life, and when it either begins, or is increased, in a human Body, the Strength and vital Motions forthwith fail and are destroyed, as we evidently see in Plagues, malignant Fevers, and Mortifications of the internal Parts; for this Reason Remedies prepared of *Balsamics* are justly stiled the *Balsams*, the Waters, and Spirits of Life, since they have such a direct and immediate Influence upon it.

Since then *Balsamics* convey Motion, Strength, and Tone, to all the Parts of the Body, we may easily see, that these Medicines must be singularly efficacious in those Disorders and Indispositions, where the Strength and vital Motions are impaired, or where the Viscera and other Parts are too much relaxed, and deprived of their due and proper Tone. For this Reason, they will never frustrate the Expectation of the Physician, who prudently exhibits them in Weaknesses of the Brain and Nerves, Imbecillity of the Memory and Senses, a Palsy of the Members, and Privation of Voice, a Hemiplegy, Inappetencies, Loathings of the Food, Vomitings, Diarrhæas, and Gripings of the Belly; in Cases where Flatulencies prove uneasy, in Langours of the whole Body, in Faintings, and in all cold catarrhous

De-

Defluxions, in Coughs that are too moist, a Coryza, a Fluor Albus, a Gonorrhæa, a moist Asthma, and in a Word in all Cases where the Parts are to be strengthened. Then again, as the best and most valuable Balsamics convey Strength and Energy to the solid Parts of our Bodies, especially to the Heart and muscular Fibres, which move and impel our Fluids, hence it follows, that they are the surest and most efficacious Preservatives against all Kinds of Diseases, as will sufficiently appear from the following Considerations. As long as the Blood and Humours are quickly and uninterruptedly carried thro' the Ducts and Vessels of the whole Body, and what is superfluous and recrementitious is carried off thro' proper Strainers and Emunctories, so long the whole Body, and each particular Part of it, are in a State of Health, and duly perform their respective Functions: But as soon as this Motion is disturbed, or interrupted, in the whole Body, or any of its Parts, or when the necessary Secretions are not duly made, a sure Foundation is, by these very Means, laid for Diseases. Now nothing is of more Efficacy for preserving the vital Circulation of the Humours, and carrying on the necessary Business of Perspiration, than those Substances which strengthen and corroborate the Heart, the principal Part of the Body, with their *balsamic* Qualities. But our noble *Balsamics* are particularly and singularly useful as Preservatives with uncommon Success, when epidemical Disorders rage; they are, also, very properly joined with Alexipharmics in the above-mentioned Disorders, because they resist Putrefactions, recruit the Strength, and promote a due Circulation of the Humours; and since they so powerfully guard against Putrefaction, which is so prejudicial to Life, they

are, for this Reason, very properly and successfully used in the venereal Disease, which is truly of a putrid Kind, and in those Scurvies which are the Result of an impure Air, and unwholsome Aliments; for the Decoctions, Elixirs, and Essences of the Woods, derive their Virtues and Efficacy from the *balsamic* Qualities of the Ingredients. Besides, *Balsamics*, especially of the fragrant Kind, have this singular Advantage attending them, that they becalm the exorbitant Motions of our Fluids, and allay Pain. For this Reason, in violent Head achs, Tooth-achs, and Pains of the Ears, they often afford great Relief, even when only externally applied. Neither is it to be forgotten, that *Balsamics* prove excellent Correctors to all the more violent and drastic Medicines, especially Evacuants and Anodynes; for they remarkably qualify their Virtues, by their Qualities. For this Reason *Balsamics* are very happily joined, with almost all evacuant and anodyne Medicines. From all these Considerations it appears, how proper and efficacious *Balsamics* are, for the Cure of a large Number of Diseases.

But as nothing is in every Respect perfect and compleat, as there is no Medicine however valuable in itself, but what produces bad Consequences, when imprudently exhibited, there is no doubt to be made, but this is also the Case with *Balsamics*; for when there is in the Body too large a Quantity of hot and fervid Blood, when its Motion is too much accelerated, and the Pulse quick and vehement, Nature has, in these Cases, more need of a Check than a *Stimulus*; for which Reason we must neither attempt to excite, nor augment the Motions of the Fluids. Besides, fragrant Substances have this Disadvantage attending them, that when the Brain, in Consequence of some

some Weakness, with Difficulty transmits the Blood, and the Vessels of the Head are become turgid with Humours, they occasion a greater Derivation of Humours to it, and sometimes increase the Pains, Torpors, Vertigos, and Oppressions of the Senses. I must here add, that Physicians have not as yet sufficiently discovered the Virtues and Efficacy of *Balsamics*, in the Practice of Medicine, since they are far more powerful and efficacious than is commonly believed. The spurious *Balsams*, which are commonly sold, and which ought to be made of the purest, ethereal, aromatic and cephalic Oils, are for the most Part sophisticated and adulterated, so that Physicians have no Reason to be surprised, if they do not produce the Effects they would do, if they were pure and genuine. I must in the last Place observe, that Physicians are very faulty in drowning, as it were, *Balsamics* in spirituous Liquors, since they almost always either mix them with Spirit of Wine, or join them with it by Distillation, by which Means the Virtues of the *Balsamics* are infringed, and it assumes a violently hot Nature. The more then their genuine Natures are retained, the more efficacious and useful they are.

CHAP. X.

Of EMMENAGOGUES.

Emmenagogues are Medicines which promote the menstrual Flux, tho' *Hoffman* includes under this Name, those Remedies which cause a Discharge of Blood from the hæmorrhoidal Veins.

Among those which best and most commodiously answer this Intention, we may reckon the Roots of Birthwort, Zedoary, and the five aperient Roots, the Herbs Mugwort, Calamint, Feverfew, Pennyroyal, Baum, Savin, Poly Montain, Rue, Marjoram, Rosemary, Wallflowers, Saffron, Bay-berries, Juniper-berries; the Gums Bdellium, Galbanum, Opoponax, Sagapenum, and Amber: Among purgative Substances, Aloes, Rhubarb, and Bryony; as also Aromatics, and animal Salts, Castor, and Chalybeate Preparations, which excel all others of the mineral and chymical Kind.

The more these Excretions are subservient to Life and Health; the more it were to be wished, with *Hippocrates*, that we had certain and efficacious Medicines for regulating them, and by that Means preventing and curing several very terrible Disorders. But as these Excretions are principally the Work of Nature, and in Women appear, return, and end at certain Periods, but are neither incident to all Men, nor so periodical as the *Menses*, and as a certain Redundance of Blood, together with a certain State of the Vessels of the Anus and Uterus, disposed to a spontaneous Evacuation, are requisite in order to these Discharges, and as these Evacuations may be obstructed, or totally destroyed by various Causes, it must of Course be a difficult Task, to fall upon effectual Means

of

of reftoring thefe Evacuations when ftopt, or inlarging them when impaired; neither of which Ends can ever be attained, without knowing the Caufe from which the Misfortune proceeds.

But fuppofing that there is a Redundance of Blood, the principal Caufe of this Evacuation; fuppofing alfo, that the Veffels of the Uterus and Anus are fo difpofed, that they may be diftended, by a large Quantity of Blood flowing to them, and be capable of difcharging this Blood; yet if the Excretions are not duly carried on, either on Account of Obftructions, or fpafmodic Conftrictions of the fmall lateral Veffels of the Arteries, in Confequence of this, the Blood does not circulate naturally; or on Account of a Diminution of the fpirituous Principle of the Blood, and the elaftic contractile Force of the Heart and Arteries, then the above enumerated Medicines afford the defired Relief: For the capillary Veffels are excellently opened, and Obftructions removed, by the five aperient Roots, Birthwort, Rhubarb, Briony, and Wallflowers, efpecially if exhibited by Way of Decoction with fome faline Stimulus, fuch as Borax. This Invention is, alfo, excellently anfwered by the Gums exhibited with Aloes, and other Purgatives, in the Form of Pills. The fmall capillary Ducts, when fpafmodically conftricted, or preternaturally contracted, are excellently relaxed and opened by Mugwort, which is of a demulcent Nature, as alfo by Yarrow, Saffron, and Caftor. In order to reftore the fpirituous Principle of the Blood, ftrengthen the Solids, and confirm the Tone of the Fibres and Veffels, fuch Corroboratives are to be ufed, as operate by their fine volatile and oleous Salt, among which we may reckon all Aromatics, Myrrh, the Berries of the Bay, and Juniper Trees,

Rofemary, Penny-royal, Baum, Savory, Savin, Wall-flowers, Calamint, Amber, Filings of Steel, Chalybeate Tinctures, and volatile oleous Salts.

When the Evacuation is impaired, or rendered flow, by a Redundance of Blood, which too powerfully refifts the Elafticity of the Veffels, the Emmenagogues already mentioned, efpecially thofe of the hotter Kind, are by no Means to be exhibited; for by thefe the Blood is thrown into violent Commotions, and a Train of formidable Symptoms is frequently brought on; in this Cafe, therefore, Venefection is the firft to be recommended, fince by Means of that alone thofe falutary and critical Evacuations are often happily reftored.

Nor are the Emmenagogues already enumerated proper, in Cafes where there is a Deficience of Blood, and laudable Juices, as in Perfons recovering from the Shock of a Difeafe, thofe whofe *Primæ Viæ* are loaded with vifcid Sordes, or thofe whofe villous Coats of the Stomach are lined with a vifcid Mucus; by which means Digeftion and Chylification are unduly carried on; in Cafes of this Nature, the principal Intention of the Phyfician ought to be, not only the Regeneration of good and laudable Blood by nutritive, gelatinous Subftances, and Broths eafily convertible into Blood and Juices, but alfo, if neceffary, the Reftitution of the Digeftion, and Elaboration of the Chyle by Emetics, gentle Purgatives of a faline aperient Nature, and bitter Stomachics.

Thefe Evacuations are frequently ftopt, by Obftructions and Infractions of the vafcular Subftance of the Anus in Men, and the internal Part of the Uterus and Vagina in Women; in Confequence of which they admit no Blood however ftrongly propelled

pelled to them. In these Cases forcing Remedies are not only superfluous, but pernicious, unless the indurated and infracted Vessels are previously relaxed and softened, by proper Medicines. And this Intention can be neither more speedily, nor efficaciously answered, than by Baths and Fomentations, or Vapour-Baths, so contrived that a Vessel full of warm Water, impregnated with Mugwort, Penny-royal, and Chamomile Flowers, may be placed under the Abdomen in such a Manner, that the Steam may ascend, and penetrate into the Uterus and adjacent Parts. This is to be done in a warm Room, with the Patient's Body well covered; and in order to keep the Water warm, red hot Flints are now and then to be put into it. Frictions of the Legs and Thighs with warm Cloaths, especially after bathing with sweet Water, also, contribute very much to the Production of this Effect.

But in Disorders arising from Suppression, a Defect, or Irregularity of the Menses, or hæmorrhoidal Discharges, nothing is more certain, safe, and effectual, than a prudent Use of proper mineral Waters: By these all the Intentions of Cure are excellently answered; for by drinking these Waters, the viscid Humours are attenuated and evacuated, and the Obstructions of the capillary Vessels removed, whilst by Bathing in others, the Stricture of the Parts is removed, and the Vessels so enlarged, as readily to admit the Blood, and again discharge it.

As in Medicine 'tis a difficult Task to keep the menstrual Discharges in due and natural Order, so it is still more difficult to manage the hæmorrhoidal, when a large Quantity of Blood attempts its Discharge by the Veins of the Anus, but does not find them disposed for its Evacation; but the Discharges of this Kind are most powerfully promoted, by Pills prepared of Aloes, which by their highly subtile, resinous, and sulphureous Particles, not only excite a violent Orgasm in the whole Mass of Blood and Humours, but also by stimulating the Coats of the Colon and Rectum by their tenacious viscid and resinous Parts, excite a greater Afflux of Blood to those Parts: Yet when the Blood, after it has arrived here, cannot make its Way through the Vessels, it partly protrudes them, like so many Tubercles accompanied with Pain, and partly stagnating between the nervous Coats of the Intestines, and pressing them, produces violent Inflations, Spasms, and other terrible Disorders of the Abdomen. A Discharge, therefore, of Blood from their Vessels is to be attempted, by Insessions over a Vessel filled with hot Water, in such a Manner, that the Vapour of the Water may arrive at the Region of the Anus; for by this Means the Vessels are distended, and swell; and then the Parts are to be rubbed with Fig-leaves, or coarse Flannels, in order to sollicit a Discharge.

C H A P.

CHAP. XI.
Of VISCERALS.

VISCERAL Remedies, in general, are those which impart Strength and Firmness to the sanguineous Viscera, such as the Liver, Spleen, Uterus, Kidneys, and Lungs; by which Means they are render'd capable of more happily and expeditiously performing their respective Functions. To this Class we may, therefore, commodiously refer hepatic, splenetic, pneumonic, uterine, anti-cachectic, anti-hydropic, anti-icteric, anti-hysteric, and anti-phthisical Medicines: But the most considerable Viscerals are, the Roots of Gentian, long and round Birthwort, Succory, Zedoary, Fern, true Rhubarb, and Rhapontic, Turmeric, and Rest Harrow, Peruvian Bark, Winters Bark, the Bark of Tamarisks, the Ash, and Capers, together with Cloves, the Herbs Wormwood, the lesser Centory, Fumitory, Carduus Benedictus, Marsh Trefoil, Golden Trefoil, Baum, Spotted Lungworth, Spleen Wort, Agrimony, Horehound, Dodder, Pauls Betony, Scabious, Spurge, Maidenhair, and Mouse Ear. The Viscera are, also, excellently strengthened by some of the resinous Gums, such as Myrrh, Aloes, Bdellium, the Gum of the Ivy-tree, Gum Ammoniac, Olibanum, Sagapenum, Opponax, and Asa Fetida. Some Minerals are, also, excellent Viscerals, such as the Flowers of pure common Sulphur, Filings of Steels, and all Preparations of that Mettal. Some Chymical Preparations are, farther, powerful Viscerals, such as the Salts of Herbs ob-

tain'd by Incineration, the Terra Foliata Tartari, Cream of Tartar, Sal Polychrestum, Antimoniated Nitre, Spirit of Sal Ammoniac, the Tincture of Mars extracted with Spirit of Wine, the Tincture of Tartar the Tincture of Antimony, the Elixir Proprietatis, the Essence of Soot and others, of a like Nature. To the Class of Visceral Medicines, also, belong Mineral Waters, especially such as contain a certain subtile Chalybeate Principle, such as those of *Pyrmont*, *Spaw*, and others; and much more those which contain a large Quantity of a Chalybeate Principle.

The *Balsamic* Viscerals, partly by a sulphureous, Balsamic, and somewhat fixed earthy Principle, and partly by their alcaline, sulphureous, saponaceous, and bitter Quality, perform their Operation upon the Viscera, whose Vessels are obstructed and infarcted by gross and viscid Humours, by inciding and dissolving the tenacious Juices, and at the same time procuring a due contracting and elastic Force to the Vessels, and Fibres of the Viscera, which had lost their Strength and Tone. Hence they are of great Efficacy, both for the Prevention and Cure of those Chronical Diseases, which arise from any Disorder of the Viscera.

Though all the Viscerals agree in this, that they strengthen the Tone of the Viscera, and remove Infarctions and Obstructions, yet it is necessary to vary them according to the Diversity of the Viscera affected, and

d the Diseases thereby produced;
u, for Instance, if the Liver is
structed, and a Jaundice, Cachexy,
Scurvy produced by that Means,
e most efficacious Viscerals are those
essed of a certain saponaceous
d detersive Bitterness; such as the
e aperient Roots, Rhubarb, Tur-
eric, Opoponax, Bdellium, Venice
ap, Elixir Proprietatis prepar'd
ith an Acid, and all good Prepara-
ns of Steel. When there are too
at a Relaxation and Infarction of
e Lungs, and the Diseases by that
eans produced are present, Myrrh,
um Ammoniac, Flowers of Sul-
ur, *Pauls* Betony, Scabious, Cher-
l, Lungwort, Mouse Ear, Hore-
und and Maidenhair, are generally
ught most efficacious. When the
leen being preternaturally large
d infarcted with Blood, favours the
neration of an impure Blood, and
ecially of a Cachexy, the Barks
Tamarisk and Capers, Fumitory,
leenwort, Dodder, Spurge, the
ots of Restharrow, and Chaly-
ates, are preferrable to other Re-
dies. When from a too weak and
ued Tone of the Kidneys, Neph-
t Pains and Stones are formed,
Bark of the *Egyptian* Thorn
t, and an Infusion of it, as also
parations of Houndstongue and
uper, are in a peculiar Manner
acious. From a weak State of
Uterus, and its Vessels, and a
r Circulation of the Blood and
ours, arise numberless Chroni-
Diseases, which are efficaciously

cured by long and round Birthwort,
Mugwort, Myrrh, Feverfew, Galbanum, Bdellium, Opoponax, Amber, the fetid Pills, and other prepared
in the same Manner. If the Intestines and their Glands, the secretory
and excretory, biliary, pancreatic
and lacteal Ducts, are so deprived of
Strength, that by a copious Defluxion of Humours, excessive Fluxes
are produced, or if the Humours
stagnating in the Vessels lay a
Foundation for febrile Motions,
and Paroxysms, Rhubarb, *Peruvi-*
an Bark, Winter's Bark, Cascarilla
Bark, and the most subtile Crocus
and Essences of *Mars*, are found
more efficacious than any other Remedies.

With respect to Corroboratives in
general, it is to be observ'd, that
they produce far better Effects, if
not only before their Exhibition the
redundant Blood is lessen'd, and the
Sordes of the *Prima Via* are evacuated by proper Laxatives, but if also, in
order to render the Humours more
fluid, they are exhibited in Decoctions or Infusions, or which is still
better, with Medicinal Waters, or
Whey; by which Means, the Operation of these Corroboratives, which
are of an astringent Nature, is greatly assisted in removing violent chronical and inveterate Disorders; especially when their Use is for a considerable Time persisted in, with proper Exercise, whether by Riding or
Walking.

C H A P.

CHAP. XII.

Of ASTRINGENTS.

ASTRINGENTS are very proper to reftore a Tone and Elafticity to the animal Fibres, when debilitated by Difeafes, Intemperence, or Accident. But thefe are very feldom proper without a previous Attenuation of the Juices, and a Courfe of deobftruent Medicines, becaufe Obftructions are more firmly rivetted, and the vifcid Juices circulate with more Difficulty, when the Diameters of the Veffels are contracted by Aftringents.

Among the feveral Claffes of Corroborative Medicines, that of *Aftringents* is none of the leaft confiderable and important. The feveral Subftances which come under this Denomination, are alfo by the *Latins* ftiled *Vulnerary,* and by the *Greeks, Traumatic* Medicines. Their Virtue in general confifts in a certain fixed, and gently conftrictive Principle, by Means of which they brace up the Parts and Fibres that are too much relaxed, corroborate thofe which are weakened, and confolidate and agglutinate fuch as are corroded and wounded. The principal Medicines belonging to this Clafs are, the Roots of the Avens, Tormentil, Biftort, the greater Confound, Bugle, Saracen's Confound, Goofeberries, Agrimony, St. *John's* Wort with its Flowers, Yarrow with its Tops, Horfetail, *Pauls* Betony, Strawberries, Vervain, Moufe Ear, Male Speedwell, all Sorts of Plantain, Oak-leaves, *Jerufalem* Oak, Baum, Mint, Betony, and Lamium or the dead Nettle, the Flowers of Rofes, Balauftines, the *Peruvian* Bark, that of Pomgranates, and of the Root of the E gyptian Thorn, *Japan* Earth, Dra gons Blood, Hurtleberries, and Quin ces. Of *Spices;* the Nutmeg, of *Mi neral Subftances,* the Bloodftone, A lum, and all Species of Earths an Marles; and many *Preparations.*

The feveral Subftances now men tioned operate by Means of a conf derable fixed terreftial Principle, i Conjunction with an Acid: And by conftricting the too much relaxe Fibres, they free them from a Cong ftion and Stagnation of Humours, by bringing them into a nearer Co tact with each other, they promo their Confolidation, and Coalefceno But this conftrictive Virtue is n equally ftrong and powerful in a the Subftances we have mentioned for in the Tormentil Root, in th Biftort Root, and its Extract, in th Balauftine Flowers, the Pomgran Bark, the Oak-leaves, the Alu the Juice and Bark of the *Egyptia* Thorn, Quinces, and dried Hurth berries, this aftringent Quality much ftronger, than in what w commonly call the Vulnerary Herb which confifting of a fubtile, earth and alcaline Principle, intermix with Particles of a fulphureous, ba famic, and fomewhat fixed Natur operate more fafely and mildly, a are of fingular Ufe and Advantage the Practice of Phyfic. But that the *Vulneraries,* as well as the ftrong and more powerful Aftringents, co tain a Principle of a fubtile, diffolv ble and earthy Nature, is plain fro this, that rich Infufions of them, u on the Admixture of Vitriol of Ma even of any Chalybeate Liquor whatever, become back, and assume an inky Colour, just as they wou'd do by the Addition of Galls.

If Skill and uncommon Caution are required in the Use of any Medicines whatever, they are certainly so in the Administration of *Astringents*; for since not only the Soundness of the Body in general, and of all its several Parts, but also Life itself, is maintain'd and preserved by the perpetual progressive and circulatory Motion of sufficiently attenuated and fluid Humours, thro' the Structure of the Body, which is almost entirely vascular, and composed of inconceivably minute and slender Ducts, and since, at the same time, such are the Natures, and Properties of *Astringents*, as to inspissate our Fluids mixed with them, and brace up the Pores and Ducts of our Solids, 'tis therefore obvious, that Remedies of this Class must be unfriendly, to the very Natures and vital Motions of animal Bodies; for which Reason they are not so safe and secure as some may imagine, unless when used with the utmost Care and Circumspection: For daily Experience convinces us, that Medicines of an Astringent Quality, rashly and unskilfully applied for stopping Hæmorrhages, or Fluxes, produce numberless fatal Consequences, and generally bring on slow Fevers, Cachexies, Ædematous Swellings, Spasmodic Disorders, Cholics, and Hypochondriacal Indispositions: For this Reason we are carefully to avoid the imprudent and immoderate Use of the *Peruvian* Bark, for carrying off the Paroxysms of intermittent Fevers. Since by its Astringency, the viscid bilious and salival *Sordes*, lodged in the *Primæ Viæ*, and which ought to be discharged, are so much the longer confin'd and retain'd, by which Means a still more formidable Disorder is sometimes brought on.

If Necessity should at any time call for the Use of Astringents of this Nature, they are not to be administered all at once; but successively, in gentle Doses, and in Conjunction with a sufficient Quantity of some proper Liquid; prescribing at the same time, a due Degree of Exercise.

'Tis highly unsafe and dangerou to repress excessive Vomitings, Discharges of bloody Urine, Hæmorrhages of the Nose, Uterus, or Anus, and Spitting of Blood, by Means of Astringents; since the Patients are always sure to suffer by such a Practice, unless the Spasms on which these Discharges of Blood for the most Part depend, as much as Effects do upon their immediate Causes, are first soothed, the violent and impetuous Motions of the Fluids checked, and the exorbitant and preternatural Affluence of Humours, derived to other Parts.

The traumatic or vulnerary Herbs, and Decoctions of them, are of very singular and uncommon Service, not only in Wounds, Erosions, and Solutions of Continuity, but also in some Diseases of a chronical and violent Nature, such as a Phthisis, Scurvy, Cachexy, and Disorders arising from the Stone, when these Indispositions draw their Origins from a preternatural Stagnation of the Juices. But we ought at all Times carefully to avoid using them, in Cases when there is too great an Obstruction of the Vessels, a Constriction of the Fibres, or in a Phthisis, when the Lungs are full of hard Tumours and Tubercles. However in other Cases, Infusions of vulnerary and gently astringent Medicines, are of singular Service and produce excellent Effects, especially in preventing fabulous and stony Concretions in the Kidneys, which for the most Part arise from an Exulceration or Relaxation of these Organs. This Intention is, is, also, very well answered by Infusions of Yarrow and its Tops, of *Pauls* Betony, Ground Ivy, Strawberries, Agrimony, and the Bark of the *Egyptian* Thorn Root. In involuntary Discharges of the Urine, arising from too great a Relaxation of the Sphincter Muscle of the Bladder, whether in Children or Adults, Infusions of this Nature produce very happy Effects, applying externally, of the same Time, rectified Spirits at Wine.

In Cases where the external Parts are hurt or wounded, well rectified Spirit of Wine proves by itself, a noble and efficacious *Vulnerary*, since it puts a speedy Stop to Defluxions of the Blood and Humours, and is of singular Service, where the more sensible Nerves, and tendinous Parts, have suffered by a too great Effusion of Blood; for spirituous Liquors not only coagulate the Juices of the human Body, as we find by making the Experiment upon Blood and Lymph, but also by removing the superfluous Humidity, render the Fibres tense and rigid; and by bracing them more strongly up, prevent Stagnations. Nor is the spirituous Water called *L'Eau de Arquebusade, or Aqua Sclopetaria*, a despicable Vulnerary, (in the Opinion of *Hoffman*) since it is prepared by Distillation in *Balneo Mariæ* from some of the best Vulnerary Herbs, and Wine: But its Virtues and Efficacy are to be ascribed to the Spirit and the Wine, rather than to the Herbs whose Virtues are lodged in a fixt earthy Principle, which does not come over the Helm of the Still.

CHAP. XIII.

Of HEATING MEDICINES.

THAT the Natures and Qualities of the several Medicines coming under this Denomination may be more thoroughly understood, it is necessary to observe, that there may be Heat without the external Application of Fire; and that it discovers its Presence by numberless Effects, but in no Case more conspicuously than by the Dilatation of the Fluid in the Thermometer. The Means, then, by which Warmth is generated in Bodies, are the very same with those by which apparent Fire is produced: Where there is Heat, there also is a proportionable and correspondent Motion and Agitation of the Parts of the Body said to be hot; and, *vice versa*, where there is an Agitation of the Parts there is a proportionable Heat or Warmth.

Motion consider'd in an abstracted and metaphysical Light, does not generate Heat, since a Body moving *in vacuo* can never produce any such Effect; so that Warmth must be originally owing to a brisk and lively Attrition of such Bodies, as are naturally susceptible of Heat, and capable of communicating it. The Generation of Heat in Bodies, and its several Degrees, are determined by three mechanical Axioms, the first of which is,

That the more dense the Matter is, the Degree of Heat generated is proportionably the greater: For by the Laws of Mechanics, if two Bo-

move with an equal Degree Velocity, the Effects produced then will bear a direct Proportion their respective Densities, or Quantity of Matter.

Secondly, The greater or stronger mutual Pressure of the Parts of one upon those of another is, the Heat generated is, *cæteris paribus*, proportionably the more intense: as two Plates of Iron gently and lightly moved upon each other, do produce the same Degree of Heat, when the Attrition is stronger and her.

Thirdly, The denser Bodies are, the stronger their mutual Pressure, and quicker their Motions, the greater is the Degree of Heat produced; and in Proportion as the Velocity is raised, so the mutual resistance between the Body mov'd, and that which may be said to sustain the Motion, is augmented.

From these Considerations we come to understand, why such human Bodies as are dense, hard, ponderous, robust, accustomed to Exercise, and abound with compact Humours and Juices, are always found not only warmer, but also require larger Time to become cold, than others, since such Bodies by a vigorous Application of the Solids to the Fluids are render'd dense by Compression, may reasonably be supposed not only to generate a greater Degree of Heat, but also to retain it longer than Bodies of an opposite Make, or in another State. Hence, also, we understand, why the internal Parts of Carcases deprived of Heat, grow cold very slowly; whereas their external Parts become so very soon. On the contrary, 'tis obvious that lax, soft, languid, and weak Bodies, can never excite an extraordinary Degree of Heat in their aqueous Humours, because the Attrition of their parts being weaker, their Fluids must be less dense, and the Surfaces of

their Parts the more lax, and consequently less capable of retaining the generated Heat. *Aristotle* was well apprised how much the Density or Thinness of the Blood, flowing in the Vessels of Animals, contributed to generate or produce Heat in their Bodies, as is obvious from the following Passage *Lib. 2. Cap. 4. de part. Animal.* " That Blood, says he, " which is too much diluted is cold, " and consequently cannot become " hard: But those Animals whose " Blood abounds with a great Number " ber of gross thick Fibres, have " more of an earthy Principle in their " Constitutions, and are fierce, wrath- " ful, and furious; for Rage begets " Warmth, and solid Bodies, and " all Substances of a firm Texture, " when become hot, warm more " powerfully, than such as are of a " moist and humid Nature. Now " the Fibres of such Animals are " solid and of a terrestrial Nature; " so that by Rage, Fermentations, " and preternatural Heats are excited " in the Blood. Hence it happens " that Bulls and Boars are of a fierce, " a wrathful, and furious Disposition, " on, because their Blood abounds " more with solid Fibres, than that " of some other Animals." For the Mass of Blood consists not only of red Globules, such as come more strictly under the Denomination of Blood, but also of Serum, in which these Globules swim; and the larger the Quantity of Serum is, the thinner and more diluted the Mass of Blood must of course be, and *vice versa.* On the other Hand, the thinner the Blood is, the more faint and weak the Attrition caused by its Motion must be, and the weaker its Attrition is, the smaller the Degree of Heat generated must be; therefore the thinner the Mass of Blood is, the fainter the Heat produced by it must be, and *vice versa.* Hence the Reason is obvious, why Men of hardy, ro-

bust

buſt Conſtitutions, who have their Veſſels fill'd with a thick and rich Blood, are more ſubject to burning Fevers, and inflammatory Diſorders, than thoſe of lax and weak Conſtitution, whoſe Veſſels contain a thin and much diluted Blood. Hence, alſo, appears the Reaſon, why Veneſection is the moſt infallible Method of diminiſhing the Heat of the Body, becauſe by leſſening the Quantity of the Blood, its Attrition in the Veſſels, on which the Denſity of the Humours depends, is proportionably leſſen'd. But to conſider the Method by which Heat is generated and increaſed in the human Boby, a little more accurately: The Blood itſelf is a Body; the Heart alſo, and the Arteries are Bodies, and conſequently the Heart cannot contract itſelf without preſſing upon the Blood, and this preſſure is continued by the Arteries. When a Body moves thro' a Cylinder, the Attrition produced is little or none at all; whereas when the ſame Body moves from the Baſe towards the Apex of a conical Canal, it muſt ſtrike againſt its Sides: Hence ariſes a Repercuſſion and conſequently an Attrition. Now the Arteries of our Bodies are ſuch conical Canals, and conſequently reſiſt the Impreſſion of the Blood; therefore an Attrition muſt neceſſarily be produced; and by natural Phyloſophy we are taught, that where there is Attrition, there alſo muſt be Heat, ſo that there can be no Heat in the human Body, and what is produced by the Circulation of the Fluids; and when this Circulation is ſtopped, the Heat is of Courſe deſtroyed. Hence the Degrees of Heat in a human Body, are moſt properly eſtimated by the Pulſe, ſince the beſt Pulſe denotes an equable Heat, diffuſed thro' all the Body; whereas the Pulſe preternaturally increaſed or diminiſh'd, indicates a proportionable Increaſe or Diminution of Heat. Hence the

Reaſon is obvious, why the art Blood of the Brain is the colde any, ſince in the Arteries of the B the Syſtole and Diaſtole are faint and languid, becauſe u their entering the Cranium, loſe their muſcular Coat. This ſervation, for the ſame Reaſon, h true with regard to the Blood in Bones. The muſcular Coat of Arteries, produces a proportic Preſſure of the Parts of the Bl upon each other: Hence ariſes trition, and this Attrition ceaſin being diminiſhed, the Heat acc ingly ceaſes, or is impair'd. Fi theſe Circumſtances we are able account for the arterial Blood b hotter than the venous Blo ſince in the Arteries the Blood is ways carried from wider to narro Parts, where the Reſiſtance, Preſſure, the Attrition, and co quently the Heat, are increaſe whereas in the Veins the Bloo carried from narrower into wi Parts, where the Reſiſtance, Preſſure, the Attrition, and co quently the Heat, are diminiſh The Reaſon why ſome Men, oth wiſe in a good State of Health, w faint away upon ſeeing Phleboto perform'd, firſt become cold at Extremities, is, becauſe in th Parts, the Humours firſt begin ſtop. Since, then, all the Heat a human Body is produced by Motion of the Fluids, and ſince Exceſs of Heat, bears a juſt Prop tion to the Attrition of the movi Fluids with themſelves, and with t Veſſels in which they flow, it hence obvious, that whatever i creaſes the Velocity of their cir latory Motion, muſt of Courſe au ment the Heat of the Body; ſo th by Motion and Exerciſe alone, t Degrees of Heat are not only i creaſed in a human Body, but al bear a Proportion to the Velocity that Motion, whether it be runnin any other Kind of Exercise. The Reason why *Hippocrates* in the fifteenth Aphorism of his first Section affirms, that in Winter and the Spring the Belly is naturally hotter than at other Seasons, is, because at these Times the Blood flows thro' the Vessels braced up, and render'd narrow by the Influence of the external Cold; for if the same Quantity of any Liquid is to move thro' a Vessel or Canal, narrower by one Half than the Vessel it formerly moved in, it will flow quicker by one Half than it did in the other; hence its Attrition, and consequently its Heat, must be increased. " The Circula- " tion of the Blood according to " *Hoffman*, in *Med. Rat. Syst.* is the " immediate and productive Cause " of Heat in the human Body; and " all Substances which increase this " Circulation, produce correspon- " dent Degrees of Heat in it; " whereas such Substances as retard " its Motion, of Course proportion- " ably impair its Heat." From what has been said it is obvious, that under the Denomination of heating Medicines, all such are to be rank'd, as increase the Velocity of the Cir- culation, and produce a greater Pres- sure of the Vessels upon the Fluids; since upon this Circumstance depends the Density of the Humours, which, as it is the principal Cause, so also may it prove the Effect of an in- creased Degree of Heat. Among the Medicines of this Kind we may reckon:

Stimulating Substances, among, which are the four greater hot Seeds of Anise, Caraway, Cumin, Fennel; the four lesser hot Seeds of Bishops weed, Stone-parsley, Smallage, and wild Carrot.

To this Class also belong Astrin- gents, and such Substances as block up the Pores externally, such as im- moderate Cold, a heavy Air, cold Water, tight Cloths, or thick Bed- cloaths.

Among such things as increase the Heat of the human Body, we may also reckon muscular Motion, and principally Frictions.

In the last Place, to this Class be- longs external Heat, whether occa- sioned by the Fire or the Air; to which we may, also, refer the warm Atmosphere immediately surround- ing the Body itself, when depriv'd of all Communication with the ad- jacent cool Air; when, for Instance, the Body being cover'd close up in Bed, becomes gradually warmer by the Heat exhaled from itself. Ac- cording to *Celsus L. 1. C. 3.* " The " Degrees of Heat are increased in " the Body by Unction, by Salt " Water, especially if hot, by all " saline Substances, and by austere " Wine". The Distinction of heating Medicines according to their several Degrees, seems to bear an Air of Absurdity in it, since these Degrees cannot be absolutely determined, but are meerly relative to the seve- ral Constitutions to whom such Me- dicines happen to be exhibited. As for Heat externally applied to the Body, 'tis to be observ'd, that a dry Heat is more proper for generating Warmth in the Constitution, than a moist one; since the latter at first excites the Sensation of Heat, but af- terwards augments the Cause from which the Sense of Cold proceeds, by relaxing the Vessels, diminishing their Resistance, and consequently impairing the Pressure which ought to be made upon the Fluids. In this Sense we are to understand *Hip- pocrates*, when in the sixteenth A- phorism of his fifth Section he asserts, that " Too frequent an Use of hot " Substances is attended with Ten- " derness of the Flesh, and Weak- " ness of the Nerves."

Old Persons, and People of wi- ther'd, dry, and rigid Constitutions, seem to be proper Exceptions to this Rule, since in Consequence of the

O   Re-

Relaxation to be expected from a moist Heat, the Passages of the Humours thro' their cappillary Veffels, are render'd more free and open. The Health of such Patients is, according to *Valleſius* in his *Philoſophia Sacra*, moſt effectually conſulted by following the Example of pious King *David* in the like Circumſtances. *Langius*, in the twelfth Epiſtle of his firſt Book, among the Fomentations which afford the moſt kindly Warmth, reckons a young Puppy, or a little Boy laid in the Boſom of an old Man, and immediately ſubjoins : Thus when *David* was ſeventy Years of Age, and his native Heat ſo much exhauſted, that he could not become warm by any other Means, he, by the Advice of his Phyſicians, got *Abiſhagh* the lovely *Shunamite*, to ſleep in his Arms, that the decay'd Strength of his Stomach might be reſtored by the kindly Warmth imparted by the blooming Lady.

When the Parts are refrigerated by the external Air, provided they are not become quite rigid by the Exceſs of the Cold, and the Blood is ſtill capable of circulating, they are reſtored to their former Vigour, by being firſt immerſed in cold Water, and afterwards beſprinkled with it, upon which they begin gradually to conceive a genial Warmth.

From what has been ſaid it is obvious, that heating Medicines are not only proper, but neceſſary when thin and diluted Humours are to be inſpiſſated ; where the ſolid Parts become flaccid, are to be render'd tenſe ; and where the Circulation of the Juices is either to be promoted when ſtopt, or accelerated when too faint and languid ; the Pulſe of the Patient, in the mean Time, directing the Phyſician how far to carry on his Deſign : So that heating Medicines carefully applied, muſt be a-

dapted to what we call cold Conſti tutions, to ſuch as abound with recrementitious Mucus, to ſuch a are too much relaxed, to the Leuco phlegmatic, and conſequently t ſuch as are afflicted with œdematou Tumors. But they who practic Phyſic ought to take due Care, tha heating Medicines be exhibited gra dually, and that the Body be no warmed by their Influence all of ſudden ; leſt by that Means, th Fluids ſtagnating in the flaccid Vel ſels, ſhould be too haſtily driven in to the capillary Veſſels, and ther form the moſt dangerous Obſtructi ons. A Man, for Inſtance, who b being long accuſtomed to a ſedentar Life, and a Want of due muſculi Motion, is become pale, and h acquired a flaccid State of all his F bres, when all on a ſudden he uſe any violent Motion, or takes larg Doſes of intenſly hot Medicines c the more ſtimulating and acrid Kind he immediately begins to breath with Difficulty, and to be in Dange of a Suffocation, in Conſequence c the Humours moving too violentl thro' the Veſſels, as yet too lax, an unable to make a mutual Reſiſtanc to the Impulſe of the Fluids, whic of Courſe ruſh into the capillary Vel ſels, and diſtend them, ſometim to ſuch a Degree as to burſt them and occaſion a Diſcharge of thei Contents. Accidents of this Natur happen not only in cachochymic H bits, which abound with acrid an viſcid Humours, but alſo in pletho ric Conſtitutions, where the Juice are good, but move in too ſlow an languid a Manner. But as a tempe rate Heat is abſolutely neceſſary fo the Preſervation of Life and Health ſo, as we are told by *Hoffman* in hi *Med. Rat. Syſt.* if this Heat is in creaſed beyond its due Degree, a irreparable Loſs of the finer Fluid is ſuſtain'd, and all thoſe Diſorder

an

æ brought on, which draw their Origin from the Juices being too much inspiffated, or render'd acrid by the Diffipation of their diluting, balfamic, aqueous Parts. According to *Hoffman* in *Med. Rat. Syft.* " Heat generates Salts in the Juices " of Animals ; for which Reafon, " when the Heat is increafed, as " happens in Fevers, the Urine con- " tains a larger Quantity of Salts, " and is of a deeper Colour ; where- " as the more moderate the Heat of " the Body is, which is generally " the Cafe with thofe habituated to " a Life of Eafe and Temperance, " the fainter the Colour of the Urine " is, and the fmaller Quantity of " Salts it contains." From this Paffage we learn, that a Change in the State and Condition of the U- rine, is another Sign of the Heat of the Body being increafed or dimi- nifh'd ; by which, as well as by the ftate of the Pulfe, the Phyfician ought to be directed in the Ufe of heating Medicines. From what has been faid it is obvious, that the Ufe of hot Subftances is prejudicial in ri- gid Bodies, whofe the Juices move fickly, and with a confiderable force ; and confequently that they muft abfolutely be abftain'd from in feverifh Heats, and acute inflamma- ry Diforders. According to *Hoff-man* in his Treatife laft quoted, ' Hot Subftances, and fuch as agi- ' tate the Blood too violently, ea- ' fily convert a mild Humour into ' Poifon, and a mild Diforder into ' one of the malignant Kind." He, alfo, advifes young Men, ' and fuch as are in the Vigour of ' their Age, to abftain as much as ' poffible from fuch Subftances as ' are hot, or have a Tendency to ' throw the Blood into Commoti- ' ons, left by fuch a Piece of Im- ' prudence, they fhould be fudden- ' ly carry'd off by inflammatory

" Diforders." That heating Medi-cines ought to be fparingly and cau-tioufly exhibited to Infants, is alfo obvious, fince their Juices are eafily put into Motion, and their Veffels foon irritated ; for, according to *Hippocrates* in the fourteenth Apho-rifm of his firft Section, they who are in a growing State, contain a great deal of innate Heat. Now that heating Medicines perform the various Offices of Corroboratives, Refolvents, and Difcutients, is fuffi-ciently obvious to any one that con-fiders, that the Fibres, the Mem-branes, and the Blood Veffels, de-rive a certain Tone, and elaftic Force, from heating Subftances, by which Means the Circulation of the Juices is render'd brifk and lively. But that an Excefs of this Heat, ren-ders People weak and languid, is a Truth confirm'd by Experience. The Reafon of it feems to be, that the thin and aqueous Humours of the Body, being too much exhaufted, the Blood of Courfe will be deprived of the Matter deftin'd by Nature for the Reparation and Nourifhment of the Solids. The incomparable *Boer-haave*, after making repeated Expe-riments, by Means of *Fahrenheit*'s Mercurial Thermometers, in order to determine the greateft Degree of Heat the human Body could endure or breath in, affirms, that the vital Heat in Men amounts to ninety-two Degrees, whereas in Children it of-ten amounts to ninety-four, that a Man is always hotter than that Por-tion of the Atmofphere which fur-rounds him, and that he cannot bear a Heat in his Body, greater than an Hundred and a few odd Degrees, without a Ceffation of the Circulation, and Death ; in which Cafe the Injury is firft difcover'd by a Depravation of the feveral Actions of the Head, and Lungs.

The Learned have contriv'd many Inftruments to meafure the Degrees of Fire, or Heat. But for thofe who are ftudious of great Exactnefs, the beft feems to be *Fabrenheit*'s Thermometer defcrib'd by *Boerhaave*. It confifts of a glafs Tube with a Bulb at the lower End, fitted to a Brafs Plate, on which the Degrees are mark'd from one to fix hundred. In the greateft Degree of natural Cold, the Mercury fubfides to one, and rifes to two hundred and twelve in a Degree of Heat fufficient to make Water boil; and to about fix Hundred in one capable of melting the more eafily fufible Metals, and boiling Oil.

CHAP. XX.
Of TOPICS.

WITH Refpect to external Applications, they are ufed in various Intentions; as to ftimulate the Skin and raife Blifters, in which cafe they are called Sinapifms, or Veficatories: To induce an artificial Sphacelus, and deftroy the Part to which they are applied; and thefe are called Cauftics: To ftrengthen relaxed Parts, as is the Cafe in Aftringents: To mollify hard and contracted Parts, as when Emollients and Relaxers are apply'd: To repel Humours: To attenuate Humours ftagnated and concreted in any particular Part: To difpofe thefe to Suppuration; and to deterge and clean Wounds, and Ulcers, and remove the Obftructions to their healing.

In order to underftand how thefe operate, it will be neceffary to confider the Action of Heat, or Fire; and of Cold. Heat, therefore, produces Effects very different, in different Degrees.

Thus in a fmall Degree it relaxes the folid Parts of the Body, and attenuates the Fluids fubjected to its Action, producing that agreeable Senfation which we call Warmth. And this Effect increafes with the Degree of Heat, to a certain Point.

And after this it begins to excite a painful and difagreeable Senfation; to deftroy the Solids; and to coagulate the Fluids contained in them; and this Action increafes *ad infinitum*, in Proportion to the Increafe of the Heat, or Fire.

Cold, on the contrary, contracts, and braces up the folid Parts, and coagulates the Fluids; and therefore, when the Effects of Heat begin to be difagreeabe, Cold conveys a pleafing Senfation, which we name Coolnefs. In a greater Degree it becomes uneafy, and begins to retard the Motion of the Humours thro' the containing Veffels, both on Account of its Action upon the Solids, and Fluids; and ultimately it induces a true Gangrene and Sphacelus; as is evident in Animals, and their Parts, fubjected to the Influence of fevere Frofts.

Now it feems juft the fame, with refpect to the Effect, whether actual Fire operates immediately upon the Body, or whether fuch Subftances are applied to it, as excite Fire, or Heat in the Part, by what Means foever.

We are, alfo, farther to confider, that when any Tumor is form'd by a

Stag-

Stagnation, and consequent Inspisation of the Juices, if any moisture is applied to the Surface of the Part, which is capable of entering the Pores, and mixing with the stagnant Fluid, this will, by diluting it, dispose it to move forwards in the Vessels, and return into the Mass of Blood; or supposing the Fluid extravasated, and stagnated in the cellular Membrane, Dilution will dispose it to enter the absorbing Vessels, and facilitate its Reconveyance by the Veins, to the Mass of Humours, and thus exonerate the Part offended.

Relaxation will be another Means of promoting the Resolution of any coagulated or coagulating Humour, either in or out of the Vessels, as by Relaxation the Diameters of the Vessels of all Sorts are enlarged, and consequently rendered more capable of conveying Particles, which, during a State of Restriction, could not more forward; at the same time that the same Relaxation affects the Fluids, and disposes them to a greater Fluidity.

Farther, was it possible to convey the Particles of any Sustance to the stagnating Juices, even without Heat, which would render them more fluid, or as it is usually expressed, would attenuate them, these would dispose them to move forwards in the Circulation, and would be a great Step towards Resolution.

Astringent Applications, tho' directly opposite to those of the relaxing Kind, yet may promote the salutary End of Resolution, as it were, by Accident; because by increasing the Strength of the solid Vessels, their contractile Power is augmented, and consequently the Force by which they propel the Fluids forwards, in their Cavities; insomuch, that sometimes in recent Inflammations, when the Disease has not made too great a Progress, this alone has been found capable of bringing about a Resolution.

Now in Case of an inflammatory Tumor, Cold and Astringents will contribute to repel the Disorder, by increasing the contractile Power of the Part, with the Effects last mentioned; and strengthen it in such a Manner, as to exclude all farther Influx of Humours to the Part. On the other Hand, a moist and gentle Heat, equal to, or somewhat surpassing that of tepid Water, will have all the good Effects of such a Heat, and Moisture, as Dilution, Relaxation, and Attenuation. But a somewhat greater Degree of Heat, will excite Suppuration, or a Putrefaction of the stagnating Juices, and of the solid Parts, in which the Circulation ceases to be carried on. But a still greater Degree of Heat, causes the Epidermis to seperate from the true Skin, and rise in Blisters as if scalded; and one a little more intense, induces a true Gangrene and Sphacelus.

Hence it seems highly probable, that if we could always determine the exact Degree of Heat necessary to answer the Intentions of Resolution, and Suppuration; and could with Certainty regulate our Applications accordingly, we should not so frequently be disappointed in our Expectations; and find Matter formed, where we intended to discuss, and *vice versa.*

I cannot omit taking Notice of Vinegar, as a Topic; because many People erroneously imagine, that it coagulates the Juices; whereas in Fact, there is scarcely any known Substance that attenuates more, and in a greater Degree disposes coagulating Juices to Fluidity.

The late Dr. *Friend,* in his History of Physic, seems to be of Opinion, that Oils prevent Resolution, by clogging and obstructing

O 2   the

the Pores. But as we are not to be governed in Practice by Authority, but by Facts, it is worth while to consider, that the Poison conveyed by the Bite of a Viper coagulates the Juices, from the Part wounded even to the Heart, in Animals that die of it; and that by rubbing Olive Oil into the Part, this Coagulation is prevented, and the Animal is cured. And I see no Reason why we are not to believe it may prevent Coagulations of the Blood from other Causes. If we examine the Practice of the Antients, we shall find, that it turned much upon Unctions, especially in Disorders arising from Stricture, that is, in Inflammations: And even People in a perfect State of Health, frequently employed Unguents, after relaxing the Skin by Bathing. Now 'tis highly probable, that this was not done wantonly, and without Design; but that they found by Experience, that Unctions prevented the Coagulation of the Juices; and therefore they made Use of them not only as a Cure for, but as a Preservative against Inflammation. And we know that whatever relaxes, is attended with such Effects.

As practical Rules and Cautions, are of infinitely more Consequence in Physic, than philosophial Disquisitions on the mechanical Action of Medicines, I shall oblige my Readers with the following Dissertation on Topics, in the Words of the very eminent *Frederick Hoffman.*

Topics in general include whatever is externally applied to any Part of the Body, and consequently comprehend whatever is, laid to Wounds or Ulcers, or any Injuries of the Limbs, whether it consists in the Application of the various chirurgical Instruments, or in the Use of Ointments, Plaisters, Injections, and Tents. But we shall confine ourselves to the Consideration of those Topics used in Disorder which arise from an internal Cause and consequently belong rather to the Province of the Physician, than of the Surgeon.

Baths, then, for the Head, whether prepared of simple Water, Lixivium, or Wine boiled with cephalic and emollient Herbs, are often preposterously used by Persons ignorant of Medicine. These are generally prejudicial in all Disorders of the Head, and Weakness of the Brain, or Nerves; but they are in a particular Manner injurious in Achors, Catarrhs, and Ringing of the Ears, Dullness of Hearing, and Inflammations of the Eyes. I have often known an Epilepsy produced by a preposterous Use of Baths to Childrens Heads; and I am of Opinion that we ought totally to abstain from such Baths, and substitute in their room Frictions of the Head, and Substances of a drying and corroborative Nature; for the above-mentioned Disorders are produced by an impetuous Conveyance of the Humours from the inferior Parts to the Head, and a Fulness and Stagnation of Blood, either pure or serous, in that Organ. Now nothing more disposes the Head to receive the Force of the Humours, and retain the serous Part of the Blood, than these Baths which by their hot and tepid Moisture, render the Fibres flaccid, and hinder the congested Humours from returning thro' the Veins. But in all Disorders of the Head, or superior Parts, we are rather to bath and relax the Feet and Legs, in order to make a Revulsion, and Derivation, from the superior to the inferior Parts.

I also condemn the Use of cephalic Plaisters; when, for Instance, the whole Head is shaved, and covered with a Plaister, as is usual in violent Hæmorrhages, Epilepsies and other Symptoms, generally produced by external Causes, such as Contusions or Blows. And tho' some, upon this Occasion, make a Distinction of Plaisters prepared of Balsams and Gums, and those which consist of viscid and glutinous Substances, yet, in my Opinion, both are more injurious than useful. The Reason of this Assertion is that the freer the Perspiration of the Part affected is, the Cure always succeeds the better, Besides, the farther the Parts are removed from the Heart, the Source of Heat, or the less Blood circulates in them, of the greater Importance it is to promote Transpiration in them. Every one must, therefore, be convinced, that Plaisters must prove prejudicial, by closing the Pores of the Head.

We can, therefore, from Experience recommend in their Head, dry Powders, either sprinkled on the Head, or included in Bags, which by their subtile, mild, and sulphureous Quality, corroborate the nervous or cold Parts, and preserve a free Perspiration. But if dry Powders are contraindicated, we may substitute in their room, Bags, including cephalic Ingredients, boil'd in Wine, or Liniments prepared of such Substances as are possessed of a penetrating Quality, by Means of a volatile oleous Salt, and a balsamic Resin, among which the most considerable are the *Peruvian* Balsam, Camphire, rectified Spirit of Wine, Sal-ammoniac, or volatile Salt of Worms, strengthened by the unadulterated Oils of Lavender, Marjoram, Rosemary, or Nutmegs, and impregnated with Essence of Castor. These Liniments afford great Relief in all Disorders of the Head, whether they partake of the Nature of Convulsions, and Epilepsies, or are accompanied with Pain, and the Interception of any of the Senses.

But my Intention is not to destroy the Use of all Plaisters, which in certain Cases are beneficial, when applied to the Forehead, or Nape of the Neck; but I only speak of those Plaisters which cover the whole or half of the Head. It is, also, to be observed, that frequently powdering the Hair, especially with pounded Starch, is productive of bad Consequences. Thus a Gentleman of Distinction told me, that by the frequent and immoderate Use of such Powder in his Youth, he contracted a Weakness in his Eyes, which at last terminated in a perfect Cataract Nor is it difficult to assign a Reason for this, since such tenacious Substances, by blocking up the Pores of the Head, greatly obstruct Perspiration, so necessary to the Health and Strength of the Part.

It is a common Error in Practice, to apply various Liniments and Balsams, in most Disorders of the Head, especially a Vertigo, and Head-ach accompanied with a Sense of Weight, a Carus, an Apoplexy, a Torpor of the Senses, and an Hemicrania. Thus it is customary not only to anoint the Nostrils and Temples, but also the Crown of the Head, and Neck, with fragrant Balsams prepared of Musk, Amber, Civet, and Oil of Roses; because these are thought efficacious against Disorders of the Head. But such a Practice is not so innocent as it is imagined; for these are vaporous Medicines, and by their elastic Vaporosity insinuating themselves into the Pores of the Vessels, distend them too much, and in some Measure fix the impetuous Motion of the Blood, and by their sedative and anodyne Quality dispose to Drowsiness. Hence every one must perceive, that we are to deal cautiously with Medicines of this Kind, which are not proper in Disorders of this Nature, where the

Head

Head, and its Veffels, are infarcted and diftended by the Impetus and Quantity of Blood. In this Cafe, by increafing the Expanfion of the Humours, and confequently augmenting the Danger of their Stagnation, they are experimentally found to produce Head-achs, Vertigoes, Ringing of the Ears, Drowfinefs, and greater Oppreffion and Torpor of the Mind and Senfes. What *Hippocrates*, fays in *Aph.* 28. *Sect.* 5. with Refpect to Fumigations, holds true concerning thefe Medicines, which is, that they would in many Refpects, contribute to the Production of good Effects, if they did not induce fuch a Heavinefs of the Head. For which Reafon, to the Remedies above mentioned, we prefer fuch balfamic Liniments, as only confift of highly rectified Spirit of Wine, in which Camphire, the Oils of Marjoram, Lavender, and Rue, but not adulterated with Turpentine, are diffolved ; for thefe Substances rather operate by difcuffing and opening the Pores, than by filling the Head with Vapours, and for that Reafon are always fafer in Cephalalgias, and violent apoplectic Fits.

We now proceed to the Topics generally ufed in Diforders of the Eyes ; and fo great are the Errors committed both by Phyficians and Surgeons in this Refpect, that we may juftly affirm, that more are deprived of Sight by a prepofterous Application of thefe, than by the Violence of the Diforders. Thus it is a vulgar Error, that cold Subftances are friendly to the Eyes, whereas fuch as are hot are prejudicial to them : This indeed holds true when the Eyes are found, in which cafe it is more expedient to wafh them with cold Water, than with warm; becaufe the latter by corroborating the Pores of the Coats and Sides of the Veffels, prevents

an exceffive Flux of Blood and Humours, and preferves the Eyes ferene, lively, and found. But this Rule is by no Means to be obferved in a preternatural State of the Eyes, efpecially in an Ophthalmia, in which Cafe the Ufe of cold Subftances is highly dangerous. Thus *Foreftus* in *Obf. Chirur. L.2. Obf.* 16. gives us an Account of a Woman, who labouring under an *Ophthalmia,* ufed a Collyrium of Talc and diftilled Water ; but foon after her Eyes were feized with fuch an intenfe Pain and Heat, that an Ulcer. fucceeded. When the Eyes have been afflicted with an inflammatory Heat, I have feen them rendered turbid, and the Inflammation fo greatly increafed, that within a few Days the Sight has not only been obfcured, but alfo fometimes totally deftroyed, for want of proper Management ; for as in all Inflammations fkillful Phyficians juftly condemn the external Applications of cold, aftringent, and incraffating Subftances, fo I fee no Reafon why we fhould admit their Ufe in Inflammations of the Eyes, whofe capillary Veffels are far more tender than thofe of other Part ; for the Caufe and Origin of every Inflammation is an Infarction of Blood or Humours, in the larger Veffels, on Account of the Obftruction of the adjacent fmall Veffels ; now Obftructions are by nothing more confirmed, than by Things actually cold, which deprive the Juices of their Fluidity, and render them thick and incapable of Circulation.

In inflammatory Diforders of the Eyes, we not only reject fuch Collyriums as are actually cold, but alfo, fuch as are poffeffed of an incraffating Quality, or invite a farther Afflux of the Humours to the Part affected ; fuch as all the ophthalmic Waters, the Frogs Spawn Water, for Inftance, Rofe-water, that of Plan-

Ptarmin, that with Sugar of Lead, that of Alum, the White of an Egg, and Bole, and all mucilaginous Substances. Thus *Forestus* in *Lib.* 2. *Obf.* 26. obferves, that oleous and pinguious Subftances are prejudicial to the Eyes; in Confirmation of which he tells us, that a Barber treated an Ulcer with hot Oil, till breaking into the Tunica Cornea and Uvea, it at laft degenerated into a Cataract. Greater Efficacy is to be expected from fuch Subftances, which, without any great Acrimony or Heat, are poffeffed of a difcuffive Quality, among which Camphire is the moft confiderable; becaufe, as in all other Inflammations, fo also in this, it affords inftantaneous Relief. If, therefore, the Inflammation is only flight and fuperficial, Elder flower Water in which a little Saffron is diffolved, with the Addition of a few Drops of a well faturated Solution of Camphire, applied tepid, is of fingular Service. If the Inflammation is accompanied with a faline acrid Lymph, a Mucilage of Quince feeds, or Rofe-water, mixed with Saffron and Camphire, are of fingular Efficacy. But when the Inflammation is violent, deep, and dangerous, the Eye being almoft deprived of Sight and Senfibility, I have found many happy Effects produced by tepid camphorated Spirit of Wine, mixed with Peruvian Balfam, by which Means the Senfation, Motion, Tone, and Colour of the Eyes, are gradually reftored.

It is fufficiently known, that Vitriol, in Confequence of its partaking of Copper, is among Practitioners reckoned a great Arcanum in Diforders of the Eyes; but as it is almoft promifcuoufly ufed in all Collyriums, great Misfortunes are fometimes produced by it. We are, therefore, to abftain from the Ufe of Vitriol in all Inflammations, and

faline, hot, and acid Defluxions, accompanied with Rednefs and Itching, becaufe Vitriol by its Acrimony increafes all thofe Symptoms. But Vitriol is properly ufed, either when the Humours are thick, and formed into Sordes, or when they begin to form fmall Membranes in the *Tunica Albuginea*, which frequently happens after the Small Pox and Meafles. In fuch a Cafe, therefore, furprifing Effects are produced, by one Grain of *Cyprian* Vitriol diffolved in one Ounce of Celandine-water, with which Liquor upon a Feather, the Part afflicted is to be touched frequently every Day.

But when a manifeftly corroding and burning Matter is perceived, temperating, demulcent, and mucilaginous Subftances are to be ufed; and of thefe the beft are the Mucilages of the Seeds of Fleabane and the *Sief Album* without Opium, as alfo the Powder of Sarcocolla.

With refpect to the Fat of Vipers, and of the Species of Fifh called *Umber*, which is fo greatly extolled in Wounds of the Eyes, and in that Diforder in their Corners which is generally called the *Pannus*, we are to obferve, that thefe Fats ought to be recent, fince when by Age they have contracted a Rancidity, they are not only injurious in thefe, but alfo in all other Diforders of the Eyes. Befides, Collyriums are of no Ufe, or rather hurtful, when from a Fault and Dyfcracy of the Lymph and Blood, which often happens in a Scurvy and Lues Venerea, the Eyes are red, painful, dropping and turbid. In fuch cafes Topics of all Kinds are ufelefs. We muft firft correct the Juices by internal Medicines, which is excellently perform'd by a Decoction of the Woods, and of fuch Herbs as fweeten the Blood. It alfo fometimes happens, that in Confequence of an inveterate Tumour of the Glands of the Neck, an obstructed Discharge from the Ears, an Application of Cosmetics to the Face, or the Retropulsion of an Achor in the Head, the peccant Matter fixes its Seat in the Eyes; in this case we are not to trust to Topics alone, but these are to be affisted by internal Medicines, and the Cause of the Disorder must be totally removed.

With Respect to Disorders of the Ears, innumerable Errors are also committed; for nothing is more improper than in a Dulness of Hearing to put Oils, whether expressed, as the Oil of Sweet-Almonds alone, or mix'd with cephalic Oils, into the Ears. Tho' this Piece of Practice is extolled by many Practitioners, yet I have rarely found it productive of good Effects: For a Dulness of Hearing proceeds either from a too great Relaxation of the *Tympanum,* or from an excessive Humidity of the Membrane surrounding the Organ of Hearing, that is the Labyrinth and Cochlea; so that Oils, by producing a greater Relaxation, increase the Disorder; and Oils of an hot, acrid, or too spirituous Kind, produce intense Pain and Heat in that highly nervous and sensible Membrane, which surrounds the auditory Passage. Besides, if we have Recourse to the Observations of the most skillful Practitioners, we shall find that Topics are so far from being beneficial in a Dulness of Hearing, or Ringing of the Ears, that they are rather injurious. Nor do I see by what Means the Virtues of Medicines, whether unctuous, oleous, or spirituous, can penetrate to the Seat of the Disorder, which is within the Brain, or in the most remote Recesses of the *Os Petrosum;* in such Cases I have always observed happier Effects produced by apophlegmatizing and cephalic Substances.

There are, however, some Cases, in which Topics are beneficial in Disorders of the Ears, when, for Instance, the Ear Wax is so indurat as to assume the Nature and Consistence of a Plaister, and great obstruct the Hearing: In this C tepid Oil of sweet Almonds, mo fies the indurated Ear Wax, so th it may be commodiously extract with Ear Picks. I remember so Years ago, a Mountebank pretend to a wonderful Secret for removi Deafness, which consisted of injec ing into the Ear, with a Syring Fennel-water, into which a little the Oil of Tartar had been dro ped. This Injection he cautiou made several Times a Day, and some Patients, that is those who auditory Passage was closed up wi the Ear Wax, the Experiment fu ceeded very well. The like hap Effect is sometime produced by a pid Injection of mineral Waters in the Ear; but they are only benefic when the Dulness of hearing pr ceeds from Sordes too much clo ging the Membrane of the Ty panum.

As Abscesses sometimes arise the internal Ears, 'tis to be obser ed, that these require a particul Treatment, since if they are treat in any other Manner, they frequer ly terminate in putrid and cario Ulcers, accompanied with a to Loss of Hearing. 'Tis, therefo a bad Piece of Practice to Use gestive and oleous Ointments, fu as those cold dry nervous Parts ca not bear. But such Abscesses a rather consolidated and hinder from degenerating into Ulcers, putting warm Balsamics into t Ear with Cotton, such as the Tin tures of Myrrh, Opobalsam, a Amber.

The Nostrils have also their pa ticular Topics, which when prope ly applied, are very beneficial, b no less prejudicial when prepofte ou only used; an Instance of this we have in the great Variety of Things that up the Nostrils, in order to stop excessive Hæmorrhages: And tho' the Applications of this Kind be numerous, yet few of them are useful, or even innocent in Practice. For as an Hæmorrhage generally proceeds from an internal Cause, which for the most Part is a Spasm, a violent Constriction, or Obstruction of some Parts remote from the Nostrils, and as the Blood is then impetuously conveyed to the Vessels of the Head, when this Blood is too much congested, it dilates the Orifice of the Vessels, and it last breaks the Coats of the Nostrils. Hence every one must perceive, that it is not only in vain, but also dangerous in such Cases, to use external Styptics and Repellents; for closing up the Orifices of the Vessels by Astringents, we derive the Disorder to other Parts of the Head, or perhaps to the Breast, whilst the internal Force of the Blood still remains. But if the open Orifices of the Vessels from which the Blood flows are situated pretty deep in the Fauces, so that the Efficacy of Styptics cannot reach them, and the Nostrils in the mean Time are so stopt up, as to afford no Discharge of the Blood, it falls from the Fauces upon the Aspera Arteria, sometimes not without Danger of Suffocation. Besides, as all Styptics are unfriendly to nervous and glandular Membranes, they greatly injure these Parts when thrust far into the Nostrils.

These Topics for the Nostrils are, therefore, of little or no Use, unless we previously derive the Blood from the Head by Venesections, Frictions, and Immersions of the Feet and Hands in warm Wine, or Water; as also by Diaphoretics, which without any great Motion and Heat,

propel the Blood from the Center to the Circumference of the Body; and then there is no Necessity for these cold and styptic Repellents, since the Tincture of *Terra Japonica* alone, received into the Nostrils, is far superior to them all. 'Tis customary among the Vulgar, in excessive Hæmorrhages of the Nose, to apply a Piece of silver Coin wet in cold Water, either to the Forehead, or Nape of the Neck. But these Practices cannot be used in the Beginning of the Hæmorrhages, without Danger of an Apoplexy. We do not, however, disapprove of such Epithems as are at once possessed of a discutient and corroborative Virtue, such as Vinegar of Roses mixed with Nitre, Camphire and Oil of Rose-wood, which Mixture when applied tepid to the Temples and Neck, is of singular Efficacy, and preferable to all others.

We now come to consider the Topics generally used in those putrid and carious Ulcers of the Ossa Squamosa, which are familiar to those labouring under a venereal Taint, or the Scurvy. The Topics for these Purposes are generally the Water of Roses, Plaintain, and Houseleek, mixed with red Bole, Sugar of Lead, or Magistery of Lead; or if the Ulcers penetrate to the Bones of the Fauces, or corrode or consume the Substance of the Uvula, Injections or Gargarisms are commonly used. But all these cold Preparations are of no Use, since they are by no Means fit for stopping the putredinous Corruption. Disorders of this Kind require far more powerful and more penetrating Medicines, such as Oil of Cloves, which is an excellent Preserver of the Bones, especially when mixed with *Peruvian Balsam*; *Elixir Proprietatis* prepared without an acid, Essence of Amber, or camphorated Spirit of Wine,

cau-

cautioufly injected thro' the Noftrils by Means of a Syringe, are alfo excellent for curing thefe fetid and malignant Ulcers. This Method I have often upon reflecting concluded good, and upon Trial found to anfwer my Expectations. Many venereal Patients, on Account of the Ignorance of their Surgeons, and the prepofterous Applications of Medicines, are long afflicted with fuch fordid Ulcers, which at laft corrode and confume the whole internal Structure of the Noftrils, the Uvula, and the Bone of the Palate, to the great Detriment not only of their Voice, but alfo of their Health ; but Gargarifms, tho' prepared of the moft efficacious Ingredients, are in vain applied, becaufe they cannot reach the Root of the Diforder, and the Part affected, which is above the Bone of the Palate.

Many Topics are, alfo, prefcrib'd both by Phyficians, and the Vulgar, for the Tooth-ach ; but moft of thefe generally do more Injury than good ; and tho' after the Ufe of gentle Aftringents and Anodynes, the beft of which feems to me, to be, the Tincture of *Terra Japonica* mixed with an anodyne Tincture, there is fome Alleviation of the Pain, yet it is very fmall, fhort lived, and at another Time not to be obtain'd. And as a Tooth-ach is frequently epidem.cal, and rifes from a Rheum, or an acrid eryfipelatous Defluxion infefting the carious Tooth, and generally joined with a catarrhous Fever, it is eafy to perceive how idle and ineffectual an immediate Application to the Tooth muft be. In this Cafe, if any Benefit can be expected from external Applications, the beft we can ufe are paregoric Bags, prepared of difcutient, carminative, and anodyne Ingredients : And tho' the Oils of Cloves and Origanum are excellently appropriated

to a Caries of the Teeth, accompanied with Pain, yet when in a carious Tooth, a nervous Membrane is too much diftended, or corroded by an aqueous Fluid lodged between the narrow Interftices of the Bone, we are rather to ufe the liquid apoplectic Balfam, or the Balfam of Life, received into the Noftrils ; or a tepid Decoction of Milk with Elder flowers and Saffron, kept in the Mouth, will better alleviate fuch a Pain, than any other external Application whatever. And I can affirm from Experience, that Diaphoretics alone, fuch as Bezoardic Tinctures, Sulphur of Antimony, or fuccinated Spirit of Hartfhorn, mixed with the fweet Spirit of Nitre ufed in violent Tooth-achs, with a Sudorific Regimen, after the Ufe of fuch Medicines as render the Body foluble, produce very happy Effects. Thus it is fufficiently obvious how propofterously Topics are generally ufed in Tooth-achs.

Various Errors are alfo committed, with refpect to the Cure of cutaneous Diforders of the Face and Head. Thus nothing is more cuftomary among the Vulgar, than the curing Achors, and fcald Heads in Children, with various Lotions Lixiviums, Decoctions, and Ointments prepared with Sulphur, C of Olives, and other unctuous Subftances. But I have experimental found this Method productive of the worft Confequences, fince it is generally fucceeded by Epilepfies, Inflammations, and Suppurations the Eyes, an Epiphora, a Gutta S rena, violent Peripneumonies, Afthmas, and other Diforders of the like Nature. We are, therefore, fuch Cafes, to deal very cautiou with external Applications, for fear of obftructing the Perfpiration the Parts ; nor are we ever to prefcribe them, without at the fame Time exhibiting internal Medicin for correcting the peccant Humours. We are never externally to apply moift, oleous, and aftringent Subftances ; and if Topics are indicated as proper, antimonial Balfam of Sulphur diffolved in comphorated Spirit of Wine, and mixed with Oil of fweet Almonds, will produce excellent Effects, by mollifying, difcuffing, and refifting farther Putrefaction. In venereal Puftules, and a Gutta Rofacea, we are, alfo, to deal very cautioufly with Repellents, and fuch Medicines as conftrict the Pores of the Skin; fince by their Means I have often obferved the faline, acrid Serum, precipitated to the Coats of the Eyes, and an Ophthalmy produced.

How much Topics are abufed in the Cure of an Eryfipelas, is too obvious, for certainly, this Diforder requires a cautious Application of Externals, particularly when near the Brain and Origin of the Nerves ; and it is not free from Danger, efpecially in fcorbutic Patients, as Practitioners fufficiently know. Practical Authors furnifh us with numberlefs Inftances of the bad Effects of Topics in the Cure of an Eryfipelas. Thus *Rolfinckius* in *Method. curand. Affect. Capit.* makes mention of a Quinfey produced by the unfeafonable Ufe of Repellents in the Cure of an *Eryfipelas* of the Head. *Aquapendente* in *Lib. de Tumoribus,* juftly orders, that in an Eryfipelas of the Face or Head, we are neither to ufe Topics before, nor after Purging ; for by cold Subftances, the Matter may be repell'd to the Brain, and produce a Phrenitis ; or to the Fauces, where it induces a Quinfey. In fuch Cafes, all Cataplafms, all unctuous, moift, and aqueous Subftances are highly prejudicial. But we are rather to ufe dry Subftances alone, fuch as Bags prepared of emollient and difcutient

Herbs, that the Tranfpiration may remain free. Sometimes, however, camphorated Spirits of Wine, mixed with Effence of Caftor, and Oil of Nutmegs, and with volatile Salt of Worms, Nitre, and a little Opium, ufed by Way of Ointments, produce very falutary Effects.

Thofe feem to be in a great Error, who for the Cure of a *Gutta Rofacea*, and Puftules, ufe fublimate Mercury ; fince this, when receiv'd into the Pores, greatly difpofe to violent Head-achs, Hemicranias, and Loofenefs of the Teeth. But the Intention will be far better anfwer'd by Tincture of Benjamin, and with Magiftery of Lead, Camphire, Sugar of Lead, Frogs Spawn Water, and Elder flower Water.

When the Flefh of the Gums is fo corroded, that the Roots of the Teeth appear bare, the Diforder is generally thought to proceed from a Relaxation of the Fibres. Hence it is a common Cuftom to prevent this Misfortune by the external Ufe of Aftringents, fuch as the Effences of Maftich, and Tormentil, Alum, and the Tincture of Japan Earth, which inftead of being beneficial, are rather prejudicial ; for the Diforder is an Atrophy, and proceeds from a Defect of the nutritive Juice, in Confequence of an Obftruction of the minute and numerous Arteries of the Gums. Now if this Obftruction is confirmed by Aftringents, the Gums muft be ftill more deprived of their fine nutritive Juices. In fuch Cafes, happier Effects are produced by Decoctions of Wine with Sage, Origanum, Rofemary, Camphire, Nitre, and a fmall Quantity of the Spirit of Sal Ammoniac. By wafhing the Mouth and Gums frequently with fuch Decoctions warm, the Veffels are opened, the Blood and Juices invited to the Part, the Fibres

bres of the Gums corroborated, and the Use and Vigour of those Parts restored.

We now come to consider the Abuse of Topics in Disorders of the Thorax. In those inflammatory Tumors, therefore, of the Lungs, commonly called Pleurisies or Peripneumonies, nothing is more customary than the external Use of oleous Ointments, in order to allay the Pain. But I have rarely seen happy Effects produced by this Practice, since when the Disorder might at first have been dissipated by internal Resolvents and Discutients, they hinder its Discussion, and dispose it to a Suppuration; just as in erysipelatous Disorders of the external Parts, these Ointments, by obstructing the Pores, and relaxing the Fibres, invite a farther Defluxion of Humours, and dispose the Part to Suppuration, and Exulceration. If, therefore, as it often happens, the Pleurisy is spurious, that is, if an acrid saline Serum stagnates between the Membranes of the intercostal Muscles, in which Case it is a Species of Rheumatism, the abovementioned Topics will be far more injurious than beneficial, by hindering the Transpiration and Excretion of the stagnant Matter, which, however, is absolutely necessary to the Recovery of the Patient. Some, in order to allay violent Pain, have a Custom of adding to those the Oil of Henbane, by which Means the Pain is indeed alleviated, but at the same Time a Drowsiness, a Languor of the Strength, and a difficult Expectoration succeed; which, especially in older Age, are not without Danger. Besides, in these Disorders it is customary with some, to apply Plasters, such as the Emplastrum Vigonis mixed with Mercury, Balsam of Sulphur, and Camphire. But by this Means I have found, that when the Pleurisy has been spurious, and

affected the intercostal Muscles and Membranes, but not the Lungs, the Pain has indeed been dissipated; but the Matter has been convey'd to other Parts; and I have known the Matter repell'd to the of Substance the Lungs, where it has produced Impostumations sufficiently chronical and dangerous.

In my Opinion, therefore, in all these inflammatory Disorders of the Thorax, we are either absolutely to abstain from all Topics; or if any are to be admitted, camphorated Spirit of Wine mitigated, and render'd Anodyne by an Addition of Castor, Saffron, and distill'd Oil of Nutmegs, used by Way of Ointment, seems preferable to all others. There are, however, some Disorders, in which pinguious Ointments, those possess'd of an anodyne Quality, and such as relax the Fibres, produce happy Effects, tho' they are rarely used. A Disorder of this Kind is the dry Chin-cough, in which not so much the Quantity, as the peccant Quality of a thin and acrid Matter, stimulates the pneumonic Nerves, and Thorax, to violent, convulsive, and concussive Motions; in which Cases it is necessary to allay those Motions, and relax the constricted Parts of the Thorax, not neglecting, at the same Time, to inspissate and correct the thin and acrid Humour. This Species of Cough is frequently very obstinate, and raging violently at certain Seasons, principally attacks Children and Infants. I have frequently seen good Effects produced by anointing the whole Breast with an Ointment, prepared of the *Unguentum Potabile*, Sperma Ceti, Badgers Fat, Ointment of Poplar, Oil of Anise, and Camphire.

We shall now subjoin something with regard to Topics, in a true Phthisis, or Exulceration of the Lungs: We have Instances of Phthisica ical Patients, who bear some Ointments and Plaisters well; but others not without Injury. The Nature, therefore, of every Phthisis, and its particular Cause, are to be investigated. Topics are not therefore used, when the Lungs are full of hard Tubercles, which for the most Part gradually come to Suppuration: for this Purpose the Plaisters ought not to consist of too hot Substances, or those of too tough and unctuous a Kind; for the former increase the Pain and Inflammation, and the latter hinder a free Perspiration. The best of all is *Rulandus's Emplastrum Diasulphuris*, without the Colophony. But 'tis to be observ'd, that, in Disorders of the Lungs, Plaisters are not to be applied to the Sternum, thro' which they cannot penetrate, but rather to the Back and Sides, because there the Pores are more open, the Blood more copious, and the Vessels more numerous; in Consequence of which, the subtile and salutary Parts of the Plaisters are the better received and admitted.

We now come to consider some Disorders of the Stomach, in which Topics are beneficial, provided they are duly applied. No Pain is more cruel than that which is fixed in the right and left Orifices of the Stomach, which are highly sensible, and is generally call'd a Cardialgia. In this Disorder it is customary to take internally various Remedies for mitigating the Pain, and externally to anoint the Region of the Stomach with some spiritous Liniments, or an Ointment prepared of carminative and anodyne Ingredients. But this Method does not produce the desired Effect, for since the Pain is fixed in a very small Part, that is, in these nervous Orifices, it is sufficiently obvious, that a penetrating and efficacious Medicine is to be applied as near as possible to those Parts. Now if either a Plaister, Liniment, or

Ointment, is applied to the whole Region of the Stomach, a small Quantity of any of them can only penetrate to the Orifices of the Stomach. Besides, as it is certain from Anatomy, that the superior Orifice of the Stomach is nearer the Back and Vertebræ, since it is situated hard by the Aspera Arteria, it is sufficiently obvious, that the Medicines applied to the Pit of the Stomach, can by no Means penetrate to it. Such Remedies are, therefore, to be applied to the Back, about the eighth and ninth Vertebræ, before they can affect it. But if the right Orifice is affected, we are to apply our Remedies under the Stomach, towards the right Side. But in Cases of this Nature, we are by no Means to use too volatile Substances, such as Spirits, nor unctuous and emplastic Substances, which operate too slowly; but rather a pretty thick Liniment, in the Form of a Plaister, and prepared of Treacle, Saffron, Oil of Nutmegs, Camphire, Peruvian Balsam, and Oil of Henbane. I have often found this Preparation afford Relief, and where it proves unsuccessful, nothing is to be expected from other Topics.

Practitioners well know that in Weaknesses of the Stomach, Vomitings, and Nauseas, nothing is more common than to apply Ointments, or oval stomachic Plaisters, under the Sternum. But upon dissecting Carcasses, we find that only a very small Portion of the Stomach, but the Liver, the Intestinum Colon, and the small Intestines, are situated there. The Stomach inclines rather to the left Side under the Ribs, where at least three Parts of it are situated towards the Spine. If, therefore, we only apply generous and penetrating Medicines to the spurious Ribs of the left Side, towards the Back, we shall find far more happy Effects produced on the Stomach by them.

The

The violent Pain arifing from a Stone fticking in the Beginning or Middle of the Uterus, alfo, demands the Ufe of Topics; but they muft be applied with great Caution, for 'tis fufficiently known, that a pretty large Stone, whilft lodged in the tubular Suubftance of the Kidneys, creates no Uneafinefs, but excites an intollerable Pain, when it falls into the narrow and fenfible Ureters. Hence we perceive, that Topics for this Purpofe,' ought not to be applied to the Loins, where the Kidneys are not fituated, but according to the Direction of the Ureters, that is, from the Loins to the Groin. But even in this, a violent Error is generally committed, whilft with the Ointments, moft Perfons mix hot forcing Subftances, fuch as the Oil of Amber, Spirit of Turpentine, and the Oil of Juniper, which Practice is productive of very bad Effects; many indeed intend by thefe hot Subftances, to force the Paffage of the Stone thro' the Ureters; but it is by this Means rather fixed and more violent Symptoms, fuch as a Suppreffion of Urine, Vomitings and Convulfions, are excited; for, that the Stone remains fixed in the Ureter, is not fo much owing to its Bulk as to the painful Spafm of the Ureter; and as by the Afperity of the Stone, the nervous Fibres are generally irritated, there happens an Influx of the Spirits, and Pain accompanied with Spafms and Conftrictions, and the more intenfe the Pain is, the more narrow and contracted the Paffages are; For if fpirituous hot Subftances are in fuch a Cafe applied, they excite an Influx of the Blood and Spirits, fix the Stone more firmly in the Part, increafe the Pain, and induce many terrible Symptoms. 'Tis not indeed to be denied, that where there is neither Pain nor Spafms, or where there is a certain Laxity, or want of Tone, in the nervous and membraneous Fibres of the Kidneys, fuch Things externally applied, becaufe they ftrengthen the Tone of the Parts, promote a Difcharge of Urine; but they are by no Means to be ufed, when there is any Pain or Spafm, in which Cafe we are rather to ufe emollient, paregoric, and anodyne Oils, fuch as the Ointments of Poplar, Henbane, Poppy-feeds, and white Lillies, Badgers-fat, and Camphire, which gives them a penetrating Quality. With thefe the Region of the Ureters is to be frequently rubbed, and anointed, with a warm Hand; for thefe Subftances by checking the Impetus of the Spirits, and relaxing the contracted Fibres of the Ureters, occafion a far more eafy and expeditious Paffage for the Stone. For this Reafon, fitting in a Bath is highly beneficial, and fometimes affords inftantaneous Relief.

In exceffive Difcharges of the Menfes, and involuntary Effufions of the feminal Fluid in Men, 'tis cuftomary to apply to the Lumbar Region, where the large Ramifications of Blood Veffels are fituated, and freely expofed, fuch Medicines, as in fome Meafure check the Impetus of the Blood to the genital Parts; and it is of great Importance what Medicines are ufed on thefe Occafions, and at what time they are applied; for I knew a Woman, who, in an immoderate Flux of the Menfes, had a Plaifter applied to her Loins, confifting of the Frogs fpawn Plaifter mixed with Sugar of Lead, and Oil of Henbane; but from that Time her Menfes never returned, to the great Detriment of her Health. We are, alfo, carefully to abftain from all Things actually cold, and much more Narcotics; becaufe all thefe by checking the Blood, if it tends too much to thefe Parts, produce a palliative Cure, but bring on much worfe Misfortunes, fuch as Inflammations of the Kidneys, convulfive Colics, and

and spasmodic Disorders of the Abdomen. Hence it is the safest Method, especially in Evacuations of Blood, totally to abstain from these Topics; but rather to carry on the Cure by internal Medicines.

We now come to consider some Disorders which proceed from a Relaxation, Resolution, or Want of Tone and Strength in the Ligaments; such as the falling down of the Fundament in Infants, and of the Uterus in Women. Physicians and Surgeons, in Consequence of the Relaxation, generally treat these Disorders with Astringents; and for that Purpose foment the Parts affected with astringent Decoctions. But as this *Prolapsus* or falling down, does not so much proceed from a Relaxation of the Uterus, or Intestinum Rectum, as from a Relaxation of their Ligaments, on Account of the Congestion and Accumulation of the Juices there, so every one must perceive, that this Method is idle and ineffectual, because these external Astringents, cannot penetrate to the Ligaments themselves. Hence in a falling down either in the Uterus itself, or of the Vagina, such Things immediately applied to the Uterus are of no Efficacy. But rather the inguinal Region is to be fomented with balsamic and penetrating Liniments and Plaisters, which being not so much possessed of an earthy Stypticity, as of a spirituous corroborating Quality, restore Vigour, Motion, and Tone to the moist and relaxed Parts. But 'tis here to be observed, that as in all other Cases, so also in these, Topics alone are not sufficient; but that internal Medicines are more universally necessary, in all internal, and even external Disorders of the Body. I do not, however, reject Fumigations and Fomentations of Wine prepared with aromatic Herbs, such as are possessed of a volatile

oleous Salt, and a certain earthy Principle, by which these Parts may be immediately affected, since the Force of Fumigations penetrates intimately, as do also the Effluvia arising from Baths.

With Respect to blind Hæmorrhoids, it is sufficiently known, that great Uneasiness is produced by the Tumours of the hæmorrhordial Region, arising from the too great Afflux and Stagnation of the Blood, or of a viscid Serum. For the Cure of this Disorder, Physicians and Surgeons have invented numberless Medicines, especially Topics: But how much they all fall short of their Intention, is too well known to the miserable Patients; for the Astringents recommended, rather obstruct the Humours which produce the Tumor; on the contrary, emollient and anodyne Substances relax the Parts, and invite a farther Afflux of the Humours, whilst acrid Medicines corrode the Parts, and generally dispose them to malignant Ulcers, and even Fistulas. The Skill therefore of the Physician consists in distinguishing the Use of these according to Circumstances, and knowing what he ought to do; for if the Pain is excessive, anodyne and emollient Substances are beneficial. Hence Linseed Oil alone, applied in a sufficient Quantity, excellently mitigates the Pain. If the Tumor is troublesome by its Bulk, then not so much earthy Styptics, as Corroboratives, are to be used, such as Fomentations of Wine prepared with Mastich, Amber, Rose-flowers, Balaustines, Frankincense and Yarrow. Nor are Fumigations in such Cases to be excluded, especially such as are prepared of Things impregnated with a volatile oleous Salt, the Nature and Virtues of which are to insinuate themselves deeply, to strengthen the Pores, and dissipate the excessive Humidity.

From

From what has been said, I think it is sufficiently obvious, how preposterous a Practice it would be, when the Pain is greatest to use aftringent, cold, or acrid, Subftances; or if, when there is a violent Tumour without Pain, we should apply emollient, anodyne, and relaxing Subftances.

I now come to difcufs this important Queftion, Whether in exceffive Effufions of Blood or Lymph from the Uterus, Injections may be properly ufed, especially fince we find from Experience, that they are with great Advantage prefcribed in exceffive Fluxes of the Semen? But as the Vulgar are of Opinion, that Fluxes ought not to be ftopt by Aftringents, fo nothing is more dangerous, than to attempt the checking of exceffive Difcharges of this Kind by external Injections, poffeffed of an aftringent Quality. I remember a Woman, who when labouring under an exceffive Difcharge of the Menfes, by an Injection of the Decoction of Yarrow impregnated with Alum, contracted an Ulcer, accompanied with a Confumption and hectic Fever, which proved fatal to her. We are, therefore, to deal very cautioufly with Injections, fince they frequently do more Injury than Service.

We now come to confider the Diforders of the Joints; and certainly if Topics are in any Cafes abufed, they are moft fo in arthritic and gouty Pains; for becaufe the Diforder lies in the external Parts, many are of Opinion, that the Remedy is immediately to be applied to the Part affected, that it may the fooner reach the Caufe of the Difeafe. But in this they are greatly miftaken; for Topics are not, in thefe Diforders, fo requifite, but the Pain may be mitigated without them. We learn from Experience that with-

out any Topics, by internal Medicines alone, oppofite to the morbific Caufe, the Violence of thefe Pains may in Procefs of Time, be not only mitigated, but alfo totally removed. But we are above all Things to take Care, that Repellents, efpecially in the Beginning of the Diforder, be not ufed; for thefe difturb the Motion of Nature, which is from the Center to the Circumference, repel the peccant Matter inwards, and excite violent Symptoms In the Beginning of a Gout, I knew the Application of a Plaifter compofed of the White of an Egg and Alum, in a plethoric Man, produce in one Night's time a lethargic Diforder, which deftroyed the Force of his Genius, and Strength of his Memory all his Life after. *Hagendorn in Cent.* 1. *Hift.* 28. gives us memorable Inftance of a Merchant who labouring under a fcorbutic Tumor, had an Epithem prepared of diftilled Waters, Cerufs, and Camphire, applied to it, by which his Pain was alleviated; but he loft his Speech, and the Ufe of his left Arm. With no better Succefs the prefent Practice, of anointing the external Parts with camphorated Spirit of Wine, attended. It is hardly poffible to enumerate the Misfortunes which may be produced by this Remedy, ufed without any refpect to the Patient, and his Circumftances. Thus by the Application of it to gouty Feet, I have frequently obferved Cardialgias, convulfive and epileptic Motions of the Limbs, Palfies, and other terrible Symptoms excited. 'Tis, alfo, certain from Experience, that all Medicines are not beneficial to all Patients, fince fome Topics remove Pain in fome, and increafe it in others; whilft fome are relieved by fpirituous Liniments, others by anodyne Plaifters, and others by Cataplasms prepared of Milk, and the Crumbs of Bread; whilst none of all these Remedies agree with others.

The Cause of these particular Effects, is not sufficiently adverted to, and investigated, since it is sufficiently known to Surgeons, that all Patients cannot equally bear the same thing in external Wounds. But the Cause of this is not so much the peculiar Disposition of the peccant Humours, as the tensive and tonic Constitution of the Fibres, Pores, and Vessels of the Skin; for all the Parts, especially the Emunctories and Strainers, have their peculiar Strength, Tone, Tension and Dilatation, which Species of Motion, so highly necessary to the Secretions and Excretions, principally depend upon the Influx of the animal Spirits, and the Tension of the nervous Membranes. Of what Kind, therefore, this Influx of the animal Spirits, and Tension of the nervous Membranes is, in every Patient, in all Disorders, and their various Stages, ought to be diligently consider'd by Physicians, in the Application of their Topics; for every one sees, that when the Pores are contracted by Pain and spasms, hot and spirituous Medicines are by no Means proper, but rather such Medicines as gently relax the contracted Parts. On the contrary, if there is too great a Relaxation after the Pain, which appears from the Tumor, and the Decrease of the Pain, all moist, unctuous, and anodyne Ointments, are very injurious; in such Cases we are, therefore, rather to use spirituous, nervous Liniments. And tho' Topics sometimes are beneficial in allaying Pain, and mitigating the Fever, yet they do not always produce the same happy Effects in the same Patients. In a Word, the stronger Nature is in expelling, and the greater the Strength of the Body, and of the internal Motion are, the less Danger Topics,

if prudently applied, induce. But if the Vigour of the Motions has ceased, if the Patient is old, or afflicted with a Cachexy, Topics are absolutely to be rejected; for the principal Intention of the Physician is not, by Topics, to hinder the Evaporation of the peccant Matter, but to promote it; and since great Judgment is necessary to this, it is safest to abstain from all Topics, to commit the whole Cure to internal Medicines, and keep the Parts affected in a gentle Heat.

I have also observed, that the Generation of Tophs, which principally happen in a fixed Gout, is for the most Part owing to an incautious Application of Topics, especially those of the stupifying and refrigerating Kind. Thus *Wedelius* in his *Tract. de Medicament. Facultat.* informs us, " That many arthritic Patients have suffer'd much, " have had their wandering converted into fixed Gouts, and ma- " ny Tophs formed, by using unctuous and pinguious Plaisters." To this Purpose, *Galen* in *Method. Medend. Lib.* 4. *Cap.* 3. tells us, that in the Gout, Tophs are produced by a thick and glutinous Humour, which is not gradually digested, but suddenly dried by violent Remedies. And *Fernelius* in *Consil.* 12. observes, that gouty Pains are produced by the same Means. But I am of Opinion that all Topics are not to be discarded in external Pains of the Joints; for when the Pain is inveterate, and accompanied with a certain Torpor, and Insensibility, which frequently happens in old Age, then after checking the internal Ebullition of the Blood, we are, by nervous and balsamic Liniments, to corroborate the Nerves, and invite the Influx of the nervous Fluid into the weakened Parts. We must not forget the common Practice of applying live Earth-worms to the Parts affect-

ed,

ed, in a wandering fcorbutic Gout.
Great Encomiums are beftowed on
this Remedy by practical Phyficians,
efpecially by *Wierus*. And it is certain, than on Account of the volatile, abfterfive, and nitro-fulphureous
Salts thefe Animals contain, they are
of an excellent difcutient and fedative Virtue, which manifefts itfelf not
only internally, but alfo externally,
in various Kinds of Pains, and even
in the venereal Difeafe itfelf. Yet
great Caution is requifite in the Application of thefe Animals; for tho'
in the moft cruel Pain, when the
Fluids are in Motion, and theStrength
entire, and the Patient young, thefe
Subftances produce happy Effects, yet
they produce quite contrary Symptoms in a fixed inveterate Gout.

We fhall fubjoin fomething more,
with refpect to an Eryfipelas, for
the Cure of which, moft Surgeons and Phyficians have immediate Recourfe to Topics, tho' the
Errors arifing from this Practice
have been often expofed. But I
would have it obferved as a general
Maxim, that an Eryfipelas, arifing
from an external, ought to be diftinguifh'd from that arifing from an
internal Caufe. In the former produced by Contufions, and other
Wounds, Topics are not generally
prejudicial. But when the Diforder
proceeds from an Orgafm of the Humours, and a febrile Impetus, an
heterogeneous Matter, generally of
an acrid and corrofive Nature, is
protruded to the Surface of the Body; in which Cafe we muft be very
cautious, fince the Matter is eafily
repelled; and fince by thofe Topics,
which, in other Cafes prove beneficial, we may do an irreparable Injury to the Patient, by repelling into
the internal Parts the peccant Matter,
which then acquires the Nature of a
Poifon. Nothing is more common
than by Aftringents, fuch as the
White of an Egg mixed with A-

lum, to render a flightEryfipelas fixed
and profound, and to excite malignant Ulcers, Inftances of which daily
occur in Practice. Hence thofe Phyficians act prudently, who treat all
the Species of Eryfipelas with Inter-
nals, apply only externally Bags full
of paregoric Herbs, which by their
mild Influence, keep the Pores open,
relax fuch as are conftricted, and
cherifh the Parts.

We muft, alfo, obferve, that Surgeons commit a terrible Error in applying hot Cataplafms, prepared of
Bean-meal, Liquorice-root, emollient and difcutient Herbs, and certain Waters, to an Eryfipelas; for
fince by the Heat the Moifture is dried up, and the Matter is more firmly
impacted in the Skin and Pores, fo
that it can hardly be removed by a
Knife, the Bufinefs of Tranfpiration
is greatly injured, and the Eryfipelas,
which by proper Meafures might
have been difcuffed, is by thefe converted into an Abfcefs or an Ulcer.
We are, therefore, to endeavour to
preferve a free Refpiration of the
Parts affected, which can never be
obtain'd under a cold State of the Air,
an intenfe Heat, or a great Load of
Cloaths, but under a moderate Heat,
which excellently encourages Perfpiration.

In like Manner, Topics ought to
be cautioufly applied to Buboes; becaufe by Repellents they are render'd
malignant. Much lefs are we to apply Topics of an aftringent and refrigerating Kind to malignant and
critical Buboes; becaufe, fuch a
Practice is highly dangerous. Critical Buboes, when the Humours are
convey'd to the Glands, are known
by the Patients retaining hisStrength,
by their happening on the critical
Days, and by the previous Signs of
Concoction in the Urine. At this
Time all Repellents are highly prejudicial; for as *Hippocrates* juftly obferves, in a perfect *Crifis*, no Change

of the Patient's State is to be attempted; but the whole Bufiness is to be left to Nature. Sometimes a Bubo arifes from a Redundance of Blood, in which Cafe, according to *Avicenna*, *Oribafius* and others, we are by no Means to ufe Repellents. But when a Bubo tends to Suppuration, nothing is more beneficial than the Application of the Diachylon Plaifter with the Gums, mixed with Opoponax.

'Tis juftly to be doubted, whether Topics are proper in the Small Pox. We can affirm in general, that as this Diforder is a critical Evacuation, great Caution is requifite. However if before the Eruption the Patient is afflicted with a Delirium, we may with Advantage apply to the Forehead, Spirit of Rofes mixed with Camphire. But during the Eruption and Suppuration, I am of Opinion, that we ought to abftain from all Liniments. In the Decline, and at the Time of the Exficcation of the Difeafe, when the Force of the Diforder is fubdued, I cannot difapprove of Oil of Sweet Almonds, mixed with Camphire and Sperma Ceti, in order to prevent the Defedation of the Skin, and correct the Acrimony which generally lies pretty deep. For this Reafon we are cautioufly to proceed with Topics of this Kind, fuch as Spirit of Wine impregnated with Myrrh, and Sugar of Lead mixed with Rofe Water.

The Itch, which is a puftulous Erulceration of the Skin, more or lefs moift, is generally thought incurable without the Ufe of Topics. Hence neglecting all internal Remedies, they forthwith have Recourfe to various fulphureous and mercurial Liniments, which they apply either to the whole Surface of the Body, or only to the Joints, tho' frequently with very confiderable Danger both to Life and Health; for it is never fafe by Topics to cure external Diforders proceeding from an internal Caufe; but as Nature expels the he-

terogenous and morbid Matter, the Phyfician ought to do the fame, and never counteract the Intentions of Nature, which is generally done by Repellents externally applied. Hence I am of Opinion, that the Cure of thefe cutaneous Diforders, ought not only to be begun, but alfo finifhed by fuch internal Medicines, as correct and difpofe the peccant Matter to Excretion, and at the fame Time eliminate it. To this Clafs of Medicines belong not only Diaphoretics, emollient and laxative Infufions, but alfo if the Itch is inveterate and malignant, Preparations of Mercury and Antimony. Then, for the better Confolidation of the Skin, and the Reftitution of its Beauty, we may ufe Baths, and drying, fulphureous, and faturnine Ointments. But we are always to abftain from external mercurial Liniments, which can never be ufed without Danger, as is obvious from numberlefs practical Obfervations.

As for mercurial Ointments and Fumigations ufed to excite a Salivation in the venereal Difeafe, it is fufficiently known what violent Symptoms are brought on by thefe Means, and how precarious this Method of curing fo obftinate a Diforder is. I am certain from Experience, that the venereal Difeafe, may be happily removed by proper Preparations of Mercury and Antimony, and Decoctions of the Woods, exhibited internally in a due Manner, without any external mercurial Applications, and often without exciting a Salivation, or any Train of uneafy Symptoms.

With refpect to Topics applied to paralytic Parts, tho' thefe excellently affift the Operation of internal Remedies, yet they ought to be properly chofen, and cautioufly applied. Thofe are, in my Opinion, greatly miftaken, who think that Fats, Lards, and unctuous Liniments ought to be applied, either immediately to the

Parts affected, or to the Spine of the Back; for these Substances obstruct the Pores, and still more relax the Fibres, whose Tone is already destroyed; by which Means they dispose the Parts to a Tumor. On the contrary, spirituous, hot, and etherial Oils alone, do not produce the desired Effect, since most of them, in Consequence of the Subtility of their Parts, fly off in the Air, and leave the nervous and muscular Fibres too rigid. This Intention is better answered by Ointments prepared of the Fats of Animals, and the distilled Oils, such as those of Rue, Marjoram, Lavender, Juniper, Cloves and Rosemary. For the Tone of the nervous Parts ought to be render'd natural; so that there be neither too great a Relaxation, nor Constriction; too great an Humidity nor Dryness. Besides, 'tis to be observed, that in a Palsy arising from a Disorder of the Spinal Marrow, and Origin of the Nerves, these Medicines are not to be applied to the Parts destitute of Sensation, and Motion; but to the Source of the Disorder, which is lodged in the Spinal Marrow. But it is quite otherwise in that Species of Palsy in which the Motion, but not the Sensation, of the Part is destroyed, which happens frequently to Miners, in which Case 'tis of no Use to anoint the Spinal Marrow, but the Part affected is to be frequently fomented with the abovementioned Medicines.

With respect to oedamatous Tumors, which frequently seize the Feet, great Caution is, also, requisite as to the Application of Topics, since they who treat them with Baths, commit a terrible Error. Thus I have seen cachectic Persons, by immersing their Feet in warm Water, contract, in one Night's Time, a considerable Tumor of them, which could not after-

wards be easily removed. The Reason of this is obvious; for these Baths by their Moisture, which by Means of the Heat insinuates itself into the Pores, render the weaken'd Fibres still more lax; so that the Humours flow down, and are not quickly receiv'd again into the Veins and lymphatic Vessels. The same Effects are, also, produced by those who attempt to dissipate such Tumors by Ointments and Plaisters, for a Reason easily deduced from what has been said. Some have a Custom of tying discutient Herbs about the Feet, such as the greater Celandine, Fumitory, Wormwood, and Rue; but if these are moist and cold, they often increase the Tumor, instead of removing it. 'Tis, therefore, better to abstain from all these, and apply proper Bandages to the Feet, especially towards the Evening, when such Tumors are always observ'd to increase, that by this Means the Fibres may be corroborated and strengthened. Fomentations of strong Vinegar, mixed with Essence of Amber, and pour'd upon ignited Bricks, have often been found productive of happy Effects.

'Tis customary in various Disorders, to apply Epithems and Plaisters to the Pulse in the Wrists. This Practice, tho' not to be discouraged in itself, is nevertheless often abused, especially by Nurses, and the common People, who, whether a Disorder is of the cold or hot Kind, commonly have recourse to the celebrated *Aqua Carbunculi*, which they think of incredible Efficacy to restore Strength. But every one must perceive, that this is by no Means proper in a burning or acute Fever, or in the Heat of an intermittent Fever, in which Cases, rather penetrating Acids, such as Lemon-juice, and Vinegar of Roses are proper. Epithems and Plaisters are, also, applied to the Wrists, in order to remove the

febrile

febrile Paroxyfms in Intermittents; for which Purpofe they mix A-lum, Vinegar, Rue, the greater Houfeleek, and Spiders webbs. They, alfo make a Plaifter of Tur-pentine, Alum, and Powder of Spi-ders, which are often of great Ser-vice in mitigating the Paroxyfms, and even in totally removing them, f the greater Part of the febrile Mat-er is evacuated.

The Manner in which thefe Medi-cines operate, is fomewhat difficult to be conceiv'd; and fuch an Experi-ment, in my Opinion, illuftrates the Generation of Fevers of this Kind; for the Heart and Arteries, which have their proper Nerves and fyftal-tic and diaftaltic Motions, are the Inftruments, by which the intenfe Motion of the Fluids is performed. Hence fuch Things, as in fome Mea-fure check and hinder the exceffive Motion of the Spirits to thefe Parts, when immediately applied to the Ar-teries, muft neceffarily for fome Time, ftop the febrile and intenfely hot Motion of the Blood.

The End of Second B O O K.

THE NEW
Englifh Difpenfatory.

BOOK III.
Of the Simples *us'd in* MEDICINE.

CHAP. I.
Of VEGETABLES.

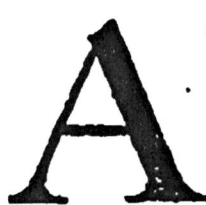*BIES*, the *Fir-Tree*. There are three Kinds of this commonly us'd in Medicine. The Firft of thefe is the *abies offic, a-bies conis furfum fpeEtantibus, C. B. Pin. Abies taxi Folio, fruEtu furfum SpeEtant. Boerb. Ind. Alt. Plant.* commonly call'd the *Silver-Fir*. The Tops of this Species boil'd in Ale or Water, and mix'd with Wine, are faid to afford a Drink, in rheumatic, arthritic, and fcorbutic Cafes, not inferior to Decoctions of the exotic Woods; efpecially if three or four Ounces of it are drank for a Month's Time, before Meals, with proper Exercife; for by exciting a Sweat, it frees the Blood from heterogeneous Particles; but if there is a Plethora, this muft be diminifh'd, before its Exhibition;

becaufe by. its balfamic Quality, it excites fome Commotion in the Blood. 'Tis faid that a confiderable Quantity of the Leaves and Tops of this Species of Fir, enters the Compofition of *Brunfwick* Mum, and that a Decoction of the Wood, or Sawduft, is much us'd by the Inhabitants of fome northern Countries for the *Fluor Albus*, and all Diforders of the urinary Paffages. The *Strawfburg* Turpentine is the Product of this Fir, and is call'd its liquid Refin, in Contradiftinction to its dry Refin, which refembles Frankincenfe.

The fecond Species of Fir ufed in Medicine is the *Abies tenuiori folio, fruEtu deorfum inflcxo, Abies mas Theophrafti. Picea Latinorum,* and *Abies tenuiore Folio, FruEtu deorfum fp.Etante, Boerhaave Ind. Alt. Plant* or the common Fir which produces white Refin, Tar, common Pitch, and

and *Burgundy* Pitch. This agrees, pretty much in Virtue with the former; and 'tis reported that the *Laplanders* prevent the Scurvy, by procuring a copious Discharge of Saliva, by chewing its Resin; as also that they remove the Uneasiness produced by intemperate drinking, by twisting the tender Twigs of this Tree round their Heads.

The third Species is the *Abies Canadensis, Abies Minor pectinatis Foliis, Virginiana, Conis parvis Subrotundis* Pluck Phytog. or *Canada* Fir Tree, which yeilds a valuable Resin call'd the Balsam of *Canada*, which is used in cleansing and deterging internal Abscesses, previously mixing it in the Quantity of two or three Drams, with Broth prepared with Flesh, Oil of Sweet Almonds, or the Yolk of an Egg.

Abrotanum, Southernwood, of this Authors have mentioned several Kinds but the most considerable are the *Abrotanum mas Officinarum, Abrotanum mas Angustifolium majus, C. B.* and *Boerh. Ind. Alt. Plant.* Male Southernwood. This Plant is so very common, and so well known, that it does not require a Description. It is justly extolled on Account of its heating, stimulating, inciding, subastringent, and discutient Qualities; for which Reason it is esteemd among the uterine, emmenagogue, diuretic, sudorific, anthelminthic, and anti-septic Medicines. *Galen* says, it diminishes the Fit of an intermittent, if the Patient is rubbed with it before its Invasion. It is used in aqueous and vinous Infusions, but it may also be exhibited in Decoctions against Worms, since in such Cases highly bitter Medicines are required. Externally it is used for uterine Baths, and Fumigations. The distilled Water of the Plant is, also, possessed of the above-mentioned Virtues, and the Oil procured from it by boiling is used externally

for Pains of the Abdomen and Intestines, as also against Worms. Hence we may understand, in what Sense this Plant is said to be good against the Bites of Serpents and other Poisons. As also why it is said to prove a Stimulus to Venery. The dried Leaves are prescribed in the *Fotus Communis* of the last College Dispensatory.

The other *Abrotanum* referred to by the College is, the *Abrotanum Fœmina foliis teretibus.* C. B. *Santolina Foliis teretibus Tourn. Abrotanum Fœmina Vulgaris.* Lavender Cotton. Park. The Leaves and Flowers boiled in Milk, and taken fasting are esteemed good against Worms. It is, also, commended against Poison, and the Wounds of venemous Animals; against Obstructions of the Liver, and Jaundice; and has the Reputation of promoting the menstrual Discharge, taken by Way of Infusion in Wine. It is, father, esteemed diaphoretic, and good against the Colic.

There is another *Abrotanum* mentioned as used in Medicine. This is the *Abrotanum Campestre, Boerh. Ind. A. Artemisia tenuifolia Offic.* Fine leaved Mugwort. This is sometimes substituted for the *Abrotanum mas,* and is said to mitigate Pains in the Stomach, and nervous Parts. There are many other Species, but these are the principal in Use.

Abrus Offic. Veslin *Phaseolus ruber Abrus Vocatus* Alp. Ægypt, *Phaseolus indicus ruber Bontio* Raii. Hist. This is imported from both the *Indies,* and the Seeds, of which there are two Kinds in the Shops both red are recommended for curing Inflammations of the Eyes, drying up Rheums, strengthening the optic Nerves, refreshing the Spirits, discussing cloudy Vapours of the Brain, and clearing the Sight.

Absin-

Absinthium. Wormwood, of this there are various Kinds, but the most considerable are the *Absinthium Vulgare. Offic.* Park. *Absinthium vulgare Majus. J. B.* Wormwood is accounted a Plant of great Efficacy in Medicine. Thus in *Ephemer. Nat. Curios. Decad. 1. An. 2. Obs. 2. Bartholine* informs us, that with great Success he used Sea-water, in which Woormwood had been boiled, for the Cure of a Gangrene. This Plant is possessed of oleous Principles, mixed with a large Quantity of Earth, and a small Portion of Phlegm; for which Reason, it is beneficial in all cold Disorders, such as proceed from Phlegm, Viscidity, or an Acid. It is, also, serviceable in Intentions where drying is requisite, or where the Bile is defective. It is accounted excellent for promoting an Appetite, and procuring Digestion. It is of singular Service, both as a Preservative and Curative, in Obstructions and Infarctions of the Viscera, as also against Putrefaction, for which Reason it is proper in intermittent Fevers, against Worms of the Intestines, Cachexies, oedematous Tumors, and Obstructions of the Liver; but it is highly prejudicial in Cases where Inflammations are either present or suspected. Its recent express'd Juice drank in large Quantities, by irritating the Vessels, dissipating the Water, and attenuating the viscid Humours, is of Service in Dropsies and Leucophlegmatias, arising from Langour and Cold, that is, from a Redundance of Water or Phlegm; but this Juice is no less injurious in that Species of Dropsy, which arises from a Dryness of the Liver or Spleen; since it augments the Force of the Circulation, Dryness, and Acrimony. This Plant is the princpal Ingredient in the celebrated Wine called *Vinum Absinthites,* so much extolled in the Time of the Plague. But that Wormwood used to Excess is hurtful to the Eyes, is sufficiently obvious from those who daily use Wines and Oils prepared with it. This Plant bruised with Vinegar, Wine and Salt, and applied externally, proves highly discutient; and it is often applied alone to the Soles of the Feet, in order to prevent the Formation of Tumors in them. *Ray* informs us, that green Wormwood worn in the Shoes, corrects a cold Intemperature of the Stomach. Hence we see the Reason, why Wormwood is called stomachic, anti-febrile, anti-hysteric, anthelminthic, narcotic, and good against the Colic. The Smoke of the kindled Flowers or Tops of Wormwood, generally allays the Tooth-ach, as we are informed by *Grube* in *Tr. de Simpl.* The Seeds of this Plant are said to be good against a Dysentery; and the Taste of its Root is first perceived on the Point of the Tongue, then at its Root, then in the Fauces and Gullet, so that at last it seems to warm the Stomach itself, tho' none of the Juice is swallowed. Nor is this Root ungrateful or prejudicial to the Health, as the Leaves are. Hence *Grevinus* infers, that it is justly to be reckoned among the most valuable Stomachics, which Mr. *Ray* found it to be from Experience. Wormwood affords a large Quantity of fixed Salt, of the same Virtues with other lixiviate Salts of the same Kind. Of this a lixivial Salt is directed to be made by the College; and an essential Oil is prepared from the Leaves.

The other Species of Wormwood taken Notice of in the College Catalogue is, the *Absinthium marinum Album Ger. Absinthium Seriphium Belgicum* C. B. This has been long used in the *London* Shops instead of the true *Roman* Wormwood, tho' *Dioscorides* and *Galen* affirms, that it is prejudicial to the Stomach. I dont know why the College have, in their Catalogue so far complied with Custom, as to substitute this in the Room of Roman Wormwood, when it is univer-sally agreed that the latter is much the better Medicine. The former, however, is more palatable. The College directs a Conserve of this; and it is an Ingredient in the *Aqua Alexiteria Simplex* in the *Aqua Alexiteria composita*, both with and without Vinegar; in the *Fotus Communis*, and *Oleum Viride*. This Species is gene-rally two or three Feet high, with many winged Leaves, lesser and finer than the common Wormwood. Its Flowers are small and naked as those of the other Kinds, and appear at the same Time. The Scent of the Plant greatly resembles that of Southern-wood, and its Taste is not very bitter, but somewhat saltish. It grows in great Plenty in most of our salt Marshes, and is generally sold in the Shops for the *Roman* true Wormwood.

There is also another Species of Wormwood distinguished by the Names *Absinthium Romanum* Offic. and *Absinthium Ponticum tenuifolium nicanum* C. B. Boerh Ind. Alt. Ro-man Wormwood. This Species is much smaller than the com-mon Wormwood, and has finer Leaves tho' of a lesser Size. Its Flowers grow in large Quantities on the Tops of the Branches, and appear in *July*. This Plant is with us cultivated in Gardens, and has neither so strong a Smell, nor so bitter a Taste as the common Worm-wood. *Matthiolus* informs us, that the most violent Dropsies, are cur-ed by a Conserve prepared of its Leaves. In the *Edinburgh* Dispensa-tory, the Conserve of Wormwood is directed to be made with this Spe-cies.

There is also a Species of Worm-wood called *Absinthium alpinum candidum humile* C. B. Tourn. Inst. Mountain Wormwood. This grows in the Mountains of *Savoy*, and a-grees in Virtues with the preceed-ing.

Abutilon. Offic. Boerh. J. A. *Althæa lutea.* Ger. Yellow Mallow. This Plant is cultivated in Gardens, and flowers in *July*. It is esteemed aperient, and vulnerary. The Leaves applied externally are said to cleanse Ulcers; and the Seeds to provoke Urine, and expel the Gravel.

Acacia. The Species of this men-tioned by the Compilers of the last *London* Dispensatory is the inspissa-ted Juice of the immature Fruit of the *Acacia Foliis Scorpioidis Leguminosa* C. B. which is also said to produce Gum Arabic. It is called *Acacia* Offic. Alpini, and *Acacia vera*, Raii Hist. Tourn. Inst. and Boerh. Ind. Alt. *The Egyptian Thorn.* It is used for strengthening the Eyes, and preventing Inflammations there-in, for curing Ulcers of the Mouth, and Fissures of the Lips, for fastening the Teeth, and strengthening weak Joints, as also for stopping Hæmorrhages and Fluxes. It is brought into *Europe* in Blad-ders containing globular Masses weigh-ing between four and eight Ounces. The best, which is that expressed from the green Pods and inspissated, is externally of a blackish, but inter-nally of a shining brown Colour, hard, brittle, and of an austere Taste. It is exhibited when the Humours are to be inspissated, and the solid Parts corroborated. It is given internally in the Form of Pills, Bo-luses, or Solutions in some proper Liquor. Externally it is used, dif-solved in Fomentations, and may prove beneficial in Disorders of the Eyes, where there is only such a slight Inflammation, as does not con-traindicate the Use of Astringents, and Repellents. Tho' *Alpinus* thinks the external Application of it bene-ficial in the Gout, yet his Opinion will never be admitted by those who know

know the prejudicial Nature of Repellents in such Cases; tho' it may be used internally for corroborating a lax and flaccid Constitution, and by that Means correcting the remote Causes of a Gout. The Dose, according to *Boerhaave*, is from four Grains to a Dram.

There is also another *Acacia*, called *Acacia Germanica* or *German Acacia*, which is no more than the expressed Juice of unripe wild Sloes, inspissated in a Bath-heat. It is black like the common Juice of Liquorice, is esteemed an Astringent, and used as such. The Dose, according to *Boerhaave*, is from six Grains to a Dram and a half.

There are some other Plants which are called by this Name as the *Acacia Indica Farnesiana*. Raii. Hist.

The Gum Arabic is said to flow from this Tree, as well as from the true *Acacia*.

The *Acacia filiquis Compressis*. Ind. Med. *Gumm. Seneca*. Offic.

The Gum called *Senegal* resembles Gum Arabic, but is imported to us in Lumps, which are rough externally, but clear and transparent within. It is sometimes whitish, and sometimes of a red Colour, of an insipid aqueous Taste, viscid and without any Smell. It is brought from *Guinea*, and as some think receives its Name from the River *Senega*. The *London* Apothecaries use the whitest and purest Parts of this Gum instead of Gum-arabic.

Acanthus, or *Branca Ursina*, Offic. *Acanthus Sativus*, or *Mollis Virgilii* C. B. This Plant grows spontaneously in *Italy*, *Spain*, and the Southern Parts of *France*, but is with us cultivated in Gardens, and Flowers in *July* and *August*. It is rarely used except in Clysters, and Baths intended to remove Obstructions, and alleviate Pains arising from the Stone and Gravel. It is said to be diuretic and to stop Diarrhœas. *Boerhaave* says, that it is possessed of an emollient and aperient Virtue, and that it is of a very soft Nature, somewhat saponacious, like the Mallow, and entirely insipid. Its glutinous and demulcent Juice is an Ingredient in emollient Clysters, and Cataplasms. It is excellent for Combustions. The Root is accounted good for Persons who spit Blood after a Bruise.

Acetosa, Sorrel. This is the *Acetosa Vulgaris*, *Oxalis* Offic. *Acetosa Pratensis* C. B. Common Sorrel is a Plant, which has many Virtues ascribed to it in Medicine; for it is of an aperient, moderately refrigerating, and corroborating Nature. Its Leaves and Roots boiled in recent Whey, prove an excellent Remedy in chronical Diseases, where there is a Tendency to Putrefaction. A Decoction of Sorrel with Whey, drank in the Morning in the Month of *April*, excellently purges the Body from the Feces collected during the Winter. But the principal Virtue of this Plant consists in its anti-scorbutic Quality; since if it is used recent, it carries off the Putrefaction of the Gums, and fixes the loose Teeth. Thus in *Hist. Acad. Royale des Sciences*, we are told, that a great many scorbutic Patients were cur'd by boil'd Sorrel and Eggs. All Patients whose Blood is too fluid, and who on that Account are disposed to a Phthisis, or Spitting of Blood, are cured by the frequent Use of the Juice of this Plant. Hence *Boerhaave* justly commends Sorrel, for Patients of hot, lax, putrid, and bilious Constitutions. Externally, the Leaves roasted under the Ashes, are of great Service for suppurating Tumors. The Leaves, also, when reduced to a Poultice with fresh Butter, prove beneficial to sordid Ulcers. The native or essential Salt of Sorrel, in Taste resembling that of Cream of Tartar, is stimulating, purgative, astringent tingent, corroborating, and proper in all Fevers of the burning, continual, and putrid Kind.

Another Species of Sorrel is the *Acetosa Arvensis* Offic. *Acetosa Arvensis lanceolata.* Boerh. Ind. A. Sheeps Sorrel. This Sorrel is much less than the former, grows in dry barren Grounds, and is possessed of much the same Virtues as the common Sorrel. It flowers in *May*.

Another Species of Sorrel is the *Acetosa Romana Rotundifolia* Offic. French Sorrel. In Virtues it agrees with the common Sorrel.

Acetosella, Wood Sorrel. This is mentioned in the College Catalogue by the Name of *Lujula,* or *Oxys Alba. Ger.* and is called *Oxys Flore Albo* by *Boerb. Ind. A.* The Juice of this Plant, according to *Boerhaave,* is somewhat oleous, acid, and nitrous, for which Reason it is beneficial in all hot, putrid, and pestilential Disorders. The Herb itself boiled in Water is excellent in Inflammations, Pleurisies and other Disorders of an acute Nature. It, also, corrects hot Humours and Bile; and prevents Putrefaction, so that it is proper for Nauseas and Want of Digestion, arising from putrified Bile, or any alcalescent Humour lodged in the Stomach. It is also accounted an excellent Remedy in a Diarrhea, and Dysentery. A very good Conserve is order'd to be made of this Plant. But neither the Conserve nor the Plant are used so much as they deserve. Entire Volumes have been wrote on the Virtues of this Plant.

Acetum. Vinegar is no less universally than justly celebrated, on Account of its resolvent, anti-septic and refrigerating Qualities, for which Reason it is class'd among the Medicines of the alexipharmic and antipestilential Kind. The resolvent Nature of this Liquor is, according to *Boerhaave* in his Chymistry, sufficiently evinc'd from its colliquating the Cartilages, Bones, and Skins of Animals, which have been long boil'd in it. Besides in *Ephemer. Nat. Curios. Decad.* 1. *An.* 2. we are told, that some Children have been born without the *Epidermis,* because their Mothers, during the Time of Gestation, us'd acid Aliments, and Vinegar instead of common Drink. In the Time of pestilential Disorders, Vinegar is of all others the best Preservative for Physicians, before they visit the Infected; for which Purpose they generally drink a small Quantity of it, and apply a Spunge dipt in it, to their Mouth and Nostrils, in order to correct the bad Quality of the Air. Vinegar diluted with Water, and mix'd with Honey and Rue, is said to be an infallible Antidote against various Kinds of Poisons. Thus the celebrated *Hoffman* in *Med. Rat. Tom.* 2. tells us, " That Vinegar " and the Theriaca, by discussing " and exciting a Sweat, afford speedy " and effectual Relief against all Poi- " sons, except those of the corrosive " Kind." In all Cases where the alcalescent Acrimony of the Humours is to be corrected, or a Coagulation of the Blood to be either remov'd or prevented, Vinegar exhibited internally is of all others the most efficacious Medicine; for which Reason it is justly recommended in Fevers arising from the Stimulus of an acrid Bile, an alcalescent Salt, or a Putrefaction of the Juices. Vinegar diluted with Water, extinguishes the most violent Thirst, after other Liquors have in vain been us'd for that Purpose. Hence 'tis obvious, that it must be serviceable in acute ardent Fevers, the Small Pox, the Measles, a Scurvy arising from an alcalescent State of the Humours, hypocondriac, convulsive, and hysteric Disorders. *Hippocrates* and *Galen,* greatly extol'd Vinegar in all

Dis

Diforders of the Spleen. This Liquor, alfo, excites a gentle Stimulus in the Solids, expels Sweat, procures a Difcharge of Urine, and ftrengthens the Nerves in Perfons afflicted with Weaknefs, Languors, lethargic Diforders, and Syncopes. In *Eph. Nat. Curiof. Decad. 3. An. 1.* we are told, that it is cuftomary for young Women who are too fat, to drink it in order to render themfelves lean. But Doctor *Slare* affures us, that thofe who ufe it for this Purpofe, generally die of Confumptions. Vinegar warm'd and drawn up the Noftrils, effectually ftops exceffive Sneezing. When us'd with the Aliments, it not only creates an Appetite, but alfo promotes Digeftion. Vinegar boil'd with Wormwood, the Flowers of Elder, or Chamomile, and others of a like Nature, is by Surgeons found highly efficacious for curing an Eryfipelas, Phlegmons, and putrid Ulcers; for foftening and difcuffing glandulous Tumors; for difcuffing Suffufions, the Effects of Contufions, and Tumors of the Feet. For the above Diforders a Spoonful of Vinegar is exhibited internally, whilft a proper Quantity of it is us'd externally in Epithems, Fomentations, Baths, Clyfters, and Gargarifms. Great Caution is to be us'd in the Choice of Vinegar for internal Ufe, fince *Stahl* affirms, that diftill'd Vinegar, by its penetrating Quality, conftricts the nervous Parts. *Hippocrates* in *Tr. de Victus Ratione in acutis,* obferves, that Vinegar is more proper for Men than for Women; fince in the latter it creates Pains of the Uterus. It is hardly poffible to explain the Manner in which Vinegar exerts its Efficacy againft thofe Diforders which have their Seat in the Blood: Firft, becaufe a Drop of Vinegar convey'd into the Vein of a live Animal, immediately proves mortal to it. Secondly, becaufe the Mouths of the lacteal Veffels fo contract themfelve as to prevent the Ingrefs of all acri Subftances; and Thirdly, becaufe th Particles of Vinegar were never b *Leuwenhoek* obferved in the huma Blood. But notwithftanding thef perplexing Circumftances, it is fuf ficient for us to know from Expe rience, that Vinegar produces th Effects above afcribed to it. Vinega is directed by the College to b ufed in the *Emplaftrum Veficatoriun* he *Unguentum Tripharmacum,* an the *Linimentum Tripharmacum.*

Acinos Offic. *Acinos multis,* Boerh Ind. A. Wild-bafil. It flowers i *June.* The Herb is ufed to chec immoderate Difcharges of the Men fes, and a Diarrhæa. And the De coction of this Plant is recommend ed as a good Application for Both and an Eryfipelas.

Acmella Offic. *Akmella Abamella* Herm. Mus. Zeyl. This grow plentifully in the Ifland of *Ceyla* and is brought thence into *Europ* *Breynæus* informs us, that the Plan is diuretic, cures nephritic Pains expells the Stone from the Kidney relieves Ifchuries, Stranguries an Dyfuries, and reftores the Menf when fuppreffed. The Leaves ar accounted moft efficacious, fince b their fine and volatile Parts, the provoke Urine and Sweat, open Ob ftructions, ftimulate to Excretion expel Stones from the urinary Paf fages, and if not very hard diffolv them. For thefe Purpofes they ar ufed by Way of Tea in pretty larg Quantities, exhibiting at the fam Time fome other Liquor of an emol lient and relaxing Quality.

Aconitum. Of this there are man Species, as the *Aconitum cæruleun feu Napellus primus.* Boerh. Ind. A *Napellus* Offic. Monks-Hood. Th *Aconitum Ponticum* Offic. *Aconitun Lycoctonum luteum.* Boerh. Ind. A. Wolfsbane. Thefe are both efteem ed poifonous to Man and Beaft.

Aco

rus Verus, or Calamus Aroma-
Offic. C. B. Boerh. Ind. Alt.
. Sweet Flag. This is by some
md a Plant of singular Virtues;
is we are informed by *Clusius*
Inhabitants of *Lithuania*, to-
Muscovy, carry the Root of
Plant about with them, and
: no Water till they have ma-
id some Portion of the Root
; and *Simon Pauli* is of Opi-
that in Camps and Armies,
teries, epidemic Fevers, and
Plagues, might be in a great
are prevented by the same
*. It is certain from Experi-
that the aromatic, stimulating,
aciding Qualities of this Root,
ghly beneficial in Disorders of
tomach, arising from a cold
Cause; in Cachexies of young
en; in Obstructions of the
s; in hysteric Disorders, and
ses in which heating Medicines
roper. The Steam of Water
ich this Root has been boiled,
d into the Mouth thro' a Fun-
reatly relieves some Kinds of
s. It grows in many Parts of
d in Rivulets, and marshy Pla-
d a great deal of it is imported
broad. It produces Catkins
y and *August*. This is not
it to be the same as the Acorus
Antients. It is an Ingredient
Mithridate, and *Venice* Trea-

ther *Acorus* used in Medicine,
: *Acorus Adulterinus*; *Pseudo-
-Gladiolus luteus*. Offic. *Acorus
rius C. B. P. Acorus nostras
rus* Ger. Bastard Acorus. The
of this is astringent, drying
seful in all Sorts of Fluxes;
said to be a Strengthener of
ain and Nerves.
: third is the *Acorus Asiaticus
Acorus verus, sive Calamus A-
rus Asiaticus, radice tenuiore,*
. Ind. A. Asiatic sweet Flag.
ws both in the East and West

Indies, and agrees in Virtues with
the true *Acorus.*

Adarces. This is procured in *Ga-
latia*, and is the Concretion of a
saltish Humour bred in moist and
marshy Places by Means of an excessive Drought. Its Substance is
lax and porous like that of the bastard Spunge, so that it may properly enough be called the bastard
Spunge of the Marshes. *Dioscorides*
informs us, that it is used as a Topic
for cleansing the Skin, in Leprosies,
Sun-burning, Tetters, and Freckles
because it is of an acrimonious Quality.

There is also an *Adarces* called
Adarces Offic. Boet. Matthiol. and
Adarce J. B. It is not known
whether this is the *Adarces* of *Dioscorides*. This Species of Incrus-
tation has been observed by many
of the Virtuosi, particularly by Doctor *Lister*, in some Conduits at *Paris*; whence he conceives a bad Opinion of it, concluding that whatever lines the Cavities of Aqueducts
with a strong Crust, would probably produce the same Effect in the
Kidneys and Bladder, especially if
these Parts are previously infirm and
tender.

Adianthum. There are several
Plants called by this Name, the first
of which is the *Adianthum vulgare,
Capillus Veneris* Offic. *Adianthum Capillus Veneris* Raii. *Capillus Veneris
verus* Ger. This is the true Maidenhair; and bears Leaves resembling
those of Coriander, set alternately on
the Stalks. It is said to grow plentifully in *Cornwall*; but what is used here,
is brought from the South of *France*,
especialy *Montpelier*. It is known
that most capillary Plants abound
with a neutral saponaceous Salt,
which approaches to the Nature of
Nitre; hence we may conceive that
this Maidenhair may be possessed
of great Virtues in all Disorders
where Obstructions are either the
Cause

Cause, or the Effect. But then it must be taken in very large Quantities, and those frequently repeated, and for a long Time. The best Way of administring it is in strong Decoctions, or Infusions. The common Method of giving it by Way of Syrup, must be very trifling, because the Quantity in a Dose must be too small to produce any considerable Effect. Few Plants have had greater Encomiums bestowed on them than this. The Leaves are said to purify the Blood by reducing the Fluids mixed with it to a just Temperature. The Plant prepares and evacuates Phlegm, as also the common Bile, and what the Antients called *Atra Bilis*. It dissipates Superfluities, resolves serous Humours, and carries them off by Transpiration. It is also diuretic, suporific, and anti-septic, for which Reason it is properly exhibited in all Kinds of Fevers. It is a sovereign Remedy for all Disorders of the Hair, since it prevents its falling off, preserves it from Scurf or Filth, and is an Antidote against Baldness. It is also said to rouse the Functions of the Brain, by removing the Excess, and correcting the peccant Quality of the Humours conveyed to it. It purifies the animal Spirits, restrains hot and bilious Vapours, and renders those mild, which have a Tendency to become acid, acrid, or narcotic. For these Reasons it is accounted an excellent Medicine, for Persons afflicted with Want of Rest, comatous Disorders, Epilepsies, Phrensies, Madness, Melancholy, Cephalalgia, and all other Disorders of the Head. It is also said to brighten the Sight, and dissipate habitual Defluxions upon the Teeth, Ears, and Glands of the Neck and Fauces. By its grateful and agreeable Smell, it exhilarates the Heart, and strengthens the vital Faculties. It is good in Disorders of the Breast, purges

the Lungs, incides and evac those thick and viscid Hu which adhere to the Sides of Ramifications of the Aspera Ar Hence it is accounted an eff Remedy against Coughs, Diffic of Breathing, Asthmas, Peri monies, Pleurisies, Spittings of B fainting Fits, and the Cardi it also restores a proper Ton the relaxed Fibres of the Sto and Oesophagus. It evacuates excrementitious Matter as c Nauseas, and an Inclination to mit. It not only quenches T but also penetrates, moistens, gently purges the Stomach an testines. It cools the Liver Spleen, removes Obstructions fr in these Organs, dissolves the in the Kidneys and Bladder. both a Preservative against, Cure for, the Jaundice and G sickness. It is particularly b cial to the Parts of Generatic preventing Sterility, expelling purities, promoting the Men deficient, and restraining the too copious. It produces the happy Effects in the Fluor It is serviceable in Disorders Joints, and those of the ne System; cures Stupors, S Pandiculations, and all Dis arising from Wind lodged i Muscles. It resolves Concr formed upon the Ligaments o Joints, and is for this very R beneficial in the Gout or I dic Pains. It is by some w recommended in Tumors c Kinds, whether hot or cold, matous, Scirrhous, Inflammat Erysipelatous. It is generall counted serviceable in Wound cers, Fractures, Luxations, an taneous Disorders. This is take tice of in the Catalogue of the *burgh* Dispensatory, but it is not tioned in that of the College.

The next is the *Adiantum Canadenſis, vel Capillus Veneris Canadenſis*, Col. Med. *Adiantum Americcum*, Raii. Tourn. Boerh. Ind. A. Lawry ſays, that this is the moſt valued of all the Maidenhairs. Much the ſame Virtues are aſcribed to it as to the preceeding.

The third is the *Adiantum Album, Ruta Muraria, Salvia Vitæ*, Offic. *Adiantum Album*, Raii. Hiſt. It is eſteemed pectoral, good for an Aſthma, and other Diſorders of the Breaſt ; to provoke Urine, and expel Gravel. It is a very ſmall Plant, ſeldom growing above three Inches high, and with crenated Leaves ſomewhat reſembling thoſe of Rue.

Another is the *Adiantum nigrum*, Offic. J. B. *Adiantum foliis longioribus, Pulverulentis, Pediculo Nigro*, Boerh. Ind. A. Common black Maidenhair. It grows in ſhady Places, at the Roots of Trees, and upon Rocks. It agrees in Virtues with the common Maidenhair.

The laſt is the *Adiantum, & Polytrichum Aureum*, Offic. *Adiantum Aureum Majus*, Raii. Hiſt. *Muſcus coronatus major pileolo Villoſo aureo*. Boerh. Ind. A. *Dale* ſays the Decoction of this Plant is recommended for a Pleuriſy. In other Reſpects the ſame Virtues are aſcribed to it as to the other Maidenhairs.

Ægilops. Thus diſtinguiſhed, *Cerrus Mas majore Glande*, Park. Holme Oak, with great Acorns. But there are alſo other Vegetables, called by the Name of Ægilops as the *Feſtuca avenacea ſterilis elatior*, C. B. *Ægilops Matthiolo*, J. B. Great wild Oat-graſs, or Drank. This grows by Hedges, Paths, and the Sides of Fields. A Decoction of its Root in Wine drank for ſome Days together, is by *Tragus* greatly commended againſt Worms in Children. *Dioſcorides*, in *Lib.* 4. C. 139. ſays, that the

Herb applied with Meal by Way of Cataplaſm, cures the Ægilops and diſcuſſes Hardneſſes. Meal wet with the Juice and afterwards dried is kept for the ſame Purpoſe.

Another Sort is the *Ægilops Narbonenſis*, Lob. or *Feſtuca Italica*, Ger. Haver Graſs. This is an Aſtringent and Drier without much heating. The Seed made into Malt with other Corn, communicates an intoxicating Quality to the Beer.

Æthiopis, Offic. Ger. Emac. *Sclarea Æthiopica, ſive Æthiopis, laciniatis, & non laciniatis foliis*, Park. Theat. Æthiopian Clary. It is cultivated in Gardens and flowers in Summer ; its Root is the Part in Uſe. A Decoction of the Root, relieves the Sciatica, Pleuriſy, Spitting of Blood, and Hoarſeneſs. It is exhibited with Honey in the Form of a Linctus.

Agallochum, Offic. C. B. Pin. *Agallochum verum*, Ephem. Germ. Dec. 11. An. 3. and *Lignum Aloes Vulgare*, Ger. Aloes Wood. This Wood is imported to us from *India* and *Arabia*, and is, like the *Thya*, marked with Spots. It is odoriferous, of a bitteriſh aſtringent Taſte, and ſomewhat mottled. It is called *Calambac* in the Country where it grows, and is brought over to us in ſmall Pieces. It is of an hard ſolid Texture, firm and ponderous, of a yellowiſh brown Colour, with ſeveral black or purple coloured reſinous Veins interperſed, of a bitteriſh, hot, aromatic Taſte, but of no ſtrong Smell till it is burnt. Moſt Botaniſts take the *Agallochum* of the Antients to be the Aloes Wood of the Shops; others ſuppoſe the Aſpalathum to be the ſame, and others, eſpecially the *Arabians*, make ſeveral Kinds. *Caſpar Bauhine* divides this Wood into three Sorts, the firſt he calls the

fineſt

finest Agallochum which is reserved for the Use of the *Indian* Kings. The second is what is sold in the Shops; and the third the wild Agallochum. *Pomet* tells us, that there are several Sorts of it, but the best is the Agallochum of the *Indies*, which comes from *Calecut*. The finest is the black Kind, of a changeable Colour, full, heavy, solid, and thick, which cannot be whitened, and is with Difficulty set on Fire. Others affirm, that we cannot have the true Aloes Wood, because it was swept away by the Deluge; whereas others assert that we cannot have it, only because it grows in Deserts, and on inaccessible Rocks and Mountains. But this is absolutely false, since the Wood is brought in great Quantities from *Surat*. It is observable that the Trunk of the Tree is of three Colours. The Wood which lies immediately under the Bark, is of a black Colour, solid, heavy, and almost like Ebony. The second, which is a light veiny Wood, and of a tanned Colour, is what we call Calambac, or true Aloes-wood. The third Sort which is the Heart, is very scarce and dear. *Dioscorides* in *Lib.* 1. *Cap.* 21. informs us, that chewing this Wood, or rinsing the Mouth with a Decoction of it, makes the Breath sweet; and that when dried and powdered, it serves as a Perfume for the whole Body, and is used in Suffumigations instead of Frankincense; that the Weight of a Dram, drank in some proper Liquor, cures the excessive Humidity, Relaxation, and burning Heat of the Stomach, commonly called the *Heart-burn*; and that when drank in Water, it relieves those afflicted with Pains of the Side or Liver, or labour under a Dysentery or Gripes.

Agaricus sive Fungus Laricis, C. B. *Agaricus ex Larice,* Park. *Agaricum,*
J.B. Agaric. This is a kind of Fungus growing on the Larch Tree, which produces the *Venice* Turpentine. It is imported from *Italy, France,* and especially *Dauphiny,* and the southerly Parts of *Germany;* but that is accounted best which grows in *Tartary.* It requires a whole Year to acquire its due Bulk, and is taken off the Bark of the Tree when it begins to become dry, and chop'd; after which it is exposed to the Sun for two or three Weeks, in order to be whitened. Then it is beaten with Sticks, that no Chinks may appear in it. Sometimes it is rubbed over with Starch, or well triturated *Agaric,* but this is by most looked upon as a bad Sign. It is generally sold in Lumps as big as the Fist, of a Kind of a round angular Form, covered with a callous Bark, white within, at first of a sweetish, but soon after of a bitter, acrid, nauseous, and gently astringent Taste. This Species is called the Female in Contradistinction to the male or spurious *Agaric.* It cannot without Difficulty be reduced to a Powder; and before it can be duely triturated, requires an Admixture of the Gums. When immersed in an Acid, it produces an Effervescence, and is converted into a cretaceous Earth. *In Hist. Acad. R. des Sciences An.* 1714. we are informed, that it contains a subtile acrid Salt, mixed with viscid Particles, so that because it remains long in the Intestines, its Virtues are conveyed to the Chyle and Blood; for which Reason, if a Decoction of it in Ale is given to Nurses, it purges the Children whom they suckle. For this very Reason, also, the Antients successfully used *Agaric* in all Diseases of the Head, arising from a cold Cause. It is ranked among the phlegmagogue Purgatives, and is particularly recommended in Coughs and Asthmas,

mas, where purging is expedient. But as it produces long continued Nauseas, and adheres to the Stomach on Account of its Viscidity, it is rarely exhibited by itself without being previously corrected with Aromatics, as Ginger, Cinnamon, Mace, and others of a like Nature. Besides, as it operates slowly, it is generally assisted by the Addition of other Purgatives. The most common Method of using it, is in Form of Troches or Pills; which ought always to be recent, otherwise they lose a great Deal of their Efficacy. *Prosper Alpinus,* in *Med. Ægypt. Lib.* 4. *Cap.* 15. informs us, that the *Ægyptians* with Success exhibited *Agaric* with a certain Portion of Myrrh, in a Decoction of Penny-royal. As the male or spurious *Agaric,* and the other Species of it, are rarely or never used in Medicine, we shall take no farther Notice of them.

Ageratum, Eupatorium Mesues, Off. *Ageratum foliis serratis,* C. B. Boerh. Ind. Alt. *Ageratum plerisque, Herba Julia quibusdam,* J. B. *Ageratum Vulgare, sive Costus Hortorum Minor,* Park. Maudlin. The whole Plant has a strong tho' not an ungrateful Scent. It is a Native of *Italy,* and the warmer Countries, but with us only grows in Gardens, and flowers in *July,* and *August.* It is of a bitter Taste, of a warming and drying Nature, beneficial in Disorders of the Stomach, serviceable in the Jaundice and Obstructions of the Menses, diuretic and anthelminthic. *Boerhaave* informs us, that it is possess'd of the Virtues of Costmary and Tansey, and is an Ingredient in all carmal Compositions; that its Seeds have been exhibited with Success instead of Worm-seeds; that its distilled Water and Spirit, diffuse a most fragrant Smell, and that the Plant is used in Syrups, Oils, Infu-

sion, Decoction, Powder and Pills. But Mr. *Boyle* observes it to be prejudicial to the Eyes. *Dioscorides* in *Lib.* 4. *Cap.* 59. informs us, that a Decoction of this Plant is highly beneficial in Fomentations, and that the Steam of it when burnt, provokes Urine, and mollifies Indurations of the Uterus. *Oribasius* in *Med. Collect.* 1. *Lib.* 15. *Cap.* 1. informs us, that the *Ageratum* is a Digestive, and gently mitigates Inflammations. The other Kinds of Maudlin are not used in Medicine, and therefore need no farther Notice.

Agnus Castus, Vitex, Offic. *Agnus folio non serrato,* I. B. Raii Hist. *Vitex Agnus Castus,* Rand. Ind. *Vitex foliis angustioribus, Cannabis modo dispositis,* C. B. Boerh. Ind. Alt. Chaste-tree. It grows in the warmer Climates, as *Italy, Naples,* and *Sicily,* and flowers in *August. Dioscorides* informs us, that this Shrub, received the Name of Αγνος, or Chaste, because the Matrons who liv'd chaste during the *Thesmophoria,* or Feasts of *Ceres,* used to lie upon it. Not only the Seeds, but also the Flowers and Leaves, are of an acrid and moderately astringent Taste. The Antients highly extolled it for repressing the Violence of venereal Inclinations, as also on Account of its heating, drying, and de-obstruent Qualities, and accordingly employed it, as one or other of these Intentions was to be pursued. But the Moderns generally look upon these Recommendations as ill grounded. *Hippocrates,* indeed, in *Lib. de Morb. Mulier.* recommends the Seeds of this Shrub for bringing away the Secundines. Some of the Moderns, also, extol it, as beneficial in a great Variety of Disorders; but as Experience has given it no considerable Sanction, the more skilful Physicians seldom use it in their Practice.

As the Seeds of this Shrub are of an heating and stimulating Nature, they should rather seem to augment venereal Inclinations, at least in coldPatients; for we observe that Persons languid in this Respect are to be stimulated and roused; so that it only seems to be possessed of an antiphrodisiac Quality, in so far as it is an excessive Drier in hot Subjects. *Kæipius*, in his *Regnum Vegetabile*, gives the following just Account of the Virtues of the *Agnus Castus*. " It operates by its volatile and as " it were camphorated Salt, whence " it is discutient; excites the Men- " ses, by Incessions mitigates the " Disorders of the Pudenda, discus- " ses the venereal Fomes in hot " Subjects, and by drying removes " it, in so far as it volatilizes the " oleous Parts of the Semen, and " causes them to transpire. It also " represses the Flatulences joined to " the Semen in the same manner as " Camphire and Rue do."

Agrifolium, Offic. Ger. Emac. *Aquifolium baccis rubris*, Boerh. Ind. Alt. *Agrifolium sive Aquifolium*, Park. Theat. The Holly-tree. The Berries of Holly are hot and dry, of thin Parts and expel Wind. They are recommended for the Cholic, inwardly taken they bring away by Stool thick phlegmatic Humours. Holly beaten to Powder and drank, is good for all Fluxes of the Belly, as the Dysentery and the like.

Agrimonia, Eupatorium Græcorum, Offic. *Agrimonia Vulgaris*, Park. Theat. *Agrimoniæ Officinarum*, Boerh. Ind. Alt. *Eupatorium veterum seu Agrimonia*, C. B. Pin. Agrimony. This is the *Eupatorium* of *Dioscorides, Galen*, and the antient *Greeks*. It grows in Hedges and the Borders of Fields, and flowers in *June* and *July*. Some think it received the Name *Agrimony*, from the large Quantity of it produced *in Agris* in

the Fields, and the Appellation of *Eupatorium* either from King *Eupator*, or from the first Discoverer of its Virtues. But be this as it will, 'tis certain that Agrimony is possessed of many singular Virtues. It contains a subaustere, subastringent and aromatic Juice; and is justly recommended for its aperient, detersive, vulnerary, corroborating, and mildly operating Qualities. Hence it is deservedly dignified with the Epithets of hepatic and visceral, for by restoring the Tone and Strength of the Fibres, it removes Obstructions arising from too great a Relaxation of the Vessels. Hence a Decoction of it is highly beneficial in Scurvies arising from Relaxation, hepatic Fluxes, bloody Vomitings, and internal Hemorrhages, where Astringents are proper. It is by some singularily extol'd in Discharges of bloody Urine, accompanied with Ulcerations of the Kidneys. *Riverius* gave the Herb reduc'd to a Powder, in Incontinencies of Urine. An Infusion of recent Agrimony with Water, is accounted a Medicine which acts by a gentle aromatic Stimulus, without any astringent Quality, and which when drank every Morning, proves beneficial to hypocondriac and hysteric Patients; is a good Reviver of the Spirits, and by its resolvent Quality, removes that peccant Matter, which adhering to the Hypocondria, is the Cause of Flatulences, Anxieties, and Sighs. If Whey, in which the recent Herb has remain'd for some time, is constantly us'd during the Summer, it is accounted an excellent Purger of the Body, and a Preservative against many Diseases; for it is more grateful and less weakening than Whey alone. The express'd Juice of this Plant boil'd, is a grateful and excellent astringent Medicine. Tho' its distill'd Water seems only to have a gently

gently aromatic Quality, yet *Morison* in his *Historia Plantarum Universalis,* informs us, that Cardinal *Bembo* found nothing more beneficial than its continual Use, for expelling Sand from the Kidneys. *Dolæus's* Assertion of its being a Specific in Madness, is sufficiently confuted by Experience, as is shewn by *Garidel* in his *Histoire des Plantes,* &c. The Plant is beneficially applied externally to any Part to be strengthen'd by astringent Medicines. Hence a Decoction of it in Form of a Cataplasm, contributes to the Resolution of inflam'd Tumors and Contusions. Cataplasms of it boil'd in Vinegar or Wine, and applied to the Scrotum, are highly celebrated in Inflammations of the Testicles.

Alaternus. The Name of a Plant, of which there are four Species, the first of which is the *Alaternus,* Offic. *Alaternus major & minor,* Park. Theat. *Alaternus,* 1. *Clusii, & Minori folio,* Boerh. Ind. A. Evergreen Privet. It grows in Hedges, and is cultivated in Gardens. It contains much Oil and Phlegm, and but little Salt. It is of a detersive, astringent, and cooling Nature, and is used in Gargarisms for Inflammations of the Mouth, and for the Quinsey. The Root moderately binds the Belly.

The second Sort is the *Alaternus Hispanicus, Celastrus dicta,* Boerh. Ind. A. *Celastrus,* Offic. *Celastrus Theophrasti,* Ger. Emac. Park. Theat. The Staff-tree.

The third Sort is the *Cassina,* Offic. *Herba Cassiana famem sitimque retardans,* J. B. Cassiny. It grows in *Carolina.* It is accounted a very good Medicine for the Small Pox, and restraining immoderate Fermentation of the Blood, without putting too great a Check upon the expulsive Faculty. It promotes Ex-

pectoration, preserves the Lungs, and keeps off the Small Pox from the Head and Throat.

The fourth Sort is the *Perygua,* Officinar. Mant. The Cassio-Berry-bush. It is found in *Carolina.* The Fragments of the dried Leaves, and the Powder of the Stalks, are used. Sometimes it purges, at other times excites Vomiting, or promotes insensible Perspiration, still acting as Nature inclines. It is accounted an excellent Specific in the Diabetes. A Tea made of the Herb is good in the Nephritic Colic.

Alcanna, Offic. *Ligustrum Orientale, sive Cyprus Dioscoridis & Plinii,* Park. Theat. *Baccifera Indica baccis oblongis in umbellæ formam dispositis,* Raii Hist. Eastern Privet. This is the *Kenna* of the *Turks* and *Moors.* Its medicinal Virtues are emmenagogue and hysteric, and accordingly is used in the Eastern Countries, to cause Abortion, and to bring away dead Children. The Leaves have an astringent Quality, by which they heal Ulcers in the Mouth, being chewed therein; and are good for Carbuncles, and other fiery Inflammations if applied in a Cataplasm. The Decoction of them is good for Burns. The Flowers bruised in Vinegar ease Pains of the Head, being applied to the Forehead.

Alcea, Offic. *Alcea Vulgaris,* J. B. Raii Hist. *Alcea vulgaris major, flore ex rubro roseo,* Boerh. Ind. Alt. Vervain Mallow. This Species of Mallow differs from the common Kind in having its Stalks more hairy and growing more erect; the lower Leaves are smaller and roundish, serrated about the Edges, and growing on long Foot-stalks; the higher they grow the Foot-stalks are the shorter. The upper Leaves are cut into five deep Segments; the Flowers are larger, paler, and not streaked like those of the common

Mal-

Mallow. The Cheese-like Seed-Vessel is larger and blacker; the Root is hard, woody, and spreads in the Ground. It grows in uncultivated Fields and Hedges, and near High-ways. It flowers in *July* and *August*, and in Autumn produces Seeds; it is possess'd of the Virtues of the common Mallow, and its Root, Leaves, Flowers, and Seeds may be us'd as Emollients. Its Root is particularly celebrated against Dimness of the Eyes by Empirics, so that some foolishly believe that a Portion of it suspended about the Neck, quickens and preserves the Sight. But this hardly seems credible. In Inflammations and Dryness arising from them, this Plant proves beneficial as other emollient, mucilaginous, laxative, moistening, and demulcent Medicines. Hence 'tis obvious that its Root, drank in Wine or Water, proves beneficial against Gripes, and Erosions of the Intestines.

Alchimilla, Offic. Ger. Raii Hist. *Alchimilla Vulgaris*, C. B. *Alchimilla Major Vulgaris*, Park. Ladies Mantle. It grows in Meadows and pasture Grounds, flowers in *May* and *June*, and in *July* and *August*, and produces its Seeds. On Account of its astringent, viscid, and glutinous Juice it is class'd among the vulnerary Plants, both applied externally with other Substances, and exhibited internally in vulnerary Potions, and Decoctions; for it inspissates the thin Blood, and is for that Reason highly beneficial in the *Fluor Albus*, and immoderate menstrual Discharges. A Decoction of it is useful for washing Wounds, which may, also, be advantageously cover'd with a Cloth dipt in the same Decoction. *Bauhine* informs us, that this Plant is of so powerful a conglutinating Quality, as to cure Ruptures of the Intestines, especially in Children; for which Purpose the dry Powder is ex-

hibited in the Decoction, or the distill'd Water of the Plant. The same Powder exhibited in a Spoonful of Wine or Broth for fifteen or twenty Days, is successfully prescrib'd for Women whose Sterility proceeds from an excessive Moisture of the Uterus, on Account of which the Semen cannot be retain'd. From what has been said 'tis obvious, that this Plant is proper in consolidating Clysters for the Cure of Dysenteries. Women in order to render their lax and flaccid Breasts firm and solid, apply to them a Cloth dipt in the Decoction of this Plant.

Alectorolophus, Offic. *Chrifta Galli*, Ger. Emac. *Pedicularis sive Chrifta Galli lutea*, Park. Theat. *Pedicularis pratensis lutea, vel Chrifta Galli*, Boerh. Ind. A. Yellow Rattle. It grows in barren Sorts of Pastures, flowering in *June*; the Seed is ripe in a short Time. It is accounted good for a Cough boiled with husk'd Beans and sweeten'd with Honey. It cures Dimness of Sight by putting a whole Seed into the Eye, where the Seed causes no Disorder, but takes off the Mist or Cloud upon itself. It changes Colour, and from black begins to turn white, then swells and comes out of itself.

Alkekengi Halicacabum, Offic. *Alkekengi Officinarum*, Boerh. Ind. Alt. *Solanum veficarium*, C. B. Pin. *Solanum Halicacabum Vulgare*, J. B. Winter Cherry. It grows with us in Gardens, where it is easily propagated, flowers in *July* and *August*, and bears ripe Fruit in *September*. The Taste of the Leaves is acrid and bitter, whereas that of the Fruit is acid, and afterwards somewhat bitter. The Seeds are, also, acrid and somewhat bitterish. The whole of the Fruit is esteem'd a celebrated Remedy against nephritic Pains, and calculous Disorders; it lubricates the urinary Passages, expels Stones, and

and Gravel ; contributes to the Cure of exulcerated Kidneys, temperates the Acrimony of the Urine, removes the Strangury and Dyfury ; and is for thefe Reafons mix'd in a great many Compofitions, appropriated to Diforders of the Liver, Bladder, and Kidneys. *Gafpar Hoffman* informs us, that its diuretic Quality is fo well known to the poor People of *Germany*, that for that very Purpofe they devour large Quantities of it. According to *Dioſcorides*, an Infufion or Decoction of it with Whey is an effectual Remedy againft the Epilepfy. When reduc'd to a Powder and taken in white Wine, or that of Juniper, it is highly efficacious in exciting a Difcharge of Urine, and relieving thofe afflicted with the Dropfy, Jaundice, Gout, or Colic. Both the Leaves and Fruit are with great Advantage applied to eryfipelatous Diforders of the malignant Kind. Thefe Effects fufficiently evince that it is of an aperient Quality, which when the Medicine is us'd internally, operates principally by Urine. There are various Methods of ufing this Remedy. Thus *Tournefort* exhibits five or fix of the bruis'd Berries, in an Emulfion. *Arnaldus de Villanova*, who is faid to have reviv'd the exploded Ufe of this Plant, found the Efficacy of a Wine prepar'd from it, in a Retention of Urine, which would yield to no other Medicines. A proper Quantity of the Seeds alone, bruis'd and drank with Coffee or Tea, is highly extolled for purging the Kidneys. Quacks and Mountebanks, as we are inform'd by Dr. *Freind*, pretend, that they can collect all the peccant Humours fluctuating in the Body, by rubbing any particular Part with *Alkekengi*, and when by this Means they have excited an Heat and Inflammation; they demand their Reward as if the Difeafe was cur'd by them, but the Part being anointed with Oil, is forthwith freed from the Pain.

Alliaria , Offic. Ger. Park. C. B. Pin. *Hefperis allium redolens*, Boerh. Ind Alt. Sauce-allalone, or Jack by the Hedge. It grows in Hedges and Bank-fides, and flowers in *May*. This Herb attenuates, incides, and greatly refifts Putrefaction. Infufions of it internally us'd, are far preferable to the Bezoar Stone as a Diaphoretic, and the Herb itfelf makes an excellent Ingredient in Spring Sallads. When applied externally after it is bruis'd, efpecially with Salt and Oxycrate, it is highly beneficial againft a Tendency to Putrefaction in carcinomatous Ulcers, and Gangrenes, in which Cafes it fupplies the Place of *Scordium*, tho' it is fomewhat lefs efficacious. There is but little Virtue in the dried Herb, for which Reafon it is to be gather'd in the End of *April* or the Beginning of *May*, and after it is dried a Day or two in a Shade, cut fmall and the Juice forthwith exprefs'd, either in a Mortar or Prefs. This Juice when put into Bottles with a little Oil upon it, may be kept for three Years. It may, alfo, be infpiffated over a Fire, and kept for feveral Years for the fame Purpofes. *Fabricius Mildanus* informs us, that this Juice, whether fimple or infpiffated, is an excellent Ingredient in Ointments deftin'd for Gangrenes, and other putrid, fordid, and malignant Ulcers. Hence we juftly deduce, that it is of a refolvent Quality ; for if the recent Herb is triturated in any proper Liquor, it proves diuretic ; when drank in *Hydromel*, it digefts and attenuates thick and vifcid Humours in the Breaft. For inveterate Coughs, it is us'd as a Linctus, with Refin and Honey ; and it is faid to prove highly beneficial to afthmatic Patients. Some put its Leaves into Clyfters defign'd for removing either Colic or nephritic Pains,

Pains, in the former of which it remarkably diffipates the Flatulences; and in the latter, furprifingly mitigates the Pain. The Juice of the Plant, or the Powder of its Seeds, blown up the Noftrils, by exciting a Sternutation in epileptic and comatous Patients, reftores them to themfelves. Externally, the Seeds bruis'd with Vinegar and applied by Way of Plaifter to the Abdomen, roufes Women under hyfteric Suffocations. The Seeds alfo put into a Linencloth, and us'd by Way of Peffary, are faid to produce the fame Effects. Upon a chymical Analyfis this Plant yields an acid Phlegm, a concrete volatile Salt, a fix'd lixivial Salt, and a large Quantity of Oil and Earth.

Allium, Offic. Ger. *Allium fativum,* C. B, Boerh. Ind. Alt. and *Allium vulgare & fativum,* J. B. Garlick. The whole Plant, and efpecially the Root, is of a ftrong and offenfive Smell. Garlick is an acrid Plant abounding with volatile Salt, efpecially its Roots, whofe diftinct Portions, generally call'd Heads or Bulbs, are by Phyficians, for the moft Part prefcrib'd in Number; and not according to their Weight. Garlick is proper when the Intentions of ftimulating, heating, refolving, and difcuffing are to be purfued: Hence the crude Root is generally us'd when the Stomach is cold or diforder'd by an inactive Mucus, or by Crudities of the vifcid and acid Kinds: This Root when boil'd, becomes milder, and is recommended againft Worms of the Inteftines, and if boil'd in Milk is faid to be a powerful Alexipharmic, when any poifonous Quality of the Air is apprehended. This Plant is by fome call'd the *Theriaca* of the Country People, to whom it is not only grateful, but alfo by its volatile Salts, attenuates the Crudities of the *prima via,* affifts Concoction, and promotes infenfible Per-

fpiration. Hence *Pliny* juftly afferts, that it guards againft the Misfortunes arifing from the Changes of Waters and Climates, and that it renders the Body of a frefher and more blooming Colour. Soldiers and Sailors often experience the happy Effects arifing from the due Ufe of this Plant, as we are inform'd by *Portius in Lib. de Sanitate Milit. Tuenda.* From what has been faid, 'tis fufficiently obvious, that Garlick is of great Efficacy in exciting an Appetite, and procuring Strength to the Stomach. Hence, as are we told in *Lettres edifiantes & curieuf. de quelques Miffionaires,* it prov'd a fovereign Remedy in a Lyentery, or Excretion of the Food without any Change. *Fr. Hoffman,* alfo, *in Med. Rat. Tom.* 2. informs us, that it is an inftantaneous Remedy for Dyfenteries produc'd by eating putrid Flefh. In the *Ephimerid. Natur. Curiof. Decad.* 2. *An.* 8. *Obf.* 202. we are affur'd, that it prov'd effectual for diffolving Milk coagulated in the Stomach. In flatulent Colics arifing from cold, acid, or vifcid Caufes, it has often prov'd beneficial, efpecially when a Soop is prepar'd of it with Oil of Olives, and a little pure Wine. *Galen* gives us an Account of a labouring Man, who being feiz'd with the Colic, cloth'd himfelf warm, eat fome Garlick with Bread, and work'd at his ufual Bufinefs the whole Day; by which Means he was freed from his Diforder. *Ramazzini* in his Treatife of the Difeafes of Tradefmen, informs us, that long protracted Quartans have been cur'd by the Ufe of Garlick, and a large Quantity of unmix'd Wine. In a Word, Garlick is properly exhibited in Cafes where the Body requires a Stimulus, or where the Vifcidity of the ftagnant Humours produces the Difeafe; in exciting the Menfes, for Inftance, provoking Urine, and removing Coughs. The judicious *Sydenham*

in,

nforms us, that Dropfies have been ur'd by the Ufe of Garlick alone, without the Affiftance of any other Evacuants. Many afflicted with the Stone, find fingular Relief from three, four, or five Bulbs of Garlick, taken with a Glafs of Brandy, which Remedy fome order to be repeated every Month, at the new Moon; others a Day before the new Moon, and others every Week, on the Day immediately preceeding the Quadratures of the Moon, as we may find by confulting the *Ephimerides Natur. Curiof. Cent.* 1. *Obf.* 55. *Vol.* 2. *Bartholin. Epift. Cent.* 3. and *Hoffmen de Remed. Domeft.* Garlick bruis'd with green Coriander, and drank in unmix'd Wine, is faid to prove a Stimulus to Venery; for which Reafon *Carolus de Aquino* in his *Nomenclator Agriculturæ*, informs us, that the *Athenians* us'd to give it to their Cocks before they began to fight. Travellers, alfo, ufe it in order to render themfelves more brifk and vigorous; for which Purpofes it is alfo given to Horfes. It is us'd internally, not only boil'd and in fpirituous Liquor, but alfo crude. *Zacutus Lufitanus* gives us an Account of an old Man, who in the Winter Time having travell'd thro' the Snow, till the innate Heat of his Stomach was almoft extinguifh'd, fell dangeroufly ill. But as the hotteft Remedies were of no Efficacy in reftoring this Heat, *Zacutus*, according to *Avicenna*'s Directions, gave him dry Garlick cover'd with Honey, by which Means he became confiderably better in four Days, and by perfifting in its Ufe for a Month, had his Health perfectly recover'd. The external Ufe of Garlick is alfo highly recommended in many Cafes, fince by its ftimulating Acrimony, it refolves, opens, and attracts. Garlick when reduc'd to the Form of an Ointment with Oil of Olives, is extoll'd for refolving cold Tumors, and removing Corns on the Feet. According to the celebrated *Profper Alpinus*, the *Egyptians* drop the warm Juice of Garlick into the Ears, in order to remove inveterate Deafnefs, and Ringing. With recent Garlick bruis'd they, alfo, cure recent Wounds. They alfo apply burnt Garlick with Honey for the Cure of Scald-heads. Infeffions in Decoctions of dry Garlicks with its Stalks, are highly beneficial in exciting the Menfes, and the *Egyptians* frequently procure an Expulfion of the Secundines, by ordering the Steam of the Decoction, or the Smoak of the Root burnt upon Coals, to be receiv'd into the Uterus. *Arnaldus de Villanova* tells us, that in Head-achs, arifing from Phlegm, Garlick bruis'd, heated upon a Tile, and applied to the Part affected, removes the Pain; and that when boil'd and fried with a little Pennyroyal and Pepper with Oil, it removes an *Hemicrania*, when applied to the Part affected. Hogs lard form'd into an Ointment with Eggs and two or three Heads of Garlick, is faid to prove an almoft immediate Cure for Hoarfenefs, if it is applied warm at Night to the Soles of the Feet, before a brifk Fire, taking Care to keep the Feet warm in the Night Time; for this Purpofe the Loins are alfo to be anointed with the fame Ointment, after the Patient is in Bed. Obftinate intermittent, and even quartan Fevers, when all other Means have fail'd, are often happily remov'd by applying bruis'd Garlick to the Wrifts, where it produces a Blifter, which being open'd, the peccant Matter is in fome Meafure eliminated. But according to *F. Hoffman*, this Practice is not to be us'd without the greateft Circumfpection; becaufe the Garlick produces violent Inflammations, which may be productive of Symptoms more terrible than the original Diforder. The

The same Observation is also made in *Eph. Nat. Curiof. Dec.* 2. *An.* 9. *Obf.* 127. where there is also Mention made of a Tooth-ach, considerably mitigated by exciting a Blister on the Elbow, by Means of bruis'd Garlick. According to *Platerus,* Garlick is to be applied to the Wrist on the same Side with the affected Tooth. *Bartholine* informs us, that the wandering Pains of scorbutic Patients are dissipated by rubbing their Joints with the Juice of Garlick. *Bartholine* also, informs us, that Garlick with Oil of Scorpions, is us'd by Way of Cataplasm to expel the Stone, and Urine. *Etmuller* says, that a Decoction of this Plant in Milk, us'd by Way of Fomentation to the Anus, brings away the Worms of the Intestines, and that the *Hungarians* in the Camp-Fever, take a Bulb of Garlick, which they saturate with Spirit of Wine, and bruise. With this Poultice, they strongly anoint the Patient's Body, then disposing him to sweat by laying a large Quantity of Cloths upon him, he is forthwith reliev'd. *Sydenham* says, " That among the various Medicines which make a " Revulsion or Derivation from the " Head, none seems to operate " so powerfully as Garlick appli- " ed to the Soles of the Feet.—— " In Adults, therefore, labouring " under the Small Pox of the con- " fluent Kind, I generally apply " slic'd Garlick wrapt up in a Cloth, " to the Soles of their Feet, from " the eighth Day till the Dif- " ease is no longer dangerous. This " Application is to be renew'd every " Day ;" for by its strongly stimulating Quality, it augments the Motion in the Part to which it is applied, makes the Humours tend towards it, and by exciting Blisters elimi- nates the acrid and foreign Mat- ter, which being mixed with the Mass of Blood, creates such Com-

motions in the Body. Hence the Reason is obvious, why Garlick is successfully us'd as a Cataplasm, for maturating pestilential Buboes. But Garlick not only sometimes fails to produce the desir'd Effects, but also, when immoderately or un- seasonably us'd, proves highly inju- rious to Health. Thus in *Ephim. Nat. Curiof. Vol.* 4. we are inform'd, that an immoderate Use of it brought on a *Cholera* and a *Cardialgia,* and *ibid. Dec.* 4. *An.* 6. *Obf.* 8, we are told, that eating it to Excess produc'd a Discharge of Blood by the urinary Paffage. In *Act. Med. Berol. Dec.* 2. *Vol.* 9. unufual Tumors of the Hands and Feet, are observ'd to be excited by an Infufion of Gar- lick in Malt Spirits, frequently ap- plied externally in the wandering Gout. As Garlick throws the Hu- mours into violent Commotions, and strongly stimulates the Solids, so 'tis fufficiently obvious; that it ought ne- ver, without the greatest Precaution and Circumfpection, to be recom- mended to Perfons of hot Conftitu- tions, thofe whofe Humours are eafi- ly put into Commotions, and thofe, the Compages of whofe Solids is weak. Hence we underftand in what Senfe the Antients are to be taken, when they afferted that Gar- lick was prejudicial to the Head, Eyes, and Kidneys. There is ftill another Quality in this Plant which renders its Ufe, efpecially when raw, improper for weak Perfons; which is the Vifcidity of its Juice, which requires a ftrong Stomach in order to fubdue it; for which Reafon we may juftly affirm, that it affords little or no Nourifhment to the Bo- dy. Its Vifcidity is fufficiently e- vinc'd by the Experiments of *Du Ha- mel,* who found its Juice to cement and join the divided Parts of Glafs and China. Its Tendency to gene- rate Flatulences, feems alfo to de- pend upon its Vifcidity. The mo- derate

derate Use then of Garlick, is only to be permitted as a Sauce, or a Medicine, but not as a daily Aliment; for it is not without Reason, that B. *Swalve* in his *Querela Ventriculi Renovata*, represents the Stomach as making the following Complaints. ' How much Labour have I from ' Garlicks, Onions, and Leeks, ' whilst I hardly ever receive any ' Advantage from them, except ' when oppress'd with thick and ' viscid Humours?" When therefore Heat is not to be increas'd in the Body, the Acrimony and Strength of Garlick are greatly to be suspected; for in other Cases, as *Hippocrates* observes in *Tr. de Vict. Rat. in Ac.* " Garlick produces Heat, and ' Flatulences about the Thorax, ' Heaviness of the Head, Anxiety, ' and if there is any previous Disorder it augments it." It is probably at all Times safer to use Garlick boil'd, than crude. From what has been said, we understand, that the Antients only call'd Garlick Purative, because it resolv'd the viscid and tenacious Matter in the *Primæ Viæ*, and by that Means dispos'd it for Evacuation. *Hippocrates* recommends the eating of Garlick, either when a Person is drunk, or inclin'd to go a drinking; in the former Case, because by promoting Perspiration, it dissipates the Intoxication; in the latter, because by strengthning the Stomach, it subdues the Liquor, and expels it either by Urine, or the cutaneous Pores. A Syrup, and an Oxymel, are directed to be made of Garlick, in the last *London* Dispensatory.

Besides the common Species of Garlick, *Botanists* have taken Notice of many others, as the *Ophioscorodon, &c. Allium sativum alterum, sive dispersum caulis summo circumvolu-* Boerh. Ind. A. Vipers Garlick, or Rocambole. This is cultivated in Gardens, and flowers in *July*. The

Root and Kernel are us'd in Medicine, and are said to agree in Virtues with the preceeding; but this is somewhat milder.

The *Scorodoprassum*, Off. *Allium sphæriceo Capite, folio latiore, sive Scorodoprassum alterum.* Boerh. Ind. A. Wild Leeks. This Species agrees in Virtues with the other, but is milder.

The *Ampeloprassum*, Off. *French Lack.* This flowers in *June*, and the Root is recommended by *Dioscorides* against the Bites of Serpents. *Dale* thinks this the true *Ampeloprassum*.

The *Victorialis*, Off. *Allium latifolium montanum maculatum*, Boerh. Ind. A. Broad-leav'd Mountain Garlick, or spotted Ramsons. It flowers in *June*, and agrees in Virtues with the other Species.

There is also the *Allium Sylvestre*, Off. Crow Garlick, to which the same Virtues are ascrib'd, as to common Garlick.

The *Moly*, Off. *Allium angustifolium umbellatum album*, Tourn. *Moly angustifolium umbellatum*, Boerh. Ind. A. Moly of *Dioscorides*. Dioscorides recommends this made into a Pessary, in Relaxations of the Uterus.

The *Moly Theophrasti*, Off. *Moly latifolium liliflorum*, Boerh. Ind. A. *Allium latifolium, liliflorum.* Tourn. Inst. Moly of Theophrastus. The Virtues are the same as those of the preceeding.

Alnus, Offic. Ger. *Alnus Vulgaris*, Park. Theat. J. B. *Alnus Rotunda folia glutinosa viridis*, C. B. Pin. Boerh. Ind. Alt. The Alder-Tree. It grows in moist and marshy Soils; the Wood becomes black in a Solution of Vitriol. *Alder* then is possess'd of the astringent Property of Galls, and may for that Reason be us'd in making Ink. But this astringent Quality is most considerable in the Fruit, and especially in the Bark, which when

when macerated in Water with old rusty Iron, or the Scoriæ of Iron, serves to tinge Leather with a black Colour. In the *Ephim. Nat. Curiof. Vol. 3. Obf.* 16. we are told, that if the yellowish Bark, not only of the Roots, but also of the Branches, is boil'd in common Water, it is of singular Efficacy in carrying off the Water of dropsical Patients. *Pliny* in *Lib.* 24. *Cap.* 10. informs us, that the Leaves taken out of boiling Water and applied, are an effectual Cure for Tumors. But this Observation can only hold true in Cases, where Repellents and Aftringents are proper. *Barbarus* in Comment. on *Vitruvius* informs us, that some cover the Floors of Rooms with its Leaves befprinkled with Dew, in order to deftroy Fleas; for the Leaves when budding, contain a Kind of pinguious tenacious Humours, to which the Fleas adhering, as it were to Bird-Lime, are killed. *Tournefort* in his *Plant. Paralip. Tom.* 2. informs us, that the Leaves of this Tree, are in the Alps us'd in paralytic Cafes, especially when the Diforder has proceeded from external Caufes, as lying in the Fields or damp Houfes. For this Purpofe fome Sackfuls of the Leaves dried either in the Sun, or in an Oven, are fpread for the Patient to lie upon, being fufficiently cover'd therewith, and with warm Cloths, till he has fweated plentifully. This Remedy is, alfo, accounted good for the Rheumatifm, Sciatica, and other Diforders of a fimilar Nature.

There is another Species of Alder, called *the black Alder-tree,* by *Dale* diftinguifhed thus. *Frangula, alnus Nigra,* Offic. *Frangula,* Boerh. Ind. Alt. *Frangula five Alnus Nigra Baccifera,* Park. Theat. Raii Synop. It grows in fuch Woods as are thick and moift, flowers in *May,* and produces ripe Fruit in *September.* The inner Bark of this Tree,

which is of a yellow Colour, and tinges the Spittle like Rhubard, is faid to purge ferous and bilious Humours, and is greatly commended for the Dropfy and Jaundice, but it ought to be corrected with proper Aromatics, otherwife it will produce violent Gripes and Vomitings. When bruifed in a Mortar, and mixed with Vinegar, it is accounted good for the Itch, the Parts affected being wafhed with it.

Aloe, Offic. C. B. Pin. Boerh. Ind. Alt. *Aloe Diofcoridis,* Colum. *Aloe Diofcoridis & Aliorum,* Sloan Cat. Jam. Aloes. From this, and fome other Species of the Plant, is obtained the *Aloes of the Shops,* which is a concreted brownifh or blackifh Juice, of a bitter Tafte and difagreeable Smell. It is imported into *Europe* in Sheeps-fkins, or large Gourds. According to *Garidel* from *Hermannus,* the pureft, or what is called the Succotrine Aloes, is the Juice gently preffed from the entire Leaves feparated from their Roots; and infpiffated in the Sun after it has depofited its moft feculent Part. This Sediment when poured into another Veffel, and infpiffated in the Sun, acquires an harder Confiftence than the former, and is called *hepatic Aloes.* And the Sediment of this fecond Species, when infpiffated, is called *Caballine* or *Horfe-aloes.* But other Authors are of Opinion, that thefe different Sorts of Aloes, are produced o different Species of the Plant. Th beft Aloes is that which is pingu ous, of a dark Colour, in fome Mea fure friable, in Smell refembling th of Myrrh, and which when pound ed yields a Powder of a golde Colour. In Confequence of its bi ter Tafte, it is called the *Gall* Nature, and alfo refembles the Bi in this, that when it is diffolved Water, it becomes vifcid, and

w a

ays tinges the Feces with a yellow Colour. But according to *Boerhaave* it loses the Bitterness after it has undergone Fermentation. Aloes consists of two Substances, one resinous which may be extracted by Spirit of Wine, and the other of a gummy Nature, which may be dissolved in Water. The purer Aloes is, the more of a gummy Portion it contains, whereas the more impure it is, the more resinous Parts it contains. The Caballine-aloes is, also, contaminated by a large Quantity of terrestrial Matter. In Consequence of this Combination of a gummy and resinous Substance, Aloes has experimentally been found not only abstersive and eccoprotic, when exhibited in a small Dose, but also attenuating and resolvent, and consequently aperient, emmenagogue, cholic, and calculated for provoking the hemorrhoidal Discharge, whether exhibited internally, or appiled to the Anus. It is, also, of a balsamic Quality, and resists Putrefaction. Aloes operates by resolving, a Consequence of its saponaceous Virtue, and by stimulating in Consequence of its heating Nature. When, therefore, pituitous Humours are to be expelled, Aloes prove an highly powerful and efficacious Medicine. Hence it is above all Things beneficial in Disorders of the *primæ viæ*, for which Reason it is by Way of Eminence stiled the *Soul of the Stomach*, since by its balsamic, corroborative, and laxative Virtues, it absterges and eliminates the viscid Humours; corrects such as are acid and vapid; and by corroborating the relaxed Tone of the Stomach, removes the Spasms and Flatulences of the *Primæ viæ*. Aloes has constantly been accounted one of the most considerable of the purgative Medicines. But the Dose ought at most to be no more than half a Scruple, since it always pro-

duces better Effects in small, than in large Quantities. Hence we justly infer, that the Ancients were in the wrong for prescribing a Scruple and more of this Medicine, since by this Means it excites too violent Commotions in the Humours, as is observed by *Simon Pauli. Quadr. Bot. Eph. Nat. Curiof. Dec. 2. An. 5. Obf. 218. Lemery Chym. Stahl ad Harv.* Aloes is an Ingredient in almost all the laxative Compositions, and most celebrated Pills of the Ancients. We are by no Means to exhibit Aloes, to Persons whose Vessels are tender or putrified, since it is only proper for those of moist, cold, and mucous Constitutions, and such are disposed to the Generation of Acids. Hence it is not to be recommended to old Persons, unless they are of dry Constitutions, because it is remarkably heating and drying; for which Reason it is less friendly to Persons of a dry, than to those of a moist Constitution. In *Aĉta Hafnienfia, Tom. 2. Obf. 64.* we are told, that a Discharge of bloody Urine, was produced by an immoderate Use of Aloes. Aloes, also, generally procures an hemorrhoidal Discharge whilst by its acrid Resin it stimulates the Veins of the Anus, and excites an Orgasm and Commotion in the Blood. *Hoffman* informs us, that by an excessive Use of Aloes, *Calvin* was seized with ulcerous Hemorrhoids, and a Spitting of Blood. Too much, therefore, was attributed to Aloes, by the Authors of that Maxim, *Qui vult Vivere Annos* NOE, *fumat Pilulas de* ALOE, the Man who wants to live as long as NOAH, ought to use Pills of ALOES. In the *Ephimerides Nat. Curiof. Decad. 2. An. 5. Obf. 218.* we are told, that Aloes is Poifon to a great many brute Animals, as well as some other bitter Subftances. In Consequence of its balfamic abftergent and anti-septic Qualities, it is externally

ternally used for the Cure of Wounds, extracted with Spirit of Wine in the Form of a Tincture, to which is generally added a due Quantity of the Tincture of Myrrh and Amber. 'Tis certain that its balsamic Virtue is so great, that Animalcules may be preserved in it for Ages, upon which Account it is used in embalming human Bodies. It is good against Worms, both internally and externally, so that anthelminthic Pills and Plaisters are prepared of it. As it has been observed that the purgative and resolvent Quality of Aloes is lodged principally in its gummy Part, and its balsamic Virtues in its resinous Principle, hence 'tis obvious, that the lucid succotrine Aloes is most proper for purging internally, whereas the hepatic Aloes is best accommodated for external, and chirurgical Purposes. Hence if the purgative Quality of Aloes is desired alone, it must be dissolved, and the filtrated Solution, evaporated to the Consistence of an Extract, which is called *prepared or washed Aloes.*

The *Barbadoes* Aloes is by some said to be procured from the *Aloe,* Offic. *Aloe Vulgaris, sive sempervivum Marinum,* Ger. Emac. The Horse-aloes from the *Aloe Guineensis Caballina, vulgari Similis sed tota Maculata.* Commel. Prælud. Bot. And the succotrine Aloes from the *Aloe Succotrina,* Offic. *Aloe Succotrina Angustifolia Spinosa Flore Purpureo,* Breyn. Prod.

An Extract and a Resin are ordered to be made from Aloes in the New Dispensatory; and it is an Ingredient in the *Extractum Catharticum.* The *Vinum Aloeticum Alcalinum.* The *Tinctura Sacra.* The *Balsamum Traumaticum, Elixir Aloes, Hiera Picra, Pil. Aromat. Pil. e Colocynthide cum Aloe,* and the *Pil. Rufi.*

Alsine, Offic. *Alsine minor,* Park. Theat. *Alsine Media,* Boerh. Ind.

A. *Alsine minor five media,* Ger. Emac. Chickweed. It grows in watery Places, by the Sides of Hedges and Paths. The Herb is in Use: It refrigerates and moistens, and has the Virtues of Pellitory of the Wall, only it has no Astringency. It is reckoned nutritive, and therefore a wholesome Food for Persons in an Atrophy or Phthisis. It is of an herby Taste, a little saltish, its Salt resembles the Salammoniac, the distilled Water of Chickweed, or the Infusion of it in Wine, restores those who are emaciated, after long Diseases. *Shroder* commends it for the Phthisic. It is good for Convulsions in Children, and they give a Dram of its Root for the Epilepsy. Its Powder being laid on the Piles, stops their immoderate Flux, and assuages the Pain. Its Juice is vulnerary and detersive, good to cleanse the Mouth, and take away Inflammations. This Herb put into an Omelette instead of Parsley is good for Spitting of Blood. Applied to the Breasts, it dissolves curdled Milk.

Althæa. This is the *Althæa Bismalva, Ibiscus,* Offic. *Althæa Dioscoridis & Plinii,* C. B. Boerh. Ind. Alt. *Althea Vulgaris,* Park. Marsh-mallows. It grows in Salt Marshes and maritime Places, flowering in the Months of *July* and *August,* producing Seeds in *September* and *October.* The whole Plant contains a Juice, which is glutinous, highly soft, free from all Acrimony, and proper where there is an excessive Exsiccation, Rigidity, or Contraction of the Fibres; or where there is an Acrimony, or too violent a Motion of the Blood. We use the Leaves or Herb, which is one of the five emollient Herbs, the Flowers, the Seeds, and most frequently the Root, because it is more mucilaginous than the other Parts. These are all used both internally and externally, mally, in Decoctions, Clyfters, Balfams, Fomentations, Cataplafms, Ointments, and Plaifters, whenever the Intention is to mollify, mitigate, and allay. In preparing Decoctions for internal Ufe, the Marfh-mallows is to be added towards the End, laft they fhould become too thick and glutinous. The Plant is moft commended in violent Diforders of the Breaft and Kidneys, as in an Heat and Retention of Urine, and nephritic Colics. It is alfo an Ingredient, in pectoral Troches. *Hippocrates;* " ordered thofe who were wounded or afflicted with Thirft in Confequence of a Defect of Blood, to drink the Juice of boiled Marfh-mallows, and the Plant itfelf to be applied with Honey and Refin to Contufions, Luxations, and Tumors, whether in the Joints, or in mufcular, or nervous Parts. He alfo ordered afthmatic and dyfenteric Patients to drink this Plant in Wine." The Root of this Plant is alfo prefcribed to be chewed in the difficult Dentition of Infants. It is alfo ufed for rubbing the Teeth, in order to cleanfe them, but in order to difguife, it is tinged with a red Colour, by boiling it with red Sanders and Alum, or with red Wine. Sometimes the Mucilage of the Roots and Seeds is ufed; for which Purpofe thefe two Parts of the Plant are macerated in Water to become glutinous, then the Mucilage is expreffed thro' a linnen Cloth, and has a proper Quantity of Sugar mixed with. The external Ufe of this Preparation, is highly efficacious in Fiffures of the Nipples, and Womens Breafts, and all other Excoriations. *Carnufert* is of Opinion, that the fmall Ulcers appearing on the *Penis* of Men labouring under the Stone after the Application of the Root of this Plant bruifed and boiled in Simple Water, is not owing to the acrimonious, but rather to the emollient Nature of Marfh-mallows, by which Means an Afflux of the acrid Humours is procured to the relaxed Parts. It is ufed in the *Syrupus ex Althæa, Pulvis Tragacanthæ compofitus,* and the *Oleum è Mucilaginibus.*

There is alfo another Sort of *Althæa* diftinguifhed thus, *Althæa Theophrafti, flore luteo, Abutilon Avicennæ,* Yellow-Mallow. This is an annual Plant, and poffeffes the Virtues of the common Mallow.

Alypum, Offic. *Globularia fruticofa Myrti folio tridentato,* Tourn. Inft. 467. Herb Terrible. It grows on Hills flowering in the Spring; the Herb is ufed, and is faid to be a violent Purgative. According to *Clufius* the Decoction has been given with good Succefs in the Venereal Difeafe.

Allyffum, Madwort. There is one Sort of Alyffum mentioned by *Diofcorides,* another by *Pliny,* and a third by *Galen.* That of *Galen* is by *Dale,* thought to be the *Marrubium album, foliis profunde incifis, flore cæruleo* of *Morifon,* of which *Galen* informs us, that the Dofe to a Perfon bit by a mad Dog, is the twelfth Part of a Pint in a Quarter of a Pint of Water and Mulfum, for forty Days together, from the firft Day. The fame Author afferts, that it is of a moderately drying and degeftive Quality, and fomewhat aftringent, for which Reafon it clears the Skin from the Vitiligo and Sunburns.

The Alyffum of *Pliny, Dale* takes to be the *Mollugo vulgatior* of *Parkinfon* or Baftard Madder. This according to *Pliny,* prevents the Madnefs arifing from the Bite of a mad Dog, if it is drank in Vinegar, and a Portion of it bound about the Part affected.

The

The *Alyssum* of *Dioscorides* according to *Dale* is the *Alyssum incanum Serpilli Folio Minus*; *Thlaspi alysson dictum Campestre minus*, C. B. or lesser Madwort. The Decoction of this drank, is by *Dioscorides* said to cure those Hiccups which are not accompanied with a Fever. It has the same Effect if held in the Hand or smelled to; bruised with Honey it cures Freckles and Sun-burning. When pounded and eaten with Food, it is thought to cure the Bite of a mad Dog.

There is also an Alyssum distinguished thus. *Alysson vulgare, Polygoni folio, caule Nudo*, T. 217. *Bursa Pastoris Minor loculo oblonga*, C. B. Pin. This and the *Alysson vulgare, Polygoni folio, loculo rotundo* are known by the Name of Whitlow-grass, and are possessed of the same Virtues with Scurvy-grass, and Water-cresses.

There is another Alysum thus distinguished, *Alysson Segetum, foliis auriculatis acutis, Myagrum Sativum*, C. B. Pin. Corn Mad-wort with auriculated sharp pointed Leaves; and another thus, *Alysson Segetum foliis auriculatis acutis fructu majori*, Corn Mad-wort with auriculated sharp pointed Leaves and a larger Fruit. These two last are called the *German* Sesamums, and the Myagra of the Shops. Bruised and drank to the Weight of three Ounces, they are sudorific and stomachic, and an excellent Remedy against cold Disorders.

Alysson montanum incanum luteum Serpilli folio majus, Thlaspi montanum luteum Serpilli folio majus, C. B. Pin. This according to *Lemery* is esteemed aperient and good against the Bite of a mad Dog. There are various other Species of the Alyssum mentioned by *Boerhaave*, all of which are endowed with a very subtile penetrating and diaphoretic Virtue by which they expel Poison.

Amaranthus flos Amoris, Offic. *Amaranthus maximus*, Boerh. Ind. A. Flower gentle. It is cultivated in Gardens, and flowers in *August*. The Flowers only are used, which both cool and dry; they are moderately astringent, and therefore used in all Fluxions, Spitting of Blood, Diarrhæas, Dysenteries, and Uterine Fluxes.

Ambrosia, Offic. *Ambrosia hortensis*, Park. Oak of Cappadocia. With us it is cultivated in Gardens. The Herb is used, which is esteemed of a repressing and repellent Quality. *Galen* says it is astringent. The Plant is of a most agreeable Scent, and abounds with heating and aromatic Virtues, and is therefore classed among the Cardiacs and Cephalics.

Ammi, Bishops-weed. Of this there are two Species, the antient and the modern, the latter of which is thus distinguish'd, *Ammi Vulgare*, Offic. Ger. Raii Hist. *Ammi Majus*, C. B. Pin. Boerh. Ind. Alt. Common Bishops weed This Plant is cultivated in Gardens, flowers in *June*, and *July*, and decays after it has perfected its Seed, which is the only Part of the Plant in Use. The Seeds are of a drying warming Nature, and consequently good to expel Wind and prevent the Colic. They are also diuretic and excite a menstrual Discharge.

The Ammi of *Dioscorides*, or that of the Antients is thus distinguished, *Ammi verum*, Offic. *Ammi Creticum*, Ger. *Ammi alterum semine apii* C. B. Pin. True Bishops-weed, by some called the *Ethiopian* Cummin but the Seed of this Herb, is much less than Cummin-seed, and of the Taste of Origanum. The Seed of this Plant come from *Alexandria*, and *Crete*, they are of a aromatic, heating Nature, and are greatly extolled against Difficulty of Urine, and the Bites of venomous Animals; for which Re fon it is they are an Ingredient in the *Theriaca* ; they are, alfo, recommended for exciting the menftrual Difcharge, but efpecially for removing Sterility in Women, and curing the *Fluor albus*. *Diofcorides* in *Lib.* 3. *Cap.* 70. informs us, that if mixed with Veficatories of Cantharides, thefe Seeds prevent the Strangury generally excited on fuch Occafions, and that applied with Honey, they take off the livid Marks of Blows on the Face.

Amomum. According to the learned *Salmafius*, there is fo great Variety of Opinions with Refpect to this, that 'tis hardly poffible for a Man to fix his Judgment ; fince *Pliny* affirms that Amomum is extreamly brittle and friable, whereas *Diofcorides* afferts, that it is foft to the Touch. The former gives it the Leaves of the Pomegranate Tree, and the latter thofe of Briony. So that amidft fo great Uncertainty, we fhall not pretend to Infallibility, but give the moft approved Accounts of the two Species of Amomum moft in ufe. The firft of thefe then is thus diftinguifhed, *Amomum*, Offic. *Amomum verum*, Raii Hift. *Amomum maximum*, Park. Theat. *Amomum racemofum*, C. B. Pin. True Amomum. The Tree on which this grows, and which is called the Amomum-tree, has Leaves which are long, ftrait, and of a pale green Colour. Its Flowers refemble thofe of the white Stock Gilly-flower. Its Fruit is pretty like the Mufcadine Grape in Colour, Bulk and Shape ; it is not fo full of Grains, and is fo juicy. Its Pods, which have Pedicles, are crowded together, and glued as it were, on a long Nerve, which they furround to the very Top, and which ferves as a Support to them. In the inner Side of thefe Pods, are found purple coloured Grains of an almoft fquare Fi-

gure, diftinct and covered with flender white Membranes. The Tafte of thefe Grains is fharp and acrid, whilft their Smell is extremely penetrating and aromatic. The neweft Amomum is always beft, and ought to have its Pods round, of a whitifh flaxen Colour, whereas that whofe Pods are black or fhriveled, is little or not at all efteemed. The Fruit of this Tree, is an Ingredient in the *Theriaca*, and is fometimes mixed with ftrong Purgatives, in order to qualify and mitigate them. It is alfo accounted carminative, alexipharmic, and ftomachic. According to *Lemery*, it is inciding, digeftive, refifts Poifons, difperfes Wind, ftrengthens the Stomach, creates Appetite and Strength, and provokes the Menfes.

Another *Amomum* is thus diftinguifhed, *Amomum*, Offic. *Sifon*, Mor. *Sifon five Officinarum Amomum*, Raii Hift. *Sifon quod Amomum Officinis Noftris*, C. B. Pin. Boer. Ind. Alt. Baftard Stone Parfley. It grows in Ditches, Banks, and moift Places, flowers in Summer, and in *Auguft* bears ripe Seeds, which are the only Parts of it ufed. Thefe Seeds are hot, dry, attenuating and good for removing Obftructions and cleanfing the Kidneys from Gravel. They are alfo diuretic, emmenagogue, and alexipharmic, for which laft Quality they are fometimes put into the *Theriaca Andromachi*, as a Succedaneum to the true Amomum.

Amoris Pomum, Offic. Ger. *Pomum majus amoris fructu Rubro*, Park. *Solanum Pomiferum fructu rotundo, Striato Molli*, C. B. Pin. Raii Hift. *Lycoperficon Galeni*. Boerhaav. Ind. Alt. Love Apples. It is fown in Gardens, and flowers in *July*. The Fruit is ripe in *September*, and perifhes with the firft Frofts. In *Italy* the Love Apples are eaten with Oil and Vinegar as Cucumbers are in *England*. They are fometimes ufed externally

R

ternally in cooling and moistening Applications for Inflammations and an Eryfipelas. The Juice is by fome greatly commended in hot Defluxions of Rheum upon the Eyes. But in general it is fo little ufed, that it deferves no further Notice to be taken of its Diftinctions and Virtues.

Amygdalus amara & dulcis, Offic. J. B. *Amygdalus fativa,* C. B. Raii. Hift. *Amygdalus fativa, fructu majore,* Boerhaav. Ind. Alt. The Almondtree. They grow fpontaneoufly in the warmer Climates, as *Spain, Barbary, Italy,* and *France*; they flower early in the Spring, and the Fruit is ripe in *Auguft.* Sometimes Trees which before bore Sweet Almonds, begin to bear thofe of the bitter Kind; whilft thofe laft often bear Sweet Almonds, if tranfplanted into a better Soil, or cultivated with more Care. Bitter Almonds, prove mortal to many Animals, Quadrupeds, and Birds. In Storks, Doves, Cats, and Dogs, they excite Convulfions, as is obvious from the Experiments recounted in *Wepfer de Cicut. Aquat. Bonet. Sepulchr. Anatom.* and *Eph. Nat. Curiof. Dec.* 3. *An.* 1. *Obf.* 156. But to Mankind they afford a proper Medicine on many Occafions, tho' they are rarely eaten on Account of their Bitternefs. They are of a ftimulating detergent, aperient, and diuretic Quality. *Hoffman ad Poter.* fpeaks of them in the following Manner: " I cannot fufficiently re-" commend the Ufe of bitter Al-" monds, for preventing the Gene-" ration of the Stone, if three or four " of them are eaten every Morning. " It is hardly credible how benefi-" cial they are in calculous Difpo-" fitions, fince they expel the U-" rine, and eliminate the Sand, " which is the Element of the Stone, " as I have found from frequent " Experience." Many recommend them before drinking, in order to

prevent Intoxication, after the Example of the Emperor *Claudius. Simeon Sethi* tells us, " that in Confe-" quence of their attenuating Quality, " they are proper for removing Ob-" ftructions of the Liver and Spleen, " and diffolve Stones of the Bladder " and Kidneys. It is alfo faid, that if " a Perfon eats them fafting, he will " not be drunk that Day." But this laft Affertion is by *Brown* in his Vulgar Errors fhewn to be falfe. Oil of Bitter Almonds expels the Urine, becaufe it opens the Paffages and relaxes the fpafmodically conftricted Parts; for which Reafon it is alfo accounted a carminative Medicine, whether taken by the Mouth or injected by the Anus. It operates more powerfully than Oil of Sweet Almonds, becaufe it is of a more penetrating Quality. Hence *Schulzius in Praelect.* tells us, that " it is refolvent and difcutient. It is " dropt into the Ears of thofe afflic-" ted with a ringing and humming " Noife. It is alfo applied to the " Pubes in Retentions of Urine, " with Lilly Roots, and Honey; it is " commended for removing Freckles " and Afperites of the Skin." In the Diforders of the Ears, it proves effectual, if they proceed from impacted Sordes, which generally happen to thofe who remain long in the Cold, and among Duft. But we are by no Means to ufe it in too large a Quantity, left by that Means, the *Tympanum* fhould be preternaturally relaxed, which greatly injures the Hearing; for which Reafon fome mix with it a fmall Quantity of Spirit of Wine, in order to diminifh its relaxing Quality. *Diofcorides* tells us, of the Gum of the Tree, " that it is heating and aftringent; " beneficial to thofe who vomit " Blood, if drank in a proper Li-" quor; and fit for removing an " Impetigo, if ufed as an Ointment " with Vinegar. It alfo cures an " inveterate

" inveterate Cough, if drank in " weak Wine." The judicious *Hoffman* tells us, " that the Gum is a- " stringent, so that it is hardly pro- " bable that it can break the Stone, " tho' it may, like Gum-arabic, so " incrustate the pain'd Parts, as that " they may not feel the Force of " the Gravel or Sand. By the same " Means also it affords Relief in sa- " line Defluxions. It also restores " the Tone of the Kidneys." Bitter Almonds are much used as a Cosmetic, in order to beautify the Hands, and render them white. An Oil of Bitter Almonds is directed in the last College Dispensatory.

Sweet Almonds if recent, are of a grateful Taste, especially if macerated in Water, and freed from the Membrane which covers them. They abound with an oleous Juice, are nutritive, and fit for making Emulsions. The Oil of recent Sweet Almonds, is highly temperate, and proper both internally and external-ly, in all Cases where Acrimony is to be corrected, Rigidity softened, or Stricture relaxed. Hence they are with great Advantage prescribed in Emulsions for emaciated, hectic, and pleuritic Patients. The unripe Fruit before the Shells are hard, if boiled in Water, and prescribed in Sugar, rouse and restore the Strength of sick Persons. The expressed Oil of Sweet Almonds is an excellent In-gredient in lenitive and emollient Liniments, and Ointments. It is, also, highly beneficial for internal Purposes; for as we are informed by *Hoffman in Tr. de Remed. Domest.* if any one has swallowed an acrid caustic Poison, it so lubricates the Sto-mach, as to prevent the Effects of the Poison, if it is taken immediately after. It is, also, an excellent Anti-spasmodic and Sedative, if exhibited to those afflicted with griping Fluxes. In Hoarseness, Coughs, Asthmas, Pthisics, and all Disorders of the

Breast, it is highly beneficial; espe-cially if mixed with Sperma Ceti, and Sugar Candy. A few Spoon-fuls of this Oil, exhibited in Broth prepared with Flesh, are highly ser-viceable in spasmodic Colics, in vio-lent gravel Pains, and in those Gripes, which generally accompany a Suppression of the *Lochia*. An Oil is ordered to be expressed from Sweet Almonds, which is a prin-cipal Ingredient in the *Sapo A-mygdalinus* of the New Dispensato-ry. That Oil of Almonds is best which is white, pellucid, and expres-sed a little before it is used. Some Authors assert, that Oil of Bitter Al-monds keeps longer free from Cor-ruption, than that of the sweet Kind. Sweet Almonds are a principal In-gredient in the *Emulsio Communis*:

Amylum. Starch. This is a Drug well known to every one, on Account of its domestic Uses. It is made of Wheat macerated in Water, till it is soft, and then the white Pulp is pressed out, and dry'd. *Dioscorides* says it is good for Rheums of the Eyes, hollow Ulcers, and Pustules; that it stops Vomiting of Blood, and mollifies the Parts about the *Aspera Arteria*, taken in Milk, or with o-ther Food. *Oribasius* recommends a sorbile Liquor, that is a Decoc-tion of Starch in Water, in a Fe-ver attended with a *Diarrhœa*; he farther says it is excellent in a Dysentery, taken either in Milk, Water, or alone. And I believe Ex-perience confirms what he advances. *Clutton,* in a Treatise on Fevers, lays great Stress on a Solution of Starch, given by way of Clyster, in a Diarrhœa, accompanied with a Fe-ver, or without one; and advises to make the Confection of Starch very thick, and to add to four Oun-ces of this, one of *French* Brandy. In boiling, *Oribasius* directs ten Drams of Starch, in four Pints of Water.

Anacar-

Anacardium, Offic. Ger. *Arbor, Indica fructu cordide, cortice pulvinato, nuclium unicum, nullo officulo tectum claudente;* Raii Hist. The Anacardium or Malacca Bean-tree. The oriental Anacardium is a Seed growing at the Top of a conical East *India* Fruit. It is in Shape and Colour like a Bird's Heart, covered with a tough Skin including a spongy Substance, full of an hot caustic Oil underneath, in which inclosed in another Skin lies the Kernel, which tastes like an Almond. *Matthiolus ad Dioscorid. & Boerhaave in Instit. Med.* reckon *Anacardiums* among the Class of Poisons, which are manifestly acrid. Others account them highly beneficial to the Brain and Memory. Some call the Confection of Anacardiums the *Confection of Wise Men.* But others, with better Reason, think that it ought to be call'd the Confection of Fools, because the Use of it brings on Madness; as we are informed by *Schulzius in Prælect.* The inspissated Juice of Anacardiums is recommended externally for dissipating hard Tumors. Some also order it to be exhibited internally, for cold and moist Disorders of the Brain. But all the Preparations of Anacardiums, are justly now disused in the Shops, because they are unsafe.

There is also an occidental Anacardium thus distinguished, *Anacardium occidentale* Jons Dendr. *Acajou.* Boerh. Ind. Alt. The Cajou or Cassu-tree. This in Form and Bulk resembles a Hare's Kidney; the Out-side is covered with a tough ash-coloured Bark. It contains a large Quantity of caustic burning Oil, and under that in a soft Shell, a white pleasant Kernel. The caustic Oil is good for curing Warts and Corns. The Fruit is said to be proper for removing Freckles and Sun-burn from the Face, but Women ought not to use it during Menstruation,

because at that Time it often produces an Erysipelas, which however may be removed by a Wash prepared of Brandy and Water.

Anagallis. There are three Species of this Plant used in Medicine. The *Anagallis mas, fæmina,* and *aquatica.* The first of these is thus distinguished, *Anagallis terrestris mas,* Offic. *Anagallis mas,* Raii Hist. *Anagallis flore Phœniceo,* C. B. Pin. Boerhaave Ind. Alt. Male Pimpernel. It flowers in *May* and *June,* and is to be found in Corn Fields.

The second is the *Anagallis terrestris fæmina,* Offic. *Anagallis fæmina,* Raii Synop. *Anagallis cæruleo flore,* Boerhaav. Ind. Alt. Female Pimpernel. The Virtues of both these Species are nearly the same. The whole of this Plant is greatly celebrated; for a Decoction of it drank, is not only commended against the Plague, the Bites of a Viper, and mad Dog, but has also been found a Specific in Madness, after the previous Exhibition of an Emetic. When boiled to a Cataplasm with Urine, it is said to afford great Relief in the Gout. It is, also, asserted, that it is beneficial in stopping Hemorrhages of all Kinds; thus 'tis said to stop immoderate Fluxes of the Menses, when suspended on the Pit of the Stomach, and to stop the Discharge of Blood from a Vein, if held in the Hand till it becomes warm. The Herb is acrid, and acts by stimulating the Vessels and resolving the Humours, like a true Soap possessed of a subastringent Quality. Hence its Juice is proper where the Purposes of Abstersion are to be pursued, in the Scurvy, and atrabiliarious Disorders; so that if it cures Maniacs, it produces its Effect by resolving and fusing the thick and viscid Humours. If it is beneficial

ficial againſt the Plague, and the Bites of venomous Animals, it muſt be on Account of its reſolvent and abſtergent Qualities. Hence the Reaſon is obvious, why its Decoction, or expreſſed Juice, with Honey, are beneficial in removing Dimneſs of the Sight, becauſe it is reſolvent, aperient, and procures free Paſſages to the ſtagnant Humour, if it is not too deeply impacted, in which Caſe more powerful Remedies are hardly of any Efficacy. The Decoction of the Plant is recommended for provoking the Menſes, becauſe it is of a reſolvent Quality.

The third Species is the *Anagallis aquatica, Becabunga,* Offic. *Anagallis aquatica minor, folio, ſubrotundo,* C. B. Pin. *Veronica aquatica major, folio Subrotundo,* Boerh. Ind. Alt. Brook-lime. It grows in Rills, and Ditches of running Water, flowers in *June,* and retains the Leaves all Winter. The whole Plant is uſed; and is a good deobſtruent and antiſcorbutic, abounding with volatile Parts; very good for the Scurvy, and therefore uſed as an Ingredient in the antiſcorbutic Juices and Dietdrinks. It is alſo deterſive, cleanſing, and uſeful in Obſtructions of the Kidneys, by Gravel or ſlimy Humours, as alſo for the Stone and Dropſy.

Anagyris, Offic. *Anagyris fœtida,* Ger. Boerh. Ind. A. Stinking Bean Trefoil. This is a Shrub which grows in warm Countries, the Leaves of which are ſaid to be reſolutive, and the Seeds emetic.

Ananas. The Pine Apple. This Fruit is now pretty commonly known, being much cultivated in the Gardens of the Curious, at a conſiderable Expence. It grows ſpontaneouſly in the warmer Parts of the *Eaſt* and *Weſt Indies,* and is a moſt delicious Fruit. It is eſteemed cordial, and analeptic;

and is ſaid to raiſe and exhilarate the Spirits, to cure a Nauſea, and provoke Urine. But 'tis ſubject to cauſe a Miſcarriage, for which Reaſon Women with Child ſhould abſtain from it.

Anchuſa. There are various Species of this Plant, mentioned by Botaniſts, but the moſt conſiderable is that thus diſtinguiſhed, *Anchuſa,* Offic. Chab. *Anchuſa puniceis floribus,* C. B. Pin. Boerh. Ind. Alt. *Bugloſſum perenne minus, puniceis floribus,* Hiſt. Oxon. *Alkanet.* This Plant grows ſpontaneouſly in *Languedock, Italy,* and *Spain.* It is alſo found in the warmer Parts of *Germany,* but the beſt is that of *Conſtantinople,* from whence its Roots are brought, almoſt as thick and as long as a Perſon's Arm, compoſed as it were of long, broad, and contorted Leaves, of an obſcure red Colour, intermixed with a little Violet and White. The Root was formerly more uſed than at preſent, eſpecially in Decoctions, where Aſtringents were judged proper in Diarrhœas and Hemorrhages, and externally to dry Wounds. When infuſed in Petroleum, it is recommended by *Ray in Hiſt. Plant.* to be uſed by Way of Ointment in recent Wounds and Punctures. It is more frequently uſed by Dyers, and was in early Times employed by the Inhabitants of the Eaſtern Countries, to tinge the Nails with a red Colour, as is obvious from the Nails of the Mummies which are always red, as we are informed in *Eph. Nat. Curioſ. Decad.* 2. *An.* 6. In *Spain* it is ſtill uſed for painting the Face, and tinging Wax and Oil. Apothecaries uſe it to colour their Ointments, but for this Purpoſe it muſt be boiled in Oil; becauſe it does not readily give a Tincture to Water.

Androſace annua, ſpuria, Ger. *Androſace vulgaris latifolia, annua,* Boerh.

Boerh. Ind. Alt. Summer Navel Wort. It grows in maritime Places, amongst Corn, and in Woods, and is esteemed aperitive, good for Retention of the Urine, for the Dropsy, and Gout.

Androsæmum, Offic. *Androsæmum maximum frutescens*, Boer. Ind. Alt. Tutsan, or Park Leaves. It grows in Hedges and Thickets, and flowers in *July* and *August*. The Flowers, Leaves, and Seeds are used, which agree in Virtues with those of the *Hypericum*, being vulnerary, and resolvent, both internally and externally used.

Anemone. Of this Plant there are two Species used in Medicine. The *Anemone Hortensis*, Offic. Garden Anemone. And the *Anemone Sylvestris*, Offic. Wild Anemone. Both are esteemed detersive, inciding, vulnerary, and drying, but are too acrimonious for internal Use, and therefore only employed externally.

Anemonoides Flore albo, Boerh. Ind. Alt. *Anemone Nemorum alba*, Ger. Wood Anemone. This Plant is hot acrimonious, and will raise Blisters on the Skin.

Anethum, Offic. Ger. Raii. Hist. *Anethum hortense*, C.B. Pin. Boerh. Ind. A. Dill. It is sown in Gardens, and if permitted, renews itself annually by the Seeds which fall from it. *Hippocrates, in lib. 2. de Diæta* informs us, " that Dill is hot, produces Co- " stiveness, and when smelled to, " stops Sneezing." The Moderns affirm, that Dill is possessed of a somniferous Quality, for which Reason this Plant is often suspended in the Beds of those who cannot sleep. With some 'tis also customary to place a Decoction of Dill, in the beds of sick Persons, after they are closely covered with Canopies, or enclosed with Curtains, as we are informed by *Simon Pauli* in *Quadripartit. Botan. Bruyer in lib. 8. c. 29.*

informs us, that the Ancients in their Feasts, used to crown themselves with Dill in order to procure Sleep. This Plant is of an aromatic, volatile, and vaporous Nature, for which Reason, when smelled to for a considerable Time, its Exhalations may fill the Head, and induce Sleep, as is also observed of Saffron, in which, however, this Quality is stronger. That the Steam of its Decoction should promote Sleep, is by no Means surprising; since the Steam of Water alone removes the Causes of Watching, such as excessive Dryness, Acrimony, and an accelerated Motion of the Fluids, arising from a Stricture of the Solids, as we are informed by *Boerhaave in Institut. Med.* As Dill is possessed of an aromatic Quality, it will stimulate the Solids, and consequently rouse the Stomach, which when corroborated will digest the Aliments better. Hence arises the greater Quantity of Chyle, and consequently an Increase of Milk in Nurses. The common People are sufficiently acquainted with this Virtue of Dill; since they mix it with the Food of Cows, in order to increase their Milk. Dill is, perhaps, better against Flatulences than most other Aromatics; because its Acrimony is temperated by a large Admixture of an oleous Principle. For this Reason it is a laudable Custom to pickle Cucumbers with the Umbels or Tops of Dill. Since, therefore, Dill is of an aromatic heating, corroborating, discutient, and consequently resolvent Quality, the Reason is obvious why a Decoction of it is useful for exciting Urine and removing the Strangury, and Dysentery; especially when proceeding from Coldness and Relaxation. Hence we find a Decoction of Dill in a sufficient Quantity of Water and Oil, greatly recommended against the Iliac Passion, arising

from

from an Induration of the Feces. It is easy to conceive, that an Hiccup arising from a cold Cause, may be suppressed by smelling Dill. Whatever Effects the Plant performs, when reduced to Ashes, are owing to the Acrimony of these Ashes. But the Ashes of the Roots, are more acrid than those of the Seeds; because the former have a smaller Quantity of Oil mixed with them. The excessive Use of it is said to procure Sterility, and render the Sight dull, which Effects it produces by heating and drying, as all other hot Substances do. The Herb or its Tops, are at present most frequently used in Clysters against flatulent Colics, but rarely in Decoctions for internal Use. The Seeds are preferable to the Tops, because the former are more aromatic, and may be kept for three Years, tho' they are the better to be renewed every Year. The Root is not at present prescribed. In *Ephemer. Nat. Curios. Decad.* 2. *An.* 1. *Obs.* 146. we have an Account of the surprising antaphrodisiac Effect of Dill Water; for a certain Man after a Fall, finding his Arm seized with a Kind of Atrophy, washed it frequently with this Water, from which he preceived considerable Relief; but at the same Time observed Impotency brought on, which was not removed till he desisted from the Use of the Water. Oil of Dill is mixed with Ointments and Plaisters, of an emollient, discutient, and resolvent Nature. It is, also, added to emollient and carminative Clysters, and is properly used as an Ointment for the Temples, in a Cephalalgia, and in order to procure Sleep. *Simeon Sethi* informs us, " that it alleviates Inflammations, " procures Sleep, and maturates " crude Humours; when used as " an Ointment, it also, discusses

" Flatulences of the Abdomen, and " proves beneficial to those who " are fatigued with hard Labour; " but some affirm, that it is injurious to the Kidneys." The Oil obtained from the Seeds, is an excellent Remedy, especially in *Eleosaccharums*, against Flatulences of the Stomach. An essential Oil is directed by the College, to be drawn from the Seeds; and a Water,

Angelica. Botanists enumerate various Species of this Plant, but that most used in Medicine is thus distinguished, *Angelica*, Offic. *Angelica Sativa*, C. B. Pin. Raii Hist. Boerh-Ind. Alt. Angelica. It flowers and produces Seeds in *June* and *July*, the Root perishing after the ripening of the Seeds, which is the second Year. This is a Plant of an highly penetrating and aromatic Nature; its Seeds and Roots are in a particular Manner resolvent and stimulating, and consequently sudorific, alexipharmic, and proper to expel the pestilental Poison by Sweat. The Root is thought best, which when chewed, has the Taste and Smell of Ambergrease and Musk mixed together, and spreads a Kind of penetrating Gratefulness all over the Mouth, without exciting any Inflammation. Hence an Infusion or a gentle Decoction of it, is commended against a fetid Breath, and when used in the same Manner, it is said to be beneficial in Coughs arising from Cold, or a viscid Mucus; because it renders Respiration more free and easy. From what has been said we may know, why the whole Plant is classed among the carminative Medicines, and for what Reason some recommend a Dram of its dried Powder, taken with Wine, or Rob of Elder, in intermittent Fevers. In Medicine the Root is more frequently used than the Seeds, whilst the Leaves are entirely neglected,

glected. According to *Valent. Muf.* Wormwood keeps the recent Root free from Rottenness. The Root macerated in Vinegar, is in the Plague reckoned a great Preservative by many, who keep a Piece of it in their Mouths, when they go to visit the Infected. The Root and Stalks preserved answer the same Intention, and a Confection of the Seeds is highly proper for those who would guard against the Injuries of a malignant Air. The Water distilled from the Roots and Seeds of Angelica, contains the volatile Parts of the Plant, is gently stimulating and diaphoretic, and may be properly used as a Vehicle for many Remedies. It is externally ordered against the Bites of venomous Animals, and some recommend it as an Ointment to be used by those afflicted either with the Gout, or Ischiadic Pains. *Bauhine* informs us from *Dodonæus*, that the Inhabitants of some of the northern Countries, eat the Stalks after taking the Bark off them, by which Means they are rendered very grateful and well tasted. The Inhabitants of *Lapland*, according to *Linnæus*, chew the Roots instead of Tobacco, and use them against a violent Species of Cholic, which rages among them. It is an Ingredient in the *Aqua Alexiteria simplex*, the *Aqua Alexiteria Spirituosa*, the *Aqua Alexiteria Spirituosa cum Aceto*, and the *Aq. Sem. Anisi Composita*.

Another Species of Angelica is the *Angelica Sylvestris*, Offic. *Angelica Sylvestris major*, Boerh. Ind. Alt. The Virtues of this are esteemed the same as those of the former, but weaker.

A third is the *Angelica Sylvestris minor, seu erratica.* Boerh. Ind. Alt. *Herba Gerardi*, Offic. Ger. *Podagraria vulgaris*, Park. It flowers in June and July, and is much recommended for the Gout.

A fourth is the *Angelica Scandiaca, Archangelica Tabernæmontani, quæ Umbella est flava, Semine rotundiore,* Boerh. Ind. Alt. This agrees in Virtues with the former.

Anisum, Offic. Ger. *Anisum Herbariis*, C. B. Pin. *Apium Anisum dictum, Semine Suaveolente*, Boerh. Ind. Alt. Anise. It flowers and bears Seeds in *July*, the Root dying every Year after it has yielded the Seeds. It is cultivated in *Germany*, but the best Seeds, which are of a smaller Size, come from *Spain*. Those Seeds are best, which when chewed remove a fetid Breath, and render it agreeable. On Account of their aromatic Qualities, they are used in Cases where Flatulencies are to be discussed, and the Stomach corroborated. In Consequence also of their aromatic Nature, they are recommended as a Stimulus to Venery, as good for provoking Urine, procuring Milk to Nurses, stopping the *Fluor albus*, and Diarrhœas arising from Relaxation and an unactive Mucus. In Disorders of the Breast arising from Refrigeration, they are proper for resolving the viscid and tenacious Matter. In purging Medicines, especially Infusions of Senna, they are used to prevent Gripes. As by Means of their aromatic Nature, they heat the Body, they are placed among the four greater hot Seeds. Hence *Pliny* was in the right when he said, they procured an Appetite. In Medicine they are used in Infusions and in Powders; many, both for the agreeable Taste, and in order to avoid too great a Relaxation of the Stomach, by the warm Water, put them into Coffee and Tea, which thus prepared, afford Relief in cold Disorders of the Breast and Stomach, to such as are not accustomed

ed

ed to thefe Liquors. Powder of Anifeeds with Crab's Eyes, is very properly exhibited to Children, a-gainft a peccant Acid in the *Primæ viæ*; as alfo to Nurfes, for the fame Intention. *Heurnius in Comment. in lect. 3. Aph. 24. Hippocrat.* fays, ' for Gripes in Children generally ' give a Scruple of Anifeeds, pow-' dered grofly in the firft Spoonful ' of their Pap, by which they are ' purged in the fame Manner as A-' dults are by Rhubarb; " for by refolving the Mucus, and ftimulating he Fibres, they expel that which eing impacted in the fmall Inteſ-ines, had produced the Gripes and flatulences. *Pliny* affirmed, that A-nife was ufelefs to the Stomach, xcept when inflated, becaufe it would prove too hot and drying, ftimulate the Fibres, and throw the Humours into Commotions. Diftilſ-ed Oil of Anife, contains the moft excellent Virtues of the Seeds; it highly penetrating and proves urminative, if the Abdomen is a-ointed with it. In order to expel Urine, it is alfo applied to the Re-ion of the Kidneys, and the Pubes. The Subtilty of this Oil is obvious rom this, that two Drops of it will convey the Tafte and Smell of A-nife, to a large Veffel full of Wa-ter. The beft is that which is white, fwims upon Water, and in a moſ-trate Cold is concreted like *Sperma-ceti*, but again becomes fluid by a gentle Heat. An effential Oil is rdered to be drawn from the Seeds. is a principal Ingredient in the *Sem. Anifi Compofita*, and en-rs the Compofition of the Mithri-te, and *Theriaca Andromachi*.

Anonis, Ononis Arefta, Bovis, Offic. *onis Spinofa flore purpureo,* C. B. n. Raü Hift. Boerhaave. Ind. Alt. llharrow. It grows in wafte rounds and by the Road fide, wering in *June* and *July*. The Root is one of the five fmaller ape-rient Roots, of a penetrating Tafte, and commended for its inciding, re-folvent, aperient, and diuretic Virtues. The Bark of the Root according to *Simon Pauli in Quadreport Botan,* is a powerful Medicine for diffolv-ing the Stone in the Kidneys and Bladder. The Root is ufed in De-coctions, in Cafes where Phlegm is to be incided, and a Difcharge of U-rine excited. *Scultetus* and *Matthio-lus* give us Inftances of Perfons cur-ed of a Sarcocele, by the continued Ufe of the Powder of this Root in common Broth, together with the Application of fome Topics. But neither this nor any other Remedy has hitherto been found fuch a Spe-cific in thefe Diforders, as to prevent the Neceffity of cutting, as we are informed by *Freind. Kænigius* alfo obferves, that the Root is not diure-tic in all Patients, and in moft ex-cites Cardialgias and Diforders of the Stomach. The Root boiled in Water and Vinegar, makes a Col-lution for the Mouth, highly com-mended againft Tooth-achs, and the exulcerated Gums of fcorbutic Perfons.

Anthora is thus diftinguifhed, *Aco-nitum falutiferum,* Boerh. Ind. A. *An-thora flore luteo Aconiti; Contrayerva germanica, Napellus Mcyfis.* Wholfome Woolfs-bane This Plant is extoll'd as an Alexipharmic, and an excel-lent Medicine againft the Bites of venomous Animals. The Ufe of the Root reduced to a Powder, is by fome greatly fufpected, becaufe it purges violently, and excites a Vo-miting, whilft others think that it is not the worfe upon this Account, fince the purgative and emetic Quality of Ipacacuana, does not deprive it of the Title of a fafe A-exipharmic, In fuch a Va-riety of Opinions, Experience is to decide who are in the right, and who

who in the wrong. Thus the judicious *Hoffman* tells us, " that if we " consult Experience, we find that " this Root instead of being an ex· " cellent Alexipharmic, is highly " unsafe, because it contains an " highly acrid, caustic, penetrating " Salt, which vellicates the Tongue " when tasted. —— I remember a " *Westphalian* Apothecary used to " give the bezoardic Powder, with " this Root, in a great many Cases, " in most of which it excited a vio- " lent Perturbation of the Stomach " accompanied with Heat, Thirst, " and Anxiety of the Præcordia ; for " this Root contains a caustic and " inflammatory Salt ; so that it is an " highly suspected Medicine, espe- " cially if exhibited in large Do- " ses."

Anthyllis prior, Offic. *Medicago Vulnerariæ facie hispanica*, Boerh. Ind. Alt. Sea Kidney Vetch. *Dioscorides* recommends this taken in Oxymel in an Epilepsy.

Anthyllis Leguminosa, Vulneraria, Offic. *Vulneraria Rustica,* Boerh. Ind. Alt. Kidney Vetch, or Lady's Finger. *Dioscorides* says, this Herb is good in a Difficulty of Urine, and Disorders of the Kidneys. And that both Kinds bruised, and applyed by Way of Pessary with Oil of Roses and Milk, assuage Inflammations of the Uterus, and are good Vulneraries.

Antirrhinum, Offic. *Antirrhinum Arvense majus,* Boerh. Ind. Alt. Snap Dragon, or Calves Snout. *Pliny* recommends this by Way of Pessary, with Honey, and Oil of Roses, in a Strangulation of the Uterus, (Hysterics) and Difficulty of Menstruation.

Aparine, Offic. Ger. *Aparine vulgaris,* Boerh. Ind. A. Cleavers, or Goose Grass. It grows in the Fields, especially about the Roots of Bushes, and Hedges. It is of a subtile Nature, opens, expels, purifies and dries. Boiled in Water, and drank, it removes Obstructions of the Liver and Kidneys, cures the Dysentery, and is beneficial in a simple Gonorrhœa. Its Juice, depurated and mixed with white Wine, may with Success be drank for the Dropsy. Its Juice taken in Wine, cures the Bites of venomous Animals, and also Pains of the Ears when warmed and dropped into them. The Herb itself boil'd with Salt, cures Excrescences, applied to them by Way of Plaister. Reduced to Powder, it cures Wounds and Ulcers, and stops Hæmorrhages. *Tragus* recommends its distilled Water for the Jaundice and Dysentery. It is also very efficacious in Disorders of the Kidneys. It eases racking Pains of the Breast and Hypochondria,.

Apium. The Species of this Plant most in Use, is thus distinguished, *Apium vulgare ingratius,* J. B. *Apium palustre sive* Offic. Raii Hist. *Apium palustre & apium,* Offic. C. B. Pin. Boerhaav. Ind. Alt. Smallage. It flowers and bears ripe Seeds in the Summer. It grows spontaneously in *Italy* and *Spain,* and delights in moist Places, Ditches, the Brinks of Rivulets, and the Sea Shore. When transplanted into Gardens, and carefully cultivated it becomes milder, more grateful, and is called Celery. *Hippocrates* in *Lib. de affectionib.* informs us, " that " Smallage, both boiled and crude " is diuretic, but the wild more so " than the Garden kind." The Plant itself is of an highly penetrating, aromatic, and stimulating Quality, and is therefore accounted anti-scrobutic, aphrodisiac, aperient, abstergent, and diuretic. According to *Tournefort,* it contains a large Quantity of volatile oleous Salt dis

solved

ved in a great Deal of Phlegm, d united to a confiderable Portion Earth, as alfo an urinous Spirit, d a fmall Quantity of a concret-volatile Salt. The Root is one of : five great aperient Roots, and is d both in diuretic Decoctions, and Cataplafms and Fomentations th Coriander and Vinegar, for ninifhing the Quantity of Milk in : Breafts of Women. The Water tilled from the Roots, is by the mmon People, thought excellent iinft the Dropfy. The expreffed ice of the Plant, is by fome great, recommended in intermittent Fe-rs. The Seeds which are among : four leffer hot Seeds, have the ne Virtues with the Root, but are re efficacious. Thofe who love tallage, ought not to ufe too large iantities of it; becaufe it is pre-icial, efpecially to weak and epi-tic Patients.

Aquilegia Cærulea, Ger. *Aquile-* : *Sylveftris*, C. B Pin. *Aquilegia* re *fimplici*, J. B. Raii. Hift. Co-nbines. It grows fpontaneoufly noft every where in *England*, and cultivated in Gardens on Account its Flowers, which it bears in me. The Plant is poffeffed of a mulating Quality, and confe-ently is accounted diuretic, and imenagogue. The Eruption of e Small Pox and Meafles is great-promoted, by half a Dram of e Seeds, either alone or with an mulfion prepared of Elder Flower 'ater, or a Decoction of Figs. A ram of the Seeds powdered with ffron, and mixed with Wine, is ought good againft the Jaundice, the Patient waits for a Sweat in d. Emulfions of Columbine Seeds epared with a Decoction of Grapes Figs, are by fome greatly extol-l in malignant Diforders. The eds bruifed and exhibited in Wine, e accounted good for difficult La-ars. *Camerarius* extols the Seeds,

incruftated with Sugar, as excellent againft the Cholic and Vertigo. The triturated Seeds are frequently ufed externally, for correcting the fcorbutic Putrefaction of the Gums and curing Ulcers of the Mouth and Fauces. According to *Ray* the Leaves are often ufed in Collutions and Gargarifms, intended to remove hot Diforders of the Fauces, and Afpera Arteria. In *Spain*, the In-habitants after long fafting, eat the Root, in order to expel Stones from the Kidneys. The Water diftilled from the Flowers, or from the whole Plant, is faid to remove Gripes, and expel Poifons. According to *Tourne-fort*, the Water of Columbines, is an excellent anti-fcorbutic Medicine, fit for deterging Ulcers, and for ren-dering the Gums firm, if ufed as a Collution.

Areca, Offic. The *Indian* Nut. *Areca, five faufel.* The drunken Date Tree, Ger. *five Faufel avellana In-diana verficolor.* The difcoloured fmall *Indian* Nut. This according to Mr. *Geoffroy* is the Fruit of a Spe-cies of Palm Tree produced in the *Eaft Indies.* The outward Cover-ing is of the Bulk and Shape of a Pullet's Egg, and confifts of numer-ous fine Filaments, running Length-ways from the Stalk to the Head, under which is contained the Fruit or Nut, externally of a brownifh Colour, fhaped like a Nutmeg at one End, but flattifh at the other, with a Kind of Navel towards one Side. Within it is white, and like a Nutmeg marbled with purplifh Veins; but it is of very little Tafte. The *Indians* chew this Nut wrapt up in a Petel-leaf, in order to affift Di-geftion, and ftrengthen the Gums, as we are informed by *Kæmpfer.* When frefh, it is gently aftringent, and of this Fruit is made that Ex-tract which in the Shops is called *Terra Japonica.* To this Extract they fometimes join that of another

Plant,

Plant, called *Lycium*, as also calcined Shells.

Argentina, is thus distinguished, *Pentaphylloides Argenteum, alatum, seu Potentilla.* Tour. Inst. Boerh. Ind. Alt. *Potentilla anserina*, Offic. *Pentaphylloides argentina Dicta*, Raii Synop. Wild Tansey. It grows in moist and barren Places, and where Water has stood all the Winter, flowering in *May*. *Tournefort* informs us, that it is astringnet, vulnerary and deterfive, that it is an excellent Ingredient in Ptisans and Broths for Looseness, Bloody Flux, and Hemorrhages, and that he has seen wonderful Effects produced by it in the *Fluor albus*, especially if seven or eight Craw-fish are added to each Decoction of wild Tansey; that it abates Inflammations of the Kidneys and Bladder, and temperates the Heat of the Urine; and that its distilled Water is good for Blearedness and Ulcers of the Eyes, as also for Tanning or Redness of the Face. Mr. *Ray in Hist. Plant.* informs us that it is an excellent Lithontriptic, and very serviceable in the Cure of Wounds and Ulcers; that externally it is much used for the Tooth-ach, putrid Gums, and allaying Heat in Fevers, for the last of which Purposes, it is to be bruised and applied to the Soles of the Feet or the Wrists; that *Agricola* found the Juice of this Herb with the Powder of common *Colchicum*, to be a Cure for the Disease of the Anus called *Marisca*; and that according to *Castor Durantes*, those who labour under Dysenteries, Fluxes, immoderate menstrual Evacuations, and even Hemorrhages from the Nose, are cured by wearing it in the Shoes. *Boerhaave* tells us, that it is possessed of the same Virtues with the Peruvian Bark; since if the Herb is bruised, and its Juice taken an Hour before the Paroxysm of an intermittent Fever, it removes it with one

or two Doses, if the Disorder is of the kindly Sort, but if there be any Malignity in the Fever, it is to be applied externally. Internally it is of Service in all Disorders consisting in the Openings of the Vessels, and Evacuations of the Fluids.

Arisarum, Offic. *Arisarum angustifolium, Dioscoridis forte*, Boerh. Ind. A. Friers Cowl. It grows in *Italy* and *Dalmatia*. It heats, dries, incides, absterges and digests.

Aristolochia. Birthwort. Of this there are three Kinds used in Medicine, the first of which is the *Aristolochia vera rotunda major*, Offic. *Rotunda, flore ex purpura Nigro*, C.B. and *Aristolochium*, Hippocrat. Round Birth wort. It grows in *Spain, Italy*, and the Southern Parts of *France*, flowering in *May*. The Root is greatly extolled for exciting the Menses, and expelling the Foetus and Secundines. When taken internally, by its hot and penetrating Bitterness, it pervades the whole Body, and puts all its Parts into Motion. Hence, by stimulating, heating, drying, and resolving, it is beneficial in many Diseases, as Dropsies, cacochymic and leucophlegmatic Cachexies, and violent Obstructions. According to *Du Hamel*, its Root infused for a Night in white Wine, cures the Jaundice, if the Patient use it three Days succeffively, fasting. *Simon Pauli* in *Quadr. Botan.* informs us, that it is highly beneficial to Persons subject to scorbutic Asthmas, if it is mixed with antiscorbutic Potions and Infusions. It is greatly extolled against Diseases of the Joints, and for this Purpose a celebrated *German* Physician constantly prescribed a Decoction of the Root of this Plant in Conjunction with Succory and China-root. But in *Holland* an Infusion of the Root in Spirit of Wine obtained a greater Reputation. In *Ephemerid. Nat. Curios.*

riof. Cent. 5. we are told, that the celebrated *Klauuig* prepared from the Root, an highly faturated Tincture, fty Drops of which he exhibited Ale, or fome other Vehicle, or in ſtead he ordered fifteen Grains of the refinous Extract of the Root in the Form of Pills, being perfuaded that all the Virtue was owing to the refinous Part, of which about two Ounces are contained in a Pound. *Æmilius Macer* recommends againſt the Gout; but 'tis hardly probable that it will prove benefi- al to all arthritic Patients; fince by drattic Quality, it excites violent Heat in the Body. Where there is Lentor and flow Motion of the Blood, this Root may prove an excel- nt Prefervative, if fparingly ufed ther in Decoctions, Tinctures or Pills. Hence 'tis obvious why, and what Occafion, the Root proves a good Ingredient in Clyfters againſt lethargic Diforders. Externally ap- ied, it is good for refolving Tu- mors, and cleanfing Ulcers. The Powder of the Root, and its Extract with Spirit of Wine, are ufed in Li- ments, defigned for cleanfing inve- rate, fordid and malignant Ulcers. Another Species of *Ariſtolochia* uſed in the Shops, is thus diſtin- guiſh'd: *Ariſtolochia longa,* Offic. B. *Langa vera,* C. B. Park. *Al- te Radice pollicis Craffitudine,* Cæ- p. Long-rooted Birthwort. This cording to *Raii Hiſt.* grows among the Corn, and in fome Vineyards of *France,* flowering in the Beginning the Spring. In Virtues it agrees with the round Birthwort, tho' ac- cording to *Hoffman,* the former is of ſtronger Nature than the latter. *von Pauli* with the Powder of this ſpecies of Ariſtolochia boil'd in Wa- of Paul's Betony, and applied in a en Cloth, in a few Days, happily confolidated a malignant Ulcer, the Cure of which had in vain been at- tempted by a Surgeon, for a whole

Year. As the Root is of a ſpongious Nature, fome ufe it inſtead of Genti- an, for Tents to dilate Fiſtulas.

The third Sort is, the *Ariſtolochia longa Noſtras,* Offic. *Ariſtolochia te- nuis,* Koker. Cat. Hort. Med. Har- mel. *Clematitis Recta,* C. B. *Clema- titis Vulgaris,* J. B. and *Ariſtolochia altera radice tenui.* Creeping Birth- wort. The Moderns have found this Species to be aromatic, penetrating, aperient, fudorific, detergent and vulnerary. The Root, either in Powder or Extract, is recommended in the hyſteric Paffion, leucophlegma- tic Cachexies, Aſthmas, and intermit- tent Fevers, where the Intentions of Heating and Refolution are to be purſued. According to *Grimmaldus* in *Eph. Nat. Curiof. Decad.* 2. *An.* 3. *Obf.* 207. the Leaves are accounted a Specific againſt Coughs and Aſth- mas, and the Oil obtain'd from the Roots by Diſtillation is of great Ser- vice in facilitating Labours. The learned *Heldius* in *Eph. Nat. Curiof. Cent.* 6. gives us an Account of the ſignal Virtue of the Root of the creeping Birthwort againſt the Gout.

Armeniaca Malus, & Præcocia, Offic. *Armeniaca Malus Major,* Ger. Emac. The Apricock Tree. It flowers in *March* and *April,* the Fruit being ripe about *Midfummer.* They create an Appetite, provoke Urine, are cordial, pectoral, and pro- mote Expectoration. An Infufion of them is good to allay the Heat of Fe- vers, and the Kernels are recom- mended to kill Worms. They are good in hot Weather, for young People that have good Stomachs, and of a bilious and fanguine Com- plexion. Yet People ought to be cautious of this Sort of Food, which contains a vifcid and thick Juice, and fometimes caufes Wind and crude Humours. They contain a confiderable Quantity of Oil and ef- fential Salt, and much Phlegm.

Armeria. The Name of a Plant which

which is thus diftinguifh'd. *Arme-rius pratenfis*, Ger. Emac. *Lychnis plumaria fylveftris fimplex*, Raii Hift. *Flos Cuculi*, *Odontis quibuf-dam*, J. B. Meadow Pink. It grows in watery Places, flowering in *May*; the Flowers are in Ufe. It is a good Alexipharmic, and commended againft Poifon.

Armoracia, Offic. *Raphanus fyl-veftris*, Ger. Emac. *Rapiftrum al-bum articulatum*, Park. Theat. *Raphaniftrum flore albo ftriato, filiquâ articulatâ ftriatâ minore*, Boerh. Ind. A. Wild Radifh. It grows among Corn, flowering in *June*. The Root is ufed. It warms and dries. It incides mucilaginous tartareous Concretions; it attenu-ates, refolves, opens Obftructions of the Vifcera, is diuretic, lithontrip-tic, and antifcorbutic.

Artemifia, Offic. *Artemifia Vulga-ris Major, caule & flore Purpuraf-centibus, & Albicante*, Boerh. Ind. A. Mugwort. It grows in Hed-ges and wafte Places and flowers in *June*. The Leaves or Tops are us'd in Decoctions, Infufions and Baths for the Feet. *Valentinus* in his *Pandectæ Medico-legales* informs us, that the Faculty of Phyfic at *Leipfic*, being appealed to judicially, in an alledged Cafe of Murder, whether Abortion could be procur-ed by a Decoction of red Mugwort and Cherry Tree Bark in Ale, an-fwered, that Mugwort alone was fufficient to provoke the Menfes, and confequently produce that Ef-fect. But as the Quantity of the Mugwort was not fpecified, and as the Woman accufed had alfo ufed other Plants, a formal Verdict was fufpended. *Baubine* greatly extols a Decoction of Mugwort edulcerated with Sugar or Honey, for mitigat-ing Coughs, attenuating vifcid Hu-mours about the Præcordia, and ex-pelling Stones from the Kidneys and Bladder. *Simon Pauli* affirms, that

he happily cured Patients whofe ner-vous Syftems were difordered, who were obnoxious to flatulent Spafms, or who complained of a Wearinefs of their Limbs after chronical, and fometimes after acute Diforders, by ordering them to fit in a Veffel, near full of the Decoction of Mug-wort, and then in the Decoctions of Sage, Agrimony, Chamomile and fine Flower. I know, fays he, an old Woman, who after large œdematous Tumors had feized both her Knees, happily removed them, by fumigat-ing them with folded Linen Cloths over kindled Mugwort. *Baubine* informs us, that Pains and Coldnefs of the Nerves and Joints, are remov-ed by fomenting them with a De-coction of the Flowers of Mug-wort, Chamomile, and Eupatorium. The fame Author from *Arnoldus* in-forms us, that the Flowers of Mug-wort, boil'd and applied to the Head after wafhing it with the De-coction, are of great Efficacy in re-moving an Hemicrania. *Ray*, from *Parkinfon*, informs us, that the recent Herb, or its Juice drank in fome proper Liquor, is of all others the moft efficacious Remedy for thofe who have taken too much Opium. In *Ephemerid. Nat. Curiof. Vol. 2.* we are told, that a certain Prince learned from *Tabernæmontanus* that Mugwort both internally in Decoc-tions, and externally in Capaplafm and Powders was of great Efficacy in Burns by Gun Powders, and Gun Shot Wounds, and that the faid Prince, had at the Siege of a cer-tain Town cured Numbers by it Means. Thefe Effects are produc-ed by the attenuating, refolvent an confequently aperient Virtues of th Plant. *Julius Pontedera* in his Dif-fertations informs us, that Mugwor is good againft Vertigoes, and In-farctions of the Lungs. There a many fabulous Reports with Refpe to this Plant, such as that it prevents Weariness in Travellers, and that under its Root is found a Coal capable of removing the Epilepsy: But these and other Stories relating to this Plant, are justly looked upon as so many Indignities to human Reason, which is never so much debased as when it yields to Superstition.

Arthanita, Cyclamen, Offic. _Cyclamen orbiculato folio inferne purpurascente,_ C. B. Pin. Boerh. Ind. Alt. Sow-Bread. With us this Root is cultivated in Gardens, but grows spontaneously in the _Alps,_ and Mountains of _Asturia_ and _Styria._ The Root is of a forcing Nature, and principally used to expel the Birth and Secundines, and excite the menstrual Discharge. The Juice is by some commended as an Errhine against vertiginous Disorders of the Head. It is also of Service against cutaneous Eruptions.

Another Sort of _Arthanita_ is the _Cyclamen, Arthanita,_ Offic. _Cyclamen Hederæ folio,_ Ger. Emac. Boerh. Ind. A Common Sowbread. This Species agrees in Virtues with the preceding, and is the Sort which is kept in our Shops.

Arum, Offic. J. B. Raii Hist. _Arum maculatum, maculis candidis vel nigris, & non maculatum,_ C. B. Pin. Boerhaav. Ind. Alt. Cuckow-Pint, or Wake-Robin. It grows in Hedges and Ditches, flowers in _May,_ and produces ripe Berries in _July._ Tho' _Boerhaave_ in _Instit. Med._ and _Lanzonius_ think that _Arum,_ on Account of its phlogistic and caustic Acrimony is to be classed among the Poisons, yet the Root is used in the Shops, for the Purposes of inciding, resolving Mucus, exciting Appetite, and curing intermittent Fevers; but it is not generally exhibited till it is previously macerated in Wine, Vinegar, or Bran, and afterwards dried. They

who desire strong Effects from this Root, and are not fond of rendering it milder, by disjoining the Spicula of the acrid Salts, use it only simply dryed, after taking off its external Covering or Pellicule. The Powder of the Root prepared in both these Manners, is highly extolled as a powerfully stimulating, resolvent, aperient, diuretic and sudorific Medicine, in Disorders of the inveterate and mucous Kind. As Arum, in Consequence of its Acrimony, acts by resolving and inciding, 'tis sufficiently obvious, that it is proper in many Diseases arising from inactive pituitous and mucous Humours. Thus in a violent Scurvy arising from the Inactivity of the Juices, and in a moist Asthma, the Root triturated and reduced to Pills, is of great Service in resolving the viscid Humours. According to _Helmont,_ the Root boiled with Vinegar, is highly efficacious in resolving Coagulations of Blood brought on by Falls from Eminences. According to _Boerhaave,_ Arum is safest in Decoctions and Infusions; Wine also corrects its Acrimony, and it becomes milder by being boiled. Arum, according to _Bauhine,_ reduced to a Powder, and mixed with Sugar, is good for those afflicted with a Phthisis, since it incides the thick and viscid Phlegm, assists Expectoration, removes Disorders of the Lungs and Breast, and is useful against a Cough. The Root, whether recent or dry, bruised and exhibited, is highly purgative. The Leaves and Root of Arum used in warm Infessions, cure a falling down of the Anus, and some other Disorders of that Part. _Pliny_ in _Lib._ 24. _Cap._ 16. tells us, that the Leaves whether recent or dry are beneficial in the Gout. It is an Ingredient in the _Pulvis Ari Compositus._

Another Species of _Arum_ is the _Arum maximum Ægyptiacum, quod vulgo_

vulgo Colocasia, C. B. *Arum Ægypt. rotunda,* & *longa Radice, vulgo Colocasia dicta,* Park. The whole Plant is acrimonious like the common *Arum,* but more mild, and is therefore used in Food. *Bontius* says, it is of a venomous Nature, and requires three Days Maceration in Water, to render it eatable.

Arundo. The Reed. Of this there are several Sorts, the first is the *Arundo,* Offic. *Arundo vallatoria,* Ger. Emac. *Arundo vulgaris, sive Phragmites Dioscoridis,* Boerh Ind. A. *Harundo vulgaris sive vallatoria,* Park. Theat. Common Reed. It grows by River Sides, and in Marshes, and agrees in Virtues with the following.

The Second is the *Arundo Donax,* Offic. Park. Theat. *Arundo Cypria,* Ger. Emac. *Arundo sativa, seu Donax Dioscorides,* Boerh. Ind. A. The great Reed. Its Root attracts any Matter lodged in Wounds, if reduced to Powder, with Wine, and applied to the Wound. It removes Pains arising from Dislocations of the Limbs, and carries off Pains in the Hips. When bruised, and applied to any Part that akes, it is of wonderful Service. *Hier. Mercurial. Med. Pract. L.* 4. *C.* 2. If it is boiled in any Lixivium, and the Head frequently washed therewith, it causes the Hair to grow; and cures scal'd Heads. *Julius Cæsar Claudinus, Ep. Vincenzo Tanar.* says, that the Root of the *Arundo* produced the same Effect in Rheumatisms and Catarrhs, with the Peruvian Bark. It is good for Consumptions. *Actius* says, it is of a drying and warming Nature, and is therefore of Service to dropsical Patients, *Serm.* 10. *C* 32. It brings Apostems to Suppuration, *Lev. Lemn. de Herb. Biblic. C.* 27. The green Leaves cut and applied, carry off the Wild-fire and

Erysipelas. Poor People boil the Flowers in Water, or in Beer, which they mix with Honey, and drink, after having filtrated it, in order to cure Coughs, Oppressions of the Breast, and Consumptions.

The third is the *Arundo Tabaxifera,* Offic. *Canna ingens Mambu vel Bambu dicta,* Park. Theat. *Tabaxir sive Bambu Arbor;* J. B. The Bambu Cane. The *Indians* use it for Wounds of the Testes and Penis. It is efficacious in choleric Affections, and the Dysentery. It is used in burning Heats, internal and external, and in bilious Fevers and Dysenteries; especially in bilious Fluxes, the Strangury, and bloody Urine. A Decoction of the Leaves and Bark, being drank, purges Wounds of Blood retained in them, and is proper for Women in Child-bed, to cleanse the Uterus after the Birth. These Canes grow in the Sand of the Sea Shores.

Asa fœtida, Offic. C. B. *Asa fœtida,* Offic. J. B. *Abith seu Asa fœtida, Javanis* & *maliais Hin Dicta* Bont. Devil's Dung. *Dioscorides,* in *Lib.* 3. *Cap.* 94. ascribes so many and so powerful Virtues to this, that one would be tempted to think, that all the Disorders incident to human Nature, might be removed by it. But without running into such exaggerated and ill grounded Encomiums, we shall confine ourselves to what we know to be true. *Asa-*fœtida, then, is a gummy Resin, brought to us in Lumps of different Colours, white, yellowish, blew or brown, which last is the worst of all. It has a very strong, fetid Smell, and the Tree producing it is accurately described by *Kempfer.* *Asa* fœtida is justly accounted an excellent Remedy, in all hysteric Disorders, whether smelled to, or mixed with such other Substances as are exhibited internally. It is also said to be good for exciting Sweat and ad corroborating the Stomach. The Dose is from twelve Grains half a Dram. But for the Sake of the Stomach it is often neceſſary give it in ſmaller Doſes. Exterally it is a good Reſolvent, and with at View is made an Ingredient in the *Ceratum de Galbano*. It is an ingredient in the *Spiritus Volatilis, inctura fætida, Tinctura Fuliginis, ulvis è Myrrhâ compoſitus,* and the *ilulæ Gummoſæ.*

Aſarum, Offic. Ger. C. B. Pin. iii. Hiſt. Boerhaav. Ind. Alt. *Nar- s Ruſtica,* Hoffman. Flo. Altorff. *Aſarabacca.* It is planted with us Gardens, and flowers in *June,* t the dried Roots are generally imported from *Leghorn.* This Plant of an acrid and very bitter Taſte, nauſeous and gently aſtringent. It of an emetic and purgative Qua- y, tho' it does not always operate theſe two Manners, but different- according to the Method of its eparation. The crude Root re- ced to a Powder, and exhibited, her in a Bolus, or in ſome proper quor, proves a powerful Emetic d Purgative; but according to *smaller* it muſt be carefully tritu- ed or reduced to a very fine Pow- , otherwiſe it only proves pur- ive. Half an Ounce of this Root, uſed for a Night in Wine, is an etico-cathartic Medicine, highly alled againſt intermittent Fevers, Dropſy, the Gout, Iſchiadic ns, and eſpecially Dyſenteries and urrhæas. But if a whole Ounce of Root is digeſted with ſixteen nces of Water, it no longer proves etic, but operates as a Diuretic. *smaller* informs us, that a De- tion of Aſarabacca with Water ll boiled is very diuretic, and a werful Diaphoretic, in chronical orders, eſpecially thoſe ariſing m ſome Fault in the Primæ viæ. m what has been ſaid 'tis ſuf- dly obvious, that the Uſe of

this Plant is proper, in all Caſes, where the languid Veſſels require a Stimulus, and where tough and viſcid Humours are to be reſolved. Hence it is an excellent Remedy in Obſtructions, not only of the Primæ Viæ, but alſo of the other Viſcera, whether by Way of Infuſion, when vomiting and purging are neceſſary; or in Decoctions, when the Cure is to be performed without producing great Commotions in the Body. Hence the Reaſon is alſo obvious, why Aſarabacca has often proved effectual againſt the Jaundice, inter- mittent Fevers, and Obſtructions of the Menſes. Externally a Decoction of the Plant, uſed by Way of Fu- migation, or dropt into the Ears, is good againſt Obſtructions of the au- ditory Paſſage by Sordes, or a Ring- ing of the Ears.

Another Species of *Aſarum* is the *Aſarum Virginianum & Serpentaria nigra,* Offic. *Aſarum Virginianum Piſtolochiæ foliis ſubrotundis, Cycla- mini more maculatis,* Raii Hiſt. Black Snake-weed. The Roots of this Snake-weed are brought over a- mong the true *Serpentaria Virgini- ana,* and are promiſcuouſly uſed with them being diaphoretic, and alexi- pharmic. It is an Ingredient in the *Pulvis Sternutatorius.*

Aſclepias, a Plant thus diſtinguiſh- ed, *Vincetoxicum, & Hirundinaria,* Offic. *Aſclepias flore albo,* Ger. Emac. Park. Theat. Boerh. Ind. A. Swallow-wort. The Roots are bitter, acrid, and give a faint red Colour to the blue Paper; the Leaves are ſaltiſh, and dye the Paper of a faint red Colour. A Pound of its Roots macerated in Wine, and boiled to a third Part, provokes Sweat, and is recommend- ed for the Dropſy. A Decoction of this Plant operates both by Urine and Tranſpiration, renders the Hu- mours volatile, and is preferable to that of *Scorzonera,* in malignant

Fevers and the Plague. The Herb, applied as a Cataplasm, dissolves Tumours of the Breasts, and the Powder of the Root is reckoned a great Counter-Poison, both against the bad Effects of *Apocynon*, and other poisonous Herbs, and against the Bites of venemous Animals. It is also commended against the Jaundice. It grows with us only in Gardens, and flowers in *June*.

Ascyrum, Offic. Ger. Emac. *Ascyrum vulgare*, Park. Theat. *Hypericum Ascyrum dictum caule quadrangulo*, Boerh. Ind. A. St. *Peter's*-wort. It grows in watery Places, and flowers in *July* and *August*. The Herb, Flowers, and Seed are used: The Herb and Flowers have the same Virtues as *Hypericum* or St. *John's*-wort. The Seeds are useful in the Sciatica, and purge bilious Humours by Stool. If used in a Cataplasm, they are good against Burnings.

Aspalatus is thus distinguished *Lignum Aspalathi & Rhodium Lignum*, Geoff. Tract. Róse-wood, or Rhodium. This Tree is by *Herman* and others thought to be a Kind of *Cytisus*. It is according to *Geoffroy* brought from the *Morea*, is very resinous and of a grateful Smell resembling that of Roses. It is much esteemed in *China*, where an Infusion of it in Water, is believed highly efficacious, both in curing and preventing many Diseases. An essential Oil is obtained from it, which has so much the Smell of Roses, as to be often substituted for their essential Oil ; the Smell of the former, is never so strong as that of the latter.

Asparagus, Offic. Park. *Asparagus Sativa*, C. B. Pin. Boerh. Ind. Alt. *Asparagus hortensis*, J. B. Sparrow-grass. It grows spontaneously in some Parts of *England*, as in *Cornwall* and near *Bristol*, but the best is cultivated in Gardens. The Root of this Plant is one of the five aperient Roots. Sparrow-grass must be quickly and slightly boiled, otherwise they become viscid and glutinous. *Fridewallis* informs us, that it is by some used, in order to prove a Stimulus to Venery. When eaten they render the Urine fetid, and when used to Excess, prove so great a Diuretic as to bring on an Incontinence of Urine. *Lister* speaks in the following Manner. " 'Tis surprising that " the Smell of the Urine is immediately changed by eating Asparagus. This denotes a very expeditious Concoction of the Kidneys, on Account of the septic Quality of the Herb ; for which Reason it is by some said to corrode the Bladder." *Etmuller* is of Opinion that Sparrow-grass is injurious to Patients disposed to nephritic Disorders. That the copious Use of them is prejudicial to the Urinary Passages, we are informed by *Lanzonius* in *Eph. Nat. Curios. Vol.* 1. *Obs.* 92. where he gives us an Instance of a Discharge of bloody Urine by the Abuse of them. In *Eph. Nat. Curios. Dec.* 2. *An.* 5. we are told, that a Woman of a sound healthy Constitution, was rendered barren by the too frequent Use of Sparrow-grass, but became prolific when she desisted from the Use of them. *Dioscorides* affirms, that Sparrow-grass is purgative and diuretic, whereas *Hippocrates* says, that they are dry and produce Costiveness. But this is a Point to be decided by every one's own Experience, since such are the Peculiarities of different Habits and Constitutions, that what proves purgative to one, frequently produces the opposite Effect in others. Upon the whole it may be asserted that Sparrow-grass is inciding, stimulating, aperient, and principally disposed to act upon the urinary Passages, for which Reason it is classed among the diuretic

Me

Medicines. On Account of its diuretic or rather aperient Quality, it is fit for exciting the menstrual Discharge, and perhaps this is the Reason, why the excessive Use of it, brought on Sterility in the Woman before mentioned, because by resolving the Blood, and promoting a too copious menstrual Discharge, it might by that very Means prevent Conception. The inciding and resolvent Virtues of Asparagus, are by *Simeon Sethi* described in the following Manner: 'Sparrow-grass is good against Colies and nephritic Disorders produced by Phlegm. It augments the Inclination to Venery, and passes sooner into the Blood, than other Pot-herbs. It excites the Menses, is good against Palpitations of the Heart, and proves beneficial to the Teeth.' The Roots are used in Decoctions, and their principal Efficacy is thought to be lodg'd in their Bark.

Another Sort of *Asparagus* is the *Asparagus sylvestris*, Diosc. *Asparagus sylvestris, tenuissimo folio*, C. B. Pin. Boerh. Ind. A. Wild Sparrow-grass. This only differs from the preceding by Culture, its Root is glutinous and sweetish like the former, and gives a faint Tincture of red to the blue Paper, which makes it probable that its Salt resembles vitriolated Tartar, so that it is dissolved in a great deal of Phlegm, thicken'd with some Earth and Sulphur, by which the Root is an Aperitive, a little temper'd.

Another Kind is the *Asparagus petræa & corruda*, Offic. *Asparagus petræa*, Ger. Emac. *Asparagus petræus, sive Corruda aculeata*, Park. Theat. Rock Sparrow-grass. The young Shoots and Roots of these, are used in the same Intentions, as those of the *Asparagus sativus*.

Asperula, Aspergula, Offic. *Asperula seu Rubeola montana odorata*,

C. B. Pin. *Asperula odorata flore albo*, Boerh. Ind. A. Wood Roof. It grows in Woods and Copses, flowering in *May*. It is esteem'd a good Hepatic, and is recommended for Inflammations of the Liver, and Obstructions of the Gall Bladder, and the Jaundice. The *Germans* use it in their Wine, as we do Borrage and Burnet, as a great Cordial and Comforter of the Spirits. The green Herb bruised, is made use of by some Country-Folks to allay hot Tumors and Inflammations, and is apply'd to fresh Cuts.

Asphodelus verus albus, Offic. *Asphodelus albus ramosus mas*, C. B. Pin. Boerh. Ind. Alt. White Asphodel. It grows spontaneously in *Italy*, *Spain*, and the Southern Parts of *France*; but with us is cultivated in Gardens, and flowers in *May*. The Root, according to *Dioscorides*, in heating, diuretic, and emmenagogue. A Decoction of the Roots in the Lees of Wine us'd externally, cures sordid and spreading Ulcers of the Breasts, Inflammations of the Testicles, Tubercles and Boils. From what has been said it is obvious, that Asphodel proves beneficial, in Consequence of that Acrimony, by which the nervous and fibrous Parts are put in Motion, and the viscid and tenacious Humours incided, and resolv'd; so that *Galen* seems to have been in the Right, when he asserted, that Asphodel as well as Asarabacca and Arum, was of an astringent and discutient Nature. According to *Fernelius*, the Juice of the Root, boil'd with Oil, cures Chilblanes, and the Root itself bruis'd and applied is, by *Forestus*, said to cure the Kings Evil.

Another Species of *Asphodel* is the *Asphodelus verus luteus, Hasta Regia*, Offic. *Asphodelus luteus, & flore & radice*, Boerh. Ind. A. Kings Spear. It is call'd by some *Anthericum*, which according to the Fiction of *Lucian*, the Ghosts of the damn'd

eat

eat in Hell. It grows in many Parts of *Italy*, *France*, and *Spain*. The Root is principally used, which is hot and of a strong bitter Taste. *Fallopius* reckons it among the best of the milder Cathartics. It is of a warming, drying, opening, discussing, purgative and cleansing Nature. It excites a Discharge of the Urine and Menses; is good for Spasms, cures Ruptures, Jaundice and the Dropsy. The Root boiled in Wine or Water, and sufficiently triturated when dry, cleanses and cures old corrosive and fetid Wounds and Ulcers, Swellings of the Breasts, and *Pudenda*, as also bloody Ulcers; it cures scrophulous Swellings being bruis'd and laid upon them, and heals Chilblanes, whether exulcerated or not. Washing the Body with Vinegar, wherein the Root of this Plant has been boiled, cures the Itch, and other scorbutic Eruptions. Some roast the Root in hot Ashes, and rub their Faces and Hands with it, in order to remove all Blotches, and purify the Skin. The Root, also, makes the Hairs grow fast and curl. This Root reduc'd to Powder, and mix'd with calcin'd Alum, corrodes the fungous Flesh of foul Ulcers, if apply'd to them. If this Root be put into the Water which Swine drink, it prevents their being affected with a pestilential Leprosy; or if they are so, it restores them to their natural State It also produces the same Effect, if they are frequently washed with such a Water.

Asplenium, Ceterach & Scolopendria, Offic. *Asplenium five Ceterach*, Ger. Emac. Spleenwort or Miltwast. It grows upon old Stone-Walls, and Buildings, especially in the West of *England*. It is one of the five capillary Plants, taking its Name from curing Diseases of the Spleen, removing Swellings thereof, and preventing its too great Largeness, whence also it is called *Miltwast*; it opens Obstructions of the Liver,

alleviates the Jaundice, and is recommended for the Rickets in Children.

Aster Atticus, Offic. Ger. Emac. *Aster luteus, foliolis ad florem rigidis*, C. B. *Astericus annuus foliis ad florem rigidis*, Boerh. Ind. A. Golden Starwort. This Plant is found in the Gardens of Botanists, and flowers in *May*. Its Leaves, are of a vulnerary Nature, though seldom prescribed in Practice. The Leaves and the Herb is of Service in preternatural Commotions and Heats of the Stomach, Inflammations of the Eyes, the falling down of the Fundament, and Tumors, in the Groins. The Water distill'd from its Flowers, if drank, is of Service in Quinsies, and the epileptic Fits of Children.

Astragalus, Offic. *Astragalus syriacus*, Ger. Emac. Park. Theat. The Silk Vetch of *Dioscorides*. It grows in windy and shady Places and where much Snow falls. Its Root, drank in Wine, stops a Looseness, and provokes Urine; dried to a Powder, it is with good Effect sprinkled on old Ulcers, and stops Bleeding. Its Root is sweetish, astringent, and gives a deep Tincture of red to the blue Paper; the Leaves give it scarcely any, they are bitter and smell like Elder, which shews that the fetid Oil is found in greater Quantity in the Leaves, and that it involves the acrid Salt and Earth. An Infusion of this Plant in Wine, is given for the Gravel, by some Botanists at *Paris*.

Astrantia nigra, Offic. *Astrantia major, corona floris purpurascente*, Boerh. Ind. A. Black Masterwort. This Plant is cultivated in the Gardens of Botanists, and flowers in *July*. Its black and fibrous Roots are only used. It is said to purge melancholic Humours; and *Dodonæus* thinks that it resembles the *Veratrum nigrum* of *Dioscorides*, both in its Form and Qualities. *Hildanus*

1

prescribes it for the Cure of a Scirrhous Spleen.

Atractylis, Offic. Ger. Emac. *Cnicus Atractylis lutea dictus,* Boerh. Ind. A. Distaff Thistle. It grows in *Italy* and *Greece,* and flowers in Summer. The Leaves only of this Thistle are used. It is aperitive, sudorific, a good Antidote against Poison, and is particularly recommended against the Stinging of Scorpions.

Atragene, Offic. *Viorna,* Ger. Emac. *Clematis Sylvestris latifolia,* Boerh. Ind. Alt. Travellers Joy. This Plant is found under Hedges, flowering in *July.* Its Flowers, Bark, Seeds and Root, are of a caustic Quality. The Bark applied to the Skin raises Blisters.

Atriplex There are various Species of this Plant, but that most in Use is distinguished thus, *Atriplex,* Offic. Chab. *Atriplex alba hortensis,* J. B. Raii Hist. *Atriplex hortensis alba, five pallide virens,* C. B. Pin. Boerhaav. Ind. Alt. White Orache. *Galen* informs us, that this Herb is but little nutritive, and at the same Time proves injurious to the Stomach. *Pythagoras,* according to *Pliny,* was of Opinion, that it was not only concocted with Difficulty, but also brought on Dropsies, Epilepsies and Paleness. *Hippocrates* says, that Orache is of a moist Quality, without being purgative. This Herb when boiled is not only safe, but also beneficial, when the Body requires Refrigeration and Humectation. It is one of the five emollient Herbs, and frequently used, especially in moistening, emollient, and refrigerating Clysters. *Morison* tells us, that the Seeds of the Plant are said to be emetic and purgative, for which Reason *Dioscorides* seems to have affirmed, that if drank with Hydromel it cured the Jaundice.

Another Species of Orache is the *Atriplex olida,* Offic. Ger. Raii Hist.

Atriplex fœtida, C. B. Pin. *Chenopodium fœtidum,* Boerh. Ind. Alt. Stinking Orache. It grows on Dunghills and waste Places. This Herb is in a peculiar Manner appropriated to the female Sex, being aperient, deobstruent, beneficial in uterine Disorders, good to promote the menstrual Evacuations, to expel the Secundines, alleviate Child-bed Purgations, appease Strangulations of the Uterus, and remove hysteric Fits. It is generally exhibited in Decoctions.

Avena, of this there are various Species, but the most common, and at the same Time the best for Use is thus distinguished *Avena,* Offic. *Avena alba,* J. B. Raii Hist. *Avena vulgaris seu alba,* C. B. Pin. Boerh. Ind. Alt. Oats. This Grain is of singular Use, not only for Food, but also for various medicinal Purposes. Thus *Hoffman in Tr. de Remed. domest. Præstant.* when treating of the Decoction of exorticated Oats, speaks thus: " Among all the " domestic Remedies, none is more " valuable than this, which is high- " ly proper in all Disorders ari- " sing from an Acrimony of the " Blood, or of the Humours in " the Primæ viæ, as in Coughs, " Catarrhs, Coryzas, purple Fe- " vers, Measles, Small-pox, bilious " and choleric Fevers, Diarrhæas " arising from a Redundance of a- " crid Bile, and Erosions of the In- " testines. I have frequently, in the " above Disorders, with great Suc- " cess, ordered a few Pugils of com- " mon Chamomile Flowers, to be " boiled in this Decoction, which is " also commodiously injected as a " Clyster in the same Disorders." A Decoction of entire Oats, is also an excellent moistening Medicine against febrile Heats, because it resists the Alcalescence of the Humours, by Means of its great Tendency to Acidity. *Hoffman* also in the

the fame Treatife, tells us, that a Decoction of Oats in Water, with the Addition of Succory-Root, Nitre, Honey, and Poppy-Flowers, is of all others the moft efficacious Drink, in all acute Difeafes, Pains efpecially of the gouty Kind, and for purifying the Blood in fcorbutic Patients. Various other Subftances, may be added to this Decoction, according to the different Intentions to be purfued. *Boeclere* highly extols a Jelly of Oats, in hectic Cafes, taken in the Broth of Oyfters and River Crabs. Oats are no lefs ufeful for external Purpofes; for when put into a Bag, and warmed, they are fuccefsfully applied againft Gripes of the Abdomen, for diffipating the Flatulencies of hyfteric Women, and mitigating various Pains, efpecially of the nephritic Kind, arifing from Cold. *Galen* affirms, that Oats nourifh little, whereas *Ray* afferts, that thofe who live upon them, are healthy, and live to a great Age. But notwithftanding this, *Galen*'s Opinion was not without Foundation; fince Oats afford but little Nourifhment to fuch as are weak, becaufe they are not eafily digefted by them; for concocted and not crude Subftances, only prove nutritive. *Hoffman* orders Oats to be carefully freed from the Darnel or Tares mixed with them, by which Means the Liquors prepared from them will have no bad Influence on the Head, which is found from Experience to proceed from the Darnel.

Aurantia. A Fruit Tree thus diftinguifhed, *Malus Aurantia*, Offic. Ger. Raii Hift. *Malus Aurantia major*, C. B. Pin. *Aurantia vulgaris*, Boerhaave Ind. Alt. The Orange Tree. This grows in great Plenty in *Italy*, *Spain* and *Portugal*, and bears Flowers and Fruit all the Year, but the Fruit is principally

gathered in *October* and *November*. The Sevil Orange is only ufed in Medicine. The yellow Rind of Orange Peel, is of a ftimulating, heating, and confequently ftomachic Quality. It is, alfo, carminative, corroborative and cardiac. Recent Orange Peel put up the Nofe, in the Morning before eating, as alfo in the Evening, excites Sneezing, and purges the Head, without producing any bad Effects. A Scruple, or half a Dram of the Peel, reduced to a Powder, and exhibited in any proper Liquor, is beneficially exhibited in Flatulences and Gripes proceeding from a cold Caufe, as alfo againft Worms of the Inteftines. When taken in Wine it produces the Effects of an Alexipharmic, in the Time of the Plague. In difficult Difcharges of Urine, it is exhibited in Chervil or Parfley Water. The Peel reduced to a Powder with Honey and Alum, is greatly extolled as an Ointment for the fpreading Ulcers in the Mouths of Children, called *Aphtha*. According to *Schulzius in Praelect.* an Effence obtained from dried Orange Peel with Spirit of Wine, is an excellent ftomachic, carminative, and analeptic Medicine. The white Pulp of the Peel, is of an aftringent Nature. The acid bitterifh Juice of the Fruit, is refrigerating, gently aftringent, and confequently proper for corroborating the relaxed Fibres of the Stomach, and correcting the alcalefcent State of the Humours. *Labat* in his Hiftory of *America* informs us, that the Juice of the Fruit is there ufed externally for the Cure of inveterate and venereal Ulcers. The Leaves and Flowers are alfo ufed for feveral medicinal Purpofes. It is an Ingredient in the *Conferva Flavedinis Corticum Aurantiorum. Succus Scorbuticus, Aqua corticum Aurantiorum, fimplex & fpirituofa, Aqua Raphani compofita, Infufum Amarum fimplex,*

&

& *purgans*, *Vinum Ipecacuanbæ*, *Tinctura amara*, and in the *Syrupus e Corticibus Aurantiorum*.

Auriculæ Judæ & *Fungi Sambuci*, Offic. *Fungus Membranaceus auriculam referens, sive Sambucinus*, C. B. Pin. Raii Hist. *Agaricus auriculæ forma*, Boerhaav. Ind. Alt. Jews Ear. This is a Sort of Fungus adhereing to the Trunk of the Elder Tree, generally of the Form and Bulk of a Man's Ear, sometimes larger and sometimes smaller. It is a membranous, cartilaginous Substance, of a blackish grey Colour, and according to *Lemery* it contains a great Deal of Oil and volatile Salt. When immersed in Water it becomes soft and turgid like a Sponge. When boiled in Milk, or macerated in Vinegar, it is ordered as a Gargarism in Quinseys, and other Tumors and Inflammations of the Throat. When boiled in Wine, it is by some recommended in an Anasarca, but others assert, that its internal Use is unsafe. When previously macerated, it is by some ordered to be applied to Parts affected with the Gout.

Auricula Ursi, Offic. *Auricula ursi flore luteo*, Boerhaav. Ind. Alt. Raii Hist. Yellow Bears Ears. This Herb grows in great Plenty about *Utrecht, Styria, Tyrole*, and *Switzerland*, about the Middle, and on the Tops of large Mountains, and in many other Places. The Leaves are recommended for their vulnerary, abstergent Qualities, whether taken internally or us'd externally, or their Juice apply'd externally in Ointments and Plaisters. The Juice of the Flowers is said to remove Freckles and render the Skin white. According to *Gesner*, the Root if chewed, alleviates Tooth-achs, especially such as arise from cold Defluxions, proves beneficial to the nervous Parts, and heals putrid Ulcers. The Juice instilled in Chops of the Skin produc-

ed by Winds and Cold, is said to heal them in a short Time.

Azedarach, & *Pseudo Sycomorus*, Offic. Boerh. Ind. A. The Bead-Tree. The Flowers of this Tree are said by some, to be aperient and de-obstruent; but others say they are poisonous.

Balaustia, Offic. Ger. Emac. *Malus Punica Sylvestris major, sive Balaustium majus*, Park. Theat. *Punica flore pleno majora*, Boerh. Ind. A. The Balaustine Tree. *Balaustines* are of an earthy Nature, very astringent, inspissating, refrigerating and drying; whence they are very often used for all Kinds of Fluxes, as the Diarrhœa, Dysentery, the uterine Flux, and others; and for stopping of Hæmorrhages from Wounds. It is an Ingredient in the *Pulvis e Succino compositus*.

Balsamina. There are two Sorts of this Plant, the first of which is the *Balsamina* & *Momordica*, Offic. *Momordica vulgaris*, Boerh. Ind. A. Male Balsam Apple. It is cultivated in Gardens, and flowers in *August*. The Fruit, which is the Part used, is of a refrigerating and somewhat drying Quality, a Vulnerary, and mitigates Pains, especially of the Hæmorrhoids. Outwardly it is good for Wounds of the Nerves, Herniæ, and Combustions.

The other *Balsamina* is thus distinguished, *Balsamina lutea, sive Noli me tangere*, Boerh. Ind. A. *Persicaria siliquosa*, Offic. Quick in Hand, Touch me not. It is cultivated in Gardens, and the Herb is used, which is so forcible a Diuretic as to induce a Diabetes, and is thought to be of a pernicious and deleterious Quality.

Balsamita mas, Costus Hortorum, Offic. Ger. Emac. *Balsamita major*, Boerhaav. Ind. Alt. *Mentha hortensis corymbifera*, C. B. Costmary. The whole Plant is of a soft pleasant Smell, is cultivated in

Gardens, and flowers in *July*. The Leaves are principally used, being of a warm and drying Nature, good to heat and corroborate the Stomach, and to alleviate Head-achs arising from any Disorder of it, to expel Wind, and prevent acid Eructations. This Plant is said to refolve Obstructions of the Liver and Spleen; and is good against the Dropfy and Jaundice. Externally it is used in heating Fomentations for corroborating the Limbs.

Balsamum Capivi. This is obtain'd by making an Incision in a Tree thus distinguish'd. *Capivus*, Offic. Pharmacopol. *Copaiba*, Raii Hist. *Balsamum Copaiba*, Geoff. The white American Balsam Tree. The Balsam of Capivi is produc'd in *Brasil*, and brought to us from *Rio de Janeiro, Fernambouc,* and St. *Vincent* in earthen Vessels. There are two Sorts of it, the one very limpid and the other pretty thick, and of the Consistence of Turpentine; but this Difference depends upon the different Seasons of gathering it. The limpid Kind, according to *Hoffman*, is most esteem'd both for internal and external Purposes; for when diffolv'd in Tincture of Tartar, it is succefsfully exhibited for a *Fluor albus, Gonorrhæas*, and Diforders of the Kidneys and Bladder. Externally it is an excellent Liniment for the Consolidation of Wounds and Ulcers, and for corroborating the nervous Parts, which have been weakened by the Shock of any Difease. Nor is it lefs beneficial when applied to Parts weaken'd and become unfit for Motion in Consequence of gouty Pains; *Hoffman* has in his *Obf. Chym.* fhewn, that excellent pectoral and vulnerary Balsams, for internal Use, may be prepar'd by mixing this with other Ingredients, and that it may be more commodioufly used than Turpentine for increasing the Quan-

tity of etherial Oils in Distillation.

Balsamum e Mecha. This is obtain'd from a Tree distinguish'd, *Balsamum indicum, Gileadense, e Mecha verum, et opobalsamum, seu oleum Balsami, sive Balsamelæon,* Offic. *Balsamum verum;* J. B. The true Balsam Tree. The Antients call'd the Wood of this Tree Xylobalsam, its Fruit Carpobalsam, and its Juice or Tears Opobalsam. Many are of Opinion, that there is now no fuch Thing as the true Opobalsam, and that the genuine Species, of old produc'd in *Egypt* is not to be met with in any Part of the World; but *Hoffman* is of a different Opinion, becaufe the Balsam of *Mecha* is of equal Efficacy with the Opobalsam of the Antients; for which Reason he concludes that to be the fame. According to *Pomet*, it is an excellent Diaphoretic in malignant Fevers, and of great Efficacy in deterging Ulcers of the Lungs, Kidneys, and Bladder. But the Ufe of it ought to be avoided in inflammatory Difpofitions of thefe Parts, even tho' ulcerated. Neither ought it ever to be exhibited where there is an Eryfipelas in any Part of the Body. It is ufed with Succefs in *Gonorrhæas* and the *Fluor albus*, being given from ten to twelve Drops in the Morning fafting, the Patient's Body being duely prepar'd, and the Running having continued for fome Time. It is ufed externally as a Detergent, in Wounds not attended with Contufion.

Balsamum Ipecueba. This is obtain'd from a Nut in *Brafile*, call'd Becuiba which is as large as a Nutmeg, and of a brown Colour. It confifts of an oleous Kernel, inclofed in a brittle woody Hufk. The Balsam drawn from it is, according to *Geoffrey*, much efteem'd in rheumatic and paralytic Cafes.

Balsamum peruvianum. Peruvian Balsam.

Balfam. Of this there are two Kinds, the white and the black. The former is thus diftinguifh'd. *Balfamum peruvianum album, feu Styrax alba,* Ind. Med. *Balfamum album,* Park. Theat. *Balfamum peruvianum album,* Geoffr. White Peruvian Balfam.

The black Peruvian Balfam is thus diftinguifh'd: *Balfamum peruvianum,* Offic. *Balfamum peruvianum nigrum,* Park. Theat. *Balfamum ex Peru.* J. B. The natural Balfam Tree. Peruvian Balfam is brought form *America* and *Mexico* in *New Spain*; but the white is accounted beft and is by Way of Eminence call'd *Balfam of Incifion,* becaufe according to *Monardus* it flows fpontaneoufly from a Tree of a large Size, upon making an Incifion in it. This Species is limpid, of the Confiftence of Turpentine, of a fragrant Smell, and much fcarcer and dearer than the black Sort; but it is often adulterated with Venice Turpentine. The black Sort, of which large Quantities are imported to us, is according to *Clufius* prepar'd by boiling the Branches, Bark, and Leaves of the Tree. But this Species is alfo often adulterated, probably with liquid Storax. The adulterated Sort is thick and coagulated, wants the penetrating Smell and Tafte, and is with great Difficulty diffolv'd in Spirit of Wine, but remains like a thick and oleous Magma. When one Part of genuine Peruvian Balfam is intimately mix'd in a Mortar, with an equal Weight of Salt of Tartar, and highly rectified Spirit of Rofes 'pour'd upon it, by being fubjected to Diftillation in a fand Heat, it affords a fragrant and delicate Spirit, which is of fingular Efficacy, efpecially if exhibited in a Solution of Amber or Mufk. This Medicine if ufed internally, reftores loft and impaired Strength, and being very friendly to the nervous Syftem, pow-

erfully contributes to remove thofe Diforders which arife from its Weaknefs. An extemporaneous balfamic Syrup of many and great Ufes, may be prepared by mixing an Ounce of it with one Pound of Rofe-water and Sugar. This Syrup is commodioufly mixed with ftomachic and cephalic vinous Spirits. If *Peruvian* Balfam is diftilled with the Worm and Refrigeratory, it not only gives the Water a grateful Smell like that of the Balfam, but alfo renders it nervine and diuretic. This Water if liberally drank, is of excellent Service in chronical Diforders, arifing from the Scurvy, and a Weaknefs of the Nerves.

The black *Peruvian* Balfam, according to *Geoffroy,* is of a warming and ftrengthening Nature, comforting the Brain and nervous Syftem; proves beneficial in Afthmas, the Colic, and Pains of the Stomach and Inteftines. Externally ufed it corroborates the Nerves, alleviates the Cramp, relieves all Kinds of Convulfions, and Contractions of the Sinews, old Achs and Pains. It is, alfo, ferviceable in Cuts and green Wounds. The celebrated *Hoffman* in his *Obferv. Phyfico-chym.* has given an Account of fome Medicines of fingular and uncommon Efficacy, obtained from the Peruvian Balfam by Means of various chymical Proceffes. It is an Ingredient in the *Pilulæ aromaticæ.*

Balfamum Tolutanum, Balfam of Tolu. This is the Produce of a Tree thus diftinguifhed, *Balfamum Tolutanum,* Offic. *Balfamnm Tolutanum foliis Ceratiæ Similibus, quod candidum,* C. B. Pin. The Balfam Tree of *Tolu.* This Balfam is imported from *Tolu* in the *Weft Indies,* is of a tough refinous Confiftence, growing dry and friable by Age, of a yellow brown Colour, of an highly fragrant Smell, and aromatic Tafte. This is an excellent Pectoral

toral Medicine, and consequently of great Service in all Disorders of the Lungs, as Coughs, Asthmas, and Consumptions; but what renders it still more valuable is, that it has no nauseous oleaginous Taste, as most other native Balsams have. With Sugar and the Yolk of an Egg it makes an agreeable Emulsion. It is also said to be restorative, to strengthen the Vesiculæ Seminales, and stop old Gleets, and Strains, in either Sex. Externally applied, it deterges and consolidates Wounds, resists a Gangrene, strengthens the Nerves, and is good against a Rheumatism and Sciatica. Its Dose, according to *Geoffroy*, is from six to eight Grains. It is an Ingredient in the *Syrupus Balsamicus*.

Banana, Offic. *Ficoides, seu Ficus Indica, longissimo, latissimoque folio, caule macculato, fructu minore*, Boerh. Ind. A. The Banana Tree. It grows in *America*. The Virtues ascribed to the Fruit of this Tree, are to nourish much, to excite Urine, and provoke to Venery.

Bangue, Offic. Raii Hist. *Bangue Cannabi similis exotica*, C. B. Pin. Bangue. The Leaves are like those of Hemp, and have an insipid earthy Taste. The *Indians* use the Seeds and Leaves of this Plant for various Purposes especially for procuring an Appetite, and rendering them vigorous in their Amours, for making them forget their Cares, and enjoy a sound Sleep, and agreeable Dreams. Mr. *Ray* from whom this Account is taken, says he learnt from Sir *Hans Sloane*, that it was a different Plant from Hemp. It grows in *Indostan*, and other Parts of the *East Indies*, where it is principally in Use.

Banilia, is thus distinguished, *Vanilia, Banilia*, Offic. *Volubilis siliquosa, mexicana, foliis Plantaginis*, Raii Hist. Vanelloes, or Banilas. They grow in *New Spain*, and other Parts of the *West-Indies*, whence they are brought to us. In *Britain* they are only used as an Ingredient in Chocolate, to which they give a pleasant Flavour. By *Hernandez* in *Descr. Rer. Medic. Nov. Hispan.* they are said to be grateful to the Stomach and Brain, to expel Wind, to provoke Urine, to promote the Birth, and bring away the Secundines, to resist Poison, and cure the Bites of venomous Animals.

Barbarea, Offic. Ger. Emac. *Barbarea flore simplici*, Park. Theat. *Sisymbrium Erucæ folio, flore luteo*, Boerh. Ind. A. Winter Cresses. It grows in the Fields, and is cultivated in the Kitchen Gardens for Sallad. It contains a great deal of essential Oil and Salt. It is detersive and vulnerary, excites Urine, and is recommended for the Scurvy, Diseases of the Spleen, and for the nephritic Colic, either used internally or externally. The expressed Juice of the Herb cures a Defluxion of fœtid and scorbutic Humours in the Mouth, and Looseness of the Teeth, and Excrescences of the Mouth, if the Gums are rubbed with it. The Herb boiled in Wine or Milk, cures sciatic Pains, if Lint is soaked in it, and applied hot to the Part afflicted. The Seed provokes Urine, and expels the Stone. And may also be used in Sinapisms and Vesicatories.

Bardana, the Name of a Plant of which there are several Species; the first is the *Bardana major*, & *Lappa*, Offic. Ger. Emac. *Lappa major Arcium Dioscoridis*, Boerh. Ind. A. J. B. Burdock. It grows almost every where by the Way-side and flowers in *June* and *July*. The Roots, Leaves, and Seeds are used. The Roots are sudorific, alexipharmic, and good in malignant Fevers for which Reason they were an Ingredient in the *Aqua Theriacal*. They are, also, used against the

Go

Gout and Pains in the Limbs. The Leaves boiled in Milk, and applied as a Cataplasm, also, answer the same Intention. They are good for Burns and Inflammations, and for that Reason were ordered the *Unguentum populneum.* The common People frequently apply them to the Feet and Wrists in Fevers. The Seeds reduced to a Powder and exhibited in white Wine, are good to provoke Urine and alleviate Fits of the Stone.

Bardana arctium, Offic. *Lappa major montana, capitulis tomentosis, seu arctium,* C. B. Boerh. Ind. Alt. Woody - headed Burdock. This grows about ruinous Buildings, and the Way-sides, and flowers in *July.* According to *Dale* the Roots and Seeds are used in Medicine, and have the same Virtues with the former. A Decoction of them in Wine, held in the Mouth, mitigates the Tooth-ach; when used as a Fomentation, it removes Burns and Chilblanes, and when drank in Wine, is good for the Sciatica and Strangury.

Bardana, Offic. *Lappa Minor, Xanthium Dioscoridis,* C. B. *Xanthium,* Boerhaav. Ind. Alt. Louse-Bur. This is a much smaller and lower Plant than common Burdock, but is little used in Medicine, tho' some commend it in scrophulous Tumours, the Juice being taken inwardly, and the Leaves applied to the Swellings. *Matthiolus* extols it much as a Plant of singular Efficacy against the Leprosy.

Basilicum. This is the *Ocinum Basilicum,* Offic. *Ocinum vulgatius,* C. B. Pin. Boerh. Ind. Alt. Common Basil. It is sown in Gardens, flowering in *July* and *August.* The Ancients condemned the inward Use of Basil, as hurtful to the Sight. *Schroder* says it clears the Lungs of Phlegm, and provokes the Menses.

Battata Virginiana, Offic. Park. Theat. *Solanum tuberosum esculentum,* Boerh. Ind. A. *Virginia,* commonly called *Irish*-Potatoes. They are Emollient, good to prevent and cure Disorders proceeding from, or attended with a Rigidity or Stricture of the Fibres, and are therefore proper Food for those who use much Exercise.

Bdellium, Offic. Park. *Bdellium omnium auctorum,* Raii Hist. *Bdellium gummi,* Ind. Med. Gum Bdellium. According to *Pliny in lib.* 12. *cap.* 9, The Tree which produces this Gum is prickly, black and as high as the Olive Tree, bearing Leaves which are ever green, and greatly resemble those of the Oak. There are terrible Disputes about the Parts of the World in which this Tree is produced; since some will have it the Native of the *Saracens* Country, others of *Petra,* and others of still different Parts; so that among such a vast Variety of Sentiments, it seems hard, if not absolutely impossible, to distinguish Truth from Error. In the mean Time, forgetting the Speculations of the Curious, we shall confine ourselves to what is certain and evident. The Gum Bdellium, then, is of a reddish brown Colour, deeper than that of Myrrh, and of a more tough and tenacious Consistence. It is with Difficulty dissolved in any Liquor, has a bitterish Taste, and a Scent next to that of Myrrh, tho' not so pleasant. What is imported from *Turky* and the *Indies* is accounted best. There is, also, another Sort brought from *Guinea,* which is whiter, in large round Lumps, and of little or no Smell, but this Species is less esteemed than the other. This Gum is of an hot and drying Nature, and is said to be beneficial against Coughs and Imposthumations of the Lungs, to provoke Urine and the Calamenia, and to expel the Secundines. Externally it is used as an Ingredient in dissolving and discuti-

ent

ent Plaisters. According to *Diosco-rides in lib.* 1. *cap.* 80. when diluted in fasting Spittle, it discusses Tumours about the Throat, and an Hydrocele, used as a Pessary, or by Way of Suffumigation, it relaxes the Vessels of the Uterus and evacuates all Kinds of Humidity. Being drank in some proper Liquor, it is said to dissolve the Stone, and cure those who are bitten by venomous Animals. It is also good in Ruptures, Convulsions, Plurisies, and erratic Flatulences.

Becuiba Nux. This is a Nut of a brown Colour, and as large as a Nut-meg. It consists of an oleous Kernel, inclosed in a woody brittle Husk. There is drawn from it an excellent native Balsam, highly esteemed in rheumatic and paralytic Cases.

Bedeguar, the spongy Excrescences of the *Rosa Sylvestris* are thus called by some Writers on the *Materia Medica.* The Ashes of these burnt, are said to be effectual against the Gravel, and Dysury, and to incline the Person who lies upon them to sleep.

Behen album, Geoff. Tract. *Jacea orientalis patula, Carthami facie, flore luteo magno,* Tourn. Inst. *Serratulæ affinis, capitulo squamoso luteo, ut & flore,* C. B. Pin. White Bean of the Antients. White Bean is a Root, which *Rauwolfius* found at the Foot of Mount *Libanus,* and *Tournefort* brought from the lesser *Asia.* It is cordial, antispasmodic, and good to kill Worms.

Behem album, Offic. Ger. *Behem album,* Offic. J. B. *Lychnis Sylvestris, quæ Behem album vulgo,* C. B. Pin. Spattling Poppy, or white Ben. The Root of this is the only Part used in Medicine, and is accounted cordial, cephalic, alexipharmic, and a Provocative to Venery. It flowers in Summer, and is frequently to be met with in Meadows, and Corn Fields.

Behem rubrum, Limonium, & Behem rubrum, Offic. *Limonium majus vulgatius,* C. B. Boerh. Ind. Alt. Sea Lavender. It grows in Salt Marshes, and flowers in *July* and *August.* It is imported in round Slices. It is supposed to have the same Virtues, as the white Ben of the Antients, and moreover to be astringent. The Root and Seed is of Service in a Diarrhœa, Dysentery, and against excessive menstrual Discharges and the *Fluor albus.*

Belladonna. This is the *Solanum lethale,* Offic. Ger. *Belladonna majoribus foliis & floribus,* Boerhaav. Ind. Alt. Deadly Night-shade. It grows among Rubbish, and by Highways, and flowers in *June* and *July.* The Fruit of this Plant taken internally is highly dangerous, as appears from many Observations which occur in the Works of practical Authors. The Leaves are said to be great Sweetners and Resolvents. Externally they are applied to the Piles and Cancers. Some boil them with Whey, or make Use of its Juice. Mr. *Ray* greatly extols the Leaves in carcinomatous Ulcers and Indurations of the Breasts. Notwithstanding the deleterious Nature of this Plant, some have ventured to give an Infusion of it in Wine, as a Cure for a Dysentery; and others have given a small Quantity of its Juice boiled up to the Consistence of a Syrup, with Sugar, as a Narcotic; but this Practice is rather empirical than rational, and at best very hazardous. *Gerard* informs us, that at *Wisbich* in the Isle of *Ely,* three Children eat the Berries of this Plant, by which Means two of them died, whilst the third was recovered by drinking Honey and Water till he vomited plentifully. Mr. *Ray* from *Hœchstetterus* informs us, that a mendicant Friar at *Rome* by drinking in Infufion of this Plant in Wine, loft his Senfes, but was brought to himfelf by drinking a Glafs of Vinegar. I know an Inftance of a Man and his Wife, Child, and Father, who were rendered mad by eating this Plant boil'd as Greens; and a Dog who laped the Broth in which they were boiled had the fame Fate. The Dog recovered the fame Day; the Man and his Wife, the next; the Child in two or three Days; and the old Man in a Fortnight.

Benzoin, Benzoinum, Offic. *Benzoinum,* Offic. C. B. Pin. *Benzoinum, cujus arbor folio citri,* J. B. The Benjamin Tree. This grows in the *Eaft-Indies* to a confiderable Height and Thicknefs, and bears long Leaves like thofe of the Citron and Lemon-trees, tho' fmaller, and not fo green. The Gum produced by this Tree, commonly known by the Name of Benzoin, is a refinous inflammable Subftance, fometimes of a reddifh, fometimes of a pale Colour, and generally very foul. When it is covered with white Spots it is called Benzoinum Amygdaloides. It is of an agreeable Tafte, a little acrid, and is much ufed in Perfumes. It is brought us from the *Philippine Iflands, Siam,* and *Sumatra.* The Druggifts, according to *Savary,* keep two Kinds of Benzoin, that in Tears as it is called, and another Sort. The true Benzoin, which was brought into *France* by the Ambaffador of *Siam's* Retinue, was externally of a yellowifh gold Colour, but white internally, with fmall clear white and red Veins diftributed thro' it. It was friable and without any Tafte, but of a very agreeable, and highly aromatic Smell. It differed very much from that Benzoin in Tears, which is commonly fold, and which is of a clear tranfparent Mafs, of a reddifh Colour, and mixed with whitifh Tears, refembling Almonds, for

which Reafon it is called Amygdaloide Benzoin. This laft Species ought to be chofen with Qualities as much approaching to the former as poffible, and it ought above all Things to be pure and free from Dregs, a Property with which it is very rarely to be found. The other Sorts of Benzoin is the moft common of all, and very often counterfeited by a Fufion of feveral Gums together. The beft of this Kind is pure, of an agreeable Smell, refinous, and intermixed with a great many whitifh Tears, that which is black, and without any Smell, is abfolutely to be rejected. According to *Geoffroy,* Benzoin is very proper in Afthmas, to attenuate the Phlegm which oppreffes the Lungs, and deterge and cure pulmonary Ulcers; but the Flowers of Benzoin are preferred for internal Ufe. Moft Authors feem to agree that this Gum is of a warming, drying, difcuffing, diffolving and purifying Nature, refifts Putrefaction, is good againft Difeafes of the Breaft and Lungs and cures Oppreffions of the Thorax. *Amatus Lufitanus* informs us, that he cured an obftinate and inveterate Cough, by Means of the Flowers of Benzoin, and thofe of Sulphur. *Fabricius Bartoletus lib.* 5. *de Dyfpnæa, cap.* 1. fays a great deal concerning its Efficacy in Diforders of the Breaft and Defects of Refpiration, and calls it the Balfam of the Lungs. But *Marcus Banzer,* in *Controver. medico mifcellan. Dec.* 4. *Thef.* 7. endeavours to demonftrate the contrary, and afferts, that the Flowers are prejudicial in a Phthifis and other Diforders of the Lungs. Externally it is ufed in all fragrant Compofitions; for it proves cordial by its agreeable Smell, fortifies the Senfes by its Steam, dries up the cold Humours of the *Cerebellum,* diffipates Defluxions, and cures Toothachs; however in burning Benzoin,

we

we ought to take care not to swallow a great Deal of the Smoke, because it not only quickly affects the *Cerebellum,* but also acts with such Force upon the Breast and Lungs, that it is apt to destroy Respiration. It is an Ingredient in the *Balsamum Traumaticum,* and *Elixir Paregoricum.*

Barberis, Oxyacantha, Galen, Offic. *Barberis Dumetorum,* C. B. Pin. Boerhaav. Ind. Alt. The Barberry or Pipperidge-bush. It flowers in *April* and *May,* and the Berries are ripe in *September.* The Inner Bark, the Berries and the Seeds are used. The first is opening and attenuating, and is accounted a Specific against the Yellow Jaundice, taken either by way of Infusion or Decoction. The Fruit is very cooling and restringent, and good to moisten the Mouth and extinguish Thirst in burning Fevers. The Conserve is beneficial in all Kinds of Fluxes, and the Yellow Jaundice. The Seeds are binding and astringent, tho' they are but rarely used.

Beta alba, Offic. Ger. Emac. White-Beet. The Root, Leaves, and Seed are used in Medicine, which are somewhat nitrous, and loosen the Belly. It is sometimes employed in Errhines and Clysters. The Beet is one of the five emollient Herbs.

Beta rubra, Offic. Ger. Emac. Red Beet. Its Virtues and Uses are the same with the *Beta alba.* A Decoction of this, together with Lentils, is sometimes used to check a Diarrhœa.

Betle, Offic. *Betre, Betlo, Betele, five Bethle.* Park. Theat. Betle. It grows in all the Provinces of the *Indies* on the Sea Coast. It strengthens the Gums, corroborates the Heart and Stomach, and Brain; if chewed in the Morning, immediately after Breakfast, it renders the Breath agreeable, but blackens the Teeth; and according to *Bontius* not only corrodes, but makes them fall out. In the Morning, the Afternoon, the Evening, and the Night time, the *Indians* chew the Betle, and carry it continually about in their Hands; but they do not use it alone upon Account of its Bitterness, but wrap up the *Indian* Nut, and a little Lime, made of calcined Shells in the Leaf of the *Betle,* which they affirm to be a Mixture of a very grateful Taste. Others mix *Lycium* with the *Betle.* The Rich and Opulent use it with Camphire of *Borneo,* and some others with Aloes Wood, Musk, and Ambergrease.

Betonica, Offic. Ger. Emac. Wood Betony. Betony grows in Woods and Thickets, and by Hedge-sides, and flowers in *May* and *June.* The Leaves and Flowers are used. The Leaves of this Plant have an herby Taste, and a little saltish and aromatic, and give no Tincture of red to blue Paper. The Flowers and Roots, which are very bitter, stain it very little. Betony is full of Sulphur, mixed with a little oily, volatile Salt, and Earth. By the chymical Analysis, it affords a great deal of Oil, a little Earth, and fixed Salt; no concreted volatile Salt, but a little urinous Spirit. Betony is aperitive, diuretic, sweetening, good for the Diseases of the Brain, and lower Belly; a Tea of the Leaves is good for the Vapours, Sciatica, Gout, Pains in the Head, Jaundice and Palsy: The Ptisan of its Leaves, a cold Infusion of them in Water, the Conserve of its Flowers, the Syrup of the Flowers and Leaves, and the Juice and Extract of these Parts, have the same Virtues: They promote Expectoration and bring away purulent Matter; they consolidate internal Ulcers, and remove Obstructions in the Bowels: The Roots purge both upwards and downwards. A Decoction of Herniaria nizria and Betony is commended for the Stone in the Kidneys and Bladder. Others advise a Decoction of Betony to stop an immoderate Flux of the Lochia. The Surgeons mix it in their Cephalic Cataplasms. They make a Plaister of the Leaves for Wounds, especially those of the Head.

Betula, Offic. Ger. Emac. The Birch-tree. It grows in woody Places in several Places in *England.* The Leaves, Bark, and Tears obtain'd from a Perforation made in the Trunk of the Tree, in the Spring of the Year, are us'd. The Leaves which are bitter, are heating, attenuating, drying, abstergent, resolvent, aperient, and fit for evacuating Serum ; for which Reason they are of singular Service in Dropsies and the Itch. As the Bark is of a bituminous Quality, it is heating, emollient, and proper for Fumigations destin'd to correct a bad Air. The Tears are recommended for diminishing Stones of the Kidneys, and Bladder, and for removing Spots of the Skin. A Wine is made of the Sap or Juice of the Birch, which is recommended for the Gravel and Stone.

Bidens, Offic. *Eupatorium aquaticum fæmina,* Ger. Emac. Water Hemp Agrimony. It grows in watery Places, and flowers in *August.* The Herb is in Use, which is esteem'd Hepatic and Vulnerary.

Bislingua, Hippoglossum, Uvularia, Offic. *Hippoglossum mas & fæmina,* Ger. Emac. Double Tongue. This Plant is commonly cultivated in the Gardens of Botanists, and is said to be of a vulnerary Quality.

Bistorta, Offic. Ger. Emac. Bistort or Snakeweed. It grows in several moist Meadows, and flowers in *May.* The Root is mostly used in the Shops, and is of a heating, astringent Quality, especially in Dysenteries, bloody Fluxes, Dysente-

ric Exulcerations of the Intestines, and Vomitings of Blood. It cures an excessive Flux of the Menses and Hæmorrhoids, and removes violent Vomitings. It quenches Thirst. The principal Way of using it is to mix it with other proper Herbs, for the Cure of the Dropsy. It is affirm'd, that it kills Worms in the Intestines. It is used in Defluxions, and Pains of the Head, malignant Fevers, Small-pox, Measles, and the Plague. It proves a Check to the too violent Ebullition of the Blood, and prevents the overheating of its more spirituous Parts. It prevents Miscarriages, and cures Wounds and Ruptures. And when any Vessel in the Abdomen is broken, it is often made an Ingredient in vulnerary Drinks. The Root powder'd, and thrown into recent Wounds, stops the Effusion of Blood, and cures them. A Decoction of the Root, also, with Wine and Vinegar, stops immediately the most violent Effusions of Blood from Wounds, if washed with it. Some take two Parts of the Root reduc'd to Powder, and one Part of quick Lime, and mix them with Wine and Vinegar, and after having evaporated the Humidity, use the Powder which remains in the Vessel, for curing the Cancer. The Root mix'd with some Water proper for Disorders of the Mouth, cures Toothachs, fixes loose Teeth, and hardens the Gums, by preventing a Fluxion of Humours to them. Some distill a Water from the Root, Leaves, and Flowers. Other prepare a Syrup from the Root, which they call *Syrupus Colubrinus.* Both these Medicines are accounted excellent against the Plague, Dysentery, Fluxes, Vomitings of Blood, immoderate Discharges of the Menses, and Vomitings. The Water cleanses and heals all old Ulcers and Cancers, if they are washed with it, and some of the Powder of the Root is sprinkled upon them. It is confidently affirmed, that it banishes all Insects from a House. It is an Ingredient in the *Species è Scordio sine Opio.*

Blitum album, Offic. Ger. Emac. White Blite. It is planted in Gardens, and flowers in *July.* The Leaves, which are only used, and but seldom, are cooling and emollient; and are sometimes put into Clysters. The Seeds are good in Dysenteries, and immoderate Fluxes of the Menses, and according to *Tabernæmontanus,* the Seeds of it are boiled like Millet in *Silesia,* and afford the common People a grateful Food. The Juice of the Herb express'd, cures Corns in the Feet, if applied to them. A Fumigation of the Herb promotes the Menses, when stopp'd; and expels false Conceptions, and the Secundines. According to *Casp. Schwenkf. in Catal. Stirp.* the Country People use it as a Remedy against Hæmorrhages in their Cattle: And *Tabernæmontanus* informs us, that its Juice, exhibited in Wine, cures the Bites of Scorpions and Spiders.

Blitum rubrum, Offic. Ger. Emac. Red Blites. The Virtues of this are much the same as those of the preceeding.

Boletus, Offic. *Tubera Cervina,* Park. Deers Balls. These are digged out of the Earth, and the whole of them are used, which are as large as a Walnut. It is rarely used, tho' some recommend it as a powerful Stimulus to Venery, and a Medicine very proper for increasing Milk. Its external Use is recommended in hysteric Disorders, and hard Labours.

Bombax, Offic. *Gossipium sive Xylon,* Ger. Emac. The Cotton Bush. It is cultivated in *Greece, Turkey, Sicily,* and *Malta;* and flowers in *June.* In the Shops the Seeds and Wool of this Shrub are used. The Wool burn'd, and reduc'd to

Powder, stops the Effusion of Blood from Wounds, if put into them. The Seeds are good for Disorders of the Kidneys and Liver, but prejudicial to the Head and Stomach. They are also esteemed excellent for those who are afflicted with a Cough, or Difficulty of Breathing. They are good for the Stone, yield a wholesome Nourishment, strengthen the Constitution, and cure the Dysentery; for by their lenitive Quality, they obtund the acrid and exulcerating Humours. The Oil expressed from the Seeds removes Spots of the Skin, and cures running Sores of the Head. In *Egypt,* according to *Prosper Alpinus,* they extract a Mucilage from the Seeds, just as they do from those of Fleabane and Quinces, which is of Use in burning Fevers, and corrosive Coughs. They, also, restrain all immoderate Fluxes of the Menses. The Inhabitants of *Malta* fatten their Cattle with the Seeds of this Herb, which have a Taste resembling that of an Acorn.

Bonduch, Offic. *Arbor spinosa Indica, muricatis siliquis,* Park. Theat. *Lobus Echinatus,* Ger. Emac. Molucco Nuts, Marsao, Bezoar Nuts. It grows to a Man's Height, and is a Native of both *Indies;* the Parts in Use are the round Beans, which are of an Ash-Colour, white on the Inside, extremely bitter, and tasteless. They are good in Hernias, discuss Flatulencies, ease the Colic, comfort a weak Stomach, provoke the Menses, and expel the Stone.

Bonus Henricus, Tota Bona, Mercurialis, Offic. Ger. Emac. *Lapathum unctuosum, sive Bonus Henricus,* Park. *English* Mercury. It grows in waste Places, and among Rubbish, and flowers in the Spring. It is of a detersive cleansing Quality. The young Shoots, before they come to Seed, boiled as Spinage or Asparagus, are pleasant to the Palate, cooling, soluble, and good for the Scurvy.

rvy, and a Provoker of Urine. is ufed in Clyfters, and the Leaves de into a Cataplafm alleviate the nt.

Borago, Offic. *Borago Hortenfis,* r. Emac. Borrage. It grows in ardens, flowering in *June* and *Ju-* The Root, Herb, and Flowers ufed, and are efteem'd Cordial. is faid to fortify the Heart, to cure inting, to relieve Melancholy, and depurate the Blood. *Boerhaave* mmends the exprefs'd Juice, in all ammatory Difeafes, as the Gout, renitis, Paraphrenitis, and Perieumony. The Flowers are one of four cordial Flowers.

Botrys, Offic. Ger. Emac. *Chepodium Ambrofioides folio finuato,* erh. Ind. A. Oak of *Jerufalem.* grows by the Sides of Precipit, and Banks of Torrents. This erb is of a bitter Tafte, and a ftrong, but not difagreeable ell. It is of a heating, drying, folving, opening, cleanfing, and rgative Nature. It refifts Putrection, and is fingularly efficacious Oppreffions, Coughs, and all cold iforders of the Breaft, and Diffities of Breathing. It is alfo very efctual, for diffipating vifcid Matter dged in the Thorax. It opens Obuctions of the Liver, Kidneys, d Matrix; cures the Jaundice, events Dropfies, promotes a Difarge of the Menfes and Lochia, d cures Pains of the Uterus and elly. The *Venetian* Women find e Botrys to be a fure and infallible emedy againft hyfteric Fits, both fed internally and externally. Fumigations of the Herb itfelf, are excleent for provoking the Menfes, d expelling dead Foetufes: The eaves dried, reduced to Powder, d mix'd with Honey, are excelnt for Vomitings of Blood, and iforders or Ulcers of the Lungs. *Matthiolus* informs us, that by this edicine, he cured Patients, who

had fpit up Pieces of their Lungs. A Decoction of the *Botrys,* with Syrup of Violets, is recommended, as good for Abfceffes, by *J. Heurn. L. 2. Meth ad Prax. C.* 8. In the foreign Shops there is a Conferve made of the young Leaves, and a Water diftill'd from the whole Plant when it flowers: Both thefe are very good Medicines in Oppreffions of the Breaft, and in Pains of the Belly. A Lohoch of the *Botrys* is recommended as an excellent Medicine for all Diforders of the Breaft, by *P. Foreftus* and others; and the *Syrupus Diabotryos* is faid to be an excellent Medicine for thofe who are phthifical. The Herb itfelf, boil'd in any Lixivium, kills Vermin, and carries off other Sordes of the Head, if wafh'd with it. *Tabernæmontanus* informs us, that the Seeds of this Herb, if fown with Corn, kill the little Worms which prove fo hurtful to it.

Another Species of the *Botrys* is the *Botrys Mexicana,* Cod. Med. *Chenopodium Ambrofioides Mexicanum,* Boerh. Ind. A. Mexico Thea. This is only found in *Europe* in the Gardens of the Curious. The Herb and its Root are in Ufe; both which are faid to corroborate the Stomach, and to relieve in Afthma's and Obftructions. A Decoction of the Root reftrains Dyfenteries, difcuffes Inflammations, and is faid to be difagreeable to poifonous Animals, and therefore to keep them at a Diftance.

Brafilia, Offic. *Arbor Brafilia,* Park. Theat. Brafil-wood. It is cold and dry, mitigates the Heat of Fevers, and is a Reftringent and Strengthener, like the Wood of Sanders.

Braffica. Cabbage. A celebrated Plant among the Antients, and much in Ufe among the Moderns, upon which *Chryfippus* wrote a whole Volume, and *Dieuches* another. *Pythagoras* and *Cato* beftow'd

T great

great Encomiums on the Virtues of Cabbage.

There are feveral Species of Cabbage, the Firft of which is the *Braffica fativa, Caulis,* Offic. *Braffica capitata alba,* Ger. Emac. Boerh. Ind. A. White Cabbage, and Coleworts. This Sort of Cabbage is juftly it is faid preferable to other Pot Herbs, fince, both raw and boil'd, it is pofsefs'd of fuch falutary Qualities, as to prevent Occafions for the Medicines ufed in the Shops. For this Reafon, when a certain foreign Phyfician came into *Denmark* with a Defign to fettle, and faw the Gardens of the Country People fo well ftock'd with Cabbage, he, with good Reafon, prognofticated fmall Encouragement for himfelf in that Part of the World. It keeps the Belly in an eafy and foluble State, and a Decoction of the Tops of its tender Shoots, difcharges fuch an incredible Quantity of Bile and Phlegm, that no Medicine proves a quicker, a fafer, or a more efficacious Purge, Hellebore and Scammony not excepted. The Juice of Cabbage is of fuch a Nature as not only to afford a fufficient Supply of Nourifhment to the Body, but alfo to correct the acrid Salts of the Juices, allay the Acrimony of the Blood, cleanfe the Inteftines, and fcour the Kidneys. For this Reafon, Cabbage is highly falutary in Diforders of the Breaft. A Decoction of Cabbage, with an Addition of Raifins, is ufed by Preachers and Pleaders, in Hoarfenefs, and Defects of Voice, arifing from too long fpeaking. Its Juice is an excellent Remedy for the Scurvy. *Konigius* tells us of a dropfical Patient, who after defpairing of Relief from the Phyficians, was cured by a Quack, by Cabbage infufed in Wine, with proper Correctors. This Plant, a little boil'd, with fome Lemon Juice, and new Butter, is an excellent Remedy in phthifical and hectic

Diforders. Where Urine is to be provoked, or the Body render'd foluble, it, by its ftimulating muriatic Acid, proves effectual, with fuch as are not accuftom'd to take Phyfic. Many People ufe pickled Cabbage for diffipating the Remains of a Debauch. It has been obferved, that the Pickle of Cabbage, plentifully drank, has remov'd continued Fevers, cured Dropfies, and remov'd the moft obftinate Tertian Agues. When the Peafants of *Croatia* are feiz'd with Fevers, they fuccefsfully apply Cataplafms of pickled Cabbage, to their Foreheads. The Pickle of Cabbage, is good in Burns, Gangrenes, and the Beginnings of Inflammations in the Fauces, where the Intenfion is to refrigerate and repel. Nor is unpickled Cabbage lefs ufeful for various external Purpofes; fince it refrigerates, repels, opens, and deterges. After Veficatories are taken off, 'tis ufual to apply the Leaves of Cabbage anointed with Butter, which ought to be removed every two Hours. *Etmuller* fays, they may very properly be laid on Iffues, in order to carry on the Difcharge of the Matter, and prevent Confolidation. Nurfes apply the Leaves of Cabbage, to their Breafts, to prevent Coagulations of their Milk, and prevent it from being accumulated in too large a Quantity. Some apply them to Abfceffes of the Breaft, to hinder Inflammations, and promote the Confolidation of the Ulcer. Country People, to cleanfe Wounds and Ulcers, pour the Juice of Cabbage into them, or apply its Leaves bruifed to them. In peftilential Diforders, the Leaves, anointed with Rape Oil, are fuccefsfully applied, for the Maturation of Ulcers and Carbuncles. A Cataplafm of the Leaves with Butter, maturates and breaks Impofthumations. Warts have been taken off the Hands, by anointing them with the Juice of Cab-

Cabbage. The Leaves with Salt, applied to the Soles of the Feet, allay feverish Heats.

The second Sort is the *Brassica capitata rubra*, Offic. Ger. Emac. Red Cabbage. This Sort of Cabbage, is possess'd of a medicinal Quality; and abounds with a Juice, which, by its nitrous, sweet, emolient, laxative, aperitive, attenuating, and stimulating Qualities, promotes those Excretions, which are absolutely necessary to the Preservation of Health. For this Reason it is not only a Preservative against Diseases, especially of the Chronical Kind, but also contributes very considerably to their Cure. In the Roots of this Sort of Cabbage, cut longitudinally, when the Autumn is pretty far advanced, there is a Juice whose Taste resembles that of Honey or Manna, which flows from them when laid in a cool Place for sometime, and which is said to be of a purgative Quality. The red Cabbage is preferable to the white, in Cases where the Body is afflicted with Ulcers; since, in such Constitutions, the white soon assumes a putrid Quality, and becomes fetid. Some use red Cabbage-leaves, by Way of Plaister, in inflamed Wounds, and itchy Ulcers. When the Achors of Children are repell'd, the Leaves of the red Cabbage, apply'd to them, never fail to make the Discharge of the Matter return.

Another Sort of Cabbage is the *caulis rubra*, Offic. *Brassica rubra*, Ger. Emac. Red Coleworts. This Plant is cultivated in Gardens, and its Leaves only are in Use, a Decoction of which, sweeten'd with Sugar, is a celebrated Remedy in Asthma's.

A fourth Sort of Cabbage is the *Brassica sabauda*, Offic. Ger. Emac. Savoy Cabbage. This Sort of Cabbage is cultivated for the Kitchen in the Gardens of *England.* It is very delicate and tender, for which Reason, it is much sought after, by those who have nice Palates, and are acquainted with its agreeable Taste.

The fifth Sort of Cabbage is the *Brassica florida*, Offic. Park. Theat. The Colliflower. This Species of Cabbage is cultivated in Gardens, and is much used in the Kitchens. In Conjunction with other proper Ingredients, they add it to Pyes and Sauces, which are very agreeable both to the Sick and the Healthy.

The sixth is the *Brassica Gongylodes*. The Turnep Cabbage. The Seeds of this Cabbage, yield an Oil by Expression, very proper for Lamps, and for the Purposes of those concern'd in the woolen Manufacture.

The seventh is the *Brassica fimbriata*. The Boor-Cole. Its Seeds are of a blakish-Colour, an acrid aromatic Taste, and of a Smell sufficiently grateful, tho' not strong. Both for Food and Medicine, it is not inferior to the red Cabbage. The *Italians* put the young Tops of this Cabbage, into their Sallads, to render the Body soluble and provoke Urine. The black Seeds of this Cabbage are possess'd of an anthelminthic Quality; and when bruised, with Sugar, invigorate the Organs of Speech, and render the Voice clear, strong and sonorous.

The eighth is the *Brassica campestris perfoliata, flore albo,* Perfoliated wild Cabbage, with a white Flower. It grows spontaneously in several Countries, flowering in Summer, it is possessed of singular, if not more powerful Qualities, than the other Species of Cabbage; for which Reason it is by some called *Brassica rustica*, but is not used as Food. *Cato* affirms, that the Powder of the dried Plant, made into an Errhine, and taken up the Nose, cures all Defects, and amends the ill Scent therein. *Chryfippus* recommended it for Inflations, and melancholic Diforders ; alfo for recent Wounds, being applied with Honey, and not taken off before the feventh Day : Bruifed in Water, he orders it for ftrumous Swellings. Others fay, it checks the Progrefs of fpeading Ulcers, confumes Excrefcences, and fmooths the Skin from Scars ; being chewed it heals Ulcers of the Mouth, and Affections of the Tonfils ; three Parts of it mixed with two Parts of Alum, in Vinegar, cure the *Pfora,* and inveterate *Lepra,* if anointed therewith. *Epicharmus* faid, an Application of it was a fufficient Cure for the Bite of a mad Dog ; but it is more effectual with Lafer and ftrong Vinegar. The Seed roafted, is a Remedy againft the Venom of Serpents, and the poifonous Effects of Mufhroons, and Bull's Blood. The boil'd Leaves are good in Diforders of the Spleen. The Afhes of the Root, cure a Swelling of the Uvula, by touching it ; and, made into a Linctus, with Honey, reprefs the Parotides, and heal the Bites of Serpents.

The ninth is the *Braffica campeftris perfoliata, flore purpureo.* Perfoliated wild Cabbage, with a purple Flower. Its Seeds, Root, and medicinal Virtues agree with the former.

Braffica marina Soldanella, Offic. *Soldanella marina,* Ger. Emac. *Scottifh* Scurvy-grafs. It is produc'd in the moft fandy Parts of the Sea Coaft, in the North of *England,* and flowers in *June.* The whole Herb is in Ufe, and as it is excellently calculated for difcharging Water, it contributes very much to the Cure of Dropfies and Scurvies. It is likewife given in rheumatic Cafes. It works very roughly, and very much diforders the Stomach.

Britannica Antiquorum vera, five Lapathum longifolium nigrum paluftre, Munt. Herb. Brit. *Hydrolapathum,* Offic. *Lapathum aquaticum folio cubitali,* Boerh. Ind. A. Great Water Dock . *Muntingius* wrote a whole Treatife on the Subject of this Plant, in Quarto, and endeavours to prove this to be the true and genuine *Britannica* of the Antients. When *Germanicus Cæfar* had removed his Camp beyond the *Rhine* in *Germany,* they had only one Spring of frefh Water in that maritime Tract of Land, by drinking of which, within the Space of two Years, their Teeth fell out of their Heads, and the Joints of their Knees were enfeebled and relaxed. The Phyficians call'd thefe Diforders *Stomacace* and *Scelotyrbe.* There was a Remedy at length difcover'd, which was the Herb *Britannica,* a moft falutary Medicine, not only to the Nerves, and in Difeafes of the Mouth, but alfo againft an Angina, and the Poifon of Serpents. This we learn from *Pliny.* The *Britannica* has a thick, round, broad, juicy Root, fpongy when old, about a Hand's Breadth in Length, divided below into feveral thick Parts, and furrounded with little fibrous Roots ; the Colour of it, when frefh taken out of the Earth, is black on the Outfide, and White within, but foon alters into a reddifh Yellow, like that of the true Rhubarb ; and the Root, when dry, turns quite Brown. It has but few Leaves, but they are the longeft of all other Kinds of Docks, fituated near to one another, and feparate, pointing upwards, of about two Foot long, in Breadth three or four Fingers, being wideft in the Middle, ending in a fharp Point, of a deep Green, or fky Colour, of a dark Green above but paler underneath, with pale Green Fibres, of a pretty thick,

thick, clofe, hard, denfe, firm Subftance, the Edges a little curl'd, banding on Pedicles of a moderate Length and Thicknefs, fometimes ed near the Ground. They have an Aftringency, with fomething of an Acidity, falling off towards the End f *Auguft.* The Stalk is fingle, or multiply'd, according to the Age or bignefs of the Plant, two, three, ometimes four Feet in Length, brait, round, green, hollow, adorn'd on both Sides with leffer Leaves, which bend a little upwards as well as downwards, from whofe Ale, proceed little Sprigs, with ittle, fhort, and tender pendulous Leaves, and pale Flowers, which pen towards the End of *July,* and are thinly difpos'd about the Joints, but not in the Manner of Whorles. The three outer Petals of the Flower are confpicuous on both Sides or two hairy pale-whitifh Gemmuæ; but thefe are obferv'd in no fpecies of the *Lapathum,* but the *Virginian Britannica.* The Seed is mall, angular, and of a fpaliceous Colour. Every Part of his Herb, as the Stalks, Leaves, Flowers, and Seeds, but efpecially the Roots are powerfully aftringent, confolidating, and conglutinating; for which Reafon it reftrains and heals all Sorts of Putrefaction, as the Eryfipelas, Herpes, Phagedenic Ulcers and Gangrenes. It ftops Hæmorrhages, as alfo the Hæmorrhoids and Menfes, and is effectual for all thofe Purpofes, in which other cold Aftringents are requir'd. It cures all Manner of Difeafes of the Nerves, as Twitchings, Contractions, Tremblings, Convulfions, Palfies, febrile Heats, or Rigors. It banifhes away Serpents and other venomous Animals, and cures their Bites; for which Reafon it is reckon'd among the Alexipharmics; it is good for all Species of the Angina, Relaxation of the Uvula, Swelling

of the Tonfils, and other like Difeafes of the Mouth, Fauces and Stomach, which require Aftringents; as alfo Abfceffes, Tumours and Ulcers. It removes various Sorts of Defluxions, and laftly, Difeafes which proceed from hidden Caufes, as the *Stomacace,* the *Scelotyrbe,* (the Scurvy affecting the Mouth and Legs) and Ulcers in the Legs. The green Leaves, are apply'd to ulcerated Parts, for twelve Hours, and then changed; the Juice alfo harden'd by the Dog-day's Sun, or infpiffated by the Fire, is ufed to anoint the Sore. The Leaves of the *Britannica* are ftyptic, a little bitter, and give a deep Tincture of Red to the blue Paper. The Root gives it a little fainter; it alfo is very ftyptic and bitter. Its Bark is thick, of a flefh Colour, ftreaked; its Heart is foft, and of a pale Yellow. It is probable, that the falt of this Plant may be compofed of Alum and Sal Ammoniac, mix'd with a great deal of fetid Oil. I believe this Plant is very effectual in fcorbutic Symptoms; and am convinc'd by Experience, that it will effectually cure Bleeding of the Gums, if chew'd in a Morning.

Briza, Offic. *Zea monococcos, five fimplex, five Briza,* Park. Theat. *Hordeum diftichum, fpicâ nitida, Zea feu Briza nuncupatum,* Boerh. Ind. A. St. Peter's Corn. It is cultivated in *Germany;* and the Seed is ufed, which agrees in Virtue with the *Zea,* or *Spelta.*

Bromus, Offic. *Bromus Herba five Avena fterilis,* Park. Theat. Drank or Wild Oat Grafs. This is a Plant much like the Ægilops, being of a drying Quality. It is recommended for the Worms in Children.

Brufcus Rufcus, Offic. Ger. Emac. Butcher's Broom. This Plant grows in Hedges, and Thickets, flowering in *Summer.* The Root is

one

one of the five opening Roots, good to remove Obftructions of the Bowels, and to evacuate by Urine. It is prefcribed in Broths, Ptizans, and Apozems for the Dropfy, Cachexy, Jaundice, Stone, and Retention of Urine. A Pint of White Wine, in which a Dram of the Powder of the Root of Butcher's Broom, with the fame Quantity of thofe of Figwort and Dropwort have been infufed, is recommended for fcrophulous Tumours.

Bryonia, Bryony. There are two Sorts of Bryony us'd in the Shops, the firft of which is the *Bryonia alba*, Offic. Ger. Emac. *Vtis alba vel Bryonia*, J. B. White Bryony. It is found in Lanes, and by Hedge Sides, it flowers in *May*, and the Berries are ripe in *September*. The Root of this Plant is the only Part now ufed in Medicine, and all Authors are fufficiently agreed, that it is highly acrimonious and naufeous, provokes Urine, purges violently, and vomits brifkly. The Dofe of the Root, reduc'd to Powder, is from two Scruples, to one Dram; but when it is intended for internal Purpofes, its draftic Qualities ought to be corrected, by the Addition of a proper Quantity of Cream of Tartar. Since, therefore, this Root when us'd internally, acts by its ftimulating and refolvent Acrimony; 'tis fufficiently obvious, that it may be properly exhibited in Cafes, where heating Medicines are indicated, and when the Intention is to ftimulate the Nerves ftrongly, and give a Kind of Concuffion to the whole Syflem. To this Quality it is alfo owing, that it is fo much extoll'd in intermitting Fevers, in provoking the Menfes, curing thofe uterine Diforders to which young Women are fubject, and in killing and expelling Worms lodg'd in the Inteftines; for being poffefs'd of an highly draftic Virtue, it powerfully incides the tenacious Juices, and furprifingly removes Obftructions. Thus Mr. *Ray* informs us, that the Bulk of a Nutmeg, of the Conferve made of its Root, taken twice a Day, and perfifted in for a long Time, often proves the happy Means of removing and entirely curing epileptic and hyfteric Paffions; and that the fame happy Effect is produc'd, by continually putting a Piece of its Root, into the Cup out of which the Patient drinks. *Foreftus* from *Avicenna*, informs us, that Patients render'd delirious, by dangerous Wounds, are in a great Meafure reftor'd either by drinking Briony Root, for fome Days, in fome refrigerating and diluting Liquor, or ufing it in any proper Food, capable of obtunding and blunting its Tafte. The Root, externally applied, has in many Cafes, given inconteftable Proofs of its refolvent Qualities. Thus when newly bruis'd, and mix'd up with Salt and Vinegar, it refolves cold Tumors, and removes the difcolour'd Marks arifing from extravafated Blood, if applied to them. According to *Etmuller*, Briony Root, not only cures the Dropfy, when exhibited internally, but alfo evacuates the Waters collected in the Abdomen, when applied externally by Way of Cataplafm, to the Region of the Loins, either bruis'd by itfelf, or made up with Cows, Goats, or Pigeon's Dung. It is alfo applied to œdematous Swellings of the Feet and Legs, an Hydrocele of the Scrotum, and other Diforders of a fimilar Nature; in which Cafes it carries off the Serum, and confequently difcuffes the Swellings. It is alfo properly applied to fcrophulous Tumours, whether exulcerated or otherwife. If the Root of the white Briony is excavated in the Ground, and duely cover'd up, the Liquor collected in it proves

an

an excellent Medicine for arthritic Pains, if applied immediately to the Parts affected. The Root itself also, fresh bruised, mixed up with Linseed Oil, and applied warm, removes sciatic and arthritic Pains. This Medicine is to be repeated till the morbific Matter is resolv'd and dissipated. *Etmuller* informs us, that when the Uterus is to be purg'd, white Briony Root may either be used as an uterine Pessary, or by Way of Fumigation. As too violent Effects are to be dreaded from Briony Root in Substance, Mr. *Boulduc* in *Hist. Acad. Roy. des Sciences, An.* 1712. thinks it more safe to have Recourse to Infusions, Decoctions, and Extracts of it. He also prefers Infusions to Decoctions of it, and approves more of infusing it in Wine than in Water: When the only Intention is to discharge the Waters from the Abdomen, he maintains that Extracts from its Juice, are preferable to those obtain'd by Infusion or Decoction. Some think that an Ounce of the *Fæcula Bryoniæ*, or Powder which subsides in the express'd Juice of its Root, is a safer Medicine than the Root itself; but it is an ineffectual Preparation, unless assisted with Chalybeates, since according to *Etmuller* it is no more than a dead Calx.

Bryonia nigra, Offic. Ger. *Bryonia Sylvestris nigra*, Park. *Tamnus racemosa, flore minore luteo pallescente* Boerhaav. Ind. Alt. Black Briony. It flowers in *June*, and is found in the same Places with the white Briony. According to *Dioscorides*, the Shoots of the first Budding, are eaten as other Greens, provoke the Menses, and are good for epileptic, vertiginous, and paralytic Patients. *Ray* informs us, that it's Root incides and attenuates viscid Phlegm, especially in Disorders of the Thorax. *Lobelius* asserts, that it pro-

vokes Urine and the Menses, and discharges Sand from the Kidneys, if drank in a proper Liquor. But *Gesner* affirms, that it is possess'd of very drastic Qualities, and is said to contain something of a poisonous Nature, for which Reason, it is improperly us'd instead of the white Briony.

Buglossum, Offic. *Buglossum angustifolium majus*, Boerh. Ind. Alt. Bugloss. It is planted in Gardens, flowering in *June* and *July*. The Leaves, Flowers, and Root are used. The Roots are very glutinous, and give a deep Tincture of Red to the blue Paper; the Flowers give it but very little, and the Leaves scarce any at all. So that probably, the Sal Ammoniac in this Plant is involved in a glutinous Juice, in which the Earth and Sulphur predominate. *Bugloss* moistens, cools, and gives Relief to melancholic Persons; it is good to dissipate the Defluxions of the Breast, and an obstinate Cough. This Plant cools no otherwise than by restoring the Motion of the Blood which stagnates, and heats the Parts wherein its Circulation is retarded.

Buglossum Sylvestre, Offic. *Buglossum sylvestre minus*, Park. Theat. Boerh. Ind. A. Wild Bugloss. It grows by Hedges and among Corn, flowering in *May*. It is but seldom used, tho' it is reckon'd to have the same Virtues with the former, but in a milder Degree, and for the Want of that, this may supply its Place.

Another Sort of this Plant is the *Buglossum latifolium sempervirens*, B. *Borrago sempervirens*. Ever-green Borrage. It is said to be possess'd of an astringent Quality, which is stronger in the Roots than in the Leaves, and if drank in Wine stops Fluxes.

Bugula, & Consolida media, Offic. Ger. Emac. Boerh. Ind. A. *Bugula vul-*

vulgaris, flore cærulea, Park. Theat. Bugle. It grows in Woods and Hedges, flowering in *May.* On Account of its abstergent Qualities, it is accounted an excellent Vulnerary. In Consequence of its abstergent Virtue, it is also said to be a present Remedy in spreading Aphthæ, and Ulcers of the Mouth: And that an Ointment made of the Leaves of Bugle, Scabious and Sanicle, bruis'd, boil'd in Lard till they become dry, and then express'd, is excellent for the Cure of all Ulcers, Contusions and Wounds. *Konig* affirms, he has known it to heal scrophulous Ulcers in the Neck. From what has been advanc'd, we may easily perceive the Reason, why this Plant is said to be diuretic, and why it is recommended in Spittings of Blood, Dysenteries, and the Fluor albus; for when coarse, tenacious and viscid Substances are attenuated, and Obstructions remov'd, in Order to make Way for a free Circulation of the Juices, the Emunctories are not only open'd, but the spasmodic Contractions, which are the immediate Cause of the morbid Fluxions, being remov'd, these Disorders are cur'd. The Herb Bugle is most properly us'd in Decoctions, or its express'd Juice may be us'd, which is highly saponaceous and opening. *Poterius* recommends a Decoction of Bugle, made with Mutton Broth, as an excellent Medicine in a *Phthisis,* and internal Ulcers; affirming, that it gently relaxes the Belly, wonderfully recruits the Liver, and fortifies other Parts. *Etmuller* informs us, that the *Italians* in the Spring, cleanse the Root and Leaves of Bugle, and use them as a Sallad, which is not only grateful to the Palate, but also seems calculated to prevent Cachexies. Its Juice is an excellent Medicine in malignant Ulcers.

Bulbocastanum, Offic. *Bulbocastanum majus & minus,* Ger. Emac. *Nucula terrestris major & minor.* Park. Theat. Earth Nut, Kipper Nut, Pig Nut, and Hawk Nut. It is emollient, and inspissates the Juices, and is often recommended to those, whose Fluids are too thin, and to such as are phthisical, consumptive and extenuated. *Trallian* recommends it for Spitting of Blood. The Seeds of this Plant are of a diuretic Quality. The Root is reckon'd an Incentive to Venery.

Bulbocodium vulgatius, J. B. *Pseudo-Narcissus Anglicus vulgaris,* Park. *Narcissus sylvestris pallidus, calyce luteo,* C. B. Pin. Daffodil. It grows in Fields and Gardens, and in many other Places. The Plant abounds with Oil and essential Salt. The Root is purgative, aperitive, and evacuates viscid Phlegm. The Dose is two Drams in an Infusion: It is hurtful to the Nerves; but outwardly is said to be good for Ambustions, Wounds, and Hernia's. *Herman* says, the bruis'd Leaves are good for an *Erysipelas.*

Bulbonach, Offic. *Viola lunaris sive Bulbonach,* Ger. *Lunaria major, siliqua rotundiore,* Boerh. Ind A, Sattin or Honesty. It grows spontaneously in several Parts of *Germany* and *Hungary;* but is cultivated in Gardens in *England.* It is of a hot, bitter, and acrimonious Taste. It abstenges, heats, and provokes Urine. The Powder of the bitterest Seeds is recommended for the Epilepsy.

Bulbus, Vomitorius, Offic. *Muscari Clusii,* Ger. *Muscari obsoletiore flore ex purpura virente,* Boerh. Ind. A. Musk Grape Flower. It flowers in *April;* and the Root is us'd, which being chew'd, or drank by Way of Decoction, cures Disorders of the Bladder, and provokes Vomiting.

Buphthalmum, Offic. *Buphthalmum verum,* Ger. Emac. *Cotula flore luteo radicato,* Tourn. Inst. Ox-

Ox-Eye. It grows wild in the North of *England*, flowering in *June*, or *July*. The bruis'd Flowers with Cerate, discuss œdematous Tumours and Hardnesses, and are recommended for the Yellow Jaundice.

Buphthalmum Germanicum, Offic. *Buphthalmum vulgare*, Ger. Emac. *Buphthalmum Tanaceti minoris folio*, Boerh. Ind. A. Common Ox Eye. It is reckon'd to be aperitive, vulnerary, and good for a Jaundice, but is seldom met with in our Shops.

Bupleurum, Offic. *Auricula Leporis umbella lutea*, J. B. Hares-Ear. It grows in hilly Places; flowering in *July* and *August*. The Herb is used. It is accounted a good Drier, aperitive, and discutient; it expels Urine and Sweat, and deterges Wounds.

Bursa Pastoris, Offic. Ger. Emac. *Bursa Pastoris major vulgaris*, Park. Theat. *Bursa Pastoris major, folio sinuato*, Boerh. Ind. A. Shepherd's Purse. It grows every-where among Rubbish, Banks and Walls, flowering all the Summer. It is of an herby Taste, a little saltish and detersive. This Plant yields a great deal of concrete volatile Salt, fix'd trivial Salt, and Earth. These Principles mix'd together, render the *Bursa Pastoris* proper to dissolve the Blood, when it is thicken'd by foreign Acids, which hinder it from passing, with its ordinary Velocity, from the Arteries into the Veins; to which we may refer the greatest Part of Defluxions. Besides, the Earth, which is in this Plant, easily imbibes the Serosities, which occasion a Relaxation of the Fibres; thus, by the Consent of all Authors, it is vulnerary and astringent; it is also believ'd to be febrifuge and lenitive. The Juice of its Leaves drank, from four Ounces to six, is an excellent Remedy in all Losses of Blood, and in Defluxions attended with an Inflammation. A Handful of it boil'd in lean Broth, is used in Ptisans, Glysters, and Cataplasms. Its distill'd Water has little or no Virtue. It is also recommended for Headachs, immoderate Fluxes of the Menses, Discharges of bloody Urine, Diarrhœas, Dysenteries, Lienteries, and Gonorrhœas.

Butomus, Offic. *Butomus floresae*, Boerh. Ind. A. *Juncus floridus*, Park. Theat. *Gladiolus palustris Cordi*, Ger. Emac. Water Gladiola. It is found in the Channels of Rivers among the Mud, flowering in *June*; the Herb is only used, and is of an aperient and deobstruent Quality.

Buxus, Offic. Ger. Emac. *Buxus arborescens*, Boerh. Ind. A. The Box Wood. It grows wild, in some Parts of *Kent* and *Surry*. A large Quantity of Box Leaves infused in near a Pint of white Wine, proves, according to *Blegny*, an infallible Cure for pituitous and flatulent Colics, if the strain'd Liquor is drank warm. They distil from the Wood an Oil, which is very narcotic, and wonderfully extoll'd in Epilepsies, Tooth-achs, and Rottenness of the Teeth. A Decoction of the Flowers of Box, is reckon'd sudorific, and 'tis said that one Dram of them proves a violent Purge. *Rondeletius* don't doubt in the least, but, that the Shavings of Box, in Consequence of their sudorific Quality, would cure the venereal Disease, but adds that they are not to be used for that Purpose, because they excite Head-achs. *Amatus Lusitanus*, cured an Hemicrania, by a Decoction of Box Wood, after all other Medicines had prov'd ineffectual. The Oil distill'd from the Wood, is recommended for Fevers, Vertigoes, the Falling Sickness, and Hæmorrhoids. This Wood

Wood fubjected to Diſtillation, from a Retort in a fand Heat, yields an acid Spirit, and a fetid empyreumatic Oil, which is order'd with melted Butter for Cancers, and with Oil of St. *John's* Wort is recommended for the Gout and Rheumatiſm. And if rectified and digeſted with Spirits of Wine it makes a good Medicine for internal Uſes. The Smoak of burnt Box-wood is very much recommended for the Plague. The Leaves are bitter, have an ill Smell, and give a faint red to the blue Paper. Of this is made the *Oleum Buxi.*

Cacalia, Offic. *Cacalia incano folio,* Ger. Strange Coltsfoot. It grows on Hills and in Woods. The Root macerated in Wine, cures Coughs and Roughneſs of the *Aſpera arteria.* The Berries powder'd and made into a Cerate ſmooth the Skin, and free it from Wrinkles.

Cacao Americæ, five Avellana Mexicana, J. B. *Amygdalis ſimilis Guatimalenſis,* C. B. Pin. *Arbor Cacavera,* Piſ. Mant. The Cacao Tree. This grows to be pretty large, and is found in ſeveral Parts of the *Weſt-Indies,* tho' thoſe of the beſt Kind are ſaid to be produc'd in *Caraccao,* in *New-Spain.* What renders this Tree very conſiderable is its bearing the Cacao Nuts, twenty or thirty of which are included in a round Capſula or Pod. Theſe Nuts are externally brown, and as large as an Almond, tho' rounder and thicker. The Juice expreſſed from the mucilaginous Pulp contain'd in the Huſk of theſe Nuts, reſembles Cream, and is poſſeſſed of a grateful Taſte, and cordial Quality. It is alſo of a detergent Nature, and when uſed externally, very proper for removing cutaneous Eruptions, and Aſperities. The Nuts themſelves included in the Huſk or Shell, are ſaid to be of ſo nutritive a Quality, that one Ounce of them con-

tains more real Nouriſhment, than a whole Pound of Beef. The Cacao Nuts when ſubjected to a chymical Analyſis, beſides other Principles, yield a large Quantity of Oil, which is wonderfully pungent and penetrating, eſpecially before it is ſeparated from the volatile Salt, of which it contains a large Quantity. It is alſo highly aromatic and cordial. A certain Quantity of this Oil, diſtilled from a Cucurbit by the Heat of Aſhes, yields an unctuous Liquor, which concretes as it drops, and is call'd the Butter of Cacao. This Butter, when not rectified, may not only be uſed with Food as Olive Oil, but is alſo extoll'd as an highly anodyne Medicine, and proper for correcting the acrimonious Humours, which prove uneaſy to the *Aſpera Arteria.* Various other Virtues are alſo aſcrib'd to this Butter by practical Authors. But the Circumſtance, which of all others renders the Cacao Nut moſt celebrated, is its being the Baſis or principal Ingredient of Chocolate, a factitious Subſtance firſt brought from *America* into *Europe* by the *Spaniards,* about the Beginning of the laſt Century. Some diſſolve this Subſtance in Water, others in Milk, and others in Wine, but Water ſeems to be of all others the beſt Vehicle for it, ſince by its diluting Quality it beſt promotes the Diſtribution of its nutritive Principles. Chocolate from its component Parts ſeems to be principally proper for Perſons of cold Conſtitutions, for old People, for ſuch as have their Strength impair'd by continual Watchings, and for thoſe who travel in cold Mornings. It is, alſo, by ſome commended, in Caſes where the Digeſtion is weak, but it is of too oleous and tenacious a Nature to be digeſted by a weak Stomach; for which Reaſon *Cheyne,* in his Eſſay on Health, thinks that it ought not to be uſed by the weak and infirm, ei-

ther

ther as an Aliment or Medicine; but owns that it may produce all the falutary Effects of a wholefome Food, in vigorous and robuft Conftitutions; in which it may alfo be ufed as an Anodyne Medicine in Colics and nephritic Pains; fince by its Vifcidity it fheathes up and blunts, the faline, acrid, and irritating Humours, that thus by the brifk Impetus of the Vifcera, they may be difcharg'd through proper Paffages. It is, alfo, confirm'd by the Experience of many practical Phyficians, that in hectic, fcorbutic, and catarrhous Diforders, Atrophies, malignant Itches, and Chin-coughs, Chocolate has prov'd a divine and miraculous Remedy, and that in thefe Diforders, when other Medicines have been ineffectual, the Phyfician has been oblig'd to have Recourfe to Chocolate, as the laft and moft effectual Remedy. The celebrated *Hoffman*, in his Confultations, afferts that Chocolate prepar'd with Water, and drank at proper Times, may conduce very much to the Cure of melancholic Diforders, arifing from too weak and lax a State of the Nerves, efpecially if a few Drops of the Effence of Amber are mixed with it. As Chocolate is nutritive, and corrects the Acrimony of the Juices, fo we think, Dr. *Stubbs* in *Philofoph. Tranf.* was in the Right when he affirm'd, that well-prepar'd Chocolate was an excellent Diet, not only for fuch as are fcorbutic, afflicted with arthritic Pains, or the Stone, for Women in Labour; and for preventing Convulfions, and expelling the Meconium of Children, but alfo for hypochondriacal and chronical Diforders. A Man in perfect Health, may drink as much Chocolate as he has an Appetite for, provided he finds himfelf refrefhed, and his Stomach not over-loaded by it. But he ought to remain in a State of

Reft for Half an Hour, or an Hour, after he has drank it, left Concoction and Digeftion fhould be interrupted or irregularly carried on. He ought, alfo, to abftain from Food, for fome Time after he has drank Chocolate, left by a contrary Practice, he fhould injure his Stomach; for Chocolate is itfelf very good Matter of Nourifhment. Hence the moft proper Time of ufing it is, when the Concoctions are finifhed, whether in the Morning, or the Afternoon; and fince in an hot Air the Powers of Digeftion are fainter and more languid than in a cold State of the Atmofphere, 'tis fufficiently obvious, that Chocolate ought to be ufed in fmaller Quantities, and more rarely in Summer than in Winter. The aromatic Ingredients of Chocolate recruit the languid Stomach; but *Caldera* advifes, that if during an exceffive Heat, the Perfon who intends to drink Chocolate, is thirfty, he fhould a little before take a moderate Draught of cold Water, left the Chocolate fhould render the Thirft more intenfe than it was before. The fame Author, alfo, informs us, that any Liquor drank after Chocolate produces terrible Effects. He alfo tells us, that Chocolate cool'd with Ice or Snow, is equally virulent and dangerous with cold Poifons. When Chocolate is prefcribed as a Medicine, the Phyfician muft determine the Quantity, and fix the proper Seafons of Exhibition. Thofe who are become weak in Confequence of Inanition, may judge of the Quantity from the Senfe of Refrefhment they feel; but at the fame Time, they ought to ufe it more fparingly than thofe who are vigorous and robuft. Chocolate when moderately ufed, contributes to the Health of thofe, who are in no Danger of having their Juices ftimulated into too brifk a Motion, or their Conftitutions o-

Ver-heated

ver-heated by the Use of Aromatics. As also of those, whose Stomachs are able to concoct and subdue the pinguious Substance of the Cacao Nuts. Hence 'tis obvious, that those Persons must abstain from the frequent and immoderate Use of Chocolate, who are in the full Vigour of their Youth, whose Juices are easily thrown into preternatural Commotions, who have spare dry Constitutions, and whose *Primæ Viæ*, in Consequence, of having lost their Tone, are unfit for the due Concoction of the Aliments. *Baglivi* informs us, that in hot and sanguine Constitutions, the immoderate Use of Chocolate, by inspissating the Blood and rendering it less fit for Circulation, produces Inflammations of the Viscera, long mesenteric Fevers and Apoplexies. *Meisner* and *Jrussieu* assert, that Chocolate produces Obstructions, and *Hoffman* asserts, that the more it is drank by hypochondriac Patients, the greater Injury they sustain, since Eructations, Loss of Appetite, Pains, and Uneasiness of the Præcordia, are produced by the Inflation and Distension of the Stomach, occasion'd by it. That drinking Chocolate to Excess contributes very much to the Formation of Stones, especially in the Gall-bladder, is sufficiently attested by the Observations of some of the best practical Physicians. On Account of the large Quantity of Sugar which enters the Composition of Chocolate, its Use, and much more its Abuse, ought to be avoided by Women labouring under uterine Disorders, and by those who are subject to hypochondriacal Flatulences. The Disadvantages arising from the Abuse of Chocolate consider'd as prepar'd with warm Water, are abundantly plain to every one who reflects, that the frequent Use of warm Water, relaxes the Organs of

Digestion, and all the Solids in general, and must consequently prove pernicious.

Cactos, Offic. *Carduus esculentus*, Park. *Cinara spinosa, cujus Pediculi esitantur*, Boerh. Ind. A. The Chardon. It is found in *Italy*, and agrees in Virtues with the Artichoak.

Calamintha. There are five Sorts of this Plant made use of in Medicine; the first is the *Calamintha montana*, Offic. *Calamintha vulgaris*, Park. *Calamintha vulgaris vel Officinarum*, Boerh. Ind. Alt. Calamint. It is found in Hedges, flowering in *June* and *July*. The Antients extoll'd it for its heating, alexipharmic, resolvent, and discutient Qualities, and prescrib'd the external and internal Use of it, affirming, it kill'd Worms. It is good for phlegmatic Constitutions, and such as are afflicted with Flatulences, and is very conducive to the Relief of Women labouring under Obstructions of the Uterus, a Fluor Albus, or a catarrhous Disorder of the Womb. It is a powerful Provoker of the Menses, and even excites them in Women big with Child, and kills the Fœtus. It is said to expel the Lochia, Secundines, and Fœtus. It is an excellent Diuretic, cleanses Ulcers of the Kidneys, and cures Discharges of bloody Urine. Boil'd with Oxymel, it is of great Service in Asthmas, or Orthopnæas. It ought not to be exhibited to those, who have no Occasion for an additional Stimulus, for it acts by producing a Heat, which, tho' small, is nevertheless often found prejudicial to the Asthmatic. But where the languid and relaxed Fibres are to be stimulated, or the sluggish Humours roused into a brisker Motion, *Calamint* will be found of singular Use and Importance, and is, therefore, justly rank'd in the Classes of cordial, alexipharmic,

lexipharmic, ftomachic, carmina-tive, uterine, and emmenagogue Medicines; and is ufed in Clyfters, Cataplafms, Fomentations, and fuch Baths as are intended for the Purpo-fes of Refolution, Difcuffion, and provoking the Menfes. It is an In-gredient in the *Theriaca Andro-machi.*

The Second, is the *Calamintha magno flore,* Boerh. Ind. A. *Cala-mintha montana praftantior,* Ger. Park. Mountain Calamint. It is cultivated in Gardens, and agrees in Virtues with the former.

The Third, is the *Calamintha,* Offic. *Calamintha Odore Pulegii,* Ger. *Calamintha altera, odore Pulegii, fo-liis maculofis,* Park. *Calamintha Pu-legii odore, feu Nepeta,* Boerh. Ind. A. Field Calamint. It grows about the Roots of Hedges, and by the Sides of Fields, flowering in *June.* The Herb is ufed. and agrees in Virtues with the firft Species, to which it is a Succedaneum.

The Fourth, is the *Calamintha paluftris,* Offic. *Calamintha aquatica,* Ger. *Mentha arvenfis verticillata hirfuta,* Boerh. Ind. A. Water Ca-lamint. It grows in moift Places, flowering in *July.* The Herb is ufed. which agrees in Virtues with the *Pulegium* or Penny-royal.

The Fifth, is the *Calamintha in-cana, Ocymi foliis,* Hoary Calamint, with Leaves like Bafil. This Spe-cies is poffefs'd of the fame medici-nal Virtues as the firft Sort.

Calcitrapa, there are two Sorts of this Plant, the firft is the *Carduus ftellatus,* Offic. Ger. *Jacea ftellata, folio Papaveris erratici,* Boerh. Ind. A. Star Thiftle. It grows upon Commons, flowering in *June.* Its Leaves are bitter, and give a faint Tincture of Red to blue Paper, but the Root a deeper. It contains a Salt like the natural Salt of the Earth. It is febrifugous, vulnerary, and aperitive. Four or fix Ounces

of its Juice is recommended in an intermitting Fever, and is good to remove Webs of the Eyes. A Wa-ter diftill'd from the Flowers, or the Seeds in Powder, are good to ex-pel the Stone. The Root is good in flow Fevers, and purge the Body of ill Humours.

The Second, is the *Calcitrapa,* Offic. *Carduus folftitialis,* Ger. *Jacea ftellata, Spina folftitialis dicta, fo-liis Cyani,* Boerh. Ind. A. Saint Bar-naby's Thiftle. It is reckon'd ape-rient, deobftruent, lithontriptic, and is good to affwage the Fervor of the Blood. *Camerarius* commends it for the Jaundice, and all Sorts of Obftructions; for the Cachexy, Dropfy, Pleurify, and Sciatica.

Calendula. Of the *Calendula* there are feveral Sorts, but the Chief for medicinal Ufes, is the *Calendula,* Offic. *Caltha vulgaris,* Boerh. Ind. Alt. Garden-Marigold, the Flowers of which are only ufed in the Shops. They are of an aromatic Smell, and when chew'd, exert a penetra-ting and almoft burning Acrimony, from whence they derive their fudo-rific Virtues, in which they are fcarce inferior to Saffron. *Schulzi-us,* in his *Praelectiones,* informs us, that they have uncommon Efficacy afcribed to them, by feveral emi-nent Phyficians, in the Cure of ma-lignant and peftilential Fevers; in which Cafe they are recommended by *Ray.* They are likewife very proper, where ftimulating Medi-cines are neceffary, for which Rea-fon, a Decoction of them is often exhibited to promote the Erupti-on of the Small Pox, and accor-ding to *Ray,* a Poffet Drink impreg-nated with the Flowers, has for a long Time been ufed in *England* to anfwer the fame Intention. Their refolvent, and aperient Qualities ren-der them ufeful in Decoctions, for provoking the obftructed Menfes: and when ufed in Vapour Baths, they

they not only excite the Menses, but also expel the Fœtus and Secundines.

The second Sort, is the *Calendula arvensis*, Ger. *Caltha arvensis*, Boerh. Ind. A. The Wild Marigold. All thePreparations of this Plant, are excellent for the Jaundice, Palsy, Dropsy, Small Pox, malignant Fevers, and Green Sickness; its Leaves and Flowers are good to eat as a Sallad, especially for Children who have scrophulous Tumors. *Cæsalpinus* prescribes the Water of Marigolds for contagious Distempers; *Tragus* commends it as an excellent Remedy to cure the Redness and Inflammations of the Eyes.

Calendula palustris Populago, Offic. *Populago flore majore*, Boerh. Ind. A. *Caltha palustris major*, Ger. Marsh Marigold. The Herb is only used in the Shops, and is, by *Dioscorides*, said to be good for removing the Pains of the Loins; and according to *Boerhaave*, it is of a caustic Quality, highly acrid, and resembling Hellibore.

Camphora. Camphire. This is not mentioned by the ancient *Greeks*, and was first introduced into the *Materia Medica* by the *Arabians*. It is a Substance of a very singular Nature, dry, friable, powder'd with Difficulty, light, white, pellucid, and not unlike the Crystals of Salt, of an acrid and somewhat bitterish Taste, of a penetrating Smell, and to some greatly offensive. It flames in an open Fire, and when kindled, burns till it is totally consumed; in Water it also, burns, and sends forth a thick dark Smoak, which also produces a blackish Soot. When put into a pure glass Vessel, with an Alembic fitted to it, it melts by the Force of Fire, ascends into the Alembic, and there concretes again into the Form of Camphire, without the least Alteration. Many celebrated Chymists have taken Cam-

phire for a solid volatile oleous Salt, form'd in the same Manner as the *Offa Helmontiana*, of a saline and oleous Principle; but this Opinion is rejected by others. *Boerhaave* affirms it to be a highly perfect, most simple, and volatile Resin, or an Oil of a solid Form and Consistence. *Hoffman* affirms, that Camphire, is, as it were, a distilled Oil in a dry Form, or a most subtile volatile Oil, which seems to have in its Composition a certain subtile Acid, to which its Form is owing, and of which it may be deprived, if mixed with Salt of Tartar, and subjected to Distillation with highly rectified Spirit of Wine; for in this Case, a Spirit is yielded, whose Taste and Smell discover it to be sufficiently saturated, with the Corpuscules of the Camphire, and which, when poured into Water, does not become milky, nor is any of the Camphire precipitated, as happens with camphorated Spirit of Wine. What remains after the drawing off of the Spirit, is a well saturated Solution of Camphire. But when dropped into Water, it does not run into a thick Coagulum, like camphorated Spirit of Wine, but may without Difficulty be mixed with the Water; for the Salt of Tartar entering into the most intimate Texture and Composition of this Substance, dissolving the oleous and thick Parts, and inducing a Change on the more subtile Acid, occasions a Resolution of this Substance into highly subtile Parts, not afterwards to be coagulated; and the Change of its Colour from white to brown, is owing to the Sulphur, or phlogistic Principle, being disentangled, and set at Liberty by the Alcali. In the Truth of Camphire's being a pure inflammable Oil, in a solid Form, we are confirmed by this Circumstance, that in hot Climates, and sometimes even in *Europe*, aromatic Substances are often heated to such a Degree, that their

Oils

Oils are converted into Camphire, as happens in the Diftillation of the Oil of Anife, Cardamoms, Caraway, Fennel, Laurel, Zedoary, Cinnamon, Southernwood, and Thyme. The fame Phænomenon, is fometimes obferved to happen, when thefe Oils, dropping thro' a long narrow or cold Worm, form themfelves into a folid kind of Mafs, which blocks up the Cavity of the Worm, but may be again diffolved by Heat. But becaufe thefe camphorated Subftances, want either the Hardnefs, the Smell, or the other Properties of the common Camphire of the Shops, we fhall only here treat of that Camphire, which is produced by the *Arbor Camphorifera*, and which is called the *Camphora Japonenfis* or *Camphora Sinenfis*. If Camphire, when put upon hot Bread, becomes moift, it is a Sign of its being good and genuine; but if it becomes dry, it is a Proof of its being bad and fpurious. When it is mark'd with reddifh or black Spots, thefe are faid to be produced by handling it with impure Hands; or to be the Effects of Moifture; but this is eafily prevented, by gathering it in a linnen Cloth, and immerfing it in warm Water, with an Addition of Lemon Juice. Thus when it is well wafhed, it muft be dried in a fhady Place, by which Means it becomes white. Formerly it was the Cuftom, in order to prevent the Exhalation and Diminution of Camphire, to keep it in Linfeed, the Seeds of Fleawort or fome others of a like Nature, which by their large Quantities of Oil, might, as it were, entangle the volatile Parts of the Camphire, and prevent their flying off. Others think that the fame Effect is produced by Pepper; but what has given Rife to this Notion is fomewhat hard to determine. The beft way to preferve Camphire, is, to anoint its Surface with expreffed Oil of fweet Almonds; for the Pores being by

thefe Means block'd up, its more fubtile and volatile Parts, will not fo eafily fly off, as otherwife they would do; but as it may be well enough preferv'd in glafs Veffels well ftop'd, to prevent the Admiffion of Air, fo there is no great Neceffity for the preceeding Method. Camphire is applied to various Ufes. The *Indians* mix it with acrid and aromatic Subftances, of which they form Troches, for promoting a Difcharge of the Saliva, when chew'd; becaufe Camphire in former times was thought to be poffeffed of cold Qualities, it is likewife faid to be given to be chew'd and fmelled by the *Monks*, to extinguifh Inclinations to Venery. But the Falfity of this Opinion is now fufficiently known; for as Camphire confifts of highly volatile Parts, it is found to poffefs Virtues highly penetrating, difcutient, refolvent, ftimulating, corroborating, alexipharmic, and is proper for refifting Putrefaction; but it does not act in a ftrong and draftic Manner, becaufe it does not remain long in the Parts into which it has penetrated, but is in a very fhort Time exhaled. *Tralles* recommends it in fcorbutic Diforders. It is faid to be poffefs'd of an alexipharmic Quality, when ufed internally, againft the Wounds of Serpents. The Notion of its being poffeffed of a cold Quality, may poffibly have taken its Rife from the Obfervation of its cooling Effects, in Inflammations of the Eyes, and Burns; for it is of fingular Efficacy in removing external Inflammations, as alfo internal, and which threaten a Sphacelus and Death if they are fevere; but more efpecially if they are fituated in the membranous Parts; for anfwering which Intentions, it is moft happily exhibited with Nitre; as, alfo, in continued Fevers, which for the moft Part have fomething of an inflammatory Nature in them; likewife in moft other Kinds of Inflammations, Pleurifies,

Phren-

Phrensies, Quinseys, and Inflammations of the *Uterus*. The celebrated *Hoffman* used Camphire, with the Addition of Bezoardic Powder, with great Success; for immediately after the Exhibition of this Medicine, the burning Heat, the Delirium, the Thirst, and the Watchings were greatly abated. *Stahl* stiles Camphire, the Subduer of all Inflammations; and the learned *Werlhofus* found very happy Effects arise from three or four Grains of Camphire in nitrous Emulsions, taken every two or three Hours in acute Fevers, Phrensies, and Deliriums. The learned *Tralles* excellently demonstrates the refrigerating and antiphlogistic Qualities of Camphire, and how efficacious it is, in Conjunction with Nitre, in a Pleurisy. An Instance whereof he gives us in his Work intitled *De Remediis Terreis.* *Capuccius* an *Italian* Physician, affirms the Virtues of Camphire to be very great, both in curing and preventing pestilential Fevers, for which Purpose one or two Grains of it may be chew'd, and swallowed by itself, three or four Times a Week, unless the State of the Patient renders the more frequent Use of it necessary. *Graan*, a celebrated *Dutch* Physician, in a Phrensy, Madness, Pleurisy and Peripneumony, highly extolls Champhire with Spirit of Nitre. In Inflammations of the Kidneys he recommends Sal Prunellæ and Camphire; for allaying the Thirst in continued Fevers, he orders three Grains of Camphire to be added to proper Powders, which Medicine with the *Bezoardicum Minerale*, he also commends in pestilential Fevers. The *Philosophical Transactions* afford us some Instances, of Maniacs cured by half a Dram of Camphire exhibited in a Bolus, Morning and Evening. *Simeon Sethi* and *Rhases*, inform us, that Camphire cures the most acute Disorders, as Pains of the Head arising from Heat and Inflammations, and those especially of the Liver. *Tachenius* informs us, that *Avicenna* was the first of the practical Physicians, who observed the Virtues of Camphire in acute Disorders, and called it the *Theriaca contra Venena calida*, or the *Theriaca* against hot Poisons. *Du Verney* thinks Camphire exhibited in cordial Potions, an excellent Remedy against the Head-ach in malignant Fevers, and tells us that he himself frequently prescribed it, with that Intention. *Mindererus*, in his Work *De Peste*, ranks Camphire, among the strongest Antidotes against the Plague; and affirms, that it is more efficacious than any of the Bezoardic Preparations, as it prevents Putrefaction, and expels the poisonous Effluvia. *Hoffman*, in all putrid Disorders, and in the Plague at its Accession, and about its Crisis, recommends Camphire to be given in an acid Vehicle, as also with Balsamics, in a Gonorrhœa. In all dangerous and terrible Hæmorrhages, especially such as accompany malignant Fevers, as also in Spittings of Blood arising from internal Causes, such as the Spasms of the Viscera, Camphire is of singular Use. In Vomitings of Blood, after Venesection, *Riverius* orders half a Scruple of Camphire, to be exhibited in four Ounces of Oxycrate, or Plantain Water. *Joubert* affirms of his Master *Rondeletius*, that in all Vomitings of Blood, especially those proceeding from acrid Defluxions, he successfully used Camphire, and sometimes gave a whole Scruple of it, diluted in a Glass of Spring Water, with a little Vinegar. Camphire, when mixed with Nitre, is of the greatest Efficacy in all Hæmorrhages; besides, nothing is found more useful in promoting the accustomed Evacuations of the Blood, than Camphire, especially when exhibited in Conjunction with balsamic and an-

tis-fpafmodic Specifics. *Wedelius de Medicam. Facultat.* juftly obferves, that Camphire is of fingular Efficacy, in promoting the brifk and lively Motion of the Blood, and muft confequently be improper, when that Fluid is too much rarified, or put into an Ebullition; fince by that very Means, the Watching, the Thirft, and Heat would be increafed. *Mindererus* of Opinion, that Camphire, ought never to be exhibited, to fuch as have infirm Heads, or weak Stomachs. Hence it is, that ftudious and fedentary People, and Women f delicate Conftitutions, who cannot bear ftrong Smells, have a thorough Averfion to Camphire, and that the latter, by the Ufe of it, fall into hyfteric Fits, to which, however, puts a Stop, in more robuft Conftitutions. With Refpect to the external Ufe of Camphire, fome put a Grain or two, into a rotten Tooth, and even ufe it as a Gargarifm in the Tooth-ach. Camphire worn as an Amulet, has been experienced an effectual Remedy, againft Fevers, as we learn from the *Mifcellanea Curiofo-Medico Phyfica Academiæ Naturæ curioforum, J. Boetlerus* gives the following Account of it, " Some hang Camphire about their Necks, for the Cure of an intermittent Fever, and the Camphire is fure to fly away, but the Fever very often remains." However, this I dare affert, that Camphire hung about the Neck, in peftilential Times; fo that the Effluvia may be received into the Noftrils, is no improper Prefervative; becaufe it corrects the Atmofphere of the Body, and fo prevents the ill Effects of the contagious Air. Camphire is a ufual Ingredient in Ointments and Plaifters, for the Sake of its Stimulus, which is of Service, in mollifying and diffolving hard Tumors, and alfo opens the Way, for the Virtues of the o-

ther Ingredients to penetrate deeper thro' the Pores of the Skin. When it is to be mixed for a Plaifter, the beft Way, as *Etmuller* advifes, is to diffolve it with Balfam of *Peru*. The Water of Camphire, according to the Account given us by the *Arabians*, diftills from the Tree which produces the Camphire. But *Garcias* obferves it to be a Fable. Others, therefore, call by this Name, the Water, in which kindled Camphire has been immers'd, and recommend it to be drank by Women labouring under Hyfterics, in which it is excellent. A Water of this Kind is prefcribed in the *Pharmacopæia Pauperum*, under the Title of *Julapium Camphoratum*. *Horftius* relates, that fome Virgins, taken with a *Furor Uterinus*, met with moft Relief, by ufing for their ordinary Drink, Water, or Beer, in which kindled Camphire had been quenched. The Solution of Half an Ounce of Camphire in a Pint of highly rectified Spirit of Wine (tho' the *London* and *Edinburgh* Difpenfatories direct an Ounce of Camphire) is a very common Topic in Contufions, Luxations, and Rheumatifms; becaufe it readily diffolves the Stagnations of the Humours, in different Parts of the Veffels, and caufes them to exhale, or puts them in Motion; whence it is of extraordinary Service, not only in all Pains and Tumors, but alfo in all inflammatory and eryfipelatous Affections; reftores Warmth to the Feet and Hands benumb'd with Cold; mitigates the Pain of the Hæmorrhoids, prevents a Gangrene, and is commodioufly applied in Cafes of a beginning or confirm'd Putrefaction, a Sphacelus, fetid Ulcers, and Wounds which are putrid, or inclining to Putrefaction; as alfo the *Cholera Morbus*, the Cholic, and the Contraction or Refolution of the Nerves confequent thereto; and the like Affections both

U of

of the internal and external Parts: It may, also, be given internally, to the Quantity of twenty Drops or more, where Diaphoretics are required. *De Maets* recommends in Affections of the Head, one Dram of camphorated Spirit, mixed with an Ounce of Spirit of Wine distill'd upon cephalic Herbs, and three Ounces of Rosemary Water: Some Drops of this Mixture drawn up the Nostrils will give immediate Ease, in the Head or Tooth-ach. Observe, that the Water of Rosemary mitigates the other Ingredients, and that its Strength, is augmented or diminished, in Proportion to the Quantity of Rosemary Water.

Camphorata, Offic. *Camphorata hirsuta*, Raii Hist. *Camphorata Monspeliensum*, J. B. Stinking Ground Pine. The Herb, which is used, is of a drying and astringent Quality, strengthening to the Nerves, and serviceable in the Gout, Convulsions, Palsy, Defluxions of the Eyes, and Catarrhs. The Plant is a Cephalic, is effectual for Wounds according to *Lobelius*, and is prescrib'd, by some, in Dropsies. The Tops of this Plant are used, in Baths and Fomentations, for Disorders and Swelling of the Joints; for Cramps, Palsies, and other Affections of the Nerves.

Canella alba, Park. Theat. *Cassia lignea Laurifolia Americana, cortice albo, valde acri & Aromatico*, Pluk. Almag. *Arbor Baccifera Laurifolia, Aromatica, fructu viridi calyculato racemoso*, Philosoph. Transact. The wild Cinamon Tree. All the Parts of this Tree, when fresh, are very hot, aromatic, and biting to the Taste, not much unlike Cloves, which are often so troublesome, as to require a Remedy from fair Water. The Bark of this Tree, is what is mostly used, as well in the Plantations of the *English*,

between the Tropics in the *West Indies*, as in *Europe*, and is cured without any Difficulty, by only cutting the Bark, and letting it dry in the Shade. It likewise, in the *West Indies*, as well as in *Europe*, is thought a very good Remedy, against the Scurvy, and to cleanse and invigorate the Blood; being in *London*, both in Druggists and Apothecaries Shops, used for those Purposes, under the Name of *Cortex Winteranus*, which it is not, tho' it may very well supply its Place. It is in the *West Indies*, mixed and given with Steel, or some other Medicines; but if the Patient is of a hot Constitution, it is more prejudicial than beneficial, being of a very warm Nature. The Bark, if mixed with Water, and distilled *per Vesicam*, yields an aromatic Oil, which, like the Oil of Cloves, sinks to the Bottom of the Water. When it is mix'd with some small Quantity of the Oil of Cloves, it has been sold for it. The Bark is, also, accounted a Specific against the Scurvy, is a good nervous Medicine, useful in Palsies and Convulsions, and is of singular Service, against Diseases of the Stomach and Bowels.

Cannabis, Offic. *Cannabis Sativa*, Park. Boerh. Ind. A. Hemp. The Root boil'd, and applied by Way of Cataplasm, mitigates Inflammations, discusses Tumors, and dissolves tophaceous Concretions at the Joints. The Seed of Hemp is the only Part exhibited in Physic, which when boil'd in Milk till the Hulls crack, is esteem'd efficacious in old Coughs, as also a Specific against the Jaundice. It has been accused of rendering Persons impotent in venereal Affairs; but how inconsistent that is, will appear, not only, by its making Hens lay their Eggs in greater Plenty, if moderately given; but also the famous *Bangue*, so much extoll'd boil'd both by the *Persians* and *Indians* to promote Venery, is a Sort of Hemp.

Cannacorus latifolius vulgaris, Tournf. *Harundo florida,* Ger. The Indian Reed. This Plant grows only in warm Places, the Cold being very injurious to it; it is supposed that the Leaves, which are wrapp'd about the Gum Elemi, belong to this Reed. It is deterfive and aperient.

Cantabrica. Convolvulus minimus, Offic. *Convolvulus minimus, Spicæ foliis,* Ger. *Convolvulus Linariæ folia, assurgens & humilior.* Boerh. Ind. A. Lavender leaved Bind-Weed. It grows wild in the Fields, flowers in *June,* and is by some recommended as good against Worms.

Capparis, Offic. *Capparis Rotundiore folio,* Ger. *Capparis Spinosa, fructu minore, folio Rotundo.* Boerh. Ind. A. Capers. The Caper Bush grows in the southern Parts of *France* and *Italy,* in sandy and stony Places. Those are generally thought the best which, are imported from *Genoa;* but those brought from *Alexandria* to *Venice,* are esteem'd by some still better, tho' larger than the *Italian* Capers; for the largest are judged best as being most entire. Their austere bitterish Taste, sufficiently convinces us of their astringent and corroborating Virtues; and if we consider the Qualities they derive from the Vinegar and Salt, in which they are preserved and brought to us, we may easily conceive, that they are of a resolvent and inciding Nature. For this Reason, they are recommended, in Order to strengthen a languid Appetite, and purge the Stomach of gross pituitous Humours. They are good for Obstructions of the Viscera, especially those of the Spleen, for the Palsy, and Convulsions arising from a Superfluity of peccant Humours; nor

are they less recommended in long and chronical Fevers. *Laurentius Joubert,* in the Plague, recommends them season'd with Salt, gently boil'd in Water, and eaten with Vinegar; for as he says, " they ex-" cite an Appetite, and open Ob-" structions;" for this Reason, they ought not only to be allowed, in pestilential Cases, but also recommended, because they resist Putrefaction. Externally, says *Etmuller,* the Pickle of Capers, is applied to the Side, under the left Hypochondrium with Linen Cloths, or a Sponge, for discussing Swellings of the Spleen. If to this, Mustard Seed is added, that the Vinegar may be impregnated with its volatile Salt, it is an excellent Remedy in Disorders of the Spleen.

Caprifolium, Periclymenum Matrisylva, Offic. *Periclymenum, sive Caprifolium vulgare,* Park. Theat. Honey Suckle, or Wood Bind. It grows almost every where, flowering great Part of the Summer. The Leaves, only, of this Plant are used in Medicine; they are exhibited in Gargarisms, for sore Throats; tho' others think them not so proper for that Intention, on Account of their hot Nature. Some prescribe them for a Cough and Asthma, and to remove Obstructions of the Liver and Spleen. The Oil, made by the Infusion of the Flowers, is esteem'd very warming, and efficacious in removing Cramps, and Convulsions of the Nerves. Their Bark is acrid, saltish, styptic, and stinking. Their Salt resembles Sal Ammoniac, but contains some fetid Oil and Earth. The Decoction of Honey Suckle Leaves, is both vulnerary and deterfive, good for Diseases of the Throat, and Wounds of the Legs. The Leaves bruised, cure cutaneous Diseases; and the distilled Water of the Flowers, assuages Inflamma-

tions

tions of the Eyes, and ftrengthens Women in Labour.

Capficum, Piper Indicum, Offic. *Capficum Siliquis longis propendentibus,* Boerh. Ind. A. *Capficum longioribus Siliquis,* Ger. Guinea Pepper. It is fown every Year in Gardens, flowering in *Auguft,* and produces red Pods, towards the latter End of *September* and *October,* but perifhes with the firft Froft. A Decoction of *Guinea* Pepper with Penny Royal, is commended by fome, to expel a dead Child. The Skins boil'd, and ufed as a Gargle, help the Tooth ach. And a Cataplafm made of the Seeds, mixed with Honey, and apply'd to the Throat, is good for a Quinfey, otherwife it is not much ufed in Phyfic.

Caranna, Offic. Park. Theat. The Caranna Tree. The Caranna Tree, is a Species of Palm, and fpontaneoufly pours out its Refin or Gum, when an Incifion is made in the Bark. This Gum is outwardly of a blackifh Colour, but internally, refembles that of Pitch, and is of a bitter, pinguious, and oleaginous Tafte, of a fragrant Smell, not much differing from that of Lavender. This Gum is imported in foft Maffes, wrapt up in the Shreds of Reeds, or Bulrufhes, from *Carthagena,* a Province in the *Weft-Indies* of *New Spain,* of which that is efteemed beft, which is whiteft, efpecially if foft, and of the Confiftence of a Plaifter. In Virtues it agrees with the Tacamahac. This Gum, is of fingular Efficacy, in Pains of the Joints, to which if applied, it fpeedily removes them, thofe Cafes only excepted, where there is a Defluxion of hot Humours; it difcuffes inveterate Tumors, and ftops Defluxions of cold Humours. It is highly beneficial in all Pains of the Brain and Nerves, and without the Admixture of any other Medicine, cures recent Wounds, efpecially of the

Nerves and Joints. If applied to the Ears and Temples, it ftops Defluxions on the Eyes, and other Parts. *Etmuller* tells us, that in Cardialgias, Pains, and other Diforders of the Stomach, it is often applied by Way of Plaifter to the Region of the Stomach. *Geoffroy* obferves, that it is term'd a Gum, but very unjuftly; becaufe it is diffoluble, only in Spirit of Wine, which is the Property of refinous Subftances.

Cardamine, Offic. Ger. Emac. *Nafturtium pratenfe majus, five Cardamine latifolia,* Park. Theat. Meadow Creffes, or Ladies Smock. It grows every where in the Meadows, and flowers in *April.* This Plant, in fome Meafure refembles Water Creffes, not differing much from it in its Virtues, being both heating, warming, and good for the Scurvy. It may, where Water Creffes cannot be had, fupply their Place, tho' it is but feldom ufed in the Shops.

Cardamomum, Cardamom. We have three Sorts of Seeds in the Shops call'd by this Name. The firft of which is, the *Cardomum Maximum, Grana Paradifi,* Offic. *Cardamomum Arabum Majus,* Ger. *Melleguetta five Cardamomum Maximum, & Grana Paradifi,* Park. Theat. Grains of Paradife. They have the fame Virtues as Pepper, and are a Specific in all paralytic Difeafes. The fecond is the *Cardamomum Majus,* Offic. Raii Hift. *Cardamomum Majus vulgare,* Ger. Emac. Great Cardamums. Thefe being grown quite out of Ufe, are not to be met with in the Shops. Notwithftanding the Seeds are the Part in Ufe, which are of a heating and drying Quality, comfort the noble Parts, attenuate, difcufs Flatulences, help Concoction, provoke Urine and the Menfes, help Shortnefs of Breath, and remove Obftructions of the Liver, Spleen, and Mefentery. The third

is,

is, the *Cardomum minus*, Offic. Boerh. Ind. A. *Cardamomum minus vulgare*, Ger. Emac. Common Cardamums. This Sort is in frequent Use; being of a warming Nature; they greatly comfort and strengthen the Stomach and Bowels; they aid Digestion, and expel Wind; they are excellent in all Distempers incident to the Head and Nerves; they greatly provoke Urine, as also the Menses, and are of great Service in the Jaundice. These Seeds are us'd in the *Extractum Catharticum*; *Aqua Seminum Cardamomi*; *Infusum amarum Purgans*; *Infusum Senæ Commune*; *Tinctura Rhabarbari*; *Tinctura Amara*; *Tinctura Cardiaca*; *Tinctura Senæ*; *Tinctura Stomachica*; *Species Aromaticæ*; *Confectio Cardiaca*; *Mithridatium* and *Theriaca Andromachi*.

Cardiaca, Offic. Ger. Boerh. Ind. A. Mother Wort. It grows in Lanes and wet Places, and by Wall Sides, and flowers in *June*. This Plant is called *Cardiata*, because it relieves in Faintings, and Disorders of the Stomach, the superior Orifice of which is called *Cardia*; for according to *Shroder* in his *Pharmacopœia*, it is of singular Service, in Distensions of the Hypochondria, and Disorders of the Stomach in Children. The Herb, is of a highly bitter and penetrating Taste, a Circumstance which indicates its stimulating, inciding, resolvent, and aperient Qualities, in Consequence of which it is proper, in Diseases proceeding from a Redundance of Phlegm, or viscid Juices. Hence, it is exhibited with an Intention to provoke Urine, promote the Menses, and facilitate difficult Labours. A Decoction of Mother-wort, and the Powder of it, mixed with Sugar, are, by *Ray*, said to be Medicines of uncommon Efficacy, in Palpitations of the Heart, Affections of the Spleen and hysteric

Disorders. *Matthiolus* and *Dioscorides* affirm, that a Spoonful of its Powder, drank in Wine, is of singular Service in difficult Births. *Etmuller* informs us, that this Plant cut down, dried, and by Boiling reduced to the Form of a Cataplasm, is, in Consequence of its inciding and resolvent Qualities, very good against those Disorders of Children produced by a mucous Acid, and the Flatulences arising from it, if applied to the Region of the Stomach and Hypochondria. A Water distilled from Mother-wort, with Oak of *Jerusalem*, is used in Inflammations of the Hypochondria of Children. *Simon Pauli* in his *Quadripartitum Botanicum*, orders its Leaves to be boil'd in the Oil of Wormwood, and of bitter Almonds, and applied to the Navel, in Order to kill Worms of the Intestines.

Carduus, the Thistle. Of this Plant there are a great many Sorts, in so much that *Boerhaave* enumerates no less than thirty-three different Species; but we shall only take Notice of those to which medicinal Virtues are ascribed.

The first of these is, the *Carduus, caule crispo, capitulis minoribus. Carduus Asininus, seu Sylvestris.* Thistle upon Thistle. *Riverius* observes, that Half an Ounce of the Roots of this Thistle, boil'd with two Drams of Liquorice, is a very good Medicine, for those who are afflicted with the Stone, cleansing the Bladder and Kidneys from Sand and Gravel.

The second is, the *Carduus Hæmorrhordalis*, Offic. *Carduus Vinearum Repens Sonchi folio*, Boerh. Ind. A. *Carduus Vulgatissimus Viarum.* The common creeping Way Thistle. It grows in uncultivated Places, and flowers in *July* and *August.* It is called *Hæmorrhoidalis* (Hæmorrhoidal) from its Effects; for being boil'd in Water, and reduced to

a Cataa Cataplasm, it greatly alleviates the Pains of the Hæmorrhoids. Some affirm, that the Tubercles arising from the Bitings of Insects on the Stalks, if worn in a Bag, or tied in the Patient's Shirt, produce the same Effect; but others advise wearing the dried Heads of the Plant in a Bag.

The third Species is, the *Carduus Mariæ*, Offic. *Carduus Mariæ vulgaris*, Park. *Carduus albis maculis Notatus vulgaris*, Boerh. Ind. A. Ladies Thistle. This Plant grows upon Banks and Borders of Fields, flowers in *June*, and seems to contain a Salt, not unlike the *Oxysal diaphoreticum Angeli Salæ*, that is, an acrid Salt, abounding with Acid; thus it is both sudorific and diuretic. Four Ounces of the Juice of its Leaves, give great Relief in the Dropsy. The Seed is of a stimulating and opening Property; the Dose of which is a Dram in Powder, but it is oftener used in Emulsions, being mixed with other Seeds for that Purpose. An Emulsion prepared of the Seeds, with Honey, or a little Syrup of Violets, and drank, is highly commended in severe pleuritic Pains. *Tournefort*, for the Pleurisy, and that Species of Rheumatism which resembles it, advises an Emulsion, prepared of two Drams of the Seeds of *Carduus Mariæ*, with six Drams of the distilled Water of the Leaves. " This Me- " dicine, says *Pontidera*, gives Re- " lief under all Pains, mollifies " Hardnesses, evacuates Humours, " and maturates Pus, wherefore it is " recommended, as a present Reme- " dy for all Disorders of the Throat " and Lungs." The Seed pulverised, and taken in Wine, from one Dram to two, is recommended against an *Hydrophobia*, as being an excellent Sudorific. Externally it is accounted good for *Nomæ*, and phagedenic and corroding Ulcers.

The fourth Species is, the *Acanthium*, Offic. *Acanthium vulgare*, Park. *Carduus tomentosus Acanthi folio vulgaris*, Boerh. Ind. Cotton Thistle. This Plant never flowers till its second Year, and then continues in Bloom from *June* to *August*; but when the Seed is ripe, the Root perishes. The Root is esteem'd opening, and diuretic, carminative and stomachic, discutient and resolvent. Some commend it for the Tooth-ach, and for epileptic Disorders in Infants.

The fifth Species is, the *Carduus Eriocephalus*, Offic. Boerh. Ind. A. Wooly headed Thistle. It flowers in *July* and *August*. *Borelli* says, its Juice, or bruised Leaves, cure the Cancer of the Nose and Breast; he calls it *Ornipodon*, and recommends the Use of it in those Cases.

Carlina. The Carline Thistle. *Boerhaave* makes mention of no less than seven different Species of this Thistle. The first of which is, the *Carlina. Chamæleon Albus, Carlina.* Offic. *Carlina humilis*, Park. Theat. *Carlina acaulos magno flore*, Boerh. Ind. Carline Thistle. It grows in *Germany*, and other Parts beyond Sea, and flowers in *July*. The Root, which is the only Part used, is esteemed sudorific, alexipharmic, and efficacious against all contagious and pestilential Diseases, the Plague itself not even excepted. It is no less diuretic, helps the Dropsy, promotes the Catamenia, and is good in all hypochondriac Distempers, and is very properly exhibited, where Nature is to be irritated, and requires a Stimulus, to throw off an excrementitious Load; whence it is apparent, how proper it is, for removing Obstructions, exciting a Diaphoresis, provoking the Menses, promoting a Discharge of the Urine, and killing Worms, in Consequence of its Bitterness. The *Carline Thistle* banishes Sleep, and consequently prevents

prevents preternatural Drowfinefs. The other Species have much the fame Virtues afcrib'd to them.

Carpobalfamum, the Fruit of the Balfam Tree. *Profper Alpinus* informs us, that in *Egypt*, the Carpobalfamum is ufed in all the Intentions, for which the Balfam itfelf is applied, tho' it is not fo efficacious. The Dofe is generally two Drams, with a Decoction of Spikenard. It is alfo ufed in Fumigations, for uterine Diforders arifing from a cold Caufe. The only Ufe the *Europeans* make of the Carpobalfamum is, in the *Venice* Treacle and Mithridate, and that not much, for Cubebs and Juniper Berries, often fupply its Place.

Carthamus. Baftard Saffron. *Boerhaave* enumerates three Species of his Plant. The firft of which is, he *Carthamus Cnicus*, Offic. *Carthamus Officinarum flore croceo*. Boerh. Ind. A. *Cnicus five Carthamus fativus*, Park. Baftard Saffron. It is own in Gardens and Fields, and lowers in *July*, the Seeds only are fed in the Shops, which are accounted a ftrong Cathartic, evacuting tough, vifcid Phlegm, both pwards and downwards, and confequently, are thought to clear the .ungs, and help the Phthific; they re likewife good againft the Jaundice, tho' now pretty much out of Jfe. With Regard to their Virtues nd Efficacy, *Diofcorides* gives the ollowing Particulars. The expreffed Juice of the triturated Seeds, xhibited in Conjunction with Hoey and Water, or the Broth of a owl, purges the Inteftines; but is rejudicial to the Stomach; of this nice, with the Addition of Almonds, Nitre, Anife, and boil'd loney, are prepared Cakes, which nder the Body foluble; thefe akes are to be divided into four arts, as large as a Walnut, two or ree of which, are fufficient for a

Dofe, to be taken before Supper. *Hippocrates* in *lib. de Diæta*, informs us, that Cnicus is purgative. *Galen* affirms, that the Seeds of Cnicus, are only ufed for Purges. *Paulus Ægineta* and *Sylvius*, reckon them among the Hydragogues. *Bauhine* fays, that the Seeds bruifed and boiled in the Broth of Flefh, or Chickens, and drank, evacuate Phlegm and tough vifcid Humours. *Etmuller* prefcribed them, when the *Primæ Viæ* were loaded with a thick and vifcid Mucus, in Diforders of the Breaft, in Afthmas, and Coughs produced by thick and vifcid Matter; for which Reafon, they are ranked among the Medicines which evacuate Phlegm: The Seeds are, by Experience, found to be a draftic purgative Medicine, which by Reafon of its acrid Quality, in Conjunction with its Vifcidity, generally excites violent Gripes, with an Inflammation of the Abdomen.

Another is, the *Chamæleon Niger*, Offic. *Chamælcon niger verus*, Park. *Chamæleon niger umbellatus flore cærulco hyacinthino*, C. B. Black Chameleon. It grows in *Greece*, and flowers in *June*; the Root is only ufed, which is of fo acrimonious a Quality, that its Juice burns the Skin, but it is very efficacious in cleanfing malignant Ulcers.

Carum, Offic. *Carum Vulgare*, Park. Theat. *Carui*, Boerh. Ind. A. *Cuminum pratenfe, Carui officinarum*, C. B. Caraways. The Seed is one of the greater hot Seeds, is ftomachic, and carminative, expels Wind, and is ferviceable againft the Cholic, and Weaknefs of the Stomach, helps Digeftion, is good for Dizzinefs of the Head, and Weaknefs of the Sight, to provoke Urine, and increafe Milk in Nurfes. The Seed of this Plant is in common Ufe, tho' fome ufe the Root

U 4 *car-*

in carminative Ptisans and Glysters. The Seed is stomachic, diuretic, and very proper to dissolve the glutinous Matter, which causes the Cholic. Caraway Seeds are put into Bread, as a Preservative against this Disease. Candied Caraway-seeds expel Wind. The chymical Oil is very acrid and penetrating ; five or six Drops of it are prescribed in Oil of sweet Almonds, and some Drops of it in Spirit of Wine imbibed by Cotton, and put into the Ears, may be used in the Case of Deafness, instead of Syringing.

Caryophyllata , Offic. *Caryophillata Vulgaris.* Park. Theat. Boerh. Ind. A. Ordinary Avens, or Herb Bennet. The Roots are only used, which being infused in Wine, give it a pleasant Smell and Taste, and render it more cordial, and chearing to the Spirits ; they mitigate Pains arising from Cold, or Wind in the Intestines ; they are of a cephalic and alexipharmic Nature, and manifestly binding and efficacious in all Kinds of Fluxes and Hæmorrhages. Avens is bitter, styptic, and its Root smells like Cloves ; its Salt resembles Sal Ammoniac, but is greatly loaded with an Acid, and involved by a great deal of essential Oil and Earth. An Infusion of *Avens Root* in Wine, is stomachic, according to *Trogus,* and removes Obstructions of the Liver. The Wine is, also, very vulnerary and detersive. The Extract has the same Virtues, and is prescribed in Rheumatisms.

Caryophyllus. The Clove gilly Flower, Carnation, or Pink, of which there are many Species. As the *Caryophyllus flore simplici,* Offic. *Caryophyllus hortensis simplex flore majore,* C. B. *Betonica coronaria, sive Caryophyllus flore simplici sativus,* J. B. Single Pink. The medicinal Virtues of this Species, are the same with those of the subsequent.

Caryophyllus ruber. Betonica, Tunica; Offic. *Caryophyllus altilis major,* Boerh Ind. A. *Betonica coronaria sativa sive Caryophylleus flos.* J. B. Clove Gilly Flower. The Flowers are esteem'd cephalic and cordial, and are principally used in a Vertigo, Apoplexy, Epilepsy and other Affections of the Head and Nerves, as also in a Syncope and Palpitation of the Heart. They are good in Wounds, facilitate Delivery, and are recommended in Weakness of the Stomach, Cardialgias, and pestilential Fevers.

Caryophyllus silvestris, Offic. *Caryophyllus sylvestris vulgaris latifolius,* C. B. *Armenius latifolius flore rubro, saturo, holoserico,* Park. Wild Pinks. This Plant flowers in *June,* and is said to be good for the Stone and Epilepsy, taken with the Water of *Rest Harrow,* or *Lillies of the Valley.* Besides the Plants above mentioned, there are some Aromatics which go by this Name ; the first of which is the *Caryophyllus aromaticus fructu oblongo,* B. B. Pin. *Caryophyllus aromaticus Indiæ Orientalis, fructu clavato monopyreno,* Pluk. Almag. Cloves. They are very heating and drying, cordial, cephalic, and stomachic, stop Vomiting, strengthen a weak Stomach, expel Wind, prevent Fainting, and are good in malignant Distempers ; the distilled Oil cures the Tooth ach. They are of a heating, drying, and discussing Quality, for which Reason they are serviceable in a Lipothymy, Crudities of the Stomach, and the Vertigo, and remove malignant, uterine, and other Disorders.

Cassia Caryophyllata, Offic. *Caryophyllus aromaticus Indiæ Occidentalis, foliis et fructu rotundis, dispereis, Seminibus fere orbiculatis planis,* Pluk. Almag. *Amomum aliud quorundam et Caryophyllon Plinii Clusio suspicatum.* The Clove-berry-tree. Both as to Smell and Taste it approaches

proaches to thofe of Cloves, is cephalic, cordial, and agrees with Cloves in all their Virtues.

The third Sort is, the *Pimenta,* Offic. *Piper Jamaicenfe, quibufdam, odoratum Jamaicenfe noftratibus,* Raii Hift. *Myrtus arborofa, foliis Laurinis aromatica, Cocculi Indi Aromatici,* Muf. Regiæ Societatis. *Jamaica* Pepper, or All-Spiece. The Fruit, with Water diftilled *per Veficam,* yields a very odoriferous chymical Oil, which finks to the Bottom of Water, like Oil of Cloves; it is the moft temperate, mild, and innocent of common Spices, almoft all of which it far furpaffes, by promoting the Digeftion of Meat, attenuating tough Humours, moderately Heating, ftrengthening the Stomach, expelling Wind, and doing thofe friendly Offices to the Bowels, which we generally expect from Spices.

Cafcarilla. Cortex Thuris, Offic. *Cortex Thuris nonnullis dictus, vel Thymiama,* Raii Hift. *Kina Kina Aromatica. Palode Calenturas. Cafcarilla Cortex Elaterii, five Scacarilla Officinarum. Cortex Peruvianus grifeus, five fpurius,* Geoff. Tract. *Indian* Bark. The Cafcarilla, bears a near Refemblance to the Peruvian Bark, tho' of a fomewhat paler Brown, lefs compact, more friable, of a bitter and fomewhat ftyptic Tafte, pungent, and pretty acrimonious to the Tongue, leaving at laft a Senfation of Bitternefs, mixed with fomething of an aromatic Nature. In all probability, its refinous and penetrating Parts, divide the ill concocted, thick, and vifcid Subftance which is the *Fomes* of a Fever. This Febrifuge has this particular Advantage over the Peruvian Bark, that it acts in a fmaller Dofe, nor requires fo long a Continuation. The illuftrious *Stahl,* Phyfician to the King of *Pruffia,* extended its Ufe ftill farther; he prefcribed it for fevere and convulfive

Coughs, fuch as thofe called the *Chin cough,* in which Cafes it produces the defired Effects, by inciding, and attenuating the vifcid Matter, and confequently it is highly beneficial in thofe Cafes, where the Intention is to affift or augment Tranfpiration. The Virtues of *Cafcarilla* have been experienced in flatulent Colics, and in thofe hyfteric, and hypochondriac Diforders, commonly called Vapours. But it is to be obferved, that when the Intention is to reftore and confirm the Tone of any Parts, which have been fhock'd, agitated, or ftrain'd, *Cafcarilla* in Subftance, ought to be prefcribed, it being in this Cafe neceffary, that its earthy and ftyptic Parts, fhould perform the Office of Aftringents. *Cafcarilla* in Subftance, is of fingular Service in internal Hæmorrhoids, which flow with Difficulty, provided the Patient is of a pretty corpulent Habit of Body. This happens, becaufe in fuch a State, the Skin being relaxed, the *Cafcarilla* augments the Tranfpiration, in confequence of which, the Humours will have more Liberty, and the Hæmorrhoids be opened. Perhaps, alfo, the Cafcarilla, may contribute to make the Hæmorrhoids flow, by reftoring and bracing up the Veffels, which contain the Hæmorrhoidal Blood, of which Facts, Mr. *Boulduc* himfelf was a Witnefs. But what he obferved, as more particularly advantageous in *Cafcarilla,* was, the fingular Service it did, in the Dyfenteries which raged in the Year 1719, whether accompanied with a Fever, or not. He further obferves, that whereas *Ipecacuanha,* and other emetic Vegetables, leave a long Indifpofition and Weaknefs in the Stomach, *Cafcarilla* fpeedily reftored and confirm'd its Tone and Strength. This Bark, then, has the fame Virtues with the *Quinquina* and *Ipecacuanha,* and perhaps exerts them

them rather to a greater Advantage than either the one or the other.

Caffia Fiftula, Offic. *Caffia fiftula Alexandrina,* Raii Hift. *Quauhayohuatli five Caffia fiftula,* Hern. The Pudding Pipe Tree. The *Egyptians* never ufe the Caffia Pods, till they are four Months old; fince when young and recent, they are obferved not only to be ufelefs, but noxious. They ufe the Pulp, extracted from the Pod, in the Form of a Bolus or Potion. They are of Opinion, that Caffia exhibited internally, by evacuating and obtunding the hot and parched Parts of the Blood and Humours, cools the Blood and renders it more pure; they, alfo, by Experience find, that by its Means, the Stomach is difburthen'd of an excrementitious Subftance which may prove offenfive to it; they alfo ufe it with great Succefs, in Defluxions of hot Humours upon the Lungs, or Thorax, exhibiting it either alone, or mixed with Sugar Candy, or with Oil of fweet Almonds. They find it, likewife, fingularly beneficial to the Bladder and Kidneys; becaufe it extinguifhes any immoderate Heat of thofe Parts, fcours from thence the Humours, and difcharges them by Urine. Hence the frequent Ufe of it, prevents the Generation of Stones and Gravel. They ufe the Pulp, in Conjunction with *Agaric,* againft immoderate Coughs, Dyfpnœas, Afthmas, and Orthopnœas. They ufe it, alfo, by Way of Plaifter, to be applied to the Parts affected in hot Pains of the Joints, the Gout, and hot Inflammations. The Flowers, preferved with Sugar, make an highly beneficial Medicine, for correcting the Heat of the Kidneys, and eliminating the tough and vifcid Recrements lodged in the Ureters. Befides, the Flowers are ufed by the *Egyptians,* for alleviating Pains of every Kind, efpecially thofe of the Gout. *Bontius* informs us, that the Ufe of the Caffia Pulp, is very frequent among the *Malayans,* in Diforders of the Kidneys and Bladder, in all nephritic Indifpofitions, as alfo in Gonorrhœas contracted by impure Embraces, when it is mixed with the Powder of boil'd Turpentine. It is, alfo, proper in feverifh Heats, and extinguifhes Thirft. *Schulzius* fays, it is a Purgative; but becaufe in Subftance a large Dofe of it is to be taken, and becaufe it is obferv'd to weaken the Stomach, it is rarely exhibited at prefent with us. But if the recent Extract is to be ufed, it may moft properly be exhibited, with the Addition of fome Carminative, fuch as Anife, or Fennel. Hypochondriac and hyfteric Patients, thofe who are afflicted with a Weaknefs of the Stomach and Flatulencies, and fuch as are fubject to the Colic, ought to abftain from Caffia, as alfo pregnant Women. The *New London Pharmacopœia* introduces this into the *Electuarium e Caffia,* & *Electuarium Lenitivum.* The Caffia Lignea is a Species of Cinnamomum.

Caffumuniar, Offic. *alias Rifagon. An Zerumbeth feu Zingiber rubrum, fylveftre, Ternatenfe.* Camel. Syllab. Cafumunar. It is very much commended as an excellent nervous Medicine, and good for the Palfy, Convulfions, Colic, Griping of the Bowels, as alfo hyfteric Affections. The Root is faid to be moderately heating and aftringent; for which Reafon, it is recommended, for corroborating the Nerves, recruiting the vital and animal Spirits, ftrengthening the Stomach, and expelling Flatulences. It is prefcribed in Apoplexies, convulfive Motions, Palfies, Tremors, hyfteric and hypochondriac Diforders, Vertigoes and Gripes.

Gripes. It is highly extolled for a Loss of Memory, and esteemed a Corrector of the *Peruvian* Bark.

Castanea. There are two Species of Chesnuts, to which the same Virtues are ascrib'd, as the *Castanea,* Offic. *Castanea sativa,* Boerh. Ind. A. The Chess Nut. The other is, the *Castanea,* Ind. Med. *Castanea Sylvestris quæ peculiariter Castanea,* C. B. Pin. *Castanea vulgaris,* Park. Theat. The Wood Chess Nut Tree. Chesnuts fatten and nourish, but they bind also, and sometimes generate Wind. The Meal mixed with Honey, or the Chesnuts themselves roasted, and work'd up with Honey and Flowers of Sulphur, make a good Electuary, for those who spit Blood, or cough very much. The Decoction of *Chesnuts,* or their Shells roasted, asswage the Flux of the Belly, as does, also, the little Skin under the Shell. An Emulsion made of *Chesnuts,* Poppy Seeds, and Barley Water, asswages the Heat of Urine. *Chesnuts* are sweet, a little styptic; and, it is evident, that the Fruit partakes somewhat of the Nature of Alum and Sulphur.

Cedrus folio cupressi, major fructu flavescente, C. B. Pin. *Juniperus major Dioscoridis,* Clus. H. It is said to be of a heating and diuretic Quality, like common Juniper. According to *Dioscorides,* the Berries are moderately heating, astringent and beneficial to the Stomach. When exhibited in a Draught of a proper Liquor, they are highly efficacious against Disorders of the Breast, Coughs, Inflammations, Gripes, and the Wounds inflicted by Serpents. They provoke Urine; and for that Reason, are proper, for Patients afflicted with Ruptures, Convulsions, and hysteric Fits. The Leaves contain a certain Degree of Acrimony; for which Reason, either they themselves, or their Juice,

may properly be drank in Wine, against the Bites of Vipers, or the Parts affected may be anointed with the same Preparation. The Country People of *Provence* in *France,* apply the Leaves bruised, to Carbuncles, in Order to put a Stop to their Increase. From the Berries, or the recent Wood, boil'd in Must, is prepared the *Vinum Cedrinum,* or Cedar Wine, according to *Pliny. Dale* informs us, that he saw a Gentleman who expresly affirmed, that in *Carolina,* this Tree yielded a Gum, so like the true Olibanum, that when he accidentally mixed some Particles of it with Olibanum, brought from *Europe,* they so much resembled each other, that they could neither be separated nor distinguished. Hence he concludes, that this is the Tree, which produces the Olibanum.

Cedrus, Offic. *Cedrus Libani,* Ger. *Cedrus magna conifera Libani,* Park. Theat. Cedar of Libanus. The Wood of this Tree, is said to prevent the Putrefaction of all animal Bodies. The Saw-dust of it, is thought to be one of the Secrets, used by those *Mountebanks,* who pretend to have the Embalming Mystery. This Wood is, also, said to yield an Oil, which is famous for preserving Books and Writings; and the Wood is thought by Lord. *Bacon* to continue above a thousand Years sound.

Celery. This Plant is possess'd of the same Virtues with the *Apium of the Shops.* Those who are fond of venereal Intercourses, love Brandy distilled from the Seeds of Celery. The Root, which is extremely white, and the interior Part of the Stalk, when well wash'd and cut into Slices, are used as a Salad, and thought an uncommon Delicacy, in the Winter, and latter End of Autumn. The Root is, also, boiled with Flesh and Fish, in Order to render them

more

more delicious. Some are fond of the Seeds prepared with Vinegar.

Celtis, Offic. *Celtis fructu nigricante*, Boerh. Ind. *Lotus Arbor fructu Cerasi*, J. B. The Nettle Tree. This Fruit, is used in Medicine, and is astringent, binds the Belly, but has least of these Qualities when ripe. The Decoction thereof is good for a Dysentery, and for Women labouring under an immoderate Flux of the Menses.

Centaurium majus, Offic. *Centaurium majus vulgare*, Park. *Centaurium majus folio in Lacinias plures diviso*, Boerh. Ind. A. Great Centaury. This Plant flowers in *July*. The Root, which is the only Part used, is drying and binding, and good for all Kinds of Fluxes, stops Bleeding, either at the Nose, Mouth, or any other Part, is of great Use to heal Wounds, and according to *Pliny*, derives its Name from the Centaur *Chiron*, who when shot by an Arrow of *Hercules*, cured himself, by the Application of this Plant: It is, also, reputed to open Obstructions of the Liver, and to corroborate that Part; it is also used in Hernias.

Centaurium Minus, Offic. *Centaurium minus vulgare*, Park. Theat. *Centaurium minus flore purpureo*, J. B. Common Centaury. It flowers in *June* and *July*; and is of a very bitter Taste, and of an aperitive cleansing Faculty, opens Obstructions of the Liver and Spleen, provokes Urine and the Menses, alleviates the Jaundice and intermitting Fevers, strengthens the Stomach, and destroys Worms; outwardly, it is used in Fomentations against Swellings and Inflammations. It is an Ingredient in the *Theriaca Andromachi*.

Cepa, Offic. *Cepa vulgaris floribus, & tunicis candidis & purpurascentibus*, Boerh. Ind. A. *Cepa rubra & Alba rotunda & longa*, J. B. O-

nions. They are somewhat windy, but otherwise very wholesome, for those who abound with cold and moist Humours, and are good against Coughs and Diseases of the Breast. We are convinced by Experience, that Onions, especially when externally applied, are possess'd of very singular medicinal Virtues; for nothing is of greater Efficacy in soft'ning hard Tumours, and maturating venereal Buboes, than roasted Onions, especially when applied in Conjunction with Figs. They, also, afford speedy Relief, if applied to the Pubes of Children labouring under a total Suppression of Urine. There is, also, in the various Species of Onions, a certain subtile caustic Salt, of a highly penetrating and blistering Quality, which, when applied immediately to the nervous Parts, excites violent Pains, and sometimes an Inflammation, tho' Onions are daily used internally without producing any bad Effects. They are very diuretic.

Cerasus Rubra, Offic. *Cerasus Anglica*, Park. Theat. *Cerasus sativa fructu Rotundo, Rubro & Acido*, Tourn. Inst. The red Cherry Tree. The Fruit is cooling, drying, and astringent, and corroborates the Heart and Stomach; hence they are useful in allaying feverish Heats and Thirst; the Kernels are good to dissolve the Stone. The Gum of the Tree is likewise accounted lithontriptic. Cherries are esteem'd a very salutary and agreeable Fruit. The Juice of them, when perfectly ripe, is saponaceous and highly resolvent, and if taken in large Quantities, and those frequently repeated, especially when boil'd or baked, it is capable of curing many obstinate chronical Distempers, and taking away the obstructing Matter by a salutary *Diarrhæa*.

Cerasus acida nigricans, Ind. Med. *Cerasus fructu acido, serotino, succi sangui-*

anguinei, Tourn. Inft. *Cerasa acida nigricantia solidiora tardius matu-rescentia*, J. B. The Morello Cherry. The Fruit preserv'd, and the Rob of the Juice, are used, and a-gree in Virtues with the red Cherry.

Cerasus nigra, Offic. Ger. Black Cherry-tree. It flowers in *April*, and the Fruit is used in Medicine, which is esteem'd temperate and ce-phalic, and particularly efficacious in Disorders of the Head, as Apo-lexy, and Palsy. The Stones of black Cherries, with their Kernels baked and powdered, are said to be extremely diuretic, but the Kernels have been lately said to yield by Di-stillation, an Oil equally poisonous with that of the Laurel. Hence black Cherry Water has got into some Disrepute, tho' as far as I can learn, without any Foundation from Experience.

Padus, Offic. *Cerasus Ramosa syl-vestris fructu non edili*, C. B. Pin-*Cerasus Avium racemosa*, Park. Theat. Birds Cherry. The Fruit is used to hang about the Necks of Children, as a Cure for the Epi-lepsy.

Cerasus sylvestris amara, Maha-leb parata, Raii Hist. Rock-Cherry. This grows upon rocky Mountains, and the Kernels are said to be heating and emollient.

Chamædrys minor Repens, C. B. P. *Chamædrys vulgaris*, Park. Theat. *Chamædrys vulgo vera existimata*, J. B. Germander. The Leaves of this Plant are bitter and aromatic, and contain Principles, different from those of the small Centaury. The Salt of Germander, is not diffe-rent from that which is naturally in the Earth, which is a Mixture of marine Salt, Nitre, and Sal Am-moniac. It is acrid, very bitter, and aperitive. It is probable, that what is found in this Plant, has lost its Acrimony by the Mixture of

a great deal of essential Oil, which renders the Germander aromatic. It is febrifugous, stomachic, aperitive and diaphoretic. Some infuse, cold, over Night, a Handfull of its Leaves in a Glass of white Wine, with Half a Dram of vegetable Salt, and give the Infusion to drink Fasting, for the Green Sickness. Some also prepare an Extract of its Leaves and Flowers, and give a Dram of it, with a Drop or two of the Oil of Cinnamon, and make an Infusion of the Leaves like Tea, principally for the Gout and Scia-tica. They enter into the Compo-sition of the Powder of the Prince of *Mirandola*, which is esteemed a great Specific in such Disorders.

Chamælæa tricoccos, C. B. Pin. *Chamælæa*, Dod. Boerh. Ind. Alt. Widow-wail. *Ray* informs us, that the Virtues of *Chamælæa*, are in a great Measure, the same with those of the *Laureola*, or Spurge Laurel; but as it is dubious, whether it is really the *Chamælæa* of the Anti-ents, we shall not ascribe to it the Virtues, which *Dioscorides* and *Pli-ny* attribute to that Plant. But says J. *Bauhine*, the Juice of the whole Plant, is much used at present, espe-cially at *Montpelier*, where according to *Rondeletius*, the Apothecaries keep it, expressed and inspissated; in Imitation of whom, says he, I have often with great Success exhi-bited one or two Drams of the re-cent inspissated Juice by itself, and oftener in Conjunction with other Hydragogue Cathartics. But it does not produce so large a Discharge of the peccant Matter, nor operate with such a Degree of Violence, as the Spurge Laurel, the German Mezereon, and the Gratiola gene-rally do. Sometimes, it operates little or none at all, except when mixed with some mild and gentle Cathartics. When exhibited to Children, it neither excites Gripes nor Vomitings, but only discharges Water and Serum. When applied to the Pubes and Abdomen of dropsical Patients, no Medicine is more effectual for provoking Urine, in which Manner, says he, *Roualetius* used it with Success.

Chamæmelum vulgare, Leucanthemum Dioscoridis, C. B. Pin. *Chamæmelum vulgare,* Offic. *Chamæmelum elatius, foliis obscure virentibus, semine Nigro,* Pluk. Almag. Wild or Dogs-Chamomile. It is found in uncultivated Places and among Corn, and flowers in *June.* The Herb and Flowers, are said to be possessed of the same Virtues with those of the common Camomile. This Plant is bitter, aromatic, and seems to contain some Sal Ammoniac, loaded with a great deal of Acid, and involved by a great deal of Sulphur and Earth. It is aperitive, diuretic, lenifying and febrifugous. The Powder of its Flowers, were used in *Dioscorides's* Time, to cure intermitting Fevers. *Rivarius* prescribed it on the same Occasions, and it is still the common Febrifuge of the *Scotch* and *Irish.* The Infusion of its Tops, with those of *Melitot* give great Ease, to such as are tormented with a nephritic Colic, and Retention of the Urine. It assuages the acute Pains of Women newly brought to bed. *Simon Paulli* recommends a strong Infusion of Chamomile Flowers in Wine, taken by Spoonfulls, while a Hogs-bladder filled with a Decoction of the Herb, is applied hot, and renew'd as Occasion requires, in pleuritic Cases. It is also used in lenifying and resolving Clysters, Fomentations, Cataplasms, and Baths for the Gout, Sciatica, and the Piles. The Oil of Chamomile made by Infusion, is very good in the same Cases. A Liniment of an equal Quantity of Chamomile, and Oil of St. *John's* Wort, with camphorated Spirit of Wine, in which a folded Cloth hath been dipt, and

applied very hot to the affected Part, is good in Rheumatisms.

Chamæmelum nobile, sive Leucantheum odoratius, C. B. P. *Chamæmelum odoratissimum repens flore simplici,* J. B. Chamomile. It digests, relaxes, mollifies, alleviates Pain, and excites a Discharge of the Menses and Urine. Hence it is singularly beneficial in Colics, flatulent Spasms, and Convulsions. It is used externally in paregoric emollient and maturating Cataplasms, and in Clysters. Among all Plants none are more efficacious than Chamomile Flowers, for Baths, intended to remove nephritic Pains. Doctor *Morton* asserts, that he was told by an eminent Physician, that he had found Chamomile Flowers, reduc'd to a fine Powder, and taken at due Intervals, as infallible in curing intermitting Fevers, as the Peruvian Bark; and farther, that he himself tried it, in three Instances, in every one of which it succeeded. *Frederic Hoffman* asserts, that no Simple in the Materia Medica, is possessed of a Quality more friendly and beneficial to the Intestines, than Chamomile Flowers; for which Reason says he, I have, instead of all other Ingredients, hitherto with great Success, prescrib'd their Use in Clysters, adding when there is a Necessity for it, Oil of Sweet Almonds; and for Patients of the poorer Sort, Linseed Oil, or Oil of Turnep-seeds; or for evacuating the Fœces, a sufficient Quantity of common Salt, which for its stimulating Quality, is of more Service than the whole Train of laxative and purgative Extracts and Electuaries, which may be very well left out of Clysters. These Flowers make an excellent Cataplasm, for discussing, softening, and maturating Abscesses. When boil'd in Milk, and put into a Bladder, either alone, or in Conjunction with the Flowers of Elder, Mallows, Yarrow, or Saffron, they are highly efficacious in

alleviating Pains and softening Tumours, if the Bladder is applied to the Part affected. I have learned from long Experience and Practice, that Brandy, distill'd from the Tops of Yarrow, Chamomile Flowers, Anise-seeds, and *Ethiopic* Cumin, is of more Efficacy in discussing Flatulencies, than any of the other so much extoll'd carminative, and antispasmodic Preparations. The last *London Pharmacopœia* directs an essential Oil from this Plant, and It is an Ingredient in the *Decoctum commune pro Clystere* ; *Fotus commune* ; and *Oleum viride.*

Chamæmelum nobile, flore multiplici, C. B. *Chamæmelum repens odoratissimum perenne flore multiplici,* Inab. Double Chamomile. This possesses the same Virtues as the former.

Chamæmelum fœtidum, C. B. P. Boerh. Ind. A. *Chamæmelum annuum ramex fœtidum semine aureo,* Hist. Oxon. May Weed. This Plant is acrid and bitter, smells like Bitumen, and contains a great deal more of fetid Oil than the common Chamomile. Fomentations of May-weed are very good for the Vapours, according to *Tragus;* at *Paris* they use it to asswage the Pain of the Piles, but 'tis rarely used, tho' some Authors commend it against Vapours and hysteric Fits.

Chamæmorus, Offic. *Vaccinia Nubis,* Ger. *Chamæmorus Anglica,* Park. Theat. Knot Berries, Cloud Berries. It is most efficacious in the Scurvy, in so much that it is almost incredible what Number of Cures are perform'd by it.

Chamæpitys lutea vulgaris, sive folio bifido. C. B. P. *Chamæpitys lota arthritica,* Offic. *Chamæpitys vulgaris odorata, flore luteo,* J. B. GroundPine. The Leaves of Ground-pine, drank in Wine for seven Days together, are said to cure the Yellow Jaundice ; for forty Days together in Hydromel, the Sciatica. They are likewise prescribed for Distempers of the Liver, Difficulty of Urine, and as a Specific in Disorders of the Kidneys ; they also help the Gripes. The Inhabitants of *Heraclea* in *Pontus,* used this Herb, as an Antidote for those who had drank the Decoction of *Aconitum.* Ground-pine is hot and dry, warming and strengthening to the Nerves, helps the Palsy, Gout, Sciatica, Rheumatism, Scurvy, and Pains of the Limbs. It is a strong Diuretic, opens the Obstructions of the Womb, and powerfully promotes the Menses, in so much that it is forbidden to Women with Child, for fear of an Abortion ; it is bitter and aromatic, and contains some oily volatile Salt, loaded with a great deal of Sulphur and Earth ; for by a chymical Analysis, it yields several acid Liquors, a little urinous Spirit, and a great deal of Oil, but more Earth. It is no Wonder, then, if this Plant restores the ordinary Course of the Spirits, and Liquids in the Nerves, and capillary Vessels ; whence it is very good in nervous Affections. It is diuretic, emmenagogue, and dissipates the Cause of the Gout. Drink its Infusion in Wine, or make a Ptisan of it with Germander.

Chamæpitys Moschata foliis serratis an prima Dioscoridis, C. B. Pin. *Chamæpitys altera,* Offic. *Chamæpitys odoratior.* Park. Theat. *Chamæpitys tertia Dodonæi,* Ger. Emac. *Italian* Ground Pine. This is common in *Italy,* and flowers in *June. Dioscorides* says, that the two last, are possessed of the same Virtues as the first, tho' in a weaker Degree.

Chelidonium magis vulgare, Park. Theat. *Chelidonium majus,* Offic. *Papaver corniculatum luteum Chelidonia Dictum,* Raii Synop. Celandine. Celandine is bitter, acrid, and burning, but more especially the Root, which

yields

yields more of Orange colour'd Juice, than the other Parts of the Plant; it smells like rotten Eggs, which makes some believe, that its Juice is Phagedenic, and something like the Liquor which results from the Mixture of the Solution of sublimate, and Lime Water, or Milk which has boil'd sometime with an acrid Salt. Taken inwardly it is very aperitive and cleansing, opens all the Obstructions of the Spleen and Liver, and is of good Service in the Jaundice and Scurvy. For the Dropsy some infuse for twenty four Hours, one Ounce of the Root of Celandine, and half an Ounce of the Tincture of Steel, in a Pint of White-wine, and straining the Infusion thro' a Linnen Cloth, give the Patient three Ounces of it twice a Day.

· *Chelidonium minus.* The lesser Celandine. *Chelidonium minus,* Offic. *Scrophalaria minor sive Chelidonium minus vulgo dictum,* J. B. Pile Wort. This Herb is reckoned good for the Piles, to ease their Pains and Swellings, as also to stop their Bleeding, the Roots being taken inwardly, and outwardly applied in an Ointment made of the Leaves and Roots. Some greatly commend it for the Jaundice and Scurvy, but more especially that in the Mouth; it is reckoned a Strengthener of the Gums, and a great Preserver of the Teeth. It is also esteem'd an excellent Remedy, either internally taken, or externally applied for Hernias in Children.

China, Offic. *China Radix,* C. B. Pin. *Chinæ Radix,* Raii Hist. China Root. This is a Root of a pale red Colour externally, but white within, of a farinaceous, earthy, and somewhat astringent Taste, but without any Smell. It is supposed to be the Root of a certain *Smilax,* call'd *Lampatam* in *China,* where it grows plentifully. There is, also, in *America,* and *New Spain,* a Root

nearly similar to this, which they call *West Indian China,* but is inferior to that which comes from *China,* and the neighbouring Countries. This Root first began to acquire an uncommon Reputation in *Europe,* in the Time of *Vesalius,* which was about the Year 1535. The Decoction of the Root for the venereal Disease, became famous, and was prepared in the following Manner:

> Take an Ounce of fresh China Root, cut into thin Slices, let them maceratte for twenty-four Hours in six or eight Pints of tepid Spring-Water, which is to be boiled in a large earthen Pot close cover'd, over a slow Fire to the Consumption of a Third. Then strain the Decoction, and set it aside in a glass Vessel stopp'd, keeping it tepid for daily Use.

The Patient, being prepar'd by Purging and Bleeding, took ten or twelve Ounces of this Decoction every Day, early in the Morning, and composed himself in Bed well cover'd with Cloaths, to sweat for two or three Hours: After this, wiping off the Sweat, he was permitted to rise and walk about the Room, and after ten or twelve Days, if the Weather was mild, to walk Abroad, taking Care to keep himself warm. He was more indulg'd with Respect to Diet, than if he had used a Decoction of Guiacum; for he was allow'd to eat Chickens, or Capons roasted or boil'd without any Salt. But he was wholly to abstain from Wine, and to use nothing for his ordinary Drink, but a warm Decoction of China Root. This Regimen was persisted in for four or five and twenty Days together, after which, the Cure was thought to be perfected. If the Patient was subject to be coftive, they added fome Senna to the Decoction, or adminiftered an emollient Clyfter every other Day. What contributed greatly to raife the Character of the China Root was, its affording confiderable Relief to the Emperor *Charles* V, when afflicted with the Gout, and Cachexy. This Root, however, foon loft its high Reputation; for *Vefalius*, in a Letter publifh'd in 1542. affures us, that Decoctions of China Root, were far inferior to thofe of *Guaiacum*, for Excrefcences and Tumors of the Bones, and for the Cure of malignant venereal Ulcers. Doctor *Aftruc* informs us, that in venereal Cafes he could produce no happy Effects by Means of this Root. It is by fome thought to be of Service in the Gout, Sciatica, œdematous Tumors, King's Evil, Imbecillity of the Stomach, Hemicranias, and in Ulcers of the Bladder and Kidneys.

China Occidentalis, Pharmacop. *China fpuria Nodofa*, C. B. Pin. American China. This is poffefs'd of the fame Virtues with the former, but is not efteem'd fo good.

Chondrilla prima, Offic. *Chondrilla cærulea altera Cichorei fylveftris folio*, C. B. *Lactuca fylveftris perennis purpuro cæruleo, laciniato longo folio*, Hift. Oxon. Gum Succory. It grows in uncultivated Places in *Germany* and *Italy*, and flowers in Summer according to *Diofcorides*. *Dale* is of Opinion, that the Herb is the *Chondarilla prima* of *Diofcorides*. About the Branches of this Plant, there is a Gum found refembling Maftich, about the Bignefs of a Bean, which bruifed with Myrrh, and applied in Linen to the Quantity of an Olive, provokes the Menfes. The Herb with the Root is bruifed, and with an Addition of Honey is made into Troches, which diluted and mixed, deterge the *Alphi*. Drank in Wine it cures the Bite of a Viper, and the Juice boil'd and drank with Wine, or alone, ftops a Loofenefs, according to *Diofcorides*.

Chondrilla altera, Offic. *Chondrilla Juncea*, Ger. Gum Succory with yellow Flowers. It grows in fandy Soils, in *Germany* and *Italy*, and flowers in June. The Stalks and Leaves are faid to have a digeftive Faculty.

Cicer Album, Offic. *Cicer fativum Album*, Park. Theat. *Cicer arietinum*, J. B. White Chiches. The *Cicer* is a Kind of Pulfe, fown in *Italy*, *France*, and other warm Climates, from whence the Seed is brought to us. They flower in *June*, and the Fruit is ripe in *July*. They are, alfo, cultivated in the Gardens of the Curious, and the Seeds are ufed in Phyfic. They are efteemed flatulent, but are faid to ftimulate to Venery; they deterge, open, incide, digeft, and are faid to diffolve the Stone; but are prejudicial when the Bladder or Kidneys are exulcerated. The Decoction is faid to be good in a Jaundice, to deftroy Worms, to provoke the Menfes, and to expel the Fœtus. In Cataplafms they are efteem'd efficacious in the Cure of Tetters, Ringworms, and Parotides, to difcufs Inflammations of the Tefticles, and to confolidate malignant Ulcers.

The *Cicer nigrum*, and *Rubrum*, differ in nothing from the *Album* but in the Colour of the Flower, which is of a Purple Colour, and the Fruit of a reddifh Brown.

Cicer Sylveftre, Offic. *Cicer fylveftre majus*, Park. Theat. *Aftralagus luteus perennis, filiqua gemellâ, rotunda veficam referente*, Boerh. Ind. A. Wild Chiches. They grow wild in Fields, and in uncultivated Places in *Italy*, and other Countries, and flower in the Summer; the Seed is ufed, which is of a heating, drying, deterfive and aperient Quality, and

X

agrees

agrees with the preceding Cicers in Virtues.

Cichorium latifolium, five Endivia vulgaris, Boerh. Ind. A. *Endivia scariola, Intybus,* Offic. *Intybus sativa latifolia, five Endivia vulgaris.* Endive. It grows in Gardens, flowers in *June,* and when the Seed is ripe the Root perishes. Endive is much used in Salads. It is cooling and moistening, opens Obstructions of the Liver and Spleen, is efficacious against the Jaundice, provokes Urine, and greatly cools a hot Stomach; its Seed is one of the lesser cold Seeds.

Cichorium sylvestre five Officinarum, C. B. *Cichorium agreste sylvestre,* Offic. Wild Succory. It grows in Lanes and Hedge Sides, and flowers rather later than the *Garden Succory.* The Virtues of the *Wild* differ but little from those of the *Garden Succory.* A Water distilled from the Flowers, is esteem'd good in Inflammations of the Eyes. The Roots and Leaves, are aperitive, diuretic, and cooling. They seem to cool only by removing the too long obstructed Humours of the Bowels. They are prescribed in Broths, Ptisans, Apozems, and Clysters. The Juice procures Expectoration in Defluxions of the Breast. The Extract, has the same Virtues and purifies the Blood. The simple or compound Syrup, is a good Aperitive, especially if two Drams, or half an Ounce of Tincture of Steel be mixed with an Ounce of it. The Conserve of its Flowers is used on the same Occasions, in aperitive Boluses and Electuaries. These Electuaries are of great Service in the Cachexy, Dropsy and hypochondriac Disorders, intermitting Fevers, and troublesome Heats of the lower Belly.

Cichorium, Ger. Garden Succory. It is planted in Gardens, and flowers in *June.* The Root, Leaves, Flo-

wer and Seeds are used, its Seed is one of the four smaller cold Seeds. The ancient *Botanic* Writers generally affirm, that Succory is cold, but its Bitterness manifestly shows it to be hot; however it is aperitive and diuretic, opens Obstructions of the Liver, and is good for the Jaundice. It provokes Urine, and cleanses the urinary Parts of slimy Humour that may stop their Cavities.

Cicuta, Offic. Ger. *Cicuta major vulgaris,* Park. Theat. Hemlock. It grows in Fields and by Hedge Sides, and among Rubbish, and flowers in Summer. Hemlock is used outwardly, in Swellings and Hardness of the Liver and Spleen. Its Leaves are very lenifying and resolvent; when boil'd with Milk, they are apply'd with good Success to the Piles, and the Parts afflicted with the Gout. A Cataplasm of Hemlock Leaves bruised with some Snails, and work'd up with the resolvent Meals, is excellent for Inflammations of the Testicles, for the Gout and Sciatica. The Hemlock Plaister is a good Resolver of scirrhous Tumors.

Cicuta latifolia fœtidissima, Seseli Peloponnense, Offic. *Seseli Peloponnesi acum recentiorum,* Park. Theat. Great broad leaved Hemlock, or Bastard Hemlock. It grows plentifully in the Country of the *Grisons.* The Root and Seed is in Use. *Dale* says, that this Plant is possessed of the same Virtues as the *Seseli Massilense,* according to *Dioscorides.* But as Botanists agree, that this Plant is erroneously taken for the *Seseli Peloponnense* of *Dioscorides,* we must not attribute the Virtues of the former to this.

Cinara hortensis foliis non aculeatis, C. B. Pin. Offic. The Artichoak. Artichoaks have the Reputation, of promoting venereal Inclinations, to a very great Degree. The Stalks preserv'd in Honey, are said to be an excel-

excellent Pectoral, but they should be first blanched, like Celery. The common Leaves boil'd in white Wine Whey, are much commended in the Jaundice, as also the Juice of these Leaves

Scolymus sylvestris, Offic. *Scolymus Dioscoridis*, Park. Theat. *Cardus sive Cinara sylvestris latifolia*, Hist. Oxon. Wild Artichoak, or Cardonet. This grows in *Italy* and *France*. The Part in Use, is the Flower, which is thought, by the Vulgar, to prevent Sterility, and to preserve the Foetus in the Womb, to the just Period of Maturity. The Flowers coagulate Milk.

Cinnamomum, Offic. Park. *Cinnamomum sive Canella Zeilanita*, C. B. Pin. Raii Hist. The true Cinnamon Tree. What is at present called Cinnamon in the Shops, is an aromatic Bark, of a reddish Colour, woody, friable, in Pipes of a different Thickness and Length; of a sweetish, hot, pungent, and somewhat astringent Taste; of a fragrant Smell, appropriated to various Uses, both in Medicine and Cookery, and gather'd from the *Arbor Cinnamomifera Zeilanica*. These Trees grow in several Parts of the *East Indies*, but none yield such good Bark, as those of *Zeilan*. From an Incision made in the Root of this Tree, there drops a Liquor, which smells like Camphire. Besides, Camphire, now-and-then ouses from the Bark of this Root, in Form of white Drops, which insensibly coagulate into white Grains. This Species of Camphire, by the *Indians* call'd *Baru*, is also obtain'd by Distillation, from the Bark of the Root dried, bruised, and immersed in Water. The Physicians of *Zeilan*, use this distill'd camphorated Water with Success, exhibiting a Spoonful of it at proper Intervals, as a Sudorific, in continual and malignant Fevers. They, also, mix it with common Water against Defluxions. Externally, it is applied with Linen Cloths, for discussing œdematous and watery Tumors. The Leaves of the Tree, in Distillation, yield an Oil, of a bitterish Taste, resembling Oil of Cloves, to which a little of the Oil of Cinnamon has been added. This is call'd *Oleum Malabathri*, and is celebrated as an instantaneous Remedy, against Pains of the Head and Stomach, and several other Disorders. The Oil of the Leaves, made by boiling them with common Oil, is on Account of its healing, anodyne and resolvent Quality, highly recommended for chirurgical Intentions, in the Composition of Liniments, for Instance, Cataplasms, and Clysters; as, also, in Colics, Gripes, Tympanies, and other windy and watery Tumors. From the Flowers, is obtain'd by Distillation, a fragrant Water, which when exhibited by Spoonfuls, at proper Intervals, corroborates the Stomach, and immediately alleviates colic Pains, arising from Cold. A Conserve is, also, made of the Flowers, which is highly commended against Diseases arising from a cold Cause. From the Kernels of the ripe Fruit, is expressed an Oil, which in some Measure resembles Suet, and is made up in Cakes. This is by the *Indians* used for several Disorders, both internally and externally. In the Shops, that Cinnamon is generally accounted best, which is lately gather'd, of a yellowish Red externally, and internally of a somewhat darker Colour; which is smooth, easily broken, of a fragrant Scent, and pungent Taste. That which is small, is preferable to the large Kind, and the long Pipes are esteem'd more valuable than the short. Some adulterate it with the Bark of the Caper Bush, Tamarisk, or the Cassia Lignea; but this Piece of Fraud is easily detected.

tected. *Bauhine* expresly affirms, that whatever Virtues the Antients ascrib'd to their Cinnamomum and Cassia, justly belong to our Cinnamon; since it is of an aromatic, stimulating, and corroborative Quality. Hence it is classed among the stomachic and uterine Medicines, affords singular Relief to Women afflicted with a Loss of Strength, a lax State of the Fibres, or a Suppression of the Menses. Tho' Cinnamon is an excellent Cordial, and highly beneficial in Palpitations of the Heart; yet it has, by being too often used, been found to bring on the same Disorder, in which Case, Acids are the most effectual Means of Relief. Tho' 'tis highly proper, in some Disorders incident to pregnant Women; yet in these Cases *Etmuller* justly advises the cautious Use of it; because it powerfully irritates the Uterus, to discharge and expel the Fœtus. Of half an Ounce of the best Cinnamon, infused in a close stopp'd Vessel, with two Pints of boiling Water, is prepar'd an highly grateful Drink, which recommends itself, not only on Account of its Smell and Taste, but, also, on Account of its analeptic, stomachic, and moderately astringent Quality in Fluxes, as, also, in a Weakness of the Heart, and Stomach. The styptic Quality of the Decoctions of Cinnamon, is sufficiently evinc'd by Doctor *Hales*, in his *Statical Essays.* The essential Oil is yielded with the Water, in Distillation, and subsides to the Bottom, as being specifically heavier. It is of an inflammatory and corrosive Nature, whether externally applied, or internally exhibited. It is by Reason of its acrid and caustic Nature, highly celebrated as an excellent Medicine in a deep seated Caries of the Bones. *Juncker*, in his *Conspectus Therapiæ*

Generalis, tells us, that distill'd Oil of Cinnamon, is an excellent Medicine, for stopping the Progress of Mortifications. *Tulpius*, also, in *Obs. Med.* informs us, that in Order to separate the carious Parts of Bones, he never knew a more effectual Medicine, than Oil of Cinnamon, mix'd with Oil of Sublimate. *Boerhaave* informs us, that it is of a restorative Quality, in Cases where Strength is impair'd, in Women during Gestation, hard Labour, or after Delivery, when there is no Inflammation nor Rupture of the Vessels. He, also, says, that it is good in Disorders of the Uterus, arising from a cold and mucous Phlegm. It may, also, be added to Purgatives, not only with an Intention to render them more palatable, but, also, to prevent Flatulences and Gripes. It may, also, be very properly added to Ointments and Balsams, not only for its fragrant Smell, but, also, on Account of its resolvent, discutient, and heating Qualities. Six Drops of it may be given in Substance, either in a poach'd Egg, sweet Wine, or Broth prepar'd with Flesh, but more properly dropp'd upon Sugar. It is used in the *Aqua Cinnamomi*; *Aqua Spirituosa Cinnamomi*; *Spiritus Lavendulæ compositus*; *Vinum Chalybeatum*; *Tinctura Thebaica*; *Tinctura Aromatica*; *Tinctura Cinnamomi*; *Tinctura Japonica*; *Tinctura Stomachica*; *Syrupus Cydoniorum*; *Syrupus Scilliticus*; *Syrupus e Spina Cervina*; *Confectio Alkermes*; *Pulvis Ari compositus*; *Pulvis e Bolo compositus sine Opio*; *Pulvis e Sena compositus*; *Species Aromaticæ*; *Species e Scordio sine Opio*; *Confectio Cardiaca*; *Confectio Paulina*; *Mithridatium*; *Theriaca Andromachi*; *Emplastrum Stomachicum.*

Another Species of the Cinnamomum, is called *Cassia Lig-*

sia, Offic. Hern. *Caßia Lignea*, Officinarum, Park. Theat. *Canella Malabarica & Javenßs*, Jons Dendr. The Caßia Lignea Tree. This Bark of the Cinnamon bearing Tree, produced in *Malabar, Sumatra, Java,* and the *Philippine Islands,* is brought into *Europe,* in small Pipes, like the *Ceylonian* Cinnamon, but is of a darker and more rusty Colour, more hard and compact Texture, of a more languid Smell, of a sweet mucilaginous and less hot Taste. That Sort of this Bark, is reckon'd best, which is small, of a purplish Colour, easily broken, fragrant, acrid, of a sweetish Taste; because it then abounds with a volatile oleous Salt, sheath'd up in a vast Quantity of mucilaginous Substance, and therefore operates less powerfully on the human Body, and is greatly proper, where the Intention is only moderately to heat, open, resolve, and strengthen. It, also, obtunds the Acrimony of the Humours, by its mild and balsamic Mucilage. An Infusion of it, is by some recommended in Disorders of the Throat, and is also, said to be beneficial in Diseases of the Uterus. Its Virtues, are the same with those of the *Ceylonian* Cinnamon, tho' somewhat weaker and less aromatic. It is rarely prescribed by Physicians, in any other Preparations than those which come under the Denomination of Antidotes.

A third Species, is the *Caßia Lignea communis*, Pharmacopolis. *Caßia Lignea fusca Aromatica,* C. B. Pin, *Arbor canellifera Indica cortice accerrimo, viscido seu mucilaginoso, qui Caßia Lingea,* Officinarum, Breyn. Prod. The common Caßia Lignea. This Bark is somewhat thicker than Cinnamon, and is of a fainter Smell and Taste, of a more reddish Colour and harder Substance. It is brought from the *East Indies,* and is frequent in the Shops.

Citreum. Of this there are two Species. The *Citreum vulgare*, Tourn. Inst. *Malus Citria*, Offic. *Malus Medica sive Citria*, Park. Theat. The Citron Tree. And the *Citreum, Medulla dulci.* The first of these, is principally used in Medicine. It is esteem'd beneficial, in Cases where mortal Poisons have been drank, and in Order to sweeten the Breath; for if any one squeezes the Juice of the Citron Peel into his Mouth, and swallows it, after being boil'd in Broth, or any other Liquor, it procures a sweet Breath. The dry'd and fresh Citrons used before Meals, are said to resist all Poisons. *Dioscorides* says, that the Seeds of the Citron, drank in Wine, resist Poison, render the Body soluble, procure a sweet Breath, and that they are principally used by Women, against that Species of Disorder, call'd *Malacia.* *Pliny* tells us, that the Seeds when exhibited in Vinegar, are good against a Weakness of the Stomach. The Flowers of this Tree, are preserved in Sugar, and used as a Sweetmeat, they are of a cordial Nature, and generally prescribed in Electuaries. *Gui Patin,* a celebrated Physician, highly extolls this Fruit, gives it the Preference to some of the Shop Cordials, and affirms, that in all malignant Disorders, putrid and pestilential Fevers, more infallible Relief is to be expected from a few Citrons, than from all the various Preparations of the Oriental Bezoar.

Citrullus, Offic. *Citrullus folio Colocynthidis secto, semine Nigro quibusdam Anguria,* J. B. *Anguria sive Citrullus vulgatior,* Park. Theat. Citrul, or Water Melon. It grows spontaneously in hot Climates, and though it is sown in more northern Countries, it never arrives at perfect Maturity. The fungous Pulp or Marrow is a grateful Ali-

ment

ment, not very nourifhing, aqueous, but juftly celebrated for its moiftening, laxative, diuretic, and refrigerating Qualtities. The Seeds are by Phyficians claffed among the four greater cold Seeds. They provoke Urine, but lefs powerfully than the Seeds of the Pompion. They are principally ufed in cooling Emulfions.

Clematis, five Flammula furreƐa, alba, J. B. *Flammula Jovis,* Offic. *Flammula Jovis furreƐa,* Park. Theat. Upright Ladies Bower. This flowers in Summer; the Herb with the Flower is ufed, and are of a hot burning Quality. The Flowers, Seeds, Bark and Root, have a cauftic Virtue; rubb'd with the Fingers and then held to the Noftrils, it ftrikes them, in an Inftant, with a ftrong and moft vehement Smell. It yields a Water as hot as Spirit of Wine, and which is found to be very effeƐual, as *Matthiolus* tells us, in the coldeft Difeafes, but doubtlefs it cannot be taken inwardly with Safety, unlefs it be well mixed and temper'd with other Waters, to prevent its injuring the Vifcera. Some commend the Oil for the Sciatica, for Difficulty of Urine, and the Stone in the Kidneys, to be rubb'd on the Parts hot, or mixed with Clyfters.

Clematis cærulea vel purpurea repens, C. B. Pin. *Clematis Altera,* Offic. *Clematis peregrina flore rubro vel purpureo fimplex,* Park. Theat. Virgins Bower. This is thought to be the *Clematis* of *Diofcorides,* who informs us, that the Seeds, taken in Water, or Hydromel, purge Phlegm and Bile, and that the Leaves applied to the Part affeƐed, cure a Leprofy.

Clinopodium Origano fimile, elatius, majore folio, C. B. Pin. *Clinopodium,* Offic. *Acinos five Clinopodium majus,* Park. Theat. Great white

Bafil. It grows frequently in Hedges. The Herb and its DecoƐion are taken as an Antidote againft the Bites of venomous Animals, and as a Remedy for Spafms, Contufions, and Stranguries. It facilitates Delivery, provokes the Menfes, and cures penfile Warts, call'd *Acrochordones,* if taken for fome Days. It ftops a Diarrhæa, boil'd to the Confumption of one Third, and then drank. It muft be boil'd in Wine, in Cafe of a Fever, but in Water if there is no Fever.

Cnicus fylveftris, hirfutior, five Carduus BenediƐus, C. B. Pin. *Carduus BenediƐus,* Offic. *Carduus luteus, procumbens fudorificus & amarus,* Hift. Oxon. Holy Thiftle. *Pauli* after *Cæfalpinus* obferves, that the Head of this Herb, is of a fragrant Smell, refembling that of the Mufcadel Pear; but *Cæfalpinus* compared it to that of Mufk itfelf. This Cnicus, is faid to have been firft imported from the *Indies,* by Way of Prefent to the Emperor *Frederick* the Third, at which JunƐure it was highly celebrated, either ufed in Aliments or Drink, as an excellent Prefervative againft that Species of Head-ach, call'd *Hemicrania.* It flowers in the Summer, and in the Autumn its Seeds become ripe. *Hoffman* gives us the following Account of the medicinal Virtues of this Plant: " Its Virtues are nearly " the fame with thofe of Worm- " wood. DecoƐions of it, efpeci- " ally in Wine, are of fingular Ef- " ficacy, when the Patient is not " feverifh. It is lefs efficacious " when exhibited in Powder, and " the diftilled Water is much lefs " fo. It is highly extolled in all " pituitous Diforders of the Head, " Hemicranias, Deafnefs, Verti- " goes, Epilepfies, Defluxions on " the Breaft, Dropfies, Quartan Fe- • goes "vers, and those of long standing, " as these Disorders draw their Ori- "gin from Obstructions. It is, " also, celebrated as an excellent " Medicine in Colies, nephritic and " sciatic Pains, as it partly discusses " the peccant Matter, and partly " derives it to the urinary Passages. " But its Efficacy, is principally ce- " lebrated in that formidable Dis- " temper the Plague, against which " it is used; both internally and " externally. Internally it is exhi- " bited, both with a preservative " and curative Intention; since it " powerfully excites a Diaphoresis. " Externally it is applied, for brea- " king and opening pestilential Bu- " boes, with which Intention, it is " also applied to other Imposthuma- " tions. In the Opinion of the " common People, a Wine pre- " pared of it in the Autumn, is " possessed of so powerful Quali- " ties, that it is little less than a " *Panacea,* or universal Remedy. " It is preferable to the Wine of " Wormwood, because, in Conse- " quence of its analeptic Quality, " it does not prove offensive to the " Head, whilst, at the same Time, " it is equally, if not more benefi- " cial to the Stomach; for it is " proper both for bilious and pi- " tuitous Patients. As it is a power- " ful Astringent, it is used in stop- " ping Hæmorrhages."

There is another Species of *Cnicus,* which is the *Carduus pinea,* Offic. *Carduus Creticus humillimus integris & Augustis foliis,* Hist. Oxon. *Chamæleo albus Apulus purpureo flore gummifer,* Raii Hist. The Pine Thistle. The Country People of *Apulia* who attend the Flocks, ga- ther the Gum produced in the Head, and between the Leaves of the Cup. This Gum they call *Ce- ra di Cardo,* because when it is concreted, it becomes hard like Wax. They use it as a drawing

Topic. Whilst it is recent, its Parts cohere like those of Bird Lime, and may be drawn out into a Thread of a whitish Colour; for it originally consists of a milky Juice, which, when collected, becomes thick like Wax, and when handled assumes a blackish Colour. These Accounts are given by *Colonna.*

Cocculus Indus, Offic. *Cocci Orien- tales,* Ger. *Solanum racemosum In- dicum arborescens, Cocculos Indos fe- rens,* Raii Dendr. Indian Berry. This is a little Berry, about as big as a Bay Berry, but more of a Kid- ney Shape, having a wrinkled Out- side, with a Seam running Length- ways from the Back to the Navel. It is of a bitterish Taste, being the Fruit of a Tree described in the se- venth Volume of the *Hortus Mala- baricus,* under the Name of *Natsia- tam. Crondronchius,* who has wrote a Treatise concerning these Ber- ries, informs us, that he has often found from Experience, that a small Quantity of their Powder mixed with Hogs Lard, a boi- led Apple, or some Substance of a like Nature, applied to the Heads of Children, kill Lice more effectually than Staves-acre, and with less Danger than Quick- silver.

Coccus de Maldiva, Offic. *Coccus de Maldiva, sive Nux Indica ad venena celebrata,* Raii Hist. *Palma Naldivensis, aliis Maidivensis,* Jons Dendr. The Maldiva Nut. This is of so high a Value among the Na- tives at *Malabar,* that as *Acosta* as- sures us, not only the common Peo- ple, but even their Princes have Re- course to it as a sovereign Remedy, under almost all Kinds of Diseases, and it is accounted in particular, an excellent Alexipharmic. Under this Persuasion, they make drinking Cups of it, and let a Piece of the Pulp hang by a Chain in the Water which they drink, being

Confident that no Poison can hurt those who drink out of those Cups. But some affirm, that they have found by Experience, that this Medicine is more injurious than beneficial. As to its specific Quality, says *Piso*, of promoting and facilitating Delivery; and of resisting the Fits of an Epilepsy, we have it confirm'd by more than one Experiment, and those made by some of our most eminent Physicians, who have used it with all the desired Success.

Cochlearia folio cubitali, Tourn. Instit. *Raphanus sylvestris*, Offic. *Raphanus sylvestris, seu Armoracia multis*, J. B. Horse Rhadish. It grows wild in several Places, near River Sides, and is planted in Gardens for the Sake of the Root, which is only used. It is heating, drying aperitive, and frequently used in Sauces to create an Appetite. It is of great Use against the Scurvy, Dropsy and Jaundice, and is often put into Diet Drinks for those Purposes. The expressed Juice, being suffered to putrify, affords an alcaline volatile Salt, like that of Urine, which is the Reason why it is so highly beneficial in the Scurvy, arising from an acid State of the Fluids. In the other Kind of Scurvy it is very pernicious, in which Case, I have known it to procure a Rupture of the Liver. But where there is a Defect of Heat, and a Coldness and Viscidity of the Juices, it is very proper. In a Scurvy attended with a hot Fever and a Putrefaction, it would destroy the Patient. So, also, in a Dropsy, if it proceeds from a cold Cause, this Plant is proper to be used, otherwise not. This Root, taken in a large Quantity, excites Vomiting. The Juice drank to the Quantity of two Ounces, it is good for those who are afflicted with pituitous Sordes in the Stomach, and if

this be attended with Vomiting, it will beproper to drink plentifully of warm Water after taking the Dose. This Herb in Conjunction with Sorrel, makes an excellent antiscorbutic Medicine; but where its Acrimony is to be feared, it must be temper'd with Milk, Whey or Raisins. It is used for Gargarisms, in Putrefactions of the Gums, and yields a noble Spirit and Tincture. It is used externally in Sinapisms, and is an Ingredient in the *Aqua Rhaphani composita.*

Cochlearia folio subrotundo, C. B. Pin. *Cochlearia Batava, rotundifolia, hortensis*, Offic. *Cochlearia major rotundifolia, sive Batavorum*, Park. Theat. Garden Scurvy Grass. It grows wild in several Parts of the North of *England*, by the Sea Side, but is very much cultivated in Gardens, and flowers in *April*. *Scurvy Grass* abounds with fine volatile Parts, and therefore the Herb infused, or the Juice expressed, is more prevalent than a Decoction, the volatile Parts flying away in the Boiling. This is accounted a specific Remedy against the Scurvy, purifying the Juices of the Body from the bad Effects of the Distemper, and cleansing the Skin from Scabbs, Pimples, and foul Eruptions. It must be remember'd, that these warm alcalescent Plants, are only proper in an acid Scurvy, but that in a putrid alcaline Scurvy, they are Poisons.

Cochlearia, folio sinuato, C. B. Pin. *Cochlearia Britannica marina*, Offic. *Cochlearia Britannica folio sinuato*, Hist. Oxon. Sea Scurvy Grass. It grows in salt Marshes, and particularly by the *Thames* Side, all the Way below *Woolwich*, and flowers rather later than the preceding Species. In scorbutic Remedies, the *Sea Scurvy Grass* is often used, mixed with the *Garden* Sort. It wants the fine volatile Parts, and is not so efficacious, but as it abounds
much

much more in faline Particles, it may with good Succeſs be uſed as a Diuretic.

Coffee, Offic. *Jaſminum Arabicum, Caſtaneæ folio, flore albo odoraſſimo, cujus fruĉtus Coffy in Officinis cuntur*, Boerh, Ind. A. The Coffee Tree. This is a low ſhrubby Tree or Buſh, which grows in *Arabia Felix*. It is a Species of Jaſmine, according to *Commelin*, having very ſweet odoriferous Flowers, like thoſe of Jaſmine. Coffee, is eſteem'd efficacious for the Cure and Prevention of comatous Diſorders, ariſing from Phlegm, or a too viſcid Blood, and by its Chylification and Sanguification increaſes the Quantity of the animal Spirits, and repairs the Loſs of them ariſing from preternatural Watching. By its volatile Salts it removes Obſtruĉtions of the Brain, dries up its ſuperfluous Moiſture, and conſequently reſtores a due Degree of Elaſticity to its Membranes and Veſſels. Is is an infallible Secret for removing that Species of Head-ach, which in Conſequence of a bad Digeſtion, ariſes ſome Hours after Dinner. Coffee in general, ſeems more proper for Perſons of phlegmatic Conſtitutions, than for Patients of choleric Habits. In moſt Diſorders of the Head, ſuch as a Cephalalgia, Vertigo, Lethargy, and Catarrh, when the Habit is plethoric, the Conſtitution cold, the Blood aqueous, the Brain too moiſt, and the Motion of the Spirits too ſlow and languid, Coffee is of great Advantage. On the contrary, thoſe who are lean, of a bilious or melancholic Conſtitution, whoſe Blood is acrid or retorrid, whoſe Brain is hot, or whoſe animal Spirits are ſtimulated to too briſk and irregular Motions, ought entirely to abſtain from this Liquor. *Hoffman* in his Diſſertation, *de Remediorum benignorum Abuſu* ſays, " no one will eaſily "believe, that Coffee is prejudicial to "his Health; ſince not only with the "*Turks*, but with our Countrymen, "nothing is more common than to "drink liberally of it, both faſting "and after Meals. Yet Proofs are not "wanting to manifeſt the Conſequen-"ces ariſing from a too frequent and "immoderate Uſe of this Liquor, "eſpecially to weakly Perſons, but "more particularly Women, whoſe "Nerves and Strength is conſiderably "impair'd by it, and either in Child "Birth, or on the Attack of an Diſ-"eaſe, ſo conſiderable a Languor is "brought on, that their Strength is "hardly able to ſurmount the Symp-"toms with which they are afflicted." *Stenzelius* in his *Toxicologia* ſays, Coffee often proves a temporary Poiſon, when uſed too frequently, in too large Quantities, or promiſcuouſly by Perſons of every Conſtitution, eſpecially in the Afternoon; for by the roaſting, its ſaline volatile Parts are carried off, and there are only left a narcotic Oil and an Earth, which produce Obſtruĉtions and Coſtiveneſs. In the Year 1695, it was in the Schools of *Paris* defended as a Theſis, that the daily Uſe of Coffee rendered both Men and Women unfit for Procreation but no one will affirm this, who conſiders, that as numerous a Progeny is brought into the World, ſince the daily Uſe of this Liquor in *Europe*, as before. Coffee made very ſtrong, is eſteem'd by ſome an excellent Remedy for a nervous Aſthma, and is ſaid to attenuate the Blood, and to be diuretic. *Geoffroy* affirms, that its Uſe endangers a Miſcarriage.

Colchicum commune, C. B. Pin. *Colchicum*, Offic. J. B. *Colchicum purpureum & Anglicum album*, Ger. Meadow Saffron. It is found in fat and rich Meadows. The Root is the Part uſed, and is mortal to thoſe who eat it after the Manner of Muſhrooms, by ſuffocating them

them. The Root is by some supposed to be the Hermodactyl of the Shops. It is of a poisonous Quality, but recommended, externally applied, in the Gout.

Colchicum Chionense, floribus Fritillariæ instar tessellatis, foliis undulatis, Hist. Oxon. *Hermodactylus,* Offic. *Colchicum minus malignum, sive Hermodactylus Officinarum,* J. B. Hermodactyls Authors greatly differ with Respect to the Plant of which this is the Root. Some affirm it to be the Root of a *Colchicum,* or *Dens Caninus,* others that of the tuberous Iris, and others, of a Species of Cyclamen. It is a very strong Cathartic, and purges serous and phlegmatic Humours from the Joints, and is therefore highly recommended in the Gout, and rheumatic Pains in the Limbs.

Colocynthis, Offic. *Colocynthis vulgaris,* Park. Theat. *Colocynthis fructu Rotundo minor,* C. B. Pin. Coloquintida. The Pulp of this Fruit is bitter and purgative, but the Seeds have neither of these Qualities, in so great a Degree, except they have touch'd the Pulp; for then they become very bitter. *Coloquintida* taken in a large Dose, is one of the most violent Purges now known. It not only brings away pure Blood, but produces violent Convulsions, Ulcers in the Intestines, and fatal Hypercatharses. When the Pulp is taken in Substance, it sticks to the Coats of the Stomach and Intestines, and therefore it has been judged convenient to divide it as much as possible. Thus being reduced to a fine Powder, it is made up into Lozenges, called *Trochisci Alhandal,* but even these, are hurtful to Persons of weak abdominal Viscera. When it is thought proper to give it in Clysters, it ought to be boil'd in a Linnen Bag, that no large Pieces of the Pulp may mix with the Decoction. These Clysters are often ordered in apoplectic Cases. Some say, that Coloquintida will purge Children, by being reduced to a Paste with Oxes Gall, and applied to the Navel.

Colocynthis fructu Rotundo major, C. B. Pin. *Colocynthis major Rotunda,* Park. Theat. The greater Coloquintida. This Plant is imported from the *Levant,* and is said to agree with the preceeding in Virtues.

Colutea vesicaria, C. B. Pin. *Colutea,* Offic. *Pseudo-Senna, sive Senna Europæa,* Boerh. Ind. Alt. Bastard Sena. It grows wild in several Parts of *Italy,* but with us only in Gardens, and flowers in *July.* The Leaves of this Plant, but more especially the Seeds, purge most violently, both upwards and downwards, and consequently ought only to be exhibited to Persons of very strong and robust Constitutions, nor even then without good Correctives.

Contrayerva, Offic. *Contrayerva Hispanorum sive Drakena Radix.* Park. Theat. Counterpoison. The Contrayerva Root, was called *Drakena* by *Clusius,* because it was first imported into *England* in 1581, by Sir *Francis Drake,* on his having finish'd his Voyage round the World. From its Smell and Taste, it seems to be composed of a moderate Portion of a volatile, oleous, and aromatic Principle, wrapt up in earthy Parts. Hence we may account for its aromatic Qualities, that is, those by which it stimulates, incides, attenuates, corroborates, resists Poison, and increases the Motion of the Humours. Hence it becomes proper, in Cases, where Perspiration is to be augmented, or the Body heated, and in Fevers, in which Coldness is to be surmounted, and the Causes of the Disorder eliminated thro' the cutaneous Pores. *Clusius* informs us, that the Inhabitants of *Peru,* esteem it highly as an Alexipharmic; that it strengthens the Heart and vital Faculties, if the

Powowder of it is taken in a little Wine the Morning; and that in Water contributes to allay feverish Heats. *Monardus* says, that the Powder of *Contrayerva* exhibited in white Wine, a speedy and efficacious Remedy against Poisons of all Kinds, Sublimate only excepted, (which can only be cured by copious Draughts of Milk) since it either throws it up, or evacuates it by a Diaphoresis. The Powder of *Contrayerva*, is said to dislodge Worms from the Intestines. Tho' it is esteem'd a very good Counterpoison, yet, because it seems to act by stimulating, resolving, and putting the Humours into Commotion, we cannot hence reasonably conclude, that it is an universal Antidote. This to *Wedelius* seems too hyperbolical an Assertion, since different Poisons require Remedies of different Virtues. It is certainly very efficacious against most malignant Disorders, and in Cases where the Intention is to excite a Diaphoresis. *Paulus Neucrantzius* affirms, that he has found it highly efficacious in purple Fevers, in which it carries off the peccant Matter by a Diaphoresis, but rarely operates by Vomit. Some, in intermittent Fevers, exhibit the Powder of *Contrayerva*, with double the Quantity of *Peruvian* Bark, and against Dysenteries, in Conjunction with *Ipecacuanha*. *Contrayerva* is an Ingredient in the *Syrupus Contrayervæ*, and the *Pulvis Contrayervæ compositus*. The *Contrayerva Nova*, commonly called *Mexicana*, was imported into *Europe* after the preceding Species, and is thought to be a Native of *Mexico*; it is of a sweet aromatic Taste, and differing but very little from the ancient *Contrayerva*, to which it is not thought inferior. On Account of its alexipharmic, diaphoretic, and antifebrile Qualities, it is prescribed in Conjunction with Absorbents, for the

Cure of malignant and petechical Fevers, Measles, and the Small Pox.

Conyza Mas Theophrasti, major Dioscoridis, C. B. *Conyza major*, Offic. *Conyza pulicaria*, Chab. Greater Flea Bane. It grows in *Italy*, and other Places, near the Highways, where it flowers in *July* and *August*. The Fume of the Leaves when burned, is said to drive away Gnats, Fleas, and other troublesome Insects.

Conyza Media, Offic. *Conyza media Asteris flore luteo, vel tertia Dioscoridis*, C. B. *Conyza media Matthioli, flore magno luteo, humidis locis proveniens*, J. B. Common Flea Bane. It grows in moist and watry Places, and flowers in *July* and *August*. Some prepare an Ointment of the Leaves and Root of this Plant, which is recommended for the Itch. The Leaves taken with red Wine, are said to be good against a Dysentery and Jaundice, to be effectual in promoting the Menses, and curing a Strangury. The Decoction of the Herb, has the Reputation of being diuretic.

Conyza minor Vera, Offic. *Conyza fœmina Theophrasti, minor Dioscoridis*, C. B. *Virga aurea minor foliis glutinosis & graveolentibus*, Tourn. Inst. Small true Flea Bane. It agrees in Virtues with the first Species.

Corallina, Offic. *Muscus Maritimus, sive Corallina Officinarum*, C. B. Sea Coralline. White Wormseed. It grows upon Rocks of the Sea, and often on Oysters and other Shell Fish; and is only used to destroy and expel Worms from the Bowels, when reduced to Powder.

Corallium Album, Offic. *Corallium album majus*, Park. White Coral. It is found upon the Rocks, in the *Tuscan* and *Sicilian* Seas. It is good in all Fluxes, Cardialgias, and Disorders proceeding from an Acid.

Corallium

Corallium rubrum, Offic. *Coralli-um Rubrum majus,* Park. Red Coral. It grows in the Sea, and is found with the White, than which it is more ufed. It is drying, refrigerating, and aftringent, fweetens the Blood, 'frees the Stomach, from acid Juices, greatly ftrengthens the Liver, and ftops all Fluxes. This is an Ingredient in the *Pulvis e Chelis Cancrorum compofitus.*

Corallium nigrum, Raii Hift. *Corallium Nigrum five Antipathes,* J. B. *Keratophyton arboreum Nigrum,* Boerh. Ind. A. Black Coral. It is found fometimes in the *Italian,* but more frequently in the *American* Sea. It agrees with the other Corals in Virtues.

Another Species is, the *Aftroites, Stellaris, & Stellæ Lapis,* Mont. Exot. *Lapidis Aftroitidis five Stellaris primus genus,* Boet. *Stellarius Lapis,* Laet. de Gem. Star Stone. It is found in the Sea near *Jamaica,* and has the fame Virtues as the preceeding Corals.

Coriandrum, Offic. *Coriandrum majus,* Boerh. Ind. A. Coriander.. It is fown in Fields, and flowers in *June.* The whole Plant, whilft green, has a naufeous ungrateful Smell; but the Seed when dry, is of a pleafant agreeable Scent, and is ripe in *July* and *Auguft;* the Seed is the only Part in Ufe, and is efteemed ftomachic, fuppreffes thofe Vapours which offend the Head, and produce Eructations, and is a goodCorrector of draftic Medicines. Yet *Diofcorides* writes, that being drank, it caufes Hoarfenefs, with a Difturbance of the Brain and Reafon, like that excited by exceffive drinking of Wine *Simeon Sethi* fays, that the Juice drank, is a mortal Poifon, and makes the whole Body fmell of *Coriander.* Several of the *Arabians* have afcribed to this Plant a cold narcotic Quality, producing a Stupor, Difturbance of the Senfes and fatal Dif-

orders. To this *Matthiolus* adds, that the Seed ought never to be ufed in Food or Medicine, without a previous Maceration for three Days in Vinegar. Yet *Lobel* and *Alpinus* affure us, that the *Egyptians* very commonly ufe the green Herb in Food. *Bauhine,* is of Opinion, that we ought to be very cautious in the Ufe of this Plant, efpecially if unprepared. It is an Ingredient in the *Aqua Calcis magis compofita,* and the *Electuarium Lenitivum.*

Coris, Offic. *Hypericordes Coris quorundam & Coris legitima cretica,* J. B. Baftard St. John's Wort. It flowers in *June,* and the Seed is the only Part in Ufe, which provokes Urine and the Menfes, is good againft the Bite of the *Phalangium* (a poifonous Spider) and for that Species of Convulfion, called *Opifthotonos;* for which the Oil muft be impregnated with the Plant, and applied externally.

Cornus, Offic. *Cornus Mas,* Ger. *Cornus fativa five domeftica,* J. B. The Cornelian Cherry. It grows in Gardens, and flowers in *March* and *April.* The Fruit is the Part ufed, which is cooling, drying, and aftringent, ftrengthens the Stomach, ftops Fluxes and Loofenefs, and is good in Fevers, efpecially when attended with a *Diarrhæa.*

Corona folis Tabernæmontani, Elem. Bot. *Flos Solis,* Offic. Sun Flower. It is thought, to be of the Number of the vulnerary Plants, in Confequence of the terebinthinaceous balfamic Liquor, with which it abounds. *Etmuller* fays, that the feed Veffels, when the Seeds are almoft ripe, if cut and boiled, afford a copious Gum, which reduced into the Form of a Plaifter, is a moft fingular Vulnerary. Some fay they are Incentives to Venery.

Coronopus hortenfis, C. B. Pin. *Coronopus,* Offic. *Coronopus five Cornu Cervinum vulgo Spica Plantaginea,*

June,

, B Buckſhorn Plantain. It grows in ſandy Places, and flowers in June. It agrees in Virtues with the other Plantains, and is ſaid to be very efficacious in the Cure of a *Hydrophobia*.

Cortex Maſſoy, Mont. Exot. This is a warm aromatic Bark, found in *New England,* but not in our Shops. It is alexipharmic, opening, carminative, cephalic, cordial and ſtomachic. It is ſaid to warm very much, to eaſe pungent Pains and Gripes, and to be poſſeſs'd of a very grateful Fragrance.

Cortex Winteranus, Offic. *Cortex Vinteranus, Cortex Megallanicus,* Mont. Exot. *Cortex Winteranus aris, ſive Canella alba,* J. B. Winter's Cinnamon. It grows in the *Streights* of *Magellan,* very plenifully. The Bark is reſolvent, diſcutient, and ſubaſtringent; for which Reaſon, it is ſucceſsfully preſcribed in Diſorders of the Stomach, Crudities, Nauſeas, Diarrhæas, exceſſive Vomitings, and Colics; as, alſo, in the Declenſion and End of intermittent Fevers, with a View to corroborate the Stomach. It is, alſo, ſaid to be highly beneficial to ſcorbutic Patients, and ſuch as labour under Obſtructions of the Viſcera, Cachexies, and Irregularities of the Menſes; but it neither cures quartan nor petechical Fevers, nor affords any conſiderable Relief to paralytic Patients. The wild Cinnamon, is not the true *Cortex Winteranus,* for which, it is commonly ſold in the Shops. But tho' they are the Barks of different Trees, growing in very diſtant Places, and by their outward Appearance, ſeem quite different from each other, yet their Taſte is much the ſame, and they may be uſed as a Succedaneum to each other, tho' the true is much to be valued beyond the falſe (which is now generally ſold in the Shops) being far

more aromatic. It is an Ingredient in the *Tinctura Sacra,* and *Hiera Picra,* of the *London* Pharmacopœia.

Cortuſa, J. B. *Cortuſa ſanicula montana,* Offic. *Sanicula alpena ſive Cortuſa Mattbioli,* Park. Theat. Bears Ear Sanicle. It grows in mountainous Places, and flowers in the Spring. The Leaves promote Expectoration.

Coſtus, Offic. *Coſtus Arabicus Dioſcoridis,* C. B. Pin. *Iridem redolens ejuſdem amarus,* Officinarum, ſeu *Helenium, & Comagenium Dioſcoridis ejuſdem, dulcis Officinarum, Centaurio magna Cognatus ejuſdem,* Raii Hiſt. Sweet and bitter Coſtus. It is reckoned hot, dry, and comforting to the Head and Stomach. It helps vertiginous Diſorders, is a good Deobſtruent, opens Obſtructions of the Uterus, and procures the Catamenia. It is alſo eſteemed a good Hepatic, and of Service in Obſtructions of the urinary Ducts and againſt the Colic, Dropſy, and Palſy. It is an Ingredient in the *Confectio Paulina, Mithridatium, & Theriaca Andromachi.* According to ſome there are three Species of Coſtus in the Shops, *viz.* The *Arabian,* the *Bitter,* and the *Sweet;* hence *Caſpar Baubine* and other Botanic Authors, have divided it into four Species. But *Bontius* rightly informs us, that it is one and the ſame Root differing only either by *Place, Age,* or *Corruption. Garcias ab Horto,* together with *Acoſta* and *Cluſius,* believe there is but one Species, who ſay that when it is freſh, it is Sweet and of a whitiſh Colour, but that when it begins to corrupt by Age, it contracts a Bitterneſs, and grows black.

Cotinus Coriaria, Boerh. Ind. A. *Cotinus,* Offic. *Coccigria, ſive Cotinus putata,* J. B. *Venice* or red Sumach. It is found in *Italy,* flowers in *May,* and the Fruit is ripe in *Auguſt.* The Fruit is thought to be extremely treemly drying and aftringent; Gargarifms are prepared of a Decoction of the Leaves, which are good for Ulcers of the Mouth and Tongue, and are ufed againft Relaxations of the Uvula and Glands in the Fauces. The Fruit is particularly ferviceable, in Ulcers of the Fauces and Pudenda, and reftrains Diarrhœas, and a too copious Difcharge of the Menfes. According to *Matthiolus* the Leaves dried and powdered, and then fprinkled on the Belly, after anointing it with Vinegar of Rofes, ftop any Flux of the Belly.

Cotyledon major, C. B. Boerh. Ind. A. *Umbilicus Veneris,* Offic. Navelwort. It grows upon old Stone-Walls and Buildings in *England,* and flowers in *May.* The Leaves are the only Part ufed, which are gently cooling, moiftening, refrigerating, and aftringent. They are ufeful in hot Diftempers of the Liver, provoke Urine, and take off the Heat and Sharpnefs thereof; the Juice outwardly applied helps the Shingles, and St. *Anthony's* Fire, the Pain and Inflammations of the Piles, and is likewife ufeful in Kibes and Chilblains.

Cotyledon, Offic. *Cotyledon radice tuberofa longa repente,* Elem. Bot. *Sedum luteum umbilicatum, fpicatum radice repente,* Hift. Oxon. Creeping Navelwort. The Leaves are ufed with the fame Intentions as the former.

Couhage, Offic. *Phafeolus filiqua hirfuta,* Park. Theat. *Pafcolus Zurratenfis filiqua hirfuta pungente,* Hift. Oxon. Couhage or ftinking Beans. They grow in the *Eaft-Indies,* from whence they are brought to us. The Bean is the Part ufed by the Inhabitants of *Barbadoes* for a Dropfy.

Cratægus, folio laciniato, Boerh. Ind. A. *Sorbus torminalis,* Offic. *Sorbus torminalis feu Vulgaris,* Park. Theat. The Wild Service or Sorb Tree. The Fruit of this Tree is fubftituted for the *Sorbus Sativa,* or true *Sorbus,* being of the fame Nature or rather more aftringent and binding. It is good for all Kinds of Fluxes, either of Blood or Humours when ripe it is pleafant and grateful to the Stomach, promotes Digeftion, prevents the too hafty Paffage of the Food to the Bowels, and is commended in Fevers attended with a Diarrhæa.

Crithmum, five fœniculum maritimum majus, Boerh. Ind. A. *Crithmum fœniculum marinum herba Sancti Petri,* Offic. Samphire. The whole Plant has a warm aromatic Smell and Tafte, growing upon the Rocks by the Sea fide in many Places in *England.* It ftrengthens the Stomach, procures an Appetite, provokes Urine, opens Obftructions, is good for the Jaundice, and is extoll'd as a Diffolver of the Stone and Promoter of the Menfes.

Crocus Sativus, C. B. Pin. Boerh. Ind. Alt. *Crocus,* Offic. Ger. Saffron. This is a Simple fo well known that no Defcription of it feems neceffary. *Hoffman in Differt. de Remed. Domeft. Util.* informs us, that Saffron in Confequence of its mild, anodyne, and vaporous Sulphur, is excellently calculated for alleviating Pains and Spafms, and that by Means of its acrid and volatile Salt, it contributes to open and remove Obftructions. *Newman* deduces the narcotic Virtue of Saffron, from its highly attenuated, rarified, and vaporous oleous Parts. Lord *Bacon* advifes Saffron to be mixed with Medicines, intended to prevent the Effects of old Age; for continues he, Saffron conveys Medicines to the Heart, cures its Palpitation, prevents Melancholy and Uneafinefs, revives the Brain, renders the Mind cheerful, and generates Boldnefs. *Boerhaave,* in his Chymiftry, calls Saffron a true and genuine Roufer of the animal Spirits, becaufe it is poffeffed of aromatic, ftimulating, and heat-

heating Qualities, and is therefore difcutient, refolvent, aperient, and corroborating. *Diemerbroeck* in his *Treatife de Pefte* informs us, that Saffron is not to be exhibited in Plagues, becaufe it affects the Head, and when exhibited in large Quantities, induces a Droufinefs or Delirium, both which Symptoms, are highly to be dreaded in peftilential Diforders. It is by fome, fuccefsfully exhibited in order to purge the Lungs from vifcid Phlegm. *Camerarius*, in his *Hortus Medicus*, affirms, that it is fo beneficial in Diforders of the Thorax, that fome exhibit a Scruple and an Half of it, with Half a Grain of Mufk, to be drank in warm Wine for curing Afthmas. He alfo affirms, that it greatly contributes to remove the Effects of a Perfpiration obftructed by Cold. *Paulus de Sorbait* informs us, that if we want to protract the Life of a phthifical Patient, for fome time, we muft exhibit to him, Half a Scruple of Saffron. In the Cure of a Dyfentery, Saffron acquired a great Reputation after *Bontius* affirmed, that no more efficacious Remedy could be found, and that the Extract of Saffron was the moft genuine Antidote in this Diforder, tho' of the moft obftinate and virulent Kind. *Bauhine*, from *Matthiolus*, informs us, that Children who continually cry, are weak, and difcharge fabulous Concretions in their Urine, are greatly reliev'd by a little Saffron, exhibited with Milk. The Cafes related by practical Authors, of Children tinged in their Mothers Bellies, fufficiently prove that Saffron has a peculiar Influence on the Uterus, and that its emmenagogue and ecbolic Virtues are to be deriv'd from this Circumftance Lord *Bacon* informs us, that a certain Gentleman, who ufed to be exceffively fick at Sea, had his Naufeas prevented by wearing a Bag of Saffron on the Region of his Stomach. Externally, it is commended as an excellent Ingredient in Medicines calculated for Diforders of the Eyes. According to *Bauhine*, Saffron mixed with Milk, Oil of Rofes and a little Smallage, alleviates the intenfe Pains of a Gout, arifing from a hot Caufe. In arthritic Pains and Eryfipelas, a linen Cloth impregnated with Saffron, is faid to be a divine Remedy. *Etmuller* informs us, that Spirit of Wine impregnated with Saffron, and applied with a linen Cloth to the Toes and Fingers, when fo injur'd by the Cold, that a Gangrene is apprehended, is an excellent Remedy. *Weaelius* in his *Opologia*, informs us, that Nurfes, in Order to remove obftinate Watchings in Children, put a Bag of Saffron under their Heads. But *Fricius* fays, that this Bag fhould be taken away as foon as the Child is afleep. Saffron is often ufed in Conjunction with Opium; but *Geoffroy* juftly doubts, whether it either corrects, or augments the Effects of the Opium. *Borelli*, in his *Obfervationes Medico-Chymicæ*, informs us, that a certain Woman, by wearing Saffron on the Pit of her Stomach, was cur'd of Melancholy, and a perpetual Inclination to weep. *Schulzius* in his *Prælectiones*, informs us, that the exhilarating Virtues of Saffron, are fufficiently confpicuous in young Children, who are fet a laughing, by applying to their Noftrils, an empty Phial, in which Effence of Saffron has been. But the celebrated *Juncker*, is of Opinion, that its internal Ufe, efpecially in a large Quantity, is far from being faic, tho' he thinks that its external Ufe is eftablifhed upon furer Foundations; for, fays he, it is highly proper for an Eryfipelas, and inflammatory Tumors, efpecially for difpelling the ferous Matter lodg'd in them, and alleviating the Pains with which
they

they are accompanied. *Hoffman,,* in *Diſſert. de Remed. Domeſt. Præ-ſtant.* ſpeaks thus of it: " In obſti-" nate Coughs and Difficulties of " Breathing, an Infuſion of Saffron " in the Water of Paul's Betony, " with the Addition of a ſufficient " Quantity of Sugar Candy, is " found to be of ſingular Efficacy. " An Infuſion of it with Cinnamon " Water, is highly beneficial for " provoking the Menſes, facilita-" ting difficult Labours, expelling " the Secundines, and promoting " the Lochia; eſpecially, when at " the ſame Time, Oil of ſweet Al-" monds is now-and-then exhibited. " Externally, Saffron, boil'd with " Milk, the Flowers of Elder and " Chamomile, and the Crumbs of " Bread, and applied by Way of " Cataplaſm, wonderfully alleviates " arthritic Pains." I have alſo " known the ſame Remedy applied " with Succeſs, for removing the Pain " of the blind Hæmorrhoids. Saffron " put into Roſewater, with the Addi-" tion of a little Camphire, cures " Inflammations of the Eyes, in the " Meaſles and Small-Pox. But, tho' " numerous Virtues are aſcrib'd to " Saffron;" yet *Galen* in *Tr. de Simpl. Med. Facult.* claſſes Saffron among theſe Subſtances, which when libe-rally uſed, either deſtroy the Pati-ent's Reaſon, or procure his Death. Beſides, *Geoffroy, Borelli, Friccius, Amatus Luſitanus, Caſpar Hoffman, Simon Pauli,* and other practical Au-thors, furniſh us with Inſtances, in which Saffron has produced Death, Deliriums, ſo immoderate Diſ-charges of the Menſes, as to prove mortal, and other very terri-ble Symptoms; ſo that as the mo-derate Uſe of Saffron is highly be-neficial in ſeveral Diſeaſes, it is e-qually obvious, that when exhibited unſeaſonably, in too large Doſes, or for too long a Time, it proves high-ly prejudicial to Health. For this

Reaſon, *Boerhaave* plac'd it among the narcotic Poiſons, and its Anti-dotes are aqueous, oleous, acidu-lated Vomits, and ſuch as have Honey for an Ingredient. It is alſo obvious, that Saffron is better a-dapted to thoſe of cold and leuco-phlegmatic, than thoſe of hot and bilious Conſtitutions. With Re-ſpect to the Doſe of Saffron, Au-thors are by no Means agreed; ſince as *Geoffroy* obſerves, ſome af-firm, that Half a Scruple, and o-thers a Scruple and an Half, may be ſafely exhibited internally. Ac-cording to *Etmuller,* the Inhabi-tants of *Poland,* are ſo accuſtom'd to the Uſe of Saffron, that they often mix an Ounce of it with their Aliments. But this is purely owing to the Force of Cuſtom, the Power of which is ſufficiently obvious, from thoſe who gradually habitua-ting themſelves to Opium, can at laſt bear a Quantity, which would have at firſt prov'd infallibly mor-tal. But upon the Whole, it ſeems that Saffron may be ſafely pre-ſcribed in Subſtance, from Half a Scruple to a whole Scruple, or e-ven Half a Dram; tho' the largeſt Doſe, for ſuch as are not accuſtom'd to it, ought not to exceed Half a Scruple. It is an Ingredient in the *Vinum Aloeticum Alkalinum; Vinum Croceum; Tinctura Rhabarbari; Tinctura Rhabarbari ſpirituoſa; E-lixir Aloes; Syrupus Croceus; Pilu-læ Rufi; Pilulæ e Styrace; Confectio Cardiaca; Mithridatium;* and the *Theriaca Andromachi.*

Cruciata, Offic. *Cruciata vulga-ris,* Park. Theat. *Gallium, Cruci-ata quibuſdam flore luteo,* J. B. Croſswort. It grows in Hedges and Borders of Fields, and flowers in *July.* The Leaves and Tops are uſed; this Plant is claſſed among the vulnerary Herbs, in Conſe-quence of its drying and aſtringent Qualities, but chiefly is extoll'd in

Swellings

wellings of the Scrotum, occasioned by the falling down of the Intestines. *Camerarius* highly recommends a Decoction of this Herb, or promoting the Expectoration of iscid Humours.

Cubeba, Offic. *Arbor baccifera Braliensis, fructu piper recipiente*, Raii list. *Arbor Bisnagarica Myrti amlioribus foliis, per Siccitatem nigris, abebæ sapore*, Pluk. Almag. Cuebs. They are brought to us from he Island of *Java*, and are recommended in a Hoarseness and Loss of Voice, especially when the Tonsils are stuffed and obstructed. They re both heating and drying, coroborate the Stomach, expel Wind, nd, are particularly useful in all Disorders of the Head.

Cucumis sativus vulgaris, C. B. 'n. *Cucumis hortensis*, Offic. *Cumis sativus*, Park. Theat. Cuumber. This is common in Garlens, and flowers in *June*; the 'ruit and Seed, which is one of the our greater cold Seeds are used; The seeds are esteem'd refrigerating, bstergent, and opening; they provoke Urine, and are frequently used n antipleuritic and antinephritic Emulsions.

Cucurbita, Offic. *Cucurbita lanaria major*, Park. Theat. The Gourd. It grows in Gardens, tho' eldom, and flowers in *July*. The Seed, which is the only Part used, is one of the four greater cold Seeds, and allays Thirst, provokes Urine, and extinguishes Inclinations to Venery.

Cuminum sylvestre, Offic. *Cuminum sylvestre primum valde odoratum, globosum*, J. B. *Umbelliferis affinis, capitulis globosis & villosis*, Hist. Oxon. Wild Cumin. This Plant grows principally in *Crete*. The Part used in Medicine, is the Seed, which is recommended against Flatulencies, for curing the Hiccup, removing Sugillations, and repelling Inflammations of the Testes.

Cuminum, Offic. *Cyminum siv Cuminum sativum*, J. B. *Fœniculum Orientale Cuminum dictum*, Tourn. Inst. Cumin. This Plant grows in great Quantities, in the Islands of *Malta* and *Sicily*, from whence it is brought to us. The Seed is the only Part in Use, and is one of the four greater hot Seeds; it is of a very warming Quality, and powerfully expels Wind from the Stomach and Bowels; for which Purpose, it is often exhibited in Clysters, as, also, sometimes in Powder mixed with Wine. Externally applied, it is very efficacious in removing Pains of the Breast, Sides, or Bowels. This is an Ingredient in the *Oleum Cymini*; *Mel Solutivum*; *Emplastrum e Cymino*; and *Cataplasma e Cymino*, of the last *London* Pharmacopœia.

Cuminum Siliquosum, Offic. *Hypecoi altera Species*, C. B. Pin. *Hypecoum siliquis propendentibus, non articulatis, bivalvibus incurvis*, Hist. Oxon. Codden wild Cumin. This Plant grows in *Spain*, flowers in *May*, and is said to have the same Effect as the Poppy.

Curcuma, Offic. *Crocus Indicus, Arabibus Curcum, Officinis nostris, radix Curcuma dicta*, Bon. *Cannacorus radice crocea sive Curcuma Officinarum*, Boerh. Ind. A. Turmeric. It grows in the *East Indies*, from whence it is brought to us. Of this Plant there are two Species, the *Long* and *Round*; but the first is best; its Virtues are said to be abstergent, attenuating, opening and discutient; it provokes the Menses, facilitates Delivery, opens all Obstructions of the Intestines, provokes Urine, expels the Stone, and is a Specific in all icteric, dropsical, and cachetic Disorders.

Cuscuta, Offic. Park. Theat. *Cuscuta major*, C. B. Pin. Raii Synop. Tourn. Inst. *Cuscuta sive Cassuta*, J. B. Dodder. This Herb grows in Thickets, and is said to be

Y   excellent

excellent against Disorders of the Liver and Spleen. It is also abstergent, subastringent, and aperient. It corrects melancholic Humours, and is beneficial in the Itch and black Jaundice.

Cuscuta minor, is thus distinguished. *Epithymum*, Offic. Park. Theat. *Epithymum sive Cuscuta minor*, C. B. Pin. Raii Hist. *Cuscuta minor*, Tourn. Inst. Dodder of Thyme. The whole Plant is used. It gently purges melancholic and serous Humours. It is principally used in the Itch, Ulcers, melancholic Disorders, and Obstructions of the Hypocondria and Spleen. *Tournefort* informs us, that the Species brought from the *Levant* under the Name of *Venetian* Dodder, does not purge, but is rather aperient and stomachic.

Cyanus major, Offic. Ger. Raii Hist. *Cyanus major vulgaris*, Park. *Cyanus hortensis*, Boerh. Ind. Alt. Great Blew-bottle. This is cultivated in Gardens, and flowers in *June* and *July*. The Leaves and Flowers are used, and are said to be of an alexipharmic and uterine Nature. They are cold, temperate, and consequently of a repelling Quality. They are also said to be beneficial in an Erysipelas, the Jaundice, Palpitations of the Heart, and Suffocations of the Uterus.

Cyanus minor, Offic. *Cyanus Segetum*, C. B. Boerh. Ind. Alt. Small Blew-bottle. This grows among the Corn, and flowers in *June*. The Leaves and Flowers are used. The distilled Water of the Flowers is said to be beneficial in Dropsies, and in Inflammations, Redness and Lippitude of the Eyes. In *Saxony* it is customary to give a Glass of Beer, in which an Handful of it has been boild, to those who labour under the Jaundice, or a Retention of Urine. *Camerarius* used to bathe the Gums of Infants, with the distilled Water of the *Cyanus*, mixed with the Juice of

Cray-fish, in order to make the Teeth cut easily: The Powder of this Plant, according to the same Author, resolves a St. *Antony*'s Fire in the Face. A Decoction of the Flowers is diuretic and emmenagogue.

Cyclamen is thus distinguished. *Arthanita Cyclamen*, Offic. *Cyclamen*, Schrod. *Cyclamen orbiculato folio inferne purpurascente*, C. B. Pin. Boerh. Ind. Alt. Sow-bread. This is cultivated in the Gardens of the Curious, and flowers in *September*. The only Part of it used is its Root, which is highly inciding, aperient and proper for Errhines. It is principally used in Obstructions of the Menses, and for expelling the Foetus, but internally it ought to be used with great Caution.

Cyclamen artanita, Offic. *Cyclamen hederae folio*, Raii Hist. Boerh. Ind. Alt. Common Sow-bread. This is frequent in Gardens, and flowers in *September*. Its Root is used and is possessed of the same Virtues with the former. This is the Species found in the Shops.

Cydonia thus distinguished. *Malus Cydonia, Cotonia*, Offic. *Malus Cydonia*, Boerh. Ind. Alt. The Quince Tree. This is cultivated in Gardens and green Houses, and flowers in *April*. The Fruit and Seeds are used, the former being stomachic, refrigerating, drying, and astringent. They are principally used in Vomiting, Fluxes, Hiccups, and Relaxations of the Stomach. The Seeds are cooling, and moistening, and by their Mucilage correct and obtund Acrimony.

Cynoglossa, Offic. *Cynoglossum*, Raii Synop. *Cynoglossum majus vulgare*, C. B. Pin. Tourn. Inst. Houndstongue. This grows on the Road sides and flowers in *June*. The Root and Leaves are used, and are of a refrigerating and drying Nature. They are recommended for

stopping

...pping Fluxes, Gonorrhæas, Catarrhs, and Hemorrhages. They are scrophulous and strumous Disorders, and are serviceable to Wounds and Ulcers of all Kinds. Some, also, ascribe a narcotic Quality to this Plant. But Dr. *Fuller* says, he could never discover any such Virtue in it. This Plant, when subjected to a chymical Analysis, gives strong Indications of an acrid Salt and Sulphur. Thus the Root of it is proper to stop all Sorts of Defluctions, and to correct acrid Humours. The Leaves of the Plant are vulnerary and detersive.

Cyperus longus, Offic. Ger. *Cyperus odoratus radice longa sive Cyperus officinarum,* C. B. Pin. Boerh. Ind. Alt. Long-rooted Cyperus. It grows in marshy Places, but is very rarely to be met with. The Root is used, and is said to be stomachic and uterine. It is principally recommended for exciting a Discharge of Urine, and the Menses, for consuming the Crudities in the Stomach, curing a windy Dropsy, removing the Colic and Vertigo, and for rendering the Breath Sweet.

Cyperus rotundus, Offic. *Cyperus rotundus orientalis major,* C. B. Pin. Round rooted Cyperus. This is brought to us from *Egypt,* and its Root is used for the same Purposes with the former.

Cyperus esculentus, Raii Hist. *Cyperus rotundus, esculentus angustifolius,* C. B. Pin. Boerh. Ind. Alt. *Cyperus niloticus vel Syriacus maximus papyraceus,* Hist. Oxon. Sweet Cyperus or Rush-nut. This grows in *Egypt,* and *Syria.* The Stalks are commended as useful for relaxing Fistulas, and the Water distilled from such as are recent, is good against Catarrhs, Dimness of Sight, and other Disorders of the Eyes.

Cupressus mas & fæmina Plinii, Tourn. Inst. Boerh. Ind. Alt. The Cypress Tree. This is cultivated in Gardens. The Wood, Tops, and Nuts are used. The Wood is refrigerating, drying, and astringent. The Tops and Nuts are moderately heating, drying, and highly astringent; for which Reason they are principally recommended in Spittings of Blood, Diarrhæas, Dysenteries, and involuntary Discharges of Urine. They are, also, used, both internally and externally in curing Hernias.

Cytiso-genista Scoparia vulgaris, flore luteo, Boerh. Ind. Alt. *Genista,* Offic. Ger. *Genista vulgaris et Scoparia,* Park. Theat. Common Broom. This grows in Fields and Commons, and flowers in *April* and *May.* The Flowers and Stalks are used, and are said to be aperient, hepatic, and proper for removing Obstructions of the Spleen. They provoke Urine, and infused in common Drink are good for the Dropsy; the Flowers pickled with Salt and Vinegar, are esteem'd wholesome for the Stomach and good against Diseases of the Spleen and Liver. This Plant is accounted excellent in a Dropsy.

Cytisus, Offic. *Cytisus incanus, siliquis falcatis,* C. B. Pin. *Medicago trifolia frutescens incana,* Boerh. Ind. Alt. Shrub Trefoil. It grows in Gardens, and flowers in Summer; the Leaves are only used, and are said to refrigerate, and discuss Tumors, and a Decoction of them is recommended for provoking Urine. Though ancient Authors, mention but one Species of the *Cytisus,* and that but very imperfectly, yet more modern Botanists have found several Plants to which they give that Name, tho' this Plant may more justly than any other assume the Name of the *Cytisus* of *Dioscorides. Volckamerus* says, that it is at this Time in daily Use among the *Turks,* so that if it is not a Native of that Country, it is certainly well known to the Inhabitants.

Pfeudo-Cytifus, Offic. *Cytifus Hifpanicus arboreus,* Park. Theat. *Cytifus foliis fubrufa lanugine hirfutis.* C. B. Pin. It grows in *Italy* and *Sicily,* the Leaves are only ufed, and anfwer the Intentions of the other Species.

Afpalathus altera, Offic. *Afpalathus fecunda trifolia quæ Acaria fecunda, Matthiolo trifolio,* J. B. *Cytifo-Spartium aculeatum, Acacia trifolia dictum,* Pluk. Almag. Trefoil Acacia. It grows in *Sicily* and *Italy,* and the Juice is only ufed, which is aftringent. *Diofcorides* fays, it is a good Medicine for the Eyes.

Daucus, Carrot. Of this there are various Species, three of which are only ufed in Medicine. The firft of thefe is *Daucus vulgaris,* or *Wild Carrot,* which is thus diftinguifhed by Botanifts. *Daucus vulgaris,* Boerhaav. Ind. Alt. *Paftinaca Sylveftris tenuifolia Diofcoridis, vel Daucus officinarum,* C. B. Pin. The Seed infufed in Ale is efteemed no defpicable Diuretic, and excellent to prevent the Stone, and alleviate its more violent Fits. It alfo expells Gravel and provokes Urine, and the Menfes; nor is it lefs beneficial in all uterine and hyfteric Diforders. *Helmont* fays, that he was acquainted with a Lawyer, who every fifteen Days was troubled with a Fit of the Stone, and was for feveral Years freed from the Racks of that violent Diforder, only by an Infufion of two Drams of this Seed in fome clear Malt Liquor; an Infufion of two Drams of this Seed in white Wine drank, cures hyfteric Paroxyfms. *Tragus* as well as feveral others, highly recommended the fmall Purple Flowers which grow in the Middle of the Umbels, as an infallible Antidote againft an Epilepfy.

The fecond Species ufed is the *Daucus fativus, radice atrorubente Paftinaca, tenuifolia, fativa, radice atrorubente,* C. B. P. *Paftinaca fativa, five Carota rubra,* J. B. Dark

red rooted Garden Carrot. The Virtues of the Seeds and Herbs differ nothing at all from thofe of the *Daucus officinarum.* By *Schroder* they are efteemed a Specific in hyfteric Fits. The Roots are frequently ufed in Food, tho' they are flatulent. They are thought to render the Body foluble and contribute to the Cure of a Cough. *Quercetan* affirms, that Half a Dram of the Seeds, of white Carrot, dried, reduc'd to a Powder, and exhibited with Baum Water is a Specific againft hyfteric Fits.

The third Species is the *Daucus Maritimus Lucidus,* T. *Gingidium folio Chærophilli,* C. B. P. Boerh Ind. Alt. In the Hiftory of Plants afcrib'd to *Boerhaave,* we are inform'd, that the Root is much celebrated, for its Efficacy againft the Stone and nephritic Diforders, and for provoking the Menfes; that the Seeds gather'd in a proper Seafon, are poffeffed of a certain Acrimony, and when infufed in Beer, are highly beneficial in the forementioned Diforders. Empirics rafp the Root, and boil the Rafpings in Milk which they fweeten with Honey, and exhibit in all Diforders of the Breaft and in Quinfeys. They alfo order externally, to hinder Ulcers from contracting a Cruft. They give it in Child-bed Pains, Colics and Stranguries.

Delphinium hortenfe flore majore fimplici, Tourn. Juft. Boerh. Ind. A. Larks-Spur. This is cultivated in Gardens and flowers in July. The Root, which is the only Part ufed is vulnerary, being of a confolidating and conglutinating Nature It is alfo faid to quicken and corroborate the Sight.

Dens Caninus, Offic. *Dens Caniore rotundioreque folio,* C. B. Raii Hift. Dogs-tooth Violet. This is found at the Foots of fome Mountains, and flowers in *April.* The Root, which is the only Part ufed mitigates

itigates colical Pains, is beneficial epileptic Children, expells Worms, a Stimulus to Venery, and nourishes the Body.

Dens Leonis Taraxacum, Offic. *Dens Leonis latiore folio*, Tourn. Inst. Boerh. Ind. Alt. Dandelion. This found every where in Gardens and Pasture Grounds. It flowers thro' the whole Summer. The Root and Leaves are used, and agree in Virtues with Endive, tho' they operate more powerfully. It is principally described in putrid and inveterate Fevers, as also in a Phthisis, Consumption Scurvy, and Cachexy.

Another Species of this is the *Dens Leonis tuberosa radice*, Tourn. Inst. *sorbcum bulbosum*, Raii Hist. Bulbous Succory. This grows on the Sea Coast. The Bulbs of the Roots are used, being accounted Anodyne and proper for removing the Kings-vil.

Dentaria, Offic. Ind. Med. *Dentaria beptaphyllos*, C. B. Pin. Raii Hist. Tooth-wort. This is frequently to be found in the Gardens of Botanists, flowers in *April*, and is thought to be of a drying and astringent Nature.

Dentillaria, Offic. Ind. Med. *Ledum Dentillaria dictum*, C. B. P. Toad-wort. This grows spontaneously in *France* and *Italy*, and flowers in *August*. The Herb itself is used, being of a caustic Quality and thought proper to remove the Tooth-ach if applied to the Wrists or only held in the Hand.

Dictamnus. Dittany, of this there are two Species, The first of which is the *Dictamnus Creticus*, Offic. C. B. P. Park. Theat. Boerh. Ind. A. Dittany of Crete, or Candy. The true Dittany grows chiefly in the Island of *Crete* or *Candy*, and flowers in *June*, the Leaves being only used. *Jeffrey* informs us, that the Leaves have always been looked upon as an excellent Vulnerary, a powerful Cor-

dial, as also an Emmenagogue and Diuretic. They have all the Virtues of the Garden *Pulegium* or Penny-royal, but in a much greater Degree, for not only when drank, but also when barely applied or used in Fumigations they expel the dead Foetus. The Herb applied draws out Splinters from the Soles of the Feet, or any other Parts of the Body, and is good against Pains of the Spleen by diminishing that Part. It accelerates the Birth, and the Juice drank in Wine relieves those who are bit by venomous Animals, which are driven away by the bare Smell of the Herb, but killed by the Touch. The Juice instilled into venomous Wounds or Bites, and drank at the same Time is a present Remedy. It is cordial, alexipharmic, uterine, cephalic, and kills Worms in the Body. It is an Ingredient in the *Pulvis e Myrrha Compositus*, *Species e Scordio sine Opio*, *Mithridatium* & *Theriaca Andromachi*.

Digitalis, Offic. *Digitalis purpurea*, *folio aspero*, C. B. Pin. *Digitalis vulgaris purpurea*, Park. Theat. Fox Glove. It grows in Woods and Hedges and flowers in *June*. This Plant is emetic and vulnerary and agrees in Virtues with the *Pilewort*. The Ointment of Fox Glove is very resolvent, and the Decoction of it purges very powerfully both upwards and downwards.

Dipsacus sylvestris, aut virga Pastoris major, C. B. *Dipsacus sylvestris, sive labrum Veneris*, Offic. *Dipsacus sylvestris*, Park. Wild Teasel, it grows upon Banks and in the Borders of Fields and flowers in *June* and *July*.

Dipsacus sativus, C. B. *Dipsacus sativus*, *Carduus Fullonum*, Offic. Manured Teasel. This Plant is cultivated in Fields and flowers in *July*. The Wild and Manured Teasel agree in their Virtues. They cure the Scrofula and resist Putrefaction, and when boiled in Wine they purge by Urine as effectually as Asparagus.

The

The Root bruised and mixed with Honey, has been found of extraordinary Virtue in Confumptions, which have been regarded as desperate.

Dipfacus fylveftris, capitulo minori, vel virga Paftoris, C. B. Boerh. Ind. A. *Virga Paftoris,* Offic. Shepherds Rod. It grows in moift and watery Places, by the Sides of Hedges, and flowers in *July.* The Leaves are only ufed in Medicine, the Water of which *Ægineta* commends for a depraved Appetite in Women ; and a Dram of the Powder is exhibited for Spitting of Blood.

Doria Narbonenfium, Boerh. Ind. A. *Virga aurea major, carnofis fucculentis foliis ad caulem latis;* Hift. Oxon. *Herba Doria,* Offic. Dorias Woundwort. It grows on the Banks of Rivers, and flowers in *July* and *Auguft.* It is an excellent Vulnerary, and in Virtues agrees with the Golden Rod.

Doria quæ Jacobæa Alpina, foliis longioribus ferratis. Boerh. Ind. Alt. *Solidago faraccnica vera, falicis folio,* Park. *Confolida faracenica, Solidago,* Offic. Saracens Confound. It flowers in *September,* and the Leaves are only ufed, which are an excellent Vulnerary, and may be properly exhibited both internally and externally. They heal Fiftulas, and cleanfe and confolidate malignant Ulcers.

Doronicum, Offic. *Doronicum vulgare,* Park. *Doronicum majus officinarum,* Ger. Leopards Bane. It grows in many Places upon the *Alps* and flowers in *May* and *June.* The Root is the only Part ufed, tho' but very feldom. It is likewife produced in the Gardens of the Curious, and is heating, drying, difcutient and alexipharmic.

Doronicum minus, Offic. *Doronicum plantaginis folio,* C. B. *Doronicum folio fere, Plantaginis oblongo,* J. B. Leffer Leopards Bane. The Part in Ufe is the Root which differs

nothing in Virtues from the former, and is indifcriminately taken for it.

Doronicum radice dulci; C. B. Pin. *Doronicum Brachiata radice, Doronicum radice repente,* Creeping Leopards Bane. The Huntfmen and Shepherds who live in the Mountains, call this Plant by the Name of *Wild Goats Root,* and account it, together, with the largeft Sort of *Doronicum,* as effectual a Remedy againft the *Vertigo,* as the *Auricula Urfi* with a yellow Flower, and affirm it to be of extraordinary Ufe for confirming their Strength.

Draba, Offic. *Draba multis flore albo,* J. B. *Draba Lepidium humile incanum arvenfe,* Tourn. Inft. Arabian Muftard, or Turkey Creffes. This is cultivated in Gardens, and flowers in *June.* The Herb and its Seeds are ufed. In *Cappadocia,* the Herb is boil'd in Pulfans ; and the Seeds when dried, are ufed inftead of Pepper, for feafoning Aliments.

Draco herba, Boerh. Ind. Alt. Raii Hift. *Dracunculus,* Offic. *Abrotanum Lini folio acriori & odorato,* Tourn. Inft. Tarragon. This is cultivated in Gardens, and flowers in *July* and *Auguft.* As this Plant is poffeffed of a great Degree of Acrimony, fo it powerfully heats, dries, attenuates, and digefts; for which Reafon, according to *Matthiolus,* it is good for a cold Stomach ; it alfo excites the Appetite, diffipates Flatulences, ftrengthens the Limbs, provokes Urine and the Menfes, and opens Obftructions.

Draco arbor, Park. Theat. C. B. Pin. *Palma foliis Longiffimis pendulis abfque pedunculo ex caudice glabro Enatis,* Boerh. Ind. Alt. The Dragon Tree. This grows in *Porto Santo,* which is one of the *Canaries,* and in *Madera.* Dragon's Blood, is the Gum of this Tree. This is a Refin of a redifh Colour, eafily melted by the Fire, and kindling into Flames, *when*

when thrown into it. There are two Sorts to be met with in the Shops, which only differ in being more or lefs pure. The Curious, generally take the Dragons Blood of the Moderns, for the Cinnabar of *Diofcorides.* This Gum is a powerful Drier, Aftringent and Repellent, but is principally ufed externally, for drying up Defluxions, ftopping Hemorrhages, conglutinating Wounds, and faftening loofe Teeth. The late *Helvetius,* melted it with powder'd Alum, and then made them into Pills, for ftopping Diarrhœas, Hæmorrhages, and the like; but the Patient ought to be prepar'd, by Bleeding, and other proper Management.

Dracontium, Offic. *Dracontium majus,* Ger. Raii. Hift. *Dracunculus polyphyllos,* C. B. Pin. Boerh. Ind. Alt. Dragons Blood. This is cultivated in Gardens. The Herb and its Root are ufed, and are faid to be alexipharmic and fudorific. They are principally recommended in the Plague, malignant Fevers, and the Bites of venomous Animals.

Dracunculus major, Offic. *Dracunculus Biftorti folia,* C. B. Pin. Great Dragons. This grows fpontaneoufly in *Virginia.* Its Root is heating, drying, and beneficial againft Orthopnœas, Ruptures, Convulfions, Coughs and Defluxions.

Dryopteris, Offic. *Dryopteris adverfariorum,* Ger. *Felix Querna,* C. B. *Felix minor non Ramofa,* Tourn. Inf. Oak-fern. This grows in marfhy and putrid Soils. This Plant triturated, is ufed for banifhing Fleas. But *Rondeletius* affirms, that it is prejudicial, when put into Medicines, inftead of the Polypodium. In fome of the Shops, it is found under the Title of the Adianthum Album.

Ebenus Æthiopica, Offic *Palma Americana fpinofa,* C. B. Pin. Raii Hift. The Macow or Ebony Tree. What

we have grows in *America,* and is from thence brought to us; the Part only in Ufe is the Heart or medullary Subftance of the Wood, which is black and extreamly hard, and was by the Antients accounted good for the Eyes. The Powder of it according to *Pliny,* is efteem'd a Specific for the Eyes, and the Wood triturated with *Paffum* is faid to cure Dimnefs of Sight. *Zacutus Lufitanus* fays, it is of Service in flatulent Convulfions. Ebony, according to *Diofcorides,* has a deterfive Virtue, in cleanfing the Pupil of the Eye from whatever darkens the Sight, and is good for inveterate Rheums and Puftules in the Eyes. If it is ufed inftead of a Stone in Triturations for preparing of Collyria, thefe Medicines will have the better Effect. An excellent Ingredient in Collyria is prepared of the Duft or Shavings of Ebony macerated a Day and a Night in *Chian* Wine, and then carefully triturated. They burn it alfo according to *Diofcorides* in a crude and unbaked earthen Pot, till it is reduced to Coals, and then wafh it in the fame Manner as burnt Lead. When thus prepared it is very effectual in dry and fcurfy Ophthalmies.

Echinopus major, J. B. Boerh. Ind. A. *Crocodilion,* Offic. Globe Thiftle. This Plant is cultivated in Gardens, and flowers in Summer. The Root and Seeds are ufed in Medicine. The Root drank excites a copious Hæmorrhage at the Nofe, and is given with good Succefs in all Diforders of the Spleen, and the Seeds provoke Urine.

Echinopus, folio Acanthi aculeati tenuiter laciniato, flore albo, Boerh. Ind. A. *Spina Alba,* Offic. *Carduus Sphærocephalus capitulo longis fpinis armato,* C. B. Prickly Globe Thiftle. With us this Plant is cultivated in Gardens, and flowers in Summer. The Root and Seeds are both ufed in Medicine. The Root is efficacious

cacious in the cæliac Paffion, provokes Urine, and us'd in a Decoction
cures the Tooth-ach. The Seed helps
Convulfions in Infants, as alfo the
Bites of Serpents.

*Echinopus folio Acanthi aculeati te-
nuiter laciniato, flore albo,* Boerh. Ind.
Alt. *Spina Arabica,* Offic. *Carduus
Spinofiffimus Sphærocephalus rigidis
aculeis armata,* C. B. *Carduus Spinofiffimus Sphærocephalus Cardui arabici
Nomine miffus,* Park. Theat. *Arabian* Thiftle. It grows in Gardens
and flowers in Summer, the Root and
Leaves being ufed. The Leaves as
well as the Root are good in ftopping Hemorrhages, the Menfes, and
other Fluxes.

Echinopus minor, J. B. *Ritro,* Offic.
*Carduus Spærocephalus cærulæ mi-
nor,* C. B. Little Globe Thiftle.
It grows in Gardens and flowers in
June. The Root is only ufed, and
agrees in Virtues with the foregoing.

Echium, Offic. *Echium vulgare,* C.
B. Pin. Boerh. Ind. A. Vipers Buglofs. This is found by Path-ways and
the Sides of Roads, and flowers in
June. Some prefcribe the Roots in
an Epilepfy, and perternatural Heats,
and *Diofcorides* fays, they are good
in Pains of the Loins.

*Echium Egyptiacum, ferox, flore al-
bo,* Boerh. Ind. A. *Lycopfis,* Offic.
Echium Orientale longioiribus floribus,
Hift. Oxon. Wall Buglofs. This
is an *Afiatic* Plant, and the Root is
ufed in Medicine, which when made
into a Cataplafm with Oil is a good
Vulnerary, and when mixed with
Barley Meal is a good Topic in an
Eryfipelas. When triturated and ufed
by Way of Unction with Oil it provokes Sweat.

Elæagnus, Offic. *Gale frutex odoratus feptemtrionalium. Elæagnus,*
Cordo Raii Synop. *Rhus myrtifolia
belgica,* C. B. Pin. Dutch Myrtle,
or Gaule. This grows in marfhy

Places. Its Leaves are ufed, which
dry, difcufs, and kill Worms.

Elaterium, Offic. *Cucumis Sylveftris, afininus dictus,* Boerh. Ind. Alt.
Cucumis Sylveftris five afininus, Raii
Hift. Wild Cucumber. This Plant
is one of the moft draftic Hydragogues in all the *Materia medica;* for the
Elaterium of the Shops, is no more
than a certain Preparation of its expreffed Juice. In order to render
the Preparations from this Plant
more mild and gentle, Mr. *Boulduc*
has been at incredible Pains, and in
the Courfe of his Experiments found,
that this Plant has fcarcely any fulphureous Principles, becaufe Brandy
and Spirit of Wine, hardly act upon it at all, and becaufe the Principles they draw from it, are only
Salts diffolved, and carried off not
by the Sulphur of thefe Menftruums,
but by the Phlegm they always retain. The wild Cucumber, then,
only contains faline Parts, in which
its Virtues confift; and as it is a ftrong
Purgative, we may from this Circumftance conclude, that Salts are
as properly Purgatives as Sulphurs;
tho' this Quality is not fo generally
afcribed to the former as to the latter. But after an incredible Number of Experiments, fometimes on
one and fometimes on another Part
of this Plant, Mr. *Boulduc* found,
that an Extract from its dried Root,
was the beft Preparation he could
obtain from it, fince it was at
once a mild and powerful Hydragogue. The Dofe is from twenty-
four to thirty Grains, in Conjunction with a few Grains of Mechoacan or Rhubarb, and Salt of Wormwood incorporated with Extract of
Juniper. The fame Author dried
the wild Cucumber very well, and
reduced it, together with its Seeds to
a Powder, which he found a very
good Hydragogue. There are two
Sorts of *Elaterium* mentioned by
the

he Antients. That of *Theophraftus* which is green, and in all probability made of the inner Subftance of he Pulp of the Fruit, and that of *Diofcorides* made only of the thin and waterifh Parts, which is white, and or that Reafon accounted beft by him and *Mefue.* The Green, is not half fo ftrong, in promoting any Evacuations, either by Vomit or Stool, as the White; one Grain of which diffolv'd in any Liquor, operates very powerfully on People of weak Conftitutions. This Medicine powerfully eliminates aqueous, and vifcid Humours, collected about the Joints. The Juice of the Root produces the fame Effect, and is, therefore, properly ufed in Clyfters, or laid as a Poultice, to the Parts affected, in fciatic Pains. This Juice, alfo, when boil'd with Wormwood, in Water and Oil, cures inveterate Megrims, if the Temples are frequently bath'd with it, and fome of the Leaves and Roots, beaten together, and applied to them as a Poultice. When this Juice of the Root, is injected into the Noftrils with Milk, it is faid to produce the fame Effect; when mix'd with Goat's Dung, and applied by Way of Plaifter, to any Tumors or hard Swellings, it is faid powerfully to refolve them. According to *Mefue,* the Juice not only of the Fruit, but alfo of the Root, or a Decoction of either, if drank, affords Relief in the Dropfy, Jaundice, and all Obftructions of the Liver and Spleen. *Diofcorides,* for the Cure of a Dropfy, orders Half a Pound of the Roots to be bruifed, and put into three Quarters of a Pint of ftrong Wine, three Ounces of which, are to be exhibited for three or four Days, till the Dropfy is remov'd, which it carries off without creating any Uneafinefs to the Stomach. According to *Caftor Durantes,* a few Grains of Elaterium, mix'd with

Conferve of Rofes, will produce the fame Effect. The Powder of the Root, mix'd with Honey, removes the Marks of Sugillations. The Root, boil'd, or fteep'd in Vinegar, cures the Morphew, and removes Specks and Freckles. The Powder of the dried Root, according to *Diofcorides,* cleanfes the Skin of the Face, from all Scurf, and the unfeemly Remains of Scars. The Juice of the Leaves dropt into the Ears, removes Pains, Noife, and Deafnefs. In the Shops, the Root of the wild Cucumber, is generally ufed as a Succedaneum, for that of the Coloquintida, or bitter Apple, fince the latter is not fo eafily obtain'd as the former. Mr. *Soam* informs us, that a certain Empiric ufed to give two Pills, of the Size of Chiches, compofed of wheaten Meal, and the Juice of the wild Cucumber, to Patients labouring under a Dropfy. After this, with a Lotion for the Legs, made of a Decoction of the Stalks, he drew the Matter downwards, and then exhibited another Dofe of his Pills, and by this Means, perform'd many Cures.

Elemi. A Gum bearing the fame Name, and produc'd by a Tree thus diftinguifh'd. *Arbor brafilienfibus Gummi Elemi fimile fundens, foliis pinnatis, fufculis verticillatis, fructu Olivæ, figura & Magnitudine,* Raii Hift. The Gum Elemi Tree. This Gum heats, mollifies, digefts, refolves, maturates, alleviates Pain, and is beneficial in Diforders and Wounds of the Head and Nerves; and in particular, it is a Specific for Wounds of the Cranium. It is, alfo, good for Contufions of the Joints, and provokes Urine and the Menfes.

Emerus, Offic. *Emerus minor,* Tourn. Inft. Scorpion Sena. This grows in mountainous Places, and flowers in *June.* Its Leaves are ufed, but *Boerhaave* fays, he knows

of

of no medicinal Virtues afcrib'd to them. But according to *Ruppius*, the common People fubftitute them, in the Room of Sena Leaves.

Empetrum, Offic. *Thymelea foliis Kali lanuginofis, falfis*, Raii Hift. *Sanamunda altera Clufii*. Sea Heath Spurge. It grows fpontaneoufly on the Coafts of *Bætica*, or *Andalufia*. The Root, is the Part ufed in Medicine, a Dram whereof taken in a Decoction of Chiches, purge pretty much.

Ephedra, Offic. *Ephedra maritima major*, Boerh. Ind. *Equifetum Polygonoides bacciferum majus*, Hift. Oxon. Sea Grape, or fhrub Horfe Tail. It grows in *Sicily*, and other maritime Places. The Fruit is ufed in Medicine, which drank in Wine, helps the Cœliac Paffion, and Women labouring under uterine Fluxes.

Ephemerum, Offic. Deadly Saffron. It grows in Woods and fhady Places. A Decoction of the Root, is a great Prefervative for the Teeth, if they are wafh'd with it, and the Leaves boil'd in Wine, difcufs Tumors, and Tubercles, which have as yet contracted no Moifture.

Epimedium, Offic. Boerh. Ind. *Epimedium quorundam floribus purpureis, cum apicibus luteis*, Chab. Barren Wort. With us, it is cultivated in Gardens. The Leaves and Root are ufed, both of which, effectually caufe Abortion.

Equifetum paluftre brevioribus foliis, polyfpermum, C. B. Pin. *Polygonum fæmina*, Offic. *Equifetum alterum brevioribus fetis*, Park. Theat. Female Horfe Tail. It grows in Lakes and Pools, and by the Sides of Rivers, and is efteem'd a vulnerary Plant.

Equifetum majus, Offic. Ger. Raii Hift. Great wild Horfe Tail. This grows in Marfhes, and watery Soils. The Stalks and Leaves are ufed, and agree in Virtues with the *Equifetum arvenfe longioribus Setis*.

Equifetum arvenfe longioribus Setis, C. B. Pin. Boerh. Ind. Alt. *Cauda Equina minor & Equifetum minus*, Offic. Corn Horfe Tail. It grows among Corn, in moift Places; it is Vulnerary, infpiffating and aftringent; and is principally ufed in ftopping Hæmorrhages, proceeding from an *Anaftomofis*, or a *Diærefis*; as, alfo, Exulcerations of the Kidneys and Bladder.

Erica, Offic. *Erica vulgaris humilis, femper virens, flore purpureo & albo*, J. B. *Erica vulgaris glabra*, Boerh. Ind. Alt. Common Heath. It is common in Thickets, and flowers in *June*. The Flowers is the Part ufed, the diftill'd Water whereof, takes away Rednefs of the Eyes, and eafes their Pain, and is with Succefs exhibited in the Colic. Fomentations, and hot Baths made of the Flowers, are faid to cure gouty and paralytic Patients.

Erigerum, Senecio, Offic. *Senecio vulgaris*, Park. Raii Hift. Groundfel, or Simfon. This grows in Fields and cultivated Grounds, and may be had at all Seafons of the Year. The Herb itfelf is ufed, and faid to be beneficial in the Cholera, Jaundice, Intemperature of the Blood, fciatic Pains, and exceffive menftrual Difcharges. Externally, it is applied to remove Inflammations of the Breafts, Scald Head, King's Evil, Pains of the Stomach, Retention of Urine, the Gout, and Wounds.

Eruca, Offic. *Eruca latifolia alba fativa Diofcoridis*, C. B. Pin. *Eruca major fativa, annua, flore albo, ftriato*, J. B. Garden Rocket. It is planted in Gardens. The Seeds are the Part ufed, which are warming and drying, and are chiefly ufed to provoke Venery, and in Anti-apoplectic Medicines.

Eruca

Eruca Sylvestris, Offic. *Eruca syl-*
vestris major lutea, caule aspero, C.
. Pin. *Eruca sylvestris major, vul-*
nior foetens, Hist. Oxon. Wild
acket. It grows upon old Walls,
nd flowers in *June.* The Seed is
e Part used; it violently expels U-
ne, and is much more acrid than
he Garden Sort.

Ervum verum, Tourn. Inst. Oro-
us, Ervum, Offic. *Orobus sativus sive*
ervum semine impuloso, siliquis inter
ernua Junctis, Hist. Oxon. Bitter
Vetch. It grows, tho' seldom, in
ur Gardens, and flowers in *June,*
ut is much more common in *Italy,*
nd some Parts of *France.* The
Parts in Use, is the Seed, which is
n angulous, roundish, brown, red-
lish Grain, of a leguminous, bitterish, and disagreeable Taste, and
contains a farinaceous Substance, not
unlike Fenugreek, as, also, a diuretic Salt; in Consequence whereof, it
is recommended for expelling the
Stone.

Eryngium, Offic. *Eryngium mari-*
timum, Boerh. Ind. Alt. Hist. Oxon.
Eringo. It grows in sandy Places,
by the Sea Side, and flowers in *June*
and *July.* The Root only is used,
which is hepatic, nephritic, and a-
lexipharmic; it is chiefly used in Obstructions of the Menses, and Urine,
and of the Liver, Gall, Spleen, and
other Parts; and consequently, is effectual in the Jaundice and Colic.

Eryngium vulgare, Offic. Boerh.
Ind. Alt. *Eringium mediterraneum,*
seu Campestre, Park. Theat. Common Eringo. This Plant, is rarely
found in *England,* tho' common e-
nough beyond Sea; it flowers in
June. Its Root is the Part used,
and agrees in Virtues with the foregoing.

Eryngium trifolium, Offic. Trefoil Eringo. It grows in the Gardens of the Curious. The Root,
which is the Part used, provokes

Urine, and is a Stimulus to Venery.

Erysimum, Offic. *Erysimum vul-*
gare, Boerh. Ind. Alt. Hedge Mustard. It grows near Hedges and
old Walls, and flowers in *June.*
The Plant, as well as the Seed, are
used, which are heating, drying, attenuating, aperient, help to expecto-
rate viscid Phlegm from the Lungs,
and are good against an habitual
Cough. *Riverius* commends a Decoction of it in Wine, against a Colic.

Erysimum latifolium, Offic. *Erysi-*
mum Monspessulanum Sinapios foliis,
Raii Hist. Broad leaved Hedge Mustard. The Herb is used, and agrees
in Virtues with the preceding.

Euonymus, Offic. *Euonymus vul-*
garis granis rubentibus, Boerh. Ind.
Alt. *Euonymus multis, aliis Tetrago-*
nia, J. B. The Spindle Tree. It is
frequent in Hedges, and flowers in
May. The Fruit is used, which
provokes Vomiting, and purges by
Stool; the whole Plant is noxious,
and taken inwardly not without
Danger; outwardly applied, it is
emollient and resolvent, kills Lice,
and deterges furfuraceous Disorders
of the Head.

Eupatorium cannabinum, C. B.
Pin. *Eupatorium Avicennae, Eupato-*
rium cannabinum, Offic. *Eupatorium*
Cannabinum vulgare foliis trifidis
profunde dentatis. Hemp Agrimony.
It grows by the Sides of Rivers, and
flowers in *July.* The Herb is used,
which is hepatic and vulnerary, and
is principally used in a Cachexy,
Catarrh, and Cough; it is likewise
efficacious, in a Stoppage of the
Urine and Menses. According to
Schroder, externally applied, it is
one of the most noble Vulneraries,
and the Root purges, like White
Hellebore, according to *Gesner.*

Euphorbium, Offic. *Euphorbium*
verum Antiquorum, Raii Hist. Boerh.
Ind. Alt. The Euphorbium Tree.

It

It grows in the *Eaft Indies.* The Part in Ufe, is the Juice, which is. call'd *Euphorbium,* and is a gummous and refinous Subftance, which moft powerfully purges, and expels all ferous and watry Humours from the whole Body, but muft not be given to dropfical Patients unlefs fuch as are of a very ftrong Conftitution, it is with good Succefs applied externally in a Caries of the Bones, but great Care muft be taken never to apply it to Ulcers of the Fauces, Nofe, Palate, or Tongue; applied to the Nofe it provokes Sneezing.

Euphrafia, Officinarum C. B. P. Boerh. Ind. A. *Euphrafia vulgaris,* Park, Eye Bright. It grows in Meadows, and flowers in *July.* The Herb is ufed, which is Ophthalmic and Cephalic; it is principally ufed in all Diforders of the Eyes, and a decayed Memory.

Faba, Offic. *Faba Bona major.* Hift. Ox. *Faba flore candido, lituris nigris confpicuo,* Tourn. Inft. Garden Beans. They are fow'd in great Numbers in our Gardens for the Ufe of the Kitchens. The Flowers, Pods, and Beans are ufed; its Virtues confift in its being adhefive, refrigerating, drying, incraffating, and extergent; it is ufeful internally applied in a Diarrhæa and Lientery; externally applied it removes Freckles and other cutaneous Diforders; the Water of the Pods mitigates the Gripes in Children.

Faba minor feu Equina, C. B. P. The fmall or Hcrfe Bean. They are fown in Fields, and flower and ripen fomewhat later than the Garden Bean, and are confiderably fmaller, they are externally applied for the fame Purpofes as the preceeding, but are moftly confumed in Food for Horfes.

Faba fancti Ignatii, Offic. *Igafur, feu Nux vomica legitima Serapionis Camelli, Faba fancti Ignatii vulgo,* Raii Dendr. *Nux Pepita, feu Faba fancti Ignatii.* Act Philof. Lond. St. *Ignatius's* Bean; this Fruit is brought to us from the *Eaft Indies.* It refifts Poifon, cures quartan Fevers, provokes Urine and the Menfes, induces a Vertigo, and excites Vomiting.

Faba Ægyptia, Offic. *Faba Ægyptia Diofcoridis et Theophrafti cujus radix Colocaffia dicebatur,* Park. Theat. *Nymphæa glandifera Indiæ paludibus gaudens, foliis umbilicatis, amplis, pediculis fpinofis, flore rofeo purpureo, et flore albo,* Pluk. Almag. Ægyptian Bean. It grows in *Ægypt;* the Root is only ufed, which has an aftringent Faculty, is good for the Stomach, and is very efficacious in Dyfenteries, and the Cœliac Paffion. The Root triturated and mixed with Sugar in the Form of a Conferve is efficacioufly exhibited in the Hæmorrhoids. The extracted Juice of the Flowers ftops an immoderate Flux of the Menfes.

Fagopyrum, Offic. *Fagopyrum vulgare erectum,* Elem. Bot. *Fagotriticum,* J. B. Buck-wheat or Brank. It is fown in Fields and flowers in *July.* Its Seed is only ufed, which affords lefs Nourifhment than Barley or Rye, yet more than Panic or Millet, Broths and Ptifans made of the Flour are eafily digefted, and they greatly help Coughs and a Difficulty of Urine.

Fagus, C. B. Pin. B oerh. Ind. A *Fagus Latinorum Oxya Græcorum,* J. B. The Beech-tree. It grows frequently in Woods and Hedges in the Southern Parts of *England,* tho' *Cæfar* in his *Commentaries* denies it to be of *Englifh* Growth; the Maft is in Ufe, and has the fame Properties and Virtues which the Chefnut is poffeffed off. Its Fruit and Seeds expell the Gravel and Mucus from the Kidneys. The Water found in the Clefts of old Beech Trees, as *Tragus* affirms, cures Scabs, Itch, Tetters, and all other cutaneous Itchings. The frefh Leaves of the Beech

Beech bruised and applied hot to Tumors, discuss them, and corroborate the Limbs when affected with a Numbness. Chew'd they are an excellent Remedy for the Disorders of the Lips and Gums. Mixed with Hogs-lard and applied hot to the Region of the Loins, they are said by some to be excellent for the Stone. The Mast eaten plentifully, especially when green, are said to disturb the Head like Lolium or Darnel.

Ferrum Equinum, Offic. *Ferrum equinum Germanicum filiquis in Summitate*, C. B. Pin. *Ornithopodio affinis, vel potius Soleæ aut Ferro Equino herba*, J. B. Tufted Horse shoe Vetch. It grows in Chalky Places and flowers in *June*, the Herb is in Use, which is esteem'd astringent and stops Bleeding.

Ferula fruticosa semper virens, foliis Anisi, Galbanifera, ex qua Galbanum, Offic. Par. Bat. Prod. *Galbanifera Planta*. Offic. *Oreoselinum Anisoides, arborescens, Ligustici foliis et facie, flore luteo Capitis bonæ Spei*, Breyn Prod. The Galbanum Plant. It grows in the Gardens of the Curious; from this Plant distills the *Galbanum* of the Shops.

Ferula Africana, Galbanifera frutescens Myrrhidis folio, C. Comm. Hort. Amst. Another Galbanum Plant. This Plant as well as the former, being wounded emits a milky Juice, which concretes into a Substance in every respect resembling Galbanum.

Ferula Galbanifera, J. B. *Ferula latiore folio*, Park. Theat. *Ferulago latiore folio*, C. B. Pin. Small Fennel Giant. It grows in most Physick Gardens. *Lobelius* says, that it was first produced from a Seed found in the Tears of Galbanum at *Antverp*.

Ferula, Offic. *Ferula major seu fæmina Plinii*, Boerh. Ind. A. *Ferula tenuiore folio, seu fæmina Plinii*, Hist. Oxon. Fennel Giant. It grows

in Physick Gardens, and flowers in *June*. The Parts used in Medicine, is the Medullary Substance of the Stalks, the Seed, and Juice or Gum called *Sagapenum* in the Shops. The Pith of the green Ferula drank is good for Spitting of Bloods, and helps those that labour under the Cæliac Passion, stops Eruptions of Blood, and eases the Head-ach, the Seed drank relieves the Gripes, the Stalks which are commonly pickled, eaten as Food, produce a Head-ach.

Ferula minor ad singulos Nodos umbellifera, Boerh. Ind. A. *Panax Asclepium*, Offic. *Libanotis quibusdam, flore lutro, semine Ferulæ*; J. B. The All-Heal of *Æsculapius*. It grows in *Istria*, and flowers in Summer, the Parts used in Medicine are the Flowers and Seed, which when bruised and applied with Honey are excellent against Phagedenic and other Ulcers and Tubercles; they are also effectual against the Bites of Serpents, when drank in Wine.

Ficus, Offic. *Ficus vulgaris*, Park. Theat. *Ficus communis*, Boerh. Ind. The Fig-tree. It grows frequently in Gardens and Orchards in hot Climates; the Fruit is used both green and dried, they are both moistening and pulmonary, are good for Coughs, cure the Gravel in the Kidneys or Bladder, and resist Poison, they are of singular Use in the Small Pox and Measles, they are maturating, emollient and drawing, whence they are efficacious against all pestilential Buboes.

Ficus sylvestris Discorides, C. B. Pin. *Caprificus*, Offic. *Ficus sylvestris sive Caprificus*, Jons Dend. The Wild Fig-tree. It grows in Greece and other warm Countries, the Fruit is used, which possesses the same Virtues as the Garden Species.

Ficus Indica, Offic. *Ficus Indica arcuata*, Chab. *Ficus Indica foliis mali cotonei similibus, fructu ficubus simili ex Goâ*, C. B. Pin. The *Indian*

Fig-

Fig-tree. It grows in the *East-Indies*, the Fruit is used, and agrees in Virtues with the common Fig.

Ficus folio Mori, fructum in Caudice ferens, C. B. Pin. *Sycomorus,* Offic. *Sycomorus sive Ficus Ægyptia,* Park. Theat. The *Ægyptian* Sycamore; it is found in *Ægypt* and some other Places, the Parts used are the Fruit and Gum; the Fruit is refrigerating, moistening, and laxative, and cures hard Tumors. The Gum is good against the Plague and Poisons.

Ficus Cypria, Offic. *Ficus sylvestris cretica folio non diviso, leviter crenato,* Tourn. *Sycomorus altera sive Ficus Cyprica,* Park. Theat. The Cyprian Sycomore-tree. Its Name shows it a Native of *Cyprus,* the Fruit is only used which has all the Virtues of the preceeding Species.

Filago seu herba Impia, Tourn. Just. *Gnaphalium,* Offic. *Gnaphalium vulgare capitulis rotundis sessilibus ad angulos floridum,* Hist. Oxon. Common Cudweed. It grows in dry Places and flowers in *June.* The Leaves are used, the distilled Water whereof is good against Cancers in the Breast, they are drying and astringent, and consequently good against all Hæmorrhages, Dysenteries, too great a Discharge of the Menses, and also a Quinsey.

Filago alpina capite folioso, Tourn. Inst. *Gnaphalium alpinum,* Ger. Lion's Foot. It grows in mountainous Places, and flowers in *July.* The Herb bruised and boil'd in Oil, is apply'd to Sugillations and Bruises.

Filipendula, Offic. *Filipendula vulgaris, an Molon Plinii?* C. B. Pin. Boerh. Ind. A. Dropwort. It grows in Fields and Meadows, and flowers in *June.* The Root and Herb are both used, the Plant is diuretic, and is principally used when a tartareous Mucilage affects the Lungs, Reins, and Joints; in a flatulent Colic, and Fluor Albus, or too copious Fluxes of the Lochia. *Tabernæmontanus*

greatly commends the Powder and Juice against an Epilepsy, and *Boerhaave* advises the Leaves infused or boil'd, against a Jaundice.

Filix non ramosa dentata, C. B. Pin. Boerh. Ind. A. *Filix-mas,* Offic. Common Male Fern. It grows in Hedges and shady Lanes; the Root is only used, and has the same Virtues as the *Osmund Royal,* for which it is often sold by the Herb-women. It is thought to be hurtful to the Female Sex, and to cause Abortion. It has a peculiar Efficacy against the Rickets, expels Worms and the Stone, and relieves those who labour under a Swelling of the Spleen.

Filix fæmina, Offic. *Filix ramosa major pinnulis obtusis, non dentatis,* C. B. *Filix ramosa repens vulgatissima,* Hist. Oxon. Female Fern, or common Brakes. It grows very frequent upon Commons and Heaths, the Root is used which is deem'd antisplenetic, astringent, and opening; it is chiefly used in Obstructions of the Bowels, as also of the Spleen and Uterus; outwardly applied it is reckoned good for Burns. The distilled Water of this Plant is esteem'd a specific Remedy against Worms, especially those of the flat Kind.

Flos Adonis, Offic. *Flos Adonis vulgo, aliis Eranthymum,* J. B. *Adonis hortensis flore minore atrorubente,* C. B. Pin. Boerh. Ind. A. Red Maithes. This grows in the Fields, but is rarely to be met with. It flowers in *June* and *July.* The Flowers are used, and according to *Parkinson,* are good for alleviating the Pains of the Colic and Gout.

Flos solis, Offic. Raii Hist. *Chrysanthemum indicum maximum, annuum, non Ramosum,* Hist. Oxon. *Helenium indicum maximum,* C. B. Sun-Flower. This is cultivated in Gardens, and flowers in *August.* The Buds of the Flowers are used, and when boil'd, are said to be a Stimulus to Venery. The Seeds are

are accounted pectoral and good for extinguishing excessive Heat, but when eaten plentifully excite a Pain of the Head. This Plant is also said to be a Vulnerary.

Fœniculum, vulgare, Germanicum, Boerh. Ind. Alt. *Fœniculum,* Offic. *Fœniculum vulgare,* Raii Hist. Pennel or Fenicle. Tho' this Plant grows spontaneously in some Places on the Sea Coast, as also at *Woolwich* and *Gravesend,* yet it is most generally cultivated in Gardens, and flowers in *June.* The Leaves, Root and Seeds are used. The Root is one of the five aperient Roots, and the Seeds are classed among the great carminative Seeds. *Simon Pauli* informs us, that in putrid Fevers, attended with Malignity, there is no Plant more aperient and sudorifie, than Fennel; whence nothing is more proper in the Small Pox, and Measles, than a Decoction of the Herb, or of its Seeds, or Roots. Distill'd Fennel-water dropt into the Eyes is by several Authors, said to be an excellent Preserver and Restorer of the Sight. The Seeds corroborate the Stomach, cure a Nausea, and Loathing of Food, and are an excellent Carminative. These Seeds are also possessed of an alexipharmic Quality, and when mixed with other Pectorals afford singular Relief in an Asthma. The Roots provoke the Menses, and Urine, are supposed to open Obstructions of the Liver and Spleen, and to cure the Jaundice.

Fœniculum dulce, Offic. C. B. Boerh. Ind. Alt. *Fœniculum dulce, majori et albo semine,* Tourn. Inst. Sweet Fennel. This is imported from *Germany,* the Seeds are used, and are possessed of the same Virtues with those of the former. This is the Species of Fennel referr'd to in the last Colledge Dispensatory, in which a Simple Water is order'd to be drawn from it, and it is an Ingredient in the *Aqua Juniperi Composita.* De-

coct. Commun. pro Clyf. The Oxymel ex allio, Mithridate and the *Venice* Treacle.

Fœniculum sylvestre, Offic. *Fœniculum sylvestre perenne, Ferulæ folio breviori,* Tourn. Inst. *Seseli perenne, folio glauco breviori,* Boerh. Ind. A. Bastard Spignel. This grows in dry mountainous Places, and flowers in *June.* The Root is used, and when dried is extremely hot and emetic. Externally, it is accounted escharotic.

Fœniculum tortuosum, J. B. Raii Hist. Boerh. Ind. Alt. French Hartwort. This is found in the Gardens of Botanists, and flowers in *August.* The Seeds are used, which are white striated, and of an aromatic Taste, attended with some Degree of Acrimony. They are hot and dry, provoke Urine and the Menses, and enter the Composition of the *Theriaca Andromachi.*

Fœniculo simile millefolium aquaticum umbelliferum, Chab. *Millefolium aquaticum umbellatum capillaceo, brevique folio,* C. B. Pin. Water Fennel. This grows in marshy Places. The Herb itself is used, and thought to be vulnerary.

Fœnum Græcum sativum, C. B. P. Boerh. Ind. Alt. *Fœnum Græcum,* Offic. Fenugreek. It is sown in Fields and flowers in *June.* The Seed is used, which is emollient, digestive, maturating, discutient, paregoric, and are frequently used in emollient Clysters. It mitigates Ischiadic Disorders, and discusses Tumors in the Breasts; triturated and made into a Cataplasm with Hydromel boiled, it is effectual against all internal and external Inflammations. Made into a Cataplasm with Nitre and Vinegar it extenuates the Spleen. The Decoction of Fenugreek used by Way of Insession is effectual in Female Disorders, proceeding from an Inflammation or Obstruction of the Uterus; made into a Pessary with the

Fat

Fat of a Goofe it mollifies and dilates the Parts about the Region of the Uterus, the green Herb ufed with Vinegar is accommodated to fuch Parts as are relaxed and exulcerated. The Decoction is excellent in a *Tenefmus* and Dyfentery, when attended with fetid Difcharges. It is an Ingredient in the *Oleum e Mucilaginibus.*

Fragara, Offic. *Fragara major,* J. B. *Cubebis affinis Fragara major,* C. B. Pin. This is found in the *Philippine* Iflands. The exterior Bark of the Berries, which is black, tender and of an aromatic Tafte, being broken, exhibits a fhining folid Seed which is heating and drying, and ufeful in cold Diforders of the Stomach and Liver. It alfo promotes the Concoction of the Aliments, but induces Coftivenefs.

Fragaria, Offic. *Fragaria vulgaris,* Boerh. Ind. Alt. *Fragaria ferens Fraga alba & rubra,* J. B. The Strawberry. This Plant grows in Woods Gardens and Hedges, and flowers in *May.* The Leaves and Fruit are both ufed; the Herb is diuretic, and frequently ufed in a Jaundice, and is often an Ingredient in Gargarifms, Baths, and Cataplafms; the Fruit is cooling and moiftening, good in fplenetic and nephritic Diforders, and refifts Poifon. In tertian and quartan Fevers, it is ufed inftead of the *Peruvian* Bark; the Seed is a good lithontriptic Remedy. One Inconvenience often attends the Ufe of Strawberrys, which is, that Toads and venomous Serpents greatly delight to be among them, and often poifon the Fruit with their Saliva, Urine, or Breath; infomuch that they are faid to have proved fatal to many. The Decoction of the Herb and immature Fruit is ftrengthening and aftringent; the ripe Fruit is emollient, nutritive, relaxing, cooling, aperitive, and corrects Acrimony, and confequently is proper in burning Fevers,

under the higheft Degree of Inflammation; the Fruit eaten cures a Gonorrhæa. The Pulp applied in a Cataplafm is excellent for all external Inflammations. *Gefner* obferves, that thofe Strawberries which grow upon Hills and mountainous Places, are far preferable to thofe which grow in thofe which are low and watery.

Fragaria fterilis, C. B. Pin. *Fragarioides,* Offic. *Fragaria non frugifera vel non Vefca,* J. B. Barren Strawberry. It grows in barren Ground, and flowers in *May,* the Herb is aftringent. It is faid to agree in Virtues with the preceeding.

Fraxinella, Ger. Emac. Tourn-Inft. Boerh. Ind. *Fraxinella vulgaris,* Park. Theat. Baftard Dittany. This is cultivated in Gardens, and flowers in *July.* The Bark of the Root is ufed and accounted cordial, alexipharmic, uterine, cephalic, and anthelminthic. It is principally ufed in malignant Diforders, Epilepfies, and other Difeafes of the Head, as alfo in Obftructions of the Uterus.

Fraxinus, Offic. *Fraxinus excelfior,* C. B. Pin. Boerh. Ind. Alt. Common Afh-tree. It is common in Woods and Hedges, the Bark, Wood, Leaves, and Seed are ufed. The Bark is drying and attenuating, and foftens the Hardnefs of the Spleen, it is diuretic and lithontriptic, and is of Service in intermittent Fevers, and it provokes Sweat. The Leaves dry powerfully, and cure the Bite of Serpents. The Seed is warming, greatly drying, and is ferviceable in hepatic, pleuritic and nephritic Diforders. The Wood is a good Vulnerary, and is by fome commended in the venereal Difeafe, and fupplies the Place of the *Lignum fanctum.*

Fraxinus folio rotundiore, C. B. Pin. *Mannifera Arbor,* Offic. The round leaved Afh. It grows in *Calabria*

and

d *Italy*, the condenfated Juice
hereof is *Manna*.

Fucus maritimus, vel Quercus ma-
tima, veficulas habens, C. B. Pin.
xerh. Ind. Alt. *Quercus marina*,
ffic. Common Sea-wrack. The
erb is ufed, which is cooling, and
not only efficacious againft the
out, but alfo in all Inflammations.
Fucus, Offic. *Fucus marinus Ro-*
lla Tinctorum dictus, Alga Tinctoria,
B. *An Fucus, five Alga membra-*
tea purpurea parva, R. Synop.
irple Sea-wrack. It is found in
e *Mediterranean. Nicander* advifes
e Ufe of this Herb againft the Bites
f Serpents.

Fucus folliculaceus ferratus, Sarga-
, Mont. Exot. *Vitis marina &*
eticula Marina, Offic. *Lenticula*
vina ferratis foliis, Park. Theat.
a Lentils. It is found upon Rocks
r the Sea-fide, the *Portuguefe* and
utch ufe it for a Dyfentery.

Fuligo, Soot. This is fo well
own, that it requires no Defcrip-
n. The Soot of Vegetables, up-
i a chymical Analyfis yields a large
antity of tranfparent Water, a
llow volatile Salt, and a thick
ack Oil. By confidering the Ana-
fis of Soot, we may learn what
arts of Vegetables are volatile, and
hat not, and be convinc'd that
en Earth which appears fo fix'd in
e moft violent Fire, after being
parated from the other Principles,
et when mix'd with the reft, is ei-
er by the Force of Flame or Fire
rown to a great Diftance thro' the
ir, in the Form of a thin Cloud.
ills compofed of dry Soot, and gild-
d, are recommended for the Cure
f cold Diftempers. The volatile
alt of Soot is ufed with the fame
uccefs as that of Animals. *Hart-*
man recommends the Salt which rifes
aft for giving Relief in Cancers ;
But the Soot produc'd by Oak-wood
lone, the common *Dutch* Tufts, or
ommon Pit-coal, appear different,

upon a chymical Analyfis; and that
again, would be very different, which
fhould be collected from the Chimney
of a public Kitchen, which is continually fill'd with the Fumes, not only
of the Fewel, but alfo of all Kinds
of boil'd, roafted, and fry'd Aliments.

Fumaria, Offic. *Fumaria purpurea*,
Ger. *Fumaria Officinarum & Dios-*
coridis, C. B. Fumitory. It grows in
Fields and cultivated Grounds, the
whole Plant is ufed. It is good againft
fplenetic and hepatic Diforders, it
attenuates and expells ferous, bilious,
and aduft Humours, it conftricts the
Vifcera; and when fo conftricted,
corroborates them and purifies the
Blood, in confequence whereof it is
fpecifically good in the Scurvy, and
all Diforders of the Spleen and Mefentery, in a Jaundice, the Itch and
all Diforders of the like Nature. The
diftilled Water dropt into the Eyes,
is faid to cure Dimnefs of Sight.

Fumaria lutea, C. B. Pin. *Fuma-*
ria lutea montana, M. H. *Fumaria*
quæ Split *Dicitur*. J. B. Yellow
Fumitory. It is gather'd on the
Mountains of *Befuia*, in a ftrong
Soil. It is of Service in all cold
Affections of the Nerves, comforts
the Brain, gently purges, provokes
Urine, and opens Obftructions of the
Mefentery and Liver.

Fumaria bulbofa, Offic. Schrod.
Fumaria radice cava major, C. B. P.
Tourn. Inft. The hollow Root.
This is cultivated in Gardens and
flowers in *April*. The Heart is ufed,
and is heating, drying, abftergent,
fubaftringent and aperient It is hepatic, uterine, alexipharmic, fudorific, diuretic and vulnerary. It is
principally ufed in exciting a Difcharge of the Menfes and Lochia.
It expels the dead Fœtus. cures the
Jaundice, cleanfes the Blood, and
confequently carries off the Itch.
Externally it is recommended for
cleanfing and confolidating old and
fiftulous Wounds. it is recommend-

ed for removing arthritic Pains arising from a cold Cause, for resolving coagulated Blood in Contusions, and for curing a Putrefaction of the Mouth. Some of the Shops fraudulently use this instead of the *Aristolochia rotunda.*

Fungus, Offic. *Fungus esculentus,* Park. *Fungus Pileolo lato & rotundo,* C. B. Tourn. Inst. The Mushroom, or Champignon. This grows in barren pasture Grounds and is found in the Autumn. The whole Plant preserv'd in Vinegar is used in Kitchens, but rarely or never found in the Shops.

Fungus ovatus, Park. *Fungus rotundus orbicularis,* C. B. Puff-balls, Bull-fists, Molly-puffs. This is found almost every where in pasture Grounds in the Autumn. The whole Plant is used, and as it is of a drying and astringent Nature, when sprinkled in recent Wounds it stops the Hæmorrhage, dries inveterate Ulcers, and stops the hemorrhoidal Discharge; but it is thought prejudicial to the Eyes.

Fungus maximus rotundus pulverulentus, J. B. *Lycoperdon alpinum maximum Cortice lacero,* Great Dusty Mushroom. This is found in fat pasture Grounds, and near Dunghills. The whole Plant, which is sometimes as large as a Man's-head, is used for checking dangerous Hæmorrhages, for which Purpose the Barbers use it in many Parts of Germany.

Fungus Phalloides, J. B. *Phalloides,* Offic. *Fungus virilis penis Effigie,* Ger. Emac. This Species of *Fungus,* according to some is of singular Service in intolerable arthritic Pains, and the Country People in *Saxeny,* apply it externally in all Pains of the Joints.

Fungus typhoides coccineus, Offic. *Fungus typhoides coccineus Melitensis,* Raii Hist. Scarlet Mushroom. It is found on a Rock near the Isle of *Malta,* and is esteem'd a very great Astringent. The Quantity of a Scruple, or a little more is given in Wine, or Broth, or any other Vehicle, in Order to stop Hæmorrhages.

Galanga major, Offic. Ger. Emac. Park. Theat. Great Galangal. It grows spontaneously in *Java* and *Malabar,* and is from thence brought to *Europe.* The Root, is the Part used in Medicine, which is good in all Disorders of the Stomach, Head, and Uterus; it incides and opens; hence it is good in all Crudities and Inflammations of the Stomach, a Vertigo, and all other Diseases, proceeding from cold and flatulent Causes.

Galanga minor, Offic. J. B. C. B. Pin. Common Galangal. It grows common in *China,* and is from thence transported to us. It has the same Virtues ascrib'd to it as the former, tho' this is the most esteem'd. It expels Wind, provokes Urine and the Menses, and helps Digestion; it abounds with a volatile oleous Salt, immersed in mild viscid Parts.

Galbanum. This is the Juice, or Gum of the *Ferula,* a Plant growing in *Syria,* and by some, according to *Dioscorides,* call'd *Metopium.* The best, is what resembles Frankincense, is grumous, pure, pinguious, free from Chips, retaining some of the Seeds, and of the Plant, of a strong Smell, not very moist, nor yet quite dry. This Gum is of an heating, drawing, and discutient Quality. When used by Way of Pessary, or for a Suffumigation, it provokes the Menses, and expels the Fœtus; drank in Wine, with Myrrh, it resists Poison, and expels the Fœtus, when dead. It is applied in Pains of the Sides, as also to Boils. The Smell of it raises those who labour under an Epilepsy, or hysteric Fits. When burnt, its Smoke drives away venomous Animals.

als. This Gum, when rubb'd on the Body, preserves it from the Bites of Serpents. A little of it put into the Cavity of a putrid Tooth, alleviates the Tooth-ach. It is an excellent antihysteric, emmenagogue, and forcing Medicine. When applied by Way of Plaister to the Navel, it is said to cure hysteric Convulsions. It is sudorific, when taken internally, and when externally applied, softens and digests Tumors, and brings them to a Suppuration. For internal Use, it ought to be strain'd, but not for external. It is an Ingredient, in the Species e scordio cum Opio; *Pilulæ Gummosæ*; *Confectio Paulina*; *Mithridatium*; *Theriaca Andromachi*; *Emplastrum commune cum Gummi*; & *Cataplasma maturans*, of the last *London* Dispensary.

Galega, Ruta capraria, Offic. *Galega vulgaris floribus cæruleis*, Park. Inst. Boerh. Ind. Alt. Goats Rue. It grows by River sides, and marshy Places, in several Parts of *Italy*, but with us only in Gardens; it flowers in *June* and *July*. It is a most celebrated Alexipharmic and Sudorific, and most powerfully discusses pestilential Poison; its principal Use is in expelling pectoral Eruptions, and other pestilential Diseases, and in curing the Plague itself; it is good in the Measles, and Epilepsies of Children, and the Stings of Serpents, and destroys Worms, even by external Application.

Galeopsis, Offic. *Galeopsis procerior ætida spicata*, Tourn. Inst. *Galeopsis sive Urtica iners magna fætidissima*, J. B. Hedge Nettle. It grows by Hedges, and flowers in *July* and *August*. The Leaves and Seeds are used, which dissipate all Hardnesses, Ulcers, Kings Evil, Pains, and Parotides; it is highly commended against Putrefaction, Gangrenes, and

phagedenic Ulcers. It is the best Plant in the World for uterine Suffocations, according to *Boerhaave*.

Galeopsis Angustifolia fætida, J. B. *Galeopsis palustris, folio Betonica, flore variegato*, Boerh. Ind. Alt. *Panax Coloni*. Offic. Clowns all Heal. It grows near Rivers, and in watry Places, and flowers in *July*. The Herb, is a most celebrated Vulnerary, beaten into a Cataplasm, with Hogs Lard; it likewise stops all Hæmorrhages; and *Cæsalpinus* affirms, that it cures tertian Agues.

Gallium, Offic. *Gallium luteum*, Boerh. Ind. Alt. *Gallion verum*, J. B. Cheese Reping. It grows in dry Places, and flowers in *June* and *July*. The Herb is used, which whole or in Powder, stops Hæmorrhages and Fluxes of Blood, which it effects, by its coagulating and incrassating Quality; the Decoction of the Herb, is esteem'd good for the Gout, and in a Bath, it removes Weariness. It coagulates and stops Fluxes, and is a Soporific.

Gambogium. See *Gutta Gambu*.

Genista juncea, Boerh. Ind. Alt. *Genista Hispanica*, Offic. *Spartium arborescens: seminibus lenti similibus*, C. B. Pin. Spanish Broom. It is common in Gardens, and flowers in *June* and *July*. The Branches, Flowers, and Seeds are used; it is more efficacious than the common *Genista*, being a potent Expeller of pituitous and serous Humours, both by Vomit and Stool; it is effectual in Dropsies, the Sciatica, and Gout; provokes Urine, and breaks the Stone in the Kidneys; the Oil of the Flowers discusses Tumors of the Spleen, by anointing the Part with it; the Flowers used with Honey of Roses, or an Egg, dissolve strumous Swellings. The Flowers and Seeds, work most violently by Vomit, not unlike Hellebore, but with Safety. The Juice of the Branches macerated in Water, and then bruised, are efficacious in the Sciatica and Quinfey.

Genista tinctoria Germanica, C. B. Pin. Tourn. Inft. Boerh. Ind. Alt. Green Weed, Dyers Weed. This is too frequent in Pasture Grounds, and flowers in *June* and *July*. The Herb is used, and has an aftringent Virtue afcrib'd to it. It agrees in Temperament and outward Appearance with the common *Cytifo-Geniſta*, and may be fuppofed to have the fame Qualities.

Genista-Spartium, majus, brevioribus aculeis, Tourn. Inft. Boerh. Ind. Alt. The Leffer Furz. This flowers in Autumn, and the whole Plant is ufed, which agrees in Virtues with the preceding.

Genista Spartium, majus, longioribus Aculeis, Tourn. Inft. Boerh. Ind. Alt. Furz or Gors. This Plant flowers in the Spring, and the Whole of it is ufed in Medicine, for the fame Purpofes as the two preceding.

Gentiana, Offic. *Gentiana major*, Ger. *Gentiana major lutea*, Tourn. Inft. Boerh. Ind. Alt. Gentian. This is cultivated in the Gardens of the Curious, and flowers in *June*. The Root is fo well known that it requires no Defcription. It is alexipharmic, aperient and attenuating, and is principally ufed in the Plague, malignant Diforders, and Obftructions of the Liver and Spleen. It is efteem'd a good Stomachic. From this the College direct an Extract to be made; and it is an Ingredient in the *Infufum Amarum fimplex*; the *Infufum Amarum purgans*, the *Vinum Amarum*; the *Tinctura Amara*; the *Species e Scordio fine Opio, Mithridate*; and the *Venice Treacle*.

Gentiana cruciata, Offic. C. B. Pin. Tourn. Inft. *Gentiana minor cruciata*, Park. Parad. Crofs-wort Gentian. This grows in uncultivated Places and Gardens, flowering in *July* and *Auguſt*

The Root is accounted ftomachic, febrifuge, and excellent againft the Plague, and the Bites of venomous Animals. As both the Leaves and Root are bitter, it is probable, they will produce the fame Effects with other Bitters.

Gentiana angustifolia autumnalis major, Tourn. Inft. Boerh. Ind. A. Marfh Gentian. This grows in moift Thickets, and flowers in Autumn. The Herb itfelf is ufed, and is by later Phyficians thought effectual againft peftilential Diforders, and the Bites or Stings of venomous Animals. Others highly extol it in Diforders of the Lungs and Liver. In Virtues it agrees with the common Gentian, but is much weaker.

Gentianella verna, Offic. *Gentianella verna major*, Raii Hift. *Gentiana alpina magno flore*, Boerh. Ind. Alt. Gentianel. This grows fpontaneoufly on the Tops of the Alps, is frequently cultivated in Gardens, and flourifhes in *April* and *May*. The whole Herb is ufed, and upon Account of its intenfe Bitternefs is recommended in a Jaundice and Obftructions of the Liver.

Gentianella autumnalis, Offic. *Gentiana pratenfis, flore lanuginofo*, C. B. Pin. Tourn. Inft. Baftard Gentian. This grows in mountainous, chalky, and dry pafture Grounds, flowering in *September*. It is thought to agree in Virtues with the common Gentian. It is an excellent ftomachic, a grateful Bitter, and far fuperious to the leffer Centaury, in whofe ftead the Phyficians and Apothecaries of *London* frequently ufe it.

Geranium Batrachioides, Offic. Ger. *Geranium Batrachioides, Gratia Dei Germanorum*, C. B. Pin. Boerh. Ind. Alt. Crow-foot Cranes-bill. This grows in moift Meadows and pafture Grounds, flowering in *June* and *July*. The Powder of the dried Herb, laid upon a Wound not only ly forthwith ftops the Hemorrhage, t alfo furprifingly and fuddenly nfolidates it.

Geranium Columbinum, Pes Colum-us, Offic. *Geranium Columbinum*, ii Hift. Doves-foot. This grows the Sides of Hedges, and flowers *June*. The Herb itfelf is ufed, ag accounted an excellent Vulne-y.

Geranium mofchatum, Offic. Raii ft. *Geranium cicutæ folio mofcha-*, Tourn. Inft. Mufked Cranes-l. This Herb grows fometimes rarely in the Fields, but is fre-ently to be met with in Gardens, wering in *June*. The Herb is d and accounted a remarkably od Vulnerary.

Geranium Robertianum, Gratia i, Offic. *Geranium Robertianum*, iii Hift. Boerh. Ind. Alt. Herb bert. This is every where to be md in Hedges, and flowers in y. The Herb is ufed, and is mo-rately dry in y, aftringent, and de-gent. It alfo refolves coagulated ood, and is beneficial to Wounds, which it is ufed in vulnerary Po-ns, and applied externally.

Geranium Sanguinarium, Offic. er. *Geranium fanguineum maximo* r, C. B. Pin. Tourn. Inft. Bloody-anes-bill. This grows in Thickets d Groves, efpecially of the moun-nous Kind, flowering in *July*. he Herb itfelf is ufed, and when hibited in whatever Manner, is id to ftop Hæmorrhages of all nds.

Geranium Tuberofum, Offic. Ger. aii Hift. *Geranium Tuberofum Ma-*, C. B. Pin. Knotted rooted anes Bill. This is cultivated in e Gardens of the Curious; and owers in *June* and *July*. The oot is ufed, which when drank in Vine, is faid to difcufs Inflamma-ons of the Pudenda.

Gingidium, Offic. *Gingidium fæ-iculi folio*, C. B. Pin. *Thapfia orien-tlis, Anethi folio, femine eleganter cre-*

nato, Tourn. Inft. Boerh. Ind. Alt Oriental Pick-tooth. This is found in the *Eaft-Indies*, and flowers in the Summer. The Leaves are ufed, and it is faid, that a Decoction of them in Wine, when drank, proves beneficial in Diforders of the Blad-der. The Plant itfelf, when eaten, either crude or boil'd, is accounted highly ferviceable to the Stomach,

Ginzeng & Ninzin, Offic. *Ginfeng & Genfing Quibufdam*, Raii Hift. *Aureliana Canadenfis Iroquæis Ga-rentogon, Sinenfibus Ginfeng*, R. P. Lafiteau. The Root of this Plant is white, fomewhat knotty, about thrice the Thicknefs of the Stem, and which goes tapering to the End; a few Inches from the Head, it fre-quently parts into two Branches, which gives it fome Refemblance to a Man, whofe Thighs the Branches reprefent. This Plant bears a Kind of reddifh Berries, which grow in a circular Clufter, but are not good to eat. It dies away every Year, and the Number of its Years may be known from that of the Stalks it has fhot forth, of which there always remain fome Marks. This Plant is found be-tween the thirty-ninth and forty-feventh Degree of Northern Lati-tude, and between the tenth and twentieth Degree of Eaftern Longi-tude, reckoning from the Meridian of *Peking*. There is here a long Tract of Mountains almoft inaccef-fable, on Account of the thick Fo-refts which cover and encompafs them. The Ginfeng is found on the Declivities of thefe Mountains and in the Forefts amidft a thoufand other Plants. This Circumftance, renders it highly probable, that if it is to be met with any where, it may be found in *Canada*, where the Forefts and Mountains exactly re-femble thofe now mention'd. Ac-cordingly, Father *Lafitau*, induc'd by a Letter, from Father *Jartoux* in *China*, concerning the Ginfeng, fought for it in the Forefts of Ca-

nada, and believ'd he had found it, because it was exactly like what Father *Jartoux* had describ'd. The *English,* also, discover'd this Plant in *Maryland.* But notwithstanding its Scarceness every where, we have some Reason to comfort ourselves for the Want of it, since as Mr. *Rentaume* in *Hist. de l'Acad. Royale,* assures us, the *Hepatica Nobilis Tragi,* a common Plant in Medicine, but less esteem'd than it deserves, is endued with all its principal Virtues. The most eminent Physicians in *China,* have wrote whole Volumes upon the Virtues and Qualities of this Plant, and make it an Ingredient in almost all the Medicines they prescribe for the Nobility, since it is too dear for the common People. They affirm, that it is a sovereign Remedy for all Weaknesses, occasion'd by excessive Fatigues, either of Body or Mind; that it dissolves pituitous Humours; that it cures Weakness of the Lungs and the Pleurify; that it corroborates the Stomach, and helps the Appetite; that it dispels Fumes and Vapours; that it fortifies the Breast, and is a Remedy for Shortness of Breath; that it strengthens the vital Spirits and increases Lymph in the Blood; that it is good against Vertigos and Dimness of Sight, and that it prolongs Life to extreme old Age. It is impossible, that the *Chinese* and *Tartars* should set so high a Value upon this Root, if it did not produce the most salutary and happy Effects. Those who are in Health, often use it in Order to render themselves more vigorous and strong. It is certain that it subtilizes, increases the Motion of, and warms the Blood; that it helps Digestion, and invigorates in a very sensible Manner. The green Leaves when chew'd, also remove Weariness in a very remarkable Manner. The Root of this Plant is to be boil'd, in Order to extract its Virtues, as is practis'd

by the *Chinese,* when they give it to sick Persons, on which Occasion they seldom use more, than the fifth Part of an Ounce of the dried Root. But as for those who are in Health, and only take it for Prevention or some slight Indisposition. Father *Jartoux* advises them not to make less than ten Doses of an Ounce, and not to use it every Day. The Root is to be cut into thin Slices, and put into an earthen Pot well glaz'd, and fill'd with about a Pint of Water. The Pot must be well cover'd, and set to boil over a gentle Fire, and when the Water is consum'd to the Quantity of a Cupful, a little Sugar is to be mix'd with it, and it is to be drank off immediately. After this, as much more Water is to be put into the Pot, upon the Remainder, and to be boil'd as before, in Order to extract the whole Juice and spirituous Parts from the Root. One of these Doses is to be taken in the Morning, and the other at Night.

Gladiolus, Offic. *Gladiolus floribus uno Versu dispositis major, floris colore purpureo rubente.* C. B. Pin. Boerh. Ind. Alt. Corn Flag. It is cultivated in our Gardens, and flowers in *June.* The Root which is the Part used is of an attracting, discutient, and drying Quality. It is commended as an Alexipharmic, and against the Pestilence. It is accounted by the ignorant and superstitious Vulgar a Charm against Witchcraft, and a Spell to render the Body invulnerable.

Glans unguentaria, C. B. Raii Hist. *Nux unguentaria,* J. B. *Nux Ben sive Glans unguentaria,* Park. Theat. The Ben Nut, Nephritic Wood. This grows in both the *Indies.* The Fruit is used. The Wood, which is of a darkish Colour, solid, hard, and heavy, is in the Shops, call'd Nephritic Wood. The Nuts are heating, drying, detergent, emetic, and purgative. They, also, evacuate Bile and Phlegm, and cure
the

: Itch and Impetigo. The Oil of
is extracted from the Kernels,
d imported to us from *Italy*. The
ood is heating and drying. It is
ncipally recommended for Difor-
s of the Kidneys, and difficult
fcharges of Urine, and may be
ounted proper in Obftructions of
Liver and Spleen.

Glaftum, Offic. *Ifatis fativa vel
ifolia*, C. B. Pin. Tourn. Inft.
ftum fativum, Ger. Woad. This
own in the Fields, and flowers in
e. The Herb is ufed; being of
rying and aftringent Nature. It
n excellent Vulnerary, congluti-
s Wounds, and ftops Hæmor-
ges, and immoderate Difcharges
the Menfes.

Glaucium flore luteo, Tourn. Inft.
erh. Ind. Alt. *Papaver Cornicula-
*, Offic. Yellow horned Poppy.
fcorides fays, this Plant is diuretic,
d *Galen* looks upon it to be vulne-
y and deterfive, without confider-
g that it muft only be ufed to eat
y the fungous Flefh of Ulcers.
vertheless, they give an Infufion
Half an Handful of it in White-
e, to thofe who are fubject to
Stone. In *Provence*, they ufe
fame Leaves bruifed, for Ulcers,
d efpecially for the Wounds of
orfes.

Glaucium, Offic. *Argemone Mexi-
*, Tourn. Inft. Boerh. Ind. Alt.
paver Spinofum, Raii Hift. Pur-
g Thiftle. This is cultivated in
Gardens of Botanifts, and flow-
in *July* and *Auguft*. The Juice,
hich bears the Name of *Glaucium*,
the Part ufed; and being, as *Dio-
rides* fays, of a refrigerating Qua-
y, is beneficial in recent Diforders
the Eyes. *Dale* and *Bauhine*
nk, that the *Glaucium*, is the
ice expreffed from the laft-menti-
ed Plant, being induc'd thereto by
e Defcription *Diofcorides* gives of

Glaux, Offic. *Glaux*, Diofcoridis,

Glaux Hifpanica, J. B. The Milk-
Wort of *Diofcorides*. This grows
in hilly and chalky Grounds, flowering in *June*. The Herb is ufed,
which, according to *Diofcorides*,
when boil'd in Barley-Water, is effectual for reftoring Milk in Women's Breafts, when it is loft. There
is a Difpute among Botanifts, about
the *Glaux* of *Diofcorides*, fome taking it for one, and others for another Plant.

Glaux vulgaris, Offic. *Aftragalus
luteus perennis, procumbens vulgaris
feu Sylveftris*, Raii Synop. Tourn.
Inft. Liquorice-vetch. This grows
in Bufhes, and on the Borders of
Fields, flowering in *July*. The
Herb is fometimes fraudulently fold
in the Shops for *Galega*. The Root
is fweetifh, aftringent, and gives a
deep Tincture of Red to the blue
Paper. The Leaves, hardly give it
any, but are bitter, and fmell like
thofe of Elder, which fhews that the
fetid Oil is found in greater Quantity in the Leaves, and that involves
the acrid Salt and Earth. This
Plant is not much in Ufe, tho' an
Infufion of it in Wine is given with
Succefs for a Retention of Urine,
and the Gravel, by fome Botanifts at
Paris.

Globularia vulgaris, Tourn. Inft.
Boerh. Ind. Alt. *Globularia*, Offic.
Bellis cærulea Monfpeliaca, Ger.
French Daify. This is found in the
Gardens of the Curious, flowering
in Summer. The Herb itfelf is
ufed, and is of a vulnerary Nature.

Glycirrhiza Siliquofa vel Germanica,
C. B. Pin. Boerh. Ind. Alt. *Glycirrhiza, Liquoritia*, Offic. Liquorice. This
is fo well known that it requires no
Defcription. The Roots, which are
the only Parts ufed, are pectoral, and
of great Ufe in Diforders of the
Lungs, as Coughs, and Shortnefs of
Breathing. They, alfo, mitigate
the acrimonious Particles which caufe
Sorenefs in the *Afpera Arteria*, and

Hoarfe-

Hoarseness. They are, also, good in nephritic Disorders, as the Stone, Gravel, Heat and Retention of Urine, and Ulcers in the Kidneys. There are two Kinds of the inspissated Juice sold in the Shops, one made in *England,* and prepared of the Decoction of the Roots, mix'd with the Pulp of Prunes, and made up into Balls; the other is imported from *Spain,* being made near *Tortosa* in *Catalonia,* and brought to us in beautiful, shining, brittle Lumps, wrapp'd up in Bay Leaves. It is a good Emollient and Healer, and fit for promoting Expectoration, because the viscid Parts which it contains, sheath and blunt the acrid Salts. It is to be used in small Quantities, and often repeated, otherwise it proves disagreeable to the Taste. *Tragus* prefers the Root and its Juice before Sugar. Every one, says he, knows, that bitter Things and Sugar excite Thirst, which this sweet Root and its Juice extinguish. The Bark, according to *Dodonæus,* has something of a Bitterness, and is of an hoter Quality than the other Parts, and therefore ought to be scrap'd off. But *Caspar Hoffman* says, we are not to regard this Direction, because the Bitterness gives it an abstersive Quality. Liquorice boil'd in Water with a little Cinnamon is by some used for their ordinary Drink, and after Fermentation intoxicates no less than Beer. This is an Ingredient in the *Decoctum pectorale;* the *Aqua Calcis minus Composita;* the *Aqua Calcis magis Composita;* the *Syrupus Pectoralis;* the *Pulvis e Tragacantha Compositus;* the *Trochisci Bechici Albi & Nigri;* the *Electuarium Lenitivum,* and *Venice Treacle.*

Gnaphalium Alpinum, Ger. *Gnaphalium Alpinum pulchrum,* Raii Hist. *Leontipodium,* Offic. Lion's Foot. This grows in mountainous Places, and flowers in *July.* The Root is said to discuss Tubercles; and the Herb when boil'd, and bruised with Oil is by Country People effectually applied for removing hard Marks, Contusions, and the Effects of Blows.

Gnaphalium maritimum, C. B. Pin. *Gnaphalium marinum seu Cotonaria.* Park. Sea-Cudweed, or Cotton-Weed. This Plant is detersive, desiccative, and very restringent.

Gossipium sive Xylon, Ger. *Bombax,* Offic. *Xylon sive Gossipium herbaceum,* Raii Hist. Boerh. Ind. Cotton-Bush. This grows in the Island of *Malta,* and several other Countries. The Seeds which are black and round are used, and thought beneficial in Disorders of the Lungs, Coughs and Asthmas. They are, also, believ'd to augment the Quantity of the *Semen.*

Gramen Arundinaceum, Offic. *Gramen Dumetorum panicula acetosa, Semine papposo,* Raii Hist. Reed-Grass. This grows in moist woody Places. The Root is used, and in Virtues agrees with the common Reed.

Gramen Caninum, Ger. *Gramen Caninum arvense, seu Gramen Dioscoridis,* C. B. Pin. Quick-Grass. This grows in the Fields, and is cultivated in Gardens. Its Root, which is the only Part used, is of a refrigerating, drying, aperient, subastringent, and penetrating Quality. This is the celebrated *Chien-dent* of the *French,* which they constantly use as an Ingredient in all their Ptisans. The Root is cold and dry, but the Herb refrigerates, though weakly, and is in a middle State between Humidity and Dryness. The Root is possess'd of a pungent Quality, consists of subtile Parts, and has often been fonnd effectual for dissolving the Stone. It is, also, moderately aperient and lenitive, and removes Obstructions of the Viscera, without producing any bad Consequences. By a Chymical Analysis, great deal of Oil, Earth, and several acid Liquors, as, also, a little r'd but no volatile Salt is obtain'd on this Root. So that, probably, it is by a Salt analagous to that of oral involv'd in a large Quantity Sulphur.

Gramen Dactylon, Offic. *Dactylon folio Arundinaceo majus*, C. B. Pin. ock-foot Grass. This grows in elds, Vineyards, and sandy Places. Root is used, and its Virtues are arly the same with those of the quick Grass.

Gramen Leucanthemum, Offic. *Alx pratenfis gramineo folio ampliore*, ourn. Init. Stitch-wort. This is very where found in Woods, Thickets, and Hedges, flowering in the Spring. The Herb is used, and of a refrigerating and drying Quaty. It is, also, said to be beneficial in Inflammations of the Eyes.

Gramen Manna, Offic. *Gramen lannæ esculentum*, Ger. Manna Grass, Russia Seed. This grows in rmany and *Poland*. The only Parts . Use are the Seeds, which are nall, oblong, pellucid, white, of a int Taste, and when decorticated, ot unlike Rice. The Seeds are offeffed of the same Qualities with ice, are moderately aftringent, resolve hard Tumors of the Breast, and then used as Aliments are moderately nutritive. They are, also, said to be highly efficacious for the Cure of Rickets in Children.

Gramen Parnaffi, Ger. Emac. Raii Hist. *Parnoffia paluftris & vulgaris*, Tourn. Inft Boerh. Ind. Alt. Grass of Parnaffus. This grows in marshy and putrid Soils, flowering in *Auguft*. The Root, Herb and Seeds, are used. The Juice of the Leaves, and a Decoction of the Roots are accounted excellent Medicines for Disorders of the Eyes. The Seeds are extremely diuretic, and stop Vomiting and Diarrhœas.

Grana Tiglia & Lignum Moluccenfe,

Offic. *Palma Chrifti Indica*, Tourn. Mat. Med. Purging Nuts. This is the Fruit of a Tree cultivated in *Malabar* and elfewhere, whofe Wood is fpongious, light, rare, pale, cover'd with a cineritious Bark, of an acrid, hot, and naufeous Tafte, but without any Smell. The Fruit is oblong, oval, gibbous in one Part, and depreffed in another, of a blackish Colour, and of an acrid, hot and naufeous Tafte. Both the Fruit and Wood heat, incide, and attenuate, but as they are of too cauftic a Quality they are rarely found in the Shops.

Granata malus, Mont. Ind. *Malus Punica*, Raii Hift. *Punica quæ malum Granatum fert*, Tourn Inft. Boerh. Ind. Alt. The Pomegranate-tree. This grows fpontaneoufly in hot Countries, and flowers in *May*. The Flowers, Fruit, Bark of the Fruit, and Seeds are ufed. The Fruit is good for the Stomach, but yields very little Nourifhment; they are acid, cold, aftringent, and ftomachic, and are chiefly ufed in bilious Fevers, a Gonorrhæa, depraved Appetite of pregnant Women, correcting Putrefaction in the Mouth and the like. The Flowers are of the fame Nature as Balauftines. The Bark which in the Shops is call'd *Malicorium*; has the fame Virtues as the Flowers, efpecially in ftopping Fluxes of the Hæmorrhoids, Noftrils, and Uterus; the Seeds are refrigerating and aftringent.

Gratiola, Offic. Ger. Emac. *Gratiola vulgaris*, Park. Theat. *Digitalis minima*, *Gratiola dicta*, Boerh. Ind. Alt. Hedge-hyffop. This is cultivated in Gardens, and flowers in *July*. The Herb is us'd and accounted a Specific for evacuating aqueous, vifcid and bilious Humours, for which Reafon it is much us'd in the Dropfy and Jaundice. It is alfo faid to kill Worms.

Groffularia Spinofa fativa, C. B. Pin.

Pin. *Grossularia, Uva crispa,* Offic. *Grossularia,* Park. Theat. The Gooseberry Bush. It grows in Gardens, flowers in *April,* and produces its ripe Fruit in *July.* The Fruit is us'd. The unripe Berries are good for the depraved Appetite of pregnant Women. They procure Appetite, and stop all Fluxes of the Belly. The Berries boil'd in proper Liquors are advantageously exhibited to feverish Patients. The ripe Fruit is esteem'd good for the Stomach.

Guaiacum, Offic. Ger. Emac. Raii Hist. *Guaiacum, sive Lignum Sanctum,* Park. Theat. *Guaiacum magna Matrice,* C. B. *Fructus Guaiaci putatus & folia,* J. B. *Guaiacum,* or Pock-wood. There are two Species of Wood adapted to the Cure of the venereal Disease; one of them solid, dense, resinous, blackish, consisting of variously complicated Fibres, of an acrimonious, bitterish aromatic Taste, and of a fragrant Smell. This the *Americans* call *Hiacan,* or *Huiacan,* whence comes the European Name *Guaiacum.* The other very much resembles this in Denseness, Complication of Fibres, Taste and Smell, but is of a more whitish or rather yellowish Colour. This the Natives call *Hoaxecan,* and we *Lignum sanctum,* on Account of its extraordinary Virtues. The Bark of both is ligneous, thin, hard, of an acrimonious and bitterish Taste, but almost entirely void of Smell. Both these Species are now common in the Leeward Islands, and all that Part of *America,* which lies under the Torrid Zone. The antient Method of preparing the Decoction of *Guaiacum* was to take a Pound or twelve Ounces, of the thin Chips or Raspings of the Wood, and infuse them in eight, ten, or twelve Pints of Water, for four-and-twenty Hours, in a new earthen Pot. Then the Vessel being well stopp'd, they boiled it by setting the Pot in a Furnace full of Water, to the Consumption of a fourth or third Part, or even of an Half, as they thought most agreeable to the Strength and Temperament of the Patient, or the Violence of the Disease. Then they strain'd the Decoction, and letting it cool, bottled it up for Use. To the Wood left in the Pot they pour'd the same Quantity of Water as before, and boil'd it over a gentle Fire, to the Consumption of a fourth Part, then strain'd it and set it aside. This second Decoction was bottl'd for ordinary Drink. When these Decoctions were got ready, the Patient being prepar'd by some gentle Cathartic, and a spare Diet, for some Days, was closely confin'd to his Chamber, which was kept very warm, and well secur'd against the Air and Cold. The Patient lying in Bed, took every Morning, very early, a Glass which held eight or ten Ounces of the first Decoction warm. Then covering himself well up with the Bedcloths, he compos'd himself to sweat for two or three Hours. Then the Sweat being absterg'd, and the Body dried, four Hours, at least, after taking the Decoction, he had two or three Ounces of Biscuit, with a few Raisins, Almonds, or Pistaches offer'd him to eat, and he was order'd to drink plentifully of the second Decoction. Four Hours after he took eight or ten Ounces of the first Decoction, sweated three Hours as before, and after wiping his Body, was allowed to eat two or three Ounces of Biscuit, with some Raisins, Almonds, or Pistaches, and to drink some Cups full of the second Decoction. But if the Patient was then extenuated, or of a weakly tender Constitution, and unlikely to support so great Abstinence, a larger Quantity of Raisins and Biscuit was allow'd, or even some Chicken-Broth. Some Days after, perhaps, he had Half or a Quarter of a small Chicken

Chicken roafted or boil'd in pure Water, without Salt, allow'd him. In this Method they perfifted for fifteen Days, in which Time, if the Patient was coftive, an emollient Clyfter was injected every fecond or third Day. After the firft fifteen Days, the Patient was purg'd with fome gentle Cathartic, as the Pulp of Caffia, Manna, Tamarinds, and the like ; and on fuch Occafions he drank nothing but the fecond De-coction for that Day. When this was over, he enter'd upon the fame Courfe of Medicine as before, till the thirtieth or fortieth Day ; but had a little larger Quantity of Food gradu-ally allow'd him ; and, after the twenty-fifth or thirtieth Day, if his Strength was fufficient, he was per-mitted now-and-then to get out of Bed, and being well cloth'd, to take a Turn or two about the Chamber, provided he was free from the leaft Sweating. Towards the End of the Cure he was again purg'd, and after that, he had the Liberty of walking out of his Chamber, not indeed into the open Air , but into another Room, till he was able to bear the Air. They were alfo very cautious with Refpect to fudden Changes, fince they requir'd a Month longer to bring the Patient by Degrees to his ufual Method of living, during which he obferv'd a proper Regimen, ab-ftain'd from Wine, and us'd the fe-cond Decoction for his ordinary Drink. By this Method the ftrong Decoction of the *Guaiacum*, entering into the Lacteals, exhaufted, by Ab-ftinence, and pervading all the Parts of the Body, diffolved, attenuated and freed the Globules of Blood and Lymph, which were harden'd and infpiffated by the Contagion, and ei-ther altered or corrected the obvious contaminated Fluids, or expell'd and eliminated them by Urine or Sweat. The Vifcera, alfo, in all their Parts, and Veffels, being for forty Days ma-

cerated in this acrimonious Lixivium, had all their Obftructions and Infrac-tions infenfibly remov'd, fo that the Virulence of the venereal Contagion being fubdu'd, and eliminated, the Patients were reftor'd to their former Health. Of the Truth of this *Ulric Hutten* was a memorable Inftance, who for many Years, labouring un-der the venereal Difeafe, attended with fevere Pains, numerous Exoftofes, an ulcerous Caries of the Bones, an extreme Emaciation, and a dange-rous Marafmus, underwent a Saliva-tion eleven Times to no manner of Purpofe ; but by the foleUfe of the De-coction of *Guaiacum* for 30 Days toge-ther, was reftor'd to perfect Health. The *Guaiacum* was at firft thought to be innocent and fafe ; but in a fhort Time it was found from Experience, that by the Strictnefs of the Regimen, the Acrimony of the Decoction, and other concurring Symptoms, Perfons of tender, hot, bilious Conftitutions, thofe labouring under Diforders of the Lungs, Liver or Kidneys, and thofe difpos'd to Confumptions, were fo exhaufted and attenuated, as to fall into an incurable Phthifis. To avoid Misfortunes of this Nature, it was thought expedient to mitigate the Severity of the Regimen, and render the Decoction weaker, by which Means the Virtues of the Remedy were fo far deprefs'd, that it was no longer effectual for the Cure of the Difeafe ; fo that *Guaiacum*, which was at firft receiv'd with fo much Applaufe, began to lofe much of its Reputation, till the celebrated *Boer-haave* in his Preface to the Collec-tion of Authors, on the venereal Difeafe, endeavour'd to revive its Ufe in the Cure of venereal Dif-orders, and gave it this great En-comium, that it will perform a Cure where a Salivation has fail'd, where-as if *Guaiacum* fails, it is in vain to try a Salivation. Befides, the Ufe of *Guaiacum* in venereal Cafes, it is

said

aid in general, to be hot and drying, and therefore a great Promoter of infenfible Perfpiration, rather than of Sweat. On this Account it is reckon'd an excellent Sweetener and cleanfer of the Blood, and therefore is much prefcrib'd in cutaneous Diforders of all Kinds. On Account of its hot and penetraring Quality, it is alfo efteemed good in the Gout, by diffipating and infenfibly wafting the Humours thrown upon the Joints; as alfo in Dropfies and Catarrhs, by drying up and confuming the fuperfluous Humidities. In a word, daily Experience evinces its Ufe in all Diforders arifing from a Redundance. In making the Decoction of *Guaiacum*, it is to be obferv'd, that the Rafpings of the frefh and green Wood are much better than thofe which are old and dry, and that the longer it is boil'd, the better it is. *Boerhaave* informs' us, that if the Tincture of *Guaiacum* prepar'd with pure Alcohol, and infpiffated to an Half, is mixed with four Times its Quantity of the Syrup of the five aperienr Roots, and taken upon an empty Stomach, in the Morning, lying in Bed, it prefently diftributes itfelf over the whole Body, which it warms, promoting at the fame Time a copious Sweat. And hence it is commended in the venereal Difeafe, when it has feiz'd upon the fubcutaneous Parts. *Hoffman*, in *Obfervat. Phyf. Chym.* informs us, that when a Decoction of *Guaiacum* is infpiffated over a gentle Fire, there remains at the Bottom a refinous Subftance, which is of a balfamic Nature, grateful Smell, and fomewhat acrid Tafte, and which when reduc'd to a Powder, and receiv'd into the Noftrils, by ftimulating the glandulous Coats which cover the Bones of the Noftrils, fo powerfully colliquates and evacuates the Phlegm lodg'd there, that from ong Experience it appears preferable to all other Errhines; for, befides its ftimulating Quality as an Errhine, it

is alfo poffefs'd of a corroborating Virtue, which is highly friendly to the nervous Parts of the Head. *Guaiacum* is of late much come into Practice in the Rheumatifm. In the laft *London Pharmacopœia*, an Extract, a Tincture, and a Balfam, are directed to be made of *Guaiacum*; and it is an Ingredient in the *Oleum Capaivæ compofitum*, the *Aqua Calcis magis Compofita*, and the *Pilulæ Aromaticæ*.

Guaiacum propemodum fine Matrice, C. B. P. *Lignum Sanctum*, Offic. *Palum Sanctum Indiæ Occiduæ*, Park. Theat. Holy wood. This is a firm compact Wood, fomewhat whiter than the former and poffefs'd of the fame Virtues. From thefe Trees is obtain'd the Gum *Guaiacum*, which is poffefs'd of the fame Virtues with the Wood, but is accounted more efficacious. It is thought greatly to promote infenfible Perfpiration, and for that Reafon to be good to remove fuch cutaneous Diforders as proceed from an Obftruction of the perfpirable Matter in the miliary Glands. It is very warm and deterfive, and therefore good in Gleets, and all Exulcerations, whether internal or external. In Gonorrhæas it is by fome deemed a Specific. It, alfo, frequently proves beneficial in the Gout, not only by deterging and cleanfing the Joints and mucilaginous Glands from tartareous Matter, but alfo by warming and ftrengthening the Fibres, it enables them to move with fuch Vigour as to fhake off, and prevent the Adhefion of fuch Particles to them.

Gummi, Gum. A concreted Vegetable Juice, which tranfudes thro' the Bark of certain Trees, and hardens upon the Surface. The Chymifts only allow thofe to be properly Gums, which are diffolvable in Water; thofe which are only diffolvable in Spirit they call Refins; and thofe of a middle Nature, Gum Refins. *Geoffroy* fays, that Gums are fome-something between Acid and Oil, being an acid Salt so fix'd in Earth, as that the greatest Part of it is changed to an Alcali, the other into Oil; so that the Mixture arising from thence is an oily Salt, resembling the saponaceous Concretes of the Chymists, made of Oil of Olives, and a Lixivium of Tartar, or the mucilaginous Bodies form'd of Spirit of Wine, and the volatile Spirit of Urine. And thus we see, that all Seeds which are oily when Ripe, are in the Beginning only a Mucilage, or imperfect Oil. In the antient Writers *Gummi* (κόμμι) put absolutely, imports Gum Arabic. *Gummi Ammoniacum.* Gum Ammoniac. *Pliny* tells us, that, in that Part of *Africa* which borders on *Ethiopia*, amongst the Sands, distills the Tear of Hammoniac, taking its Name from the Oracle of *Hammon*, near which grows the Tree call'd *Metopion*, whence it flows in manner of a Gum or Resin. There are two Kinds of this *Hammoniac*, one called *Thraustin* like Male Frankincenoe, and which is most valued; the other is fat and resinous and named *Phyrama*. It is adulterated with Sand, as if it were contracted in its Growth; for which Reason, that which is in the smallest and purest Lumps bears the highest Price, which is forty Asses (about three Shillings) the Pound. This Gum is of an opening, cleansing and attenuating Nature, proper to clear the Lungs of viscid Phlegm, for which Reason it is greatly recommended in Asthmas, and Shortness of Breath. It is also good in nervous, hysteric and hypochondriac Disorders; externally used, it is suppurating, ripening and dissolving. It is proper for Hardness of the Spleen, Liver and Mesentery, good for opening Obstructions of the Menses. This Gum contains Plenty of essential or volatile Oil, some Phlegm and Earth.

Gummi Anime. A Sort of Gum of which there are several Sorts taken Notice of by Authors, but that principally in Use is thus distinguish'd *Gummi Animi*, Offic. *Gummi seu Resina Animæ*, Schrod. *Gummi Aminea*, Serap. *Minea*, Galeni. *Aminea, Myrrha*, Cæf. *Aniimum*, Amat. This Gum is brought to us from *America*, and flows from an Incision made in a Tree, of a moderate Bigness, the Leaves of which resemble those of the Myrtle. It contains a great deal of Oil and essential Salt, and is greatly recommended to soften and dissipate Cold, Painful, Rheumatic, flatulent Affections of the Head, Nerves and Joints. It is also good to strengthen the Brain, by applying it to the Top of the Head. The best Gum Anime is that which is of a white, Colour, dry, friable, clean, of a good Smell, and which soon consumes when thrown into the Fire.

Gummi Arabicum, Gum Arabic. This Gum is thought, by some to be the Gum of the *Acacia foliis Scorpioidis Leguminosa*. It is of a white Colour, inclining to yellow, pale and pellucid, of an insipid taste, and viscous; it exsudes spontaneously from an Incision made in the Tree. That is best which is pellucid like Glass, unmixed and in the Form of small Worms. It heats and moistens, inspissates, stops the Pores of the Skin, and blunts the Acrimony of Medicines. From its soft, glutinous Quality, it is serviceable against Coughs, Hoarseness, and Disorders of the Aspera Arteria, is a proper Ingredient in Applications to the Eyes and Arteries, and is of great Efficacy in the Dysuria, or Heat of Urine, and the Diabetes.

Gummi Bdellium. This is already taken Notice of under the Article of Bdellium.

Gummi Caranna. This is already taken Notice of under the Article of Caranna.

Gummi

Gummi Cerasorum. This is mention'd under the Article of *Cerasus rubra.*

Gummi Copal. The Name of a Gum thus distinguish'd, *Resina Copal,* Offic. *Rhus Virginianum Lentisci foliis,* Raii Hist. This Gum is brought from the *Spanish West Indies,* being taken by our latest Authors for the Gum of Virginian Sumach. The Natives of *America* give the Name of *Copal* to all odoriferous Gums, which are transparent. The Gum we call by that Name is not much used in Physic, but is greatly used by the Varnishers, who dissolve it in *Oleum Spicæ,* tho' it has sometimes been employ'd in Fumigations for violent Defluxions of the Head, and is still by some People recommended in the Palsy and other Weaknesses of the Nerves.

Gummi Elemi, See *Elemi.*

Gummi Guajaci, See *Guajacum.*

Gummi Hederæ, See *Hedera Arborea.*

Gummi Juniperi, See *Juniperus.*

Gummi Senegalense. This is already taken Notice of under *Acacia.*

Gummi Tacamahaca. Tacamahac. This is a resinous Substance, of which there are two Kinds, one in Shells, the other in Dumps. The first is the best, being sometimes called *Tacamabaca sublimis.* It is of a very agreeable Smell, resembling that of Lavender and Angelica. It is brought from *Madagascar* and *New Spain,* being the Product of a Tree called *Tacamabaca Populo similis, fructu colore Pæoniæ simili,* J. B. *Tecomahoica,* Hernand. It is used externally in the same Intentions with the *Gummi Caranna.* It resolves Tumors, strengthens the Nerves, being spread upon Linen and put behind the Ears, it represses all Manner of Defluxions from the Head apply'd to the Temples, it is good for all Rheums of the Eyes and other Parts of the Face, and put into an hollow putrid Tooth, it

cures the Pain thereof. Being apply'd to the Nostrils, or burnt upon Coals, it gives immediate Relief in Hysterics. It is also recommended in arthritic Pains.

Gummi Tragacantha, Gum Tragacanth, or Gum Dragon, is a Gum which bursts forth from the *Tragacantha,* Offic. *Tragacantha Massiliensis,* J. B. Goats Thorn. It is brought to us from *Turkey* in Pieces of different Sizes. Externally used it is of Efficacy in the Dysentery; and dissolved in Milk or Rose-water, is good for the Redness, and acrimonious Rheums affecting the Eyes, and for Asperities of the Eye-lids. Dissolv'd in Water, its Mucilage is very convenient for the Formation of Troches, and other Forms of Medicines. It is moistening, lenient, emplastic, corrects Acrimony, and incrassates, Hence it is of Efficacy in Hoarsnesses, Spitting of Blood, Asperities of the Fauces, and the Strangury; four or six Grains of it exhibited in Milk or Water, are effectual in voiding of Blood by Urine.

Gutta Gamba. This is said to be produc'd from *Cambogium,* Offic. *Carcapuli,* Park. Theat. *Coddam Pulli, seu Ota-Pulli,* Hort. Mal. Gamboge. There are many Opinions concerning the Generation of this Gum: Some will have it to be natural, others factitious; some refer it to the *Esula: Bontius* to an *Indian* Plant, near a Kin to the *Esula,* others to the Flowers of the *Indian Riciuus,* and its Colour to the *Curcuma;* and some again endeavour to derive it from the *Tithymalus* and *Scammony.* We take it to be the concreted Juice of the Trees abovemention'd. *Boulduc* is of Opinion, that this ought to be esteem'd a resinous Juice, because it is inflammable, and will flow in the Fire, and be almost entirely dissolv'd in Spirits of Wine; but, on the contrary, in aqueous Menstruums, spreads

itself

itfelf into a milky Subftance like Scammony, and afterwards precipitates. The fame Author endeavour'd to get Flowers from Gamboge, like thofe from *Benjamin,* but without Succefs. He made Trial on it with Spirit of Wine, a Lye of alcaline Salts, and Water: The Spirit of Wine diffolv'd all, except about a fixth Part; the Remainder, which the Spirit would not touch was eafily diffolv'd by a Solution of Salt and Tartar. This, fays he, may be efteem'd the faline Part of Gamboge; and tho' it had no purgative Virtue, was very Diuretic. The Refin, which was made by the Spirit of Wine, purg'd more violently, and with greater Irritation, than the Gamboge itfelf. This Gum was entirely diffolv'd by an equal Quantity of Salt of Tartar, and a fufficient one of boiling Water, excepting fome few terreftrial Parts. The Liquor filtrated, and evaporated by a gentle Fire, gave a Sort of grey Salt, which eafily flow'd in the Air, if not kept clofe ftopt in a Phial. This faline Extract purg'd with lefs Irritation, and in a fmaller Dofe, than the Gum; but caus'd a great Acrimony and Heat in the Throat, in fo much that it was intolerable, and ought, therefore, to be inveloped in fome other convenient Subftance when it is given. This Gentleman obferv'd before, that Water would not diffolve it, but only made it flow into a milky Subftance of a yellow Colour, which foon precipitated, and left the Water clear above it. This Refidue dry'd, differ'd in nothing from the Gum, only was more pure. By cafting diftill'd Vinegar on this milky Subftance, it became clear; Oil of Vitriol, on the contrary, made it again turbid, and Spirit of Wine gave it a golden Colour. There are many ways, this Author obferves, of correcting it, but he things that by alcaline Salts the beft. However, he

gives one of his own, which, as it is different from any other hitherto ufed, he alfo continually practifed with Succefs. The Manner is, by tying the Gum in a Rag, and putting it into a hot Loaf, as it comes out of the Oven, where it muft remain for twenty-four Hours; afterwards it is to be powder'd, and this muft be repeated four or five Times. By this Management, he fays, he always found it freed from its great Violence, as well Purgative as Emetic. He farther obferv'd the Crum of Loaves thus ufed to have both a purgative and emetic Quality. It purges very well in the Quantity of four Grains, but from fix to eight Grains, it Purges and Vomits violently. It is reckon'd particularly ferviceable in Dropfies, by evacuating the watery Parts of the Fluids; and, as it has no Tafte, a very fmall Dofe of it, fuch as a Grain or two, diffolved and mixed with Sugar is very fit for Children. It is worthy Obfervation, that tho' this Gum is fo very Purgative, yet the Fruit of the Tree, to which it belongs, is perfectly harmlefs, and is eaten in the Country like Oranges.

Halimus, Offic. *Halimus latifolius five fructuofus,* C. B. *Halimus latifolius, five Portulaca marina incana major,* Park. Sea-Purflane. It grows in Hedges near the Sea, and flowers in Summer. The Roots help Contufions, and the Gripes. The Quantity of a Dram in Hydromel procures Plenty of Milk; the Leaves are boil'd for Food.

Harmala, Ger. *Ruta Sylveftris Harmel.* Offic. *Ruta Sylveftris Syriaca five Harmala,* Park. Theat. Wild Rue. It grows in Phyfick Gardens, and flowers in *July.* The Herb and Seed are ufed. The *Arabian* Authors fay, that the Seeds are fo inebriating, as to make Men fleep a long Time; but that they are good in Melancholy Diforders. It partakes much of
the

the Nature of Garden Rue, and provokes Urine.

Hedera arborea, Offic. *Hedera arborea sive Scadens & Corymbosa nigra,* Park. Theat. *Hedera communis major,* J. B. Ivy. It grows in many Places. The Leaves and Berries are us'd; as also the Gum, or Tear, which is a resinous, dry, hard and compact Substance, of a spadiceous Colour, somewhat inclining to a Yellow, and shines like Glass, but is not like that pellucid, and is of a sharp subastringent, and sweet Taste. The Herb is heating, drying, and subastringent. It is seldom exhibited internally, being tho't noxious to the Head and Nerves. Externally it is often applied to dry and cure Achors, and Ozænas. The Berries purge upwards and downwards, whence it is by the Vulgar given against Fevers. The Gum is a celebrated Caustic, and kills Nits.

Hedera terrestris Chamæcissus, Offic. *Hedera terrestris vulgaris,* C. B. Pin. *Calamintha humilior folio rotundiori,* Tourn. Inst. Ground-Ivy. It grows by Hedges, and flowers in *April.* The Herb is us'd, which is deem'd a good Vulnerary. It is frequently us'd for inciding and resolving the gross tartareous Matter of the Lungs, Kidneys, and other Parts, and consequently is efficacious in all Obstructions thence proceeding; as also in the Jaundice. The Syrup made of this Plant is good against a convulsive Cough; but chiefly against spitting of Blood, and bloody Urine.

Hedysarum Clypeatum, Mont. Indr *Hedysarum Clypeatum flore suaviter rubente,* Boerh. Ind. A. *Onobrychis major perennis filiculis articulatis, asperis, clypeatis, recta Junctis, flore ruberrimo,* Hist. Oxon. French Honey-Suckle. It grows in Gardens, and flowers in *July.* The Herb is us'd which is deobstruent and vulnerary.

Helenium, Ger. *Enula Campana Helenium,* Offic. *Helenium sive Enula Campana,* J. B. Elecampane. It grows in watery Fields, and Meadows, and flowers in *June* and *July.* The Root is the Part us'd, which is both pulmonic and stomachic, alexipharmic and sudorific. Is is chiefly us'd in Coughs, Asthmas, Crudities of the Stomach, in opening the urinary Ducts; in the Plague, and other contagious Distempers. Externally it is recommended in the Itch, Spasms, and Ischiadic Pains.

Helianthemum Vulgare, Park. Theat. *Panax Chironium Helianthemum,* Offic. *Chimæcistus Vulgaris flore luteo Panax Chironium sive flos Solis,* Merc. Bot. Dwarf-Sun Flower. It grows in dry, chalky, and mountainous Places, and flowers in *June* and *July.* The Root and Herb are both used; the Root resists the Poison of Serpents, and other venomous Creatures; the Plant is vulnerary; a Decoction thereof, is successfully exhibited in Diarrhæas, Hæmorrhages, and Disorders of the Fauces; it is astringent, hence in all Disorders where there is too great a Flux, it may be used in the Room of Cumfrey.

Helichrysum seu Chrysocome angustifolia vulgaris, Hist. Oxon. *Stæchas Citrina,* Offic. *Elichryson sive Stæchas citrina angustifolia,* Boerh. Ind. Alt. Goldy Locks. It grows in Gardens, and flowers in *May.* The Flowers are used in Obstructions of the Liver, Kidnies, Spleen, and the Menses; they resolve coagulated Blood, dry up Catarrhs, kill Worms, and are said to cure the Jaundice.

Helichrysum sive Chrysocome caulibus deciduis latiore folio Germanica, Hist. Oxon. *Stæchas citrina Germanica,* Offic. *Stæchas citrina Germanica latiore folio,* J. B. German Goldy Locks. It is found in *Germany,* and flowers in *July.* The Herb and Tops are used; it is heating, drying, aperient,

perient, and abſtergent, and is celebrated for its Uſe in all Diſeaſes of the Brain proceeding from a cold Cauſe.

Helichryſum Orientale, C. B. Pin. *Chryſocome*, Offic. *Stœchas citrina floris magnitudine & colore ſpecioſa*, J. B. Oriental Goldy Locks. It is found in the Iſland of *Crete*, and flowers in *July.* The Root is uſed, which is heating and aſtringent, and is good for thoſe who labour under an Inflammation of the Liver and Lungs.

Helichryſum montanum flore rotundiore candido, Boerh. Ind. Alt. *Pes Cati*, Offic. Cats Foot. It grows in mountainous and chalky Places. The Herb is uſed, which is drying and aſtringent; the Syrup is highly eſteemed in Exulcerations of the Lungs, and Spitting of Blood; it is recommended in convulſive Coughs of Children.

Heliotropium majus, Offic. *Heliotropium majus Dioſcoridis*, C. B. Pin. Boerh. Ind. Alt. Turnſole. It grows in Gardens, and flowers in Summer. The Herb and Seeds are uſed; a Decoction of it potently evacuates all pituitous and bilious Obſtructions by Stool, and is good againſt the Bites of Scorpions; the Seed repreſſes all fleſhy Excreſcences, makes penſile Warts wear off, provokes the Menſes, and facilitates Delivery.

Heliotropium minus, Offic. *Heliotropium minus ſupinum*, Tourn. Inſt. *Heliotropium humi fuſum, flore minimo, ſemine magno*, Tourn. Small Turnſole. It grows in Gardens; the Herb is uſed, which has all the Virtues of the proceeding aſcrib'd to it.

Heliotropium tricoccum, Offic. *Heliotropium minus quorundam; Heliotropium tricoccum Plinii, Verrucaria*, Chab. *Ricinus humilis Althææ folio, fructu verrucoſo rotundo*, Hiſt. Oxon. French-Turnſole. This Plant grows in ſeveral Parts of *Languedoc*, and flowers in *July* and *Auguſt.* The Natives of *Languedoc* expreſs the Juice of the Berries of this Plant, with which they ſtrongly impregnate Linnen Rags, and it is thus brought to us, and ſold in the Shops for the Uſe of the Dyers. It is, alſo, uſed in Medicine, and is a moſt powerful Remedy againſt carcinomatous and gangrenous Ulcers, and ſtrumous Tumors, according to *Matthiolus.*

Helleborine, Offic. *Helleborine latifolia montana*, C. B. Pin. Boerh. Ind. Alt. Baſtard Hellebore. It grows in Copſes, Woods, and ſhady Places, and flowers in *May.* The Herb is uſed, and is thought by ſome to poſſeſs the ſame Virtues as the white Hellebore, but it is ſeldom or never found in our Shops.

Helleborus albus, Elleborus, Offic. *Helleborus albus, flore ſubviridi*, C. B. P. White Hellebore. It grows in mountainous and craggy Places, principally in *Germany.* The Leaves, Roots, Stalk, or Flowers of white Hellebore, applied to the Skin of a living Perſon, excoriate the Part, and produce an Exulceration: They alſo burn the Tongue. The true white Hellebore of *Hippocrates* is celebrated on many Accounts. This Plant has a Cauſtic and burning Juice, which attracted into the Noſtrils, after the Manner of Snuff, excites an invincible Sneezing, whence it appears to be a Ptarmic in the higheſt Degree. Taken into the Stomach it purges upwards and downwards with ſevere Gripings. *Hippocrates* ſays, that it purges the moſt remote Parts of the Blood, and therefore, before its Adminiſtration, he cauſed his Patients to bathe, and ordered them to drink Oil and Honey for ſome Days; by which Means all the Parts being relaxed, he then adminiſtered white Hellebore, and directed Geſtation, either on Horſeback, or in a Ship; When the Medicine began to work, he ordered his Patients reſt. The

ſame

same Effect would indeed, in some Measure, follow from a right Use of our white Hellebore. But *Salmasius* writing of the *Veratrum*, or white Hellebore, says, that its Leaves are very finely jagged, which makes it doubted whether it be the same with ours. White Hellebore is much stronger than black Hellebore, and sometimes excites Convulsions, unless exhibited with great Prudence: Hence it is never given in Substance, but to Persons of the most robust Constitutions; and in melancholy and maniac Cases; and then with great Caution. It is also exhibited in quartan Fevers; in which an Ounce of the Decoction, taken inwardly, has often surprising Effects. It is a Plant, however, more adapted to Horses than Men; though used as a Sternutatory in soporous Diseases, as the Apoplexy and Lethargy. White Hellebore has been celebrated, even to a Proverb, for the Cure of Maniacs, and *Hippocrates* particularly recommends it in many Cases, and mentions a μαλθακὶς ἐλλέβορος, *soft or soften'd Hellebore*, which was probably Hellebore prepar'd in such a manner as to render its Operation milder, and in most Cases he directs it after Supper, intending by that Means, probably, to mix it with the Aliments in the Stomach, that it might operate more gently and safely. *Hesophilus* is also said to have entertain'd a very great Opinion of this Cathartic. *Aretaus* asserts, that it is not only a Vomit, but, also, the most efficacious and powerful Purge of all others: This good Service it does, he says, is not owing to the great Discharge of Humours it makes; nor in the Cholera Morbus, there is the same Sort of Evacuation; nor is it owing to the violent Efforts it causes; for sailing upon the Sea excites more violent Efforts: But it is owing to a particular Virtue in it, which cannot be enough admired;

for though sometimes it purges but little, yet it nevertheless cures. In old Disorders, where all other Remedies have failed, Hellebore has succeeded. To those that breathe difficultly, it renders Respiration easy; to such as are pale it gives Colour, and makes those plump that were before emaciated. But notwithstanding all those Encomiums, white Hellebore by some Means lost its Reputation, and was but little used for many Years, till about the Year 500 *Asclepiodorus* a Physician, as we learn from *Photius*, revived its Use, curing many obstinate Distempers by it, and thereby acquiring great Reputation. At present I don't know that it is much used, except as an Errhine, and an Ingredient in Ointments for the Itch. But I have known it given by *Empirics*, in very large Quantities, without exciting any violent Symptoms, and even alone without any Corrector; and I also know that it has been given in Maniacal Cases, in the Quantity of eighteen Grains, together with twelve Grains of Castor, and in such a large Dose, without any Operation that was terrible, and with very great and good Effects to the Patient. I do not recommend this Practice, but rather leave it to the Consideration of proper Judges. Mean Time in Maniacal Cases, or others, where a violent Stimulation is necessary, as in Apoplexies, in which last Case it is recommended by *Celsus*, Hellebore either in Clysters, or taken into the Stomach, will certainly answer the Intention of stimulating in a very great Degree.

Helleborus niger, Offic. *Helleborus niger flore roseo*, C. B. P. Black Hellebore. It is cultivated in Botanic Gardens, flowering in *January*. The Root, especially the fibrous Parts of it, is used, and is said by almost all Authors, to purge powerfully melancholic Humours; but that which we make

make Use of in *England*, is so far from operating violently, that it scarcely purges at all, tho' given from fifteen Grains to two Scruples. It is particularly recommended in Madness, in the hypochondriac Passion and Elephantiasis, Herpes, Cancer, Quartan, Vertigo, Epilepsy, Apoplexy, and the Itch; but its great Excellence consists in promoting the Menses, and carrying off the Waters in a Dropsy. It is given either in Substance, Infusion, Decoction, or Tincture. M. *Balduc* gives some Experiments, which he made upon this Root, in the *Memoirs of the Academy of Sciences*, for the Year 1701. We shall not take Notice of those made by Distillation, because he himself believ'd them to be of no Consequence. The Extract which he procured with Spirit of Wine was very little in Quantity, because this Root contains few resinous Parts. And I am, says he, the more confirmed in this, since from what remained I was able to get a great Quantity of an Extract with Water. He also made an Extract of the Root with Water, wherewith was drawn all that could be extracted; for from the Residue there was nothing to be got, by Means of Spirit of Wine. Whence it seems reasonable to conclude, that the saline Parts are able so to dissolve its few resinous ones, that both may be drawn off by Water, without the Aid of Spirit of Wine. He further remark'd, that the first Extract, which was purely resinous, and made with Spirit of Wine, purged little, and with Irritation; that the Extract made of its Remainder, with Water, purged not at all, but was very diuretic; and, that, on the other Hand, the Extract made first with Water, and without Spirit of Wine purged gently. And this, he says, he has observed of most Purgatives: Whence he thinks, that the Extract, made by Spirit of Wine alone, ought

to be suspected; since, being depriv'd of its proper Salts, which, when joined to the Ferment of the Stomach, open, divide, and attenuate the Resin, it happens that its thick and sulphureous Parts adhere to the Fibres of the Stomach, and cause Gripings, and, by remaining undissolved sometime, excite a Tenesmus. And this is confirm'd by Experience; for the most able practical Physicians correct the Resin with Salt of Tartar. He confesses that to be a good Method in these Cases; but supposes one may do without it, by leaving to those resinous Extracts the proper Salts which Nature has endued them with. Whence he affirms, that the Way of making the Extract with Water is preferable to the common Way of doing it by a sulphureous Menstruum; since thereby the Substance is freed from its terrestrial Parts, without depriving it of any of its natural Principles. He takes Notice, that the Hellebore which is brought from *Switzerland*, is preferable to that which comes by the Way of *England*. This latter, whether it is spoiled by keeping, or losing its Virtue in Transportation, he found to have little or no Effect. So that, there is Reason to suspect very much, that our Hellebore falls greatly short of the Goodness of that used by the Antients; since we find there is so great a Difference between it, and what so near Neighbours as the *French* have in Use among them at this Time. Of ours, according to *Quincy*, fifteen or twenty Grains, in Powder, are frequently given as an Alterative and a Sudorific; and in Tincture, where the Root has been one Part, and the Menstruum three, it may be given to sixty, or one hundred Drops to a Dose. Its Virtues are best drawn, by rubbing a little Salt of Tartar with it in a gross Powder, and letting it lie till the Air makes it run; for that so penetrates

into

into the very Substance of the Root. that its Parts immediately join with the Menstruum, as soon almost as put into it. Small Wine is the best, as most likely to take up all the Parts of any medicinal Efficacy.

Helleborus niger hortensis, flore viridi, C. B. P. *Helleboraster,* Offic. *Helleboraster minor flore viridante,* Park. Theat. Bears Foot. It grows in mountainous Places, flowering in *March* and *April.* The Parts used in Medicine are the Root and Leaves. The Leaves taken in Beer are recommended for the Small Pox, and against contagious Distempers. The Root has the same Virtues with that of the black Hellebore, and may be taken instead of it ; it purges the lower Belly, evacuating Phlegm, and yellow Bile. Farriers and Graziers put a great deal of Confidence in this Herb, against the Murrain among their Horses and Cattle. Their Method is to thrust a Bodkin thro' the Dewlaps of their black Cattle, thro' the Skin under the Neck of their Horses, and through the Ears of their Sheep, and then put a Fibre of the Root into the Wound; whence it is called *Peg Root.* The same is described by *Columella,* one of the *Rei Rusticæ Scriptores,* who wrote under the Empire *Claudius.*

Helleborus niger fætidus, C. B. P. *Helleborastrum,* Offic. *Helleboraster maximus, five Consiligo,* Park. Theat. Setter-Wort. It grows in woody Places, though but rarely, flowering in *February* and *March.* The Leaves are used, which, being dried and pulveriz'd, are exhibited in small Quantities to Children affected with Worms; and are esteem'd, by the common Sort of People, a most potent and certain Remedy : But *Tragus* very well observes, that it is not to be used internally, but avoided as a most pernicious Herb. How dangerous a Medicine it is, may be understood by the following Accident, related by

Dr. Martyn. Some Years ago, when the Ground was cover'd with a very deep Snow, a Flock of Sheep, in *Ox-Mead,* near *Fulbern* in *Cambridgeshire,* finding nothing but this Herb above the Snow; eat plentifully of it. They soon appear'd terribly out of Order, and most of them died, a few being saved, by timely giving some Oil, which made them cast up this Herb. Some of those which died, being open'd, were found to have their Stomachs greatly inflam'd. I myself once was Witness of the deleterious Effects of this Plant. A strolling Quack, sold a Worm Powder to an elderly Gentlewoman in the Country who kept an Inn, which she gave to several Grand Children who lived with her, with good Success ; but one Dose being left, she took that herself, and about an Hour after, was very much disorder'd ; I happen'd at that time to be talking to a Gentleman on the other Side of the Street, and was press'd by one of her Domestics to visit her immediately, which I did directly, but she dy'd before I could get up Stairs.

Hemionitis, Offic Boerh. Ind. Alt. *Hemionium five Hemionitis quibusdam Splenium,* Chab. Mules Fern. It is said to grow in *Italy.* The Herb is used, which taken in Vinegar, according to *Dioscorides,* consumes the Spleen. *Bobart* says, it is a splenetic Herb, and possesses the same Virtues as the Harts-tongue; and *Boerhaave* esteems it an astringent, vulnerary, and pectoral Plant, efficacious in splenetic Disorders, as also Spittings of Blood

Hepatica trifolia cæruleo flore, Boerh. Ind. Alt. *Trifolium aureum, Hepatica nobilis,* Offic. *Trifolium Hepaticum five Trinitatis Herba flore cæruleo,* J. B. Noble Liverwort. It grows in Gardens, and flowers in the Spring. The Leaves only are used, which by modern Physicians are thought vulnerary ; they corroborate

rate the Stomach by their aftrin-
at Quality, and therefore are e-
xm'd good where there is too
eat a Relaxation, and confequently
e ufeful in vulnerary Drinks, in a
abetes, Spittings of Blood, or bloody
rine, they are much extolled in
ernias; the Leaves pulverized are
od in Dyfenteries. A Decoction
the Leaves is effectual againft
: Jaundice, Itch, fetid Ulcers, and
e Quinfey. The whole Plant is
ry good in Obftructions of the
idneys, Bladder, and Liver. The
uch make it an Ingredient in the
rup of Succory.

Herba Paris, Offic. Boerh. Ind.
k. *Solanum quadrifolium bacciferum*,
. B. Pin. Herb Paris. It grows in
ady Places, and flowers in *May*;
d the Berries, which are ufed in
ledicine, are ripe in *July*. Thefe
ken internally, are alexipharmic;
e Leaves bruifed, and reduced into
Cataplafm, and applied, are good
all peftilential Buboes, and other
x Tumors; the Plant is very good
ainft Madnefs. *Tachenius* recom-
ends it as good in Sciatic Pains;
elmoat in livid Contufions; and
xbaum, adminifter'd it with Suc-
is in hyfteric Diforders. This
lant was formerly accounted poi-
nous, and rank'd among the Aco-
ites, which is thought to be owing
) *Fuchfius*'s calling it *Aconitum Par-
alianches*, yet more modern Au-
hors attribute quite different Effects
) it, efteeming it a Counter-poifon,
ad Alexipharmic, and good in ma-
ignant and peftilential Fevers.

Hermodactylus, Offic. Park. Col-
hicum radice ficcata alba, C. B. P.
Hermodactyls. According to the
Hiftory of Plants afcribed to *Boer-
have*, this Plant purges moft power
ully both upwards and downwards,
n Confequence whereof, it is re-
ommended in the Gout as a pow-
aful Cathartic; it is, alfo, commend-
d as a Specific in the *Gutta Serena*;

on Account of its Vifcofity, it is
mixed with Ginger, being greatly
fubject to excite Gripes.

Herniaria, Offic. *Herniaria glabra*, J. B. *Millegrana major five
Herniaria vulgaris*, Park. Theat.
Rupture Wort It grows in fandy
Places, and flowers in *June* and *July*; the whole Plant is ufed in Medicine, and is refrigerating and drying;
it is chiefly ufed in the Cure of Ruptures, it provokes Urine, breaks the
Stone in the Kidneys and Bladder,
incides Mufcofities in the Stomach
and other Parts, expels Bile and
Water, and confequently is efficacious in the Jaundice.

Herniaria Alfines folio, Tourn.
Inft. *Arenaria*, Offic. *Anthyllis marina incana Alfine-folia*, Ger. Emac.
Sea Chick-weed. It grows in maritime Places, and Vineyards, and
flowers in Summer. The Herb,
which is the Part ufed in Medicine,
cures a *Paronychia*, and the *Favi*, being rubbed thereon.

Hefperis, Offic. *Hefperis hortenfis
flore purpureo & albo*, Boerh. Ind.
A. *Hefperis flore purpureo albo &
vario, five Viola Matronalis*, Park.
Theat. Dame Violets. They grow
in Gardens, and flower in *May* and
June. The Plant and Seeds are ufed,
which, as *Clufius* fays, cure Coughs,
and Difficulties of Breathing. *John
Bauhine* fays they provoke Urine,
and Sweat, that they incide, abfterge,
and digeft. *Dodonaus* fays, that as
it taftes like Rocket, fo it feems to
be poffeffed of much the fame Virtues.

Hieracium minus, Offic. *Hieracium folio Chondrilla, caule viminco
levi*, Boerh. Ind. A. *Hieracium minus praemorfa radice*, Park. The
Leffer Hawkweed. It grows almoft
in all Pafture Grounds, and flowers in
June and *July*. The Leaves are ufed, but the Juice feldom or never;
it fharpens the Sight taken inwardly, and expells black Bile.

Hieracium,

Hieracium, Offic. *Hieracium dentis Leonis obtuso folio mojus*, C. B. Pin. *Hieracium macrocaulon junceum five minus primum Dodonæo*, J B. Long rooted Hawkweed. It grows in Pasture Grounds, and flowers in *June, July*, and *August*. The Leaves are commonly used, which have the Virtues of the other Species of this Plant, the Herb taken internally is a Remedy for Pains in the Sides.

Hieracium Clusii, Ger. *Hieracium alpinum, latifolium, maculatum, hirsutie incanum, flore magno*, Boerh. Ind. A. *Herba Costa*, Offic. Hungarian Hawkweed. It grows on Chalky Hills, and flowers in *June*; the Herb is used, which is greatly extolled in all Diseases of the Lungs. It is of singular Use in Consumptions.

Hippocastanum vulgare, Boerh. Ind. A. *Castanea equina*, Ger. *Castanea equina folio multifido*, J. B. Horse Chesnut. It is cultivated in Gardens and Walks, and flowers in *May* and *June*; the Fruit is used which is esteemed Errhine, it is likewise said to be good for broken winded Horses.

Hippophaes, Hippophæstum, and *Hippomanes*, Offic. *Hippophaes Anguillaræ & Dodonæi, sive Spina purgatrix*, J. B. Purging Thorn. It grows in the *Morea*; the Juice of this is said to carry off by Stool all pituitous Humours.

Hordeum, Offic. *Hordeum distichum*, Ger. *Hordeum distichon quod Spica binas ordines habeat Plinio*, C. B. Pin. Boerh. Ind. A. Barley. It is sow'd in the Spring in Fields. The Seed is used, which is refrigerating, drying, abstergent, aperient, digestive, and emollient; it is also diuretic and nutritive. *Bartholine* cured an epidemical Pleurisy only by a Decoction of Barley. It is an Ingredient in the *Decoctum Pectorale*.

Horminum Sylvestre Lavendulæ flore, C. B. P. *Oculus Christi*, Offic. *Gallitrichis affinis Maru, si non Genus*

aliquod, Sclarea Hispanica, J. B. Wild Clary. It grows in gravelly Places and flowers in *June* and *July*. The Seed is chiefly used, one of which if put into the Eye cleanses it of any Thing that is offensive, and takes away Redness, Specks, or Inflammations.

Horminum sativum, Offic. *Horminum sativum genuinum Dioscoridis* Park. Theat. *Horminum Coma purpuro-violacea*, J. B. Purple spiked Clary. It grows in the Gardens of the Curious, and flowers in *July*. The Seed is used, which drank in Wine is esteem'd a potent Stimulus to Venery. Mixed with Honey it clears the Eyes from white Specks. It stimulates the Nerves, and inebriates, and its heating Quality renders it very serviceable in the Dropsy.

Horminum sylvestre, Offic. *Horminum sylvestre latifolium verticillatum*, C. B. Pin. *Horminum Germanicum humile*, Park. Theat. Wild Clary. It grows frequently in *Germany*, and flowers in Summer, the Seed is used, and is said to possess all the Virtues of the preceding Species, but in a higher Degree.

Hyacinthus, Offic. *Hyacinthus Anglicus*, Ger. *Hyacinthus oblongo flore cæruleus major*, C. B. Pin. Hare Bells. They grow in Woods and Hedges and flower in *April*. The Root is used, which stops Fluxes of all Kinds, provokes Urine, and is of Service in the Jaundice.

Hyoscyamus, Offic. *Hyoscyamus major*, Ger. *Hyoscyamus major vel vulgaris*, Boerh. Ind. A. Henbane. It grows in uncultivated Places, amongst Rubbish, and by Ditch Sides, and flowers in *June*. The Parts used in Medicine are the Root and Herb. It is refrigerating and wonderfully emollient, induces Sleep, mitigates violent Pains, and Acrimony, but disturbs the Reason, whence it is but very seldom exhibited internally, yet is sometimes so administred to ease

Spitting

Spitting of Blood. The Seeds are exhibited in Hæmorrhages; from the Seeds is prepared an Oil which induces Sleep by anointing the Temples therewith, it is used in a Gonorrhæa and too copious Fluxes of the Menses applied to the Region of the Loins and the Perinæum.

Hyoscyamus albus, Offic. *Hyoscyamus, albus major, vel tertius Dioscoridis, & quartus Plinii,* Boerh. Ind. A. Hift. Oxon. White Henbane. It grows, tho' but seldom, in Botanic Gardens. The Seeds are only introduced into Medicine, which are exhibited to cure Spitting of Blood; they are of a milder Nature and consequently safer in the Administration, than those of the preceeding Species. The Juice of this Species is very good in an inveterate Cough, proceeding from a Defluxion of saltish acrimonious Humours, the dreadful Forerunner of a Pthisis, in order to prevent which the *Egyptians* before they betake themselves to rest, take a Spoonful of the Seeds, finely triturated with an equal Quantity of powder Sugar, by which they procure considerable Relief, by its blunting and sweetning the Acrimony of the saltish Humours, and inducing Sleep; their Women do the same, for an immoderate Flux of the Menses. The Juice expressed from the green Stalks, Flowers and Seeds, or the dried Plant, macerated in warm Water and then bruised, mitigates acute Pains especially of the Eyes, for which purpose Collyriums were prepared of it, and the same Preparation was used, for violent Pains in the Ears, tho' in the Opinion of modern Practitioners, all those Medicines which take away the Sense of Pain, and which were called *Narcotics* cannot but be pernicious if too frequently used, for what takes away the Sense of Pain, must diminish the sensitive Faculty.

Hypecoum, Offic. *Hypecoum latiore folio,* Boerh. Ind, A. *Hypecoum siliquosum,* J. B. Horned Wild Cummim. It grows in *Provence* and *Languedoc,* and flowers in *May.* The Herb and Juice are used. According to *Dioscorides,* it possesses the same Virtues as the Poppy, nor do the modern Accounts differ any thing from his. *Herman* says, that its Juice induces Sleep as well as *Opium.*

Hypericum, Offic. *Hypericum vulgare, five perforata caule rotundo, foliis glabris,* J. B. *Hypericum vulgare, perforata, Fuga Dæmonum,* Merc. Bot. St. *John*'s Wort. This grows in Hedges and Thickets, and flowers in *July.* The Herb, Flowers and Seeds are used; they consist of subtile Parts, are Diuretic and Vulnerary. They are chiefly used in cleansing and consolidating Wounds, in resolving coagulated Blood, in dissolving the Stone in the Kidneys, and killing Worms. Outwardly applied it is reckon'd good in Contusions, especially those of the Nerves, as also in Tremors and Wounds. The Tincture of the Flowers is good in Maniac Disorders. It is an Ingredient in the *Mithridate,* the *Theriaca Andromachi,* and the *Oleum Hyperici.*

Hypocistis, Offic. *Purpurea flore candicante & flore luteo,* T. Coral, *Minor a Cisto Nascens,* Hift. Ox. Rape of Cistus. The Juice is used, which is refrigerating, drying, most powerfully astringent and condensating; it is chiefly used in stopping Fluxes of any Kind, Diarrhæas, Dysenteries, Lientery, immoderate menstrual Discharges, Vomitings, and Hemorrhages. It is an Ingredient in the *Pulvis e Succo compositus, Mithridatium,* and *Theriaca Andromachi.*

Hyssopus, Offic. *Hyssopus vulgaris,* Park. Theat. *Hyssopus officinarum cærulea five spicata,* Boerh. Ind. Alt. Hyssop. It grows in Gardens, and flowers in *July* and *August.* The

Herb

Herb is used, which is attenuating, aperient, and abstergent. It is chiefly used in all tartareous Disorders of the Lungs, Coughs, and Asthmas. It is often externally applied in Sugillations of the Eyes, to cleanse the Uterus, to remove Noise in the Ears, and to cleanse the Mouth. Some prefer it to Wormwood for fortifying the Stomach.

Jacea, Offic. *Jacea nigra pratensis latifolia,* C. B. Pin. *Jacea nigra vulgaris,* Park. Knapweed or Matfellon. It is too frequent in Pasture Grounds, flowering in *July* and *August.* The Herb is used, which is good against Tumors of the Tonsils, Hernias and Wounds.

Jacea foliis Cichoraceis, altissima, flore purpureo, Tourn. *Stoebe,* Offic. *Stoebe major foliis Cichoraceis mollibus lanuginosis,* C. B. Silver Knapweed. It grows with us in Gardens, and flowers in *July.* The Herb and Seed are used, which are both astringent, wherefore a Decoction is good for those who labour under a Dysentery. It is likewise instilled into purulent Ears; a Linctus prepared of the Leaves, removes Lividness, occasioned by Blows about the Eyes, and stops violent Eruptions of Blood.

Jacobæa, Offic. *Jacobæa vulgaris laciniata,* Boerh. Ind. A. *Jacobæa vulgaris major,* Park. Ragwort, or Seggrum. It grows in watery Places near Path Ways, and uncultivated Places, and flowers in *July* and *August.* The Herb is used, which has the same Virtues as Groundsel. It cures all Wounds, Inflammations, and Fistulas ; applied in the Form of a Cataplasm, it is good against the Gripes from a violent Dysentery ; of it is prepared an excellent Gargarism against the Quinsy, and Inflammations of the Tonsils.

Jalapium Mechoacana nigra, Offic. *Convolvulus Americanus, Jalapium dictus,* Raii Hist. *Bryonia Mechoacana nigricans,* C. B. Pin. Jalap. The Root is used, which is brought to us from the *Indies,* the Root only is used which powerfully purges all noxious, but more in particular, all serous Humours. *Wepfer* in his Treatise *de Cicuta Aquatica* says, it is one of the best Cathartics we have, and wonders it is so little used, since it wants no Corrector on one Hand, nor any thing on the other to promote its Operation, which can hardly be said of any other Purgative; as one Part of the Root may abound more with the purgative Quality than an other the Dose of the Resin is much more certain.

Jasminum, Offic. *Jasminum album,* Ger. *Jasminum sive Gelseminum flore albo,* J. B. White Jasmine, or Jessamy. It is cultivated in Gardens, and flowers in Summer, the Flowers are used, which are digestive, heating, emollient, and aperient ; its internal Use is principally to heat and relax the Uterus, and to cure a Schirrus; it promotes Delivery, is good for a Cough and Difficulty of Breathing, Pleurify, and Pains of the Stomach, Intestines, and Uterus.

Ilex aculeata cocciglandifera, C. B. Pin. Boerh. Ind. Alt. *Ilex aquifolia sive Coccigera,* Park. Theat. The Scarlet Oak. The Produce of this Plant used in Medicine, is the *Kermes.*

Ilex folio rotundiori molli modiceque sinuato, sive Smilax Theophrasti, C. B. Pin. *Smilax Arborea,* Offic. *Smilax Arcadum glandifera, major,* Park. Theat. The great Scarlet Oak. This is frequent in *Italy* and *Languedoc,* the Bark Leaves, and Acorns are used, which are esteem'd more astringent than those of the Oak.

Imperatoria major, C. B. P. Boerh. Ind. A. *Imperatoria & Astrantia,* Offic. Master Wort. It is cultivated in Gardens, and flowers in *August.* The Part used in Medicine, is the Root which is both Alexipharmic and Sudorific ; it is chiefly used in contagious

tagious Diftempers and Contufi-
s, in phlegmatic Diforders of the
ead, Palfy, Apoplexy, and in Cru-
ties of the Stomach, and the Colic;
is a moft divine Remedy in the
olic, and flatulent Diforders, ac-
rding to *Hoffman.*

Indicum, Offic. *Emerus America-
u Siliqua incurva,* Tourn. Inft.
Polygala Indica frutefcens Hermanni,
aii Hift. Blue Indigo. This is a
ell known Preparation from a Plant
hich grows in Brafil, to the Height
f two or three Feet, refembling
Rofemary. This Preparation is ge-
erally thought to be of an attenuating and penetrating Nature, in
Confequence of which it is faid to be
beneficial in a Jaundice. It furpri-
ingly ftops Fluxes, becaufe it is a
ftrong Aftringent. In *Ephimer. Ger.
Ann. 11. Obf.* 113. it is recommended for ftopping immoderate Difcharges of the Lochia, and for curing a
falling down of the Uterus and A-
nus. *Indigo* was formerly thought
to be poffeffed of a poifonous Quality, and according to *Paulus Ammanus,* it was once accounted of fo
corrofive a Nature, that, the Elec-
tors of *Saxony,* prohibited the Im-
portation of it into their Territories.

Ipecacuanha, Offic. Pomet. *Ipecacuanha Brafilienfibus,* Raii Hift. *Pe-
riclymeno, accedens Planta, Barfi-
liana, flofculis congeftis albis,* Brafilian
Root. This is the Root of a Plant
produced in *Brafil, New Spain,* and
various other Parts. There are generally three Kinds of it found in the
Shops, the Grey, the Brown, and
the White; the Grey is generally reckon'd beft, and moft commonly
ufed, when it can be had. Great
Care ought to be taken in our Choice
of this Root, fince according to Sir
Hans Sloan, in his natural Hiftory of
Jamaica, there is a poifonous *Apocynum* whofe Root greatly refembles
it. Mr. *Boulduc* after reiterated chymical Analyfes, of thefe three Kinds
of the Root, found that their Vir-

tues confifted not only in their Refin,
but alfo in their faline Parts. This
curious Gentleman alfo found Means
to deprive this Root of its emetic
Quality, the Difference between this
and other violent Purgatives having
encourag'd him in this Refearch;
the other draftic Cathartics as Scammony and Coloquintida, however
prepar'd or corrected, leaving too
often, fatal Marks of their Action,
whereas Ipecacuanha, tho' it may
appear very brifk in its Operation,
leaves generally behind it no more
than an Aftriction of the Part it had
before opened, and fatigued. He
made a refinous Extract with
Spirit of Wine, and then drew
out the faline Particles with
Rain-water, and found by Experience that its Violence, as in moft
other Purgatives, was owing to its
Refin. For the Effects of the Refin
were more violent than thofe of the
Root itfelf, leaving little or no A-
ftriction afterwards; but the faline
Extract, was diuretic, purg'd gently, with little or no Naufea, and in
fhort was poffeffed of the fpecific
Quality of the Root in curing Dyfenteries. The Root is given from
fifteen Grains to half a Dram, and
we ought never to exceed a Dram.
It never fatigues the Stomach, and
is the beft Succedaneum for emetic
Tartar. It is the beft Specific in Dyfenteries hitherto known, acting in
fuch Cafes, not only as an emetic,
but alfo deterging Ulcers in the Inteftines by a Mucilage contain'd in it,
like that of Marfhmallows, by which
it in fome Meafure fupplies the villous Coat of the Inteftines, when
corroded and deftroy'd by the Difeafe. It alfo powerfully agitates and
evacuates the Glands of thefe Parts.
Its moft celebrated Effects are thofe
produc'd in cold Dyfenteries after
many other Medicines have been
tried, and the Body has by thefe been
fufficiently prepared. Then the firft
or fecond Dofe, generally produces
vifibly

visibly happy Effects, or if it should happen otherwise, it ought to be continued every Day, in the Quantity of three or four Grains, acting in that Case as an Alterative. This Root has at once an emplastic and detersive Quality, and tho' it does appear sensibly, acrid, yet it produces, in those who powder it, an Oppression of the Thorax, Difficulty of Breathing, and Spitting of Blood. It is likewise offensive to the Eyes, increases the Discharge of the lachrymal Glands, and when the Tears do not find a ready Vent, produces a Swelling of the Eyes. These Effects are probably owing to the mucilaginous Quality of the Root. It is used in Substance, reduced to a fine Powder, either mixed with a Liquid, or incorporated with some proper Syrup into an Opiate. It may likewise be given in Infusion, Decoction, or Tincture.

Iris vulgaris nostras, Offic. *Iris vulgaris,* Raii Hist. Common Flower-de-Luce. This is by Transplantation into Gardens render'd more beautiful, flowering in *May.* The Root when recent is of a drying Nature, and is used as an Hydragogue, and Errhine. It is principally employ'd in evacuating the Waters of dropsical Patients. Externally it is used in Impetigos, and for removing other Defedations of the Skin.

Iris florentina, Iris Illyrica, Offic. *Iris alba florentina,* C. B. Tourn. Inst. Florentine Orris. This is cultivated in Gardens, and flowers in *May.* Its Root is of a fragrant Smell, and possessed of an inciding, attenuating, expectorating, digerent, abstergent, and emollient Quality. It is principally used in Obstructions and Infarctions of the Lungs, Coughs, Asthmas, Obstructions of the Menses, and Gripes in Children. Externally it beautifies the Skin, removes Freckles, and sweetens the Breath.

Iris fœtida, spatula fœtida, Xyris, Offic. *Iris fœtidissima seu Xyris,* Tourn. Inst. Stinking Gladdon. This grows in Hedges and Thickets, flowers in *June,* and is rarely to be met with. The Root is used, which is of a drying Nature, and principally recommended in the King's Evil, hysteric Passion, Orthopnœa, and hypocondriac Disorders.

Iris humilis seu Chamæiris angustifolia graminea, Herm. Cat. *Iris angustifolia prunum redolens major & minor,* C. B. Pin. Tourn. Inst. Grass-leaved Flower-de-Luce. This is cultivated in Gardens, and flowers in *May.* The Herb itself is used, and is said to agree in Virtues with the first mention'd Species.

Jujuba, Offic. *Ziziphus sive Jujuba major,* Raii Hist. *Ziziphus,* Tourn. Inst. Boerh. Ind. Alt. The Jujube Tree. This is cultivated in the Gardens of *Spain* and *Italy.* The Fruit is used, being moderately heating and moistening. It is principally recommended in Asperities of the Lungs, Coughs, Pleurisies, Acrimony of the Urine, Effervescence of the Blood, and Erosions of the Kidneys and Bladder.

Oenoplia, Offic. *Oenoplia spinosa & non spinosa,* Ger. Emac. Raii Hist. The Great Jujube. This grows in *Egypt, Crete,* and some other Countries. The Fruit is used, and when immature is of an astringent Quality, removing the Relaxation of the Stomach and Intestines. The Juice of the ripe Fruit purges the Stomach of Bile.

Jujuba Indica, Raii Hist. *Jujuba Indica, rotundifolia, spinosa, foliis majoribus, subtus lanuginosis & incanis.* Breyn Prod. Commel. flor. Mal. The Lacca Tree of which only the Gum is used in the Shops. This Gum is distinguish'd into three Kinds. First, the *Stick-lack,* which is a resinous, hard and friable Substance, of an unequal granulated Surface, of a red Colour, a resinous Taste, and of a grateful Smell

smell whilst burning. Secondly, The *seed lac*, which consists of resinous, and and friable Grains, of a reddish Colour, pellucid, and of the same Taste and Smell with the preceeding. Thirdly, *Shell-lac*, which is made of the purest Grains melted into a Mass, of a reddish Colour and almost tranf- arent. This Gum is heating, atte- nuating and aperient. It also puri- fies the Blood, excites Sweat, and is diuretic. It is principally recom- mended in Obstructions of the Spleen, Gall Bladder, Liver and Lungs, for which Reason it is accounted benefi- cial in the Dropsy and Jaundice.

Juncus vulgaris, Offic. *Juncus læ- vis, panicula sparsâ, major.* C. B. Pin. Boerh. Ind. Alt. Common Soft Rush. This grows in marshy Places.

Juncus acutus capitulis Sorgi, C. B. Pin. Raii Hift. Boerh. Ind. Alt. Pricking large Sea-Rush. This grows in maritime Places, and the Herb and its Seeds are us'd.

Juncus aquaticus maximus, Ger. Emac. Raii Hift. Boerh. Ind. Alt. Bull-Rush. This grows in Rivers and large Fish-Ponds. The whole Plant is us'd. The Seeds of these three Species when roasted stop Fluxes and the excessive menstrual Discharges of Women. They also provoke U- rine and procure Sleep. The Plant when tender, is applied externally against the Bites of the Phalangium, a Sort of highly venomous Spider.

Juncus odoratus sive Aromaticus, C. B. Pin. *Gramen ad Junceum acce- dens Aromaticum mojus Syriacum*, Hift. Oxon. Camels-Hay. This is brought from *Arabia*. Its Top and Leaves are us'd, being of an acrid, bitterish, and as it were sweetish Taste, and of an highly grateful Smell. It is heating, subaftringent, attenuating and difcutient. It is principally us'd in Obstructions of the Menfes, of the Liver and Spleen, in Inflations of the Stomach, Vomitting and Hiccup; in Difficulty of Urine,

and Pains of the Kidnies, Bladder and Uterus.

Juniperus, Offic. *Juniperus vulga- ris fruticofa*, C. B. Pin. Tourn. Inst. Boerh. Ind. Alt. The Juniper-Tree, or Bush. It grows in Thickets, and the Wood, Berries, and Gum are us'd. The Gum, which is the Gum-*San- darac* of the *Arabians*, is a resinous, dry, whitish, pale Substance, con- creted into Drops, of a resinous Taste. By a chymical Analysis we obtain from Juniper a fix'd Salt, loaded with a great deal of more Acid than is necessary to saturate it. Thus by a chymical Analysis of Ju- niper, we obtain several acid Liquors, and a fix'd, but no volatile Salt. 'Tis to be obferv'd, that the Plant is in- volv'd in a great deal of Sulphur, and fome terreftrial Parts. Juniper- wood yields, befides the etherial Oil, a great deal of Oil thicken'd to the Confiftence of a Syrup. Its Berries yield a great deal more, and its Tops a little lefs. It is no hard Matter to perceive that all thefe Principles fhould render the Juniper good to reftore the Functions of the Stomach, to diffipate Wind and other Sub- ftances which produce acute Pains, to clear the Lungs, and evacuate that grofs Lymph, which often occafions Difficulty of Breathing. The Plant is alfo sudorific, cephalic, and anti- hyfteric. It provokes the Menfes, removes Obftructions of the Vifcera, reftores their Elafticity, and gives a free Paffage to the Urine. The Wood, the Tops and Berries are us'd. A Decoction of the Wood volatilizes the Blood, and purifies it by infenfible Perfpiration, much after the Manner of *Guoiacum*. A Semi- cupium prepar'd with this Wood, gives great Eafe to thofe afflicted with the Gout. The Wine in which the Tops of Juniper have been boil'd is very diuretic. *Tragus, Matthiolus, Hartman*, and *Simon Pauli* affirm, that they have cur'd fome Perfons of

a Dropfy

a Dropſy, by Means of this Wine. The Honey of Juniper, which is no more than the Berries boil'd with Honey, is excellent in Clyſters for the Dyſentery and Teneſmus. It is cuſtomary to burn the Fruit of this Plant in order to remove a peſtilential Air, and an Infuſion of it in Vinegar is us'd in the Time of the Plague to waſh Letters, Linen, and common Utenſils. The celebrated *Frederic Hoffman*, in *Tr. de Præſtantia Remed. Domeſt.* ſpeaks in the following manner, " The " whole of the Juniper Tree is poſ- " ſeſs'd of a medicinal Quality, be- " cauſe the Whole of it is balſamic. " Its Wood is ſo far from being in- " ferior to the exotic Woods Guai- " acum and Saſſafras, that it may " not only be commodiouſly us'd as " a Succedaneum to them; but, is " alſo preferable to them in my " Opinion, in all Diſorders ariſing " from an impure State of the Hu- " mours. Its Berries in Conſequence " of the large Quantity of balſamic " Oil they contain, whether uſed in " Subſtance, reduc'd to a Rob, or " toaſted and uſed with Water by " Way of Coffee, are highly effica- " cious in all thoſe Diſorders which " ariſe from Obſtructions of the " Viſcera, or a thick and viſcid Con- " dition of the Blood; for which " Reaſon they are of great Service, " in Aſthmas, Cachexies, the Jaun- " dice, the Colic, the Stone of the " Kidnies and Bladders, as alſo in " Crudities of the Stomach. Some " Phyſicians of no inconſiderable " Character inform us, that large " Numbers of dropſical Patients " have been cured by a Lixivium " of the Aſhes of this Tree, exhibi- " ted in Wine."

Juniperus major, Offic. *Juniperus major Baccâ cæruleâ.* C. B. Pin. Tourn. Inſt. The Black Juniper. This grows in *Greece.* The Wood and Berries are uſed, agreeing in Virtues with the former Species.

Juniperus Alpina, C. B. Raii Hiſt. *Juniperus minor montana folio latiore, fructuque longiore*, C. B. Pin. Tourn. Inſt. Dwarf-Juniper, Wild-Savine. This grows on Mountains; the Herb itſelf being uſed. A Decoction of its Tops, or its expreſs'd Juices, is ſaid to be good for deſtroying that Species of Vermin called Bots, which are ſometimes lodg'd in the Stomach and Inteſtines of Horſes.

Jupicai Braſilienſibus. A Species of Graſs which grows in *Braſil.* Piſo informs us that this Plant rub'd upon the Part affected, is highly beneficial in an Impetigo, and eaſes the troubleſome Itching.

Kali, Offic. *Kali Cochleatum majus*, Park. Theat. *Kali majus cochleato Semine*, Raii Hiſt. Tourn. Inſt. Boerh. Ind. Alt. Glaſs-wort. The Herb is uſed and grows in ſaltiſh Soils, and on the Sea-Coaſt. There are various uſeful Preparations of this Plant; ſuch as, 1ſt, *Pot-aſh*, which is no more than a Quantity of this Herb burnt to Aſhes, and concreted into a blackiſh cineritious Maſs. This is acrid, pungent, cauſtic, and poſ- ſeſs'd of the ſame Virtues with the Plant itſelf, tho' ſtronger. 2dly, *Salt of Glaſs*, or *Sandiver*; this is a Kind of Salt of a cineritious Colour and of an acrid, pungent Taſte. It is poſſeſs'd of the ſame Virtues with the Pot-aſh, and is uſed by Farmers for cleanſing the Eyes of Horſes. It is alſo uſeful for cleanſing the Teeth, drying running Ulcers, and curing the Herpes, Impetigo and Itch; 3dly, The *Lixivium*, Offic. or *Soap-Lye*, which is a Solution of the Pot-aſh in Water. This is poſſeſſed of an acrid, corroſive and cauſtic Quality. This is uſed for removing Spots on the Skin, as alſo for curing Alphi, Freckles,

is, and Sun-burn; but it should be
utioufly ufed left it should corrode
e Skin. Of this Lixivium is pre-
red that celebrated Cauftic known
the Shops by the Name of *Lapis
'rnalis*; 4thly, the *Sapo*, Offic.
p, which is of three Sorts; 1ft,
mmon Soap, which is prepared of
arfe Oil, Suet and Pot-afh, boil'd
a proper Confiftence, and if to
s a proper Quantity of Soot is add-
, black Soap is produced; 2dly,
ftile Soap, which is prepared in the
ne manner with the former, only
ftead of common Oil, that of O-
res is ufed, and the Mafs ting'd
ith Indigo or fome other Subftance,
f a blueifh Colour. 3dly, *White* or
nice Soap, which is prepared much
i the fame manner with the others.
oap is aperient, digeftive, detergent,
d diuretic. It alfo opens Ob-
ructions of the Liver and Spleen,
d expels Sand and Gravel. Exterally applied, it attracts, and cures
urns when not exulcerated, efpeci-
lly the Black-Soap, which alfo de-
troys all Kinds of Lice, and efpeci-
lly Crab-Lice. It is however to be
bferv'd, that the Lixivium of the
hops may be prepared not only of
Pot-afhes but alfo of the Afhes of
ny burnt Wood. 5thly, *Sal Alka-
ï*, Offic. or *Alcaline Salt.* Tho'
this properly-fpeaking is the Salt extracted from Pot afhes, yet in a more
extenfive Senfe, it comprehends. 1ft,
The volatile Salts obtain'd from the
Parts or Excrements of Animals, as
Salt of Hartfhorn, and that of Urine.
2dly, The fix'd Salts obtained from
the Afhes of Plants, fuch as the Salt
of Kali and that of Wormwood.

Kali Hifpanicum, Cod. Med. *Kali Hifpanicum, fupinum Annuum, Sedi
foliis brevioribus*, Act. Reg. Par. An.
1719. Alicant Glafs-wort; which is
employ'd in preparing *Alicant*-Soap.

Kina Kina, vel Cortex Peruvianus,
Offic. Ind. Med. *Arbor febrifuga
Peruviana, China Chinæ, & Quin-*

quina, & Gannanaperide dicta, Raii
Hift. The Jefuits-Tree. This is a
pretty large high Tree like the Lime-
Tree, growing in the Inland Parts of
Peru, on the Mountains near *Loxa*,
or *Loja*, in the Province of *Quito*.
Its Bark is uneven and thick, with
a Colour refembling that of Cinnamon, Coffee, or Ruft of Iron. The
Spaniards fay, that the Ufe of this
Bark, was difcover'd in the follow-
ing Manner. Near the Town of
Loxa was a Lake furrounded with
Quinquina Trees, before the *Spaniards* fettled in that Country. Thefe
Trees being by fome Accident thrown
into the Lake communicated a bitter
Tafte to the Water, fo that the Inhabitants who before ufed to drink
it, could ufe it no longer. An *Indian*, however, who had a violent
Fever upon him, and confequently
an intenfe Thirft, finding no other
Water, was forced to drink of this,
by which he was perfectly cured.
He related this Accident to fome of
his Neighbours, who having made
the fame Experiment were alfo cured.
Upon this they fet themfelves to difcover what had given this febrifugous
Quality to the Water of the Lake, and
found in the firft Place, that a great
Number of Trees had fallen into
it; and fecondly, that after a certain
Time, thefe Trees being rotted in the
Water, it loft its bitter Tafte, and at
the fame Time its Virtue; whence
they concluded, that its Virtue was
owing to the Trees. Then they infufed all the Parts of thefe Trees in
Water, and thus difcover'd that their
whole Efficacy refided in the Bark.
This Medicine, however, remain'd
as a Secret to the *Spaniards* till 1640,
when it was difcovered by a Soldier,
who, by its Means had the good
Fortune to cure the Vice-Queen of
Peru, of an intermittent Fever, which
had fo far baffled the Skill of the
Phyficians, that her Life was defpair'd of. This was a Circumftance
of

of so striking a Nature, that the *Spaniards* afterwards used it with uncommon Success, and in 1649, Father *de Lugo*, a Jesuit, then Procurator General of his Order, and afterwards a Cardinal, brought it into *Rome*, upon which the Society of Jesuits began to bring it into Reputation in *Europe*, by which Means they got a great deal of Money in a short Time, since they sold it for more than its Weight in Gold, and never parted with it but in Powder, in order to disguise it the better. Two Drams were at that Time thought sufficient for the Cure of any intermittent Fever, because they never gave it till after many other Medicines had been made Trial of. At this Juncture the Physicians were greatly divided with respect to the *Peruvian* Bark, some looking on it as a divine Medicine, whilst others believed it dangerous, and even fatal in many Cases. But notwithstanding the Opposition it met with, it at last acquir'd a great Reputation, by Means of the judicious and successful Experiments made by the *English* Physicians. The Enemies to this Medicine, who still have their Abettors, pretended from their own Experience, that it was not only attended with violent Relapses, but also brought on new and incurable Diseases; such as Cachexies, œdematous Tumors of the Feet, Dropsies, obstinate Costiveness, Oppression of the Præcordia, hypocondriac and hysteric Disorders, slow and hectic Fevers, accompanied with a Loss of Strength and Appetite, Consumptions, and some Times Convulsions and Epilepsies in Children. *Baglivi* affirms, that Fevers cured by the Bark either return in a few Days, or are succeeded by Asthmas, Dropsies, slow Fevers, Consumptions and other dangerous Disorders. Many learned and eminent Physicians object against the Bark, that its a-

stringent and corroborating Qualities, suspend the febrile Commotions of Intermittents, but do not remove the Fever, which afterwards induce Relapses, or perhaps more terrible Disorders. But, it is certain, that the Bark, exhibited duly and in Conjunction with other suitable Remedies, has a Tendency to remove the Causes of Fevers by promoting Perspiration and restoring the due Tone of the Solids. Besides, the Bark is possess'd of a bitter Quality, which is universally allow'd to be a proper Remedy for Fevers, since almost all Bitters, such as Wormwood, Carduus Benedictus, Fumitory, the lesser Centaury, and others of a similar Nature, are esteem'd excellent Febrifuges. Some alledge that it is certain from Experience, that many Persons afflicted with Fevers, have by this Medicine been hurried into dangerous and incurable Diseases, as slow and hectic Fevers, Cachexies, and others of a similar Nature. But it is to be observed, that before the Fever, the Humours and Viscera are generally disposed to these Diseases, and that the bad Regimen of the Patient may contribute to their Production. Besides, it is sufficiently evident, that the most efficacious Remedies, such as Venesection, Purgatives, Emetics, and Opiates, if used without Judgment, are equally pernicious and fatal; so that the Bark, tho' on some particular Occasions improper, is yet so far from being in general an unsafe and dangerous Remedy in Fevers and other Distempers, that it is highly safe, efficacious and innocent, especially in the Hands of a Physician who administers it with Judgment and Reason, since its bad Effects do not proceed from the Medicine itself, but should be deservedly attributed to the improper Use of it, the Errors of the Patient, or a Neglect in removing the peccant Reliques. But however noble a Febrifuge the Bark rk may be, yet it is by no Means be exhibited till the Primæ Viæ : cleanfed from the Collection of cant Humours with which they ound. Nor fhould it be prefcrib'd, ecially in a confiderable Quantity, he abdominal Viscera are obftruc- or infarcted with Blood and Hu- ors, before thefe Obftructions are en'd, and the Infarction remov'd. r is the Cure of intermittent Fe- s to be undertaken with the Bark manifeftly plethoric, cacochymic, hectic, and hypocondriac Patients, when critical Evacuations of Blood fuppreffed. Great Caution is alfo ceffary, if the Patients to whom is Febrifuge is to be given, have eir Strength and Blood exhaufted; they are obnoxious to exorbitant ffions; if they are cold, and if e Fevers themfelves approach to a ntinual hectic, or a flow Fever; there is a continual Coftivenefs; the Urine is limpid and without a- Sediment; if the Hypocondria e tumid, or an Autumnal, or Win- r Fever has already been long pro- cted; for in fuch Cafes it is bet- r to moderate the febrile Commo- ns by gently evacuating and cor- borating Medicines, till at laft, as it quently happens, the Fits fponta- oufly ceafe, either by a Change of lace, a more exact Regimen, or he Influence of a ferene and warm ir. It is of great Importance to e proper and falutary Ufe of the ark in what Form, Dofe, Seafon, d under what Regimen it is to be xhibited. As to the Form, it is oft commodioufly given in Sub- ance in a proper Vehicle without ny Addition. But if the Stomach aufeates it in this Form, there are everal Methods of preparing it in a ore agreeable Manner. As to the Dofe of the Bark, it ought never to be given in large Quantities, as a Dram or more at a Time. But it is more advifeable to give at different

Times, one or two Scruples only on the intercalary Day, after the Fit, every three Hours, drinking after a fufficient Quantity of Water, De- coction, Broth or Beer. As to the Time, we ought to perfift in this Method of Cure, at leaft for a Week; then the Fever being gone, and the Appetite returning, a Dofe fhould be taken once every Day, and after that every other Day. Befides the pecu- liar febrifuge Quality of the Bark, it is alfo of fingular Service, not only in ftopping the Progrefs, but alfo in perfecting the Cure of begun Gan- grenes and Mortifications.

Knawel, Offic. *Polygonum Germa- nicum five Knawel Germanorum*, Park. *German* Knot Grafs. It grows in fandy Fields. The Herb is ufed, which is drying, aftringent, and vul- nerary; and by fome is efteem'd Li- thontriptic.

Lachryma Jobi, Offic. *Lithofper- mum Arundinaceum forte Diofcoridis*, C. B. P. Job's Tears. It is cultiva- ted in Gardens, the Seeds are ufed, which take their Name of *Lachryma Jobi*, from their refembling Tears: They are detergent and aperitive, and therefore good for the Stone in the Kidneys and Bladder.

Lactuca, Offic. *Lactuca fativa*, Boerh. Ind. A. Garden Lettuce. It is fown in Gardens, the Leaves and Seed are ufed. *Galen* in the Decline of his Age fuffer'd very much, by want of Sleep, for which Diforder he ufed in the Evening to eat a Lettuce, which was his only fovereign Reme- dy. For a Phrenfy, Delirium, burn- ing Fever, and other like Diforders, *Simon Pauli* recommends a double or treble linnen Cloth, well moiften- ed in Water of Lettuce, in which purified and cryftallized Nitre, or *Sal Prunellæ* have been diffolved, in the Proportion of half an Ounce to a Pint, to be applied to the Temples the Coronal Suture and the Wrifts. *Athenæus* and *Conftantine Cæfar* fay, thus this Plant was by the *Pythagoreans* call'd the *Eunuch*; and the Ancients fabled, that, after the Death of *Adonis*, *Venus* lay upon a Bed of Lettuces, in order to repress her lewd Inclinations; and for this Reason, some of the *Pagans* made a religious Scruple of eating them. Lettuces in general are esteemed, emollient, refrigeratting, saponaceous, resolvent, diuretic, and somewhat laxative; but are better raw than boil'd.

Lactuca sylvestris, Offic. *Lactuca sylvestris major odore Opii,* Ger. Wild Lettuce. It grows in Hedges, flowering in *June.* The Herb and Seeds are used, and are effectual for mitigating Pain.

Lactuca sylvestris Costa Spinosa, C. B. Pin. *Lactuc sylvestris laciniata,* Park. Jagged leaved wild Lettuce. It grows in Hedges, flowering in *June.* The Herb and Seeds are used. It agrees in Virtues with the former.

Ladanum. This is a Gum oozing out of the *Cistus Ladanifera,* Offic. *Cistus, Ledon Cretense,* C. B. Pin. This Gum mollifies, digests, maturates, and attenuates, and externally used is Anodyne, and good for the Tooth-ach. Alopecia, Heart-burn, Pains of the Stomach, and hysteric Fits. In *Dioscorides's* Time, this Gum was gathered from the Hairs of the Goats, which fed among the Trees which produce it, but at present, according to *Tournefort,* the *Greek* Monks gather it from the *Cistus Ladanifera,* with a Sort of Rakes. It is an excellent Balsamic in Dysenteries and Hoarseness.

Lamium rubrum, Offic. *Galeopsis, five Urtica iners, flore & folio minore,* J. B. Red Archangel. It grows in Hedges by Highways. The Leaves and Flowers are used. The Flowers are good to stop a Dysentery, and Hæmorrhages from Wounds. The Herb bruised is said to discuss Tumors, and to be serviceable to Wounds,

putrid Ulcers, and Inflammation and is recommended for an Excess the *Catamenia.*

Lamium album, Urtica mortua, O fic. *Galeopsis five Urtica iners, flori bus albis,* J. B. White Archangel It grows by Hedge Sides, flowering in *April* and *May.* The Flowers are used. The Plant is emollient inciding, diuretic, and lithontriptic and good against hysteric Fits. The Root is recommended against the Jaundice, and the Flowers are accounted a Specific against the *Fluor Albus.*

Lampsana, Offic. *Soncho affinis Lampsana domestica,* C. B. P. Nipplewort. It is found in Gardens and Fields, flowering in *June* and *July.* It is said to be drying, detergent and digestive, and is esteemed excellent for curing ulcerated Nipples, from whence it derives its Name *Nipplewort.*

Lapathum Alpinum folio subrotunda, Boerh. Ind. A. *Hippolapathum,* Offic. Bastard Monks Rhubarb. This agrees in Virtues with the *Lapathum hortense latifolium.* This is what the Herb Women of *London* frequently sell for the true Monk's Rhubarb.

Lapathum hortense latifolium, C. B. P. *Rhabarbarum Monachorum,* Offic. *Hippolopathum sativum,* Ger. Monk's Rhubarb. It is planted in Gardens, and grows wild in several Parts of *France, Italy,* and *Germany.* A Dram of this powder'd with a Scruple of Ginger, and taken in a Morning fasting, in warm Broth, is good to purge off the yellow Bile and serous Humours. The Juice of the Root. with Sulphur, cures the Itch, and with the Meal of Lupines, cures Pimples, Freckles, the *Alphus,* and other cutaneous Disorders. The dry'd Powder taken in Wine, is said to expel the Stone from the urinary Passages; and taken with the Juice of Horehound, is good for the Jaundice.

Lepa-

Lapathum acutum, Oxylapathum, Offic. _Lapathum folio acuto, plano,_ C. B. P. Sharp-pointed Dock. It grows in moist Places, and among Ruins and Rubbish. The Root and Seed are used. _Willis_ recommends the Roots of this Dock in a Diet Drink, as a most excellent Antiscorbutic. And they are said by others to be effectual in a Jaundice, and to cleanse and purify the Blood, and are good for the Scurvy and Rheumatism, and all Manner of Scabby, Itchy Eruptions. The Seeds taken in Powder, corroborate the Liver, and stop all Sorts of Fluxes.

Lapathum folio acuto, crispo, C. B. P. _Lapathum, acutum crispum,_ J. B. The Root of this Plant is very bitter, astringent, of a pale Yellow, giving a pretty deep Tincture of Red to blue Paper; its Leaves are sourish, giving the same Paper a lively Tincture of Red, which gives Reason to conjecture, that they contain more acid Salt. The Salt approaches that of Nitre; for it does not blacken the Tincture of Galls, any more than that of Sorrel. The Root of Dock is generally used at _Paris_ in Broths, and aperitive Ptisans. The Root bruised is apply'd to Ulcers of the Legs, and is an Ingredient in Ointments for the Itch.

Lapathum sanguineum, Offic. _Lapathum folio acuto, rubente,_ C. B. P. Bloodwort. It is cultivated in Gardens, flowering in _June._ The Leaves and Seeds are used. The Leaves taken in Broth, loosen the Belly; and the Seed powdered, and taken in any astringent Liquor, are recommended as effectual for stopping too profuse menstrual Discharges, and over uterine Fluxes.

Laserpitium, foliis latioribus, lotis, Boerh. Ind. A. _Gentiana alba,_ Offic. _Libanotis Theophrasti minor,_ &c. The lesser Herb Frankincense of _Theophrastus._ It grows on the Mountains of _Switzerland,_ and

the _Pyrenees,_ flowering in _July._ The Root is alexipharmic, and good in uterine Disorders.

Laserpitium Gallicum, C. B. Pin. _Laserpitium, e Regione Massiliæ allatum,_ J. B. Laserwort. It is cultivated in Gardens, flowering in the Summer. The Root is used, which is heating, and good against Sugillations, strumous Swellings, Tubercles, Ischiadic Pains, and Excrescences about the Anus. It is said to repress venereal Inclinations.

Lathyrus, Offic. _Lathyrus latifolius,_ C. B. P. _Clymenum Dioscoridis quibusdam._ Peas Everlasting, or Chichling Vetch. It grows in Woods and Thickets, flowering in the Summer. The express'd Juice of the whole Plant, together with the Root, being drank, is effectual against Vomiting of Blood, and the Cœliac Passion, and to restrain Hæmorrhages of the _Uterus,_ and from the Nose. The Leaves and Pods bruised, and applied to Wounds, promote their Cicatrization.

Lathyrus sylvestris, flore luteo, Park. Theat. _Lathyrus sylvestris luteus foliis Viciæ,_ C. B. P. Everlasting Tare. This grows in Woods and Thickets, flowering in _June._ The Herb is reckon'd a good Astringent.

Lavendula, Offic. _Lavendula latifolia,_ C. B. P. _Pseudo-Nardus, quæ vulgo Spica,_ J. B. Greater Lavender. It is planted in Gardens, but is rarely met with in _England._ The Herb and Flowers are used, being of fine Parts, and friendly to the Head and Nerves. It is principally used in Catarrhs, Palsies, Convulsions, the Vertigo, Lethargy, and Trembling of the Limbs; it provokes Urine, the Menses, and expels the Fœtus; and is good for the Gripes, proceeding from Flatulences. Outwardly it is of Service in _Lixivia,_ for the Head and Members, and in Masticatories.

Lavendula angustifolia, C. B. P.

B b

Spica

Spica Lavendula vulgaris, Offic. *Pseudo Nardus quæ Lavendula vulgo,* J. B. Common Lavender, or Spike. This grows wild in the Southern Parts of *France* and *Spain,* but is cultivated with us in Gardens, flowering in *July.* It takes its Name *à Lavando,* Washing or Bathing, because it was used in Baths on Account of its Fragancy: It is, also, called *Spica,* Spike, because among all the verticillated Plants, this alone bears a Spike: Many call it *Nard,* and perhaps, this is the true Nard of the Antients, which we will not dispute, since we cannot arrive at any Certainty in the Matter. It is the principal of all the Cephalic Plants, being very comfortable and reviving, under Faintings; whence it is very proper in Lethargies, Apoplexies, Palsies, and Epilepsies, and is recommended in Disorders incident to Virgins. The Plant is, also, an Emmenagogue, and a great Promoter of the Lochia, after the Birth. That Lavender is far more potent and penetrating, and of greater Efficacy, in cephalic, uterine, and nervous Disorders, than the Flowers of Rosemary, appears from the Oil of it distilled, and from the Salivation excited by the Leaves and Flowers in chewing; whence it is much commended in soporific and catarrhous Disorders. Lavender given in a Phrensy, proceeding from an Inflammation, infallibly destroys the Patient; but it is good for vertiginous old Persons, and Distempers owing to Dulness and Want of Spirits. It is outwardly used in warming and strengthening Fomentations.

Laurocerasus, Offic. Boerh. Ind. A. *Cerasus folio Laurino,* C. B. P. *Padus exotica folio amplo, crasso, sempervirenti,* Rupp. Flor. Jen. Laurel, or Cherry Bay. It has been customary to mix the Water distill'd from the Leaves of Laurel with Brandy or other spirituous Liquors, in order to impart to them the Taste of *Ratafia;* and it has been very common to use Laurel Leaves in Cookery in order to give the same Sort of Taste to Custards, and some Sorts of Sweetmeats. But some Years ago, some People at *Dublin* were manifestly poison'd by drinking Laurel-water; and it has been since found by repeated Trials upon Dogs, that this Laurel-water is the most deleterious Poison perhaps known, killing almost *in Instanti.* There is a full Account of these Accidents and Experiments in the *Philosophical Transactions,* which the Curious may consult. It is said, that the Villainy of some Dealers in Medicine has been destructive to some People, by substituting the Water of Laurel, instead of that of black Cherries, on Account of the Resemblance in the Smell of each; and this is not at all unlikely. Hence black Cherry-water has fell into some Disrepute, however innocent, for I am satisfy'd it is as harmless as any of the other Simple Waters, and may be used as safely, if Experiments made upon Animals with a View of discovering the Truth can be depended upon, provided it is only made of the usual Strength. The Berries of the *Laurocerasus* are esteem'd a good Antiscorbutic.

Laurus, Offic. *Laurus vulgaris,* C. B. P. *Laurus mas & fœmina,* Ger. The Common Bay Tree. It is planted in Gardens, flowering in *March* and *April.* The Leaves and Berries are used. They are heating, drying, emollient and revolvent. The Berries are principally used to provoke Urine, and the Menses, for Disorders of the Nerves, Palsy, and Colic, for Pains after Birth, and for Crudities of the Stomach. The Leaves are recommended for the Stinging of Wasps, to soften Tumours, nours, to provoke the Menses, to mitigate Pains, and to give Relief in the Tooth-ach.

Laurus Alexandrina, Offic. *Laurus Alexandrina fructu folio insidente,* C. B. P. *Ruscus latifolius fructu folio insidente,* Boerh. Ind. Alt. Laurel of Alexandria. This grows in the Gardens of the Botanists. The Herb is used, which is esteem'd vulnerary and diuretic.

Laurus latifolia, Offic. *Platytera Dioscoridis,* C. B. P. *Laurus major, sive latifolia,* Park. The broader-leaved Bay Tree. It grows in *Spain.* The Leaves are used which agree in Virtues with the common Bay Tree.

Laurus Tinus, Offic. *Laurus sylvestris Corni fœmina foliis subhirsutis,* C. B. P. *Tinus prior Clusii,* Boerh. Ind. Alt. Wild Bay. It is a Native of *Portugal,* flowering in *July* and *August.* The Berries are used, and taken internally purge by Stool, with great Disorder and Perturbation of the whole Body, and being held in the Mouth, soon burn the *Fauces,* and are sometimes given in the Dropsy with singular Success, being a very strong Cathartic. It is a very dangerous Medicine, and inflames the Intestines to a very great Degree; and indeed may more properly be call'd a deleterious Poison, however some People who have taken it may have escap'd.

Lens, Offic. *Lens vulgaris,* C. B. *Lens major & minor,* Mer. Pin. Lentils. They are sown in Fields, flowering in *May,* and the Seed is ripe in *July,* which is the Part used. They dull the Eye Sight, are difficult of Digestion, incommode the Stomach, and generate Flatulencies, both in that Part, and the Intestines: They stop a Looseness, and are prejudicial to the Nerves, Lungs, and Head.

Lenticula palustris vulgaris, C. B. P. *Lens palustris,* Offic. *Lenticularia minor mononrhiza foliis subrotundis*

utrinque viridibus, Mich. Nov. Gen. Duck's Meat. This is found in watery Places. The whole Plant is used, which is of a cooling, mollifying Nature, and is recommended in Inflammations, the Gout, and St. *Antbony's* Fire, and is by some commended for the Jaundice.

Lentiscus, Offic. *Lentiscus ex Chio, ex qua fluat Mastiche,* Ind. Med. Tourn. Itin. The Mastich Tree. It grows plentifully in the Island of *Scio* or *Chios,* in the *Archipelago,* flowering in *March* and *April.* The Parts used, are the nodous and brachiated small Branches, which are of the Thickness of a Man's Finger, white on the Inside, but cover'd with an Ash-colour'd Bark, and of a resinous Taste and Smell. The other Part in Use in Medicine, is the *Resina Mastiche,* Offic. Mastich. It is dry, transparent, and of a pale yellow Colour. It flows from an Incision made in the Bark of the abovemention'd Tree, and is brought to us in small, and almost pellucid Drops, and is of a resinous and astringent Taste, and of a fragrant Smell. That is to be esteem'd which is of a sweet Smell, bright, shining, dry, friable, and unadulterated. The Wood is drying and binding, good for all Sorts of Fluxes, and for a falling down of the Anus and Uterus; it is good to stop phagedenic Ulcers, to provoke Urine, and to fasten loose Teeth. The Gum is heating, drying, emollient, and a good Strengthener of the Stomach; it stops Vomitings and Nauseas. It blunts and corrects the Acrimony of Cathartics, strengthens the Head, and the nervous System; and cures Coughs and Spitting of Blood.

Leontopetalon, Offic. Boerh. Ind. A. *Leontopetalon quorundam,* J. B. Black Turnep. It grows in *Apulia,* flowering pretty late in the Year; the Root is used which cures the Bites of Serpents. *Galen* ascribes a digestive, geftive, heating, and drying Quality to it.

Leontopodium. This is already taken Notice of under the Article *Gnaphalium.*

Lepidium, Piperitis, Offic. *Lepidium latifolium,* C. B. P. *Raphanus fylveftris Officinarum, Lepidium Ægineta Lobelio,* Ger. Emac. Dittander. It grows in moift Places near Rivers, flowering in *June* and *July.* The Leaves are ufed, which are efteem'd good for the Sciatica, and being chew'd they caufe a great deal of Rheum to come from the Mouth, and are therefore recommended for fcrophulous Tumors in the Throat. The *Suffolk* Women give them to haften the Birth boil'd in Ale.

Leucanthemum vulgare, Boerh. Ind. A. *Bellis major,* Offic. *Bellis fylveftris caule foliofo major,* C. B. Ox Eye Daify. It grows in Fields and Meadows, flowering in *May.* The Leaves and Flowers are ufed. A Decoction of the whole Plant being drank is recommended as a fingular Remedy for an Afthma, Phthifis, and Orthopnœa. They are alfo good for Wounds and Ruptures.

Leucas montana, Offic. *Lamium luteum,* Ger. Emac. *Galeopfis five urtica iners flore luteo,* J. B. Yellow Archangel. It grows in Woods and Thickets, flowering in *May,* and is faid to refift the Poifon of venomous Animals, particularly thofe of the Sea Kind.

Leucoium album, Offic. Ger. Emac. *Leucoium incanum majus,* C. B. P. Stock-gilly-flower. It grows in Gardens, flowering in Summer. The Flowers are ufed, which are recommended by *Diofcorides,* for Ulcers and Chaps in the Fundament, and Inflammations of the Matrix. *Galen* affirms, that they provoke the Menfes and haften Birth.

Leucoium luteum, Cheyri, Offic. *Leucoium luteum vulgare,* C. B. P. *Keyri five Leucoium vulgare luteum,*

Park. Theat. *Viola lutea,* Ger. Emac. Wall Flower. It grows upon old Walls and Buildings, flowering in *June.* The Flowers are ufed, which are efteem'd cordial, good to mitigate Pains, provoke the Menfes, and to expel the Secundines, and give Relief under the Palfy and Apoplexy. There is fcarce a more effectual Remedy known, than the Wall Flower, taken twice every Day in warm Beer for the Jaundice.

Levifticum, Offic. *Ligufticum vulgare,* C. B. P. *Levifticum vulgare,* Ger. Emac. Lovage. It is cultivated in Gardens, flowering in *June.* The Roots, Leaves and Seeds are ufed; and in every Refpect, agrees as to Virtues with Angelica and Mafterwort. It is alexipharmic, diuretic, and vulnerary.

Libanotis, Offic. *Libanotis Ferula folio five Cachryfera, five Cachrys vera,* Park. Theat. Fennel Herb Frankincenfe. It grows on the Mountains of *Italy* and *Sicily,* flowering in *May.* The Root and Seed are ufed, which are by fome of the Ancients recommended for their heating and drying Qualities, and are faid to be good for the Epilepfy.

Lichen, Hepatica vulgaris, Offic. *Lichen petræus cauliculo pileolum fuftinente,* Boerh. Ind. A. Liverwort. It grows in moift and fhady Places, and by the Banks of Rivers. The whole Plant is ufed, which is an extraordinary Hepatic, and is principally ufed in Obftructions of the Liver and Bladder; whence it becomes of Service in hectic Diforders, the Jaundice, the Itch, Lichen, Gonorrhæa, and Fevers, outwardly applied, it ftops Hæmorrhages in Wounds.

Lichen Arboreus pullus, Offic. *Lichen cruftæ modo arboribus adcrefcens pullus,* Boerh. Ind. A. Tree Liverwort. It grows to Trees. The whole Plant is ufed inftead of the *Mufcus Pulmonarius.*

Lichen

Lichen cinereus, Offic. *Lichen cinereus terreſtris*, Raii. *Lichen pulmonarius, ſaxatilis digitatus major cinereus*, Boerh. Ind. Alt. Ground Liverwort. It is found upon dry barren Places. The whole Plant is uſed being accounted a Specific againſt the Bite of a Mad Dog, given with Pepper ; but Experience convinces us, that many Dogs and ſome Men have dy'd after taking it in due Time, and with all imaginable Regularity.

Lichen petræus ſtellatus, C. B. P. *Hepatica ſtellata*, Offic. *Lichen ſive Hepatica vulgaris*, Park. Star Liverwort. It grows in moiſt and ſhady Places. The whole Plant is uſed, which agrees in Virtue with the common Liverwort. This is more in Uſe among the common People, than among the Phyſicians.

Lignum Aloes. This is already taken Notice of under *Agallochum.*

Lignum Aquila, Ind. Med. Eagle Wood. It is uſed in the Shops at *Paris* inſtead of the following.

Lignum Aſpalathum, Pharmacop. *Aſpalathum*, Offic. Geoff. Tract. *Agallochum præſtantiſſimum*, C. B. P. Calambac Wood. This Wood is brought from the *Eaſt Indies* in Pieces thicker and leſs ſolid than the *Lignum Aloes*, of a paler Colour, and fainter Smell, bituminous, fat and reſinous, and of a bitteriſh Taſte. It agrees in Virtues with the Log *Agallochum*, for which it is often ſold, but it is weaker.

Lignum Campeſcanum, Offic. J. B. *Tſiam Pangam.* Hort. Mal. Log-Wood. It grows in the *Eaſt* and *Weſt-Indies*, and the Wood is uſed, which is eſteem'd aſtringent, good to fortify the Stomach, and is much celebrated of late for its Virtues in curing a Dyſentery.

Lignum Carabaccium, Bagliv. de Fibra Motric. This Wood has the Taſte of Cloves, but very mild, and quite grateful, and is of a Colour very much reſembling that of Cinnamon. It is imported from *India*, but is as yet unknown in our Shops. Bagliuj affirms, that he very ſucceſsfully preſcrib'd a warm Potion of the Decoction of this Wood for correcting the Acrimony of the Lymph.

Lignum Cedrinum. This is already taken Notice of under the Article *Juniperis.*

Lignum Colubrinum, Snake Wood. This Wood is ſaid to grow in *Ceylon* and *Timor.* The Root is woody, and as thick as a Man's Arm, with a dark colour'd Bark mark'd with Aſh-colour'd-Spots; the Wood underneath is ſolid, ponderous, of an acrid bitter Taſte, but no Smell. It is ſaid to be hot, dry, and abſtergent, and to cure the Bites of Serpents. It operates by Stool, and ſometimes by Vomit; and is by ſome recommended in Tertians, and Quartans, and for the Worms. But it is more generally agreed, that this Wood has a virulent, and malignant Quality ; and that it is ſo extremely narcotic, as to induce a Tremor and Stupidity.

Lignum Moluccenſe. This is already taken Notice of under the Article *Grana Tiglia.*

Lignum Nephriticum. This is already mention'd under *Glans Unguentaria.*

Lignum Pavanum. This is a Name for the Saſſafras Wood.

Lignum Rhodium. This is ſpecify'd under *Aſpalatus.*

Lignum Sanctum, is *Guaiacum.*

Liguſticum, is the *Leviſticum.*

Liguſtrum, Offic. Ger. Emac. *Liguſtrum Germanicum*, C. B. P. Privet. It grows in Hedges, flowering all the Summer. The Leaves and Flowers are uſed, which are cooling, drying, aſtringent, and inciding, and good for Inflammations, Putrefactions and Exulcerations of the Mouth and Fauces, and for a Relaxation of the Uvula, and Bleeding of the Gums.

Lilium album, Offic. Ger. Emac. *Lilium album vulgare,* J. B. White Lilly. It is sown in Gardens, flowering in *June.* The Root, Seed, and Flowers are used. The Root is seldom internally used, but often applied for softening and ripening of Tumors, for removing Corns of the Feet, being mixed with old Lard, for mollifying the *Pudenda* in Labour, and for Burns, and the like Cases. The Seeds exhibited in Vervain-water are good to facilitate the Birth. The Flowers are emollient, suppling, and anodyne.

Lilium rubrum, Mont. Ind. *Hemerocallis,* Offic. *Lilium aureum,* Ger. Emac. *Lilium purpureo croceum majus,* C. B. P. Red Lilly. It is cultivated in Gardens, flowering in *June* and *July.* The Roots and Leaves are used. The Root drank, or made into a Pessary with Honey and Wool, expels Water and Blood. The Leaves bruised mitigate Inflammations of the Breasts, contracted after Child-birth, and Inflammations of the Eyes. The Root and Leaves are successfully applied by Way of Cataplasm to Burns.

Lilium montanum minus, Ger. Emac. *Martagon,* Offic. *Lilium floribus reflexis, montanum,* C. B. P. Martagon, or *Turks* Cap. It is cultivated in Gardens, flowering in *June.* The Root which is used, is substituted, in our Shops, in the Room of the Yellow Asphodel. The common People hang it about the Necks of Infants, to facilitate Dentition.

Lilium Convallium, Offic. *Lilium Convallium flore albo,* Park. Lilly of the Valley. It is found in Woods and shady Places, flowering in *May.* The Flowers are used, which are esteem'd cephalic; and are principally used in cold Disorders of the Head, as the Apoplexy, Palsy, Vertigo, Epilepsy, and in fainting Fits.

Limonia malus, Offic. Park. Theat. *Malus Limonia acida,* C. B. P. Li-

mon *vulgaris,* Tourn. Inst. The Lemon Tree. It grows in *Italy* and *Spain.* The Fruit is used, which is cooling, and grateful to the Stomach, allaying Thirst, and promoting an Appetite, and is good for both common, malignant and pestilential Fevers. Lemons provoke Urine, and the Juice being mixed with Salt of Wormwood stops Vomiting, and strengthens the Stomach. Of late Years, the Juice of Lemons, perfectly neutralized with Salt of Wormwood, has been very much given in Fevers, and with very good Effect, in the Quantity of about half an Ounce, repeated at due Intervals.

Limonium, Sea Lavender. This is already taken Notice of under the Article *Behen rubrum.*

Linaria, Offic. *Linaria lutea vulgaris,* Ger. Emac. *Linaria vulgaris lutea, flore majore,* C. B. P. Toad Flax. It grows upon Banks and Hedges, flowering in *June* and *July.* The Herb is used, which is diuretic, and is principally used in the Jaundice, Dropsy, Obstructions of the Liver, and in a Difficulty of Urine. It is accounted an excellent Remedy for the Piles; and an Ointment made of it is used with Success externally in the same Complaints.

Linaria, Cymbalaria dicta, Raii Hist. *Cymbalaria,* Offic. *Linaria hederacea folio glabro, seu Cymbalaria vulgaris,* Tourn. Inst. Ivy-leaved Toad Flax. It is found about old Walls and Quarries. The Herb is used, which is of an astringent Nature, and in *Italy* this Herb is used in the Room of the *Umbilicus Veneris,* and is said to have the same medicinal Virtues ascrib'd to it.

Lingua Cervina, Phyllitis, Offic. *Phyllitis sive Lingua Cervina vulgaris,* Park. Harts Tongue. It grows in shady Places, and among Stone Buildings. The Leaves are used, and are principally recommended in a tuminmified Spleen, and for a Spitting of Blood. Externally apply'd it cleanses Wounds and Ulcers. Exhibited in Powder, it is good for the Palpitation of the Heart, for a Suffocation of the Uterus, and for Convulsive Motions. Boiled in Wine it is good for the Bite of a mad Dog, and Obstructions of the Viscera. It is also given in the Rickets and to scorbutic Habits.

Linum, Offic. *Linum sativum*, C. B. P. Flax. It is sown in Fields, flowering in *June*. The Seed is used, which is usually called Linseed, and is digesting, emollient, and ripening, and is principally recommended in Coughs, Pleurisies and Consumptions. Externally apply'd it ripens Tumors, mitigates Pains, and expels the Fœtus. Flax infused in Water, as in Ponds or Rivers, as it is practised in order to rot the Stem, and procure the Bark for mechanical Uses, communicates to the Water a very poisonous Nature, insomuch that Cattle, which drink of it die; and the Fish in such Waters, are poison'd. The Seed of this Plant, afford an excellent Medicine, since from them is expressed an Oil, which is anodyne, demulcent, and extremely adapted to all Manner of Asperities; it relaxes, and involves Acidities, whence it is of extraordinary Service in the most desperate Colics. The stiff and rigid Limbs, being anointed with this Oil, are relaxed and render'd flexible. This Oil, when fresh drawn, and taken at the Mouth, is very good in a Pleurisy, and a Cough, to help Expectoration; and, injected in Clysters, is very proper in the Hæmorrhoids, and indurated Fœces, whence proceeds the Colic; mixed with sealed and Japan Earth, it is a great Arcanum in the Dysentery, and is a very good Remedy in the Stone: This Oil boiled with Honey, clears the Skin and Face of Spots, and all cutaneous Blemishes.

Linum Catharticum, Offic. *Linum sylvestre Catharticum*, Ger. Emac. *Linum pratense flosculis exiguis*, C. B. P. Purging Flax or Mill Mountain. It grows upon dry, hilly and chalky Places, flowering in *June* and *July*. The Herb is used, which is possess'd of a Cathartic Quality. It cures Tertians, and is recommended in the Gout. I once knew an Instance of a Man, who took a Purge from a Quack, of an Infusion of this Plant; which in a few Hours, swell'd him to such a Degree, that his ordinary Cloaths were not by much sufficient to cover him; and it was with some Difficulty, that he was recovered by more gentle Evacuations.

Liquid-Ambar, Offic. C. B. P. *Xochiocotzo Quahuitl, seu Arbor Liquid-Ambarum Indicum*, Hern. *Styrax Aceris folio*, Raii Hist. *Platanus Virginiana Styracem fundens*. Herm. Par. Bad. Prod. Liquid Amber. It grows in *Virginia, New-Spain*, and other Places in the *West-Indies*. The Part used is the Resin, which is a fat Liquid Substance, of the Consistence of Venice Turpentine, Yellow, inclining to Red, of an acrimonious Taste, aromatic and fragrant. It heats and moistens, resolves and opens Obstructions; and is an Emollient and Ripener. Its principal Use is in Obstructions and Hardness of the Womb, in hard Tumours, &c. It is employ'd in Suffumigations, and the like. *Hernander* says, that this Balsam distils from a Tree, either spontaneously, or from a Wound. Some break up the Branches into small Bits, and boiling them, skim off the Oil that rises on the Liquor, which they sell for the true Balsam; and this Liquor is thought by some to be the liquid Storax commonly sold by the Apothecaies and Druggists.

Liquiritia, Liquorice. This is already taken Notice of under the Article *Glycirrhiza*.

Lithospermum sive Milium Solis, Offic. *Lithospermum vulgare minus,* Park. Theat. Gromwell. It grows in Fields and by the Path ways, flowering in *May* and *June.* The Herb and Seeds are used It expels the Stone, cleanses the Kidneys, and provokes Urine. Boil'd in Wine or Water it is of Service in a Gonorrhœa. The Plant gives hardly any Tincture of red to the blue Paper; the Fruit stains it a little.

Lolium, Offic. *Lolium album,* Ger. Emac. *Gramen Loliaceum Spica longiore,* C. B. P. Darnel. It grows among Corn. The Seed is used, which is heating, drying, attenuating, discussing and cleansing. Darnel mix'd with Malt promotes Drunkenness. It hurts the Eyes, and creates a Dimness, by the acrid Vapours it elevates to the Brain. *Hippocrates* recommends bruis'd Darnel in Uterine Disorders, in form of a Fomentation.

Lolium rubrum, Ger. Emac. *Phœnix,* Offic. *Gramen Loliaceum folio & Spica angustiore,* Tourn. Inst. Ray Grass, Darnel Grass. It grows in Pastures, and by Path Ways, it is astringent and drying; stops a Looseness and the Menses; and restrains the Urine. It is sown in some Places as Food for Cattle.

Lonchitis, Offic. *Lonchitis altera foliis Polypodii,* J. B. *Polypodium angustifolium folio vario,* Boerh. Ind. Alt. Rough Spleenwort. This Plant grows in moist Woods, rough, and uncultivated Places. The Herb is good to agglutinate Wounds without suffering an Inflammation to come on. Drank in Vinegar it consumes the Spleen. The Root is aperient and diuretic.

Lotus Hæmorrhoidalis, Park. Theat. *Trifolium Hæmorrhoidale,* Offic. *Lotus Pentaphyllos siliquosus villosus,* C. B. P. Pile Trefoil. It grows in *Sicily* and *France.* The Seed is used which is recommended in the Hæmorrhoids.

Lotus corniculata, Ind. Med. *Lotus sive Melilotus pentaphyllos minor glabra.* C. B. P. *Trifolium siliquosum minus,* Ger. Emac. Birds-foot Trefoil. It grows in Pastures, flowering in *June.* The Herb is used which is esteem'd anodyne, emollient, maturating and good for Burns.

Lotus urbana, Trifolium odoratum, Offic. *Lotus hortensis odora,* C. B. P. *Melilotus major, odorata, violacea.* Boerh. Ind. Alt. Sweet Trefoil. It is sown in Gardens, flowering in *June.* The Herb and Seed is used. It is alexipharmic, anodyne, diuretic, and Vulnerary.

Lujula. A Name for the *Acetosella,* or Wood-Sorrel.

Lunaria, Offic. *Lunaria minor,* Ger. Emac. *Osmunda foliis lunatis,* Boerh. Ind. Alt. Moon-wort. It grows on hilly Places. The whole Plant is used, which agrees in Virtues with the *Ophioglossum.* The People in *Wales* apply an Ointment of this Plant, to the Reins, which they esteem as a certain Remedy for a Dysentery. It stops the Menses, and suppresses a *Fluor Albus.*

Lupinus, Offic. *Lupinus sativus, flore albo,* C. B. P. Lupines. It is sown in Gardens, flowering in *June.* The Seed is used, which ground to a Meal, affords a good Food, and is emollient, nutritive and anodyne, but internally taken, it binds the Belly; for which Reason it is given with a little Muscadine, in the worst Dysenteries. Lupines bring down the Menses, and expel the *Fœtus.* Externally us'd they are of Service in Achors, Pustules, Gangrenes and and malignant Ulcers.

Lupinus sylvestris, Offic. *Lupinus sylvestris flore cæruleo,* C. B. P. Wild Lupines. It is sown in Gardens, flowering in *July.* The Seeds are used, which agree in Virtues with the Former.

Lupulus, Offic. *Lupulus mas & fœmina,* C. B. P. *Lupus salictarius,* Ger.

Ger. Emac. Hops. They grow in Hedges, flowering in *July* and *August*. The Leaves, Flowers, and Tendrils are used. The Flowers are of a bitter Taste; and are esteem'd anodyne and discutient. *Hops* are principally used in Obstructions of the Liver and Spleen, they cure a Jaundice, are recommended in Hypochondriacal Disorders, and provoke Urine and the Menses. Externally used they asswage Pains, and are serviceable in Contusions, Luxations, and Tumours. The Tendrils are good to purify the Blood, and are recommended for the Itch, but an excessive Use of them creates a great Pain in making Water. The Herb is reckon'd a good Epithem in intermittent Fevers, being apply'd to such Parts of the Body where the Vessels are most expos'd.

Luteola, Ger. Emac. *Struthium*, Offic. *Luteola Herba Salicis folio*, C. B. P. Dyers Weed. It grows upon Walls and ruin'd Places, flowering in Summer. The Herb is used, which is sown principally for Dyers Use, to dye of a Yellow Colour, tho' it is by some accounted a good Vulnerary, and of Use against the Jaundice. It is frequently sold by the Herb Women for *Glastum*, or Wead.

Lychnis coronaria, Offic. J. B. *Lychnis coronaria Dioscoridis sativa*, C. B. P. *Lychnis coronaria vulgaris*, Park. Theat. Rose Campion. It is cultivated in Gardens, flowering in *June*, the Seed is used, which purges Bile by Stool, and heals the Sting of the Scorpion.

Lychnis sylvestris, Offic. *Lychnis sylvestris sive aquatica purpurea simplex*, C. B. P. *Ocymoides purpureum multis*, J. B. Red Wild Campion. It grows by Hedges, flowering in Summer. The Seed is used which agrees in Virtues with the former.

Lycium, Offic. *Lycium Buxi foliis*, C. B. P. *Lycium sive Pyracantha*, Ger. Emac. *Lycium Italicum*, J. B. Box Thorn. It grows in hot Coun-

tries. The Nob or concreted Juice of the Leaves and Branches are used, the Preparation of which is as follows. The Branches with the small Roots are bruised, and being macerated for many Days, are boil'd; then the Wood being thrown away, the Liquor is again boiled to the Consistence of Honey. *Lycium* is adulterated by putting *Amurca*, or the Juice of Wormwood, or Ox Gall, into the boiling Liquor. In the same manner is *Lycium* prepared of the expressed and insolated Seed. The best *Lycium* is what will burn, and, when quenched, shews a red Spume; is black on the outside; but, when broken, red within, which has nothing of a rank Smell, but a bitterish astringent Taste, and is of the Colour of Saffron. It is of an astringent Quality, and deterges whatever darkens the Pupil of the Eye, and cures the Ulcerations, Itchings, and inveterate Rheums, affecting the Eyelids. It is effectual, also, in Purulencies of the Ears, in Exulcerations of the Gums, and Tonsils, Tissures of the Lips, or *Rhagades* of the Anus, and Abrasions, the affected Parts being anointed therewith. Exhibited either in Potion, or by way of Clyster, it is very proper for the Cæliac Passions, and the Dysentery. For an *Hæmoptoe* or Cough, it is given in Water; and to those who are bit by a mad Dog, it is prescrib'd to be swallowed in Pills or drank in Water. It renders the Hair yellow, cures a *Paronychia*, *Herpes*, and putrid Ulcers; applied in a Pessary, it stops the Menstrual Flux; and drank in Milk, or taken in Pills, it relieves those who are bitten by mad Animals. There are two Species of *Lycium* mentioned by *Dioscorides*; one is produced from a Plant growing in *Greece*, which is our present Subject, and is called simply *Lycium*; the other is prepared of an *Indian* Plant which is the following. But since the *Lycium* is unknown to the Moderns, there

ae

are different Opinions about it. The Shops, as *Schrader* writes, commonly make their *Lycium* of the Berries of the *Periclymenum*, or Honeysuckles, others of the Fruit of *Ligustrum*, or Privet, and others of wild Plums. But they might have provided a better *Succedaneum*, as *Caspar Bauhine* or *Matthiolus* observes, from the *Oxyacantha*, or the *Rhamnus*.

Lycium Indicum, Offic. *Lycium Garciæ sive Cate*, J. B. *Lycium foliis Ericæ*, C. B. P. *Arbor spinosa, unde Cate sive Lycium exprimitur*, Bont. *Indian* Thorn. It grows in the *East Indies*. The inspissated Juice is used, which is called *Cate*, and which strengthens and fastens the Teeth and Gums. Whether the *Cate* of *Bontius*, and the *Terra Saponica*, or *Catechu*, be the same, is not easy for the Learned to determine. From the Nearness of the Name *Cate* and *Catechu*, I am inclined to think they are the same thing. But since *Helbigius* affirms, that the *Catechu* is taken from that Tree, whose Fruit the Natives eat with Lime and Betle, which, *Bontius* assures us, is the Fruit of the *Areca* or *Fausel*, I cannot (says *Dale*) but give Credit to so great a Man, especially, considering he lived many Years in that Country. And since there is so great a Variety, both in the Colour and Weight of *Terra Japonica*, I don't see why they may not be the Product of different Plants, tho' called by the same Name.

Lycoperdon. A Species of Mushroom. See the Article *Fungus.*

Lycopersicon. A Name for the *Amoris Pomum.*

Lycopodium, Offic. *Muscus terrestris repens sive clavatus*, C. B. P. *Plicaria & Cingularia*, Polonis. Club Moss. It grows on Heaths and hilly Places, flowering in *July* and *August*. The whole Plant is used, and the Flower or yellow Powder of the Clubs. It refrigerates and dries; its principal Use is in expelling the Stone, and in Fluxes of the Belly. Outwardly it is of Service in fastening loose Teeth, and in drying and consolidating Wounds; and in extirpating the *Plica Polonica.* The Flower is very serviceable in the Epilepsy of Children, and in the Heart-burn, and flatulent Gripes, with which they may be affected. It is also recommended in pulmonary Disorders. The Country-women in the *Ukraine*, when labouring under an excessive Flux of the Menses, with Pains and Strangulations of the Uterus, prepare a Girdle of it, which they wear next their Skin; and bind it about their Heads as a Diadem, to repress an Hæmorrhage from the Nostrils.

Lycopsis. Wall Bugloss. This is already specify'd under *Echium.*

Lycopus, Offic. *Lycopus palustris glaber*, Boeth. Ind. Alt. *Marrubium aquaticum*, Ger. *Marrubium palustre glabrum*, C. B. P. Water Horehound. It grows in watery Places, flowering in *July*. The Plant is used, which is ranked in the Class of Astringents.

Lysimachia, Offic. *Lysimachia lutea major, quæ Dioscoridis*, C. B. P. *Blattaria spuria altera lutea*, Volck. Flor. Nor. Yellow Willow Herb. This Plant is called *Lysimachia* from *Lysimachus* the Son of a King of *Sicily*, who is said to be the first who discovered it. It grows by River Sides, flowering in *June*. The Herb is used, which is vulnerary, and is said by some to be possess'd of an astringent Quality, tho' it is seldom used.

Lysimachia purpurea, Salicaria, Mont. Ind. *Salicaria vulgaris purpurea foliis oblongis*, Boeth. Ind. Alt. *Lysimachia spicata purpurea forte Plinii*, C. B. P. Spiked Willow Herb. It grows in marshy Places, and by the Banks of Rivers, flowering in *July*. The Herb is used, which is an Opthalmic. The distill'd Water is a present Remedy for Wounds, Punc-

...nctures and Sugillations of the Eyes, as well as Dimness of Sight, and all other Infirmities incident to those Parts. It is a Specific in Inflammations, and a Decoction of the Herb is an excellent Remedy for the Epidemic Diarrhœa of _Ireland_.

MACER, Diosc. Theoph. _Macer Veterum_, C. B. P. _Macer Dioscoridis & Græcorum_, J. B. The Grecian Macer, It is brought from _Barbary_; the Bark is used, which is of an astringent Taste, and is recommended by _Dioscorides_ as good for spitting of Blood, the Dysentery and Fluxes.

Macis, Mace. See the Article _Nux Moschata_.

Majorana, Amaracus, Sampsuchum, Offic. _Majorana vulgaris_, C. B. P. Sweet Marjoram. It grows in Gardens, flowering in _July_. The Herb and Seed are used. It is cephalic and uterine, and principally used in Disorders of the Head and Nerves, as well as of the Uterus and Stomach. It provokes the Menses, used in a Pessary; comforts the Brain, and discusses Flatulencies, that molest it. Dr. _Nicholas Chesneau_ of _Marseilles_, commends the following Errhine, in the Head-ach : Take of the Root of white Hellebore, half a Dram; of the Leaves of Sweet Marjoram, two Pugils; boil them in six Ounces of Water, to the Consumption of a third Part. When you use it, fill your Mouth with Water, and putting some of the Decoction, a little warm, in the Hollow of your Hand, draw it up your Nostrils, when the Pain is very violent, for it exasperates a slight one. The Water of Sweet Marjoram helps a Catarrh, if, instead of an Errhine, you fill your Mouth with Wine, or pure Water, and taking some of the Water of the Herb in the Hollow of your Hand, you stop one Nostril, and draw it up the other as far as the Root of the Nose, or the _Os Ethmoides_. If

you don't take this Method, the Errhine will not ascend to the aforesaid Place, but will be diverted and drawn back upon the _Fauces_, or _Narium Foramina_. This Errhine (says _Simon Pauli_), my Father used with the highest Reputation in the Case of Prince _Walenstein_, who was afflicted with a Rheum. If the Sides of the Nostrils, or the Space between the Eyebrows, be anointed with the Balsam of this Plant, it has a wonderful Effect in a Catarrh, or rather a Rheum. The Nape of the Neck and the Temples, are usually anointed with the same Balsam, not only in the aforesaid Disorder, but in other cold Distempers of the Head. Being chew'd or apply'd, it eases the Tooth Ach.

Majorana Oleracea, Offic. _Majorana hortensis viridis_, _tenuior_, C. B. P. Pot Marjoram. It is cultivated in Gardens among other Culinary Herbs, flowering in Summer, and agrees in Virtues with the following.

Majorana Sylvestris, Park. Theat. _Origanum_, Offic. _Origanum sylvestre, Cunila bubula Plinii_, C. B. P. Wild Marjoram. It grows in Hedges and Thickets, flowering in _July_; the Herb is used, which is opening and abstersive; and principally in Obstructions of the Lungs, Liver and Uterus. It is of great Service in a Cough, Asthma, and Jaundice. It increases Milk, and expels ichorous Excrements by Sweat. Externally used, it is frequently put in Baths for the Head and Uterus, and for the whole Body, under the Itch.

Majorana tenuifolia, C. B. P. _Majorana tenuior & lignosior_, J. B. Marjoram Gentle, or Perennial. It grows in Gardens, and the Herb is used, which agrees in Virtue with Sweet Marjoram.

Malabathrum, Park. Theat. _Malabathrum & Folium Indum Officinarum_, J. B. _Tamalapatra_, Ger. Emac. _Cinna._

Cinnamomum seu Cassia crassior, Pseudo-Cassia, C. B. P. Indian Leaves. This is the Leaf of a kind of wild Cinnamon Tree, brought us from *Malabar*, and other Places of the *East-Indies*. These Leaves are distinguish'd from the true Cinnamon Leaves, by their being less aromatic. They agree in Virtues with Spikenard, particularly in powerfully provoking Urine, and correcting a *Fætor* of the Mouth.

Malicorium. The Peel of the Pomegranate is so call'd.

Malva, Offic. *Malva vulgaris flore majore, folio sinuato,* J. B. Common Mallows. It grows by way sides, flowering in *June*. The Root, Leaves, and Seed are used. The Mallow is loosening, cooling, and mollifying, it being one of the five Emollient Herbs. It mitigates Pains, and allays the Sharpness of Urine. The Herb is a proper Remedy, first, where excessive Acrimony requires Demulcents; secondly, where too great a Stricture requires Relaxation? thirdly, where Pains are to be mitigated; and fourthly under an excessive Glutinosity. Hence it is effectual for dry and rigid Fibres; for rendering the hard Intestines lubricous; and for the Vertigo in those who labour under Hypochondriacal Disorders. The Surgeons also make great Use of this Plant, and there is scarce a Cataplasm design'd for maturating, but has Mallows for an Ingredient: It is of Efficacy in Affections of the Lungs and Intestines, a Phthisis, Hoarseness and Cough. The Flowers are good for Inflammations of the Gums and Uvula; a Cataplasm of the Herb is commended for the Erysipelas, and an Infusion of the Leaves after the manner of Tea, cures an inveterate Heat of Urine.

Malva minor, Offic. *Malva sylvestris pumila,* Ger. Emac. *Malva sylvestris folio rotundo,* C. B. P. Small, Wild, or Dwarf Mallow. It flowers in *June*, and the Leaves are used, which agree in Virtues with the preceeding.

Malva crispa, Offic. *Malva foliis crispis,* C. B. P. French Mallows. It is sown in Gardens, flowering in *June*; the Leaves are used, which agree in Virtues with the other Species of Mallows.

Malva arborea, Offic. *Malva rosea folio subrotundo,* C. B. P. *Malva rosea sive hortensis*; J. B. Holly-hocks. It grows in Gardens, flowering in *June*; The Leaves and Flowers are used, which are mollifying, but in a lesser Degree than the common Mallows. It is principally used in Disorders of the Tonsils, and for a profuse menstrual Flux.

Malva arborea maritima, Offic. *Malva arborea marina nostras,* Park. Theat. Sea Mallow Trees. It grows in Gardens, flowering in *June*, and the Leaves are used, which agree in Virtues with those of the other Mallows.

Malus, Offic. *Malus sive Pomum,* C. B. P. Tho' Apple Tree. It is cultivated in Gardens and Orchards, flowering in *April.* Tho' Apples may be hurtful to a cold and humid Stomach, they are very agreeable to a hot and bilious one; and render the Body soluble. Almost all Apples have a Property in common, that, if their expressed Juice be drank with a little Saffron, it become an Antidote against Poisons, and expels Worms, or other Animals, from the Belly. A Cataplasm prepared of sweet Apples is very much recommended for pungent Pains in the Sides, and for Ambustions by Gun-powder. There is a Medicine, which frequently occurs in our Practice, which is a Poultice prepared of Apples, and apply'd to an Inflammation of the Eyes, and it is common, to apply a putrid Apple to all sorts of Tumours and Inflammations of the Eyes. *Gesner* with good

good Success, advised a roasted Apple open'd, and fill'd with a Dram of Frankincense for a *Dyspnœa*, and other Disorders of the Lungs.

Malus Insana, Offic. *Malum Insanum folio non spinoso Solanum pomiferum fructu oblongo*, C. B. P., Mad Apples. It is cultivated in Gardens, flowering in the Summer. The Fruit is used. It induces a *Sopor* and Madness, whence it takes its Name, but is used in Sauces and Sweetmeats by the *Italians* and *Spaniards*.

Malus Sylvestris, Offic. *Mala sylvestria quæ & alba, & rubra, & majora, & minora*, C. B. P. Crab Tree, or Wilding. It grows in Woods and Hedges, flowering in *April*. Its Fruits and Juice are the *Agresta* of the Shops, called *Verjuice*, it is vehemently austere, acid, and astringent, and an excellent Application for Strains.

Mandragora, Offic. *Mandragora, fructu rotundo*, C. B. P. Mandrake. This is cultivated in Botanic Gardens, flowering in *May*. The Leaves, the Bark of the Root, and the Fruit are us'd. The Leaves are sharp-pointed, about a Cubit long, and a Palm and a half broad, of a dark green Colour and fetid Smell. The Bark of the Root is of a deep Ash Colour, white within and rough without, and of a disagreeable Smell. The whole Plant is esteem'd soporific and narcotic, and according to some of a poisonous Nature, tho' others say that the Fruit may be eaten without any ill Consequence. It is however seldom used internally; but externally the Juice is recommended against Pain, and Redness of the Eyes, an Erysipelas, hard Tumors and strumous and scrophulous Swellings. The Herb-women in *London* generally sell the Leaves of the *Hyoscyamus luteus*, for those of *Mandrake*, and these or those of *English* Tobacco, are said to be usually employ'd in

making the *Unguentum Populneum* instead of those of *Mandrake*.

Manga, Offic. *Mangas*. Park. Theat. The Mango Tree. This grows in the *East Indies*, and the Fruit is brought to us pickled, which is esteem'd to be cooling and moistening. According to *Garcias*, the Stones roasted cure a *Diarrhœa*.

Manna. This is produced from the *Mannifera Arbor*, Offic. *Fraxinus rotundiore folio*, C. B. P. The round-leav'd Ash, and is certainly a Juice flowing from the Trunk and larger Branches of this Tree, as is said, when the Sun enters the Sign *Cancer*. This Juice is every Year collected in hot and dry Weather, about, or a little before the Dog-Days, and the *August* Rains, because, when rainy Weather begins, it ceases to flow: There are three Kinds of this *Calabrian* Manna, one by the *Italians* called *Manna di Corpo*, which is the most elegant of all the others, and is either spontaneously discharged from the Trunk, and large Branches of the Tree, in form of a Crystalline Liquor, and becomes concreted into Grains, some larger, and some smaller, which are, the succeeding Day, carefully gather'd, lest they should be again melted by the Rains, or the Fogs; or about the Rising of the Sun the Bark of the Tree is divided with a Knife, and the discharg'd Liquor is receiv'd in Vessels, put upon Paper, and expos'd to the Sun, in order to be dried: The second Species, by them called *Forcata*, which is obtain'd by Art, is, by the same Trees, after they cease to drop spontaneously, yielded in the Month of *August*, from Incisions made in the Bark to the Wood. From these Incisions, the Manna flows copiously from Noon till ten o'Clock at Night, and is next Day expos'd to the Sun in order to be dried; but this Species is less esteemed, on account of its Impurity and Yellow Colour: The

third

hird Species is called *Manna di Frondi*, and is spontaneously, by way of Sweat, discharged from the Leaves of the Trees, on which the Drops are indurated; but, this last Species is not very carefully collected, because it is not, without the greatest Difficulty, to be separated from the Leaves. The *Arabians* are the first, who give us any Account, of *Manna* as a Cathartick which they call *Tereniabin*, *Siracoss*, and *Mal de Cussuram*. *Manna* is not only purgative, but, also, possessed of a correcting and temperating Quality, and therefore it is justly to be accounted a Medicine of all others the most mild, safe, and friendly to Nature; for though, especially when exhibited in large Doses, it powerfully purges the *Primæ Viæ* from all *Sordes*, and, in some Patients, procures, perhaps, twenty Stools, when three or more Ounces of it are taken; yet so wonderful and salutary are its Virtues, that it expeditiously produces its Effects, without bringing on violent Pain, Loss of Strength, Ebullition of the Blood, an Augmentation of the Thirst and Pulse, or a preternatural Heat. We may, therefore, in general, affirm of *Manna*, that it's Use is more extensive, and it's Nature better accommodated to most Persons, than that of any other lenitive or purgative Medicine; so that it is possessed of some peculiar Virtues, which are not to be found in other Purgatives. Such is the Nature of *Manna*, that it expeditiously discharges from the Body all kinds of Humours, whether serous, bilious, or acid; it corrects and sheaths up the Acrimony of the bilious Humours; and, which generally happens with other Purgatives, it is neither entanged, nor its force impared, by acid Humours, but, by correcting and subduing them, rather facilitates their Evacuation by the Anus. Besides, the Use of *Manna* is suited and adapted to all those, who, in Consequence either of their Weak-

ness, or the Delicacy of their nervous Systems, cannot bear acrid Medicines, though at the same time, their *Primæ Viæ* are to be freed from the *Sordes* lodged in them. This Medicine is calculated for Persons of all Ages, Sexes, Constitutions, and Countries. For which reason, *Zacutus Lusitanus*, gives a compendious, but just Account of the Virtues of *Manna*, in the following Words: " *Manna* may be exhibited to Per-" sons of all Constitutions; for it " purges the whole Body from ex-" crementitious Humours, and es-" pecially from Bile. It cleanses the " Breath, is of a lenitive Nature, " and, together with the thin, ex-" pels the viscid Humours from the " *Thorax*, without doing any Injury " to the Head, or nervous System. " It strengthens the *Viscera*, corrobo-" rates the Stomach, purifies the " Blood, exhilarates the Heart, ren-" ders the Breathing free, allays " Thirst, and excites the Appetite: " In a Word, every Part of the Body " receives singular Benefit and Ad-" vantage from it." *Manna* is esteem'd a most excellent Cathartic in the Disorders of Children from Acidities, for old People and even pregnant Women, and where-ever acid and bilious Juices abound, or whenever there is a great Acrimony of the Humours. It is much recommended in rheumatic, arthritic, and scorbutic Disorders, in the Chin-Cough, and is said particularly to be of very great Service in Fevers, in hypochondriac Disorders, in Colics, the Stone in the Urinary Passages, or a Suppression and Heat of Urine. Besides the Virtues of *Manna* consider'd as a Cathartic, it also sooths as it were, and relaxes, and by this Property removes Spasms and Contortions of the Fibres. *Manna* is, also, possessed of a diuretic Quality, and is upon the whole, perhaps, the very best and most universally useful Cathartic in the Shops. *F. Hoffman* as-

serts,

rts, that *Manna* is generally given too small Doses, by which means a Sordes contain'd in the Intestines is put in Motion, but not carried off, consequence of which Flatulencies are excited. He therefore advises to give it in the Quantity of three or four Ounces to Adults, and to Infants and Children from two Drams to half an Ounce; and by this means informs us, that it purges with Efficacy, Safety, and without exciting those Flatulencies, which it raises if taken in a small Dose. *Manna*, like Honey dissolv'd in Water, will ferment, and produce a vinous Liquor. And I have great reason to suspect, that *Manna* is extremely powerful in the dissolving that Inflammatory Spissitude of the Blood and Juices, which is the most general Source and Support of Inflammations and Fevers. That *Manna* is best esteem'd which is white and recent; that which is dark-colour'd and brown being old and decay'd. The Druggists sometimes adulterate it with Sugar.

Marrubium album, Prassium, Offic. *Marrubium album vulgare*, C. B. P. White Horehound. It grows frequently in publick Roads, flowering in *June*. The Herb is used, which is esteem'd healing, drying and pectoral; it is recommended in Obstructions of the Lungs, Liver, Spleen, and *Uterus*, in *Phthisis*, Spitting of Blood, difficult Labour, a Retention of the Lochia, and a Jaundice. The Leaves of this Plant, gives no Tincture of red to the blue Paper; they are very bitter, and have a penetrating Smell. It is probable, that in *Flanders* this Smell may approach to that of Musk; for *Dodonæus* affirms it does so. The bitter natural Salt of the Earth, compofed of marine Salt, Sal Ammoniac, and Nitre, feem to be united in this Plant, with a confiderable Quantity of Sulphur, Phlegm, and Terreftrial Parts. This

Plant by the chymical Analyfis, yields a great deal of acid Phlegm, Oil, and Earth: a little urinous Spirit; fome concreted, volatile, and a fixed Salt, a little lixivial. Thus it is no wonder, if the white Horehound fhould be a great Diffolver, and a good Aperitive; and excellent for thofe who have the Afthma or Jaundice. The Juice of this Plant is given to drink, from two Ounces to fix, for Rheums and ftubborn Coughs.

Marrubium nigrum, Ballote, Offic. *Marrubium nigrum fœtidum, Ballote Dioscoridis*, C. B. P. Black Horehound. It grows in Hedges, flowering in *June*. The Herb is us'd, which is efteem'd good in hypochondriacal and hyfterical Diforders. *Boerhaave* recommends it as an excellent Uterine, and fays it is good againft apopleftic, epileptic, and hyfteric Fits.

Marum, Offic. *Marum vulgare*, Park. Herb Maftich. It is cultivated in Gardens, flowering in *June*. It is fudorific, cephalic and aperient; it is of Service againft venomous Bites, and a cadaverous Breath. It is hotter than Betony, and not fo hot as *Serpyllum* and Thyme, tho' it has the fame Virtues, only is a little more aftringent.

Marum Syriacum, Offic. *Marum Syriacum, vel Creticum*, Park. *Majorana Syriaca vel Cretica*, C. B. P. Syrian Herb Maftich. This Plant grows naturally in *Candia* and *Syria*, but with us is cultivated in Gardens, flowering in *June*. It is remarkable that Cats are great Admirers of this Plant, infomuch that they will eat and deftroy it, if they can get to it, and rowl themfelves upon it with all the Marks of exceffive Pleafure. This Plant is very friendly to Nature; the Leaves, rubbed, emit an Odour, which affects the Brain like volatile Salt; but in Summer, when fcorched, and, as it were, burnt by the

the fervent Heat of the Sun, yields no Smell at all, tho' rubbed never so vehemently. Hence it appears to contain an acidulous volatile Salt, and that nothing in Art or Nature affords the like. This Salt is very good against Apoplexies, Lethargies, and hysteric and epileptic Disorders, provided they proceed from a cold Cause. The Spirit, sprinkled in any Place, diffuses amost grateful Scent; and Paper, impregnated with it, maintains its Fragrancy for a whole Year. It is a Plant of an extraordinary Use in phlegmatic Disorders, proceeding from the Stomach, the *Anasarca*, and stomachic and uterine Disorders. The Conserve, with Spirits of Wine, yields a Spirit far exceeding *Hungary* Water. It is of Service, also, in venomous Bites, a fetid Breath, and is an Ingredient in Theriacal Compositions.

Mastiche, Mastich. This is already taken notice of under the Article *Lentiscus*.

Matricaria, *Parthenium*, Offic. *Matricaria vulgaris simplex*, Park. Feverfew. It grows in Hedges, flowering in *June*. It is called *Matricaria*, from *Matrix*, because it is of singular Efficacy in Diseases of the Matrix; it is also, called *Parthenium*, from παρθενος, a Virgin, for the same Reason. It has a peculiar Smell, and is proper in all cold Diseases of the Uterus; and has a more bitter, oleous, and acrid Taste than Chamomile, as favouring somewhat of Camphire and Castor. Hence it is of Service in provoking the Menses, expelling the Reliques of the Secundines, false Conceptions, and the Lochia, when retained by a cold Cause. Its Virtues consist in an inflammable, aromatic, and highly volatile Oil: It is made the same Use of as Chamomile; and Baths for the Feet are prepared of it, in order to provoke the Menses. Feverfew in Clysters, discusses Flatulencies, and

is of excellent Service in Surgery, for discussing Tumors and Contusions. It is recommended for Impotence, and for the Dropsy; it purges by Urine, and sometimes by Stool. It is also recommended for putrid Fevers, for the Stone in the Kidneys, for a Vertigo, and for the Gout.

Mays. A Name for the *Triticum Indicum*, or Indian Wheat.

Mecaxochitl, Offic. *Piper longum humilius fructu.è summitate caulis propendente*, Cat. Jamaic. Small American long Pepper. It grows in *New Spain*, and is an Ingredient in Chocolate, but is seldom found in our Shops. It is healing and drying, and may be reckon'd as a Species of long Pepper. It is drank with Chocolate, to which it gives a grateful Taste: It is corroborative; heats the Stomach, and corrects a fetid Breath, it attenuates grofs and viscid Humours; resists Poison, and is good for the Cholic and Iliac Passion.

Mechoacana alba, Offic. *Mechoacan*, J. B. *Bryonia*, *Mechoacana alba*, C. B. P. White Mechoacan. It is brought us to from *America*, the Root is used, which purges pituitous, aqueous, and serous Humours from all Parts of the Body, and especially from the Head, and nervous System, and from the Breast. The *Spaniards* prepare from it a white *Fæcula*, called by them *Lac Mechoacannæ*, half an Ounce of which is a Dose, powder'd and mix'd in Broth. That is to be esteem'd which is recent, white, and ponderous.

Mechoacana nigra is Jalap.

Meconium. The concreted Juice of the Poppy, in which Sense it is the same as *Opium*.

Medica, Offic. *Medica major erectior, floribus Purpurascentibus*, J. B. *Trifolium Burgundicum*, Ger. Emac. Medic-Fodder. It takes its Name *Medica* from *Media*, because it was brought from thence into *Greece*, in the Time of the *Persian* Invasion, under

ler *Darius Hystaspes.* It is sown
Fields, flowering in the Summer.
e Herb is used, which is call'd
the *French St. Foin,* and *Foin de
wyogne.* In *Spain* it is constantly
d to nourish and fatten Cattle,
ich they find by Experience to
prove them beyond any other Fod-
whatever. The green Seed
de into a Cataplasm relieves those
o want Refrigeration.

Medium, Offic. *Medium Dioscori-
Rauwolfio,* J.B. *Viola Mariana, la-
atis foliis, peregrina,* C.B.P. Syrian
l-flower. It grows in *Syria,* and
ecce; the Root and Seed are used.
e Root stops the Menses, but the
ed provokes them.

Melampyrum, Triticum vaccinum,
lic. *Melampyrum, comâ purpuraf-
te,* C.B.P. Cow-Wheat. It
ows among Corn, flowering in
ne; the Seed is the Part in Use,
t has hitherto been neglected in
edicine. In *West Friesland* and
inders, where it is very plentiful,
vitiates the Bread, and renders it
ick, and those who feed on it
mplain of a Heaviness in the
ead, as if they had eaten Darnel;
t *Tabernæmontanus* often eat of this
ead, and assures us, that he found it
ry savoury, and not hurtful.

*Melampyrum sylvaticum, Cratæo-
nm,* Offic. *Melampyrum luteum la-
folium,* C.B.P. Wild-Cow Wheat.
grows in Woods and Thickets,
owering in *June* and *July;* the Seed
used, which stimulates to Venery.

Melanthium, Offic. *Melanthium
sylvestre sive arvense,* J.B. *Nigella
rvensis, cornuta,* C.B.P. It grows
mong the Corn in *Germany,* flower-
ng in *June.* The Seed is used, which
laid to attenuate and open, it is prin-
ipally used in mucilagious Infarctions
f the Lungs, to promote Expectora-
ion, to increase Milk, to excite Urine
nd the Menses, and to cure vene-
nous Bites; is is esteem'd a Specific
n Quartan and Quotidian Fevers.

Melilotus, Offic. *Melilotus Officinarum Germaniæ,* C.B.P. *Trifolium
odoratum, sive Melilotus vulgaris,
flore luteo,* J.B. Melilot. It grows
in Hedges and among Corn, flowering in *July. Melilot* takes its Name
from μίλι Honey, and λωτὸς a celebrated Plant among the Antients, not
from its sweet Taste, for the Leaves,
Flowers, and Fruit are bitter, but
because there is no Plant from which
the Bees gather sweeter Honey, or
more in Quantity. The Leaves, besides their emollient Quality, are endued with a Virtue of healing in a
very gentle Manner, by their aromatic Quality; the Flowers, are also
aromatic and emollient, and therefore, reckoned among internal Pectorals; but they are more used outwardly, as emolient, discutient, and
anodyne, on which Accounts they
are serviceable in all Sorts of Inflammations, particularly of the *Uterus,
Testes,* and *Anus,* as well as in nephritic,
and Arthritic Pains. The Seeds are
discutient, aperient, aromatic and
and Resolvent, and reduc'd to a
Meal compose a Cataplasm, which
is highly emollient and resolvent.
The Decoction of the Leaves and
Flowers taken inwardly is very good
to cleanse the Passages obstructed by
Cold. A Decoction of the Tops of
the Plant is good for Inflammations
of the Intestines, the Colic, Retentions of Urine, and the Rheumatism;
they are prescribed in Conjunction
with Chamomile Flowers, in Cataplasms, Plaisters, and Fomentations.
This Plant gives hardly any Tincture
of red to the blue Paper; it is acrid,
bitter, styptic, odoriferous, and gives
a slight Nausea, when chew'd; by
which it seems, that its Salts very much
resemble the natural Salt in the Earth,
united with a great deal of essential Oil,
and terestrial Parts. For by the Chymical *Analysis,* the *Melilot,* besides
a great deal of acid Phlegm, yields,
also, a good Quantity of Oil of Earth,

C c together

together with an urinous Spirit, volatile, concrete; and a fixed Salt very lixivial.

Melilotus vera, Offic. *Melilotus Italica folliculis rotundis*, C. B. P. Italian Melilot. It is a Native of *Italy*, but cultivated with us in Gardens, flowering in *July*. The Herb and Flowers are used, and agree in Virtues with the preceeding.

Melissa, Offic. *Melissa hortensis*, C. B. P. Baulm, Baum, or Balm. It is cultivated in Gardens, flowering in *June*. This Plant is endowed with extraordinary Virtues; for Pleasantness of Taste and Smell, no Herb exceeds it. The Leaves infused in Wine impregnate the same with its grateful Scent, and render it an highly useful and comfortable Medicine in all melancholly Affections; for it greatly exhilarates, being very cordial. The expressed Juice has, also, an Astringence, and is good for those who are subject to Melancholy, and hypochondriacal Flatulencies; and, in such Cases, it is always proper to be exhibited, though attendant on hot Disorders. The Herb fresh gathered, and infused in half Wine and half simple Water cold, or drank after the manner of Tea, affords great Relief to melancholly Patients. This Herb is an excellent Remedy for hysteric Women, since it wonderfully exhilarates the Spirits. Women subject to rumblings of the Intestines, Eructations, and Syncopes, are greatly relieved by *Baum* Leaves, bruised and held to the Nose, in the Paroxysms of these Disorders. A medicated Wine prepared of this Herb, is highly beneficial in gouty Rheumatisms, and arthritic Pains, provided it is daily used. A Decoction of the Leaves corroborates lax Gums. An infusion of it with Wine, Ale, or Water, contributes greatly to the Cure of that Species of Melancholy, which draws its Origin from a Defect of Spirits. It is com-

mended against Epilepsies, Madness, Barrenness, Apoplexies, Palsies, Vertigos, and Faintness. It is beneficial in Crudities of the Stomach, Obstructions of the Menses, and a Retention of the *Lochia*. It removes the fetid Smell of the Breath, and is serviceable to those who labour under a Retention of Urine. Externally, it is used in Cataplasms, Baths for the Feet, poisonous Stings, and other Misfortunes of a like Nature.

Melissa Fuchsii, Ger. Emac. *Pseudo-Melissa*, Offic. *Melissa adulterina quorundam amplis foliis & floribus, non grati odoris*, J. B. *Lamium montanum Melissæfolio*, C. B. P. Bastard Baum It grows in Woods, and the Herb is used, which is aperitive, and is esteem'd by some as a Vulnerary. It is greatly recommended in a Suppression of Urine.

Melo, Offic. *Melo vulgaris*, C. B. P. Musk Melon. It grows in Gardens, flowering in *June*. The Seed is used, which is one of the greater cold Seeds. It is esteem'd hepatic and nephritic, good for Coughs, Consumptions, and Fevers, and is serviceable in the Strangury, and Heat of Urine, and to allay Thirst; in other Respects it agrees with the other greater cold Seeds.

Mentastrum, Offic. *Mentastrum spicatum folio longiore candicante*, J. B. Horse-Mint. It grows in moist Meadows, flowering in *July*; the Herb is used, which agrees in Virtues with the *Mentha*, or Spear-Mint.

Mentastrum minus, Ger. Emac. *Mentastrum hirsutum*, Park. Theat. *Mentha palustris folio oblongo*, C. B. P. Cylonian Plant. It grows in watery Places, and frequently about the Sides of Rivers, flowering in *August* and *September*. The Herb is used, which is an efficacious Remedy in Deafness.

Mentha, Offic. *Mentha angustifolia spicata*, C. B. P. *Mentha Romana*, Ger. Emac. Spear-Mint. It grows

rows in Gardens, flowering in *July.* The Herb is ufed, which abounds in fubtle and fedative comforting Oil, which is highly friendly to the Nerves. But its Power of corroborating the Tone of the Stomach and Inteftines is not only owing to this Oil, but, alfo, to a fub-aftringent earthly Principle: For which Reafon this Herb, either in Subftance, or infufed in Water, Wine or Brandy, is highly beneficial, whether ufed internally, or externally, in ftoping Hiccups, Vomitings, immoderate Fluxes, and Colics. After the previous Ufe of Purgatives, inveterate *Gonorrbæas,* and a *Fluor Albus,* have been happily removed only by means of Spirituous Mint-Water, exhibited in due Quantities: It is beneficial to Patients afflicted with a-rabilarious and hyfteric Diforders. In bloody Dyfenteries, the Herb bruifed and applied to the Abdomen, is a fovereign Remedy; but is faid to deftroy that Power to which we give the Name of Virility. It is carminative, and excites copious Eructions. It is beneficial in the Scury, provokes Urine, and the Menfes. The Herb boiled with Whey, and applied externally to the Face, folliots eryfipelatous Swellings, and Inflammations of the Fauces, to the furface; and, by that means, relieves the internal Parts. Of the tender Tops are prepared an Oil, of which an *Elæofaccharum* and Balfam are made, which are highly beneficial againft Convulfions proceeding from a cold Caufe; and are excellent for the Cure of Contufions and Wounds. This Plant alfo kills Worms.

Mentha aquatica, Sifymbrium, Offic. *Sifymbrium,* J. B. Mentha rotundifolia paluftris, feu aquatica major, C. B. P. Water-Mint. It grows in moift Places, flowering in *July.* The Herb is ufed, which agrees in Virtues with the former. This Plant was by an illiterate *London* Quack

efteem'd fo powerful a Specific a-gainft the Stone, that, when he had Occafion to exhibit it for that Purpofe, he retired to his Clofet, and cut it fo fmall, that it was no eafy Matter to difcover what Plant it was. At laft a fmall Quantity of this *Arcanum* came into the Hands of Dr. *Watfon,* who fowed it in his Garden, and the Produce revealed the Secret. This Mint is juftly commended a-gainft Pains of the Stomach: For which Reafon the Water diftilled from it is by fome called Colic-Water.

Mentha Crifpa, Offic. Mentha crifpa verticillata, C. B. P. Crifped or Curled-Mint. It grows in watery Places, flowering in *Auguft.* The Herb is ufed, the Powder of which is recommended againft a Weaknefs of the Stomach, and againft Vomiting.

Mentha fufca, Offic. Mentha hortenfis verticillata Ocymi odore, C. B. P. Red-Mint. It grows in Gardens and watery Places. The Herb is ufed which agrees in Virtues with the other Species of Mint.

Mentha Piperis fapore, Offic. Mentha paluftris fpicis brevioribus & habitioribus, foliis oblongis, fapore Piperis, Raii Hift. Pepper-Mint. It is found about Ditches and watery Places, flowering in *Auguft.* The Herb is ufed, which is efteem'd a Specific in the Stone in the Kidneys and Gall Bladder. The diftill'd Water is by fome called Colic-Water.

Mentha fylveftris, Offic. Mentha fylveftris rotundiore folio, C. B. P. Round-leaved Horfe-Mint. It is produced in watery Soils. The Herb is ufed, which is efteem'd ftomachic and hyfteric.

Mercurialis, Offic. Mercurialis mas & fæmina, J. B. *French* Mercury. It grows in Gardens, flowering in Summer. *J. Bauhine* and others found fomething nitrous in this Plant; it is of an herby Tafte, a lit-

tle

tle faltifh, and gives no Tincture of red to the blue Paper. Perhaps the great Quantity of Sulphur, with which it abounds, hinders the Sal Ammoniac from manifefting itfelf; for by the chymical Analyfis it yields a great deal of volatile concrete Salt, Oil and Earth. *Hippocrates, Dioscorides,* and *Galen* agree, that this Mercury is purgative; the Syrup made with its Juice is laxative and aperitive. The Water, in which it has been macerated cold for twenty-four Hours, is given for the Dropfy, Cachexy, and Green-ficknefs: This Plant is ufed in *Semicupiums* for the Suppreffion of the Terms; for it is very emollient alfo; and they make thofe Perfons who are believed to be barren, take three Ounces of its Juice depurated, and mix'd with two Drams of Tincture of Steel. It is alfo good to foften Tumors.

Mercurialis repens, J. B. *Cynocrambe,* Offic. *Mercurialis montana tefticulata & fpicata,* C. B. P. Dog's Mercury. It grows in Woods and Hedges, flowering in the Spring. The Herb is ufed, and tho' *Prevotius, Moreton* and others, affirm it to be poffefs'd of the fame Virtues with the former, yet the Effects it produc'd on fome Perfons near *Shropfhire* fufficiently prove it to be of a foporiferous and malignant Quality. Another Species of *Mercurialis,* is the *Phyllon* or Childrens Mercury.

There is alfo another Sort of *Mercurialis,* which is the *Bonus Henricus,* or *Englifh* Mercury.

Mefpilus, Offic. *Mefpilus Germanica folio Laurino, non ferrato, five Mefpilus fylveftris,* C. B. P. The Medlar Tree. It is cultivated in Gardens, flowering in *May.* The Fruit and Seed are ufed; the Fruit is cooling, drying, and of an auftere Tafte; it is very aftringent and binding, and injurious to the Stomach, efpecially whilft hard. When foften'd, they are lefs aftringent,

not fo injurious, and quickly rot, and then only they are eatable: They are ufed both externally and internally, in Diarrheas and Dyfenteries. The Seed are accounted good for the Gravel and Stone.

Mefpilus Aronia, Offic. *Mefpilus aronia veterum,* J. B. *Mefpilus Apii folio laciniato,* C. B. P. The *Neapolitan* Medlar. It is cultivated in the Gardens of the Curious, flowering in *May.* The Fruit is ufed, which moderately binds the Belly.

Meum, & Meum Athamanticum, Offic. *Meum foliis Anethi,* C. B. P. Spignel. It grows in Meadows and Paftures, flowering in *June.* The Seed and Root is ufed, which difcuffes Flatulencies, and is principally us'd in Inflammations and Eructations of the Stomach, for provoking Urine and the Menfes, in a Suffocation of the Uterus, for the Gripes, for Catarrhs, and for expectorating the Tartar of the Lungs. The Seed has the fame Virtues as that of Fennel, but is more balfamic, and recommended in an Afthma, where there is an Adhefion of flimy and vifcid Matter, provided there be no Inflammation. They fay that no Plant is a greater Provocative to Venery than *Meum.* Chew'd in a Morning fafting, it corrects a fetid Breath, and ftrengthens the Gums.

Meum Alpinum, C. B. P. *Mutellina,* Offic. *Meum Alpinum Germanicum, illis Mutellina dictum,* Park. German, or Mountain Spignel. It grows on hilly Places; the Herb is ufed, which agrees in Virtue with the former.

Milium, Offic. J. B. *Milium femine luteo,* C. B. P. Millet. The Seed is ufed, which is of extraordinary Service in Difeafes of the Lungs, and Exulcerations of the Kidneys; made into a Cataplafm, it is anodyne and refolvent. It potently provokes Sweat and Urine.

Milium

Milium Solis. A Name for the *Lithospermum,* or *Gromwell.*

Millefolium, Offic. *Millefolium vulgare album.* C. B. P. Yarrow. It grows in Pastures, flowering in *June.* The Leaves are used. This Plant is a little acrid, bitter, aromatic, and gives a considerable Tincture of red to the blue Paper. The acid Part of the natural Salt of the Earth, disengaging itself of the other Principles thro' the Texture of this Plant, forms, with the terrestrial Parts, an aluminous Salt, united with a little essential aromatic Oil. By the chymical Analysis are extracted from Yarrow several acid Liquors, a great deal of Earth, no volatile concreteSalt, but a little urinousSpirit. Thus this Plant is vulnerary, resolvent and astringent. It is used in Ptisans, and Infusions, after the manner of Tea. Some boil its Leaves in Broths, to stop all forts of Hæmorrhages, and especially the irregular Flux of the Piles, or Fluor Albus. The Water of Yarrow is recommended by some for the Epilepsy ; and Wine or Mead, impregnated with this Plant, stops all Sorts of irregular Fluxes. Externally, it is of Service in the Tooth-Ach, Hernia, Tumors of the Penis, Head-Ach, Pterygia of the Eyes, and poisonous Stings or Bites.

Millefolium nobile, Ger. Emac. *Achillea,* Offic. *Achillea Mille-folia odorata,* J. B. Achilles Iron-wort. It grows in *Germany, Italy,* and *France,* flowering in *July.* The Herb is used, which represses all Sorts of Hæmorrhages ; and, outwardly used, is an excellent Vulnerary.

Millegrana, a Name for the *Herniaria,* or Rupture-wort.

Mirabilia Peruviana, Ger. Emac. *Solanum Mexicanum flore magno,* C. B. P. *Jalapa flore purpureo,* Boerh. Ind. Alt. Marvel of *Peru.* It is cultivated in Gardens, flowering in *August.* The Leaves and Root are used ; the former of these, when bruis'd, dissipate cold Tumors, if applied to them ; and the Water, in which an Ounce or two of the recent Roots have been boiled, is an excellent Purgative for dropsical Patients, and we are inform'd by some, that two Grains of the Root, taken internally, are highly efficacious in evacuating Waters in a Dropsy.

Mollugo, Offic. *Mollugo montana angustiifolia, vel Gallium album latifolium,* C. B. P. Bastard Madder. It grows in Hedges and Bushes, flowering in *June ;* the Root is used, which is possess'd of the same Virtues as the *Rubia Tinctorum,* or Common Madder.

Mollugo montana, Offic. *Mollugo montana, latifolia, ramosa,* C. B. P. Mountain Wild-Madder. It grows on hilly Places, flowering in *July.* The Herb is used, which is said to be aperitive.

Moly Dioscoridis. A Species of Garlick. See *Allium.*

Moly Theophrasti. Another Species of Garlick. See *Allium.*

Molybdæna. A Name for the *Dentillaria* or Lead-wort.

Momordica. A Name for the *Balsamina,* or the Male-Balsam Apple.

Monophyllon, Offic. *Monophyllon sive Unifolium,* Park. *Smilax unifolia humillima.* Tourn. Inst. One Blade. It grows in Woods and Thickets, flowering in *May* and *June.* The Flower is used, which is alexipharmic and vulnerary.

Morsus Diaboli, Succisa, Offic. *Morsus Diaboli vulgaris, flore purpureo,* Park. *Succisa glabra,* C. B. P. Devils Bit. It grows in Meadows, flowering in *August.* The Leaves, Flowers, and Roots are used. It is alexipharmic and vulnerary, and in other Respects it agrees with the *Scabiosa.* The Leaves are bitter, and give a deep Tincture of red to the blue Paper. The Root, which is bitter and styptic, stains the blue Paper with a still deeper Red.

Morsus Gallinæ. A Name for the *Alsine* or Chickweed.

Morsus Ranæ, Offic. *Morsus Ranæ sive Nymphæa minor,* J. B. *Nymphæa alba minima,* C. B. P. Frog-bit. It grows in muddy and slow Waters, flowering in *July.* The Herb is used, which agrees in Virtues with the white Water Lily, or *Nymphæa.*

Morus, Offic. *Morus fructu nigro,* C. B. P. The Mulberry Tree. It is cultivated in Gardens, and the Fruit is ripe in *August.* The Bark of the Root, and the Fruit is used, the former of which is heating, drying, and astringent, good to open Obstructions of the Liver and Spleen, and helps the Jaundice. The unripe Fruit is refrigerating and drying, and is principally used in all kind of Fluxes, as the Diarrhæa, Dysentery, menstrual Flux, and spitting of Blood, and externally used, it is good for Inflammations of the Fauces, and Ulcers. The ripe Fruit is refrigerating, drying, and somewhat loosening, it allays Thirst, and excites an Appetite, and is recommended by some for the Scurvy.

Moxa. This is a Kind of downy Substance, taken from the Leaves of the *Artemisia Chinensis, cujus Mollugo Moxa dicitur,* Pluk. Phytog. or the *Chinese* Mugwort. This is used by the *Indian* Nations, as something of the same kind was formerly employ'd by *Hippocrates,* and other ancient Physicians, in cauterizing Parts afflicted with Pain. Some Moderns highly extolled this Operation, as the most effectual Remedy for curing, and even wholly extirpating the Gout. But tho' this Operation was for some time highly commended in *Europe,* it is now entirely disused, and not without Reason; for, besides the acute Pain produced, it has often little or no Effect. Among the *Chinese* and *Japanese* however, this Opera-

tion, and Acupuncture, continue in the highest Esteem. These Cauterizations are, also, said to be at present used by the *Arabians.*

Musa, Offic. *Musa Arbor,* J. B. *Palma humilis longis latisque foliis,* C. B. P. The Plantain Tree. It grows in both *Indies,* and the Fruit is used, which is very nourishing, provokes Urine, and stimulates to Venery. The Leaves of this Tree are sometimes so large, that a Man may cover his whole Body with one of them, and are said to be those with which *Adam* and *Eve* cover'd their Nakedness; which seems more probable, than that they should make Use of the Leaves of the common Fig-Tree for that Purpose, as represented by the Painters.

Muscari. A Name for the *Bulbus Vomitorius,* or Musk Grape Flower.

Muscipula, Offic. *Muscipula viscaria sive Lychnidis Species,* J. B. Catch-Fly. It grows among Corn, flowering in *June* and *July.* The Seed is used. It agrees in Virtues with the *Lychnis.*

Muscus, Offic. *Muscus arboreus: Usnea Officinarum,* C. B. P. Hairy Tree Moss. This Moss is found hanging upon old Trees, but seldom in *England.* The whole Plant is used, which is accounted astringent.

Muscus marinus, Offic. *Muscus marinus capillaceus Dioscoridis,* Park. Sea Moss. This Plant is found in the *Adriatic* Sea. The whole is used, and is of an inspissating Quality, checks Congestions of Humours, and refrigerates the Parts affected with arthritic Pains.

Muscus pulmonarius, Offic. C. B. P. *Muscus pulmonarius sive Lichen arborum,* Park. Tree Lungwort, Oak Lungs. It grows upon Trees, and especially upon Oaks, and is of an earthy and astringent Taste. The whole Plant is used. It is drying and astringent, good to stop Bleeding, and

and to agglutinate recent Wounds; and is esteem'd by the common People good for Disorders of the Lungs.

Muscus pyxidatus, Offic. J. B. *Muscus pyxoides*, C. B. P. Cup Moss. This Moss is found upon dry barren Places. The whole Plant is used, which is esteem'd a Specific in the Whooping Coughs of Children.

Matellina. This is specify'd under the Article *Meum.*

Myagrum. This is already taken Notice of under the Article *Alyssum.*

Myosuros, Offic. J. B. *Myosuros, sive Cauda muris*, Merc. Bot. *Holosteo affinis Cauda muris*, C. B. P. Mouse-Tail. It is found in the Fields, flowering in *May*. The Herb is used, which is said to be possess'd of the same Virtues with the Plantain.

Myrica. A Name for the *Tamariscus*, or Tamarisk.

Myrobalani, Myrobalans. Of this there are five Sorts, the first is the *Myrobalanus Inda Nigra*, Offic. *Indian* or black Myrobalans. This Fruit is more slender and narrow than any of the rest, with eight Ridges upon the Superficies. They are rough, solid and hard, and black both within and without, of a subacid, rough, and astringent Taste. The second is the *Myrobalanus Citrina flava*, Offic. Citron or yellow Myrobalans. This is an oblong, round, pentagonal, rough Fruit, of a Citron Colour, including an angular Stone, under a carnous Bark. The third is the *Myrobalanus Chebula*, Offic. Chebule Myrobalans. This is an oblong rough Fruit, with five Ribs on the Superficies, including an oblong, thick, and cavernous Stone, under a carnous Bark. It is of a roughish Taste, and the largest of all the Myrobalans. The fourth is the *Myrobalanus Bellerica*, Offic. Belleric Myrobalan. This is a round and somewhat angular Fruit, about the Sieze of a large Gall, containing a

hard Stone, under a carnous Bark. It is of a subacrid and astringent Taste. The fifth is the *Myrobalanus Emblica*, Offic. Emblic Myrobalan. This is a roundish black Fruit, flat at each End, sexangular, and easily separating into six Parts, containing an hexagonal, round, white Stone, divided into six Cells. The Citrine Myrobalans, are said to purge Bile. The *Indian*, black Bile, and the other three, first Phlegm and then Bile. *Geoffroy* says, that they purge gently, and strengthen the Intestines at the same time; and therefore, are very proper in Diarrhæas and Dysenteries, and make a good Succedaneum for Rhubarb; only the Dose must be larger; and they may, likewise, be very conveniently mixed with Rhubarb.

Myrrha, Offic. C. B. P. Myrrh. This is a resinous, dry, and hard Substance, of a brown, or reddish yellow Colour, of a subacrid, bitter, aromatic Taste, and fragrant Smell. It is of a heating, drying, opening and subastringent Nature, and is said to attenuate, maturate, discuss, and resist Putrefaction. It is principally used in Obstructions of the Uterus, to promote the *Menses*, accelerate Delivery, and procure a Discharge of the *Lochia* and Secundines. It is also recommended for Infarctions of the Lungs, Hoarseness, Coughs, Quinseys, Pleurisies, Colics, and for the Worms. Externally apply'd it is said to cure Wounds and Ulcers. The Committee of the College of Physicians, employ'd to form the last Dispensatory, absolutely deny, that it is so difficult to dissolve Myrrh in Water or Wine, as is generally imagin'd; but affirm on the contrary, that boil'd in Water it dissolves freely, and while the Water is boiling hot, keeps almost entirely suspended; but when the Water is cold, about one third only, or less subsides,

much

much the greater Part remaining united with the cold Water. This Water evaporated leaves a Gum dissolvable again in Water, but will not give so much as a Tincture to Spirit: Spirit will take up a great Part of what precipitates from the Decoction, the rest seeming to be Dregs. They also assert, that macerating Myrrh with Salt of Tartar, will not enable Spirit to dissolve more of the Myrrh, than this resinous Part now mentioned; and the same Quality may be extracted by Spirit from the whole Myrrh without any such Preparation. A Quantity of Myrrh, first powdered, being divided into two equal Parts, one reserved by itself, and the other macerated with Salt of Tartar for more than half a Year, then both set in the same Heat with equal Quantities of Spirit, each of these Tinctures, by evaporating equal Portions of them, were found impregnated with the same Quantity of Resin from the Myrrh.

Myrrhis, Offic. *Myrrhis major vel Cicutaria odorata,* C. B. P. Sweet Cicely. It is cultivated in Gardens, flowering in *June.* The Leaves are used. It has the Taste of Cloves, is used in Sallads, and has the aperitive, exhilarating, diuretic and demulcent Virtues of the Clove, and is a very great Antiscorbutic, the expressed Juice being taken in Whey, to the Quantity of some Ounces. A Cataplasm prepared of the Leaves, is applied to the *Perinæum* and *Ossa Pubis,* for Bruises by Falls, and for Contusions. It is an excellent Remedy in a Suppression of Urine from a Spasm of the Bladder, or its Sphincter, and to provoke the *Menses,* or discuss Tumors. It is also discutient and resolvent, and may be exhibited in the Pleurisy, as, also, in a Peripneumony, with Whey and Honey, in order to resolve the Phlegm: It is, also, proper in hot

Distempers, as well as chronic; which, though seeming to imply a Contradiction, is nevertheless true: It potently exhilarates, and is, therefore, exhibited to melancholy Patients in Whey.

Another Species of *Myrrhis,* is the *Daucus Creticus,* Offic. *Myrrhis annua semine striato, villoso, incano,* Tourn. Inst. Carrots of Crete, or Candy Carrot. It is brought from *Candy.* The Seeds are used, which are oblong, grey, acuminated, hairy, and of a fragrant Smell and Taste. They are of singular Efficacy in Uterine Affections, and diuretic. Thus it discusses Flatulencies, and is principally used in Obstructions of the Menses, Strangulations, and Pains of the Matrix, in the flatulent Colic, Hiccup, Dysury, inveterate Cough, and the like Disorders.

Myrtus, Offic. *Myrtus communis Italica,* C. B. P. Common Myrtle. This Plant is cultivated in Gardens, flowering in *June*; both its Leaves and Berries, which are used in the Shops, are of a blackish Colour, of an oblong round Form, of an astringent Taste, and a faint and languid Smell. Both of them are refrigerating, drying, and highly astringent; the Powder of the Leaves, if sprinkled on the Axillæ and Groin, prevents their fetid Smell. These Leaves, if the Body is rubb'd with them, stop immoderate and profuse Sweats. They also, prove beneficial in catarrhous Disorders and Fluxes; they are an excellent defensive in the Herpes, heal Putrefactions of the Mouth; stop Hæmorrhages of the Nose, and cure a Polypus. The Berries mitigate Inflammations of the Eyes; and are beneficial in Luxations of the Joints, and Fractures of the Bones, and its *Rob* is good in all Disorders, which require Refrigeration and Astringency. Some derive its Name from *Myrrha,* Myrrh, because it smells

mells like Myrrh; and others will have it so called from an *Athenian* young Woman named *Myrrha*, who was beloved by *Pallas*, and after her Death changed by her into this Tree.

Myrtus Brabantica. A Name for the *Elæagnus* or *Dutch* Myrtle.

Napellus. Monks-Hood. A Species of *Aconitum*.

Napus dulcis, *Bunias*, Offic. *Napus sativa*, C. B. P. Navew Gentle. It is sown in Gardens. The Root is used in the Kitchen, and the Seeds in Phyfic, which are said to be heating, drying, abflerging, aperitive, and digeftive ; and to be Enemies to Venery.

Napus sylvestris, Offic. C. B. P. *Napus sylvestris sive Bunias*, Park. Rape. It grows amongft Corn, and on the Sides of Ditches, flowering in the Summer. The Seeds are used which agree in Virtues with the former.

Napus sylvestris Cretica, C. B. P. *Pseudo-Bunium*, Offic. Candy wild Navew. It is found in the Ifland of *Crete*. The Herb is us'd, which according to *Dioscorides* cures Gripes, Stranguries and Pains of the Sides. It alfo difcufles Scrophulous Tumors, if mix'd with Salt and Wine, and apply'd to them by way of Ointment.

'Tis a Controverfy hotly agitated among the *Literati*, whether the Seeds of the *Napus Dulcis*, or thofe of the *Napus sylvestris* ought to be used in the Compofition of *Venice Treacle*. The Seeds of the former are for this Purpofe ufed in our Shops. In this they imitate the *Greeks* ; for *Dioscorides* makes not the leaft Mention of the *Napus sylvestris*. *Andromachus* the Elder, alfo, orders the Seed of the *Napus dulcis*, and *Matthiolus*, in the fifth Book of his Epiftles to *Balbaserus* affirms, that the Seeds of the *Napus dulcis* refift Poifon more power-

fully than thofe of the *Napus Sylvestris*. *Andromachus* the Younger, when enumerating the feveral Simples which enter the Compofition of the *Theriaca*, commends the Seeds of the *Napus sylvestris*, as being more acrid, and of confequence more efficacious in promoting the Intention of the Medicine. But *Galen*, in his firft Book *de Antidotis*, differs from both thefe Opinions, and recommends the Seeds of the *Pseudo-Bunium*, as moft proper for compofing the *Theriaca*.

Narcissus, Offic. *Narcissus pallidus circulo luteo*, C. B. P. Common pale Daffodil, or Primrofe Peerlefs. It grows on Banks, and in Meadows, flowering in *April*. The Root is ufed, which taken either in Meat or Drink, is an Emetic. It is of Service in Ambuftions, conglutinates the divided Nervès, is effectual in Luxations of the *Malleoli*, and inveterate Pains of the Joints ; removes cutaneous Blemifhes in the Face, and the *Vitiligo* ; cleanfes foul Ulcers, breaks Abfcefles, and draws out Splinters from the Body.

Narcissus luteus. A Name for the *Bulbocodium*.

Nardus Celtica, Offic. J. B. *Nardus Celtica Dioscaridis*, C. B. P. Celtic Spikenard. The Roots with the Leaves are ufed. The Roots are fibrous, hairy, and black, and have upon them fmall Leaves of a green-yellow Colour, of an acrid, bitter and aromatic Tafte, and of a fragrant Smell, fomewhat weighty. As it agrees in *Genus* and external Appearance with *Valerian*, fo it feems to agree in Virtues. The Plant is heating and drying, and agrees in Virtues with the *Indian Spikenard* ; but is more effectual in provoking Urine, ftrengthening the Stomach, and difcuffing Flatulencies ; outwardly it is an Ingredient in the Compofition of *Malagmas* and Ointments.

Nardus

Nardus Indica & Spica Nardi.
Offic. *Nardus Indica vulgaris,* J B. *Nardus Indica, quæ Spica, Spica Nardi & Spica Indica officinarum,* C. B. P. *Indian* Spikenard. The Root is used, which is long, fungous, and of the Thickness of one's Finger, of a yellowish-brown Colour, of a bitter, acrid, and aromatic Taste, and of a grateful Smell. That is best which is recent, light, having long Hairs upon it, and of a bitter Taste. It is brought from the *East-Indies,* and *Alexandria.* It is heating, drying, attenuating, astringent, nephritic and stomachic. It is principally used in Inflammations, the Jaundice, and to destroy Worms. *Galen* relates, that he cured an Emperor of the Colic in his Stomach, by rubbing that Region with an Ointment of this Nard. It may be given inwardly, from half a Dram to a Dram ; and, in Infusions, from half an Ounce to an Ounce and half.

Nardus montana, Offic. *Nardus montana radice Olivari,* C. B. P. Mountain Spikenard. This is the Root of a Species of Valerian which grows in the Mountains of *Leon* in *Spain,* but we are not certain what the Ancients called by this Name. It is not much used in Physic ; but its Virtues are like those of the *Nardus Celtica.*

Nasturtium aquaticum, Offic. *Nasturtium aquaticum supinum,* C. B. P. *Sisymbrium aquaticum,* Tourn. Inst. Water-Cresses. It grows in watery Places, flowering in *June* ; the Herb is us'd, which is heating, drying, attenuating and aperitive, and is principally recommended for the Stone and Gravel, for Obstructions of the Liver, Spleen, and Menses. It is reckon'd a Specific in the Scurvy, and cures all Diseases proceeding from a Viscidity and Ropiness of Blood. This Plant gives no Tincture of red to the blue Paper. It con-

tains a Salt pretty much resembling the *Oxysal Diaphoreticum Angeli Salæ,* which is an alcaline Salt, over saturated with Acid. Besides this, there is in the Water Cresses a little Sal Ammoniac and Sulphur, and a great deal of Earth. For by the chymical Analysis we obtain from this Plant a great deal of Acid and Alcali, a little urinous Spirit and Sulphur, and a pretty deal of Earth. They affirm, that the Juice of this Plant takes away the *Polypus* of the Nose, and makes it fall off, if it be often washed with it.

Nasturtium hortense, Offic. *Nasturtium hortense vulgatum,* C. B. P. *Nasturtium vulgare,* J. B. Garden-Cresses. It is sown in Gardens, flowering in *June.* The Herb and Seeds are used. The Seeds are attenuating, opening and abstergent, and are principally used in Tumours of the Spleen, Obstructions of the Menses, and expelling the dead Fœtus ; they cut the tartarous Mucilage of the Lungs, and are good for the Scurvy and Dropsy. The Herb bruised or parched, and mixed with the Fat of an Hog, cures the Scurf, and scabby Sores of the Head, and other Parts, being anointed therewith. This Herb liquifies the Blood, and renders it acrimonious ; whence it is proper, where there is a Coldness and Viscidity ; but in hot Distempers it is Poison. It quite eradicates pituitous Diseases, is a good Pectoral for old Persons, where Phlegm hinders Respiration, and is good in hysteric and hyphondriac Cases. The Leaves newly bruis'd, and mixed with Ferment, heat, and excite a Redness of the Skin, and even a Blister, if their Application be continued for a considerable Time. Where it meets with a sweet viscid Phlegm, and none but cold Humours, with an extreme Laxness of the Solids, in all these Cases it is highly serviceable. The Seeds by a singular
Property,

bperty, are effectual in Hernia's, ither internally or externally used. *Nasturtium Indicum*, Offic. *Nasturm Indicum majus*, C. B. P. *Indian ress*. It is a Native of *Peru*, but quently cultivated with us in Gardens, flowering all the Summer. The ower is serviceable in a Weakness Pain of the Stomach, proceeding m Cold and Flatulencies; it is an gredient in Sallads, with other reens. It is also recommended r a stubborn and malignant Itch, and r recent Wounds.

Nepeta, Mentha Cataria, Offic. *Nepeta sive vulgaris*, Park. *Mentha Cattaria vularis & major*, C. B. P. Nep. It rows in Hedges, flowering in *June* and *uly*. The Herb is used, which is f fine Parts, and is principally recommended for Disorders of the terus, for Sterility, and to expel e Foetus, and is sometimes us'd to t the tartarous Mucilage of the ungs.

Nephriticum Lignum. Nephritic-Vood. See *Glans Unguentaria.*

Nerium, Offic. *Nerium sive Rhodo- indron, flore rubro & albo*, J. B. *lerium floribus rubescentibus & albis*, . B. P. Oleander, or Rose-Bay. It s cultivated in Gardens, flowering n *July*. This Plant has a Force vhich is insuperable; for its Juice xcites so great and violent an Inlammation, as immediately to put Stop to Deglutition; and, if it be received into the Stomach, that Part is render'd incapable of retaining any thing, the pernicious Drug exerting its Force, and purging both upwards and downwards. Antidotes against its Poison, are Vinegar, and all Acids.

Nicotiana, Petum, Tabacum, Offic. *Nicotiana major latifolia*, C. B. P. *Hyoscyamus Peruvianus*, Ger. Emac. Tobacco. The *Indian* Name of this Plant is *Picelt*. It is a Native of *America*, where it grows spontaneously in great Plenty; with us it is cultivated in Gardens, flowering in *June*. The Leaves are the Part us'd in Medicine, which are said to absterge, incide, and resolve; to be somewhat astringent and to resist Putrefaction. It is a strong Sternutatory, and Apophlegmatism; and is narcotic, vulnerary, and emetic. The *Edinburgh* Dispensatory has given a Syrup of Tobacco, but this Plant is in general so emetic, cathartic and narcotic, that I think the internal Use of it is never to be allow'd, tho' a Water distill'd from the green Leaves is much recommended for dislodging Stones in the Urinary Passages. *Monardes* informs us, that the *Indians* use the Leaves of Tobacco for curing Wounds; and esteem them an efficacious Remedy in the Head-Achs, *Hemicraniums*, Flatulencies, Stiffness of the Neck, a *Tetanus*, and Pains of the whole Body arising from a cold Cause, if apply'd to the Part affected. The Juice also of Tobacco is much recommended to preserve the Teeth and Gums, and to cure the Tooth-Ach. The Leaves are, farther, esteem'd effectual in Hysterics apply'd to the Navel and Region of the Uterus; and in Pains of the Joints, and œdematous Tumors, warm Leaves of *Tobacco*, or a Cloth dip'd in the Juice, are said to be very effectual. Apply'd to pestilential Carbuncles, these Leaves are said to induce a Crust, and promote a Cure, and to be a present Remedy for the Stings and Bites of Venomous Animals, and for that Poison with which the *Cannabals* tinge their Arrows. A Drop or two of the Oil of *Tobacco* put upon the Tongue of a Cat, immediately kills it. *Diemerbroek* highly recommends the Use of *Tobacco* in the Plague, asserting that both at *London* and *Nimeguen* when the Plague rag'd, those Houses that sold *Tobacco*, escap'd the Infection. We learn from the *Edinburgh Medical Essays*, that

Tobacco, beat well with Vinegar or Brandy into a Mash, and apply'd in a Linnen Bag on the Stomach, occasions strong Vomiting, and has sometimes very good Effects in removing hard Tumors of the Hypochondria. Mr. *Stedman* who communicated this Account, informs us, that he knew two Instances of its making a complete Cure: One of an old Man, who, by sleeping in the open Air, while the *Serenas,* or Night Dews fell, was taken, in the *West-Indies,* with a Numbness of his whole Body, which soon was followed with Purging and Vomiting; and these going off, he had all the Symptoms of a Jaundice, and Hardness, and Pain, under the short Ribs of the left Side. The Pain went off in a few Days, but the Tumor increased. After he had used Variety of Medicines for five Years to remove this Disease, a Sea Surgeon applied a Poultice of *Tobacco,* disguised with Green Tea, Sugar and Cochineal upon the *Epigastrium* and *Hypochondria.* After this Application had been made four or five Hours, he vomitted a great deal of purulent Matter. When the Poultice was taken away, the Vomitting ceased. He continued to apply this Mash once a Day for a Month, and was perfectly cured. The other Example was of a Boy, who was cured, much in the same Manner, of an hard indolent Tumour of the Left *Hypochondrium.* The Man had six Ounces of *Tobacco* in his Poultice; the Boy had only one, and the Quantity must always be regulated by the Age of the Patient. Smoaking and chewing of Tobacco have been esteem'd of Service in Disorders, where the Glands of the Fauces, have abounded with Lymph, or where the Constitution in general has been too much loaded with *Serum;* and the same has been said to relieve some Asthmatic Patients, which is not un-

likely, both on account of its Narcotic Quality, and because it evacuates a Part of the superfluous *Serum;* but this can be of no Reason for its habitual Use, especially in those who have no Occasion for it; for in such I apprehend it does a great deal of Prejudice, by drawing off the *Saliva,* which Nature providently prepares, to dilute, and in some Measure to dissolve the Aliments taken into the Stomach; besides, it excites a perpetual Thirst, and tempts the Person, who smoaks or chews, to drink more, than is sufficient for any good Purposes in the Constitution. I have known several People brought into Dropsies and Consumptions by too profuse Discharges of the *Saliva,* excited by smoaking or chewing Tobacco; and upon the whole I esteem it extremely prejudicial, unless when it can be made subservient to any good medicinal Purposes; and then like *Opium* it should be used when required only, and left off immediately, when the Necessity for it ceases. And the same may be said of *Tobacco,* consider'd as a Sternutatory, which may answer some Purposes as a Medicine, but it is sure to be prejudicial, when render'd habitual by way of Amusement. But the greatest Use of *Tobacco* in Medicine is in Clysters; for the Smoak of *Tobacco,* convey'd into the Intestines, either by an Instrument contriv'd on Purpose, or blown in by means of a common *Tobacco Pipe,* will stimulate strongly, so as to procure Stools, when every other Method of doing it has fail'd. Hence it is of Service in the Iliac Passions and some Species of Ruptures, attended with absolute Costiveness, and may be employ'd to very good Purposes in other Disorders where a strong and sudden *Stimulus* is requir'd. And this Method of taking *Tobacco* might, no doubt, by Habit, be render'd equally amusing, mufing, as finoaking or chewing it; and it has this to recommend it, that it is a much lefs filthy and naufeous Entertainment.

Nicotiana minor, C. B. P. *Tobacco Anglicum,* Park. *Priapeia quibuf-lam, Nicotiana minor,* J. B. Englifh Tobacco. It is fown in Gardens, flowering in *July* and *Au-guft.* The Leaves are ufed, which agree in Virtues with Henbane. The Leaves of this Plant are frequently fold by the Herb Women for the *Mandragora* or Mandrakes, and fome-times for the common Tobacco

Nigella, Gith, Offic. *Nigella flore minore fimplici, candido,* C. B. P. *Melantbium calyce & flore minore, femine nigro,* J. B. Fennel Flower. It is fown in Gardens, flowering in *July.* The Seed is ufed, which is attenua-ting and opening, and is principally ufed in refolving, and expectora-ting the Mucilage of the Lungs, for increafing Milk, for provoking Urine and the Menfes, and againft the Bites of venomous Animals; it is alfo efteem'd a Specific in quartan and quotidian Fevers. The Plant is recommended for the Stone in the Kidneys, and for deftroying Worms, the Quantity of two Ounces thereof being boil'd in Wine. This is alfo faid to cure the Colic.

Nigellaftrum, Offic. *Lychnis fege-tum major,* C. B. P. *Pfeudo-Melan-tbium,* J. B. Cockle. It grows a-mong Corn, flowering in *June* and *July.* The Seed is ufed, which is heating and drying, and being ap-plied in a Peffary with Honey, pro-vokes the Menfes. It is extoll'd by fome as a Vulnerary. A Dram of the Powder of the Seed of this Plant, given to drink in Broth, or Water, for three Mornings, is an excellent Remedy for the Vapours. *Senner-tus* and *Simon Pauli* ufed the Root of this Plant fuccefsfully, to ftop Hæmorrhages, even thofe which hap-pen in continued Fevers. They put

it under the Tongue of the Patient, and left it there for fome time.

Nuces è Barbadoes, Offic. *Ricinus Americanus major, femine nigro,* C. B. P. *Barbadoes* Nuts. This grows in *Barbadoes,* and other Parts of the *Weft-Indies.* The Fruit is oblong, oval, of the Size of a fmall Bean, having one Side convex; the other deprefs'd, including under a hard Pellicle a white Kernel. It agrees in Virtues with the *Ricinus vulga-ris.*

Nummularia, Offic. *Nummularia major lutea,* C. B. P. *Nummularia Centimorbia,* J. B. Money-wort. It grows in watery Places, flowering in *May;* the Herb is ufed, the Juice of which partakes of the Nature of *Beca cabunga;* for it has as a afponaceous, aromatic and balfamic Tafte: Hence it has the fame Virtues. It has an Acrimony, which is not ungrateful, mix'd with fomewhat aromatic, and of an aftringent acid Tafte. Hence, it works the fame Effect as *Scurvy-Grafs,* mixed with *Serrel,* which we ufe when we are apprehenfive of fpitting of Blood. For this Reafon it is proper in all Sorts of Scurvy, where the Humours are to be ren-der'd more fluid without danger of too great a Refolution, or Tenfion; for Inftance, in an exceffive Flux of the *Menfes,* where a total Stop would it fucceeded by an Inflam-mation, and yet the immoderate Evacuation requires to be reftrained, for which purpofe this Herb is very proper. A Decoction of the Leaves, in Wine fweeten'd with Honey, is good for Ulcers of the Lungs, the *Fluor Al-bus, Dirrhæa, Dyfentery, Afthma,* Spit-ing of Blood, *Hæmorrhoids,* and the dry Coughs of Infants. The Powder of the Leaves is good for an *Hernia* in Infants; and the Leaves bruifed, and applied in the Form of a Ca-taplafm, cleanfe and dry up fetid Ulcers. This Plant refifts Putre-factions,

factions, generates *Pus*, is corroborative, and cures many Diseases. For the *Arthritis*, *Podagra*, Scurvy, Dropsy, and Jaundice, take an Ounce or two of the Juice in the Morning fasting; it is opening, and purges by Stool and Urine.

Nux Avellana sylvestris, Jons. Dendr. *Avellana*, Offic. *Corylus sylvestris*, Ger. Emac. The Hazel. This is very frequent in Woods and Hedges, and there are many Species of it, which all agree in medicinal Virtues. The *Juli* or Catkins, and Shells of the Nuts, are said to be astringent and binding. The Kernels are said to load the Stomach, to be of difficult Digestion, and to render the Head heavy; some affirm, that they are binding, and consequently good in a Dysentery; others, on the contrary, assert that they are loosening. They are esteem'd pectoral, and the Oil by Expression is recommended by *Tragus* for a Cough. The Cream of these Nuts is good in the Stone and Heat of Urine. Emulsions may be made of them. *Quercetan* gave a Dram of the Powder of Nutshels, mixed with an equal Quantity of prepared Coral, in a Glass of the Water of *Carduus Benedictus*, or Corn Poppy, in the Pleurisy.

Nux Juglans, Offic. *Nux Juglans five Regia vulgaris*, C. B. P. The Walnut-Tree. The Catkins appear in *March*, and the Nuts come to Maturity in *Autumn*. The Bark of the Tree, the Catkins, the Nuts, and the stony Substance which lies betwixt the Lobes of the Kernel, and the external *Putamen* or green Hulls, are us'd in Medicine. The recent Nuts are said to heat and dry, and to be a Preservative against the Plague. The *Putamen* or green Hull is gently emetic. The internal Bark of the Tree taken off while succulent and dry, excites Vomitting pretty powerfully; and the *Juli* or Catkins, do the same, but in a milder Manner. Their principal Use is in Cholic and Nephritic Pains; they are also said to stop a Diarrhœa. The recent Nuts excite Stools; when dry they are more hot, difficult of Digestion, and exasperate a Cough. Two or three immature Walnuts preserv'd with Sugar are said to excite Stools. And the Nuts eaten in a Morning, are esteem'd a Preservative against Poisons and contagious Distempers. A *Pediluvium*, prepar'd of the Leaves, is by some recommended in the Gout; and these Leaves are also said to cure inveterate Ulcers. The fungous Substance which lies between the Lobes of the Kernel, dry'd, powder'd, and exhibited in Wine, is reported to have been of infinite Service, in an epidemical Dysentery, which rag'd among the *English* Forces in *Ireland*, and resisted all other Methods. This Substance is also recommended, in the Quantity of a Dram for a Dose, in a Pleurisy, and is reckon'd a Specific in a Cancer, if long continued. A preserv'd green Walnut, cures the Hiccups, perhaps more effectually, than any other Medicine.

Nux Moschata, Offic. *Nux Moschata*, *Nux Myristica*, *Nucista*, Mont. Exot. The Nutmeg-Tree. It grows spontaneously in the Island of *Banda*, in the *East-Indies*, in great Plenty. It is as large as a Pear-Tree, bearing fragrant Leaves somewhat resembling those of the Peach-Tree. The Fruit is about the Size of a small Peach, cover'd with a soft juicy Hull like a Walnut; immediately under this is found the Mace, which closely adheres to the subjacent hard, woody Shell, which incloses the Nutmeg. Nutmegs are heating, drying, and somewhat astringent, stomachic, cephalic, and uterine; they discuss Flatulencies, help Digestion, mend a fetid Breath, are reviving to the *Fœtus* in the Womb, are excellent in Faintings, and Palpitations of the Heart,

Heart, diminish a tumid Spleen, restrain *Diarrbæas* and Dysenteries, and stop Vomitings. The Fruit is brought to us preserv'd from *India*; but these eaten to Excess, are said to have a narcotic Quality, and to produce a Delirium, or Sort of Intoxication. The same Virtues with those of Nutmegs are ascrib'd to Mace; but because its Parts are more small and minute, it is thought to operate more effectually, and to be possess'd of a more penetrating Quality than Nutmegs. The *Oleum Nucis Moschatæ*, or as it is improperly called *Oil of Mace*, is the Oil of the Nutmeg by Expression: That is best which is brought from the *East-Indies* in *China*-Jars, of a thick and pinguious Consistence, of the Colour of Mace, and of a fragrant Smell; but this is seldom met with in the Shops; instead of it we generally meet with another Sort brought from *Holland*, in square Masses, of a harder Consistence, a paler Colour, and less fragrant Smell; but this is not near so good as the former. The genuine Oil of Mace by Expression is made in the *East-Indies*, from the Mace whilst recent, whence it is brought to us in Glass-Bottles, but it is a very rare Commodity. What is genuine is liquid, of a red Colour, smelling strongly of Mace, of a pungent Taste, and somewhat thicker at the Bottom of the Vessel than at the Top. What is commonly sold for Oil of Mace in the Shops, is a Kind of factitious Oil, or Unguent, made of Sheep's Suet, Palm Oil, and the like Ingredients, scented and colour'd with Oil of Nutmeg. This is by no Means equal to true Oil of Mace in Efficacy, and ought to be a very cheap Ingredient, as it is pretty insignificant.

Nux Pistacia, Offic. Park. Theat. *Pistacia*, J. B. *Pistacia peregrina fructu racemoso sive Terebinthus Indica Theophrasti*, C. B. P. The Pista-

chio, or Fistick Nut-Tree. This Tree grows in hot Countries. The Nuts are us'd, which are heating, moistening, attenuant, and aperitive. They are principally used in mucilaginous Infarctions of the Lungs, and Obstructions of the Liver; they strengthen the Stomach, repress a Nausea and Vomiting, excite an Appetite, and afford good Nutriment; and *Dioscorides* affirms, that if bruised and taken in Wine, they are effectual against the Bites of venomous Reptiles. Those are best which are recent, ponderous, and not rancid.

Nux Virginiana, Offic. *Prunifera, vel Nucifera, seu Nuciprunifera Arbor Americana præcelsa, angustis Lauri foliis latè virentibus, Mastichen odoratum fundens*, Sloan. Hist. Raii Dendr. The *Virginia*-Nut. It grows in *Barbadoes*, and the Fruit is us'd, which is nearly of the Shape and Size of the Kernel of a Filbert, smooth, of a brown Colour, with an Eye near one End, and containing an hard Stone; which incloses a white, globular Kernel, of a bitterish Taste, and aromatic Smell. It potently opens Obstructions, depurates the whole Mass of Blood, and corrects a scorbutic and bad Habit of Body, by impregnating the vital Liquor, the Blood, with those volatile Salts, which exalt it from its low and vapid State to a more pure and spirituous one; and by that Means, preserve it from Stagnation. It, also, clears the Skin of Spots, and all other Defedations.

Nux Vomica, Offic. Ger. Emac. *Nux Vomica, in Officinis*, C. B. P. Vomic-Nuts. These grow in *Malabar*, but are not, or at least ought not to be, us'd in Medicine, for they are extremely narcotic and virulent, exciting Inquietudes, Rigors, Convulsions, Horrors, Tremors, and an irregular Respiration. They are principally used for poisoning Dogs, Cats, Crows, and other Animals,

by

by a Barbarity peculiar to Mankind.

Nymphæa alba, Offic. Ger. Emac. *Nymphæa*, *Nenuphar*, Chab. White Water-Lilly. It grows in Rivers, and flowers in *July*. The Root, Leaves and Flowers are us'd in Medicine. The Root, refrigerates and dries, and the Leaves and Flowers, refrigerate and moisten; all are us'd in Fluxes of the Belly, nocturnal Pollutions, against Acrimony of the seminal Fluid, and too great Heat and Thinness of Blood. The Leaves are said to be a good Application for hot Tumors and Inflammations. By the chymical Analysis it yeilds a good deal of Acid, and very little concreted volatile Salt; so that it is no Wonder it should be sweetening. The Roots are frequently us'd in cooling Ptisans, for a Heat of Urine, and Inflammation of the Kidnies, and other Bowels. There is a Syrup prepar'd of this Plant, which is said to be a little narcotic. Many are very cautious of using this Plant, for fear of extinguishing all amorous Desires, and rendering themselves impotent; for it is found by Experience, they say, that the Use of the Seed and the Root, renders Persons very cold and dull as to venereal Inclinations. *Pliny* writes, that they who take it twelve Days successively, find themselves deprived both of the Seminal Fluid, and the Power of Coition. The Root of this Plant, boiled in black Wine, and drank, stops the immoderate Flux of the Menses, even when the Disorder has been regarded as desperate.

Nymphæa lutea, Offic. Ger. Emac. *Nymphæa major lutea*, C. B. P. This grows frequently in Rivers, flowering in *July*. The Root, Leaves, and Flowers are used, which agree in Virtues with those of the preceeding.

Ocymoides, Offic. *Ocymoides album multis*, J. B. *Lychnis Sylvestris flore*

albo, C. B. P. Wild White-Campion It grows among Corn, flowering in the Summer. The Seed is used. It is drying, and of fine Parts, and cures the Bites of Vipers, and other Serpents. It is good in a *Sciatica*, and being boil'd in Posset-Drink is an excellent Remedy for Convulsions in Children.

Ocymum. See *Basilicum*.

Oenanthe Petroselini folio, venenosa, Offic. *Oenanthe succo virosa, Cicutæ facie Lobelii*, J. B. *Filipendula Cicutæ facie*, Ger. Emac. Hemlock-Dropwort. It is very frequent in watery Places, especially about *Bath*, flowering in *June*. The Plant is extremely poisonous and malignant, especially the Root, which however us'd to be sold by the Herb-Women in *London*, for the Roots of Piony. The Plant is so poisonous, that if tasted, it causes immediate Death with Convulsions, as it happen'd at the *Hague*, where two Men went out a Simpling, and finding this Plant, tasted it: One of them was immediately taken with Convulsions, and died on the Spot; the other soon after. Some such Instances we have in *Stalpart Vander Wiel's* Observations, where Persons have died within two Hours, after only tasting this Plant, which affects the Brain, so as to cause Convulsions, and is so quick in Operation, as scarce to give Time for a Remedy. The Root has an acrid and unpleasant Taste; it yields at first a milky Juice, but afterwards a yellow, virulent, poisonous, and fetid one. The Plant taken inwardly, immediately excites an extreme Pain in the Stomach, with such violent Convulsions, that the Jaws become immoveable, and a frequent Hiccup succeeds, with fruitless Efforts to vomit, and a copious Hemorrhage from the Ears. The only Remedy in this Case is for the Patient to swallow great Quantities of Oil, Butter, or Milk, that the acrid Particles

les may firſt have their Points ſheath-
d, and afterwards be evacuated by
the upper or lower Paſſages.

Oenanthe aquatica, C. B. P. *Filipendula aquatica,* Ger. Emac. Water Dropwort. It grows in moiſt
Meadows, and watery Places, and is
ſaid to be reſolvent, and friendly to
the human Body; but it is very little
us'd, and I don't find that Authors
are much acquainted with its Virtues.

Oenoplia. The great Jujube is thus
call'd.

Olea, Offic. *Olea ſativa,* Ger.
Emac. The Olive-Tree. This is
a large Tree growing in hot Countries, flowering in *June.* The Leaves
are refrigerating, drying, and aſtrin-
ent, and are principally us'd in pro-
fuſe Fluxes of the Belly, and of the
Uterus; they are alſo eſteem'd a good
application in an *Herpes.* The Fruit,
or Olives, are pickled and brought to
us, being gather'd before they are
ripe. We have generally of two
ſorts, the *Spaniſh* Olives, which are
as large as a Plumb, and are ſomewhat bitter; and the *Luca* Olives,
which are leſs, but milder. Theſe
eaten at the Beginning of a Meal,
are ſaid to increaſe the Appetite, to
render the Belly ſoluble, and to dry
and comfort a Stomach when too
moiſt. An Oil is expreſs'd from the
unmature Olives, which is called
Omphacinum; which is eſteem'd refrigerating, drying, and aſtringent.
But the Oil expreſs'd from the ripe
Fruit, is of more general Uſe, being
that we call *Olive,* or *Sallad*-Oil.
It is warming, and moiſtening, e-
mollient, digeſtive and vulnerary; it
relaxes the Belly, is good for Dryneſs, and Strictures of the Breaſt,
mitigates Gripes, mollifies, and relaxes the urinary Paſſages, and ab-
ſterges and heals Eroſions. It has
lately been found by Experience, to
be an abſolute Cure for the Bite of a
Viper, if well rubb'd into the

Part wounded, before the Fire, and
is at leaſt; as effectual as the Oil of
the Viper. Now as the viperine
Poiſon, acts by coagulating the Blood
in the Veins from the Part firſt affected towards the Heart, Oil in this
Caſe muſt produce its ſalutary Effects, by preventing ſuch Coagla-
tion. This Circumſtance, together
with the frequent Uſe of Oils and
Unctions, among the antient Phyſicians, eſpecially thoſe of the methodic Sect, makes me ſtrongly ſuſpect,
that the external Uſe of Oil may be
very powerful in preventing Coagulations of the Blood, when it is diſpos'd to run into Concretions from
other Cauſes beſides the Bite of a
Viper.

Oleaſter, Offic. *Olea Sylveſtris,*
Ger. Emac. The Wild-Olive-Tree.
It grows ſpontaneouſly in *Italy, Spain,*
and many other Countries, and the
Leaves are us'd, which in Virtues a-
gree with thoſe of the preceeding
Olive.

Olibanum, & Thus maſculum, Ind.
Med. *Thus, ſive Olibanum,* Offic. C.
B. P. Frankincenſe, or *Olibanum.*
This is a reſinous Subſtance, of a
pale yellow Colour, ſomewhat hard
and pellucid, form'd into ſmall Drops
like Maſtick, of a bitteriſh reſinous
Taſte, and fragrant Smell. It drops
ſpontaneouſly from the Tree which
produces it, and is tranſported to us
from *Turky* and the *Eaſt-Indies.*
That which is in ſmall Drops, is preferable to the other Kinds. It is
heating, drying, and ſubaſtringent.
It is principally us'd internally, a-
gainſt various Diſorders of the Head
and Breaſt; as, alſo, againſt Fluxes
and Hæmorrhages of the Uterus,
Coughs, Vomitings, Spittings of
Blood, Diarrhæas, and Dyſenteries.
Externally, Fumigations of it corroborate the Head. It diſcuſſes
Catarrhs, incarnes hollow Ulcers,
and brings them to a Cicatrix. It
conglutinates recent Wounds, eſpe-

cially

cially those of the Head. It cures Chilblains, and mitigates malignant Ulcers not only of the *Anus*, but, also, of other Parts. It also, remove Redness and Inflammation of the Eyes, and carries off beginning Wars and Impetigo's. What we call the *Manna Thuris* of the Shops, are Fragments of the Frankincense, as small as Meal, produced by the Collision of the Bags with each other during the Carriage. But others by the *Manna Thuris*, mean small Portions of the Frankincense. Nothing certain is left upon Record, with Respect to the Tree which bears the Frankincense. *Theophrastus* informs us, that it is not a very large Tree; that it is about five Cubits high, full of Branches, with Leaves resembling those of the Pear Tree, and a smooth Bark, like that of the *Bay-Tree*; but, says he, others affirm it to be like the Mastich Tree; bearing similar Fruit, and a reddish colour'd Leaf, whilst others assert, that both its Leaves and Bark resemble those of the Bay Tree. *Diodorus Siculus* ascribes the Form of the *Egyptian* Thorn to the Tree which bears the Frankincense, and the Leaves of the Willow. *Garcias* informs us, that this is a low Tree, whose Leaves resemble those of the Mastich-Tree: But *Thevetus* tells us, that it resembles the Resinbearing Pines. Mr. *Ray* also says, that we are still uncertain of the true Form of this Tree.

Omphacium. The Juice of unripe Grapes. The Antients used to expose the Grapes to the Sun some Days, and then press out their Juice into large Vats; and, in the Time of *Dioscorides*, they used to let it stand in them, exposed to the Sun, till most of the Humidity was exhaled, and the Remainder inspissated into a Rob. This *Dioscorides* recommends, with Honey and *Passum*, for Ulcers and Relaxations of the Tonsils, Uvula, Mouth, and

Gums; and for Putridencies of the Bars; for Dysenteries, and Uterine Fluxes, in Clysters, or Injection. He farther says, it clears the Sight, and cures Asperities of the Angles of the Eyes; and that it is good for a recent Spitting of Blood, from a Rupture of a Vessel; But, in this Case, it must be taken in a small Quantity, because it corrodes powerfully.

Onagra, Offic. *Chamaenerium latifolium vulgare,* Tourn. Inst. Rose Bay, Willow-Herb. This grows in Mountains, flowering in *July*. The Root is said to be a good Application for malignant Ulcers.

Onobrychis, Offic. *Caput Gallinaceum Belgarum,* Merc. Bot. *Polygalon Gisneri,* J. B. Medic-Vetchling, or Cocks Head, commonly but falsly called Saint Foin. It grows in chalky Soils, and in Meadows, flowering in *June* and *July*. The Herb is used, which being bruised and apply'd, discusses Tubercles; taken in Wine, it cures the Strangury; and rubbed on the Skin with Oil, provokes Sweat.

Onosma, Offic. *Lycopsis Anglica,* Ger. Emac. *Echium alterum,* Merc. Bot. Stone Bugloss. The Leaves taken in Wine expel the *Foetus,* according to *Dioscorides.* Dr. *Sherard* is said to have found this Plant in the Island of *Jersey.*

Ophioglossum, Offic. J. B. *Ophioglossum vulgatum,* Boerh. Ind. Alt. Adders-Tongue. It grows in Meadows, and moist Pastures; and the whole Plant is used, which is esteem'd an admirable Vulnerary both internally taken and externally apply'd. It is particularly recommended in Ruptures.

Opium. This is an inspissated Juice, of a blackish brown Colour; sometimes reddish, of a bitter Taste, and a very disagreeable Smell. The *Greeks* distinguished two Kinds of it; one got by wounding the *Papaver album,* Offic. the other by Expression.

son. The Opium which we have, is of the first Kind; and as it was cultivated formerly in *Egypt*, near the City of *Thebes*, it has acquir'd the Name of *Opium Thebaicum*. If we may believe *Kempfer*, all the Opium now used in the East, is what transudes spontaneously from the Plants in *Natolia*, and other Places. But M. *Tournefort*, and several other modern Travellers, could find no such Opium among the *Turks*, all that they met with being the same with what is brought to us in soft Lumps. They, also, observe that the sober People among the *Turks*, seldom take above a Dram in a Day; and a few Grains of that Quantity are always mix'd in their Coffee. In the Empire of the great *Mogul*, Opium is sold as commonly in the Shops, as *Tobacco* with us. The Inhabitants prepare it in different Manners, and mix it with different Ingredients, such as Rhubarb, the Extract of Rhubarb, and the like. Some add to it other narcotic Substances, such as the *Datura*. This last is generally the Artifice of the Quacks, by which they who take this, are thrown into pleasing Dreams, which they take for Ecstasies, and believe to be real. *Kempfer* relates many wonderful Effects of this Preparation, which he terms the *Indian Nepenthe*. The Effects of Opium are always narcotic, whether taken inwardly, or applied externally; and it has been found to cause Sleep, when given in a Clyster, better than when taken by the Mouth. When applied to the Eyes and Ears, it has caused Blindness and Deafness; and *Galen* relates, that an *Opium* Plaister, laid on a *Gladiator's* Head by a Stratagem of his Enemy, killed him in a little Time afterwards. This Author, also, says, that he never used Opium, except in very pressing Cases. Opium does not make the Pulse quicker or harder, than it was before; but only greater, and

heats very much; which is a sure Proof, that it dissolves and rarefies the Blood; and this appears also from its causing an Itching in the Skin, and sometimes Sweat. It is observed of the *Turks*, who are killed in Battle, that as soon as their dead Bodies are removed from the Places where they fall, they begin to bleed, their Blood being made more fluid by the Opium which they take. By this Rarefaction of the Blood in the Vessels, the Nerves which lie near these Vessels, are compress'd; and thus the Course of the animal Spirits is stopt, as is, also, the Secretion of many Fluids, such as the Bile and Urine, which occasion Costiveness, and the making of very little Water. Opium, in all probability, acts by its narcotic Sulphur, which divides and rarefies, in an extraordinary Manner, the sulphureous Parts of the Blood: And accordingly we observe all Vegetables, which contain an Oil of this Kind, such as Nutmeg, Saffron, and the like, produce in the Body an Effect of the same Nature with that of *Opium*. Neither is it at all improbable, that Sulphurs should be capable of a very great Degree of Rarefaction, since the Smell of Musk, or Ambergrise, may extend through so large a Space. *Pitcairn* was of Opinion, that the Effects of *Opium* were owing to its volatile Salt; but it seems to contain that Principle in too small a Quantity for such Operations. When a Person has taken too great a Quantity of *Opium*, the first thing to be done is to empty the Vessels by copious Bleeding, if the Patient's Strength can bear it. The next Thing is to drink acid Liquors, such as Vinegar, Lemonade, Syrup of Barberries, and such like, which coagulate the Blood, and thus give the Vessels room to contract. Smelling to Vinegar, and all Aromatics, is also proper; and, if the Stupor be very great, Scarifications ought to be made, and Vinegar and Salt sprinkled upon the scarified Parts. Blisters and sharp Clysters answer the same Effect. The Rules to be observ'd in taking *Opium* are these : (I.) If the Patient be plethoric, he ought not to take *Opium*, till he has lost some Blood. (II.) It ought not to be given in the Time of the *Menses* and *Lochia* of Women, nor during the usual Flux of the *Hæmorrhoids* in Men, because it stops all these natural and healthful Evacuations. Neither ought *Opium* to be given in every *Diarrhæa*, because, if it be critical, the Stoppage thereof may be very hurtful. It must, also, be very improper in a Suppression of Urine, and the general Rule is, that, when the Suppression of any one Evacuation by *Opium* is foreseen, other Evacuations, especially by Bleeding, ought to succeed. (III.) *Opium* ought never to be taken on a full Stomach, because it hinders Digestion, and proves, commonly, emetic. The Digestion ought, therefore, to be completed at the Time of taking it; and the same thing is to be said of all other Narcotics, which given unseasonably, and for a long Continuance of Time, quite destroy the Appetite, bring on Hickups, Nauseas, and habitual Vomitings. (IV.) Persons who begin to take *Opium*, ought to venture only on a very small Quantity at first, because the Effects of the same Quantity on different Persons are very different; and there is no Way to determine, but by Experience, how much any Person can bear. Half a Grain has been found to cause Sleep for twenty four Hours together, to a Person, who, afterwards, required half a Dram to produce half that Effect. For it is a certain Observation, that they who accustom themselves to take *Opium* habitually, must often increase the Dose, otherwise it gradually looses its Effect on them;

and the elder *Geoffroy* knew a Woman who took seventy two Grains every Day, merely to ease the Pain of a cancerous Breast. The common Quantity among the *Turks* is a Dram in a Day; but some take much more. The Antients were extremely cautious in giving *Opium*; but in the Beginning of the last Century, *Felix Platerus*, a learned Physician of *Basil* in *Switzerland*, began to bring the Use of it in Vogue. *Sylvius de le Boe*, perfected what *Platerus* began; and, from that Time, many of the most famous Physicians in *Europe*, such as *Sydenham*, and others, found, by certain Experience, that it was one of the most valuable Medicines in the World, when prudently administer'd, in calming the too violent Motion of the Blood, and easing Pain. There are, however, still some very great Men, who continue Enemies to *Opium*; and among these M. *Stahl* has declared himself, in his Dissertation *De Imposturis Opii*. They are afraid to use it for the Ends just mentioned, for fear of suspending the Crises which commonly happen after violent Pains, such as those of the Gout and Rheumatism; and in acute Distempers, in which the Fluids are violently agitated, they apprehend, that by giving *Opium*, to diminish these Motions, they only throw a Veil over the Distemper, which hinders them from observing its true *Genius*, and the Tendency of Nature in the Course of it. Of this they cite Pleurisies as an Example; and they are certainly in the right, not to give *Opium* in that Disease. But notwithstanding all the Strength of these and other Reasons, against the Use of *Opium*, and the Authority of those who advance them, this Medicine is undoubtedly very proper on many Occasions, as in great Want of Sleep, too great Motion of the Fluids, occasioned by Purgative, and other Kinds of Medicines, in great Defluxions, and in stubborn Coughs. But the principal Uses of *Opium* are in a Fit of the Stone, and a Retention of the Secundines on Account of a Stricture of the Uterus. For *Opium* by removing Pain andStricture, relaxes the Part, and affords a Passage to the Body which ought to come away. *Opium* is certainly of some Use in Medicine; but the Abuse of it is very great and destructive; and a hundred times more is used in *England,* than ought to be.

Opoponax. See *Panax Heracleum.*

Opuntia, Offic. *Ficus Indica,* Ger. Emac. *Tuna Indorum,* Jonf. Dendr. The prickly Pear-Tree. The only Parts of this Tree,which are used, are the Fruit and Leaves; which are of a refrigerating and moistening Quality, and good for extinguishing burning Fevers, and allaying Thirst.

There is another Plant of this Name distinguish'd, *Opuntia maxima, folio oblongo, rotundo, majore, spinulis obtusis, mollibus, & innocentibus, obsito flore striis rubris variegato,* Cat. Jam. *Cochinillifera,* Offic. The Cochineal Tree. It grows in *America,* and is remarkable for nothing in Medicine, but giving Nourishment to those Insects, which we call *Cochineal.*

Orchis. See *Satyrium.*

Oreoselinum, Offic. *Apium montanum vulgatius,* Park. Theat. *Petroselinum montanum,* Offic. Schrod. Mountain Parsley. It grows in the mountainous Parts of *Germany,* and is found in great Plenty on the Sides of the Mountain *Gurca,* not far from *Geneva;* the Root and Seed are used. As to its Virtues, it is of an heating and drying Quality; and is alexipharmic, sudorific, diuretic and discutient. Its principal Use is in the Stone of the Kidneys and Bladder; in the Plague, Flatulencies and the Strangury.

Oreoselinum, Apii folio, majus. Tourn. Inst. *Gentiana nigra,* Offic. Germ. *Daucus montanus Apii folio major,* C. B. P. *Libanotis Theophrasti nigra,* Ger. Emac. Mountain Dauke. It grows in the mountainous Parts of *Italy,* flowering in *July.* The Seed is used, which is of an heating, opening, and inciding Quality; provokes Urine, and the Menses, expels the Fœtus, and discusses Tumours.

Origanum Creticum, Offic. Ger. Emac. *Origanum sylvestre sive vulgare,* Park. Theat. Origany of Crete. It grows in the Island of *Crete,* flowering in *June.* The Flowers are used principally in Obstructions of the Lungs, Liver, and Uterus. *Dale* remarks that in Prescriptions, the *Cretan Origanum,* is not sufficiently distinguish'd from the common *Origanum;* and farther says, when the Flowers of *Origanum* are order'd, those of the *Cretan Origanum* are understood; but when the Herb is directed, common *Origanum,* or Wild Marjoram is meant; for the Leaves, or Herb of the *Cretan Origanum* are never to be found in the Shops. The Oil of *Origuum* is extremely hot, and seldom used inwardly, except for the Tooth-ach, in which Case it is put upon some Lint, or Cotton, and apply'd to, or held near the Part affected.

Origanum Heracleoticum, Offic. Ger. Emac. *Origanum Heracleoticum, Cunila gallinacea Plinii,* C. B. P. Bastard Marjoram. It is cultivated in Gardens, flowering in the Summer. The Herb is used, which is esteem'd heating, and good against the Bites of Serpents, and according to *Dioscorides* is given in Contusions, and for Dropsies.

For an Account of common *Origanum.* See *Majorana.*

Orleana, Offic. *Achiotl seu Medicina tingendo aptâ,* Hern. *Metella*

Ameri-

Americana maxima Tinctoria, Tourn. Inst. Arnotto. This is cultivated in *New-Spain*, and *Brasil*, and the Tincture of the Fruit, or a Kind of Colour made of it, is used in making Chocolate; for this Purpose they take the ripe Fruit, and infuse it in hot Water, and make up the Sediment into Lozenges, or, dye Wool with it, which is used as a Fucus or Paint, and is called *Spanish* Wool. This Tincture of the Fruit, diluted with Water and drank, or applied by Way of Fomentation externally, is said to mitigate febrile Heat, to stop bloody Stools, and discuss Tumors.

Ornithopodium, Offic. *Ornithopodium majus & minus*, C. B. P. Birds Foot. It grows in sandy and gravelly Places, flowering in Summer; the Herb is used, which breaks and expels the Stone in the Kidneys and Bladder, and is effectual in an *Hernia*.

Ornithopodium Portulacæ folio, Tourn. Inst. *Scorpioides*, Offic. *Telephium Scorpioides*, J. B. Scorpion-Wort. It is cultivated in our Gardens, flowering in the Summer; the Herb is used, which is of a heating and drying Quality; and is, according to *Dioscorides*, a present Remedy, against the Sting of the Scorpion, being apply'd to the Part.

Orobanche, Offic. *Orobanche major*, *Garyophyllum olens*, C. B. P. *Orobanche, sive Rapum Genistæ*, Ger. Emac. Broom-Rape. It grows in gravelly and dry Places, flowering in *June* and *July*. The Herb dry'd and pulveriz'd, is a present Remedy for the Pains of the Colic, and being preserv'd, or its Syrup, it is of excellent Use in splenetic and hypochondriac Disorders; and an Ointment prepared of the same, is good to soften hard and scirrhous Tumors.

Orobus, Offic. *Orobus sylvaticus foliis oblongis, glabris*, Tourn. Inst. *Astragalus sylvaticus*, Ger. Emac. Wood-Pease, or Heath-Pease. It grows in woody Places, and in Thickets, flowering in *April*. The *Tubera* of the Root, is used by the *Scotch* Highlanders, in the same Disorders of the Thorax for which Liquorice is proper. *Hippocrates* recommends this Plant in the Pleurisy, Peripneumony, and nephritic Disorders; for which Purposes, let the Seeds be roasted and bruised, and then have hot Water poured upon them; after this, it must stand a Night, and then be supphot, with an Addition of *Oxymel*. This Liquor is said to be lenitive, and of a penetrating Virtue; but whether this be the *Orobus* of the Ancients, is a Question. The Seed of this Plant, on Account of its farinaceous and mucilaginous Quality, answers to *Fenugreek*, in mollifying and maturating Abscesses; and, by Virtue of its diuretic Salt, which it contains in common with other leguminous Plants, it is of Service in provoking Urine, and expelling Gravel.

Oryza, Offic. C. B. P. Rice. This is a Food of at least two thirds of Mankind. It is the Grain principally us'd in all Parts of the *East-Indies*, in *Persia*, in the *Mogul's* Country, in *Turky*, and all over *Africa*, besides what is now us'd by the *Europeans*, and *Americans*. By this it should seem to be an exceeding wholesome Aliment. It is somewhat restringent, and for that Reason is prescribed in Dysenteries, the Cœliac Passion, Diarrhæas, and wherever there is too great a Solubility of the Belly. It has been said, that living too much upon Rice, is injurious to the Eyes, and inclines to Blindness; but this I look upon as a vulgar Error, depending entirely upon an Observation made by the Sailors, that Fowls carry'd on Ship-Board from the *American Continent*, to *Jamaica*, which are fed on Rice during the Voyage,

Voyage, are very subject to become blind; but nothing is more common, than to ascribe Effects to wrong Causes; and this is probably owing to some other Cause, in which Rice is in no Degree concern'd; I don't however find, that the Inhabitants of those Countries, where Rice is the almost constant and only Food, are more subject to Blindness than the Europeans.

Osmunda regalis, Filix florida, Offic. *Osmunda regalis sive Filix florida,* Park. Osmund-Royal. It grows in marshy boggy Places, and in moist Woods. The Root is used in Medicine, which is blackish without, and white within, of a subacrid and somewhat bitter Taste, and grateful Smell. It is in much Esteem, in Ruptures and Ulcers, and is reckon'd a Specific in the Rickets.

Osyris, Offic. *Osyris frutescens bacciflora,* C. B. P. *Caffia Poetica Lobelii,* Ger. Emac. Poets Rosemary. It grows in *Italy,* and *France,* flowering in *May.* The whole Shrub is used, which is astringent, and is used in some Shops, instead of the *Caffia* of the Ancients, but it must have contrary Effects, as appears from its astringent Taste, and be more proper for Fluxes of the Intestines.

Othonna, Offic. *Tagetes Indicus minor simplici flore, sive Caryophyllus Indicus, sive Flos Africanus,* J. B. *African* Marygold. It is sown in Gardens, flowering in the Summer; the inspissated Juice is used, which according to *Dioscorides* is proper for the Eyes, in Cases that require cleansing; for it has a biting Quality, and absterges whatever may dim, or cast a Mist before the Pupil of the Eye.

Oxalis, Sorrel is so called. See *Acetosa.*

Oxyacantha, this is the *Spina Alba,* or Haw-thorn.

Oxycedrus, A Species of Cedar, See *Cedrus.*

Oxycoccus, Offic. *Oxycoccus sive*

Vaccinia palustris, J. B. *Vitis Idaeae palustris,* C. B. P. Moor Berries. This Plant grows in marshy, and putrid Soils, flowering in *June.* The Fruit is used, which stops a Looseness, and Vomiting, quenches Thirst, strengthens the Stomach, mitigates the Heat in Fevers, and resists the Pestilence.

Oxylapathum, Sharp-pointed Dock. See *Lapathum.*

Oxys. A Name for the *Acetosella,* or Wood-Sorrel.

Padus, a Species of Cherry. See *Cerasus.*

Paeonia mas, Offic. *Paeonia mas praecocior,* J. B. Male Piony. It grows in Gardens, flowering in *May,* and is said to take its Name, from *Paeon,* a Physician, who with this Plant, as *Homer* says, cured *Pluto,* when he was wounded by *Hercules.* The Root, Flowers, and Seeds of this Plant discover, by the Taste, an aromatic and somewhat astringent Quality, attended with a Viscidity; whence it is effectual in all Disorders, proceeding from too great Laxness of the Brain, and in nervous Affections. A Dram of this Root, given every Morning to an epileptic Person, will prevent the Fit; but, as soon as you desist from giving it, the Fit returns, for Piony has not Virtue sufficient for eradicating an Epilepsy. The Root is hung about the Necks of Children, to prevent an Epilepsy; and the Seeds, are strung as Beads, to make a Necklace for the same Purpose. This Plant is also greatly commended in all Sorts of Convulsions, Palsies, Tremblings, nocturnal Frights in Children, and Apoplexies, for Obstructions of the *Menses,* for a Retention of the *Lochia,* to mitigate After-Pains, and for Obstructions of the Liver.

Paeonia faemina, Offic. Female Piony.

Paeonia, Offic. Common Piony. *Paeonia flore albicante,* Offic. White

flowered

flowered Female Piony. These three last Species of Piony grow in Gardens, flowering in *May*, and agree in Virtues with the *Pæonia mas*, or Male Piony.

Paliurus, Offic. *Paliurus Dodonæi*, Tourn. Inst. *Rhamnus folio subrotundo fructu compresso*, C. B. P. Christ's Thorn. It is a Native of *Italy*, flowering in *May* and *June*; the Fruit being ripe in *Autumn*. The Leaves, Root, and Fruit are used. The Leaves and Root are astringent, stop a Looseness, and digest, and cure Tubercles; and the Fruit is so powerfully inciding, as to diminish the Stone in the Bladder, and promote Excretions from the Breast and Lungs.

Palma, Ger. Emac. *Palma major*, C. B. P. *Indis Mahaindi*, Herm. Mus. Zeyl. The Palm, or Date-Tree. It grows in *Egypt*, and other hot Countries. The *Vagina*, or Sheath, which incloses the Flowers and Rudiments of the Fruits, was called by the antient Writers, *Elate* and *Spatha*, and that tender and medullary Substance, which grows on the Top of the Palm-Tree, call'd by *Theophrastus*, Ἐγκέφαλ⊙, (*Encephalus*) the Brain, and by *Dioscorides*, improperly, Ἐγκάρδιον σπέρμα, (*Encardium Premnu*) the *Heart and Marrow of the Trunk*, is nothing but a large Bud, producing, as *Theophrastus* himself says, both Leaves and Fruit; if the Tree be deprived of this Part, it is rendered barren, and, in a short time, perishes. It appears, in many Places of the antient Writers, that this Part is eatable; and *Xenophon*, in his second Book of his Expedition of *Cyrus*, says, that the Soldiers, in such a Place, first fed on the Bark of Palm-Trees, which all wither'd after being deprived of it. The Date is a round longish fleshy Fruit, of a yellow Colour, but frequently reddish on one Side, of a pleasant sweet mucilaginous Taste, inclosing in a thin white Skin, an hard cylindrical Stone, having a Chink, or Furrow, running its whole Length. *Prosper Alpinus* informs us, that in the Fruit, there are three things principally used in Medicine; that is the *Spatha*, the Powder contain'd in the *Spatha*, and the Dates themselves: The *Spatha* is used both in Powder and Decoctions. The Powder, taken internally, is highly beneficial in stopping Diarrhæas, Lienteries, and Dysenteries, as, also, all other Discharges of Blood, or other Humours, especially the hepatic Flux, the Hæmorrhoids, the Menses, and a spitting of Blood. This Powder is, also, used by the *Egyptians* in stopping spreading Ulcers, removing a Relaxation of the Uvula, and fixing the Teeth, when loose. They, also, use the Decoction for all the same Purposes; but often mix the Powder with it. It, also, surprisingly strengthens such Joints that are weak, and subject to Defluxions. The white Powder found in its proper Covering in the Spring, when the Palm-Tree begins to flourish, when mixed with Sugar, is by the *Egyptians* very frequently used against Hoarseness, Coughs and Inflammations of the Eyes. This Powder, is, also, sweet, and somewhat astringent; for which Reason 'tis frequently used by the Women, for stopping immoderate Discharges of the Menses, and procuring a Retention of the Fœtus. Unripe Dates, both used in Aliments and Decoctions, are by them, also, used against spitting of Blood, and for stopping all Evacuations of Blood, Lienteries, Diarrhæas, Dysenteries, Vomitings of Blood, and the Hæmorrhoids, as, also, for curing simple Ulcers and Wounds. For the Cure of these Disorders, they, frequently use a Syrup prepared of unripe Dates. They, also, use the Dates when perfectly ripe; at which time they are highly sweet, and somewhat

what aftringent; for which Reafon they are frequently ufed in Hoarfenefs, Coughs, Dyfpnæas, Pleurifies, and Peripneumonies. A Decoction of them is, alfo, frequently ufed for promoting the Eruption of the Small Pox.

Palma Oleofa, Offic. *Palma Guinea,* J. B. *Arbor exotica fructu Dactylis fimilis,* C. B. P. The Palm-Oil-Tree. This Tree grows fpontaneoufly in *Guiney.* The only Part of it ufed is its Oil, or rather a thick Ointment of an Orange Colour, and fragrant Smell, obtain'd from the Fruit in the following Manner: To the Pulp taken out of the Kernels, they add a large Quantity of boiling Water. Then they for a long Time agitate the Pulp in a Kettle over the Fire, till it is intimately mixed. Then taking the Kettle off the Fire, they let the Matter ftand, till its more fordid Parts fubfide to the Bottom. Then they fkim off the Oil floating on the Surface of the Water; and when they have taken all the Portion then floating on it off, they repeat the fame Operation by pouring boiled Water on it again. This Oil is beft when recent, not rancid, of an Orange-colour, a fragrant Smell, and of the Confiftence of Butter. Externally ufed, it is anodyne, ftrengthens the Nerves, allays arthritic Pains, removes Wearinefs, and relaxes contracted Parts.

Palma Indica, coccigera, angulofa, C. B. P. *Coccus,* Offic. *Palma nucifera arbor,* J. B. *Nux Indica arbor,* Ger. Emac. The Coco, or Cocoa-Nut Tree. It is produced in both *Indies.* From this Tree is extracted a Liquor, by the *Indians* called *Suri,* which, when drank, intoxicates like Wine. It is of a grateful Tafte, refembling that of a Mixture of fweet, faline, and acid Subftances: When 'tis newly extracted, 'tis pretty fweet, but, in Procefs of Time, becomes more acid, and is of a whitifh, fomewhat green, or pale Colour. From this Liquor is diftilled a Water, or Spirit, which burns in the Fire. There is, alfo, a Vinegar, and a Species of Sugar, by the Inhabitants called *Jagra,* prepared from it. The Method of extracting this Liquor is accurately defcrib'd by the Authors of the *Hortus Malabaricus.* They make an Incifion in the Top of the Capfule, which bears the Flowers or Fruit, and which they call the Breaft of the Tree, and hang a Veffel to it. About four Inches below the Top of the Capfule, they make an oblique Incifion in the Bark, which they raife by way of *Beard,* as they call it, over which the *Suri* may drop into the Veffel. In the Morning and Evening, and fometimes, alfo, in the Middle of the Day, they remove the Veffels with the *Suri.* That obtained in the Morning is fweet, that in the Evening fomewhat acid, and that obtained next Day acefcent; but that on the third Day, entirely acid, without any Sweetnefs at all. In order to make Vinegar of the *Suri,* they put the Veffels, in which it is received, among Lime for fifteen Days, by which a violent Fermentation being excited, much Froth thrown up, and a whitifh Matter fubfiding to the Bottom, the *Suri* is changed into Vinegar. The Species of Sugar called *Jagra* is prepared thus: They put into the Pots a fufficient Quantity of Lime, to tinge the *Suri* diftilled into them of a reddifh Colour; then they boil this Liquor, continually ftirring it with a Spoon, till it is infpiffated. Then a red Sugar is produced, which they render white by reiterated Diffolutions and Boilings. The exterior Covering of the Nut is at firft faid to be eatable, of a pretty fweet Tafte, good for coroborating the Stomach, ftopping Diarrhœa's and curing Surfeits. The Liquor,

Liquor, or Wine of *Suri*, is said to be highly beneficial to phthisical Patients, and those who labour under any Disorders of the Kidneys, or a Difficulty of discharging their Urine. From the bruised Kernels is expressed a Milk without the Assistance of Fire, eight Ounces of which drank every Morning, with the Addition of a little Salt, are highly efficacious in killing Worms, especially in Children. The Liquor contained in the Kernel is proper for extinguishing Thirst and Fevers, for curing and cleansing the Eyes, and for washing the Skins of Women. It, also, purifies the Blood; cleanses the Stomach, and Urinary Passages, and removes Disorders of the Breast. It is of a grateful Taste, affords much Nourishment, and is an excellent Drink in Biliary Fevers.

Another Species of *Palma*, is the *Coccus de Maldiva.*

Palma Haira, The Ebony Tree. See *Ebenus Æthiopica.*

Palma Arecifera. The *Areca* or *Faufel.* See *Areca.*

Palma Christi, Tourn. Mat. Med. *Ricinoides arbor Americana folio multifido*, Tourn. Inst. *Avellana purgatrix*, C. B. P. Purging Nuts. The Tree is a Native of *America*, and the Nuts are used, which are of a whitish Colour, and one of which both vomits and purges for several Days; but if divested of its Pellicle, and divided into smaller Doses, it proves a gentle Purgative.

Palma minor, C. B. P. *Chamærrhiphes*, Offic. *Palma humilis Hispanica spinosa, & non spinosa*, J. B. Palmites five *Chamærrhiphes*, Ger. Emac. The Dwarf Palm. It grows in *Spain* and *Italy*. The Berries are used, which are of an astringent Quality, and for that Reason exhibited against all Fluxes.

Another Species of *Palma*, is the *Draco Arbor*, or Dragon Tree.

Panax Asclepium, The All-heal of *Esculapius*. A Species of *Ferula.*

Panax Chironium, Dwarf Sun Flower. The same as *Helianthemum.*

Panax Coloni. Clowns all Heal. A Species of *Galeopsis.*

Panax Herculeum, Offic. *Panax Heracleum majus*, Ger. Emac. *Panax costinum*, C. B. P. *Pastinaca Olusatri folio*, Boerh. Ind. Alt. Hercules's All-heal. It grows in the Gardens of the Curious, flowering in *June*. From the Stalk of this wounded, especially near the Root, during the Summer Months, a Juice flows which concretes spontaneously, and is called in the Shops *Opopanax*, which, if good, is externally of a yellow Colour, but internally white, or somewhat inclining to yellow, of a bitter Taste, a strong Smell, and pinguious Consistence; it easily dissolves in Water, is light, friable, and when dissolv'd turns the Water milky. It mollifies, digests, discusses Flatulencies, and purges thick and viscid Phlegm, from the remote Parts, as the Brain, Nerves, Joints, and Thorax. The Roots of this Plant are said, by those who import it, to be effectual in all cold Affections of the Brain and Nerves, for Disorders of the Breast, and tormenting Pains of the Stomach; for all Obstructions of the Viscera, and Diseases of the Kidneys, Bladder, and Womb; on which account, they are of Service in inveterate Pains of the Head, Vertigo, Epilepsy, Stupor, Lethargy, Convulsions, Palsies, Asthma, Cough, Jaundice, and Dropsy.

Panicum, Offic. *Panicum album vulgare*, Park. Theat. Panick. It is sown in the Fields of *Germany*. The Seed is used, which is drying and refrigerating, and binds the Belly. It is principally used in Spittings of Blood, and in nocturnal Pollutions.

Papaver

Papaver album, Offic. *Papaver ortense femine albo, sativum Dioscoridi, album Plinio*, C. B. P. *Papaver hortum*, J. B. White Poppy. It is sown in Gardens, flowering in *July*; the Leaves, Flowers, Heads and Seeds, together with the condensed Juice, called *Opium*, are used. The Herb, Heads and Seeds refrigerate and moisten, and are principally used to promote Sleep, in Affections of the Breast, and Lungs, particularly in a Cough, Hoarseness, and Consumption, but in the last I am afraid with very bad Effect. They are also used in Fluxes of the Belly, and are excellent Ingredients in Fomentations, intended to mitigate Pain and induce Sleep. For the most severe Pain of an Ophthalmy, *Sennertus* prescribes, as an effectual Remedy, an Emulsion of the Seeds of Poppy, with Milk, Water of Lettuce, and Decoction of Fenugreek.

Papaver nigrum, Offic. *Papaver ortense nigro femine, sylvestre Dioscoridi, nigrum Plinio*, C. B. P. Black Poppy. It is sown in Gardens, flowering in *June*. The Leaves, Flowers, Tops, and Seeds are used, which agree in Virtues with the former.

Papaver rubrum, Rhœas & erraticum, Offic. *Papaver erraticum majus genuis Dioscoridi, Theophrasto, & Plinio*, C. B. P. Red Poppy, or Corn Rose. It grows among Corn, flowering in *June*. The Flowers are used, which are greatly refrigerating, induce Sleep, and mitigate Pains. It is principally used in Fevers, and Pleurisies, for which it is reckon'd a specific, and for a Quinsey. These Flowers are glutinous, and give much of a faint red Colour to the blue Paper as the Solution of Opium, by which it seems, the Salt of the one analogous to that of the other; for, in Opium, this Salt (which seems pretty near to Sal Ammoniac) mixed with a great deal of fetid Oil, whereas, in the red Poppy, the Proportion of the Oil is much less than that of the viscous Phlegm. Thus the Flowers of this Plant are emollient, and good for Expectoration in Defluxions of the Breast, in Rheums, and in a dry Cough. They stanch Blood, and are gently sudorific.

Another Species of *Papaver* is the *Argemone*, Offic. *Papaver erraticum capite longissimo, glabro*, Tourn. Inst. Long-headed Poppy. It grows by the Sides of Ditches, flowering in *June*, and the Leaves and Juice are used in Medicine. A Cataplasm of the Leaves, as *Dioscorides* says, absterges the *Albugo*, and Films, in the Eye; and mitigates Inflammations.

Papaver corniculatum, this is already specify'd under *Glaucium*.

Papyrus, Offic. *Papyrus Nilotica*, J. B. *Papyrus Antiquorum Nilotica*, Park. The Paper Reed. It grows in *Egypt* and *Syria*, and is the Plant of which the Antients made Paper. The *Egyptian* Surgeons, as we are informed by *Prosper Alpinus*, now use the medullary Substance of the Leaves, to dilate the Mouths of Ulcers. The Trunk, burnt to Ashes, cures recent Ulcers, and prevents the Increase of Malignity in others, being sprinkled thereon; and the distilled Water of the recent Trunk is very effectual against Cataracts, and Dimness of Sight.

Paradisi Grana, Grains of Paradise. See *Cardamomum*.

Paralysis, Offic. *Primula veris odorata flore luteo simplici*, J. B. *Verbasculum pratense odoratum*, C. B. P. Cowslips or Paigles. It grows in Meadows, flowering in *April*. The Herbs and Flowers are used. It is drying and heating, and has something of an acrimonious and bitterish Taste; it is, also, somewhat astringent, and has an anodyne Virtue. The principal Uses, to which

it

it is applied, are in Cephalic Disorders, the Gout, and other Pains, and Affections of the Joints.

Another Species of *Cowslip* is the *Herba Petri,* Offic. *Paralysis altera odorato flore pallido, Polyanthos,* Park. *Verbasculum pratense aut sylvaticum inodorum,* C. B. P. Great Cowslips, or Oxlips. They grow in Woods and Thickets, flowering in *April.* The Leaves infused a Night in White Wine, are recommended against the *Anasarca.*

Pareira Brava, Offic. *Caapeba Brasiliensibus, Lusitanis Erva de Nossa sennora aut Cipo de Cobras,* Marcg. *Raiz & Erva de Nossa sennora,* Worm. Mus. *Butua sive Pareira brava Lusitanica,* Geoff. Tract. Wild Vine. This Root is commonly about the Bigness of the little Finger, tho' sometimes larger. It is of a brown Colour, wrinkled both ways on the Surface; but its inner Substance is fibrous, like the *Thymelæa.* Zanoni says, that when cut transversly it represents the Sun, and its Rays, but this Conceit is without Foundation. It is of a sweetish Taste, with a disagreeable Mixture of Bitter, and without any Smell. Authors pretend that this Root comes from *Brasil,* for this Reason, because we get it from the *Portuguese:* But it is much more probable, that it is of *East-India* Growth; for a Surgeon sent it from *Surat* to M. *de Jussieu,* by the Name of *Boutua* Root; and wrote, that it grew along the Coast of *Malabar.* This Root is much celebrated by the *Portuguese,* as an Alexipharmic, and an Antidote against all poisonous Plants. It is undoubtedly a very good Diuretic, and very proper in Nephritc Colics. The Way of using it is: Boil about a Quarter of an Ounce, scraped or rasped, in two or three Pints of Water, till reduced to a Pint; of which the Patient is to drink a Glass every half Hour, in a warm Bath, his Body

being before prepared by Bleeding and Clysters. A Small Quantity of the Syrup of the five opening Roots may be added to the Decoction, and, by this Method alone, *Geoffroy* the elder, cured the great *Abbé Bignon* of a Stone Colic, and made him void a very large Stone. When given in a large Dose, it heats considerably. It seems to act by dissolving the slimy Matter contained in the Kidneys and Bladder; and has been given with great Success, mixed with Balsam of *Capivi,* in *Gonorrhæas,* after sufficient Evacuations. The Decoction already mention'd, has, also, done Wonders in Hepatic Colics, arising from an Obstruction of the Orifice of the Gall Bladder, a Glass being drank every three Hours, to the Quantity of a Quart. The *Portuguese* use this Root powder'd for *Quinseys,* and Diseases of the *Thorax.*

Pareira Brava alba, Geoff. Tract. *Pareiræ Species secunda,* Lochn. Sched. The white wild Vine. It is said to come from *Brasil.* It is more woody than the former, composed of Fibres, of which some are Longitudinal, the rest Orbicular. The Bark of this Root is white, but the Substance within yellow, like Liquorice.

Parietaria, Helxine, Offic. J. B. *Parietaria Officinarum & Dioscoridis,* Boerh. Ind. Alt. Pellitory of the Wall. It grows upon Walls. It absterges, and is somewhat astringent and cooling; it is seldom used internally, yet some commend it in Disorders of the Breast, for the Strangury, the Dropsey and the Stone. Externally used, it is good for Tumors, the *Erysipelas,* Burns, and for Wounds. By the chymical Analysis, it yields a great deal of Oil, fix'd Salt, and Earth, and several Liquors, of which some are acrid, and the rest acid: As for the volatile Salt, there is none obtained from this Plant, that is con-

crete;

crete; but it yields an urinous Spirit. *Dioſcorides* affirms, that it lenifies and reſolves, and is good to ſtop Tetters, and ſpreading Ulcers: They applied it, in his Time, to the Parts affected with the Gout; they gave the Juice to drink in an old Cough, made a Gargariſm of it for the Diſeaſes of the Throat; and injected it into the Ears to appeaſe their Pain. *Cæſalpinus* ſays, it provokes Urine, and opens the Kidneys; *Tragus* very much commends the Decoction to remove Obſtructions of the lower Belly. *Camerarius* preſcribes it bruiſed with Vinegar, and applied hot to the *Teſtes*, in Caſe of Ruptures.

Parnaſſia. Graſs of Parnaſſus. This is already ſpecify'd under the Article *Gramen Parnaſſ.*

Paronychia rutaceo folio, Offic. *Paronychia foliis inciſis,* Park. *Sedum Tridactylites tectorum,* C. B. P. Rue Whitlow-Graſs. It grows upon Walls, and old Buildings, flowering in *May.* The Herb is uſed, which is greatly commended in ſcrophulous Diſorders. A Phyſician, whom I knew, ſays *Boyle,* was ſent for to a ſcrophulous Patient, in whoſe Throat he found a Tumor ſo large, and ſo unluckily ſeated, that greatly compreſſing the *Oeſophagus,* it render'd Deglutition exceedingly difficult, the Tumor was, alſo, hard and ſtubborn, ſo as not to be diſcuſs'd, nor brought to Suppuration; whence the Patient was put in imminent Danger of being ſtarv'd. In this Strait, the Phyſician remembring the Character I had given of Whitlow-Graſs, ſent about the Country to get all that could be procured, and firſt gave a little of it, in the Form of Infuſion, in ſuch liquid Aliments as the Patient was able, though with great Difficulty, to get down; and having by this Means, after ſome Time, gradually made the Deglutition more eaſy, he gave the Remedy in greater

Plenty, to impregnate the whole Maſs of Blood and Juices of the Body with the Virtue of the Herb, whereby the Tumor was at length diſſolved, and the Patient cured.

Parthenium, Fever-few is ſo call'd. See *Matricaria,*

Paſſulæ. See *Uva.*

Paſtinaca, Offic. *Paſtinaca latifolia ſativa,* C. B. P. Parſnep. It is cultivated in Gardens, flowering in *June.* The Root is uſed in the Kitchen, and the Seed in Phyſic. The Seeds are heating and drying, provoke Urine, and diſcuſs Flatulencies. It is the Opinion of ſome, that old Parſneps which have remain'd Years in the Ground, induce Deliriouſneſs and Madneſs; for which Reaſon they give them the Name of *Madneps,* that is to ſay, Mad Parſneps. I cannot really determine, whether this is the Caſe or not, but it is very certain, that Parſneps have frequently excited all the Symptoms abovemention'd, which go off after Sleep. *Cæſalpinus* ſays, that they who pull the Roots in Winter, muſt beware of the *Cicuta,* or *Cicutaria;* becauſe while he was at *Mompelgard,* he ſaw two Families, who were almoſt dead with eating the Roots of theſe Plants, inſtead of Parſneps; but they recover'd by the Help of Vomiting, Venice Treacle, *Pulvis ſaxonicus,* and ſome Purgatives.

Paſtinaca ſylveſtris, Elaphoboſcum, Offic. *Paſtinaca ſylveſtris latifolia,* C. B. P. Wild Parſnep. It grows by the Borders of Fields, flowering in *July.* The Root, and Seeds are uſed. It agrees in Virtues with the former, and differs only from it in its Culture.

Pedicularis, Offic. *Pedicularis pratenſis purpurea,* C. B. P. *Pedicularis quibuſdam Criſta Galli, flore rubro,* J. B. Red Rattle. It grows in Meadows and moiſt Paſtures, flowering in Summer. The Herb is uſed, which is cooling and drying, and is useful

useful in *Fistula's*, and sinuous Ulcers. It stops Bleeding, and the Menses.

· *Pentaphyllum*, & *Quinquefolium*, Offic. *Pentaphyllum sive Quinquefolium vulgare repens*, J. B. Cinquefoil, or five Fingers. It grows by Hedges, flowering in the Summer. The Root, and Herb is used. It is vulnerary, and astringent, good for all Kinds of Fluxes and Hæmorrhages: It is serviceable in spitting of Blood, and in Coughs, and is recommended for the Stone, for Hernia's, and for Fevers.

Pepo, Offic. *Pepo oblongus*, C. B. P. The common Pompion. It is sown in Gardens, and upon Dunghills, flowering in *June*. The Fruit is used in the Kitchens, and the Seed in Physic, tho' but seldom. It agrees in Virtues with the Cucumber.

Percepier, Offic. *Percepier anglorum quibusdam*, J. B. Parsley-Piert. It grows among Corn, flowering in the Summer. The Herb is used, which is said to be a speedy, and potent Provoker of Urine, and to break the Stone.

Perfoliata, Offic. *Perfoliata vulgaris*, Ger. Emac. *Perfoliata vulgatissima sive arvensis*, C. B. P. Thorow-Wax. It grows among Corn, flowering in *July*. The Leaves are used. It is vulnerary, and is principally used in recent Wounds, in an umbilical *Hernia*, and for strumous Swellings.

· *Perforata*. A Name for the *Hypericum*, or St. *John's* Wort.

Periclymenum. The Honey-suckle. See *Caprifolium*.

Periploca. The Name of a Plant thus distinguish'd, *Scammonia monspeliaca*, Offic. *Scammonia monspeliaca, foliis rotundioribus*, C. B. P. *Periploca Monspeliaca, foliis rotundioribus*, Tourn. Inst. *Italian*, or *French* Scammony. It grows in the Gardens of Botanists, flow-

ering in *August*. The concreted Juice, which is used in Medicine, requires to be given in a larger Dose than that of the true *Scammony*, it being less effectual.

Persea, Offic. C. B. P. *Persea arbor Clusii*, Park. Theat. *Pyri sive Aguacat*, J. B. Spanish Pear. It is a Native of *Jamaica*. The Leaves and Fruit are used. The Fruit is good for the Stomach, and the Powder of the dry'd Leaves stops Hæmorrhages, being sprinkled on the Part.

Persica Malus, Offic. J. B. *Persica molli carne*, C. B. P. The Peach Tree. It is cultivated in Gardens, flowering in *March*, and the Fruit is ripe in *September*. Preserved Peaches are extremely grateful to sick Persons, especially to such as are afflicted with Thirst, and Dryness of the Tongue, for they strengthen at the same time they refrigerate; whence they are of excellent Service in all hot Distempers. *Brassavola* used to give his Patient a Peach or two roasted under the Ashes. *Amatus* affirms it to be a most delicious Food, and extremely grateful to sick Persons. The Leaves, on Account of their Bitterness, being boiled in Beer, or Milk, destroy and expel Worms in Children. *Galen* says, that they work the same Effect, being bruised, and applied to the Navel. *Parkinson* affirms, that they purge gently, if taken in a sufficient Quantity; the Flowers operate in the same Manner, and more effectually than Damask Roses; for which Purpose there is prepared of them a Conserve, to be taken chiefly in the Morning fasting. The recent Flowers, says *Matthiolus*, not only purge, but provoke Vomiting; and, eaten in Sallads, prove Hydragogues in Dropsies; but not without disordering the Patient: The distilled Water is a Cosmetic. The Gum of this Tree is recommended for Fluxes of the e Belly, the Stone, *Impetigo*, Tumors of the *Fauces*, Roughness of e Wind Pipe, Spitting of Blood, isorders of the Lungs, and the yfentery. *Matthiolus* recommends e Kernels for the Gripes, and to event Ebriety, being taken to the umber of fix or feven before and; and for the *Alopecia*, being uifed, and boiled in Vinegar, to ip the Confidence. The Oil of e bruifed Kernels, being rubbed on e Temples, procures Sleep, and les the *Hemicrania*, or Megrim; lk, or ufed in Clyfters, it cures s Colic; and, taken to the Weight four Ounces, it gives Relief unr the Iliac Paffion, and the one.

Perficaria acris, J. B. *Perficaria* u *maculata*, *Hydropiper*, Offic. *Perula Lufitanis Pulgera*, Pis. Lakeeed, Arfmart, or Water-Pepper. grows in watery Places. The aves are ufed, and outwardly apl'd are good for Wounds, and inated Tumors, and for inveterate lcers. It is a very potent Diuretic, d the diftilled Water of it is comended for the Stone, and to cleanfe rdid Ulcers. It is of a very acrid d burning Tafte, and gives a liventure of red to the blue Par. It is full of acid Sulphur and arth; its Salt refembles that which fults from the Mixture of the Salt Coral, with the Sal Ammoniac, ded with a great deal more Acid an ordinary. For this Plant, by e chymical *Analyfis*, yields a great al of Acid, Oil, and Earth, and a le volatile concrete Salt. Arfmart very deterfive and vulnerary; and s ufed in Glyfters, for the Dyfenry and *Tenefmus*.

Perficaria maculata, Offic. *Perficaria mitis*, J. B. Spotted Arfmart. grows in watery, and moift Plas, flowering in *July* and *Auguft*. he Leaves are ufed, which are of n aftringent and acerb Tafte. They recommended for Inflammations

and recent Wounds. This Plant gives a pretty deep red Colour to blue Paper, which makes us conjecture, that its Salt refembles Sal Ammoniac, loaded with a great deal of Earth, and joined with a little Sulphur. By the chymical *Analyfis*, it yields a volatile concrete Salt. The Decoction of the whole Plant is good for a Loofenefs, and for the Difeafes of the Skin.

Perfonata. Bur-dock. See *Bardana*.

Pervinca. See *Vinca Pervinca*.

Peruvianus Cortex. The Jefuits-Tree. See *Kina Kina*.

Pes anferinus, Offic. *Atriplex dicta Pes Anferinus*, J. B. *Chenopodium Pes Anferinus primum Tabernamontani*, Tourn. Inft. Goofe-Foot. It grows upon Dunghills, flowering in *July*. The Herb is ufed, which is efteem'd a good Uterine, and Antihyfteric; and is faid to provoke the Menfes, and to expel the dead *Fœtus*, and the Secundines.

Pes Cati. Cat's-Foot. This is already mention'd under the Article *Helichryfum*.

Pes Columbinus, Dove's-Foot. This is the *Geranium Columbinum*.

Pes Leporinus. Hare's-Foot. A Species of *Trifolium*.

Petafites, Offic. *Petafites major & vulgaris*, Tourn. Inft. Butter Bur. It grows in watery Places, flowering in *March*. The Root is ufed, which is efteem'd fudorific, alexipharmic, and good in the Plague. It is recommended in hyfteric Fits, Coughs and Afthma's. It kills the flat Worms in the Inteftines, and excites Urine and the Menfes. Externally apply'd, it is good for *Bubœs* and malignant Ulcers.

Petrofelinum vulgare, Offic. *Apium hortenfe, five Petrofelinum vulgo*, C. B. P. Parfley. It grows in Gardens, flowering in *June*. The Root, Herb and Seeds are ufed. The Root is one of the five opening Roots, and is oblong, thick, white, of a

fubsubacrid Taste, and of a fragrant aromatic Smell. Parsley is attenuating, opening, detergent, and diuretic, and is principally used in Obstructions of the Lungs, Liver, Kidneys, and gall Bladder.

Petroselinum Macedonicum, Offic. *Petroselinum Macedonicum quibusdam,* Park. *Apium Macedonicum,* C. B. P. *Macedonian* Parsley. It is cultivated in the Gardens of the Curious, flowering in *July.* The Seeds are small, hairy, striated, of a very dark Green, of an acrid and aromatic Taste, and of a fragrant Smell. It is principally used as a Diuretic, and Emmenagogue, and sometimes as a Remedy against Diseases caused by Witchcraft.

Another Species of *Petroselinum,* is the *Selinum montanum,* Offic. *Selinum five Apium peregrinum,* Park. Theat. *Daucus tertius Dioscoridis,* Raii Hist. Stone Parsley. It is cultivated in Botanic Gardens. The Seed is used, which agrees in Virtues with the former.

Petum. A Name for Tobacco. See *Nicotiana.*

Peucedanum , Offic. *Peucedanum Germanicum,* C. B. P. *Peucedanum, Pinastrellum, Fœniculum porcinum,* Merc. Bot. Hogs-Fennel. It grows in marshy Ditches, flowering in *July.* The Root is used. It is commended by the Antients for discussing inflammatory Diseases ; for which Purpose, they prescribe a Decoction of the Root in Water, sweeten'd with Honey, and drank warm. Hence it is very proper for resolving a Pleurisy and Peripneumony, when they may be remov'd by an *Anacatharsis,* or Expectoration. They prescribe it also, for bloody Urine, and the Stone or Gravel in the Kidneys. It provokes Urine, is an excellent Resolver of Phlegm, and cleanses the Kidneys of every thing which adheres to them ; for which Purpose the Root is boiled in Wine.

It is commended as of Service in the Beginning of a Cataract, and in a Redundance of Phlegm, and as an excellent Resolver and Discusser of all Obstructions. The Root is very good for the hysteric Passion ; and is possessed of a balsamic, deterging, and gently heating Virtue ; and is of extraordinary Use for cleansing Wounds and Ulcers.

Phagus. A Species of Oak. See *Quercus.*

Phalangium, Offic. *Phalangium magno flore,* C. B. P. *Liliastrum Alpinum minus,* Tourn. Inst. *Phalangium Allobrogicum,* Park. Spiderwort. It is cultivated with us in Gardens, flowering in *June.* The Leaves, Flowers, and Seed are used, which being drank in Wine, are commended for the Bites of Scorpions, and that Species of Spider called *Phalangium.*

Phalaris, Offic. J. B. *Phalaris major semine albo,* C. B. P. Canary-Grass. It grows in *Spain,* and in the Southern Parts of *France.* The Herb and Seed are used. The Seeds and the Juice of this Herb, drank, are commended by the Antients for Pains of the Bladder.

Phaseolus vulgaris, Tourn. Inst. *Smilax hortensis,* Offic. *Smilax hortensis five Phaseolus,* C. B. P. Kidney Beans. It is sown in Gardens, flowering in *July.* The Pods are used, which are opening, digestive, and provoke Urine and the Menses.

Phaseolus, Offic. *Phaseolus erectus,* J. B. *Smilax siliqua sursum rigente, vel Phaseolus Italicus,* C. B. P. *Italian* Kidney-Beans. It is sown in Gardens, flowering in *July.* The Pod is used, which, as *Dioscorides* says, if boiled whilst green, and eaten, is good to mollify the Belly, and proper to provoke Vomiting.

Another Species of *Phaseolus,* is the *Coubage,* or stinking Bean.

Phellandrium, Offic. *Phellandrium vel Cicutaria aquatica quorundam,*

dam, J. B. _Cicataria palustris_, Ger.
Emac. Water-Hemlock. It grows
in Ditches and Ponds, flowering in the
Summer. It is sweet scented and
aromatic, and of excellent Service,
where a gentle Dissipation of Humours is required. It is of use in
Surgery, for discussing inflammatory
and cold Tumors; and is said to resist a Gangrene, and nothing can be
more safely apply'd to scirrhous and
cancerous Tumours; it is also commended for Diseases of the Breast,
being apply'd in the Form of a Cataplasm. The Leaves are commended by _Blancard_ in virulent Inflammations of the _Penis_; internally it is
an Emetic.

Phellodrys, Offic. _Phellodrys sive
Cerro-Sugaro Matthiolo_, Raii. Hist. It
grows in _Dalmatia_, and, as some
say, in _Greece_; the Leaves, Bark,
and Acorns, which are the Parts used
in Medicine, agree in Virtues with
those of the _Quercus_, or common
Oak.

Phillyrea, Offic. _Phillyrea folio
Ligustri_, C. B. P. Mock Privet. It
is cultivated in Gardens, and the
Leaves are used, which are drying,
and astringent, and are greatly recommended for Ulcers of the Mouth.

Phlomis, Offic. _Phlomis fruticosa
Salviæ folio latiore, & rotundiore_.
Tourn. Inst. _Verbascum Salviæ foliis_,
C. B. P. Yellow Sage. It grows in
Gardens, flowering in _June_: It is
astringent, and reckon'd among vul-
nerary Plants.

Phœnix. A Species of _Lolium_, or
Ray-Grass.

Phu. A Name for several Sorts of
Valerian.

Phyllitis. A Name for the _Lingua
Cervina_, or Harts-Tongue.

Phyllon, Offic. _Phyllon testiculatum
& spicatum_, C. B. P. _Mercurialis
fruticosa incana testiculata & spicata_,
Tourn. Inst. Childrens Mercury. It
grows in the Gardens of the Curious,
flowering in the Summer. The Herb

is us'd, which is much esteem'd for
the Disorders of Women in _Barbary_,
and a Decoction of it is greatly recommended for the Bite of a Mad
Dog.

Phyteuma. A Species of Rocket.
See _Reseda_.

Phytolacca, Offic. _Phytolacca Americana major fructu_, Tourn. Inst.
Solanum racemosum Americanum;
Raii Hist. Pork Physic. It is a Native of _America_, but is cultivated with
us in Gardens; the Leaves are used,
which are esteem'd an excellent Anodyne.

Pilosella, _Auricula muris_, Offic.
Pilosella major, repens hirsuta, C.B.P.
Common Mouse-Ear. It grows in
dry Pastures, flowering in _June_, and
July. It is astringent, and binding,
and is reckon'd a good Sternutatory
and Vulnerary. It stops Fluxes of
the Belly and Uterus, and cures
Hernias. Externally used as a Gargarism, it is commended for Ulcers
of the Mouth. The Powder of it
is good for Hæmorrhages of the
Nose, and its Juice is recommended for the _Herpes Miliaris_. It is
very bitter, and reddens blue Paper
a little. By the chymical Analysis,
besides several acid Liquors, it yields
a good deal of Oil and Earth, a little urinous Spirit, and no concreted
volatile Salt; which shews it to contain a Salt approaching to that of
Alum, wrapped up in a good deal of
Sulphur, and mixt with a little _Sal
Ammoniac_. Thus the Mouse-Ear is
vulnerary and detersive. An Infusion of it in Wine or Water, is
good for the Jaundice, and to prevent the Dropsy. _Pena_ and _Lobel_
say, it is admirable for the Stone.

Pimenta. _Jamaica_ Pepper, or All-
Spice. See _Caryophyllus_.

Pimpinella, & _Sanguisorba_, Offic.
_Pimpinella, Sanguisorba minor hirsu-
ta lævis_, C. B. P. _Sanguisorba minor_,
J. B. Burnet. It grows in hilly
Pastures, flowering in _June_. This

E e Plant

Plant is alexipharmic, vulnerary, and pulmonic; and is principally used in Catarrhs, Affections of the Lungs, a Phthisis proceeding from Erosion, in malignant Diseases, Looseness and the Hæmorrhoids: It prevents Abortion, and is a Strengthener: Outwardly it is of Service in all kinds of Hæmorrhages. This *Pimpinella* has the Appellation of *Sanguisorba* to distinguish it from the *Pimpinella Saxifraga*, which is of a very hot Nature; but the Plant we are now treating on, is gently astringent, aromatic, and of excellent Service in a Relaxation of the Fibres, and a too thin, and fluid State of the Blood. It is prescribed in an immoderate Flux of the *Menses*, to be eaten with Bread and Butter, or drank like Tea; and so used, it renders all manner of Poison of no Effect. This Plant, infused in Wine is commended, where a Laxness of the Part requires Adstriction; and there is scarce, among Vulneraries, a better Plant for repressing a Flux of Blood in an Hæmoptoe. It is of singular Virtue in the Dysentery, both by correcting the Acidity of the Dysenteric, or peccant Matter, and by gently astringing the relaxed Fibres of the Intestines. The Leaves infused in Wine, or common Water, are good for the Stone and Gravel in the Kidneys.

Pimpinella Saxifraga, Offic. *Pimpinella Saxifraga major, umbellâ candidâ,* C. B. P. *Saxifragia hircina major,* J. B. *Tragoselinum majus,* Tourn. Inst. Burnet Saxifrage. It grows in Woods, flowering in *June*; the Root, Herb, and Seed are used, which are possess'd of the same Qualities as the Parsley, but are more efficacious in removing and assuaging Pains.

Pimpinella Saxifraga minor, Offic. *Pimpinella Saxifraga major altera,* C. B. P. *Tragoselinum alterum, majus.* Tourn. Inst. Smaller Burnet Saxifrage. It grows in dry Pastures,

flowering in *July*. The Herb is used, which agrees in Virtues with the former, to which it may be a *Succedaneum.*

Pinus, Offic. *Pinus sativa,* C. B. P. *Pinus officulis duris, foliis longis,* J. B. The Pine Tree. It grows common in *Italy*. The Bark and Leaves of all the Species of Pine Trees are refrigerating and astringent; whence they are of Service in Dysenteries, and an immoderate Flux of the Menses. The Decoction or Infusion of Pine Tree Tops in Beer, or any other proper Liquor, is supposed to be very effectual for the Stone in the Kidneys or Bladder, and for the Scurvy, and other Affections of the Thorax. The *Nuclei*, or Kernels, are moderately hot and moist, and are maturating, lenient, agglutinating, resolvent and fatning. They are principally us'd in a Consumption, Cough, Strangury, and Acrimony of the Urine. The Resin which concretes about the Cones is of the same Use.

Pinus sylvestris, Pinaster, Offic. *Pinus sylvestris,* C. B. P. The Mountain Pine. This Tree grows in divers Parts of *Germany*; and agrees in Virtues with the former. From this Tree is got what is called, *Common Turpentine,* which is whitish, thick, and opake, like Honey, of a strong Smell, and used principally by Farriers. From this is distilled the Oil of Turpentine, the finer and more volatile Part thereof, and what comes first, being called the *Spirit*: What is left at the Bottom of the Still is the common *Rosin,* which, if taken out, before it be drawn too high, and then washed in Water by a peculiar Method, is what we call *white,* or *yellow Rosin.* The black Rosin is the same, more evaporated, and not washed at all. The common Frankincense is reputed to be the native Rosin of this Tree, or the *Resina Pini,* which is of a whitish yellow Colour, whereof some Pieces are soft, and whitish, and others hard, brittle and more yellow. There is but little of this to be got pure at present, being adulterated by common yellow Rosin, by someway that crafty Dealers have found out. The black and yellow Rosin are much of a Nature, being used in Ointments and Plaisters. It is said, that the *Pix Burgundica*, or *Burgundy* Pitch of the Shops, is made of this Turpentine, after it has been boiled sometime, and before it has arrived to the Hardness of Rosin. This is done, as is said, in *Saxony*, where the white Rosin is made by boiling the Turpentine in large Vessels, without Distillation.

Pinus maritima, Offic. *Pinus maritima major*, C. B. P. *Pinus sylvestris montana*, Ger. Emac. Sea Pine. It grows in *Provence* and *Languedoc* in *France*; the Bark, Leaves, and Rosin are used, which agree in Virtues with the former.

Piper. Pepper. Botanists distinguish two Species of Pepper, the black, and the white; but *Savary* asserts, that there are not two Species of Pepper, for Mr. *Dillon*, a celebrated Physician, and Author of the History of the Inquisition of *Goa*, assures us, that all the Difference between the white and black Pepper is, that the latter has its Skin, whereas the former wants the Skin, which is taken off by beatting it before it is entirely dry, or by suffering it, after it is dry, to soak for sometime in Water. Pepper is an aromatic Fruit, of an heating and drying Quality, produc'd in Grains commonly, and us'd in Sauces and Seasonings. This Fruit, so well known in *Europe*, is produc'd by a Plant or Shrub, which grows in various Parts of the *East-Indies*. The Plant which bears it, is weak and creeping; a Circumstance which obliges those who cultivate it, to plant it at the Foot of large Trees, such as the *Areca*, and Coco-Nut-Tree. Its

Leaves in Figure resemble those of *Ivy*, but are less green, more yellow, of a strong Smell, and pungent Taste. The Pepper comes forth in small Clusters, like our Currants; and the Grains of which these Clusters are compos'd, at first appear green; then they become red, in Proportion as they ripen; and at last black, or such as they come to us, after they are left expos'd to the Heat of the Sun for sometime. Tho' Pepper is produc'd in various Parts of the *Indies*, yet it grows most copiously between *Rajapour*, and the Cape of *Camarin*. The Pepper of *Malabar*, or that produc'd between Mount *Eli* and the Southern Extremity of the Coast, is somewhat smaller than the other: but produc'd in such large Quantities, that *Europe* is principally supplied with it. The black Pepper consumed in *Europe*, is of three sorts; that of *Malabar*, that of *Jamby*, and that of *Belipatham*. But this last is less esteem'd in *Europe*, on Account of its Smallness and Dryness; two Circumstances which recommend it to the *Indians*, who think small Pepper less hot than the large Kind. The white Pepper ought to be chosen large, well nourish'd, weighty, and without Mixture of black Grains or Rubbish; which when reduc'd to a Powder, is of a beautiful Grey or a whitish Colour. As for black Pepper, which ought to be possess'd of almost all the Qualities of the white already enumerated, we must, also, take care that the Grains be not wrinkled; that there be a large Quantity of white Grains among them; and that the largest Grains have not been separated, in Order to be whiten'd, a Practice very common in *Holland*, *Rouen*, and *Paris*. As a great Part of the Pepper, whether white or black, is sold beaten, it is easy for Persons of a fraudulent Disposition to sophisticate it, which Retailers generally do by mixing, with the black Pepper; Ma-

niguette, a Species of *African* Pepper ; the Dust of Pepper ; and the Crust of Bread. With the white Pepper they mix white Spices, or black Pepper whiten'd ; so that it is very difficult to distinguish the sophisticated from the genuine Kind ; for which Reason we ought to buy from Persons of Honesty and Skill. *Druggists* and Spice Merchants sell various other Kinds of Pepper, describ'd by Travellers in their Relations ; such as the Pepper of *Madagascar*, that of *Mascarine*, or the Island of *Bourbon* ; the Pepper of *China*, the long Pepper of the *Indies*, *Ethiopia*, and *America* ; *Guinea* Pepper, *Jamaica* Pepper, the Pepper of *Thevet*, and that of *Africa*. The Pepper of *Madagascar* is white, and grows on a Plant, which creeps on the Ground, and whose Stalks and Leaves have the same Smell with the Fruit, which ripens in the Months of *August*, *September*, and *October*. The Pepper of *Mascarine*, which is, also, produc'd in the Island of *Java*, is call'd Cubebs, or Pepper with a Tail. It exactly resembles the black Pepper, except that it is larger, and has a Tail. The Plant which produces it creeps on the Ground ; and its Fruit, which ought to be chosen large, well nourish'd, and without Wrinkles, adheres to it in the Form of Clusters. The *China* Pepper describ'd by Father *Le Compte*, is a Fruit as large as a Pea, and of a greyish Colour, mix'd with red Streaks. When it is ripe, it opens spontaneously, and contains a small Nut, as black as Jet ; after it is gather'd, it is expos'd to the Sun, in order to be dried. The Nut, which is of a very strong Taste, is thrown away, and the Husk or Bark only kept. The Smell of the Pepper Tree is so strong, that the Fruit must be gather'd at different times, lest those employ'd in that Work should be injur'd by it. The long Pepper which is a kind of Congeries of many small Grains, strongly united to each other, grows upon a Shrub, whose Leaves are slender, green, and placed upon a short Stalk. This Pepper is of three kinds, that of the *East-Indies*, that of *America*, and that of *Æthiopia*, which is called Grains of *Zelim*. But that of the *Indies*, is the only true Long Pepper, since the others bear but little Resemblance to it. Good long Pepper ought to be recent, well nourish'd, large, weighty, difficult to be broken, not rotten, without Rubbish or a Mixture of Earth. It is us'd in Medicine in various *Galenical* Compositions, and is an Ingredient in the *Theriaca*. It is, also, sometimes mixed with Spices. The *Guinea* Pepper is of a red Colour, resembling that of Coral. It is cultivated in *Languedoc*, and especially in the Villages about *Nimes*. It is commonly found in the Shops of the Druggists and Grocers. The Vinegar-makers use it for making their Vinegar. Some, also, preserve it with Sugar ; it ought to be chosen recent, in Pods, which, are beautiful, dry, sound, and very red. There are four Sorts of this Pepper: The first is called *Chilchotes* ; the second, which is very small, is called *Chilterpin* ; and these two kinds are of an acrid and highly pungent Taste. The third is call'd *Tenalchiles*, which is moderately hot, and which the *Indians* eat, like other Fruit, with Bread. The fourth is call'd *Chilpelagua*. This last is neither so pungent as the two first, nor so mild as the third ; this is the Species so much esteem'd by the *Spaniards*, and generally us'd by them in preparing their Chocolate. There is, also, another Species of this Pepper, which only grows about *Peru*, where it is call'd *Agy*. A large Quantity of this Species is cultivated in a small Plain, about six Leagues in Circumference, near the Village of *Arica*, on the Coast of *Peru*, and in the Vallies

lies of *Sama*, *Tacna*, and *Cocimba*, Tho' thefe four Places are of a fmall Extent, and there is a great Demand for this Kind of Pepper, yet they furnifh every Year, as much as draws more than fix hundred thoufand *Piafters*; which would appear incredible, if the Excrements of the Bird call'd *Guana*, with which the *Peruvians* dung their Land, did not render it fo fertile, that the Grains fown in it, and efpecially the *Agy*, yield four or five hundred for one. For an Account of the *Jamaica* Pepper, fee *Caryophyllus*. The Pepper of *Thevet*, which the *Dutch* call *Amomi*, on account of its Refemblance to the *Amomi*, or *Jamaica* Pepper, is a fmall round Fruit, as large as the white Pepper, a little roundifh, and with a Species of fmall Crown at one of its Ends. It is, alfo, called the fmall round Clove, becaufe its Tafte refembles that of the true Clove.

Piper Indicum. Guinea Pepper. The fame as *Capficum*.

Piper longum, Offic. J.B. *Piper longum Orientale*, C. B. P. *Tlatlancuaye five Piperis longi Species* II Hern. *Catta-tripali*, Hort. Mal. *Acapatli*, Laet. Long Pepper. It grows in *Java* and *Malabar*, and the immature Fruit is ufed, which is of a bitterifh Tafte, and is by fome accounted alexipharmic; good for the Stomach, to expel Wind, and promote Digeftion. See *Piper*.

Piperitis. The fame as *Lepidium*, or Dittander.

Piftacia. The Piftachio, or Fiftic Nut. See *Nux Piftacia*.

Piftolochia, Offic. *Piftolochia vulgatior*, Park. Theat. *Ariftolochia*, *Piftolochia*, C. B. P. Bufhy rooted Birthworth. It grows fpontaneoufly in *Italy*, *France*, and *Spain*, flowering in the Summer. The Root is ufed, which agrees in Virtues with the *Ariftolochia*.

Pifum, Offic. *Pifum*, *vulgare parvum album*, *arvenfe*, J. B. Common white Peas. They grow in Fields and Gardens; and the Seed is ufed, but oftner in the Kitchen, than in the Shops. Broth made with Peas, not only renders the Body foluble, but, alfo, procures a more free and copious Evacuation of the *Lochia*. It is alfo beneficial in nephritic Pains, according to *Simon Pauli*. Some alfo, with Succefs, ufe a Decoction of Peas, in order to cure cutaneous Diforders and Pimples.

Pityufa. Pine Spurge. See *Tithymalus*.

Pix. Pitch. This is a Species of Gum obtained from the Pine Tree, by making Incifions in it. It receives different Names according to its different Preparations, Colours, and Qualities. When it flows from the Tree, it is called *Barras*, but is afterwards diftinguifhed into two Sorts, which have different Names: That which is moft beautiful and clear, is called *Galipot*; and that which is more full of Fæces, and of a worfe Colour, is called *Marbled Barras*. The former of thefe, or the *Galipot*, ferves to make all the different Species of Pitch defcrib'd in this Article. The pinguious Pitch, which is, alfo, called *white Burgundy Pitch*, is *Galipot* melted with Oil of Turpentine. Some however affert, that the *Burgundy* Pitch flows naturally from Refinous Trees, in the Mountains of *Franche Comté*. Refin is, according to fome Authors, a Gum difcharged from the Turpentine Tree, the Larch Tree, the Maftich Tree, or the Cyprefs: But the Opinion of others is far more probable, who from Experience, affert, that it is *Galipot*, boiled to a certain Confiftence, and reduced to a Mafs of any determinate Weight. The beft Refin comes from *Bayonne* and *Bourdeaux*. It ought to be chofen dry,

whet,

white, free from Water and Sand. Black Pitch, which is properly that known by the Name of *Pitch*, is only *Galipot*, prepar'd in a particular Manner, by putting into it, when it is quite warm, a certain Quantity of Tar, in order to render it black. There are two kinds of it, one hard, another soft, which only differ in this Circumstance. Mr. *Wheeler*, in his Voyages, has given another Method of preparing black Pitch, used in the *Levant*, and which is not much different from that given by *Furetiere* in his Dictionary. He orders us to prepare a Heap of Earth, in which we are to make an Hollow two Ells in Diameter at the Top, but which becomes gradually narrower, as it approaches to the Bottom. This Hollow is to be filled with small Portions of such Branches of the Pine Tree, as contains much Gum, laid above each other, till the Hollow is full. Then the upper Part is to be covered with Fire, which burns to the Bottom: By which means the Pitch is discharged from a small Hole made at the Bottom for that Purpose. The best black Pitch comes from *Norway* and *Sweden*, to which that made in *France*, is by no means comparable. The Goodness of hard black Pitch consists in being of a shining black Colour, brittle, dry, and forming, as it were, Rays, when it is broken. What is called the *Pix Navalis* in Medicine, ought to be the Pitch scraped off from Ships; but 'tis certain, that most Apothecaries use the common black Pitch in its stead. From the black Pitch there is obtain'd an Oil, which, on account of its singular Virtues, is called the *Balm of Pitch*.

Pix liquida. Tar. According to *Pliny*, liquid Pitch, or Tar, was obtained by setting Fire to Billets, or old fat Pines or Firs. The first Running was Tar, the latter, or thicker Running, was Pitch. *Theophrastus* is more particular: He tells us, the *Macedonians* made huge Heaps of the cloven Trunks of those Trees, wherein the Billets were placed erect besides each other: That such Heaps or Piles of Wood were sometimes a hundred and eighty Cubits round, and sixty, or even an hundred, high; and that, having covered them with Sods of Earth, to prevent the Flame from bursting forth, (in which Case the Tar was lost) they set on Fire those huge Heaps of Pine or Fir, letting the Tar and Pitch run out in a Channel. From the manner of procuring Tar, it plainly appears to be a natural Production; lodged in the Vessels of the Tree, whence it is only freed and let loose (not made) by Burning. If we may believe *Pliny*, the first Running, or Tar, was called *Cedrium*, and was of such Efficacy to preserve from Putrefaction, that in *Egypt* they embalmed dead Bodies with it. And to this he ascribes their Mummies continuing uncorrupted for so many Ages. Some modern Writers inform us, that Tar flows from the Trunks of Pines and Firs, when they are very old; that Pitch is Tar inspissated, and both are the Oil of the Tree grown thick and black with Age, and the Influence of the Sun. The Trees, like old Men, being unable to perspire, and their secretory Ducts obstructed, they are, as it were, choaked and stuffed with their own Juice. The Method used by our Colonies in *America*, for making Pitch and Tar, is, in Effect the same with that of the ancient *Macedonians*, as appears in the Account given in the *Philosophical Transactions*. And the Relation of *Leo Africanus*, who describes as an Eye-Witness, the making of Tar on Mount *Atlas*, agrees, in Substance, with the Methods us'd by the *Macedonians* of old, and the People of *New England* at this Day. Tar was by the Antients

tients esteemed good against Poisons, Ulcers, and the Bites of venomous Creatures; also for phthisical, scrophulous, paralytic, and asthmatic Persons, and is in Reality a very good Pectoral and Balsamic. Water boiled upon Tar, so strongly recommended by the Bishop of *Cloyne*, is at present in very great Vogue, and is said to have been of great Service, as a Pectoral, Balsamic, Stomachic, Alterative, and Restorative; and it should seem, that the Encomiums bestow'd on this Medicine, are not absolutely without Foundation; for the Virtues of Balsamics are very extensive in the Practice of Physick, for Reasons given in the preceeding Dissertation.

Plantago vulgaris Septinervia, Offic. *Plantago latifolia sinuata*, C. B. P. Great Plantain. It grows by Way Sides. The Root, Leaves, and Seed are used, which are heating, and drying, hepatic and vulnerary, and are principally used in all Sorts of Fluxes. The Leaves are bitter, astringent, and give a faint red Colour to the blue Paper; the Roots give it a deeper, and are only astringent; which shews, that in the Leaves the *Sal Ammoniac*, and the terrestrial Parts of this Plant, are clogged with a great deal of Sulphur. This Plant externally used, is good for Inflammations, being apply'd to the Parts affected. It is a Plant of excellent Use in a Diarrhœa, Hæmorrhages, and Diseases of the Eyes. The bruised Leaves are good to cleanse, and consolidate old Wounds and Ulcers; their Juice is very proper in intermitting Fevers, and in a Phthisis, the distilled Water, mixed with Rose Water, is a good Remedy for Inflammations of the Eyes; the Water injected is of Service in a *Gonorrhœa*, and a Decoction of the Leaves is good for Diseases of the *Fauces*.

Plantago incana, Offic. *Plantago latifolia incana*, C. B. P. Hoary Plantain. It grows in gravelly Places, flowering in *June*. The Leaves are used, which agree in Virtues with the former.

Plantago angustifolia, *Quinquenervia*, Offic. *Plantago angustifolia major*, C. B. P. Rib-Wort. It grows in Pastures, and the Herb is used, which agrees in Virtues with the *Plantago vulgaris*. A Dram of the Powder of its Leaves given in Conserve of red Roses, is commended by *Boyle*, for the Cure of Tertians.

Plantago angustifolia albida, Elem. Bot. *Holostium*, Offic. *Plantago angustifolia albida Hispanica*, Tourn. Inst. Spanish Plantain. It grows in sandy Places, flowering in *April* and *May*. The Herb is used, which is vulnerary, and is principally used in *Hernias*.

Plantago aquatica, Offic. J. B. *Plantago aquatica latifolia*, C. B. P. *Alisma*, Dill. Cat. Giss. *Ranunculus palustris Plantaginis folio ampliore*, Tourn. Inst. Water Plantain. It grows in watery Places, flowering in *June*. It is of a penetrating and acrimonious Taste. *Schwenckfield* says, that it cures the falling down of the *Anus*, and mitigates the Redness and Inflammation of the Gout, and the Pain of the Head, proceeding from a cold Cause; and is a Remedy for Spitting of Blood, and voiding it by Urine. The Leaves bruised, and applied to the Breasts, are a sovereign and approved Secret, as *Timach* assures us, for suddenly consuming, and drying up the Milk therein.

Platanus, Offic. C. B P. *Platanus Orientalis vera*, Tourn. Inst. The Plane Tree. This Tree, so much celebrated by *Herodotus*, and other Writers is, also, called *Platanus latus*, because it extends its

Branches to such a Compass, as to be able to cover more than a thousand Men under its pleasing Shade. Under this Tree, it is reported *Hippocrates* found *Democritus*, and saluted him. It grows in *Crete*. The Leaves, Bark, and its round Knob, or Fruit, are used. Its tender Leaves, boiled in Wine, and apply'd as a ataplaſm, ſtop Defluxions upon the Eyes, and give Relief under Tumours and Inflammations. The Bark, boil'd in Vinegar, makes a Colluſion for the Tooth-ach. The green Balls or Fruit, drank in Wine, cure the Bites of Serpents.

Plumbago. Leadwort. This is already ſpecify'd under the Article *Dentillaria.*

Pneumonanthe, a Name for the *Gentiana anguſtifolia,* or Marſh Gentian.

Polemonium, Offic. *Polemonium vulgare cæruleum,* Tourn. Inſt. *Valeriana Græca,* Ger. Emac. *Valeriana cærulea,* C. B. P., Greek Valerian, or Jacob's Ladder. This Plant grows in Woods, flowering in Summer. The Herb itſelf, and its Roots, are uſed. The Root, drank in Wine, is good againſt the Bites of venomous Animals, and Dyſenteries. When drank in Water, it is beneficial in Dyſuries, and Iſchiadic Pains. A Dram of it exhibited in Vinegar, proves ſerviceable to Patients labouring under Diſorders of the Spleen. When chew'd, it mitigates Tooth-achs. The Herb is vulnerary.

Polium montanum, Offic. *Polium montanum album,* C. B. P. White Poley Mountain. This Plant is produc'd in *Italy* and *France,* flowering in Summer. The Herb is uſed, which ought to be choſen recent and odorous. It provokes Urine and the Menſes, aſſiſts dropſical and icteric Patients, and is beneficial in the Bites of venomous Animals. It is alſo of an inciding and aperient Quality.

Polium Lavendulæ folio, C. B. P. Poley Mountain with Lavender Leaves.

Polium montanum luteum, C. B. P. Yellow Poley Mountain.

Polium Menſpeſſulanum, J. B. Erect, or Mountain Poley. Theſe three laſt Species grow in the ſame Places, flowering about the ſame Time, and are endued with the ſame Virtues as the White Poley Mountain.

Polium Creticum, Offic. *Polium anguſtifolium Creticum,* C. B. P. *Teucrium calice campanulato, Stæchados facie,* Boerh. Ind. Alt. Poley of Candia. It grows very plentifully in the Iſland of *Crete,* and its Tops are uſed. It agrees in Virtues with the *Polium montanum,* for which it is often ſold in the Shops.

Polygala, Offic. *Polygala vulgaris,* C. B. P. *Polygalon multis,* J. B. Milkwort. It grows frequently in dry Meadows, flowering in *July.* The Herb is uſed. Its bitter Taſte proves it to be of an hot and drying Quality. Its Leaves, boiled in Wine, purge Bile by Stool.

Polygala vera, Offic. *Polygala major Maſſiliotica,* C. B. P. *Colutea caule Geniſtæ fungoſo,* J. B. *Aſtragalus Matthioli,* Ger. Emac. Milk Vetch. It is cultivated in Gardens, flowering in Summer. The Herb is uſed, which according to *Dioſcorides,* increaſes the Quantity of Milk, if drank in ſome proper Liquor.

Polygonatum, Sigillum Solomonis, Offic. *Polygonatum latifolium vulgare,* C. B. P. Solomon's Seal. It grows in Woods, flowering in *May.* It is vulnerary and aſtringent, good to ſtop Fluxes, and to conſolidate fractur'd Bones. The Leaves of *Solomon's Seal* are inſipid, and have ſomething glutinous in them, which gives ſlight Nauſeas. The Roots are ſweet, a little acrid, and glutinous; and give a faint red Colour the blue Paper; and the Leaves are faint. This Plant seems to contain a viscous Phlegm, mix'd with a great deal of Oil. For, by the Chymical Analysis, it yields little besides some acid Liquor and Oil; a little Earth, and fix'd, but no volatile Salt. *Schroder* affirms, that fourteen or fifteen Berries of *Solomon's Seal* provoke Vomiting; and they say, that one Dram of its Root has the same Effect. The dist'd Water clears the Face, and beautifies the Complexion. The Decoction of the whole Plant cures the Itch, and the like cutaneous Diseases.

Polygonum, Centinodium, Offic. *Polygonum latifolium,* Tourn. Inst. Common Knot Grass. It grows in gravelly Places; and the Herb is used, which refrigerates and inspissates, and is good for old Ulcers and Noma's. This Plant has an herby, glutinous Taste, and a little Acid; gives a deep Tincture of Red to the blue Paper; it is likely, that the Salt of Knot Grass resembles Alum, but is mixed with a little *Sal Ammoniac*, and a great deal of Sulphur; or, by the Chymical *Analysis* it yields a great deal of Acid, Earth, and Oil, a little volatile, concrete, and very lixivial fixed Salt. The Juice, Decoction, or Infusion of it in Wine, is given to drink for the Dysentery, Piles, Spitting of Blood, and all Sorts of Hæmorrhages. The Leaves bruised cure Wounds.

Polygonum cocciferum, Offic. C. B. P. Polonian Knawel. It grows in sandy Places, but is very rare, and has the same Virtues ascrib'd to it as the common Knawel. The *Coccum Tinctorium,* or *Polonicum,* is produc'd from the Roots of this Plant; and is an Insect.

Polypodium Quercinum, Offic. *Polypodium vulgare,* C. B. P. Polypody of the Oak. It grows upon Walls and old Houses, amongst Rubbish, and upon the Roots and Trunks of Trees; that which grows upon the Oak is most esteem'd. The Root is the Part used in Medicine, which in the Phrase of the Antients, is said to purge off adust Bile and Phlegm. It is esteem'd useful in Obstructions of the Mesentery, Liver and Spleen, and hypochondriac and scorbutic Disorders thence arising. It purges but slowly, and for that Reason is seldom given alone. It is generally given in Decoction or Infusion.

Another Species of *Polypodium* is, the *Dryopteris,* or Oak Fern.

Another Species of *Polypodium,* is also, the *Lonchitis,* or Rough Spleenwort.

Polytrichum aureum, Golden Maidenhair. This is the same as the *Adianthum aureum.*

Poma Amoris. Love Apples. See *Amoris Pomum.*

Populago. Marsh Marigold. A Name for the *Calendula palustris.*

Populus nigra, Offic. C. B. P. The Black Poplar. It grows in watery Places, and by the Sides of Rivers. The Eyes or young Buds, gather'd in *April*, are used in Medicine. It is disputed whether they are of a cold or hot Quality; but the most probable Opinion is, that they are moderately hot. The Tincture of the Buds with Spirit of Wine, is excellent for old Looseneffes, and internal Ulcers. The Dose is Half a Dram, or a Dram, taken Morning and Evening in a Spoonful of warm Broth.

Populus alba, Offic. Park. The Abele, or White Poplar. It grows in watery Places; and the Bark is used both inwardly and outwardly in the *Sciatica,* Strangury, and Burns.

Populus tremula, Offic. C. B. P. *Populus Libyca,* Ger. Emac. The Asp, or Aspen Tree. It grows in Woods, and in moist watry Places; and the Leaves are supposed to agree

gree in Virtues with those of the black Poplar Tree.

Porrum, Offic. Park. Leeks. They are cultivated in Gardens, flowering in *June*; and are much more us'd in Cookery than in Physic. The Roots, Leaves, and Seeds, are said to be very heating, drying, attenuant, aperient, inciding, and resolvent; they are recommended against the Bites of Serpents, for Burns, mucilaginous Infarctions of the Lungs; and are said to be diuretic, and to increase the Seminal Juices. This Plant contains a fetid, oily, volatile Salt. Whence its Bulb being bruised, causes a Distillation of Tears from the Eyes and Nostrils; for this Reason, it is proper in Cases where Heat is required, or where an Excess of Heat is not feared; but is injurious to those who abound too much with Blood, or whose Blood is of too loose a Contexture; as when it is voided by the urinary Passage, by an *Hæmoptoe*, or by the Hæmorrhoidal Veins; it provokes the Menses and Urine; and is very good for the Bites of Serpents and Combustions.

Porrum vitigineum, Offic. *Porrum tonsile*, Ger. Vine Leeks. They are said to grow on the Mountains of *Westmoreland*, flowering in *June*. The Leaves are used, which are said to provoke Urine and the Menses, to be good against the Bites of Serpents, and to be offensive to the Stomach.

Portulaca, Offic. *Portulaca, latifolia sativa*, C. B. P. Purslane. It grows in Gardens, flowering in *July*. The Seeds are one of the four lesser cold Seeds. This Plant affords an excellent Aliment and Medicine; its Parts are very succulent; and the Juice astringent, remarkably aperient, expulsive, and cooling in inflammatory Diseases, and very good to wash the Gums, when affected with a Gangrene. A

Decoction of the Leaves makes an excellent Gargarism for the Quinsey, and is no less serviceable in the Phrensy, Pleurisy, Peripneumony, Scurvy, and Inflammations of the *Viscera* and Intestines; it tempers Bile, and is corroborative, especially if the Plant be boiled with Whey. The Juice is somewhat acid, nitrous, and very viscid, which renders it qualify'd to correct an excessive Motion, or Volatility of the Spirits, a Putrefaction, and a Rigidness of the Fibres; whence it is of Service in all acute Diseases. Being eaten in Salads in the Summer Season, it mitigates the Bile, and prevents Disorders which may be justly apprehended from an Excess of that Humour; it destroys Worms, and is of Service in malignant putrid Fevers, Heat of Urine, and the Stone in the Kidneys. The Leaves applied to the Head, ease the Pains thereof; the distilled Water is very good for an excessive Flux of the *Menses*, and for Hæmorrhages; the Juice is of great Efficacy in a Consumption. The whole Plant is extremely full of Juice; so that if you compress and rub the Leaves between your Fingers, they will almost spend themselves wholly in Juice; so that if you bruise a Pound of the Leaves, and squeeze out all the Juice, there will scarce remain a Dram of solid Substance.

Portulaca sylvestris, Offic. *Portulaca angustifolia sive sylvestris*, C. B. P. Wild Purslane. It grows in Fallow Grounds, and by the Sides of Paths. The Herb is used, and agrees in Virtues with the preceding.

Portulaca maritima, Offic. *Halimus sive Portulaca marina*, C. B. P. Common Sea Purslane. It is commonly found in the Salt Marshes, flowering in *July* and *August*. The Leaves and tender Branches, pickled after the Manner of *Samphire*, are used by the *English* as well as the *Dutch*,

in

Sances, for exciting an Appetite.
is an hot Plant, and is by some
amended as a Cosmetic.

Potamogeiton, Offic. *Fontalis ma-*
latifolia vulgaris, Park. Pond
eed. It is frequently found in
gnant Waters and Fish Ponds,
wering in *June* and *July*. The
rb is used, which is of a refrige-
ing and inspissating Quality; it
allo, beneficial against Itchings,
veterate Ulcers, and *Nomæ*.

Potentilla. See *Argentina*.

Poterium. See *Tragacantha*.

Primula Veris, Offic. *Verbasculum*
lvarum majus, singulari flore, C.
P. Primrose. It grows in Woods
d Hedges, flowering in the Spring.
he Leaves and Flowers are used,
hich are esteem'd warm and drying,
d are recommended in melancho-
and pituitous Disorders.

Prunella, Offic. *Prunella major*
lie non dissecto, C. B. P. Self Heal.
grows in Pastures, flowering in
une and *July*; it absterges and con-
lidates; its principal Use is in
ounds, especially of the Lungs,
d in Coagulations of Blood; it is,
fo, frequently employ'd outwardly
Wounds, and in the Quinsey, and
her Affections of the Mouth and
auces. This Plant is, also, of an
ccellent Virtue in all inflammatory
iftempers, Hæmorrhages, and Dy-
nteries, and in spitting, and void-
g of Blood by Urine; it gives a
retty deep red Colour to the blue
aper; it is of an herby, styptic,
d glutinous Taste, mixed with a
ery little Bitterness; from which
e may conjecture, that the acid
art of the natural Salt of the Earth
in this Plant disengaged from a
ood deal of the acrid Part; and
hat being united with Abundance of
arth and Sulphur, it produces there
Salt which resembles Alum. *Baubine*
seems a Lotion of it for Gunshot
Wounds. It is used by Way of In-
ection in deep Wounds, and by

Way of Clyfter in the Bloody Flux;
they bathe the Gums of scorbutic
Persons with it, adding some Grains
of Mastich. The distilled Water of
the whole Plant, and the Conserve
of its Flowers may be used for the
same Purpose. *Cæsalpinus* used the
Leaves bruised, and applied in
Form of a Cataplasm to suppurate
Boils, and to heal Wounds. He
used the Juice for violent Pains in
the Head, by bathing the Temples
with it, after having mixed it with
Oil of Roses and Vinegar. *J.*
Baubine added to it a little Rose
Water, and gave it to drink to those
who had been bitten by any venomous Creature.

Prunus Brignolensis, Offic. The
Prunello. It grows principally in
Provence, from whence the Fruit
is imported to us; which is said to
refrigerate and moisten, without increasing the Number of Stools; it
is frequently given in Fevers, as a
grateful Cooler.

Prunus Damascena, Offic. The
Damask Prune. It grows in *Syria*.
The Fruit or Plums are used, which
are dried, and brought from *Syria* to
Venice. These are esteem'd much
better than the common Prunes, but
are seldom to be met with in the
Shops, the common Sort supplying
their Place; they are refrigerating,
moistening, and laxative, destroying
the Acrimony of the Humours,
moisten the Tongue, and extinguish
Thirst.

Prunus Gallica, Offic. The common Prune. This Plant is cultivated
in Gardens, flowering in *April*. It
is transported dry to us from *Pro-*
vence and *Languedoc*; and its Gum is
hard and pellucid. It is thought to
be possessed of the same Virtues as
the former.

Prunus sylvestris, C. B. P. *Pru-*
nellus sylvestris, Offic. The Sloe
or Black Thorn. It is very frequent in Hedges, flowering in *April*.
The

The Bark, Flowers, Fruit, and infpiffated Juice, commonly called *Acacia Germanica*, are ufed in Medicine. The Bark, Fruit, and *Acacia*, are drying, aftringent, and incraffating, and are us'd in Fluxes of the Belly, and Uterus internally, and externally in Gargarifms, and uterine Baths. The Flowers refolve and bring away the Gravel of the Kidneys. See *Acacia*. The Leaves of the Sloe Tree are bitter, a little ftyptic, glutinous, and give a faint Tincture of Red to the blue Paper; but the Fruit gives it as deep a Red as Alum; they are a little four, and extremely ftyptic: Thus it is likely, that the natural Salt of the Earth predominates in the Leaves, where it is mixed with a little fetid Oil; but that its acrid Parts being difengag'd in the Fruit, is united with the Earth, and forms a Salt refembling Alum. *Tragus* found by feveral Experiments, that the diftilled Water of the Sloe Tree, is an excellent Remedy for the Pleurify, and for Oppreffions of the Stomach. *Matthiolus* made ufe of the Decoction of the Fruit and Root for Ulcers of the Mouth and Throat. The Juice of the Fruit affwages Inflammations of the Eyes. The Syrup is prefcrib'd by *Witticbius*, made with feveral Infufions of the Flowers of this Tree, as a good Purgative.

Pfeudo-Acacia, Offic. *Pfeudo-Acacia vulgaris*, Boerh. Ind. Alt. Baftard Acacia. This Plant is naturally produced in *America*, but is found in the Gardens of the Curious. *Boerhaave* from *Robinus* fays, that the Leaves of this Plant when boiled and expreffed, purge in the fame Manner with *Sena*. Others recommend a Decoction of the Leaves, for its corroborating and refrigerating Quality. It is exhibited in Dyfenteries, but excites violent Pains and Flatulencies.

Pfeudo-Dictamnus, Offic. *Marrubium Pfeudo-Dictamnum dictum*, Raii Hift. Baftard Dittany. It is cultivated in Gardens, flowering in *July*. The Herb is ufed, which agrees in Virtues with the *Marrubium album*.

Pfeudo-Helleborus, *niger*, Offic. *Helleborus niger tenuifolius Buphthalmi flore*, C. B. P. Baftard Black Hellebore. It grows in mountainous Places, flowering in *April*. The Root is ufed, which is bitter and crid; and fometimes fold for the Roots of black Hellebore, by a fatal Error; for it is efteem'd a deleterious Plant. It takes off Warts like the *Ranunculus*.

Pfeudo-Ipecacuanna, Offic. *Apocynum erectum folio oblongo, flore umbellato petalis reflexis coccineo*, Raii Hift. Baftard Ipocacuanna. This Root is a Native of *America*, and is imported under the Name of the true *Ipecacuanha*. It is brown, and poifonous; and I once knew an Inftance of a Perfon, who was vomited feverely, and purged for a whole Week, after taking a Dofe of it.

There is another Species of Plant, not much unlike this in its Effects, which is the *Apocynum Syriacum*, Offic. Dog's Bane. It is fometimes cultivated in Botanic Gardens, flowering in *Autumn*; and the Leaves are ufed, but only to poifon Dogs, Wolves, Foxes, and other Animals.

Pfyllium, Offic. *Pfyllium vulgare*, Park. Theat. Fleawort. It is cultivated in Botanic Gardens; and the Seeds are ufed, which are faid to evacuate both Species of Bile, and to mitigate the Acrimony of the Humours, by its mucilaginous Quality; for this Reafon it is ufed in Dyfenteries, and Corrofions of the Inteftines; its Mucilage is good to affwage Inflammations of the Eyes. The Salt of this Plant refembles that of

Coral, but is mixed with a little Ammoniac, a great deal of Sul-ꝛr, and terreſtrial Parts. By the ꝛymical Analyſis, it yields a great ꝺl of Oil and Earth, no volatile ꝼcrete Salt, a little urinous Spirit,) ſeveral acid Liquors.

Ptarmica, Offic. Sneezewort, Baſꝺ Pelliory. It grows in Meadows, ꝼwering in *July*. The Leaves are ꝺ, which are of an hot and acrid uſte, and are therefore us'd in lads, in order to correct their Cold-ꝼ. The Powder taken by way of uff, provokes Sneezing.

Pulegium, Offic. *Pulegium latifo-*ꝼ, C. B. P. Peny-Royal. It lights in moiſt Places flowering in une. The Herb is uſed, and is ꝼeem'd good for exciting the *Menſes*, a *Fluor Albus*, for expelling the *Fa-*ꝼ, for a *Nauſea*, and Gripes, for ex-ꝼlling the Stone, and provoking ꝼrine, for the Jaundice, and for the ꝼropſy. This Plant which is very ꝼtter, acrid, and of a very pene-ꝼting Smell, gives a deep Tincture ꝼ red to the blue Paper ; ſo that it probable, it contains a volatile, ꝛomatic, and oily Salt, loaded with ꝼid ; whereas, in the artificial, vo-ꝼtile, oily Salt, this Acid is detain-ꝺ by the Salt of Tartar. Thus this ꝼlant is aperitive, hyſteric, and good ꝼr the Diſeaſes of the Stomach and ꝼreaſt, ſince it evacuates thoſe gluti-ꝼus Sordes, which fill Part of the *Bronchia*, and Veſicles of the Lungs ; ꝼpecially if it is boiled with Honey ꝺnd Aloes ; for then (as *Dioſcorides* ꝼbſerves) it purges and procures Ex-pectoration. The Juice of this Plant, ꝺears the Sight, and removes Lip-pitude. It is ſaid by ſome that a Spoonful of the Juice of Penny-Royal is a good Remedy for the Chin-Cough in Children, *Cheſneau* preſcribes a Glaſs of its Decoction ꝼor Hoarſeneſs.

Pulegium erectum, Offic. Upright Peny-Royal. It grows in marſhy

Places ; the Herb is uſed, which a-grees in Virtues with the former.

Pulegium cervinum, Offic. *Pulegium anguſtifolium*, C. B. P. Hart Peny-Royal. It is ſometimes, tho' not often, found in Gardens, flowering in *June*. It agrees in Virtues with the preceeding, but is ſaid to be ſomewhat more efficacious.

Pulmonaria maculoſa, Offic. *Symphytum maculoſum ſive Pulmonaria la-tifolia*, C. B. P. Sage of *Jeruſalem*. It is cultivated in Gardens, flowering in *April*. The Leaves are uſed ; which are eſteem'd Cardiac, and good for the Lungs, and are ſaid to conſolidate and heal. It is princi-pally uſed in Ulcers of the Lungs, Conſumptions, and Spitting of Blood. Externally it is reckon'd a good Ap-plication for Wounds.

Pulmonaria, foliis Echii, Tourn. Inſt. *Symphytum maculoſum ſive Pul-monaria anguſtifolia, rubente cæru-leo flore*, Pluk. Almag. Narrow-leav'd Sage of *Bethlehem*. It is cultivated in Gardens, flowering in *May*. The Leaves are uſed, which agree in Virtues with the former.

Pulmonaria Gallica, & Pulmonaria aurea, Offic. *Hieracium murorum ſive piloſiſſima*, C. B. P. *French*, or Golden Lung-wort. It grows in Woods, upon old Walls, and in ſha-dy Places, flowering in *June* and *July*. The Herb is uſed, which a-grees in Virtues with the *Pulmonaria maculoſa*.

Pulſatilla, Offic. *Pulſatilla vul-garis*, Ger. Emac. Paſque Flower. It grows in Gardens, flowering in *April*. The Herb is uſed, which agrees in Virtues with the *Anemone* and is vulnerary ; the Root is ſome-thing acrid, and excites Sneezing. It is alſo ſaid to be poſſeſs'd of an Alexipharmic Quality. This Plant is ſo acrid, that the mere Vapour of its Leaves, rubb'd between the Fingers, ſeems to burn the Noſe, and penetrate to the very Brain : It might

might be made use of in the Lethargy. The Leaves bruised are apply'd to Ulcers, but especially to the Wounds of Horses. By the Chymical *Analysis* this Plant yields some Marks of Acidity, a great deal of Sulphur and Earth, and a little fix'd, and no volatile concrete Salt.

Punica. The *Pomegranate.* See *Granata.*

Pyracantha, Offic. *Oxyacantha sive Spina acuta Pyri folio,* C. B. P. Ever-green Thorn. It is cultivated in Gardens. The Berries are used, which are astringent, and agree in Virtues with the white Thorn.

Pyrethrum, Offic. *Pyrethrum flore Bellidis,* C. B. P. Pellitory of *Spain.* It is imported from the Eastern Parts. The Root of Pellitory of *Spain,* held between the Teeth, helps the Tooth-Ach, by drawing forth the cold watry Rheum: It, also, helps the Palsey of the Tongue, and the Loss of the Voice consequent thereon. The Root is about a Finger Thick, hard, and of a yellowish brown Colour on the outside and whiter within, and of a very hot burning Taste.

Pyrethrum verum, Offic. *Pyrethrum umbelliferum,* C. B. P. True Pellitory of Spain. It is cultivated in the Gardens of Botanists, flowering in the Summer. The Root is about an Inch thick, of a dark-yellowish Colour, externally, and internally black of a very acrid and hot Taste. This Root held in the Mouth is excellent for removing the Tooth-Ach, by carrying off the watry Rheum which causes it, and is used in Lethargic Disorders and a Palsey, to very good Purposes.

Pyrola, Offic. *Pyrola rotundifolia major,* C. B. P. Winter-Green. It grows on mountainous and woody Places, flowering in *June.* The Herb is used, which is refrigerating, and drying, astringent and consolidating. It is an excellent Vulnerary, both externally and internally used:

Pyrola altera, Offic. *Pyrola folio mucronato serrato,* C. B. P. Smaller Winter-Green. It grows in Woods, flowering in *June.* The Herb is used, which agrees in Virtues with the former.

Pyrus, Offic. *Pyrus sativa,* C. B. P. The Pear Tree. It is frequently cultivated in Gardens, and Orchards, flowering in *April.* The Fruit is used which is cooling, and astringent.

Quercus, Offic. *Quercus cum longis pediculis,* C. B. P. *Quercus sive Robur,* Chab. The Oak. It grows in Woods and Hedges, and the Bark of the Tree, the Buds, the Leaves, the Acorns, and their Cups, and the excrementitious Tubercles called Galls, are used, which are all esteem'd refrigerating, drying and astringent, and for this Reason are recommended in Fluxes of the Belly, Uterus, and Weakness of the Genital Organs.

Quercus parva, sive Phagus Græcorum, & Esculus Plinii, C. B. P. *Phagus, Esculus,* Offic. Esculent, or Sweet-Oak. It grows in *Greece* and *Dalmatia;* and the Bark, Leaves, Acorns, and their Cups or Calyces, are used, and agree in Virtues with the former.

Another Species of Oak, is the *Cerrus, Ægilops,* Offic. *Quercus calyce echinato glande majore,* C. B. P. The Holme Oak, or Bitter Oak. It grows in *Italy,* and the Root, Leaves, Bark, and Galls are used. The Root is good for the Bites of Scorpions. The Leaves, Bark, and Galls stop Fluxes.

Another Sort also of Oak is the *Robur,* Offic. *Quercus gallam exiguam nucis magnitudine ferens,* C. B. P. The Gall Oak. It grows in *Pannonia,* and *Istria.* The *Galls* are used in Medicine. With respect to *Galls,* there are several sorts: The first and best is termed the *Allepo* Nut; or *Galla Spinosa;* the second is white; the third, smooth and round;

nd; the fourth, of an irregular ure; and the fifth has a kind of own. All these *Galls* are owing Insects, which first prick the Oak ees, and then lay their Eggs in the ound: These Eggs swell with the xrescence, and first turn to Worms; n to Flies, which having perfo ed the *Galls*, make their Escape. d as some Eggs are unfruitful, d remain in the *Gall*, they are ob v'd to yield a volatile Salt. *Galls* : very astringent, and are by some ven inwardly in Dysenteries: They ve also been recommended in In mitting Fevers; but the Founda n of their Febrifugous Quality, pends on too few Instances to be fied on. *Galls* are the principal igredient in making Ink, for if ater is impregnated with Iron, in y manner whatever, and powder'd alls is put into it, the Water turns nmediately black, and the black olour is more or less deep, in roportion as the Water is more or fs impregnated with Iron. It is r this Reason that *Galls* are used n discovering the Contents of Mi eral Waters, because if they con ain any Chalybeate Principle, they vill turn Purple, with powder'd Galls, or black if the Steel is pretty xevalent.

Quercus marina. Common Sea Wrack. See *Fucus maritimus.*

Quinquefolium, Cinquefoil, or five Fingers. See *Pentaphyllum.*

Quinquenervia. Rib Wort. A Name for the *Plantago angustifo lia.*

Quinquina. The Peruvian Bark. See *Kina Kina.*

Raditula. Radish. A Name for the *Raphanus Hortensis.*

Radix dulcis, Offic. *Glycirrhiza ca ... echinato,* C. B. P. Rough headed Liquorice. It is cultivated in Gardens, flowering in the Sum mer. The Root is used, which a grees in Virtue with the common Liquorice. The Powder of the Root is very proper to sprinkle on a *Ptery gium.*

Radix Rinzago, sive *Bengalensis.* This came in Use but very lately, for I find no Mention of it in any *Pharmacopæa* or Catalogue of Plants. As to its Virtues, it is recommend ed by Dr. *Tancred Robinson,* as a very potent Cephalic.

Radix Simarouba. See *Sima Ruba.*

Ranunculus acris, Offic. *Ranuncu lus pratensis erectus acris,* Boerh. Ind. Alt. *Ranunculus rectus non repens flore simplici luteo,* J. B. Upright Mea dow Crowfoot. It grows in Mea dows and Pasture Grounds; and the Herb is used, which is caustic; and which gathered fresh and bruised, and applied to the Skin, excites Pain and Inflammation. The Coun try People take the Root for the Cure of intermittent Fevers.

Ranunculus, Offic. *Ranunculus pratensis Repens hursutus,* Boerh. Ind. Alt. *Ranunculus Repens flore luteo simplici,* J. B. Crowfoot. It grows in Meadows, and flowers in *May.* The Herb which is quite harmless, is often boil'd with other Potherbs in *April.*

Ranunculus bulbosus, Offic. *Ranun culus pratensis radice verticilli modo Rotunda,* Boerh. Ind. Alt. *Ranun culus tuberosus major,* J. B. Bulbous Crowfoot. It grows in Meadows, and flowers in *May.* The Plant and Root are both used; the Herb is caustic; the Root, in Consequence of its burning Quality, excites Pu stules and Exulcerations, and is of wonderful Efficacy in corroding and drying hard Tumors, and pensile Warts, and other Excrescences of the like Nature; but when dried it loses all its Virtues.

Ranunculus palustris, Offic. *Ra nunculus palustris rotundifolius,* Raii Hist. *Ranunculus palustris Apii folio laxis,* Boerh. Ind. Alt. Round-lea ved Water Crowfoot. It grows in

watry

watry and marshy Places, and flowers in *June* and *July.* The Herb is used; whose Leaves, Flowers, and small Stalks, applied fresh, raise Ulcers not without Pain; in Consequence of which they remove a *Psora,* and efface Sugillations; applied in the Form of a Cataplasm, in a short Time, they cure *Myrmeciæ, Acrochordones,* and Alopecia's; and the Decoction cures Chilblains.

Ranunculus flammeus, Offic. *Ranunculus longifolius palustris major,* Boerh. Ind. Alt. *Ranunculus folio longo maximus Lingua Plinii,* J. B. Great Spear Wort. It grows in watry Places and Ditches, and flowers in *June;* and possesses all the Virtues of the foregoing Species.

Ranunculus flammeus minor, Ger. Emac. *Flammula,* Offic. *Ranunculus palustris flammeus minor sive angustifolius,* Park. Theat. Spear Wort. It grows in moist Meadows, and watry Places, and flowers in *June.* The Herb is used, which possesses the caustic Qualities of the foregoing.

Ranunculus Montanus, Offic. *Ranunculus Montanus maximus albus,* Park. Theat. *Ranunculus montanus Aconiti folio, albus, flore majore,* C. B. Pin. Mountain Crowfoot, with a white Flower. It grows in mountainous and woody Places, and flowers in *May* and *June.* The Herb is used, and possesses the same Virtues as the other *Ranunculi.*

Another Species of *Ranunculus,* is the *Thora,* Offic. *Ranunculus folio Cyclaminis, radice Asphodeli major,* Boerh. Ind. Alt. *Thora Montis Baldi sive Sabaudica,* Ger. Leopard Bane. It grows on the Mountains of *Switzerland.* Its Roots and small Bulbs bruised fresh, and applied to the Skin, cause Pains, Redness, Inflammations, excite Gangrenes, and render the Humours very acrimonious; hence it is evident that it is of a violent escharotic and caustic Qua-

lity, yet they are of good Service in those Diseases where the nervous System requires a Stimulus; such as fixed Pains of the Bones, Epilepsies, Convulsions, Spasms, hysteric Passions, inveterate Pains of the Periosteum, Gouts, old Ulcers, and ischiadic Disorders; applied to the Skin, they exulcerate and burn it, and the *Panniculus Adiposus,* quite into a Crust; and, left in open Wounds produce Fistulas; hence it is called by many *Scelerata Herba,* because with its Root and Bulbs Beggars raise Ulcers on their Children, in order to excite the Compassion of the Spectators. By others it is called *Apium Risus* which made *Guilandinus* think it was the *Apiastrum* of *Pliny* which *Dioscorides* calls *Sardonia.* It is also called *Herba Strumea,* because it discusses all strumous and scrophulous Swellings. Taken internally it is poisonous, but externally applied, it cures the Itch in Children.

Rapa, Offic. *Rapa Sativa rotunda,* Boerh. Ind. A. *Rapum sativum rotundum,* J. B. Turnep. They grow in Gardens and Fields, and the Seeds are used, but more used in *Kitchens* than *Apothecaries* Shops, they are boiled with almost all Sorts of Flesh; they are moderately nourishing, produce Wind, generate Flesh, but moist, and wanting a due Degree of Rigidity, provoke Urine, increase the seminal Juices, cure the Scurvy, and mitigate the Heat of quartan Fevers. The Juice with Sugar is good for a Cough.

Rapa Sylvestris, Offic. *Rapum Sylvestre non bulbosum,* Park. Theat. *Rapum Sylvestre Matthioli,* J. B. Wild Turnep. It grows in Fields and flowers in Summer. *Dioscorides* says the Root is an Ingredient in *Smegmata,* or detersive Medicines for cleansing the Skin of the Face, and other Parts of the Body.

Raphanus

Raphanus hortenfis, Radicula, Offic. *Raphanus fativus*, Ger. *Raphanus longus*, Boerh. Ind. A. The Radish. It grows in Gardens, and the Root and Seed are ufed, which are opening, abftergent, and attenuating; the Seed is chiefly ufed for breaking and expelling the Stone, and removing Obftructions of the Liver and Spleen. They provoke Urine and the Menfes. The *Raphanus* has the fame Virtues as the *Cochlearia*; the Root is efculent, expells Phlegm from the Inteftines, and is carminative. The Flowers, Leaves, Seeds and Roots, are antifcorbutic, and confequently good for phlegmatic Conftitutions; the expreffed Juice of the Roots and Seeds taken with Honey in a Morning, is a very wholefome Medicine, drinking after it a Draught of Whey: It cleanfes the Stomach, Kidneys, and Lungs, and is good againft an inveterate Cough, and Hoarfenefs, proceeding from Phlegm; but it is quite reverfe in Coughs proceeding from an Inflammation; or for thofe who fpit Blood. The Root contains much of aqueous and acrimonious Subftance; the drier it is the more acrid it becomes, but its Acrimony is loft in boiling. Its Aquofity renders it flatulent, on which account it is faid not to be good in Hypochondriacal Diforders: The daily Ufe of the Root, however, is of fufficient Efficacy to cure a Dropfy in the Beginning; and it is of excellent Service in the Scurvy. The Seeds are opening, but taken inwardly by themfelves, they excite a *Naufea.*

Raphanus fylveftris. Wild Radifh. See *Armoracia.*

Raphanus ruflicanus. Horfe Radifh. See *Cochlearia folio cubitali.*

Raphanus aquaticus, Offic. *Sifymbrium, aquaticum foliis in profundas lacinias divifis, filiqua breviori*, Tourn. Inft. Water Radifh. It grows in marfhy Ditches, flowering in *June* and *July.*

The Herb is ufed, which agrees in Virtues with the Horfe Radifh.

Rapiftrum, Offic. *Rapiftrum flore luteo*, C. B. P. *Sinapi arvenfis præcox femine nigro*, Tourn. Inft. Charlock. It is frequently found among Corn, flowering in the Summer. The Seed is ufed. It is of a drying, deterfive, and fomewhat digeftive Quality, and provokes Urine.

Rapum. The fame as *Rapa.*

Rapunculus, Campanula efculenta, Offic. *Rapunculus efculentus,* C. B. P. *Rapuntium parvum,* Ger. Emac. Rampions. It grows by the Sides of Ditches, flowering in *July.* The Root is ufed in the Kitchen and the Seeds in the Shops. The Seed is recommended for Defluxions of the Eyes, and the Juice for Pains in the Ears. The Root is efteem'd an agreeable Ingredient in Spring Sallads, and is faid to excite an Appetite; it is fometimes eaten boil'd. If taken with long Pepper, it has the Reputation of increafing Milk.

Regina Prati. Meadow-Sweet. See *Ulmaria.*

Refeda, Offic. *Refeda vulgaris*, C. B. P. Bafe-Rocket. It is found in chalky Soils, flowering in *June* and *July.* The Herb is ufed, which mitigates Pains, and difcuffes Inflammations.

Refeda minor vulgaris, Tourn. Inft. *Phyteuma*, Offic. *Refedæ affinis Phyteuma dicta*, C. B. P. Small Bafe Rocket. It grows about *Montpelier*, flowering in the Summer; and the Herb is ufed, which is faid to Increafe Venereal Inclinations.

Refina. See *Pix.*

Refta Bovis. Reft-Harrow. See *Anonis.*

Rhabarbarum, Offic. C. B. P. *Rhabarbarum lanuginofum five Lapathum Chinenfe longifolium*, Munt. Herb. Brit. *Rhabarbarum feu Rheum Officinarum*, Geoff. Tract. True Rhubarb. As much as Rhubarb is ufed, as efficacious as it is found in Medicine, and as large a Part of Commerce as it maintains, yet are we very little acquainted as to what it is, and the real Place from whence it originally comes. Some will have it come from *Boutan*, the Extremity of all the *Indies*, others from the Provinces of *Xensi* and *Suchen* in *China*, and thence to be carry'd into *Turky*; whilst others will have it grow on the Confines of *Muscovy*, and others again only in *Persia*. This is certain, that *Rhubarb* was unknown to the Antients; and their *Rhapontic*, which came tolerably near it, was not really the same therewith. The true Rhubarb first puts out large downy Leaves, then small Carnation-flowers in the Form of Stars, and after this comes the Seed. The Root newly drawn from the Earth is thick, fibrous, and blackish on the Surface, and of a red marble Colour within; when dried, it changes Colour, and becomes yellow without, and of a Nutmeg Colour within. It ought to be chose new, in small compact Pieces pretty solid and ponderous, of an astringent Taste, somewhat bitter, and of an agreeable aromatic Odour. When good, it will tinge Water almost like Saffron, and when broke, it appears of a lively Colour, inclining a little to Vermilion. Some Druggists have the Art of recovering their decay'd Rhubarb, by giving it a yellow Tincture; but the Cheat is easily discovered by handling it: for the Yellow Powder made use of to do it, will thus stick to the Fingers. Rhapontic is often mixed with Rhubarb, and sent over from the *Levant*; but this Imposition also may be discovered, because Rhubarb is ordinarily in Pieces, almost round, the internal Grain or Lines whereof are transverse; whereas Rhapontic is in long Pieces, the internal Lines whereof, which are reddish, growing longitudinally: and besides, Rhubarb, upon chewing it, leaves no Clamminess in the Mouth as Rhapontic does. Rhubarb is one of the best and mildest Cathartics in the whole *Materia Medica*, it operates very well on the Bile, and on all the *Viscera* of the *Abdomen*, and at the same time strengthens the nervous Fibres. On these Accounts, it is proper in weak Stomachs and Intestines. It is given in Substance from twelve Grains to half a Dram, and in Infusion, from half a Dram to a Dram and half; and in a small Dose, it becomes an excellent Alterative. It purges the Bile very effectually, and has a greater Force than any other Purgative, in opening Obstructions of the Liver. It is found by certain Experience, to evacuate the Bile, preferably to any other Fluid. On this account it is the Panacea of Children; and also because it strengthens the Stomach, and carries of all Sorts of Matter that stagnate therein. It is a very good Remedy for Worms, and is given to Children subject to Chronical Diseases, in a Ptisan, called Rhubarb Water. The Use of Rhubarb is, however, dangerous, when the Kidneys or Bladder are suspected to be inflamed, because it heats considerably; and for this Reason it is improper in Hæmorrhages. It is very good in a Looseness, because it purges and strengthens at the same time. In Cachexies, it ought to be given in small Quantities for a considerable Time.

Rhabarbarum Monachorum. Monks Rhubarb. See *Lapathum.*

Rhamnoides. A Species of Plant thus distinguish'd: *Oleaster Germanicus,* Offic. *Rhamnus secundus Clusii,* Ger. Emac. *Rhamnoides fructifera foliis Salicis, baccis leviter flavescentibus,* Boerh. Ind. Alt. Sallow Thorn. It grows in sandy maritime Places, flowering in *June,* the Fruit being ripe in *September.* An acid Rob is prepared of the Berries, which is recommended for the Dysentery.

Rhamnus Catharticus, Spina Cervi-

na.

na, Offic. *Rhamnus solutivus sive Spina infectoria vulgaris*, Park. Theat. *Rhamnus Catharticus*, Boerh. Ind. Buckthorn. It grows in Woods and Hedges, flowering in *May*, and producing ripe Fruit in *September*; it purges Bile, Phlegm, and all serous Humours, and consequently is of great Efficacy in a Cachexy, Dropsy, and Gout. The only Use of the Berries is to make a cathartic Syrup.

Rhamnus albus, Offic. *Rhamnus spinis oblongis flore candicante*, Boerh. Ind. A. *Rhamnus Cortice albo Monspeliensis*, J. B. Ram Thorn with white Flowers. It grows in *Spain*, *Portugal*, and other southern Countries, flowering in *May*, and bears its ripe Fruit in *Autumn*, a Cataplasm of the Leaves is very efficacious according to *Dioscorides* in a St. *Antbony's* Fire, and spreading Ulcers.

Rhamnus niger, Offic. *Rhamnus niger Theophrasti*, Park. Theat. *Rhamnus flore herbaceo baccis nigris*, Jons. Dendr. Black Ram Thorn. It is often found in Gardens, and flowers in *May*; the Decoction of the Fruit is good for Relaxations, and Weaknesses of the Limbs, as also for Pains of the Gout.

Rhaponticum, Offic. *Rhaponticum folio Lapathi majoris glabro Rha & Rheum Dioscoridis*, C. B. P. *Lapathum præstantissimum Rhabarbarum Officinarum dictum*, Boerh. Ind. A. True Rhapontic. It is frequent in physick Gardens, and flowers in *May*. It differs but little from the true Rhubarb, only this is somewhat more acrid, less solid, and of a somewhat deeper yellow Colour; with regard to its purgative Qualities, it is somewhat less powerful; but as to its astringent Virtues, it is much stronger. It is both vulnerary and anodyne, it is of singular Efficacy in Diarrhæas, Dysenteries, Convulsions, Ruptures, the Orthopnœa, periodi-cal Fevers, and the Bites of venomous Animals.

Rhaponticum falsum, Offic. *Rhaponticum folio Helenii incano*, C. B. P. *Centaurium majus, Rha capitatum folio Enulæ subtus incano & hirsuto*, J. B. Rapontic. This is cultivated in Botanic Gardens; the Root is thick, oblong, and dense, brown externally, and when cut transversly, of a yellowish Colour internally. It is of a bitterish and somewhat acrid Taste, sub-astringent and of a pretty grateful Smell.

Rhodia Radix, Offic. C. B. P. *Anacampseros radice Rosam spirante major*, Tourn. Inst. Rose-wort. It grows on hilly Places, flowering in the Spring. The Part used is the tuberous, and brittle Root, which is of a dark brown Colour on the Outside, and whitish within, and of a rosy Smell and Taste. This Root is heating and drying, and cephalic; its principal Use is in Pains of the Head.

Rhodium Lignum. Rose-wood. See *Aspalatus*.

Rhus Obsoniorum, Sumach, Offic. *Rhus folio Ulmi*, Boerh. Ind. A. *Sumach sive Rhus Obsoniorum & Coriarium*, Park. Theat. Common Sumach. It is cultivated with us in the Gardens of the Curious, but grows spontaneously in *Italy*, *Spain*, and *Turkey*. The Part used is the Berries; which are refrigerating, drying, and astringent; good in all Kinds of Fluxes, whether of the Belly, Uterus, or Hæmorrhoids; externally applied it resists Putrefaction and a Gangrene. It is not improper to observe, that the *Rhus Obsoniorum* of the Cooks, *Rhus Coriariorum* of the Tanners, and the *Rhus rubeum*, or Red-Rhus of *Galen*, are not different Species of Trees, but one and the same; for the *Rhus Obsoniorum* is the Fruit; the *Rhus Coriariorum*, the Leaves and small Branches; and the *Rhus rubeum* the Seed of one and the same Tree.

Rhus Virginianum, C. B. P. *Sumach sive Rhus*, Ind. Med. *Virginian Sumach*. This is a Native of *Virginia*, but is notwithstanding found with us in the Gardens of the Curious; the Berries is the Part us'd, which does not differ in Qualities from the preceeding Species.

Ribes, *Ribesia*, Offic. *Ribes Vulgaris acidus ruber*, Boerh. Ind. Alt. *Grossularia multiplici acino, sive non spinosa hortensis, rubra, sive Ribes Officinarum*, C. B. P. Red Currants. They grow in Gardens, and flower in *April*, the Berries only are used which are refrigerating, drying, and subastringent, and are very good for the Stomach; they are chiefly used in Fluxes of the Belly, and Dysenteries; they ease the Colic, and are very good in bilous Fevers; they resist Putrefaction, and allay Thirst; their Sharpness will sometimes occasion Prickings in the Stomach, but that may be easily prevented by the Addition of a little Sugar. Good Sweatmeats are made of Currants, as also a Liquor with Water and Sugar called Currant Wine, used in the Heat of Summer to cool and moisten the Body. A cooling moistning Jelly is also made of them, which is used in Physick and in Food, being very agreeable to the Taste, which, mixed with Water, is given with Success to feverish Patients.

Ribes nigra, Offic. *Ribes nigrum vulgo dictum folio olente*, J. B. *Grossularia non spinosa, fructu nigro*, C. B. P. The Black Currant. It grows by River Sides, and other Places, and flowers in *June*; the Berries only are used, which are esteemed good in a Quinsey.

Ricinus vulgaris, C. B. P. *Cataputia major*, *Ricinus*, Offic. *Granadilla Peruviana*, Pharmacop. Mexico Seeds. They are cultivated both in some Parts of *Germany* and *France*;

the Kernels which are the only Part in Use, powerfully purge Bile and Phlegm, and effectually destroy Worms in the human Body, but as we have much better Purgatives, it is no Wonder that this is seldom exhibited internally.

Ritro, Offic. *Echinopus minor*, J. B. *Carduus sphærocephalus cæruleus minor*, C. B. P. Little Globe Thistle. This is cultivated in Gardens, and flowers in *July*. The Root is us'd, and agrees in Virtues with the *Echinopus major*, or Glove-Thistle.

Robur. The Gall-Oak. See *Quercus*.

Rorella. See *Ros Solis*.

Rosa Canina, *Cynosbatos*, *Cynorrhodon*, Offic. *Rosa Sylvestris Canina*, *Cynorrhodon*, *Cynosbatos*, Mont. Ind. *Rosa Sylvestris vulgaris, flore odorato incarnato*, Elem. Bot. Common Briar, or Dogs Rose. It grows in Hedges and flowers in *June*. It agrees in Qualities with the Garden Rose, but is a greater Astringent, and consequently more esteemed in the Fluor Albus, and Profusion of the Menses; the Fruit is esteemed lithontriptic, but the Kernels when taken out more so.

Rosa Damascena pallida, Offic. *Rosa Provincialis sive Damascena*, Ger. *Rosa Damascena flore pleno*, Boerh. Ind. Alt. The Damask Rose. It grows in Gardens, and flowers in *June*, the Flowers purge choleric and serous Humours, and are generally given to Children, and Persons of weak Constitutions. It is an Ingredient in the *Conserva Rosarum*, *Aqua Rosarum*.

Rosa pallida, Offic. *Rosa maxima multiplex*, C. B. Pin. *Rosa centifolia rubella plena Hollandica dicta spinoso frutice*, Chab. The Damask Province Rose. It is common in Gardens, and flowers in *July*; it has the same Virtues as the common Damask Rose.

Rosa rubra, Offic. *Rosa rubra multiplex*,

multiplex, C. B. P. *Rosa rubra Anglica*, Park. Parad. The red Rose. It grows in Gardens, and flowers in *June*; the Flower and *Antheræ* are used, which are yellow Floscules, which adhere to the Capillaments in the Middle of the Flowers. The Flowers are powerfully astringent; they are chiefly used in Fluxes, Fevers, Thirst, and Loss of Appetite. Externally in Vomitings, Cephalalgias, Watchings, Pains of the Ears, Gums, and Anus, and in Inflammations of the Mouth, Fauces, and Eyes. The *Antheræ* dried are used in Dentrifices for astringing the Gums.

Hoffman, in his Treatise *de Præstantia remediorum domesticorum*, justly observes, that Roses are of singular Service in Medicine, for the Water distilled from them by means of its fragrant Oil is highly beneficial to Nature; whether given inwardly or externally applied, excellently calculated for recruiting Strength, and mitigating Pains and Inflammations in all hot Distempers. The Conserve of Roses in Consequence of its cordial and astringent Virtues is greatly beneficial to phthisical and hectic Patients. The Vinegar of Roses mixed with the Spirit and Water of Roses, with the Addition of Nitre and a little Camphire, makes an Epithem which when applied to the Head, he from Experience found to be of uncommon Efficacy in removing obstinate Head Achs, preventing Deliriums, as also stopping immoderate Hæmorrhages of the Nose.

Rosa alba, Offic. *Rosa Anglica alba*, Park. Parad. *Rosa alba flore pleno*, Boerh. Ind. Alt. The White Rose. This likewise grows in Gardens and flowers in *June*. The Flowers are used, which are esteemed opthalmic.

Rosa Moschata, Mont. *Rosa Moschata simplici flore*, C. B. P. The Musk Rose. It grows in the warmer Climates, but with us it is never brought into Use, it purges most potently.

Rosmarinus, Offic. *Rosmarinus hortensis angustiore folio*, C. B. P. *Libanotis coronaria, sive Rosmarinum vulgare*, Park. Theat. Rosemary. It grows in Gardens, and flowers in Spring. The Leaves, Flowers and Seed are used, which are greatly cephalic, nervine and uterine; they are of great Service in Disorders of the Head, Nerves, and Uterus, Apoplexies, Epilepsies, Palseys, Vortigoes, and a Carus. They sharpen the Sight, cure a fetid Breath, resolve all Obstructions of the Liver, Spleen, and Uterus; they cure the Jaundice, and *Fluor Albus* in Women, and greatly comfort the Heart. Rosemary, with respect to its Virtues, bears a near Affinity to *Spike* and *Lavender*, and in Consequence of its abounding with a penetrating balsamic Oil, it is very good in all Disorders of the Head, with Spirit of Lavender. *Arnoldus de Villa nova* affirms, that he has often seen Cancers, Gangrenes, and Fistulas dried up and perfectly cured, though they would yield to no other Medicine, by frequently washing them with an Infusion of Rosemary in Spirit of Wine. The Leaves bruised and made up in the Form of a Paste, and swallowed, powerfully strengthen the Stomach, and rouse the Spirits. Put into a Bath they are excellent against Barrenness; externally they strengthen the Nerves, prevent Gangrenes, and resolve cold Humours. Of Rosemary Flowers gathered in the Middle of the Day bruised with Sugar, and afterwards preserved from the Air in a Galley Pot, is made the celebrated English Conserve, called in the Shops, *Conserva Florum Antbos*, which is an excellent Remedy in Vertigoes arising from a cold Cause; as also in cold Distempers, in Consequence whereof it is an excellent Stomachic, and proper in that Disorder of the

Eyes

Eyes called *Lema Lippea*, when not Proceeding from an Inflammation.

Ros Solis, Offic. *Ros Solis folio subrotundo*, C. B. P. *Ros Solis, Rosa Solis, Sponsa Solis, Rorida & Rorella etiam dicta*, Chab. Rosa Solis. It grows in boggy Grounds, and flowers in *June* and *July*. The Virtues of this Plant are much controverted, some recommending it as good for the Phthisis, and Plague, whilst others, not without Reason, forbid the internal Use, on Account of its caustic Qualities.

Rubia Tinctorum, Offic. *Rubia tinctorum sativa*, Boerh. Ind. Alt. *Rubia major sive hortensis*, Park. Theat. Madder. It grows in Fields and Gardens. The Plant is vulnerary, and chiefly used in Obstructions of the Liver, Spleen, and particularly the Uterus; hence it is good in the Jaundice, Dropsy, Obstructions of the Urine, and Coagulations of Blood. The Dyers use it for preparing a red Colour.

Rubia sylvestris, & Rubeola, Offic. *Rubia sylvestris Monspesulana major,* J. B. Wild Madder. It grows in Hedges, flowering in the Summer; the Root is used, which agrees in Virtues with the former.

Rubia Synanchica, Offic. *Rubia Cynanchica*, C. B. P. *Synanchica Lugdunensis*, Ger. Emac. Squinancy Wort. It grows in barren and chalky Places, flowering in the Summer. The Herb is used, which is said to be of extraordinary Efficacy in the Quinsey, whether inwardly or outwardly used.

Rubus Vulgaris, Offic. *Rubus Vulgaris sive Rubus Fructu nigro*, Boerh. Ind. Alt. *Rubus Vulgaris major*, Park. Theat. The Bramble, or Blackberry Bush. It grows in Hedges and Thickets, and flowers in *May*, and produces its ripe Fruit in *August*. The Part in Use is the Leaves, tender Sprouts, and Fruit,

which are drying and strong Astringents. The Fruit is temperately heating, and subastringent; it is chiefly used in Fluxes, Vomitings, Fluxes of the Belly, and Haemorrhages of the Uterus and Nostrils; externally applied it is good in Aphthæ and other Disorders of the Mouth, as a Detergent, and is recommended as an Astringent in Wounds. It renders the Hair black, and cures the Scurvy. A Decoction of its Branches, according to *Dioscorides*, stops a Looseness, and the *Fluor albus*; its Leaves chew'd cleanse Ulcers of the Gums and Mouth, and bruised and applied to Tetters; it likewise kills them, and also cures the Piles. *Galen* made Use of the Leaves for Wounds; of the Flowers and Fruit for spitting of Blood; and of the Root for the Stone. *Tabernæmontanus* says, that a Bolster dip'd in the Juice of the Bramble, and put into the Fundament, stops the Flux of the Piles.

Rubus repens fructu Cæsio, C. B. P. *Chamæbatos*, Offic. *Rubus minor fructu cærulee*, J. B. The Dew Berry. It is found amongst Corn, and flowers in *May*, and produces its ripe Fruit in *Autumn*; the Fruit is in Use, and agrees with the *Rubus Vulgaris*, or the Bramble, or Blackberry Bush, in Virtues.

Rubus Idæus, Offic. *Rubus Idæus spinosus, fructu rubro*, Boerh. Ind. Alt. J. B. The Raspberry Bush. With us they are cultivated in Gardens, but grow spontaneously in some Parts of *Wales*, and the North; it flowers in *May*, and the Fruit is ripe in *June*, which is the only Part used; it has a pleasant grateful Smell and Taste, is cordial and strengthens the Stomach, stays Vomiting, is somewhat restringent, and accounted good to prevent Miscarriages. Raspberries are of a moistening and cooling Nature, cordial, and fortify the Stomach,

Stomach, they sweeten the Breath; they are likewise esteemed antiscorbutic and antinephritic.

Rubus Saxatilis, Ger. *Chamærubus*, Offic. *Rubus Alpinus humilis*, Boerh. Ind. Alt. Stone Bramble. It is a Native of Mountains and rocky Places, and flowers in *June*; the Berries are used, which agree in Virtues with the *Rubus Idæus*.

Ruscus. Butchers Broom. See *Bruscus*.

Ruta, Offic. *Ruta major hortensis latifolia*, Boerh. Ind. Alt. *Ruta sativa vel hortensis*, J. B. Garden Rue. Rue is planted in Gardens, and the Leaves and Seed are used. The whole Plant has a very strong Scent. This Plant was greatly esteem'd by the Ancients, which will appear by its being the principal Basis of the famous Antidote of *Mithridates*. It abounds with a highly, acid, and penetrating Oil, capable of stimulating the most languid Fibres to a brisker Motion, and consequently imparting an additional Strength to them. The Leaves of Rue mixed with recent Butter, and eaten in a Morning with Bread, are beneficial to those who abound with Phlegm, and an excellent Preservative against the noxious Influences of a moist and vapid Atmosphere, and the contagious *Miasmata* of epidemical Disorders. The Leaves bruised with Pepper, common Salt, and strong Vinegar, and applied to the Arteries of the *Carpus*, provided the morbid Matter is before duly managed, excellently check the febrile Impetus, and are often used with more Efficacy and less Danger in stopping obstinate quartan Fevers than internal Astringents, and the so much celebrated *Peruvian* Bark. Strong Wine Vinegar richly impregnated with the Juice of Rue, applied to the Mouth and Nostrils, is not only an excellent Preservative against the Contagion

of epidemical Disorders, but also more effectual in preventing Deliquiums than all the cephalic rich balsamic and apoplectic Spirits. It provokes the Menses, and expels the Lochia, Fœtus, and Secundines, and drank in the Morning instead of Tea, and the Vapour received into the Eyes, sharpens the Sight; the Seed is commended for the Worms and a Gonorrhœa, and consumes the *Semen* by its excessive Heat and Dryness; the Herb is of Service in the Small Pox, Measles, Epilepsy, lethargic Disorders, and the flatulent Colic. Externally used it is good for cold, humid, and watry Tumors. A Cataplasm is prepared of Rue bruised and boil'd with Wine which resists an Inflammation. Rue may be given inwardly in the most acute Diseases.

Ruta Capraria. Goats Rue. See *Galega*.

Ruta montana, Offic. *Ruta sylvestris major*, J. B. Wild Rue. It grows on hilly Places, flowering in *July*. The Herb is used, which agrees in Virtue with the common Rue, but is more acrid.

Ruta muraria. See *Adianthum album*.

Ruta sylvestris. See *Harmala*.

Sabina, Offic. *Sabina folio Tamarisci Dioscoridis*, Boerh. Ind. Alt. *Sabina Vulgaris*, Park. Theat. Savine. It is cultivated in Gardens, but seldom produces Fruit. The Tops are used, which are of a hot, drying, opening, and attenuating Quality, inciding and discutient; they are a powerful Provoker of the Menses, expel the Fœtus, and provoke Urine. Externally applied, they are good in all Uterine Disorders. Mr. *Ray* recommends the Juice of Savine mixed in Milk and sweetned, as an excellent Destroyer of Worms; beaten into a Cataplasm with Hog's Lard, it cures scabby Heads in Children. *Boerhaave* asserts, that a Water

prepared

Prepared from *Savine* by frequent Cohobations, is a moſt excellent Ecbolic, Emmenagogue, and Promoter of the Hæmorrhoids ; that the chymical Oil of *Savine* is a potent Provoker of the Menſes, when the Retention proceeds from Languor and Debility. A Cataplaſm of the Seeds bruiſed with *Sal Gem* and Oil, is ſaid to be excellent for an Anchyloſis.

Sabina baccifera, J. B. *Sabina folio Cypreſſi,* Boerh. Ind. Alt. *Sabina baccifera major,* Park. Theat. Berried Savine. This Species, as well as the former, is cultivated in Gardens ; the Herb is uſed, which is inciding, attenuating, powerfully provokes the Menſes, and Secundines, and kills Worms.

Saccharum. Sugar. This is produc'd from the *Arundo Saccharina,* J. B. *Arundo Saccharifera,* C. B. P. *Canna Saccharifera,* Ogilb. Chin. *Vuba & Tacomarte Braſilienſibus,* Marcg. The Sugar Cane. Sugar is an artificial Concrete, prepared from the Juice of this Cane, by boiling it gently in Copper Veſſels : this occaſions the lighter Feculencies to riſe to the Top, from whence they are carefully ſcummed off ; while the more ponderous ſubſide to the Bottom of the Veſſel. The purified Syrup is then mixed with a due Portion of Lime Water, and gently boiled ; which diſpoſes it to granulate, or form ſaline Concretions. Theſe are ſeparated from the more liquid Parts by ſuitable Contrivances. By this means, the Juice of the Cane is made to aſſume the Form of coarſe Sugar : this is ſtill further purified, by the Addition of Quick Lime, and repeated Coction When it is, by theſe means, brought to a due Conſiſtence, it is poured out into conical earthen Moulds, having a Perforation at their ſmaller End, which is placed lowermoſt : through this Hole, the *Moloſſes,* or coarſer Syrup, drains, while the purer Sugar

is left behind, in a ſolid Maſs, or Loaf. A weak Solution of Sugar, expoſed to a gentle Warmth, ſoon loſes its Tranſparency, ferments, and is converted into a genuine Wine, which upon Diſtillation yields a pure inflammable Spirit. If the Fermentation is promoted or continued for a ſufficient Length of Time, an excellent Vinegar is formed. Sugar, thrown upon live Coals, emits a copious Fume and at length burns with a clear Flame leaving behind it an earthy Subſtance. Diſtilled in a cloſe Veſſel, it yields an acid Spirit, and an Empyreumatic Oil, a black Coal remaining at the Bottom of the diſtilling Veſſel, from which, after it is thoroughly calcined, may, according to *Geoffroy,* be obtained a ſmall Portion of fixed Salt. Sugar, boiled along with Vegetables, imbibes their reſinous and mucilaginous Subſtance. Ground with diſtilled Oils, it renders them perfectly miſcible with Water. F. *Hoffman,* ſpeaking of Sugar, ſays, that as it is a temperate Salt, friendly to Nature, and capable of producing an intimate Union of oleous and pinguious Parts with Water ; hence appears the Reaſon why ſome both among the Ancients and Moderns, uſed to mix Honey, Sugar, Figs, and dried Grapes with the Food intended to fatten old Animals ; for the pinguious Parts of the Aliments, which when intimately incorporated with the moſt aqueous Parts, conſtitute the Milk and Chyle, are by this means more quickly diſſolved, united with the aqueous Parts, and form a large Quantity of Chyle, which is conveyed with the Blood to all the Parts of the Body. Hence alſo appears the Reaſon, why either Honey or Sugar mixed with Milk, prevents its Elaboration into Butter ; for the Sugar more firmly unites with the Phlegm the numerous oleous Particles in the Cream, whereas, in order to the Churning of Butter, or its

Collection into one Mass, these ought rather to be separated and disjoined from each other. Hence we may also learn, that Sugar is not so unfriendly to the Mixture of the vital Fluids, as is commonly believed, since it neither induces any Change in the Blood, Milk or *Serum*, when mixed with them, but rather by stimulating the Intestinal Fibres, facilitates the Excretion of the *Fæces* by Stool. And as it greatly promotes the Union, of the oleous with the aqueous Parts of the Aliments, hence 'tis probable, that it greatly contributes to the Generation of a large Quantity of Chyle. This accounts for the usual Method of fattening Capons and Geese, by mixing a little Honey, Sugar, or Salt with Wheaten or Barley Meal for their Food. It has been a Point much disputed whether Sugar in general is wholesome or otherwise. According to some it is temperate, heating, Emolient, Resolvent, Purgative, and calculated to resist Putrefaction, good for the Stomach, Lungs, and Breast, for Coughs and all Diseases of the *Thorax*, promotes Expectoration, softens internal Tumors, cleanses Ulcers of the Kidneys, Bladder and Inestines, and hinders all Corrosive Substances from acting easily on the internal Parts. According to others it is injurious to scorbutic, hypochondriac, hysteric, cachectic and feverish Patients, if used in considerable Quantities. Others assert, that it soon becomes acescent in the Stomach and *Prima Via*, that it weakens Digestion, and produces Flatulencies, impairs the Appetite, and generates Gripes and Dysenteries. It is also said to lay a Foundation for the Piles, and some foreign Physicians have ascribed the frequent Consumptions in *England* to the copious Use of Sugar. Some Authors affirm, that Sugar generates Worms,

others, on the contrary, are as positive that it destroys them. It is however generally agreed, that the common coarse Sugars foul the cutaneous Glands, and excite scorbutic Spots and Blotches. Sugar, in some Degree, differs in medicinal Virtues according to its Degree of Fineness; thus the *Muscovado*, or Sugar first procured from the Cane, is more relaxing and purgative, and consequently more proper in Clysters, and cathartic Syrups. The *Cassonada*, or Sugar once refin'd from the former, is something less relaxing, and more proper for internal Uses. The Loaf Sugar, or *Cassonada* still further refin'd, is said to be more detersive; they both cut Phlegm, promote Expectoration, and animate the Blood; but they excite Vapours and the Tooth-ach. They who use much Sugar are liable to Fevers, and to rotten Teeth. In *Brasil*, the Skimmings of Sugar are given to the Hogs, by which they are soon fattened, and their Flesh becomes very delicate. *Sugar Candy*, or Crystals of Sugar, is of three Kinds, white, yellow, and red, which are only the three former Sorts boiled to a due Consistence. White Sugar Candy comes from the *Loaf Sugar*, yellow from the *Cassonada*, and red from the *Muscovado*. Sugar Candy is most proper in Colds, because it melts slowly, and thereby gives Time to the *Saliva* to mix with it; and thus to blunt the Acrimony of the Phlegm.

There is another Species of Sugar called *Maple Sugar*, which is produced in *Canada* and *New England*, in which Countries the Native collect the Juice that runs from a Kind of Maple Tree, by Incision, and then evaporate that Juice to the Consistence of Sugar, which while it remains unctuous, is better for internal Use than any other Kind; and
the

the famous Syrup of Maiden Hair of *Canada* is made with it. As it is brought to us, it is of a greyish Colour, and tastes like other Sugar.

Sagapenum, Offic. Park. Theat. *Sagapenum Veterum,* J. B. This Gum is brought to us from *Alexandria*; is attenuating, aperient, and purges viscid, thick and serous Humours from the Stomach, Intestines, Uterus, Reins, Brain, Nerves, Joints, and Breasts; in consequence whereof it is good in a Dropsy, inveterate Coughs, Asthmas, Cephalalgias, Spasms, Epilepsies, Palsy, Tremors of the Limbs, in Obstructions and Tumours of the Spleen, and Colic Pains, it provokes the *Menses* and Urine, but kills the *Fœtus.*

Sagitta, Offic. *Sagitta Europæa aquatica minor latifolia,* Boerh. Ind. *Sagittaria Europæa minor latifolia,* Hist. Oxon. Arrow-head. It grows in Rivers and watry Places, and flowers in *May* and *June*; the Herb and Seed are both used, and are of a cold and moist Temperament, and possess the same Virtues as the *Plantago Aquatica.* This was the Opinion both of *Matthiolus* and *Boerhaave,* but the Smell and Taste speak it of a hot Nature.

Sagittaria Alexipharmica, Offic. *Canna Indica, radice alba Alexipharmica,* Raii Hist. *Radix quædam in Malaca quæ adversus vulnera Sagittis toxico illitis facta, præsentaneum remedium est,* C. B. P. Arrow Root, Dart Wort. This Plant grows in the Gardens in *Jamaica* and the *Charibbee* Islands, whither it was transplanted from the Island of *Dominica,* and is greatly esteem'd for its Alexipharmic Virtue, and extraordinary Efficacy against Wounds inflicted by poisoned Darts and Arrows, for which purpose it is frequently used by the *Indians,* who apply the bruised Herb to the Part afflicted.

Sagou, Offic. *Palmam referens Arbor Farinifera,* C. B. P. *Arbor Farinifera,*

Park. Theat. *Zagu seu Arbor Farinifera,* Jons. Dendr. *Todda-panna seu Monta-panna,* Commel. Flor. Mal. Sago Tree, Indian Bread, or Libby Tree. It grows in several Places of the *East-Indies,* and the Pith of the Tree is used, which being well beat in a Mortar with Water, forms an Emulsion, the *Fæcula* of which dried is *Sago.* It is a very kindly and nourishing Food, never fermenting in the Stomach, and very proper in Hectic Fevers. It is very much used in *England.*

Salicaria. See *Lysimachia Purpurea.*

Salix, Offic. *Salix vulgaris alba arborescens,* C. B. P. Common Willow. It grows in watry Places, and by the Sides of Brooks. The Leaves are used, which are refrigerating, and somewhat astringent; tho' their principal Use is in restraining venereal Inclinations. Outwardly they are of Service in Hæmorrhages from Wounds, or from the Nostrils, and the like Disorders, and are of Service in Baths for the Feet, in order to procure Sleep, and cool the Heat of Fevers. The Ashes of the Bark of this Tree are effectual for extirpating Warts and Corns.

Salix rubens, Offic. *Salix vulgaris rubens,* C. B. P. Common red Willow. It grows in watry Places? and the Leaves are used, which agree in Virtue with the former.

Salix Helice, Offic. *Salix Rosea,* Park. Theat. Rose Willow. It grows by the Sides of Brooks, and is esteemed not different from the preceding.

Salsaparilla, Offic. *Smilax aspera Peruviana sive Salsaparilla,* C. B. P. *Ivapecanga vulgo Sarsaparilla herba,* Pison. *Mecapatli seu Zarca-parilla,* Hernand. *An Cari-villandi?* H. M. Sarsaparilla. It is of fine Parts, and accounted a Specific for the *Lues Venerea, Arthritis,* Rheumatism, and the like Disorders. *Sarsaparilla* is a very noted Root, which began to be very much celebrated, about the me Time with the *China* Root, as pears from an Epiftle of *Vefalius*. is inferior indeed to *Guaiacum*, but is generally fuppofed to be much perior in Virtue to *China* Root, d even to exceed *Guaiacum* itfelf, hen after a Courfe of Mercurial unctions, and drinking Decoctions *Guaiacum*, the Patient is ftill mofted with Ulcers, *Rhagades* about e *Anus*, Tophs, Nodes, *Ganglia* d *Gummata*; but efpecially with heumatic Pains, either fixed or wanering, and owing their Original to he venereal Infection, in which later Cafe it is efteemed a Specific. t is imported from feveral Countries f *America*, and efpecially from *Peru*, *Mexico*, and *Brazil*, where it is aid to grow fpontaneoufly, and plenifully, even in the Hedges. It is generally believed to be the Root of Plant, the fame with the *Smilax Afpera*, or very near akin to the *Smilax*. Hence it is called by the *Spaniards Sarfa-parilla*, or *Zarça-parilla*, (that is, *a fmall Vine refembling the Bramble*) which is the Name they give the *Smilax Afpera*, as we are told by *Andreas Lacuna*; becaufe the *Smilax* in its Leaves, Branches, and Tendrils, refembles the Vines, but in its Thorns and Prickles the Bramble; for *Zarza* in *Spanifh* is a Bramble, and *Parilla* a little Vine. This Opinion is alfo favoured by Experience; for it is certain, that the Roots of our *Smilax Afpera* very nearly refemble in Figure thofe of *Sarfaparilla*, and almoft equal them in Virtue; fince we are affured by *Fallopius*, that he made ufe of the Roots of the *Smilax Afpera* gathered in *Italy*, with happy Succefs, and cured Multitudes of the *Lues Venerea*. *Sarfaparilla* is prepared in Decoction, after the fame Manner as *China*, that is, by cutting two Ounces of the Root into fmall Bits, and macerating them a whole Day in fix Pints of common Water;

after which they boil them over a gentle Fire, in a double Veffel well clofed with a Lid, till one third, or half be evaporated. Of this Decoction the Patient is to take a Glafs, that will hold ten Ounces, very early in Bed; what remains ferves during the reft of the Day for ordinary Drink, and this Courfe is continued for twenty or twenty four Days. As to the reft, the Patient is allowed a fomewhat greater Latitude in Diet, than under the Ufe of *Guaiacum*, and obferves in that Refpect, the fame Regimen as is prefcribed to thofe who drink the Decoction of *China*.

Salvia hortenfis major, Offic. *Salvia major vulgaris*, Park. Theat. Common Sage. It grows in Gardens, flowering in *June*, and the Leaves and Flowers are ufed. Sage is diuretic; it provokes the *Menfes*, when retained thro' Thicknefs, and moderates their Excefs; it is alfo ferviceable in Palfies, Vertigoes, Tremblings, and Catarrhs; outwardly it abuerges Aphthæ in the Mouth. It is an excellent Cephalic, and was always highly efteemed by the Inhabitants of the Eaftern Nations, who at prefent prefer its dried Leaves to Tea. In confequence of the fubtile, vaporous, and fedative Oil it contains, a Decoction or rather Infufion of it by way of Tea, is highly efficacious in Spafmodic Contractions, in Contractions of the Members, and Chronical Epilepfies. In order to allay Inflammations of the *Fauces*, and other Diforders of the Teeth and Mouth, Surgeons order a Decoction of Sage to be ufed as a Gargarifm. It takes its Name *Salvia*, from *Salvus*, found, healthy, becaufe no Plant has a greater Reputation for Healthfulnefs and Wholefomnefs, whence the Queftion in the old Verfe:

Cur moriatur Homo cui Salvia crefcit in Horto.

Why dies the Man, whose Garden Sage affords?

Sage has a very fragrant Smell, and if smell'd to for a considerable Time, causes a Sort of Ebriety, and at length a Vertigo. Drank after the Manner of Tea, it is astringent, stimulates the Fluids, and corroborates and dries the Fibres and Bones. It is justly, therefore, by *Dioscorides*, esteemed a most effectual Sudorific, Cardiac and Cephalic, and has given Occasion for the Verse in the *Schola Salernitana* above cited. It is of Service in the Gout, *Vertigo*, *Leucophlegmatia*, and *Chlorosis*, or Cachexy of Virgins. It is subject however, to one very great Inconvenience, which is, that it harbours *Toads* under its Roots; the Way to avoid which, is to plant near it Rue, which these Animals cannot endure. *Sage* indeed was by the Antients justly esteemed Alexipharmic, Sudorific, and especially Cephalic, but it was only in cold Diseases, where Phlegm abounded. The distill'd Water, and the Conserve of the Flowers were usually exhibited as Preservatives against all Sorts of Poison, by their sudorific and strengthening Virtues. A Conserve of Sage is very proper for a Weakness of the Stomach in Women, for those of that Sex who have for Years together laboured under an Infirmness, or Debility of the Stomach, are said to be cured by taking half a Dram of the Conserve.

Salvia hortensis minor, Offic. *Salvia minor aurita & non aurita,* C. B. P. Sage of Vertue. It grows in Gardens, flowering in *June.* The Leaves and Flowers are used, which agree in Virtues with the former.

Salvia folio tenuiore, C. B. P. *Salvia Indica,* Ger. Emac. Spanish Sage. It is cultivated in Gardens, and the Leaves are used, which agree in Virtues with those of the common Sage.

Salvia Vitæ. A Name for the *Adiantbum Album.*

Sambucus, Offic. *Sambucus vulgaris,* J. B. Common Elder. It grows in Hedges, flowering in *May.* Its Leaves have a Taste at first herbaceous and saltish, afterwards bitter. The Fruit is sweetish, and gives a deeper Red to the Blue than to the White Paper. Its Leaves yield, by the Chymical Analysis, beside some acid and ascaline Liquors, some volatile concrete Salt, a great deal of Earth and Oil. Thus it may probably operate by a *Sal Ammoniac*, loaded with more acid than ordinary, and joined with a great deal of Oil and Earth. The Salt of the Elder-Berries resembles Alum rather than *Sal Ammoniac.* It affords only a little urinous Spirits from these Parts, but a great deal of acid, Oil and Earth. *Bartholine* informs us, that Elder is at once more safe and efficacious, than the celebrated artificial Antidotes *Theriaca* and *Mithridate.* The Flowers and Rob of Elder are highly and justly esteemed by the common People; for the former are with great Success externally applied for alleviating all Erysipelaceous Swellings, Tooth-achs and Gouts; as also for softening Abscesses and hard Tumours, produced by coagulated Milk. The Water of these Flowers, in consequence of its Anodyne Quality, is of singular Efficacy in all Diseases, whether acute or chronical; but especially in those Disorders where Expulsion is proper, where the Pain is intense, and where there is an Inflammation of the internal Parts. The Rob prepar'd of Elder-Berries, is as it were, the *Panacea* of the Country People, who use it as the best Preservative, and the safest Medicine in the Beginning of Diseases, mixing it either with warm Ale, or Elder Flower Water; for it not only provokes the Excretions by Stool and Perspiration, but it is also possessed of

aa

an Anodyne Quality. Some, in order to render this Rob more diaphoretic, add about a Dram of calcined Hartshorn to it. If this Rob is mix'd with an equal Quantity of Sugar Candy, and a due Quantity of Brandy poured upon the Mixture, and kind'd after a sufficient Agitation, it affords a Medicine, one Spoonful of which is of excellent Service in long protracted Coughs, and before the Paroxysm of Intermittent Fevers. The frequent Use of this Rob generally mitigates, and sometimes stops the *Impetues* of these Fevers, provided the Crudities of the *Primæ Viæ* have been previously treated with Laxatives and Correctors. The middle Bark of the Elder Tree, if boil'd in Ale, Water or Wine, powerfully promotes Sweat, Urine, and the *Menses*, for which Reason, it is highly proper for Cachectic Patients. This Bark when externally applied, removes œdematous and erysipelaceous Swellings; as also Pains and Tumours of all Kinds. The Leaves and Tops are commended by *Dioscorides* in the Hysteric Passion, Inflammations, Combustions and Gout.

Sambucus humilis, Ger. Emac. *Ebulus*, *Chamæacte*, Offic. *Sambucus humilis*, *five Ebulus*, C. B P. Dwarf Elder, or Dane-wort. It grows in Path Ways, flowering in *June*. The Leaves are a little bitter, and the Fruit more so. It is styptic, and does not redden the blue Paper. By the Chymical Analysis, the Leaves and Tops yield a little acid and urinous Spirit, no concreted and volatile Salt, and a good deal of Earth and Oil. The Leaves are emollient and resolvent, and are used as a Cataplasm for the Gout, and all Kinds of Tumours. The young Shoots and Bark are purgative. Half an Ounce of its Seeds, infused in a Glass of White Wine, is a proper Remedy for Hydropical Persons. The Oil expressed from the Seed is sweetening and re-

solvent. This Herb is a *Succedaneum* to the former. For Affections of the Spleen, take of distill'd Water of Dwarf, to the Quantity of about four Ounces, for ten or twelve Days in the Morning fasting. This was an approved Prescription of *Du Val*, for Pains, Inflammations, and Obstructions of the Spleen. The Leaves of the *Ebulus* being bruised and applied, are no less effectual in curing Combustions, than those of the *Sambucus*. The Berries, as well as those of the former, dye the Hair.

Sambucus Montana, Offic. *Sambucus racemosa rubra*, C. B. P. Mountain Elder. It is cultivated in Gardens, and the Leaves are used. It is cold and soporiferous, and agrees in Virtues with the *Belladonna*.

Sampsucum. A Name for the *Majorana*, or Sweet Marjoram.

Sanamunda, Offic. *Sanamunda prima Clusii*, Ger. *Thymelæa foliis Chamælæa minoribus subhirsutis*, C. B. P. *Tarton-raire Massiliensium*, Park. Theat. Heath Spurge. It grows spontaneously in *Provence* in *France*, and the Leaves are used, which are said to be possess'd of a Caustic Quality.

Sandaracha, Offic. *Vernix Arabum*. This is a Gum Resin, which flows from the *Cedrus Lycia major*, Dodon. It is attenuant and resolvent, but it is seldom used in Physic, though very much by the Varnishers, being first dissolved in Spirit of Wine. It is sometimes confounded with Juniper Gum, and is very different from that Kind of Orpiment, which was the *Sandaracha* of the antient *Greeks*.

Sanguis Draconis. Dragon's Blood. This is already specify'd under the Article *Draco Arbor*.

Sanicula, Offic. *Sanicula five Diapensia*, Ger. Emac. Sanicle. It grows in Woods and Hedges, flowering in *May*. The Leaves are principally used as a Vulnerary, and are useful

in

in confolidating Ulcers, Fiftulas, Ruptures, and Erofions. By the Chymical Analyfis, befide feveral acid Liquors, Sanicle yields an urinous Spirit, and fome concreted volatile Salt, and a great deal of Oil and Earth. It contains fome *Sal Ammoniac,* Sulphur, and terreftrial Parts. It is deterfive and aperitive. Sanicle is greatly commended by the *French* and *Walloons,* who eat it for Inflammations. *Baubine* thinks it proper in hot Difeafes of the Kidneys. It is a ufeful Plant in a Languor, and Decays, from a Vifcoufnefs of the Humours. It is of a penetrating, Balfamic Virtue; for it has an acrid Sort of a Fragrancy, in which confifts its Virtues, and leaves an aftringent Tafte in the Mouth. It is ferviceable in *Hernias,* and Hæmorrhages, and in difcuffing Tumors, by Refolution or Diffipation, the Leaves being bruifed, and applied with Wine or Vinegar. The Decoction is taken inwardly, to diffolve grumous Blood, and is good in Fractures, where Purgation and Abftertion are required.

Sanicula Montana. Bear's-Ear Sanicle. See *Cortufa.*

Santalum. Sanders. The white and yellow Sanders of the Shops, are produced by the fame Tree; the cortical Part of which, according to many, is called white Sanders, and the medullary Part, yellow Sanders: But *Garcias* informs us, that there is fo great a Refemblance between the Trees, which bear the white and yellow Sanders, that they cannot be diftinguifh'd, except by the Inhabitants who fell them to the Merchants. Yellow Sanders, is the Marrow of a certain Berry bearing Tree, called *Sarcante,* in the Ifland of *Timor;* which, when feparated from the Integuments, is folid, thick, and of a yellow Colour, of a bitterifh aromatic Tafte, and fragrant Smell. This Commodity is brought from *China* and *Siam,* and the Tree itfelf is tall, like a Walnut Tree, but bears Fruit refembling Cherries. The white Sanders is the paler Marrow of the fame Tree, of a fainter Smell, and lefs aromatic Tafte. When thefe Trees are dried, the Marrow alone is chofen; which, if it is not fufficiently odorous, is called white Sanders. Yellow Sanders derives its fragrant Smell, and aromatic Tafte, from the tender Rofin, contained in it, and which is eafily extracted, by infufing the Shavings of it, in a fufficient Quantity of highly rectify'd Spirit of Wine. By Digeftion, a very yellow Tincture is extracted from it, which when infpiffated over a gentle Fire, after the Spirit is abftracted, conftitutes a liquid Balfam, of a darkifh Colour, and grateful Tafte, and which in Confiftence and Colour, almoft approaches to *Peruvian* Balfam. And if this Balfam is again diffolved in highly rectify'd Spirit of Wine, it makes a Balfamic Effence of fingular Virtue. This Experiment excellently illuftrates the Nature and Generation of the *Peruvian* Balfam, the Balfam of *Capivi,* and that of *Metcha,* which are nothing but liquid Refins; for if the refinous Principle of Sanders is diffolved in highly rectify'd Spirit of Wine, and the Solution infpiffated, it affumes the Confiftence of a Balfam, and is no more converted into a folid Refin, fince fome moift Particles have by this means intimately infinuated themfelves into its Compofition. The Effence of yellow Sanders, is of the fame analeptic and fedative Virtue with Amber, and is highly beneficial in Diforders, arifing from a Weaknefs, and want of Tone in the nervous and membranous Parts; for which end, it may either be ufed by itfelf, or in Conjunction with the Effence of Aloes Wood, or Amber. Both the yellow and white Sanders are refrigerating, drying, and aperitive, hepatic and cordial. Their principal Ufe is in

Lipothymy, Palpitation of the Heart, and Obstructions of the Liver, and the like Disorders. Outwardly they are of Service in Catarrhs, Head-achs, Vomiting, and the like.

Santalum rubrum, Offic. Red Sanders. It grows in the *East-Indies*, beyond the River *Ganges*. The Part in use is the Wood, or rather the Heart, separated from the outer Integuments, the Bark and Wood, and of a solid, dense, ponderous and red Substance. This Species of Sanders is refrigerating and astringent. Whatever Virtues, therefore, are by the *Arabians* ascribed to the several Sorts of Sanders, against preternatural Heats, and the like Kinds of Disorder, belong in a more special Manner to red Sanders.

Santonicum & Semen Santum, Offic. *Sementina*, Ger. Emac. *Lumbricorum Semen vulgare, & Matthi-Æ*, J. B. Wormseed. It is brought from *Alexandria*. The Seeds, which are the Part used, are small, oblong, yellow, and of an acrid, bitter, and disagreeable Smell. They seem to be formed of small Scales, inclosing each other. These Seeds are in great Reputation, for their Virtues in killing Worms.

Santonicum viride, Offic. *Abotan*, Pomet. Green Wormseed. It is like the former, but is larger, and of a green Colour, inclining to a yellow. The Virtues are the same as the former.

Saponaria, Offic. *Saponaria major levis*, C. B. P. *Lychnis sylvestris, quæ Saponaria vulgo*, Tourn. Inst. Sope-Wort. It grows near Rivers, tho' but seldom; flowering in *July*. The Herb and Roots are used. It is greatly attenuating, aperitive, and sudorific. It is used in the Asthma, to provoke the *Menses*, and in the *Lues Venerea*. Externally used, it is a good Ptarmic, and is principally used to discuss Tumors and Boyls.

Sarcocolla, Offic. C. B. P. *Sarco-* col. This is a Gum which comes from *Persia*, in small whitish Grains, with a few of a reddish Colour mixed among them, of a viscid, and somewhat bitterish Taste, with a sweetish Relish. Chuse what is recent, of a Colour inclining to Paleness, (for the old and stale is reddish) of a bitter Taste, a porous and glutinous Substance. It is healing, drying, astringent, consolidating, conglutinating, digestive, and maturating. Its principal Uses are, in exterging, and consolidating Wounds, and inducing a Cicatrix over them, whence it has its Name. It is of excellent Service in Rheums, an Albugo, or Films, affecting the Eyes: For which Purposes it is macerated five Days, in Asses or Womens Milk, and being mixed with Rose Water, with a little Sugar, is applied to the Eye-Lids. It is an Ingredient in *Anacollema*'s, for Hæmorrhages of the Nose.

Sarsaparilla. The same as *Salsaparilla*.

Sassafras, Offic. Park. Theat. *Arbor Sassafras Monardi*, Pluk. Phytog. *Arbor sive Lignum Pavanum*, J. B. *Anhuiba sive Sassafras Brasiliensium*, Pison. The Sassafras Tree. It grows in several Parts of *America*. It is principally of Use in removing Obstructions, and strengthening the internal Parts; in causing Fertility, and curing the *Lues Venerea*. It is accounted a *Panacea* or Sovereign Remedy for Catarrhs. Much about the same time, with the other anti-venereal Woods and Roots, was imported the Wood called *Sassofras*, from several Parts of *America*, but principally from *Florida*, where the Natives call it *Pahamoe*, as we are told by F. *Goreal, Voy. aux Ind. Occid.* *Sassofras* is of a reddish Colour, inclining to white, ligneous, of a light and rare Substance, contained under a thin Bark, which is ash-colour'd without, and sanguineous within, of

an

an acrimonious, sweetish, and aromatic Taste, and of a fragrant Smell; whence it is usually called *Lignum Fæniculi*, or *Fæniculatum*, Fennel Wood. There was prepared and used, a Decoction of *Saffafras*, after the same manner as the Decoctions of *China* and *Sarfaparilla*: but as *Saffafras* comes next to *China*, in Virtue of curing the Symptoms of the Venereal Disease, so it is very much inferior in that Respect, to *Guaiacum* and *Sarfaparilla*. It has been the Custom for a long time past, to take the two Woods, *Guaiacum*, and *Saffafras*, with the two Roots *China* and *Sarfaparilla*, which are all of a like Nature and Virtue; and boil them together, generally without any Cathartic, but sometimes with Leaves of Senna, which was the Fashion since the Year 1550, as we are informed by *Braffavolus, de Radicis Chinæ usu*. Of these Drugs in Conjunction, then, were prepared Decoctions and *Bocheta*, which were sometimes only diaphoretic and diuretic, but sometimes cathartico-diuretic, and very commonly known by the Names of *Ptifanæ Sudoriferæ*, or *Ptifanæ e Lignis sudorificis*. The Proportions of the Ingredients were various, according to the different Intentions which were to be answered. Generally they took two Ounces of *Lignum Guaiacum*, in Dust, or small Chips, or as many Ounces of Wood of *Saffafras*, cut likewise very small, and the like Weight of the Roots of *China* and *Sarfaparilla*, each cut into very small Bits, and infus'd them warm, in ten or twelve Pints of common Water, for twenty four Hours. After this, they added thereto, if it was thought requisite, two Ounces of crude Antimony, grosly bruised, and loosely tied up in a Nodule; and boil'd the whole over a gentle Fire, in a Vessel covered with a Lid, to the Consumption of a third Part: after which, they added thereto, an Ounce

of Scrapings of Liquorice; and if they would have it purge, half an Ounce of the Leaves of Oriental *Senna*, which were to boil a Moment. This done, when warm, they strain'd the Decoction, and set it aside in Glass Bottles, well stopped, for Use. The Custom was, to take three Draughts of this Decoction every Day, for twelve or fifteen Days together; the first in the Morning fasting, the next four or five Hours after Dinner, and the last, going to Bed; or at least two Draughts, that is to say, in the Morning and Evening; omitting the Afternoon's Draught, if it should be thought proper. During the Time of taking it, the Patient was to be kept to a sparing Diet, and to confine himself at Home, if the Season of the Year requir'd it.

Satureia, Offic. *Satureia hortensis five Cunila sativa Plinii*, C. B. P. Summer Savoury. It is sown in Gardens, flowering in *June*. The Herb is used, which is one of those hot and acrimonious Herbs, which provoke Urine and the *Menses*, and is supposed to have much the same Virtues with Thyme and Hyssop.

Satureia montana, C. B. P. *Thymbra*, Offic. *Satureia vulgaris*, Park. Theat. *Calamintha frutescens, Satureiæ folio, facie & odore*, Tourn. Inst. Winter Savoury. It is cultivated in Gardens, flowering in the Summer, and the Herb is used; which agrees in Virtues with the preceding.

Satureia Cretica, C. B. P. *Thymbra vera*, Offic. *Satureia Cretica folio rigido, brevi, crasso*, Boerh. Ind. Alt. True Savoury. It is found in the Island of *Crete*. The Herb is used, which provokes Urine, and the *Menses*; and is of great Service, being mix'd with Honey, for Coughs.

Satureia spicata, Offic. *Satureia St. Juliani, five Satureia vera Lobelio*, Tourn. Inst. Rock Savoury.

voury. It grows on Hills and Walls, flowering in the Summer; and the Herb is used, which agrees in Virtues, with the other Species of Savoury.

Satyrium mas, Offic. *Orchis morionas, foliis maculatis*, C. B. P. *Cynosorchis morio mas*, Ger. Emac. Male Satyrion. It grows in Meadows and Thickets, flowering in *May*. The Root is used, which is heating and moistening, and of a sweet Taste. Its principal Use is in restoring manly Vigour; it is believed also, to strengthen the *Uterus*, and dispose to Conception.

Satyrium fœmina, Offic. *Orchis morio fœmina*, C. B. P. *Cynosorchis morio fœmina*, Ger. Emac. Female Satyrion. It is frequently to be met with, as the former, and grows in the same Places, but is later in flowering. These two last Species are of the same Virtues. It is to be observed, that there are a Multitude of Species of *Satyrion*, or *Orchis*, which may indeed, be used promiscuously; yet our Shops have thought fit to make Choice of the last mention'd, or Female *Satyrion*, before the rest.

Satyrium vel Orchis, Offic. *Orchis prateumatica*, Ger. Emac. The *French* Satyrion. It grows in hilly Places, flowering in *June*. The Root is used, which agrees in Virtues with the two former; as does likewise the Roots of all the following Species, as,

Satyrium, Rivin. Irr. Hex. *Orchis Hermaphroditica*, Ger. Emac. Butterfly, or *German* Satyrion. It grows in Woods, flowering in *May*.

Orchis major latifolia altera, Park. Theat. *Cynosorchis*, Offic. Dog-Stones. It grows in grassy Places, about *Brasil*.

Orchis barbata fœtida, J. B. *Tragorchis*, Offic. Goats-Stones. This is produc'd in fat Soils, flowering in *May* and *June*.

Orchis spiralis alba odorata, J. B. *Triorchis*, Offic. Triple Ladies Traces. It grows in dry Pastures, flowering in *Autumn*.

Satyrium Regium palmata, Chab. *Orchis palmata*, Offic. *Palma Christi mas*, Ger. Emac. Male Satyrion Royal. It grows in moist and marshy Soils, flowering in *May*.

The *Salop* is also the Root of another Species of *Orchis*, or *Satyrion*; which grows on the Mountains of *Bursia*, near *Constantinople*. See *Setapias*.

Saxifraga alba, Offic. *Saxifraga rotundifolia alba*, C. B. P. White Saxifrage. It grows in sandy Places, flowering in *April*. It is drying, heating, diuretic, and opening, and is principally used to expel Gravel, and the Stone of the Kidneys, and Bladder. It is said to be good in Obstructions of the *Menses*. *Fuchsius* affirms, that it attenuates the dense gross Lymph, which hinders the ordinary Motion of the Lungs.

Another Species of *Saxifraga*, is the *Umbilicus Veneris alter*, Offic. *Saxifraga sedi folio angustiore serrato*, Tourn. Inst. Small Navel-wort. It grows on the Mountains of *Germany*, flowering in the Summer. The Herb is used, which agrees in Virtues with the *Semper vivum*.

Saxifraga antiquorum, Offic. *Saxifraga major Italorum Matthioli*, Park. Theat. *Caryophyllus Saxifragus*, C. B. P. The great Saxifrage of *Matthiolus*. It grows on the Top of Mount *Lupo*, flowering in *June*. The whole Plant is admirably endued, as *Matthiolus* says, with the Virtue of breaking and expelling the Stone.

Saxifraga Dioscoridis, Matth. *Saxifraga vera Dioscoridis*, C. B. Matth. The true Saxifrage of *Dioscorides*, according to *Matthiolus*. It grows on Rocks and stony Places. The Herb is used, which boiled in Wine, is good in feverish Disorders; it is also serviceable in the Strangury;

cures

cures the Hiccup, breaks the Stone in the Bladder, and provokes Urine.

Scabiofa, Offic. *Scabiofa pratenfis birfuta quæ Officinarum*, C. B. P. Scabious. It grows in Paftures, flowering in *June*. The Leaves are ufed. It is alexipharmic and pectoral; and is principally ufed in Apoftems, for the Pleurify, Quinfey, Coughs, Afthma, the Plague, and fiftulous Ulcers. It is externally ufed for cutaneous Eruptions, as the Itch, and Leprofy. Scabious is bitter, and gives a faint Tincture of red to the blue Paper, which gives us Reafon to believe, that it contains a Salt refembling Sal Ammoniac, and joined with a great Quantity of fetid Oil, and Earth; for, by the Chymical Analyfis, befide feveral acid Liquors, a great deal of Sulphur and Earth, and a little urinous Spirit, and volatile concrete Salt, are obtained from it. Scabious is good to promote Expectoration, when the *Bronchia* and Veficles of the Lungs, are ftuffed with a glutinous, and condenfed Phlegm. This is a good Remedy in malignant Fevers, Small-Pox, and Meafles, after the Ufe of Antimonial Medicines. *Tabernæmontanus* fays, that the Juice of Scabious mix'd with a little Borax and Camphire, takes away the white Spots, that are often feen upon the *Cornea* of the Eye.

Scammonium, Offic. *Scammonia Syriaca*, C. B. P. *Convolvulus Syriacus, & Scammonia Syriaca*, Tourn. Inft. Scammony. The Plant affording Scammony bears green Leaves, almoft in the Shape of an Heart, or nearly approaching to thofe of Ivy; its Flowers are white, and of a Bell Figure; which has occafion'd fome Authors to rank it among the *Convolvuli*: It creeps upon the Ground, and only rifes by the Support of a neighbouring Tree or Wall. 'Tis from the Root of this Plant, which grows plentifully in many Parts of the *Levant*, particularly about *Aleppo* that the Drug Scammony is extracted. The genuine comes from *Aleppo*; 'tis light, of a grey Colour, brittle, refinous, and grinds to a grey Powder, of a bitter Tafte, and of a weak, but difagreeable Scent. That which is heavy, hard, and black, is to be rejected; and with fuch they often fill the Infide of the Cods, or Lumps, wherein it is brought to us; this ufually being what is burnt, or otherwife damaged in the Operation; for the Juice of the Scammony-Plant is not thicken'd by the Heat of the Sun, as has long been imagin'd; but by means of culinary Fire. This concreted Juice is reckon'd one of the fureft Purgatives tho', at the fame time, one of the ftrongeft; and is therefore never given without a Corrector. Befides the *Aleppo* Scammony, there are two other Sorts commonly fold, that of *Smyrna* and the *Indian*. The *Smyrna* Scammony is black, heavy, foft, and ftony, or full of Shells, and other heterogeneous Matters. But the *Indian* is grey, light, and brittle, tho' no other at Bottom, than a Compofition of fome very ftrong purgative Powders made up with Rofin; according to the manner of fome unfair Dealers in Drugs among us in *England*. But thefe two Sorts, are rather poifonous than medicinal, as M. *Pomet* has proved by Certificate, in his general Hiftory of Drugs. The *Aleppo* Sort is a very ftrong Cathartic, and caufes great Irritation, and even Inflammations in weak Habits. It is given, in Subftance, from two to twelve Grains; but ought never to be ufed, when there is the leaft Sufpicion of Inflammations, in any Part of the *Abdomen*. It is likewife a very ticklifh, uncertain Purge; fometimes it has no Effect at all; fometimes it caufes fatal Super-purgations; and, which is moft remarkable, it fometimes does not operate at all the firft

Day.

Day, but brings on an infupportable *Tenefmus*, and *Hypercatharfis* the next. It is very proper to dilute it with fome oily, vifcid Subftance; fuch as the Yolk of an Egg, or an Emulfion, made with fweet Almonds, and the cold Seeds. Prepared *Scammony*, or *Diagridium*, is a very proper Ingredient in the *Pulvis Cornachini*, which purges, without any of the bad Effects of Scammony.

Scandix, Offic. *Scandix femine roftrato vulgaris*, C. B. P. *Pecten Veneris*, J. B. Shepherd's Needle, or *Venus's* Comb. It grows frequently among Corn, flowering in *May* and *June*, The Herb is ufed. The Decoction drank, is good for the Bladder, Kidneys, and Liver. Some affirm, that the Root, bruifed with Mallows, draws out all manner of Splinters, or other Things infixed in the Body.

Scariola. A Name for the *Cichorium latifolium*, or Endive.

Schœnanthus. Camel's Hay. See *Juncus odoratus*.

Schœnopraffum, Offic. *Porrum fectivum juncifolium*, C. B. P. *Cepa fectilis juncifolia perennis*, Tourn. Inft. Cives, or Chives. It grows in Gardens, and the Leaves are ufed; which agree in Virtues with the Onion.

Scilla, Offic. *Scilla vulgaris radice rubra*, C. B. P. *Ornithogalum maritimum*, *feu Scilla radice rubrâ*, Tourn. Inft. *Cepa maris & Squilla*, Offic. Germ. Squill, or Sea Onion. It flowers in *September*, and the Root is ufed; which is of a bitter and acrid Tafte; and is attenuating, opening, difcutient, and diuretic; and is principally ufed in Obftructions of the Liver, Spleen, and biliary Ducts, for a Suppreffion of the *Menfes* and Urine, and for mucilaginous Infarctions of the Lungs, a Dropfy, and a Cough.

Sclarea, *Horminum*, Offic. *Horminum Sclarea dictum*, C. B. P. *Gallitrichum fativum*, J. B. Clary. It grows in Gardens, flowering in *June* and *July*. The Leaves are ufed. It is heating and drying, abfterges and attenuates. If the Juice is drank, it caufes Ebriety. The Plant is antihyfteric, and ufeful in difficult Labours, Obftructions of the *Menfes*, and a *Fluor Albus*, and is thought to ftimulate in a very great Degree to Venery.

Another Species of *Sclarea*, is the *Æthiopis*, or *Æthiopian* Clary.

Scolymus. The Artichoke. See *Cinara*.

Scolymus Theophrafti, Park. Theat. *Scolymus chryfanthemus*, Tourn. Inft. *Carduus chryfanthemus narbonenfis*, Ger. Emac. *Spina lutea*, J. B. Golden Thiftle. It grows in *Italy*, and the Root is ufed, which agrees in Virtues with the *Eryngium*.

Scordium, Offic. C. B. P. *Chamædrys paluftris canefcens, feu Scordium Officinarum*, Tourn. Inft. Water Germander. It grows in marfhy Places, flowering in *June*. The Herb is ufed. It is alexipharmic, and fudorific, and is principally ufed in the Plague, and peftilential Diforders. It is recommended for malignant Fevers, for Obftructions of the Liver and Spleen, for purulent and mucilaginous Infarctions of the Lungs, and for deftroying Worms. Externally ufed, it is good to mundify Wounds and Ulcers, and to mitigate Pains of the Gout. *Scordium* is bitter, aromatic, and gives a faint red to the blue Paper: It contains an oily, volatile Salt, the *Sal Ammoniac* of which it is not entirely difengaged, but wrapped up in a great deal of Sulphur. Fomentations of this Herb, are applied as a Cataplafm, on Parts which are threaten'd with a Gangrene. Among the Antients, it was an Ingredient in all Medicines, againft the Poifons of mad Animals. A Conferve is prepared of this Plant, which is fudorific, and good for the *Afthma*, and Shortnefs of Breath, and for Virgins labouring

bouring under a *Chlorosis*, and Obstruction of the *Menses*; the Leaves infused in Wine, are serviceable in Dropsies.

Scorodonia, Salvia sylvestris, Offic. *Scorodonia sive Scordium alterum quibusdam, & Salvia agrestis,* Park. Theat. *Scordium alterum sive Salvia agrestis,* C. B. P. Wood Sage. It grows in Woods and Thickets flowering in *June.* The Herb is used, principally as a Vulnerary, and to provoke Urine and the *Menses,* and is believ'd by some, to cure the *Lues Venerea.* The bruised Leaves, with Vinegar, Litharge, and Salt, cure a Gangrene and Cancer Its Leaves are very bitter and aromatic; they have a little Taste of Garlic, and give hardly any Tincture of red to the blue Paper, which gives us Reason to believe, they contain a Salt, like that of *Germander*; but loaded with more essential Oil, and in which the *Sal Ammoniac* discovers itself but little. *Tragus* commends its Juice, for the Jaundice, and a Tertian Ague. A Glass full of the Infusion of this Plant in Wine, is very successfully used at *Paris,* for the Dropsy.

Scorodoprassum. Wild Leeks. See *Allium.*

Scorpius. Furz, or Gors. See *Genista.*

Scorzonera nostra & Hispanica, Viperaria, Offic. *Scorzonera latifolia sinuata,* C. B. P. *Tragopogon Hispanicus sive Escorzonera, aut Scorzonera,* J. B. Vipers Grass. It is cultivated in Gardens, flowering in *June.* The Root is used. This Plant is said to take its Name from its Effect on the Viper, which if but touched with the Juice of this Plant, immediately droops and sickens; and it is said, that a Person may take a Viper in his bare Hand, without receiving any Harm, if he first rubs his Hand with this Herb; for the Viper will not be able to bite, but faints and sickens. The Juice is very serviceable in inflammatory Diseases; three Ounces thereof, being taken in the Morning, fasting, are recommended against all volatile Poisons; and the Herb applied, cures envenom'd Wounds. It is a proper Herb in all Diseases, proceeding from too great a Mobility of the Humours, and which require Agglutinants and Demulcents; also, in all Disorders, arising from a putrid Blood; such as the Small Pox, Measles, Pestilence, burning Fevers, Peripneumony, and Pleurisy. The Root is an excellent Cleanser, and Corrective; for which Reasons, it is of extraordinary Use in hypochondriac Disorders, being boiled in Barley-Water. It is of good Service in Melancholy, and Pains of the Gout, and some use it with Success, in an immoderate Flux of the *Menses.* There is no Plant more commended than this, in a *Phthisis,* Extenuations, and the Jaundice.

Scorzonera subcærulea, Offic. *Scorzonera angustifolia subcærulea,* C. B. P. *Viperina angustifolia, elatior,* Ger. Emac. *Hungarian* Vipers Grass. It grows in hilly Places, and the Root is used, which agrees in Virtues with the former, and may supply its Room.

Scrophularia, Offic. *Scrophularia nodosa fœtida,* C. B. P. Fig-Wort. It grows in Hedges, flowering in *July.* The Root and the Herb are used. Its Leaves are very bitter, and stinking, even more than those of Elder, and give but a very faint Tincture of red to the blue Paper; the Root gives it a deeper, which makes us conjecture, that the *Sal Ammoniac,* which is naturally in the Salt of the Earth, predominates in this Plant, where it is united with a great deal of fetid Oil. By the Chymical Analysis, we obtain from this Plant, a great deal of volatile, concreted Salt and Oil. The *Scrophularia* is of an acrid and aperient Quality, accompanied

panied with a copious *Mucus*; whence it is an effectual Lenitive, in all Pains proceeding from a peccant Acrimony, mitigating the same, as well as diffipating any grofs Matter. A Cataplafm thereof is of univerfal Efteem, for difcuffing, refolving, and maturating, though the Humour be of confiderable Hardnefs. The Powder, fprinkled on watry Ulcers, clofes, and conglutinates them; and is proper in a Dilatation of the Hæmorrhoids. The diftill'd Water of this Plant, is good for Pimples and Rednefs of the Face. An Ointment is prepared of this Plant, which is excellent for the Gout, Piles, and Tetters.

Scrophularia aquatica major, C. B. P. *Betonica aquatica*, Offic. *Scrophularia maxima radice fibrofa*, J. B. Water Betony. It grows in watry Places, flowering in *June*. The Herb is ufed, which agrees in Virtues with the former. It is of great Service in correcting *Senna*.

Scutellaria, Offic. *Scutellaria paluftris repens cærulea*, Hift. Oxon. *Caffida paluftris vulgatior flore cæruleo*, Tourn. Inft. *Tertianaria aliis Lyfimachia galericulata*, J. B. Hooded Willow Herb. It grows in Marfhes, flowering in *July* or *Auguft*. The Herb is ufed. It takes its Name, *Tertianaria*, from its curing Intermitting Fevers. A Decoction of it is recommended by fome, for the Quinfey.

Sebeften, Offic. *Sebeftina domeftica*, C. B. P. *Myxa domeftica*, J. B. *Prunus Malabarica fructu racemofo, calyce excepto*, Raii Hift. The Sebeften. This Plant is produced in *Egypt* and *Afia*, and flowers in the *Spring*. Its Fruit, which is the Part ufed, is ripe in the *Autumn*, refembles a common Prune, is of a blackifh Colour, and under a carnous, fweet, and honeyifh Pulp, includes a Kernel. *Sebeftens* are in an intermediate Degree

between hot and cold: They moiften, foften, and obtund the Acrimony of the Humours. They are principally us'd in acrid Catarrhs, and Acrimony of Urine, bilious Fevers, and Obftructions of the Belly. In a Word, as in Figure, fo in Virtues, they refemble Damfons.

Secale, Offic. *Secale hybernum vel majus*, C. B. P. Rie. It is fown in Fields. The Seeds of Rie yield a Meal, with a proper Bran belonging to it, of which Bread is made, which is of excellent Service in Cataplafms, for difcuffing Tumors and Pains. The Cruft of it toafted, cleanfes the Teeth. The Bread is lefs nourifhing, and not fo foon digefted as that of Wheat; but it is very loofening, and good for thofe who are coftive. The bran is deterfive and emollient, and of Service in a Diarrhæa, and an inveterate Cough.

Securiduca, Offic. *Securidaca lutea major*, C. B. P. *Hedyfarum majus*, Ger. Emac. Hatchet Vetch. It grows among Corn, in hot Countries, but is cultivated with us in Gardens; and taken inwardly, is good for the Stomach, and is an Ingredient in Antidotes.

Sedum majus, Sempervivum majus, Offic. *Sedum majus vulgare*, C. B. P. Houfe-Leek. It grows upon old Houfes, flowering in *June*. The Herb is ufed, which is refrigerating, and ftrongly aftringent, and is principally ufed in bilious Fevers, to allay Thirft and Heat. This Plant being analyfed, yields a good deal of Acid and Earth, and a very little concrete, volatile Salt. It probably contains a Salt refembling Alum, mixed with a little *Sal Ammoniac*; for the Juice of this Plant, evaporated to one half, emits an urinous Smell. The diftill'd Water of Houfe-Leek, is good for the Quinfey. The Juice is ufed in Injections in the *Procidentia Uteri*, and finuous Ulcers.

The

The Leaves are applied to Corns, and the Knots of the Gout. A Pint of the Juice of this Plant is an excellent Remedy for founder'd Horses. The Leaves stripped of their outer Membrane, and macerated in Water, are commended in burning Fevers, Inflammations, Gangrenes, and Suppurations of the Stomach, and Intestines, and for *Aphthæ*. The *Africans* give ten Ounces of the new expressed Juice in a Dysentery; and with the same, cure not only this Disease, but all pestilential, and spotted Fevers. It is also, a very good Plant, for correcting the Malignity of the worst Kind of Ulcers.

Sedum minus, Offic. *Sedum minus teretifolium album,* C. B. P. *Vermicularis flore albo,* Park. Theat. Small House-leek. It grows upon Walls and old Buildings, flowering in *June.* The Herb is used, which agrees in Virtues with the preceding.

Another Species of *Sedum,* is the *Illecebra,* Offic. *Sempervivum minus vermiculatum acre,* C. B. P. *Sedum parvum acre flore luteo,* J. B. Wall Pepper. It grows on Walls and old Buildings, flowering in *July.* The Herb is used. It discusses Struma's, and is a very acrid and hot Plant. The Juice, taken with some proper Liquor, excites Vomiting, and powerfully brings away pituitous and bilious Humours; whence it is of great Use in Quartans. It is also esteem'd a good Antiscorbutic. Externally applied, it makes the Skin red, excites Blisters, and exulcerates.

Sedum Cepæa dictum, Tourn. Inst. *Cepæa,* Offic. C. B. P. Base Orpine. It is sown in Gardens, flowering in the Summer. The Herb is used. The Leaves, exhibited in Wine, cure the Strangury, and the *Scabies* of the Bladder.

Selinum segetale, Offic. *Selinum Sii foliis,* Ger. Emac. *Sium arvense, sive segetale,* Tourn. Inst. Hone-Wort. It grows among Corn, flow-

ering in the Summer. The Herb is used, which is greatly recommended for Tumors.

Sempervivum. See *Sedum.*

Semen. A Seed. The four greater hot Seeds, are those of *Anise, Caraway, Cumin,* and *Fennel.*

The four smaller hot Seeds, are those of *Bishops-Weed, Amomum, Apium,* and *Daucus.*

The four greater cold Seeds, are those of the *Citrul, Cucumber, Gourd,* and *Melon.*

The four lesser cold Seeds, are *Succory, Endive, Lettuce,* and *Purslane.* For the Virtues of all these Seeds, see them under their respective Articles.

Senecio. Groundsel, or Simson. See *Erigerum.*

Senecio Asiaticus, Jacobææ folio, radice lignosa, China Officinarum dicta nobis, Boerh. Ind. Alt. *Pseudo China, China supposita,* Offic. *Parin Chakka,* Act. Philosoph. Lond. Bastard China. It grows in *Malabar.* This is the Plant, which some Years ago, was sent to the *English Bast-India* Company at *London,* under the Name of *Parin Chakka Malabarica,* by *Samuel Brown.* Mr. *Ingram* of *Newcastle,* was cured by it of a Hectic Fever, under which he had laboured many Years, as we are inform'd by Dr. *Dillenius,* in his *Hortus Elthamensis,* and who also says, that it is called *China* Root in *Madrasspatan,* and that it is two Feet in Heighth, and has a Root like that of *China.* Some Specimens of this Plant were presented by the Company, to the Royal Society at *London,* and publish'd in the Philosophical Transactions, for the Year 1702, No. 274, with Observations. A few Years after, the famous G. *Commelin,* M. D. was presented with the same Plant, and published a Description of it, in *Hort. Medic. Amstelod.* under the Name of *Senecio Asiaticus, Jacobææ folio, radice lignosa, China Offic. dicta,* " the
" Se-

' *Senecio* of *Afia*, with a Leaf like
' that of the *Jacobæa*, and a woody
' Root, called the *China* of the
' Shops," with the following Note;
' I had the Knowledge of this Plant,
' from that skilful Surgeon *Andreas*
' *Hammel*, who brought it with him
' from the *East-Indies*, into his own
' Country." This gave Occasion to
he Authors of the *Catalogus Simpli-
um*, in the *Pharmacop. Londin.* and
he *Indices Medicamentorum* in the
Pharmacop. Paris. to commit a Mi-
take, in improperly setting down
his *China of the Shops* for the Root
of the *Plant*. *Boerhaave*, in his
Historia Plantarum, informs us, that
he famous Botanist *Switfen*, sent
him a Figure, with a Description of
he *Japonese China*; but this is quite
another Plant from what we are speak-
ng of. Its Root indeed, is very
thick, as in the other; but then it
s also tuberous, which is otherwise
n the *Senecio*, and is a scandent Plant,
like the *Clematitis* of *Canada*, or
Ivy, or Briony, which last it most
resembles; and he imagines, that
our *Senecio* is not so penetrating, as
to cure the Leprosy; for it is better
qualified for an Emollient, than an
Expeller.' But the *Japonese* is far
more acrimonious; so as perhaps to
be sufficient for the Cure of the *Lues
Venerea*, as it is said of the Root of
China; tho'I never as yet, says he, saw
any such Effect performed by it.
This Root is very dear, and for that
Reason, very often adulterated; for
when it is corroded, and exhausted
with Age, they fill up the Perforations, and sell it for good and sound;
and therefore he never prescribed it
before Examination; for there is no
trusting to it unseen.

Senna Alexandrina, Offic. *Senna
Alexandrina sive foliis acutis*; C. B.
P. *Sena Orientalis*, J. B. Alex-
andrian Sena. It is cultivated in
Syria, *Persia*, *Arabia*, and *Egypt*.
The Leaf of this *Sena* is of a pretty
strong Consistence, and shaped like
the Point of a Spear. This is the
best Sort of *Sena*. It purges Phlegm
in a particular Manner; but as it is
subject to gripe, it ought to be given
with Caution, to those who have weak
Viscera, or are of an imflammatory
Habit of Body. It is usually mixed
with Carminatives, such as Coriander
Seeds, Cinnamon, &c. or more effectually with Alcaline Salts. It ought
to be well cleansed from its Stalks,
and then the Dose in Substance, is
from a Scruple to a Dram; and in
Infusion, from two Drams to half an
Ounce. Some have endeavour'd to
correct *Senna* with the *Scrophularia
aquatica major*; but that is now left
off; common Tea having the same
Effect. Some Physicians order *Sena*,
by the Name of *Folia Orientalia*.
The Follicules, or Fruit of the *Sena*
Tree, purge in a less Degree than
the Leaves. The common Dose is
from three to six Drams in Infusion,
or Decoction

Senna Italica, Park. Theat. *Senna
Italica, foliis obtusis*, C. B. P. *Sena
Florentina*, J. B. Italian Sena. This
is distinguish'd from the former, by
the Largeness and Roundness of its
Leaves. This Leaf is also much
thinner, and more brittle than the
other. It is a very weak Cathartic,
but it gripes violently, and therefore
is seldom used.

Serapias, Offic. *Serapias sive Salep*,
Marl. Obs. *Orchis fæmina procerior
majore flore*. Tourn. Herbar. Salep.
This is the Root of a Kind of *Orchis*
or *Satyrion*, which grows on the
Mountains of *Bursia*, near *Constantinople*. The *Turks* pretend, that it
is very effectual in restoring decay'd
Strength, and exciting to Venery. It
is also, said to prevent Abortion, and
is used both in Substance, and in Infusion. The Taste of the Root resembles that of Gum Tragacanth,
but has no Smell. The *Turks* and
Persians prepare a Drink of this

Root, mix'd with Milk and Ginger, which they also call *Salop*, which they drink hot, and esteem an excellent Remedy against Venereal Disorders. *Salop*, either in the Root, or in Powder, is commonly sold at the Druggists; the Way of using it is, to dissolve a Tea-spoonful of it in cold Water, by stirring it; and then to heat it, or let it just boil; and half a Pint of this Liquor, or more, makes an excellent Restorative Liquor, taken as a Breakfast, or otherwise, with Sugar, and with or without the Juice of Lemon.

Serpentaria Virginiana, Offic. *Serpentaria Virginiana Contrayerva Virginiana, Viperina,* Mont. Exot. Med. *Radix Snagrol nothæ Creticus,* (Snake Root, *Novæ Angliæ*) Corn. 214. Virginian Snake Weed. It grows in *Virginia,* the Roots are used, which are alexipharmic. They cure the Bite of a mad Dog, and defend them from the *Hydrophobia,* and are a certain, and immediate Remedy for the venomous Bite of the Rattle-Snake. It is given as a Diaphoretic in the Small Pox, Measles, and to kill Worms. It is, also emmenagogue and diuretic. The Dose is from ten Grains to a Dram.

There is another Species of the Snake Root, called the *Senekka-Rattle-Snake Root,* which is said to cure effectually the Bite of a Rattle-Snake, if taken immediately after it. The Bite of this Snake is sudden Death, for the most part; that is, Death follows often in fifteen Minutes, sometimes sooner; and at other Times the Patient may live some Days. The Reasons of these Differences, in the Time of Death, are various, such as the Season of the Year, Constitution of the Patient, and Part bit. Those that travel or hunt in the Woods, carry this Root powder'd, in their Shot Bags, to chew and swallow as soon as they are bit by the Snake, the Stagnation of the Blood being prevented by its peculiar Activity. A Nation of the Northern *Indians,* called *Senekkas,* were the Discoverers of the Efficacy of the Root of this Plant; they observing, that the Root and Flowers resembled the Rattle of the Snake, concluded that Providence had impressed that Characteristic, to point out its Use. From that *Indian* Nation, this Root is named *Senekka Rattle Snake Root,* to distinguish it from the others called *Rattle. Snake Root;* which are much inferior in Efficacy. These *Indians* returning from a War with a Southern Nation, called *Catawbaes,* in the Year 1712, communicated the Efficacy of this Root to *William Caniko,* a Planter, in the Frontiers of *Virginia,* which he imparted to the Country about him; and so it was soon known throughout *America.* The Root of this *Senekka Rattle Snake Weed* has since been us'd, as is said, with Success, in the Epidemical Fevers of *Virginia;* in Pleurisies, Peripneumonies, Gout, and Rheumatisms, either in Decoction, Infusion, or Substance; and in these it should seem to be a good Medicine, if the Accounts we have of it could be depended on.

Serpentaria nigra. Black Snakeweed. A Name for the *Asarum Virginianum.*

Serpyllum, Offic. *Serpyllum vulgare minus,* C. B. P. *Serpyllus vel Serpyllum.* Mother of Thyme. It grows in dry Pastures, flowering in *June* and *July.* The Herb is used, which agrees in Virtues with the *Thymus,* or Thyme. It provokes Urine, and the Menses. It is a little bitter, acrid, styptic, odoriferous, and stains the blue Paper, with a pretty deep Red. It is likely that it abounds with an aromatic, and oily volatile Salt; but this Salt retains still a Part of the Acid of the *Sal Ammoniac* of the Earth; whereas in the aromatic, oily, artificial, volatile Salt, the acid Part of the *Sal Ammoniac* has been stopt by the Salt lt of Tartar, or by the Afhes. Thus the Mother of Thyme is Cephalic, Stomachic, and good for the Vapours. It deſtroys the exploſive Matter, which cauſes convulſive Moſions; it reſtores the ſpirituous Parts of the Blood, and re-eſtabliſhes the Functions of the *Primæ Viæ.* The Spirit of Mother of Thyme, and a diſtilled Water, are very good for ſoporific Diſorders, and the Vapours. The eſſential Oil is commended for the Epilepſy. The Conſerve of the Flowers and the Leaves of this Plant, relieve thoſe that are troubled with the Falling Sickneſs.

Serpyllum citratum, Offic. *Serpyllum foliis Citri odore,* C. B. P. *Serpyllum Citri odore,* J. B. Lemon Thyme. It grows in hilly Places, flowering in *Auguſt.* The Herb is uſed, which agrees in Virtues with the former.

Serpyllum verum, Offic. *Serpyllum vulgare majus,* C. B. P. Great Mother of Thyme. It is cultivated in Gardens, flowering in the Summer. The Herb is uſed, which provokes the *Menſes* and Urine, and is good for the Gripes, Ruptures, Laceratiſons, and Inflammations of the Liver; eaſes Pains of the Head, and is particularly ſerviceable in Phrenſies and Lethargies; ſtops Vomitings of Blood, and is good for the Bites of Serpents.

Serratula, Offic. C. B. P. *Serratula purpurea,* Ger. Emac. *Jacea Nemorenſis,quæSerratulavulgo,*Tourn. Inſt. Saw-Wort. It grows in Woods and Meadows, flowering in *July;* it is eſteemed vulnerary, and is ſaid to mundify Ulcers, and promote the Generation of Fleſh therein; to mitigate the Pains of the *Hæmorrhoids,* and to cure an inteſtinal Rupture. The Herb and Root are recommended in Caſe of Bruiſes in Falls from Eminences.

Seſamoides parvum, Offic. *Chondrilla Seſamoides dicta,* Park. Cata-

nance quorundam, Tourn. Inſt. Baſtard Succory. It grows in dry Places in hot Countries, flowering in *June.* The Herb is uſed; it purges Bile and Phlegm by Stool; apply'd by Way of Cataplaſm, with Water it diſcuſſes Tubercles, and œdematous Swellings.

Seſamum, Offic. *Digitalis orientalis Seſam dicta,* Tourn. Inſt. *Seſamum congentibus Gangya, Luſitanis Girgilim,* Marcg. *Gangila ſive Seſamum Africanum,* Piſon.. *Schit-Elu,* Hort. mal. *Tala,* Herm. Muſ. Zeyl. Oily purging Grain. The Seeds are uſed, which are heating, moderately moiſtening, emollient, and paregoric, and are of a viſcous, pinguious, and conſequently of an emplaſtic Quality; they diſcuſs a Hardneſs of the Nerves, being rubbed therewith, and cure the Pain of the Colic.

Seſeli Æthiopicum, Offic. *Seſeli Æthiopicum Salicis folio,* C. B. P. *Bupleurum arboreſcens Salicis folio,* Tourn. Inſt Shrub Hartwort. This is found in the Gardens of the Curious, flowering in *Auguſt.* The Seed is much more acrimonious and ſcented than that of the *Seſeli Maſſilienſe,* whence it is ſuppoſed to have ſome extraordinary Virtues.

Seſeli Creticum, Offic. *Seſeli Creticum minus,* C. B. P. *Tordylium Narbonenſe minus,* Tourn. Inſt. *Caucalis minor pulchro ſemine ſive Bellonii,* J. B. Hartwort of Candy. It is cultivated in Botanic Gardens, and the Seed is uſed, which is nephritic, uterine, and pulmonic. Its principal Uſes are in the Strangury, and Stoppage of Urine; it removes Pain, provokes the *Menſes,* and promotes Expectoration in Catarrhs.

Seſeli Maſſilienſe, Offic. *Seſeli Maſſilienſe Ferulæ folio,* C. B. P. *Libanotis Maſſilienſis Ferulæ folio,* Hiſt. Oxon. Italian Hartwort. The Part uſed is the Seed, which is of principal Service in Diſeaſes of the Head, the Epilepſy, Weakneſs of Sight,

Sight, Convulsions, and the like, and in Affections of the Breast and Lungs, Coughs, Catarrhs; also in Obstructions of the Liver, Dropsy, Crudities of the Stomach, in the Stone of the Kidneys and Bladder, and in a Stoppage of the *Menses.* It is a specific Remedy against the *Cicuta.*

Seseli Peloponnense. Great broadleav'd Hemlock. A Name for the *Cicuta latifolia.*

Seseli vulgaris & Siler montanum, Offic. *Seseli five Siler montanum vulgare,* J. B. *Ligusticum quod Seseli Officinarum,* C. B. P. Common Hartwort. It is cultivated in Botanic Gardens, flowering in *June.* It is heating and drying, provokes Urine and the *Menses,* and discusses Flatulencies.

Sideritis, Offic. *Sideritis hirsuta procumbens,* C. B. P. *Sideritis Judaica Lobelii,* Ger. Emac. Iron-wort. It grows in stony Places in *Italy,* flowering in the Summer. The Herb is used. An Application of the Leaves cures Wounds, without any Danger of Inflammation.

Sideritis, Offic. *Sideritis vulgaris hirsuta erecta,* C. B. P. Common Iron-wort. It grows common in *Germany, Italy,* and *France,* flowering in *June.* The Herb is used, which is said to be good for Wounds and Ruptures, and to be so drying as to cure a *Fluor albus.* This Species is esteemed by some only as a Variety of the former.

Sideritis Monspesulana, J. B. German Iron-wort. It grows in Meadows, flowering in *June* and *July.* The Herb is greatly used in the *German* Shops, and is said to agree in Virtues with the former.

Sideritis glabra arvensis, J. B. Iron-wort with smooth Leaves. It grows among Corn; the Herb is used, which agrees in Virtues with the other Species.

Sigillum Solomonis, Solomon's Seal. See *Polygonatum.*

Siler montanum, Common Hartwort. See *Seseli vulgaris.*

Siliqua dulcis, Caroba, Carantia, Offic. *Siliqua edulis,* C. B. P. *Ceratia, Siliqua five Ceratonia,* the Carob Tree. It grows in *Sicily,* and the Kingdom of *Naples;* the Fruit is used, which is drying and astringent, and is principally used in hot Disorders of the Stomach, and in Coughs.

Siliqua sylvestris, C. B. P. *Acacalis,* Offic. The wild Carob. It grows at *Constantinople;* the Seeds are used, which are greatly recommended at *Constantinople* for Disorders of the Eyes.

Siliquastrum, Tourn. Inst. *Arbor Judæ,* Ger. Emac. *Judaica Arbor,* J. B. *Siliqua sylvestris rotundifolia,* C. B. P. Judas's Tree. It is cultivated in Gardens, flowering in the Summer; the Pod of this Plant is esteem'd astringent.

Sima Ruba, Geoff. Tract. *Radix Simarouba,* Offic. This is the Root of a *West India* Plant, which produces the *Cayan* Wood, remarkable for being very light: the Root and Bark are said to be excellent Astringents, proper in all Sorts of Loosenesses, and especially in Dysenteries. The Dose of the Root is an Ounce, cut in small Pieces; and of the Bark two Ounces, boil'd in three Pints of Water to a Pint. This Decoction the Patient uses for his common Drink till he is cured.

Sinapi, Offic. *Sinapi rapi folio,* C. B. P. *Eruca rapi folia,* Rup. Flor. Gen. Common Mustard. It grows in Gardens, and in Ditches; the Seed is used; it heats and dries, incides, attenuates, and attracts. Its principal Uses are to excite an Appetite, promote Chylification, and purge the Head. Outwardly it is used to stimulate, being put in the Nostrils, or applied to other Parts. It breaks mature Tumors, and excites Sneezing. Mustard Seed,

by

y the Chymical Analyfis, gives a much greater Indication of an acrid than an acid Salt; but it affords a considerable Quantity of Oil, very little fixed Salt fimply faline, a great deal of Earth, a little urinous pirit, and no volatile Salt. As to the internal Ufe of Muftard, it is proper where an inert, aqueous, or phlegmatic Humour is predominant. A Girl at *Amfterdam* labouring under Convulfions, after fhe had tried all Manner of Medicines in vain, was at laft, by the Advice of Mr. *Nyfch*, cured by the Ufe of crude fuftard bruifed with Wine. The feeds are alfo of Service, whether internally or externally ufed, in hyochondriac Diforders, Inflations of the Stomach, Obftructions of the Spleen, and other Difeafes proceeding from an Acid, of which Nature are the curvy, Cachexy, Chlorofis, and fopous Affections; they alfo ftimulate to Venery, and provoke Urine. The expreffed Oil is externally applied in the Palfy and cold Difeafes; the Seeds are alfo applied in a quartan, and fometimes in a quotidian Fever. Some make a Cataplafm with Turpentine, Pidgeon's Dung and Muftard, and apply it to the Parts affected with the Gout, and even to the Jaw in a violent Tooth-ach. Muftard and other acrid Vegetables, prove excellent Medicines, when prudently given in Diftempers attended with an indolent, watery, or cold phlegmatic Habit, no way faline, where acid Humours are lodged in the firft Paffages; where the Bile is fluggifh, and where no alcaline, feid or oily Matter is lodged; but the Body remains cold, torpid, and fwelled all over; as, on the other Hand, they prove hurtful, where the Body is hot and feverifh, the Bile fharp, the Juices putrid, the Parts inflamed or wafted, or where the putrid Scurvy abounds. Oil of Muftard by Expreffion, is prefcribed

with Succefs in the fevereft Fits of the Stone; but this Oil by Expreffion, is more mild, and by no means like Oil of Muftard Seed which is procured by Diftillation, and is extremely acrid and igneous.

Sinapi album, Offic. *Sinapi Apii folio*, C. B. P. White Muftard. It grows in Fields and by the Sides of Ditches. The Seeds are ufed, which agree in Virtues with the former.

Sifarum, Ger. Emac. *Sifer*, Offic. *Sifer*, *Sifar*, *Sifarum*, Chab. *Sifarum Germanorum*, C. B. P. Skirret. It is cultivated in Gardens, flowering in *June*; the Root is ufed, which is rather of culinary than officinal Ufe, and is of a bitterifh and fomewhat aftringent Tafte. It is good for the Stomach, excites an Appetite, is diuretic and lithontriptic, affords good Nourifhment, is eafy of Digeftion, and efteem'd a fpecific Antidote againft Quikfilver. It is very proper for thofe who fpit Blood, or make bloody Urine, if they confine themfelves to eat no other Food but this; boiled in Milk, Whey, or Flefh Broth; for by fuch Means they would procure a due Laxnefs of the Belly, and a Removal of the Diforder. It is recommended alfo for the Strangury and *Tenefmus*; and is efteem'd a very good Remedy againft a Dyfentery, and Fluxes of the Belly. The Root boil'd as aforefaid, then bruis'd and taken in the Morning before the Patient rifes, is very good in a *Phthifis*, or great Extenuation of the Body; as it is alfo in all pectoral Diforders.

Sifarum Germanicum, C. B. P. *Secacul*, Offic. *Paftinaca Syriaca & Secacul Arabum quibufdam*, J. B. Syrian Skirret. It grows about *Aleppo* in *Syria*; the Root is ufed, which agrees in Virtues with the former.

Sifymbrium aquaticum, Water-Creffes. See *Nafturtium aquaticum*,

Sisyrrhinchium, Offic. *Sisyrrhinchium minus angustifolium*, C. B. P. *Crocus Italicus parvo flore, radice rostratâ*, Elem. Bot. *Bulbocodium Crocifolium flore parvo violaceo*, Boerh. Ind. Alt. Spanish Nut It grows in the Kingdom of *Valencia* and *Murcia* in *Spain*, and flowers in *March*. The Root is said, by the Inhabitants where it is a Native, to be good for the Gripes; but the Body must be exercised by Dancing after taking it.

Sium, Offic. *Sium latifolium*, C. B. P. *Sium Dioscoridis sive Pastinaca aquatica major*, Park. Theat. Water Parsnep. It grows in Rivers and marshy Places, flowering in *July*. The Leaves eaten either crude, or boil'd, are said to break and expel the Stone, to excite Urine and the *Menses*; to promote the Expulsion of the *Fœtus*, and to be good in a Dysentery.

Sium umbelliferum, J. B. *Berula*, Offic. *Sium sive Apium palustre, foliis oblongis*, C. B. P. Upright Water Parsnep. It grows in watery Places, flowering in *June*. The Leaves are used; it is esteem'd an Antiscorbutic, and agrees in Virtues with the former.

Smilax arborea. This is already specify'd under the Article *Ilex*.

Smilax aspera, Offic. *Smilax aspera fructu rubente*, C. B. P. Rough Bindweed. This Plant is cultivated in Gardens, flowering in the Summer. The Leaves, Tendrils, Root, and Berries are used in Medicine, which are said to evacuate noxious Humours by Sweat and Transpiration; to cure Disorders of the Skin; to expel Poison, and ease Pains of the Joints. It is a *Succedaneum* for *Sarsaparilla*, and is celebrated for curing venereal Disorders, taken either in Decoction or Powder.

Smilax hortensis. Kidney Beans. See *Phaseolus vulgaris*.

Smilax lævis, Offic. *Convolvu-lus major albus*, C. B. P. *Scammonium Germanicum*, Hoffm. Cat. Altdorff. Great Bindweed. It grows about Hedges, and in Gardens, flowering in the Summer. The Root, the Herb, and the Water distill'd from it, are kept in the Shops at *Hall* in *Germany*. This Plant has theReputation of purging off bilious, acrid, and serous Humours. The Root is Cathartic; whence it is call'd, by *Hoffman, German Scammony*. The Women use a Decoction of this Plant as a Preservative against Miscarriages, with an Intent to allay wandering Pains, and to prevent any sudden Frights from affecting them. *Prevotius*, in his *Medicina Pauperum*, recommends a Decoction of this Plant, as a mild Evacuant of Bile.

Smyrnium & Hipposelinum, Offic. *Hipposelinum Theophrasti, vel Smyrnium Dioscoridis*, C. B. P. *Macerow*, Chab. Alexanders. It grows upon Rocks by the Sea Side, flowering in *June*. The Leaves are used; it is aperient, diuretic, and sudorific; excites the menstrual Discharge, and promotes a difficult Birth; it is good for the Colic, Asthma, and Ischiadic Pains.

Solanum, Offic. C. B. P. *Solanum vulgare*, Park. Theat. *Nilantsiunda*, Hort. Mal. *Agnara-quiya*. Pison Nightshade. It grows by Way Sides, flowering in *August*; the Herb and Seeds are used. The Leaves give but a faint Tincture of Red to the blue Paper, but the ripe Fruit gives it a very deep one, which gives us Reason to conjecture, that the *Sal Ammoniac* in this Plant, is temper'd in the Leaves by a considerable Quantity of Oil and Earth; but that the acid Part of this Salt is very much disengag'd in the ripe Fruit; so that we must make Choice of the Parts of this Plant, as different Occasions may require. The Berries, for Example, are more cooling, but

ye

et more repellent than the Leaves, which lenify by resolving, cleansing, and absorbing. By the chymical *Analysis* they yield a great deal of volatile concrete Salt. The Juice of this Plant is very penetrating, saponaceous, and detergent, whence it s proper in Wounds where Blood is extravasated and grumous. It is, also, diuretic, expelling Gravel from the Kidneys; and sudorific, for which Reason Physicians advise a strong Decoction of the tender Branches to be drank in a *Phthisis*, where Attenuants and Cleansers are required; but where there is an excessive Thinness of Blood, which manifests itself by natural Sweats, it is prejudicial. It is a very serviceable Plant in Inflammations, and too great a Tenseness of the Fibres, and the bruis'd Leaves are good in the Hæmorrhoids: The Juice is very good in a Cancer, to wash the same; and with rectify'd Spirit of Wine, is proper in an Erysipelas, and all cutaneous Diseases. It has the Virtues of Liquorice, and the Decoction of it is highly serviceable in all Disorders from Obstructions, for it is detersive and aperient, and is commended in all Distempers of the Breast, Ulcers, external or internal, the Scurvy and *Lues Venerea.* It is very diuretic, and no Plant is more proper for a Camp, where the Soldiers have receiv'd any internal or external Hurt. Outwardly it is used in the Gout to ease the Pains. Physicians highly extol the outward Use of this Plant, and, I think, with good Reason; they take the bruis'd Leaves, and expressing the Juice, mix it with Ointment of Roses, and apply it to the Head in a Phrensy, as a Refrigerant and Anodyne, whence the Juice is said to be an Antiphlogistic. The Leaves bruis'd with Salt, or Nitre, are proper in Inflammations, Gangrenes, and Suppurations. The Plant taken inwardly, is said to mitigate unnatural Heat, to refrigerate, and comfort the internal Parts. But as many Children in the Country are seiz'd with Convulsions, and destroy'd by the Use of it, which also proves mortal to Poultry, as we are assur'd by the Peasants, this Plant is to be suspected as well as its Berries. The Leaves bruised are fit to be externally applied in Inflammations of the Hæmorrhoids.

Solanum arborescens, Chab. *Amomum Plinii*, Offic. *Solanum fruticosum bacciferum*, C. B. P. Tree Nightshade. It grows spontaneously in *Madeira*, flowering in *July* and *August*. The Fruit is used. It agrees in Virtues with the former.

Solanum lethale. Deadly Nightshade. See *Belladonna.*

Solanum lignosum, Dulcamara, Offic. *Solanum scandens, seu Dulcamara*, C. B. P. *Amara dulcis*, Ger. Emac. *Glycypicros sive Amara dulcis*, J. B. Bitter-Sweet. It grows in watry Places, flowering in *June.* The Root is used; it provokes Urine, and is good for the Dropsy.

Solanum somniferum, Offic. *Solanum somniferum verticillatum*, C. B. P. *Alkekengi fructu parvo verticillato*, Tourn. Inst. *Pevetti*, Hort. Mal. Sleepy Nightshade It grows in Botanic Gardens, flowering in *July.* The Root and Fruit are used. The Root has a somniferous Quality, but milder than *Opium.* The Fruit powerfully provokes Urine, and therefore is prescribed in Hydropic Cases. Its Decoction easeth the Tooth-ach. The Juice of the Root with Honey cures Dimness of Sight.

Solanum tuberosum. Virginia, commonly called *Irish* Potatoes. See *Battata Virginiana.*

Solanum vesicarium. Winter Cherry. See *Alkekengi.*

Soldanella. Scottish Scurvy Grass. See *Brassica marina.*

Soldanella alpina, Ger. *Soldanella alpina rotundifolia,* C. B P. Mountain Bindweed. It grows on the *Alps,* flowering in *July.* The Herb is used, which is reckon'd among Vulneraries.

Solidago. Saracen's Confound. This is already specify'd under the Article *Doria.*

Sonchus asper, Offic. *Sonchus asper laciniatus folio Dentis Leonis,* Tourn. Inst. Prickly Sow Thistle. It grows in Gardens, and upon Banks, flowering in *June.* The Leaves are used, which are sometimes in Winter employ'd in Sallad, and are esteem'd good for Difficulty of Breathing, an Asthma, and the Strangury. This Plant is refrigerating, and for that Reason a very proper Application to any Part inflam'd.

Sonchus lævis, Offic. *Sonchus laciniatus, non spinosus,* J. B. Smooth Sow Thistle. It grows upon Banks and in Gardens, flowering in *May.* The Leaves are used; it agrees in Virtues with the former.

Another Species of *Sonchus* is the *Hieracium,* Offic. *Sonchus repens, multis Hieracium majus,* J. B. *Hieracium majus Dioscoridis,* Ger. Emac. The greater Hawkweed. It grows in Fields, flowering in *July.* The Leaves are said to be cooling and moderately astringent, and to be good in Inflammations. The Herb, together with the Root, is said to be a good Topic for the Sting of a Scorpion.

Sophia Chirurgorum, Offic. *Nasturtium sylvestre tenuissimè divisum,* C. B. P. *Seriphium Germanicum sive Sophia quibusdam,* J B. Flix Weed. It grows amongst Rubbish, flowering in *June.* The Herb is used; it is drying and astringent, and stops Diarrhæas, Dysenteries, and the *Menses,* if too profuse, and is of great Efficacy in deterging malignant Ulcers, and depurating sanious ones; and for con-

solidating them, especially if used internally, as well as externally. Hence it has the Title of *Chirurgorum sapientia;* for it is of a saponaceous, as well as astringent Quality; and being applied to a Wound, conglutinates it without a Suppuration: It also provokes Urine, and is of Service in the Stone and Dropsy.

Sorbus, Offic. *Sorbus sativa,* C. B. P. The Service Tree. It is cultivated in Gardens, flowering in *April.* The Fruit is used. It is refrigerating, drying and astringent; and is principally used in Fluxes of the Belly and *Uterus.* Externally used it astringes Wounds.

Sorbus aucuparia, J. B. *Ornus,* Offic. *Sorbus sylvestris foliis domesticæ similis,* C. B. P. *Ornus sive Fraxinus sylvestris,* Park. Theat. The Quicken Tree. This Tree grows in mountainous and moist Places, flowering in *May,* and produces ripe Fruit in *September.* The Fruit is said to be a very good Hydragogue, and excellent for the Scurvy. The Liquor which distils from a Wound made in this Tree, is recommended as an excellent Antiscorbutic, and as a good Remedy for Disorders of the Spleen.

Sorbus torminalis. The Wild Service, or Sorb Tree. See *Cratægus.*

Sorghum, Offic. *Melica sive Sorghum,* Park. Theat. *Milium Arundinaceum subrotundo semine, Sorgho nominatum,* C. B. P. Indian Millet. It is sown in *Italy.* The Flowers, and the Pith in the Stalks are used. The Pith is recommended for Strumas, and the Flowers for a Dysentery, and uterine Fluxes.

Sparganium, Offic. *Sparganium ramosum,* C. B. P. *Butomus dissectâ paniculâ vulgo Platanaria quia Pilulas habet Platani Pilulis similes.* Bod. in Thoph. Hist. Branched Bur-reed. It grows on the Banks of Rivers, and in marshy Places, flowering in *July.* The Root is commended by *Dioscorides,* as excellent against

ainft the Poifon of Serpents, taken
1 Wine.

Spartium. This is already taken
otice of, under the Article *Genifta
incea.*

Spatula fœtida. Stinking Glad-
on. See *Iris fœtida.*

Spelta. See *Zea.*

Sphondylium, Offic. *Sphondylium vul-
are birfutum,* C. B. P. *Sphondylium
uibufdam, five Branca Urfina Germanica,* J. B. Cow-Parfnep. It
grows in Meadows, and at the Bor-
ers of Fields, flowering in *July.*
The Seed is commended by Dr.
Villis, from *Joannes Anglicus,* as
f excellent Service in Hyfteric Paf-
ions. It is reckon'd by *Buxbaume*
and *Schroder,* one of the five emolli-
nt Herbs.

Spica Nardi. Indian Spikenard.
See *Nardus Indica.*

Spica vulgaris. See *Lavendula.*

Spina alba, Oxyacantha, Offic. *Spina appendix vulgaris,* Park. Theat.
*Mefpilus Apii foliis, fylveftris, fpino-
fa, five Oxyacantha,* C. B. P. The
White Thorn, or Haw Thorn. It
grows in Hedges, flowering in *May.*
The Leaves and the Fruit are ufed,
and agree in Virtues with the *Mefpilus,* or Medlar.

Spina alba is alfo a Name for a
Species of *Echinopus,* or Prickly
Globe Thiftle.

Spina Arabica, Arabian Thiftle.
See *Echinopus.*

Spina Cervina, } See *Rhamnus
Spina Infectoria,* } *Catharticus.*

Spinachia, Offic. *Spinachia five
Olus Hifpanicum,* Park. *Lapathum
hortenfe, feu Spinachia femine fpinofo,*
C. B. P. Spinache. It is fown in
Gardens. The Leaves and the Herb
are ufed. Spinache, which is now
fo celebrated, and ufeful a Green,
feems unmention'd, and unknown to
the Antients. It is fo called by the
Moderns, from its fpinous Seed, tho'
there is alfo, a Species of it which
bears Seed which is fmooth. We are

not certain where it grows fpontaneoufly, but it is probably of *Spanifh*
Original, fince fome call it *Olus
Hifpanicum;* but it refufes no Soil
or Climate, and is in Ufe in almoft all Parts of *Europe.* It is
mollifying, but not nourifhing; for
if a Perfon eats a Pound of it, he
voids it all again by Stool, for the
Juice goes all off in Concoction, and
fpends itfelf in loofening the Belly.
The frefh Herb affords a thick, but
very unwholefome Juice, which mitigates the Afperity of the Lungs,
and is of Service in Inflammations
of the Inteftines. It is very ferviceable in feverifh Diforders, and is
proper for old Perfons, who are fubject to Coftivenefs.

Spiræa, Offic. *Spiræa Theophrafti
forte Clufio,* J. B. *Frutex fpicatus foliis falignis ferratis,* C. B. P. Spiked
Willow. It is cultivated in Gardens,
flowering in *July,* and the Seed is
ripe in *Auguft.* The Seed is ufed,
which is of an aftringent Quality.

Spongia globofa, C. B. P. *Spongia
marina alba,* Ger. Emac. Spunge.
This is a foft, light, porous Plant,
refembling a *Fungus,* and adhering
to the Rocks in the Sea. Almoft all
Spunges are brought from the *Mediterranean* Sea. Spunges are of Ufe
for enlarging Wounds when too fmall,
and being burnt, afford an excellent
Powder for cleaning the Teeth. There
are fometimes found in Spunges fome
very fmall Corpufcles, which by the
Help of a Microfcope, appear to be
fmall *Conchæ,* which being reduc'd
into Powder, are faid to be good for
the Sand and Gravel in the Kidneys,
and alfo for Worms in Children.
All thefe being burnt together, afford a very abforbent Powder, and
emit a Smell, like that of burnt Horn.
Spunge is a very remarkable Plant,
becaufe, when fubjected to Diftillation, it affords an urinous Spirit, exactly refembling that procured from
Animal Subftances. Calcined Spunge

is celebrated for its Virtues in curing the King's Evil, and not without Reaſon; for 'tis certain, that in this Diſtemper many remarkable Cures have been perform'd by it.

Squamaria, & Squamata, Offic. *Orobanche radice dentatâ major,* C. B. P. *Anablatum Cordi ſive Aphyllon,* J. B. Tooth Wort. It grows on the ſhady Banks of Hedges, flowering in *April.* It is conſolidating, conglutinating, and good in *Hernias,* Wounds, and various Affections proceeding from Fluxions.

Stachys, Offic. *Stachys minor Italica,* C. B. P. Baſe Hore-hound. It is cultivated in Gardens, flowering in *June.* The Leaves are uſed. It is of an acrimonious, and heating Quality. A Decoction of its Leaves being drank, provokes the *Menſes,* and expels the Secundines. This Plant has a very ſtrong and rank Smell; whence it is good in Hyſteric, Apoplectic and Epileptic Diſorders.

Staphis agria, Offic. C. B. P. *Delphinium Plataxifolio, Staphis agria dictum,* Tourn. Inſt. Staves-acre. It grows in the Gardens of the Curious. The Seeds are rough, blackiſh, triangular, of an acrid, hot, and burning Taſte, and an ungrateful and nauſeous Smell. It is only uſed externally, as in Maſticatories, as an Apophlegmatiſm, Gargariſms, for the Tooth-ach, and as an Abſtergent in Ulcers and Puſtules.

Staphylodendron, Offic. J. B. *Piſtachia ſylveſtris,* C. B. P. *Nux Veſicaria,* Park. The Bladder Nut Tree. It is found in Hedges, flowering in *May,* and the Nuts are ripe in *Autumn.* The Nuts are by ſome, ſuppoſed to agree in Virtues with Piſtachio's. From the Seeds is expreſſed an Oil of a reſolvent Virtue.

Stæbe. Silver Knapweed. This is already ſpecify'd under the Article *Jacca.*

Stæchas Arabica, Offic. *Stæchas purpurea,* C. B. P. *Stæchas ſive Spica*

hortulana, Ger. Emac. French Lavender. It grows in *Spain* and *France,* flowering in *May.* It is abſterging, attenuant, and aperitive; its principal Uſes are in Affections of the Head and Nerves, as the *Vertigo,* Apoplexy, Palſy, and Lethargy. In Diſeaſes of the Breaſt, it has the ſame Effects as Hyſſop, it alſo provokes Urine, and the *Menſes,* reſiſts Poiſons, and gives Relief under Hypochondriac Diſorders. Outwardly it is uſed in Lotions for the Head, Suffumigations, and other Ways.

Stoechas Citrina;

Stoechas Citrina Germanica. Theſe are already mention'd under the Article *Helichryſum.*

Stramonium, Offic. *Stramonia altera major, ſive Tatura quibuſdam,* J. B. *Solanum fœtidum pomo ſpinoſo, oblongo,* C. B. P. Thorn Apple. It grows in Gardens, flowering in *June.* The whole Plant is narcotic, and the internal Uſe of it dangerous. Outwardly it is refrigerating, and good for Burns.

Stramonium ferox, Tourn. Inſt. *Datura,* Offic. *Solanum fœtidum pomo grandiore ſpinoſiſſimo,* Hort. Reg. Par. Dutroy. It grows in the *Eaſt-Indies.* The Seed of *Dutroy,* pulveriz'd and drank, diſorders the Senſes, and induces a Delirium, which laſts twenty four Hours; whence, as we are told by *Garcias,* it is us'd by Thieves to mix with the Food of thoſe whom they deſign to rob And *Acoſta* tells us, that it is cuſtomary with lewd Women, to give half an Ounce of the Powder to their Gallants in Wine, or any other Liquor they like beſt. He who is ſo unfortunate as to take it, remains for a long time like one without Reaſon, either laughing, weeping, or ſleeping, and ſometimes talking, and giving rational Anſwers, as if he were in his right Senſes, tho' the contrary be true, for he neither knows whom he talks with, nor remembers a Word of what has been ſaid,

said, after he comes to himself. Some of these Women are so experienc'd in administring this Medicine, and know how to temper it in such a Manner, that its Effects shall last for a certain Time, or for as many Hours as they please. There are some Physicians among the *Pagans*, who use the Seed to provoke Urine; their Method is, first to exhibit some Emetic, then inject an acrimonious Clyster, and apply strong Ligatures to the Arms and Legs, and rub them very well; and sometimes to apply Capping Glasses to them: If these have no Effect, they find it necessary to open a Vein in the great Toe. A Dram of the Root taken in Wine, induces a profound Sleep, and strange Dreams, full of surprising and extravagant Images. The Seeds macerated a Night in Vinegar, then carefully powder'd, are good to anoint a miliary *Herpes*, and spreading *Erysipelas*. An Ointment prepared of the Juice of the Leaves, with Swine's Fat, is a most approved Remedy for a Burn by Fire, or scalding Water.

Stratiotes, Offic. *Stratiotes Ægyptia*, J.B. *Lenticula palustris Ægyptiaca, sive Stratiotes aquatica foliis sedo majore latioribus*, C.B.P. Water Teagreen. It grows about the *Nile*. The Leaves are used, which are refrigerating, stop Bleeding, and are good for Inflammations.

Struthium. Dyers Weed. See *Luteola*.

Styrax, Offic. *Styrax folio Mali Cotonei*, C.B.P. *Styrax Arbor*. J.B. The Storax Tree. It grows in *Italy*, and other Countries. The Part used in Medicine is the Resin, of which there are two Sorts to be had in the Shops, the dry and the liquid. The dry *Storax* of the Shops, *Styrax Calamita*, is a fat resinous Substance, of a yellow Colour, inclining to red, concreted into Grains of various Sizes, of a resinous, and somewhat acrid Taste, a very fragrant Smell, and flowing spontaneously from the Trunk of the Tree. Observe here,

first, that our Apothecaries and Druggists sell in their Shops a most impure *Magma*, mixed with various heterogeneous Bodies, as Chaff, Hairs, Bran, and Saw-dust, for *Styrax Calamita*. Secondly, We meet with Prescriptions, in which the *Styrax Calamita* and *Rubra* are order'd distinctly. Now what is the Meaning of *Nicolaus*, in making such a Distinction, there are different Opinions. Some by the *Styrax rubra* understand the *Thymiama*, others the the best Sort of *Styrax*, which runs into Grains; and others again will have it to be nothing but the *Styrax* grown red with Age. The learned *Commelin* writes, that there are two Sorts of *Resin*, the dry and the liquid; the dry is sold in the Shops under two different Names, the *Styrax calamita*, and the *Styrax rubra*, which differ only in Purity. And *Hoffman* tells us they are the same Gum, but different in Purity; for the *Calamita* also participates something of a Redness. But when we find in medicinal Prescriptions, the *Styrax Calamita*, we are to understand it of the *Styrax* in Grains, or of what is cleansed from Impurities; but by the *Styrax rubra*, that most impure *Magma* of *Styrax*, which is commonly sold in our Shops. Chuse what is fat, consisting of pale reddish Fragments, of a lasting Smell, and which yields a melleous Liquor when it is worked.

Storax is a very good Pectoral and Cephalic, and is very efficacious in Coughs, Irritations of the Lungs, and almost all Disorders of the Breast. It is also esteem'd a Cardiac and Alexipharmic, and is said to warm and strengthen the Stomach, and promote Perspiration, and to be a Restorative and Strengthener in Uterine Disorders, either taken inwardly, or externally by way of Suffumigation.

The *Storax liquida*, Offic. Liquid Storax, is a pinguious Liquor, of a melleous and tenacious Substance, of

H h a brown

a brown Colour, or brown inclining to red, of a ftrong Smell, and flows from the Bark of the Tree. It heats, dries, mollifies, and digefts, and is very ferviceable in Diforders of the Brain and Nerves, and cures Coughs, Catarrhs, Hoarfenefs, and the like. There are alfo great Difputes among Authors about the *Styrax Liquida*. Some will have it to be the fame as *Stacte*, that is, ftillatitious Myrrh, which appears to be a Miftake, in that the Tear of Myrrh, on account of the Similitude of Subftance, will diffolve in any aqueous Liquor; whereas the *Styrax Liquida*, like other Refins, will diffolve in none but fat and oleous Liquors. Others affirm it to be a factitious Subftance, prepared of a Solution of *Styrax Calamita*, in Oil and Wine boiled, with a Mixture of *Venice Turpentine*. When this Decoction is grown thoroughly cold, the *Styrax liquida* is faid to feparate, and fall to the Bottom, fending up a more liquid and oleous Subftance to the Superficies. Some will have it made by Expreffion, and others affert it an Oil expreffed from the Kernels of a Tree, whence the *Storax* flows; fome again will have it made by a Decoction of the Bark or Wood of the *Styrax*, others of the liquid Amber. *Hoffman* afferts, that the *Styrax calamita* and *liquida*, are the fame Gum, and different only in Purity; fo that the *Liquid* is the beft. But what is fold for *Liquid Storax* in our Shops, is a Subftance merely factitious, as feveral Apothecaries affured Mr. *Dale*. The *Storax liquida vera*, is a Kind of Bird-Lime, prepared of the Bark of the *Rofa Mallos*, boiled in Sea Water, as I am, (fays Mr. *Dale*) affured by M. *Petiver*, in the *Philofophical Tranfactions*. What Sort of a Tree the *Rofa Mallos* is, and to what *Genus* to be reduced, is quite unknown to me, and therefore I can only add, that it grows in *Cobrofs*, an Ifland in the upper *Red-Sea*, not far from *Cadefs*, which is three Days Journey from the Port of *Suet*. Whether *Cattarmija* be a Name given by the *Arabians* and *Turks* to the Tree, or the Birdlime made of its Bark, is a Thing uncertain. This Birdlime is brought to *Judda*, and from thence in the Months of *June* and *July* to *Mocha*, where in Proportion to its Goodnefs it is fold from fixty to one hundred and twenty Dollars a Veffel, which weighs one hundred and twenty Pounds. The beft is what has the leaft Mixture of Dirt or Duft, with which it is very often foiled, but very eafily purified from them by the Help of Sea-Water. It is us'd in mollifying the Nerves and Tendons, and diffolving fcirrhous Tumors.

Suber, Offic. *Suber latifolium,* J. B. †The Cork Tree. It grows in *Italy* and other hot Countries. The Fruit of this Tree is aftringent, and ferviceable in the flatulent Colic; the Bark is detergent and aftringent, and ufeful in Hæmorrhages, and a *Diarrhæa,* and burnt to Afhes, is refolvent and demulcent in the Hæmorrhoids.

Succifa, Devil's-Bit. See *Morfus Diaboli.*

Sumach. See *Rhus Obfoniorum.*

Sycomorus. The *Egyptian* Sycamore. This is already fpecify'd under the Article *Ficus.*

Symphytum, Confolida major, Offic. C. B. P. *Symphytum magnum,* J. B. Comfrey. It is found in Ditches, flowering in *May.* The Root, Herb, and Flowers are us'd. The Leaves are infipid, glutinous, and give a very faint Tincture of Red to the blue Paper; the Roots give it a little deeper, and abound with a vifcid Juice. This Plant contains a Salt very much refembling the Salt of Coral, diffolved in a very glutinous Phlegm, in which there is a little Sulphur, and a very little Sal Ammoniac; For, by the chymical Analyas it yields several acid Liquors, a great deal of Earth, very little Sulphur, no volatile concrete Salt, but a little urinous Spirit. There is but a very small Quantity of the fix'd Salt; so that it may probably act principally by its viscid Juice, which the Fire destroys. This Plant has a viscous and glutinous Juice, and is of excellent Service in Wounds and malignant Ulcers, attended with Hæmorrhages, in bloody Urine and a *Phthifis.* The Root is insipid, but very demulcent, and the Juice is very good in an *Hæmoptoe* from an excessive Tenacity, and in *Hernias.* A Cataplasm of the Root is effectual in Punctures of the Tendons. The Herb is good in a Dysentery, and an Exulceration of the Kidnies and Bladder from *Cantharides*; it is exhibited like the *Althæa,* but in a smaller Dose, because of its greater Mucofness. The Flowers bruised and boil'd, with an Addition of Syrup of *Althæa,* make an excellent Cataplasm for consolidating recent Wounds.

Symphytum minimum, Bellis minor, Consolida minima, Offic. *Bellis minor Sylvestris, spontanea,* J. B. Common Daisy. It grows in Meadows and Pastures. Its Leaves are acrid, glutinous, and give hardly any Tincture of Red to the blue Paper; which shews that its Salt is not very different from that which is natural in the Earth; that is, composed of *Sal Ammoniac,* Nitre, and marine Salt, involved in a great deal of Sulphur and Earth, which thicken the Sap of the Daisies, and render it viscous. This Plant, taken in a Ptisan or Extract, dissolves the Blood which is thicken'd by too cold an Air, as it often happens in Inflammations of the Lungs, it takes away Obstructions, facilitates the Circulation of the Blood, and restores the Fibres to their natural Elasticity; for which Reason it is thought to be very vulnerary. *Ruellius* affirms, that a Ca-

taplasm, made of Daisies and Mugwort, dissolves scrophulous Tumors, and those wherein there is an Inflammation; and gives Ease to those who are troubled with the Gout or Palfy.

Symphytum petræum, Offic. *Symphytum petræum foliis Thymi,* C. B. P. *Coris Monspesulana purpurea,* J. B. Heath Pine. It grows in maritime Places, flowering in *May.* The Herb is used, which is drying, astringent, and conglutinating: The Plant is esteem'd a good Vulnerary.

Synanchica. Squinancy Wort. See *Rubia Synanchica.*

Tabacum. Tobacco. This is already specify'd under the Article *Nicotiana.*

Tacamahaca. Tacamahac. See *Gummi Tacamahaca.*

Tagetes Indicus. African Marygold. See *Othonna.*

Tamarindus, Offic. *Tamarindus & Caranda,* Bont. *Tamarindi; Lasitanis Tamaræaxula,* Marcg. *Siliqua Arabica, quæ Tamarindus,* C. B. P. *Hijabila Tamarindus,* Herm. Mus. Zeyl. *Jutra sive Tamarindus,* Pis. *Balam Pulli sive Maderam Pulli,* Hort. Mal. The Tamarind Tree. This Tree grows plentifully in *Arabia,* and both the *Indies.* The stringy Pulp of the Fruit is us'd, which is of a dark brown Colour, and a sub-acrid and acid Taste. Tamarinds are gently laxative, and are proper in febrile Heats, where not only Coolers, but Laxatives are required: They are of Service in continual Fevers and Diarrhœas, strengthen the Stomach, and are commended in a Flux of the Hæmorrhoids, from a bilious and acrimonious Blood. The Leaves quench Thirst, and are useful in burning Fevers, and to kill Worms in Children; and an Infusion or Decoction of them, is a gentle Purge. The *Indian* Physicians, as we are inform'd by *Garcias* and *Acosta,* apply the Leaves to an *Eryspelas.*

Tamarifcus, Offic. *Tamarifcus Narbonenfis*, Tourn. Inft. *Tamarix major five Arborea Narbonenfis*, J. B. Tamarifk. It is cultivated in Gardens, flowering in *May* and *June*, and the Bark, Wood, Tops of the Branches, and the Flowers are ufed. Tamarifk is heating, drying, attenuant, aperitive, abftergent, fubaftringent, diuretic, and fplenetic. Its principal Ufe is in Obftructions and Tumors of the Spleen, and in Difeafes proceeding from black Bile, and *Serum* ; as the Itch, Itchings, black Jaundice, and the *Fluor Albus*. Outwardly applied, it cures the *Tinea* of the Head.

Tamarifcus Germanica, Offic. *Tamarix Germanica five minor fruticofa*, J. B. German Tamarifk. It grows in Gardens, flowering in *June*. It agrees in Virtues with the former.

Tamnus. Black Briony. See *Bryonia nigra*.

Tanacetum, Offic. *Tanacetum vulgare*, Park. Tanfie. It grows on the Borders of Fields, flowering in *June*. Tanfie is acrid, aromatic, bitter, and gives no Tincture of red to the blue Paper: The Roots are firft infipid, afterwards aftringent, but without Bitternefs. Tanfie contains an aromatic, oily, volatile Salt, loaded with a great deal of Sulphur. By the Chymical Analyfis, it yields a great deal of Oil, a pretty deal of Earth, a little urinous Spirit, and no volatile concrete Salt. Tanfie in Temperature and Virtues, agrees with Feverfew. It is vulnerary, uterine, and nephritic, and is principally ufed againft Worms, the Gripes, Stone in the Kidneys and Bladder, Obftructions of the *Menfes*, Flatulencies, and the Dropfy. The diftilled Water kills Worms. The Juice drank with Plantain Water, cures all Intermitting Fevers, as alfo the Itch and Rheumatifm ; and relieves thofe who labour under a *Chlorofis* and *Cachexy*. The Conferve

hereof is good for the Epilepfy, Colic, and Hyfteric Paffion, and cleanfes the Kidneys from Sand and Gravel. The Flowers dreffed in a Cake, are of excellent Service in coroborating the Stomach.

Tapfus barbatus, Mullein. See *Verbafcum*.

Taraxicum. Dandelion. See *Dens Leonis*.

Taxus, Offic. The Yew Tree. It grows in mountainous Places, in Woods and Hedges. The Berries of this Tree eaten, induce a Dyfentery and Fever. This was a very noted Tree among the Antients, for its deleterious Quality, which proved mortal, as it was pretended, to all who took it.

Telephium, Craffula, Fabaria, Offic. *Telephium vulgare*, C. B. P. *Anacampferos, vulgo Faba crafia*, J. B. Orpine. It grows in Fields, flowering in *June*. The Herb is ufed, which is vulnerary, and aftringent. Its principal Ufe is in Erofions of the Inteftines, occafion'd by Dyfenteries, in the Cure of Hernia's, and for Burns.

Terebinthina. Turpentine. Of this there are feveral Sorts, the firft of which is the common Turpentine, produc'd by the *Pinus fylveftris* which fee. Another Sort of Turpentine is the *Venice* Turpentine, a liquid Subftance of the Confiftence of new Honey, of a yellowifh Colour, an acrid and bitterifh Tafte, and a grateful and fragrant Smell. It is produc'd from the *Larix* Offic. and is efteem'd heating, emollient and abftergent. It is ufed internally to deterge and heal the Lungs, and in Gonorrhœas : It promotes Difcharges by Stool and Urine. Externally it is of great Ufe, being an Ingredient in a great Number of Plaifters, on Account of its maturating Quality. Another Kind of Turpentine is produc'd by the *Terebinthus*, Offic. *Terebinthus vulgaris*, C. B. P. The beft is imported from

the

the Iſlands of *Chio* and *Cyprus*, and is of a whitiſh Colour, clear, and almoſt tranſparent; thicker, and more tenacious than *Venice* Turpentine; of a pleaſant Smell: That which comes from *Cyprus* is browner, and fuller of Droſs. This Turpentine is of the Conſiſtence of Honey, and the beſt of all Turpentines, for internal Uſe. It gives a Violet Smell to the Urine, even when given in a Clyſter. It is an excellent Diuretic, and very proper in Ulcers of the Kidneys, Bladder and *Uterus*. In Gonorrhæas, it is commonly made into a Bolus with prepared Crab's Eyes, or any other Abſorbent. It may likewiſe be taken in the Yolk of an Egg, from half a Dram to a Dram: All theſe Precautions are neceſſary, only to avoid the diſagreeable Taſte; Sugar, and powder'd Liquorice, may be uſed for the ſame Purpoſe. It is likewiſe often given in Clyſters; being firſt diſſolv'd in the Yolk of an Egg, and then mix'd with the Decoctions. It is thus adminiſter'd in the Stone Colic; but the Inteſtines ought previouſly to be unloaded by purgative Clyſters. The Doſe in this manner, is from an Ounce to an Ounce and an half, Turpentine, like all other Balſams, is to be avoided in inflammatory Diſpoſitions of all Kinds.

But that which is eſteem'd the beſt, is the *Straſburg* Turpentine, or *Terebinthina Argentoratenſis*, which is produc'd by the *Abies*, Offic. The Silver Firr. This is of much the ſame Conſiſtence with the *Venice* Turpentine, but more tranſparent, bitteriſh, and very fragrant, and of a Taſte, reſembling that of a Citron. It is eſteem'd vulnerary and detergent, and therefore good in Abſceſſes and Ulcers, in what Part ſoever, eſpecially the Lungs, Breaſt, and Urinary Paſſages, which laſt it remarkably deterges and cleanſes, from Gravel, and mucous Concretions. It is often

given in the latter End of a *Gonorrhæa*, but this muſt be done with Caution, becauſe if exhibited too ſoon, it ſometimes diſpoſes the Teſticles to ſwell, and if given in too great Quantities, or too long continued, it weakens the Parts, cauſes Gleets, and involuntary Emiſſions. It is ſometimes boiled in Water, till it becomes hard and brittle, in order to make it leſs detergent, and more agglutinating. When mix'd with an aqueous Vehicle, it is order'd to be diſſolv'd with the White of an Egg. All the Turpentines externally apply'd, are eſteem'd very detergent, and are much us'd by the Surgeons for Wounds and Ulcers; but they ſometimes incarn too faſt, and cauſe a *Fungus*. And in general, Turpentines are ſo extremely penetrating, that they enter the Pores of the Skin, and communicate a Smell to the Urine; and even ſitting in a Room, that has been lately painted, has been often experienc'd to affect the Urine in the ſame Manner. *New England* produces ſome Turpentines, which very much reſemble the finer Balſams.

Teucrium, Offic. *Teucrium multis*, J. B. *Chamædrys fruteſcens, Teucrium vulgo*, Tourn. Inſt. Tree Germander. It grows in *Italy* and *Sicily*, flowering in the Summer, and the Leaves are uſed. It is heating and drying, cures Diſorders of the Liver and Spleen, and is effectual againſt Bites of Serpents. In other Reſpects it agrees with the *Chamædrys*, or Germander.

Thalictrum, Offic. *Thalictrum majus ſiliqua anguloſâ aut ſtriata*, C. B. P. Meadow Rue. It grows in Paſtures, and moiſt Places, flowering in *June*. The Herb and Root are uſed. It cicatrizes old Ulcers. It is aperitive, inciding, and provokes Evacuation by Stool and Urine. An Ounce or two purge like Rhubarb, whence it is called in *Germany* the *Poors Rhubarb*, and *Tartary Rhubarb*.

In some Parts of *Italy*, as *Camerarius* informs us, they use it against the Plague; and in *Saxony* for the Jaundice.

Another Species of *Thalictrum*, is the *Pseudo Rhabarbarum*, Offic. *Thalictrum majus Hispanicum*, Ger. Emac. Spanish Meadow Rue. It grows in the Gardens of the Curious, flowering in the Summer. The Root is used, which agrees in Virtues with the former, and is sold in the Herb-Shops for Rhubarb.

Thapsia, Offic. *Thapsia sive Turbith Garganicum semine latissimo*, J. B. *Turpethum Garganicum*, Schrod. Deadly Carrots. This Plant is sometimes cultivated in the Gardens of the Curious, and the Part used is the long and acrimonious Root, which is black without, and white within. *Mesue* calls it black *Turbith*, and employ'd it to evacuate thin Humours. The old Women of *Salamanca* in *Spain* used the Root to provoke the *Menses*, and with Emollients to promote other Evacuations, as *Clusius* assures us. The Antients expressed a Juice from this Plant, which they made use of when they thought violent Purging necessary; for the Juice of the Root inspissated, and given to the Quantity of an Ounce, purges upwards and downwards, so as sometimes to produce an Inflammation of the Stomach and Intestines; whence a Dysentery is occasion'd. The same is so highly acrimonious as to cause Convulsions, succeeded by very bad Symptoms, which are not to be removed but by a Draught of Vinegar, Oil and Water, for which Reason the internal Use of it is dangerous. The Root has been sold for the *Turbith* of the Antients, but with very mischievous Consequences. Externally it is used in Ointments for the Itch, and the like Disorders.

Another Species of *Thapsia* is the *Turbith cinericium, Pseudo-Turbith*, Offic. *Thapsia faeniculi folio*, C. B. P.

Seseli quae Ferulae facie Thapsia, sive Turbith Gallorum, Boerh. Ind. Alt. French Turbith. It grows in the Mountains of *Aquitain*. The Root is used, which agrees in Virtues with the former.

Thea, Offic. *The Sinensium sive Tsia Japonensibus Breynii*, Raii Hist. *Chaa Herba Japonia*, C. B. P. The Thee, or Tea Plant. There are six Sorts of Tea used in *England*. The first is called *Bohea*, which is a small blackish Leaf, which tinges the Water with a brown or reddish Colour, and renders it of a Taste like an Infusion of *Sena*; the second Sort is called *Congo*; the third *Peco*; and the fourth *Green Tea*; and, by some *Single*. This last is of two Kinds, one consists of an oblong narrow Leaf; the other has lesser Leaves, but both are equally good, and of a blueish green Colour, seem very crisp when chewed, and tinge the Water with a pale Green. The fifth is called *Imperial Tea*; this has a large loose Leaf, whereas that of the other two last mention'd is convolved, or shrivelled up: This Species is also most sightly to the Eye, of a green Colour, crisp in the Mouth, and of a pleasant Smell. The sixth Sort is called *Heysham Tea*. All these Sorts of Tea are brought from *China*, and are supposed to be Leaves of the same Tree, and distinguish'd only by the Time of gathering, and the Method of Preparation, or as they call it, *Curing*. The fresh Leaf is said to affect the Head, and to intoxicate, but it loses these Qualities when dried and prepared. The *Japonese* first bruise the dry'd Leaves in Stone Mortars, and then throw a sufficient Quantity into boiling Water, and suffer it to infuse but a very little while. The greatest Advantage of Tea, considering the Quantity of what is drank, seems to be, that it prevents the hot Weather from relaxing the Stomach to too

great

great a Degree, becauſe it is a little aſtringent : All the other Effects of this faſhionable Liquor ſeem to proceed from the hot Water. Tea boiled in Milk, in the Quantity of two Drams to a Pint, has been found to ſtop a Looſeneſs ; the Doſe being repeated two or three times. *Green Tea* being drank too freely, is prejudicial to weak Lungs. They who are ſubject to this Diſeaſe, ought therefore to chuſe *Bohea,* and to mix Milk with it, in order to make it more laxative. The Virtues which the *Chineſe* aſcribe to Tea, are : That it purifies the Blood , prevents frightful Dreams, and defends the Brain from malignant Vapours ; cures a *Vertigo,* and Pain of the Head, eſpecially when it proceeds from a *Crapula* ; is good for Hydropic Perſons, for it is a potent Diuretic ; dries up Rheums of the Head ; corrects the Acrimony of Humours, removes Obſtructions of the *Viſcera,* and reſtores decay'd Sight ; for the *Japoneſe,* I believe, make uſe of a Decoction of Tea, which they call *Tebia,* as their principal Antidote againſt a Weakneſs of the Eyes, contracted chiefly from the frequent and conſtant Uſe of hot Rice, and drinking their Liquor *Sarqui.* It tempers aduſt Humours, corrects an hot Liver, mollifies a Hardneſs of the Spleen, and prevents Sleep, eſpecially in thoſe who are not accuſtomed to it. Moreover, it renders the Body briſk and lively, quickens the Senſes, prevents a *Torpor* and Drowſineſs, exhilarates the Heart, repels Fear, cures Gripes and Flatulencies, diſcuſſes Wind in the *Uterus,* comforts and ſtrengthens the *Viſcera,* revives the Memory, ſharpens the Wit, and tempers Bile, and is eſteem'd a noble Lithontriptic. Whatever Virtues are aſcribed to Tea, or however uſeful as a Medicine, it may be in *China,* I am very certain, that either the Tea, or the Water, or both, are extremely prejudicial, as

an habitual Drink in *England* ; inſomuch, that I have known many hyſterical Caſes reliev'd, and ſome cur'd, by leaving off Tea, wi-hout taking any Remedy whatever ; and one in particular, which was attended with terrible Convulſions. A great many People upon drinking a Quantity of Tea, find themſelves affected with Flatulencies, and in Order to relieve theſe Flatulencies, are oblig'd to take Hartſhorn, Spirits of Lavender, or ſome Cordial ; and when theſe do not relieve the Lowneſs of Spirits cauſed by theſe Flatulencies, they are oblig'd to have Recourſe to Wine, and then to Drams, a ſlow, but very certain Poiſon.

Thlaſpi, Offic. *Thlaſpi arvenſis ſiliquis latis,* C. B. P. Treacle-Muſtard. It is found in Corn Fields tho' ſeldom, flowering in *June.* The ſmall, black, oblong, acrimonious Seeds are us'd, which are drying and abſtergent ; and principally us'd in breaking internal Abſceſſes, provoking the Menſes, and curing iſchiadical Affections, and the like.

Thlaſpi vulgare, Offic. *Thlaſpi Mithridaticum ſeu vulgatiſſimum, Baccariæ folio,* Park. Theat. Mithridate Muſtard. It grows among Corn, flowering in *June.* The Seeds are us'd, which enter the Compoſition of the *Theriaca,* and externally us'd cleanſe all Sorts of running Ulcers ; and are alſo, a Ptarmic. They are reckoned an Enemy to pregnant Women, becauſe they kill the *Fœtus.*

Thora, Leopards Bane. This is already taken Notice of under the Article *Ranunculus.*

Thus, Frankincenſe. See *Olilanum.*

Thuja Theophraſti, C. B. P. *Arbor Vitæ,* Offic. *Arbor Vitæ, ſive Paridiſiaca vulgo dicta odorata ad Sabinam accedens,* J. B. The Tree of Life. It is a Native of *America,* and is cultivated in the Gardens of the Curious. The Leaves are us'd as an Alexipharmic, and Diuretic. It is an opening and warming Plant, provokes the Menfes, and is good againft the *Chlorofis*; bruifed with Honey, it diffolves Tumors. The Oil is commended againft the Gout, being rubbed on the Part; for it acts like Fire, by ftimulating and opening. It cleanfes Beds from Lice and Fleas.

Thymbra. See *Saturoia.*

Thymelæa, Offic. *Thymelæa foliis Lini,* C. B. P. Spurge Flax. It is cultivated in botanic Gardens, and the Berries called *Grana Cnidia* are us'd, being of a cauftic Quality. The *Englifh* Shops, as well as fome of the moft fkilful Botanifts, take the Fruit for the *Coccus Cnidius,* or *Grana Cnidia*; but *Cordus* and *Schroder* will have the Berries of the *Mezereon* to be the *Grana Cnidia* of the Shops.

Thymelæa minor, five *Cneoron Matthioli,* Park. Theat. *Cneoron niger,* Offic. *Thymelæa affinis facie externa,* C. B. P. Rock Rofe. It grows in mountainous Places, flowering in *April.* The Bark is us'd. It agrees in Virtues with the *Chamelæa.*

Thymelæa laurifolia, femper-virens, feu Laureola mas, Tourn. Inft. *Laureola,* Offic. *Laureola femper-virens, flore luteolo,* J. B. Spurge Laurel. It grows in Woods and Hedges, flowering in *February.* The Bark, Leaves, and black oblong Berries are us'd. It is of an igneous, very acrid, exulcerating, and ftimulating Quality, exciting Fevers, weakening the Force of the Heart; and the noble Parts; and purging Bile and bilious Serofities with great Violence: It is corrected by Maceration in Acids.

Thymelæa laurifolia deciduo, Offic. *Laureola fœmina,* Tourn. Inft. *Mezereon, Chamelæa,* Offic. *Laureola flore deciduo, five Mezereon Germanicum,* J. B. Mezereon, or Spurge Olive. It is cultivated in Gardens, flowering in the Spring. The Bark,

Leaves, and red Berries are us'd, which agree in Virtues with the preceeding.

Thymus, Offic. *Thymus vulgaris folio tenuiore,* C. B. P. Thyme. It is cultivated in Gardens flowering in *June* and *July.* The Herb is us'd which is ferviceable in tartareous Affections of the Lungs and Joints, frees all the *Vifcera* from Obftructions, and excites an Appetite. It is an excellent Plant in Suffumigations to revive the Spirits; and by its extraordinary Fragrancy, is very comfortable to the Brain, and highly exhilarating to the Heart. Infus'd in cold Wine, it cures the Bites of all venomous Animals, and is recommended againft the Bite of a mad Dog. It is very effectual againft pituitous and cold Difeafes, particularly the Afthma and Cough. A little Thyme mixed with Wine gives it a moft grateful Savour, and both the Smell and Tafte of it are very penetrating; whence it becomes fudorific, inciding, penetrating, healing, and opening; and is of Service in the flatulent Colic, is properly given in difficult Labour, and removes Obftructions of the *Menfes:* Externally us'd, it is effectual againft the Pain of the Gout, and cold Tumors.

Thymus fylveftris, Offic. *Serpyllum folio Thymi,* C. B. P. *Thymbra Hifpanica Coridis folio,* Tourn. Inft. Wild Thyme. It is cultivated in the Gardens of the Curious, flowering in the Summer. The Herb is us'd, which agrees in Virtues with the preceeding.

Thymus verus, Offic. *Thymus capitatus, qui Diofcoridis,* C. B. P. *Hyffopus capitata minor, Thymi odore,* Hift. Oxon. True Thyme. It grows fpontancoufly in *Crete,* but is cultivated with us in Gardens, flowering in the Summer. The Herb is us'd, which is attenuating, inciding, and opening; and is principally us'd to provoke Urine and the *Menfes,* and to bring away the Birth and After-Birth. It

deftroys

eftroys Worms, purges pituitous Humours by Stool, difcuffes Tumors, and diffolves concreted Blood.

Thyffelinum Plinii, Tourn. Inft. *Delnizium,* Offic. Germ. *Apium fyl-veftre lacteo fucco turgens,* C. B. P. Milky Parfley. It grows in moift Places, flowering in *July.* The Root is us'd which is poffeffed of an alexi-pharmic Quality. The Plant is ape-ient and diuretic.

Tilia, Offic. *Tilia fœmina follo majore,* C. B. P. The Lime-Tree. It is planted in Walks and Areas, flow-ering in *June.* The Leaves and Flowers are us'd. The Leaves are drying and repellent, and provoke Urine and the *Menfes.* The Flowers are heating and drying, and of fine Parts, difcutient and cephalic. The *Tilia* affords us fome very good Re-medies, particularly in the Flowers, by an Infufion of which in Water, after the Manner of Tea, with long and conftant Ufe, I have known fays *Hoffman,* an inveterate Epilepfy per-fectly cured. The Water of the Flowers is a fpecific in all Difeafes where Pains or Convulfions are pre-dominant; whence it juftly deferves the Name of *Polychreftum.* The middle Bark of the Tree, reduced with Water to a Mucilage, is of in-comparable Virtue in mitigating Pains, Heats and Inflammations; whence it gives immediate Relief in Pains of the Gout. Externally the Flowers are recommended in the Form of a Cataplafm in a *Tenef-mus.*

Tilia fœmina, folio minore, C. B. P. *Tilia folio minore,* J. B. The fmaller Lime Tree, Baft, or Peper Tree. It grows in Woods and Hedges; the Flowers are us'd, and agree in Vir-tues with thofe of the preceeding.

Tithymalus. A Name for feveral Sorts of Spurge, of which the eigh-teen following are us'd in Medicine.

Tithymalus paluftris fruticofus, C. B. P. *Efula major,* Offic. *Tithy-*

malus magnus multicaulis, five Efula major, J. B. German Spurge. It is cultivated in botanic Gardens. The Root is us'd, which is oblong, an Inch thick, of a dark brown exter-nally, and within pale and turgid, with a very acrid, purging and nau-feous Milk. It is faid to purge Phlegm by Stool, but fo powerfully, as to require a great Deal of Caution in its Ufe. From the Roots, Herb, and milky Juice, an Ointment is pre-pared which has the Reputation of being effectual in curing contagious Eruptions of the Head.

Tithymalus Pineus, Ger. Emac. *Efula minor, Pityufa,* Offic. *Tithyma-lus foliis Pini, forte Diofcoridis Pityu-fa,* C. B. P. Pine Spurge. It grows frequently in Gardens. The Root, Bark of the Root and Leaves are us'd. The Root is oblong, more flender than that of the former, of a brown Colour on the Out fide, but of a whitifh Yellow within, and of a pretty acrid Tafte. It burns the Tongue and *Fauces* by its cauftic Acrimony, when but tafted; but taken inwardly it purges Water from hydropic Perfons, upwards and down-wards, with fuch Violence and Dif-order, as requires great Caution in ufing it. Both this and the former, are corrected by Maceration in A-cids.

Tithymalus latifolius Cataputia dic-tus, Tourn. Inft. *Cataputia minor, Lathyris,* Offic. *Lathyris major,* C. B. P. Garden Spurge. It grows fre-quently in Gardens, and the Parts in Ufe are the round oblong Seeds, or Grains, which are bigger than a Pea, and include under a cortical Pellicle a white pinguious *Nucleus,* or Kernel, of a fweetifh acrid and naufeous Tafte, and a violent cathartic Qua-lity; but thefe Grains, as well as thofe of the other Species of *Tithy-malus,* are feldom us'd. Twelve or fourteen Grains, bruifed, and taken in Wine, put the whole Body in a

Commo-

Commotion, purge the Belly, evacuate Bile and Phlegm, potently provoke Vomiting, and attract Phlegm, Bile and Melancholy. The Whole of this Plant abounds with a milky, highly acrid Juice, which operates violently both by Vomit and Stool. It is classed among the Poisons which are manifestly acrid and caustic, which create a Gangrene and Putrefaction, and whose Effects are to be opposed by aqueous, tepid, somewhat acrid, and pinguious Substances; as, also, by Preparations of Honey.

4. *Tithymalus amygdaloides angustifolius,* Tourn. Inst. *Tithymalo maritimo affinis, Linariæ folio,* C. B. P. *Alypum Matthioli, Tithymalo affinis,* J. B. Narrow Leav'd Wood Sage. It grows in Woods and Thickets; and the Leaves are used, which agree in Virtues with the former Species.

5. *Tithymalus,* Offic. *Helioscopius,* C. B. P. *Tithymalus Helioscopius sive solisequus,* J. B. Sun Spurge, or Wart Wort. It grows frequently in Gardens; and besides the Virtues it has in common with the other Species, is recommended against Warts.

6. *Tithymalus Characias,* Offic. *Tithymalus Characias rubens peregrinus,* C. B. P. Wood Spurge. It grows in stony Places about *France* and *Italy;* flowering in *March.* The Root, Leaves, and Seeds, are of an acrimonious and caustic Quality; and the Juice as *Dioscorides* says, is a violent Cathartic.

7. *Tithymalus myrtites,* Offic. *Tithymalus myrsinites latifolius,* C. B. P. Myrtle Spurge. It grows in *Calabria* and *Sicily;* flowering in the Summer. The Root, Leaves, Seed, and Juice are used; and are said by *Dioscorides,* to be possess'd of the same Virtues as the preceeding.

8. *Tithymalus sylvaticus lunato flore,* C. B. P. *Tithymalus sylvaticus toto anno folia retinens,* J. B. Evergreen Wood Spurge. It grows in Woods; and the Root is used. It

agrees in Virtues with the former Species.

9. *Tithymalus verrucosus,* J. B. *Tithymalus myrsinites fructu verrucæ simili,* C. B. P. Rough-fruited Spurge. It grows in Fields; and the Herb is used; which agrees in Virtues with the other Species.

10. *Tithymalus paralius,* Offic. J. B. *Tithymalus maritimus,* C. B. P. Sea Spurge. It grows in sandy Places by the Sea-side, flowering in *June.* The whole Plant is used; its Leaves are very turgid, with a lacteous Juice, of a very acrimonious Quality; it agrees in Virtues with the other Spurges.

11. *Tithymalus cyparissias,* Offic. C. B. P. *Tithymalus cypressinus,* Ger. Emac. *Esula Officinarum,* Cæsalp. Cypress Spurge. It grows in the Gardens of the Curious, flowering in Summer. The Leaves of this Plant have the Taste of Almonds, the Milk of which has been drawn by Emulsion; they are styptic, but without any Acrimony, or Bitterness; and give a pretty deep Tincture of Red to the blue Paper; but the Roots give a much deeper: They seem at first, to have the same Taste with the Leaves, but leave at last a very considerable Acrimony in the Throat. It is very likely, that there is in the Roots of this Plant, a Salt resembling Alum, but involved in a great Quantity of resinous Sulphur. This Mixture whitens the Phlegm of the Spurge much after the same Manner, as it happens to the Magistery of Jalap, or that of Scammony; this Spurge is an excellent Hydragogue; it is corrected by macerating it in Vinegar, or the Solution of Cream of Tartar: For if one swallows ever so little of this Root, it leaves a considerable Acrimony and Burning, not only in the Throat, but all along the *Oesophagus,* and sometimes in the Stomach itself. The Bark of the Roots of this

is Plant, is given in Substance from Scruple to a Dram, and in Infusion from one Dram to two. This Purtive is good for the Dropsy, Caexy, and intermitting Fevers; it ay be used in all Diseases, where is requisite to carry off the Humurs that resist the ordinary Purtives.

12. *Tithymalus dendroides*, Offic. B. *Tithymalus myrtifolius arbous*, C. B. P. Tree Spurge. It ows in the mountainous Parts of *ples*; the Leaves, Seeds, and ice are used. It is used as a Caartic; for the Weight of Half Obolus purges Bile, Phlegm, d serous Humours; it is hot d dry, and excites an Inflamation and Exulceration.

13. *Tithymalus platyphyllos*, Offic. thymalus latifolius Hispanicus, C. P. Broad-leaved Spurge. It ows in *Spain*, flowering in the mmer. The Root, Leaves, and ice are used, which have the same irtues as the other Species. *Dio-wides* says, that bruised, and rown into the Water, it kills fh.

14. *Tithymalus foliis brevibus, acuatis*, C. B. P. *Pityusa*, Offic. *Tithyalus cyparissias vulgaris*, Park. heat. Pine Spurge with sharp point-l Leaves. It grows in *Italy*. The oot is used, which operates by tool.

15. *Tithymalus rotundis foliis, non matis*, Tourn. Inst. *Peplus*, Offic. eplus, sive Esula rotunda, C. B. P. etty Spurge. It grows in Gardens, owering in *June*. The Herb and ruit are used. Taken in *Hydromel*, evacuates Bile and Phlegm; rinkled upon Meat, it excites ommotions in the Belly.

16. *Tithymalus maritimus folio ob-fo*, Tourn. Inst. *Peplis*, Offic. *Pep-is maritima folio obtuso*, C. B. P. urple Sea Spurge. It grows in

sandy Places about the Sea-shore, flowering in the Summer. The Herb is used, which agrees in Virtues with the other Species of Spurges.

17. *Tithymalus exiguus procumbens, Chamæsyce dictus*, Boerh. Ind. Alt. *Chamæsyce*, Offic. C. B. P. Time Spurge. It grows in the Vineyards and Fields of *Italy*, flowering in the Summer. The Herb is used, and is esteem'd a Cathartic, as well as the Juice, which is a Remedy against the Sting of a Scorpion, the Place being anointed therewith.

18. *Tithymalus tuberosus pyriformi radice*, C. B. P. *Apios*, Offic. J. B. Round knobbed rooted Spurge. It grows in the Island of *Crete*. The Root is used, which is purgative, and is good to take away Warts.

Tormentilla, Offic. J. B. *Tormentilla sylvestris*, C. B. P. Tormentil. It grows in Pastures, flowering in *June*. The Root and Herb are used. The Root is hard, knotty, crooked, and fibrous, of a reddish Colour and astringent Taste. It dries and astringes, and is therefore very good in all Fluxes whether of the Belly or *Uterus*. It is moreover diaphoretic and alexipharmac, and is therefore given in contagious and malignant Diseases, especially if attended with a *Diarrhæa*.

Tota-bona. A Name for the *Bonus Henricus*, or *English* Mercury.

Trachelium, Cervicaria, Offic. *Campanula major & asperior, folio Urticæ*, J. B. Throat Wort. It grows in Woods and Hedges, flowering in *July*. The Leaves are used, and are recommended for the Quinsey, and for Tumors and Inflammations of the Mouth.

Tragacantha, Offic. C. B. P. Goat's Thorn. It grows in the Gardens of the Curious. The Gum is used. See *Gummi Tragacanthæ*.

Another Species of the *Tragacantha*, is the *Poterium*, Offic. *Tragacantha altera Poterium forte Clusio*. J. B.

J. B. Small Goat's Thorn. It grows in the Kingdom of *Granada,* flowering in the Summer. The Root is ufed, which being bruifed and applied, conglutinates Wounds and Cuts, where the Nerves are divided; the Decoction, alfo being drank, is effectual in nervous Affections.

Tragopogon, Offic. *Tragopogon pratenfe luteum majus,* C. B. P. Yellow Goat's Beard. It grows in Meadows and Paftures, flowering in *June* and *July.* The Roots are ufed, which are very nutritive, and for that Reafon good for lean and confumptive Perfons. They are alfo faid to cure Diforders of the Breaft, the Cough, and Difficulty of Refpiration, and the Pleurify. They are alfo fuppofed to be good for the Strangury, to expel the Stone, for Eftuations, and lancinating Pains of the Stomach and Thorax.

Tragorchis. Goat's Stones. A Species of *Satyrium,* which fee.

Tragoriganum, Offic. *Tragoriganum Creticum,* C. B. P. Goat's Marjoram. It grows in the Ifland of *Crete,* flowering in *March.* The Herb is ufed. It is heating, provokes the *Menfes,* and is a good Strengthener of the Stomach.

Tragoriganum alterum, Offic. *Tragoriganum anguftifolium,* C. B. P. *Tragoriganum Hifpanicum,* Park. Theat. Spanifh Goat's Marjoram. It grows in the Kingdom of *Valentia,* flowering in *March.* The Herb is ufed, which agrees in Virtues with the former.

Tribulus aquaticus, Offic. C. B. P. Water Caltrops. It grows in watry Places, flowering in *June.* The Herb and Nuts are ufed. The Nuts, while new, are good againft the Stone. This Herb is refrigerating and infpiffating, good for Inflammations, and for Ulcers of the Mouth and Gums.

Tribulus terreftris, Offic. J. B. Caltrops. It grows in *Italy,* flower-

ing in *July.* The Herb and Seed are ufed. The Herb agrees in Virtues with the former. The Seed is commended againft Poifons, and reftores thofe who are bitten by Serpents.

Trichomanes, Offic. *Capillus Veneris,* Pharmacop. *Trichomanes five Polytrichum,* J. B. Englifh Black Maidenhair. It grows in ftony and fhady Places, and upon old Walls. In the *Englifh* Shops it is a *Succedaneum* for the *Adianthum verum,* or *Capillus veneris,* which grows not fpontaneoufly in *England,* and is fuppofed to have the fame Virtues, and *Tragus* afcribes the fame Effects to it. The Herb, boiled in Wine, or Hydromel, and drank, removes Obftructions of the Liver, cures the Jaundice, cleanfes the Lungs; helps Difficulty of Breathing; purges Melancholy by Urine; mollifies hard Tumors of the Spleen, and the Stone; and provokes the *Menfes.* The fame Decoction, or the Powder of the Herb, or an *Eclegma,* or Syrup prepared of it, or the diftilled Water, ftops all Sorts of Fluxes of the Belly, and cools Inflammations of the Liver. A *Lixivium* of the Leaves reftrains the falling off of the Hair, the Head being wafhed therewith, and cures the Bites of Serpents, and other Animals. Some Farmers and Graziers make a fingular Ufe of the *Trichomanes,* in curing the Difeafes of the Swine. But let the Skilful judge, fays *J. Bauhine,* whether, an aftringent, cold, and dry Herb can perform fuch Effects as are afcrib'd to the *Trichomanes.* The chief Virtues of this Plant, and which are allow'd by all, are in its being adapted to the Cure of Pulmonic Fevers, the Gravel in the Kidneys, and the Strangury.

Trifolium acetofum. A Name for the *Acetofella,* or Wood Sorrel.

Trifolium aureum. Noble Liver-Wort. See *Hepatica.*

Tri-

Trifolium bituminofum, Offic. *Trifium bitumen redolens*, C. B. P. *phaltites, five bituminofum odoratum non odoratum*, J. B. Stinking refoil. It is cultivated in Gardens, wering in *August*. The Root, aves, and Seed are ufed. The aves and Seed taken in Water, are effectual againft the Pleurify, Dyfury, ilepfy, Dropfy, and Female Difders, and provoke the *Menfes*. hey alfo cure the Bites of Serpents. he Root is alexipharmic.

Trifolium Hæmorrhoidale. Pile refoil. See *Lotus Hæmorrhoidalis*.

Trifolium Leporinum, Volck. Flor. or. *Lagopus, Pes Leporinus*, Offic. *rifolium arvenfe humile, fpicatum, ve Lagopus*, C. B. P. Hares Foot. It ows in Fields, flowering in *July*. he Herb is ufed, which is drying d aftringent. It is principally ufed a *Diarrhæa*, and Dyfentery, and ftop the too great Flux of the atamenia, and the *Fluor Albus*, and itting of Blood. It helps the Uleration of the Bladder, Strangury, feat, and Pain in making Water.

Trifolium odoratum. Sweet Treil. See *Lotus Urbana*.

Trifolium paluftre, C. B. P. *Trilium paluftre, paludofum*, Offic. *Trilium fibrinum*, Offic. Germ. *Menthes paluftre triphyllum*, Tourn. nft. *Acopa Diofcoridis*, Hift. Oxon. uck Bean, or Marfh Trefoil. It rows in watry and marfhy Places, lowering in *May*. The Herb is ufed. It is good for Difeafes of the Joints, nd for the Scurvy, and is greatly ommended againft Intermitting Fevers, Catarrhs, and the Dropfy.

Trifolium pratenfe, Ger. Emac. *Trifolium Lotus herba agreftis*, Offic. *Trifolium pratenfe purpureum*, C. B. P. Common Trefoil. It grows in Meadows, flowering in *June*. The Flowers and Seeds, boiled in Wine, are recommended by *Tragus*, to eafe acute Pains, and incide the glutinous Contents of it the Inteftines.

Trifolium purpureum, Offic. *Trifolium quadrifolium hortenfe album*, C. B. P. *Quadrifolium fufcum*, Park. Theat. Purple Wort, and Purple Grafs. It is found in Meadows, and is cultivated in fome Gardens, flowering in Summer. The Herb is ufed. The Juice expels phlegmatic Humours from the Inteftines, cures Ulcers of the Mouth and the Tongue, is a Prefervative againft the Small Pox, and is vulgarly efteem'd a prefent Remedy for the Purple Fever of Children.

Triorchis. Triple Ladies Traces. A Name for a Species of *Satyrium*, which fee.

Tripolium, Offic. *Tripolium majus & minus*, J. B. *After maritimus paluftris cæruleus Salicis folio*, Tourn. Inft. Sea Star Wort. It grows on the Sea Shores, flowering in *July*. The Root is ufed, two Drams of which taken in Wine, purge off Water and Urine by Stool.

Another Species of *Tripolium*, is the *Conyza, Pulicaria*, Offic. *Conyza minor flore globofo*, C. B. P. *After paluftris parvo flore globofo*, Tourn. Inft. Small Fleabane. It grows in Places where Water has ftood all the Winter, flowering in *August*. The Herb is ufed, which is opening, penetrating, and good to purge the Brain. It is a good Sternutatory, and kills Fleas.

Triffago. A Name for the *Chamædrys* or *Germander*.

Triticum, Offic. *Triticum hybernum ariftis carens*, C. B. P. *Frumentum, Triticum*, Chab. Wheat. This is the common Food of almoft all *Europe*. The Meal applied externally by way of Cataplafm, is ufed for mollifying and relaxing Tumors, for Inflammations and Fluxions of the Eyes ; and the dry'd Meal is applied to an Eryfipelas, and is faid to eafe the Pains of the Gout. Water, in which, when heated, Bran has been infufed for a Day and a Night, is good to deterge the *Furfur* of the Head ;

and

and a Gargarism of the Decoction of Bran, mitigates the Pain and Asperities of the Fauces. Bran boiled in Water, then put into a Bag, squeezed dry, and apply'd hot, removes the pungent Pains of a Pleurisy, if the Bag, when cooled, be heated in the same Manner, then again squeez'd and apply'd, and this Method be several Times repeated. It is certain that Bran has an abstersive Virtue, by which the Intestines are stimulated to Excretion. Bread, therefore which is made of Flour, not thoroughly cleansed from the Bran, provided it be duly fermented, seems to us to be more wholesome, and also more savoury, than what is made of pure Flour, or *Siligo.* For outward Use, Crumbs of Bread serves for much the same Purposes as Wheaten Flour. *Galen* writes, that a Cataplasm prepared of Bread, is more digestive than one of Wheat, because Bread has a Mixture of Salt and Leaven; and his Opinion seems consonant to Reason, and is confirmed by Experience.

Triticum Indicum, Offic. *Frumentum Indicum Mays dictum,* C. B. P. *Mays Granis aureis,* Tourn. Inst. Indian Wheat. It is a Native of the *West Indies.* The Fruit is used, which enters the Composition of Chocolate. This is nutritious like the former, but somewhat heavier, and with more Difficulty raised into a Fermentation: for which Reason the Peasants in *France* usually roast, or parch it, by which Means it loses its Viscidity; it is very aperitive, and therefore proper in the Nephritic Colic. The Meal is of Service in emollient and suppurating Cataplasms; for, by its Viscidity, it obstructs the Pores, and is very proper for suppurating Imposthumes.

Another Species of *Triticum,* is the *Triticum spicâ Hordei Londinensibus,* Tourn. Inst. *Zeopyrum,* Offic. *Zeopyrum seu Tritico-speltum,* C. B. P.

Hordeum nudum sive Gymnocrithon, J. B. Naked Barley. It is sown in *Germany,* where it serves to make Bread, and other Sorts of Food, and is no less used than Barley. It is of a refrigerating Quality, like the *Hordeum,* or Barley, being administered in Broths to extinguish Thirst.

Triticum vaccinium, Cow Wheat. See *Melampyrum.*

Tubera, Offic. J. B. *Tubera terræ Edibilia,* Park. Truffles, or Trubs. These are more used in Cookery than in Physic, but however have the Reputation of stimulating to Venery; boil'd and made into a Kind of Plaister, they are recommended as an external Application in a Quinsey.

Tulipa, Offic. *Tulipa præcox lutea,* C. B. P. The Tulip. It grows in Gardens, flowering in the Spring. The Root is used, which is said by some to be possess'd of the same Virtues as the Potatoes, or Parsnips.

Tunica, a Name for the *Caryophyllus ruber,* or Clove Gilly Flower.

Turbith & Turpethum, Offic. *Turpethum repens foliis Althææ, vel Indicum,* C. B. P. *Convolvulus Indicus, Alatus, Maximus, foliis Ibisco nonnihil similibus, angulosis,* Raii Hist. Turbith. It grows plentifully in *Ceylon* and *Malabar,* in the *East Indies.* The Root is used. Turbith is a pretty strong Cathartic, purging tough serous Humours from the remote Parts; and thereby helps the Dropsy, Gout and Rheumatism; and is put into several of the stronger purging Compositions.

Turbith Gallorum, French Turbith. This is already specify'd under the Article *Thapsia.*

Turritis, Offic. *Turritis vulgatior,* J. B. *Brassica sylvestris sive Brassicæ affinis Turritis dicta,* Pluk. Almag. Tower Mustard. This grows in sandy Hillocks, flowering in *June.* The Herb is used; the

Juice

Juice of which is by some, recommended for Ulcers of the Mouth, and for killing Worms.

Tuſſilago, Farfara, Offic. *Tuſſilago vulgaris,* C. B. Colts-Foot. It grows in moist Places, flowering in *February* and *March.* The Flowers, Roots, Stalks, and Leaves are used. They are of a penetrating, heating, and lenitive Quality; for which Reason, they incide thick and pituitous Humours contained in the Lungs; and are good in Coughs, Consumptions, and Pleuriſies. The recent Leaves bruiſed in a Mortar, and boiled with double the Quantity of Sugar, are excellent in a *Phthiſis*; an Exulceration of the Kidneys; a long continued ulcerous *Gonorrhæa*; and Diſorders of the Stomach ariſing from Phlegm. Colts-Foot is accounted *alexipharmic,* becauſe it excites Sweat. The recent Leaves, applied externally, are beneficial for the Cure of Ulcers and Inflammations. Its Juice drank for ſome Days, is ſaid to cure Quartan Agues. The Leaves are bitter, glutinous, and a little ſtyptic; they have the Taſte of an Artichoak, and give but a very faint Tincture of Red to the blue Paper. There ſeems to be in this Plant a Salt reſembling that of Coral, involved in Sulphur, and a great deal of viſcous Phlegm. A ſtrong Decoction of the Leaves is eſteem'd excellent in the King's Evil, if duly perſiſted in.

Typha, Offic. *Typha paluſtris major,* C. B. P. Cat's Tail, or Reed Mace. This is found in Marſhes, and on the Brinks of Rivulets. The Flowers are uſed, which when mix'd with well waſhed Hog's Lard, cure Burns.

Vaccaria, Offic. *Lychnis ſegetum Rubra foliis Perfoliatæ,* C. B. P. Cow Baſil. It grows among Corn, flowering in *June* and *July.* The Seeds are uſed. It is heating, and drying; and provokes Urine.

Vaccinia, Offic. *Vaccinia nigra fructu majore,* Park. Theat. *Vitis Idæa foliis ſubrotundis exalbidis,* C. B. P. The great Bill-berry. It grows in mountainous Places, flowering in *May.* The Berries are uſed, which are ſaid to be poſſeſs'd of an inebriating Quality; whence they are call'd by the *Germans Tunckel Becren.*

Vaccinia nigra, Myrtillus, Offic. *Vitis Idæa foliis oblongis, crenatis fructu nigricante,* C. B. P. Black Whortles. It grows in ſtony Places, flowering in *May.* The Berries are uſed, which are cooling, and drying. with a manifeſt Aſtriction. They are good for a hot Stomach, quench Thirſt, mitigate the Heat of burning Fevers, bind the Belly, ſtop Vomiting, and are effectual in the *Cholera Morbus.*

Vaccinia Urſi, Park. Theat. *Vitis Idæa,* Offic. *Vaccinia Urſi, ſive Uva Urſi apud Cluſium,* Ger. Emac. Spaniſh Whortles. They grow in *Italy,* and other Southern Countries, flowering in *May.* The Fruit is uſed; which is ſaid by *Dioſcorides* to be good for exceſſive Fluxes of the Belly, Menſes, and all Kinds of Hæmorrhages.

Valeriana Græca, a Name for the *Polemonium,* Greek Valerian, or Jacob's Ladder.

Valeriana major, ſive Phu majus, Offic. *Valeriana hortenſis,* Ger. Emac. Garden Valerian. It grows in Gardens, flowering in *June.* The Root and Leaves are uſed. It is a lexipharmic, ſudorific, and diuretic. It is principally uſed in Weakneſs of the Sight, Peſtilence, Aſthma, inveterate Cough, Pleuriſy, Obſtructions of the Liver and Spleen, Stoppage of the Ureters, Hernia, and the Jaundice; and is by ſome accounted a good Vulnerary, and Antiſcorbutie, and is effectual in all Diſorders proceeding from cold, viſcid, and aqueous Humours, and to be effectual in an Epilepſy.

Va-

Valeriana minor, & Phu minus, Offic. *Valeriana minor pratenfis vel aquatica,* J. B. Small Valerian. It grows in moift Meadows, flowering in *May.* The Roots and Leaves are ufed, which as they refemble thofe of the following in outward Appearance, fo are they fuppofed to agree with them in Virtues, tho' in an inferior and milder Degree.

Valeriana fylveftris, Offic. *Valeriana fylveftris magna aquatica,* J. B. Great wild Valerian. It grows in Woods and Thickets, and alfo about watry Places, flowering in *May, June,* and *July.* The Root is ufed; the Powder of which, to the Quantity of Half a Spoonful, in Wine or any other proper Liquor, is a certain Remedy for the Epilepfy. They exhibit it in Milk, in a fmaller Dofe for Boys, and young People. It is good for Ruptures, Convulfions, and for Bruifes receiv'd from Falls. It is alfo good for Inflammations and Exulcerations of the Mouth and Gums, and for *Aphthæ.* It cures a Tertian Fever. The Leaves of this Plant have no Smell, but an herby, faltifh, bitter Tafte; and give a pretty deep Tincture of red to the blue Paper; the Roots ftain it a little; they are bitter and ftyptic, of an aromatic penetrating Smell, and fomething difagreeable.

Valerianella, arvenfis præcox humilior, femine depreffo, Tourn. Inft. *Lactuca agnina,* Offic. *Locufta Herba prior,* J. B. Lamb's Lettuce, or Corn Sallad. It grows among Corn, and in Gardens, flowering in the Spring. It is cooling and moiftening; being in Temperament and Virtues, not unlike Lettuce, and fupplies its Room in Winter, and the Beginning of Spring. It is eaten among Sallads, and is reckon'd the beft Ingredient among them.

Vanilia, Vanelloes. See *Banilia.*

Veratrum. White Hellebore, See *Helleborus albus.*

Verbafcum, Tapfus barbatus, Offic. *Verbafcum mas latifolium luteum,* C. B. P. Mullein. It grows by the Sides of Ditches, flowering in *July.* The Leaves and Flowers are ufed. The Leaves are of an herby Tafte, a little faltifh and ftyptic; they fmell like Elder; and give a pretty deep Tincture of red to the blue Paper: The Flowers give it a deeper: They are alfo ftyptic, but fweet. It is probable that the Salt of this Plant, in fome meafure, refembles that of Coral. The Leaves bruifed, and applied to any Part affected with Pain, remove the fame: They are of a demulcent Quality; for which Reafon they are an Ingredient in Decoctions, Clyfters, and Cataplafms, in all Diforders where Acrimony offends; being of great Service by their infipid, vifcous, emollient, and faponaceous Juice. Of the Flowers, with a Solution of Oil of Olives is prepared Oil of *Verbafcum,* which is very good to confolidate Wounds, and to mitigate Pains; and taken inwardly is a Laxative. The Flowers are made into a Conferve, which is excellent againft all Hæmorrhages, Spitting of Blood from Contufions, bloody Urine, immoderate Fluxes of the *Menfes* or *Lochia,* the *Tenefmus,* Dyfentery, and the falling down of the *Uterus* and *Anus.* The Decoction of the Leaves is effectual in the Colic, *Diarrhæa* and Dyfentery, and a Decoction of the Flowers makes a good Gargarifm in the Quinfey, and a violent Cough: The Leaves boiled in Milk, are effectual in the *Tenefmus* and *Hæmorrhoids.* The Juice of this Plant is of great Efficacy in the Gout. The Decoction of the Leaves in Water is ufed in Clyfters, as an Emollient for the *Hæmorrhoids;* and may alfo be injected into the *Uterus,* for the Purpofe of mollifying. The Plant, in fhort, is emollient, aperient, and

and relaxing; and therefore enters the Composition of all emollient Clysters and Cataplasms. Outwardwardly the Leaves and Flowers are useful Topics, in mitigating all Kinds of Pains, particularly in Tumors of the *Anus*, and in the *Hæmorrhoids*.

Verbascum album, Offic. *Verbascum Lychnitis flore albo parvo*, C. B. P. Mullein with white Flowers. It grows in several Places by Path-ways, flowring in *August*. The Leaves are used, which agree in Virtues with those of the preceeding.

Verbascum nigrum, Offic. *Verbascum nigrum flore ex luteo purpurascente*, C. B. P. Black Mullein. It grows by the Sides of Ditches, flowering in *July* and *August*. The Root, Leaves and Flowers are used. The Root is astringent, and of Service in a Looseness. The Leaves and Flowers agree in Virtues with those of the common *Verbascum*.

Verbena, Offic. *Verbena communis flore cæruleo*, C. B. P. Vervain. It grows in Highways, flowering in the Summer. The Root and Herb are used. It is cephalic, alexipharmic, and vulnerary, and is principally used in Pains, Affections of the Head, inveterate Coughs, Obstructions of the Liver and Spleen, the Jaundice, and Dysentery, to break and expel the Stone, and for Tertian Fevers. The Root is accounted by some as an effectual Amulet against scrumous Tumors; and is hung about the Neck, by some old Women, as an efficacious Medicine for those Purposes. The Powder of the Leaves is good for the Dropsy. The Leaves bruised, and applied in the Form of a Cataplasm, is a very good Resolvent in Pains of the Sides, and the Pleurisy. The distilled Water, as well as the Juice, cure Inflammations of the Eyes, and all Sorts of Wounds, increase Milk in Women who give Suck, and give Relief under a flatulent Colic. This Plant yields

by the chymical Analysis, several acrid Liquors, a great deal of Oil, and a pretty deal of volatile concrete Salt and Earth: Thus it may contain some *Sal Ammoniac*, united with a great deal of Sulphur.

Veronica fœmina, *Elatine*, Offic. *Elatine folio subrotundo*, C. B. P. *Veronica fœmina Fuchsii sive Elatine*, Ger. Emac. Female Fluellin. It grows in Fields, flowering in *July*. The Herb is used, which is vulnerary. The express'd Juice either internally taken, or externally applied, is said to be good for sordid and cancerous Ulcers. The Leaves boiled are good for a Dysentery. The Leaves are very bitter, a little styptic, and have a Smell a little oily; they hardly give any Tincture of red to the blue Paper. Whence we may conjecture, their Salt very much resembles the natural Salt in the Earth, being joined with a great deal of Sulphur, and terrestrial Parts.

Veronica mas, *Betonica Pauli*, Offic. *Veronica mas supina & vulgatissima*, C. B. P. Male Speedwell. It grows in dry Pastures. The Herb is used. It is commended for subduing Phlegm, for deterging the first Passages, for pulmonic Diseases, the Scurvy, *Phthisis*, and Stone, being boiled with Liquorice. Infused in Water, it impregnates it with the Smell, Taste, and all the Virtues of the *Chinese* Tea, and has the same Effects. It relaxes with a moderate Astriction, whence it is recommended in a Scurvy, proceeding from Relaxation; it is proper also, in spitting of Blood, because it has an astringent and somewhat of an aromatic Virtue; it heats, dries, strengthens, and resists Putrefaction. It is very penetrating; for, if it be tasted, it affects the whole Mouth, as if it were set on Fire. It affords not much Salt, but a very copious Humour; and has the Virtue of resolving the Humours. The Decoction of the Herb in Whey, daily drank, cures the Scurvy, as we are assured by *Eugalenus* and *Sennertus*, and resolves scorbutic Tumors ; it is good, also, against the *Scabies.* The Juice drank for a long time together, is effectual against the Gout ; for let the Patient take but two or three Ounces every Day for a Month together, and all the morbific Matter will be discharged out of the Blood by Urine, as is said. The Juice may be preserved a long time in Winter, if to the Quantity of one Ounce you put four Drops of the Spirit of Sulphur by the Bell. It incides viscid Phlegm molesting the Lungs, and is good in Coughs, Colic, *Nephritis, Phthisis,* and the Itch : It is excellent in Clysters for the Colic. The Infusion of it in Wine is effectual in the *Chlorosis ;* and the Powder, according to *Cæsalpinus,* cures the Dropsy. The Juice cures Intermittent Fevers ; the distilled Water depurates the Eyes ; and a Gargarism, prepared of a Decoction of the Leaves, cures the Quinsey. The Use of it, after the manner of Tea, is effectual in Obstructions of the Spleen, Pancreas, and Mesentery ; it is of excellent Use in the Head-ach and *Vertigo,* is of Service in the *Fluor Albus,* and all cutaneous Diseases, as well as a Cancer. I have cured, says *Boerraave,* in his *Hist. Plant.* a hundred Diseases with this Plant; for it has the Virtue of dissolving pituitous, viscous, oleous, and almost all other Kinds of Humours. An Infusion of *Veronica,* is recommended by *Heister,* to be used warm, as a Resolvent in an *Epiphora,* or *Oculus Lacrymans ;* he further observes, that this Infusion is highly commended by *Schobinger,* a Disciple of St. *Yves,* for an incipient *Fistula Lachrymalis.* The Leaves of this Plant are bitter, and give a pretty deep red Colour to the blue Paper, which gives us Reason to believe, that their Salt very much resembles

that of Coral ; but that of the Speedwell is charged with a great deal more Acid than the ordinary Salt of Coral, and is joined besides with a great deal of Sulphur : For, by the Chymical Analysis, we obtain from this Plant, a great deal of Earth, Acid and Oil.

Veronica Teucrii facie, Park. Theat. *Chamædrys spuria angustifolia,* Offic. J. B. *Veronica supina,* Ger. Emac. Germander Speedwell. It grows in Botanic Gardens, flowering in *June.* The Herb is used, which agrees in Virtues with the preceeding.

Veronica minor, Hist. Oxon. *Chamædrys spuria latifolia,* Offic. J. B. Bastard Germander. It is cultivated in Gardens, flowering in *June.* The Herb is used, which agrees in Virtues with the Male Speedwell.

Vetonica. A Name for the *Caryophyllus ruber,* or Clove Gilly Flower.

Viburnum, Offic. *Lantana vulgo, aliis Viburnum,* J. B. The Wayfaring Tree. It grows in Hedges, flowering in Summer, and the Berries are ripe in *September.* The Leaves and Berries are used, and are drying and astringent ; whence they are commended for Inflammations of the Tonsils and Throat, the falling down of the *Uvula,* the Looseness of the Teeth, and Fluxes of the Belly.

Vicia, Offic. *Vicia vulgaris sativa,* J. B. Common Tare. It is sown in Fields. The Seeds are used. Tares are heating, drying, cleansing, abstersive, and astringent.

Vicia alba, Offic. *Vicia sativa alba,* C. B. P. White Tare. It is sometimes sown in Gardens. The Seeds are used, which agree in Virtues with the preceeding.

Vicia lutea, foliis Convolvuli minoris, C. B. P. *Aphaca,* Offic. Yellow Vetchling. It grows among Corn, flowering in *June.* The Seeds are used, which are possess'd of an

astrinftringent Quality, by Virtue of which they ftop Fluxes of the Belly and Stomach, if roafted.

Vicia fylveftris, Aracus, Offic. *Vicia femine rotundo nigro,* C. B. P. Strangle Tare, or Wild Vetch. It grows in Hedges, and among Corn, flowering in the Spring. The Herb is ufed, which agrees in Virtues with the other Species.

Victoralis. Spotted Ramfons. A Species of *Allium,* which fee.

Vinca pervinca, Offic. *Vinca pervinca vulgaris,* Park. Theat. *Pervinca vulgaris anguftifolia flore caruleo,* C. B. P. Periwinkle. It grows in Fields, flowering in *May.* The Herb is ufed. It is vulnerary, and is principally ufed in Fluxes of the Belly, a Dyfentery, Hæmorrhoids, fpitting of Blood, Hæmorrhages of the Nofe, and for an Excefs of the *Catamenia.*

Vinca Pervinca Officinarum, Buxb. *Pervinca vulgaris latifolia flore caruleo,* Tourn. Inft. The greater Periwinkle. It grows by the Sides of Ditches, flowering in *April.* The Herb is ufed, which agrees in Virtues with the preceeding.

Vincetoxicum. Swallow-wort. See *Afclepias.*

Viola, Offic. *Viola Martia purpurea,* J. B. Purple Violets. They grow in Hedges, and about the Sides of Ditches, flowering in *March.* The Leaves, Flowers, Seeds and Roots are ufed. The Leaves are emollient and laxative, and are ufed in Fomentations, Cataplafms, and Clyfters. The Flowers have an Anodyne, demulcent and antiphlogiftic Virtue ; they are infufed in the pureft Rain Water, from whence by often repeating the fame, is prepared the *Syrupus Violarum fine Coctione,* by adding four times the Weight of Sugar. This Syrup is very palatable, gently opening, corrects every thing acrimonious, and loofens the Belly. The Seeds are potent Hydragogues, but

are feldom ufed except in Obftructions of the Kidneys, and the Nephritic Colic. The Root purges upwards and downwards. This Plant is pectoral and cordial, and proper in Coughs, Drynefs of the Tongue, and Afperities of the *Fauces,* as alfo, in Catarrhs, *Phthifis,* and the Pleurify. It is principally ufed to mitigate the Heat of Fevers, and for the Head-ach. The Root of this Plant is a little faltifh, glutinous, and deterfive ; neither it, nor the Leaves, which are infipid, and pretty glutinous, give any Tincture of red to the blue Paper ; the frefh Seeds give it a little, and are falter than the Roots. There is a glutinous Sap in the Violets, which clogs the other Principles, and hinders their Motion : For, by the Chymical Analyfis, we obtain from this Plant feveral acid Liquors, a great deal of Oil, a pretty deal of volatile, concrete, and fixed lixivial Salt.

Viola tricolor, Offic. *Viola tricolor hortenfis repens,* C. B. P. *Jacea tricolor five Trinitatis flos,* J. B. Heart's Eafe. It grows in Gardens, flowering in *May.* The Herb is ufed, which agrees in Virtues with the preceeding. Dr. *Baynard* fays it is a Cure for Madnefs.

Viola Lunaria, Offic. *Viola lunaria major filiquâ oblongâ,* C. B. P. Sattin Flower with long Pods. It flowers in *May.* The Leaves are ufed. A certain *Swifs* Surgeon, as *Camerarius* fays, prepared a good vulnerary Ointment of the bruifed Leaves of this Herb and Sanicle.

Viola Mariana, Offic. *Viola Mariana Dodonæi quibufdam Medium,* J. B. *Campanula hortenfis folio & flore oblongo,* C. B. P. Coventry Bells. It is cultivated with us in Gardens, flowering in the Summer. The Root, which is feldom ufed in Medicine. is as a Food, efteemed refrigerating, drying, and aftringent.

Viperaria. Viper's Grafs. The fame as *Scorzonera.*

Virga aurea, Offic. *Virga aurea vulgaris latifolia,* J. B. Golden Rod. This Plant, as we are told by *Tournefort,* is a Native of *Canada,* but is now common throughout *Europe,* becaufe the Seeds brought from that Country have diffufed themfelves thro' all the *European* Regions, and grow without Difficulty. It flowers in *August.* This Plant is fo acrimonious, that no Pepper can be compared with it, tho' it leaves not the leaft Relifh of Acridnefs in the Mouth, but proceeds thro' the whole Body. It is like the *Ranunculus acris* of the Shops, and is of a moderately or fomewhat aftringent Tafte, which at firft is not unpleafant, but leaves an ungrateful Relifh in the Mouth. *Barclay* in his *Satyricon* fays, that he cured a Perfon of Quality, to whom he was fent on an Embaffy, of the Stone, and a Suppuration of the Kidneys, with the Powder of the dry'd Leaves. Three or four Ounces of the Plant macerated in Water, are a good vulnerary Dofe, and proper for internal Hæmorrhages, the Dyfentery and *Diarrhæa.* Externally it depurates Wounds, abfterges Putridnefs of the Gums, faftens loofe Teeth, and cleanfes malignant Ulcers and Fiftulas. I have often exhibited it, (fays *Boerhaave* in his *Hift. Plant.*) with great Succefs, in all Sorts of putrid, vifcid, and cold Indifpofitions. The Leaves duly dry'd, and infus'd after the manner of Tea, and drunk with an Addition of Honey, are highly corroborative and deterfive, and of extraordinary Efficacy in Ulcers of the Lungs, and Wounds of the Breaft, and other Parts. Golden Rod is ftyptic, bitter, and gives no Tincture of red to the blue Paper. It is likely that its Salt refembles that which is natural in the Earth; but it is mixed with a great deal of Oil, and terreftrial Parts.

Virga Pastoris. Shepherd's Rod. See *Dipsacus.*

Viscum, Offic. *Viscum baccis albis,* C. B. P. *Viscus quercus & aliarum arborum,* J. B. Miffel, and Miffeltoe. It grows upon feveral Trees, but efpecially upon the Oak, which laft is moft efteem'd. The Wood, Leaves, and the glutinous Matter which is found in the Berries, and Bark, called Birdlime are ufed. The Wood is of principal and fpecific Ufe in the Epilepfy ; it is alfo prefcribed for the Apoplexy and Vertigo, taken inwardly, or hung about the Neck : For thefe Diforders it is acknowledged to be effectual, by the unanimous Confent of antient and modern Phyficians. We know fome, fays *J. Bauhine,* who have made ufe of the Wood of *Viscum,* macerated in Wine, with Succefs againft the Vertigo. The Powder of *Viscum,* efpecially what grows upon Oaks, not only cures the Epilepfy, but provokes the *Menfes.* It is alfo an *Arcanum* againft a Pleurify, being taken once, and again, and a third Time, in Water of *Carduus* and Poppy. *J. Bauhine* writes that he has feveral Times advifed the Ufe of *Viscum,* bruifed and macerated in proper Waters, againft Worms of the Inteftines in Children. The Powder of the *Viscum* which grows on the *Oxyacanthus,* being infufed in white or *Spanish* Wine, and given two Hours before the Paroxyfm, or Fit, and the Dofe repeated, if neceffary, has often removed, and perfectly cured a Quartan. The Leaves after they have been chewed, and ground by the Teeth of labouring Beafts, and Cows, are by our ruftic People, efteemed effectual for expelling the *Secundines.* The Birdlime, or Glue, ufed for Fowling, was much employ'd by the Antients in Medicine. It has the Virtue of mollifying and difcuffing Tumors, the *Parotides* and Abfceffes, being mixed with Rofin, and

an

an equal Quantity of Wax; it also cures the *Epinyctides,* and, as *Pliny* says, dries up strumous Ulcers, and cures the Epilepsy. It is good for many other Disorders, according to *Dioscorides, Pliny,* and *Galen.*

Visnaga, Offic. J. B. *Gingidium umbella longa,* C. B. P. *Fœniculum annuum, umbellâ contractâ, oblongâ,* Tourn. Inst. Spanish Pick Tooth. It is cultivated with us in Gardens, flowering in Summer. The Leaves are us'd. The Pedicles or Footstalks, of the Umbellas, on account of their Stiffness, and sweet Scent, serve for Tooth-picks, with many Persons, especially among the *Spaniards,* whence we call it *Spanish Pick Tooth.* It agrees in Medicinal Virtues with Fennel.

Vitex. The Chaste Tree. See *Agnus Castus.*

Vitis, Offic. *Vitis vinifera,* Commel. Plant. Usual. The Vine. This is a Vegetable too well known to require any Description. The Leaves and the Tendrils of the Vine are refrigerating and astringent, and are us'd in Dysenteries, Vomiting, a *Pica,* Spitting of Blood, and other Hæmorrhages. The Juice which distils from the young Shoots when cut, taken internally, has the Reputation of breaking and expelling the Stone: Externally it is said to cure Dimness of the Sight, Redness of the Eyes, and cutaneous Eruptions. The immature Grapes are refrigerating, drying and astringent, and are us'd to excite an Appetite, and check a Diarrhœa. The ripe Grapes, and their unfermented Juice, are extremely saponaceous, resolvent and detergent, and if taken in pretty large Quantities, will excite a *Diarrhœa,* with very good Effects, if not carry'd too far. The *Acini* or Grape Stones, are esteem'd astringent, and are recommended in Vomitings and Fluxes. Wine, Vinegar, and

Tartar, are produc'd from the Juice of the Grape after Fermentation, and these are taken Notice of under their respective Articles.

Vitis Corinthiaca, sive Apyrina, J. B. *Uva Passa minores, Passulæ,* Offic. *Corinthiacæ;* Park. Theat. The Currant Vine. It is cultivated in *Zant* and *Cephalonia.* The ripe Fruit dry'd, is used. It is cooling, mitigates febrile Heat, allays Thirst, and purges the Belly.

Another is the *Uva passa major,* Offic. *Uva passa major, Βημας Grœcis forte,* C. B. P. Raisins of the Sun. They are brought to us from *Spain,* and are hot or temperate, lenient, loosen the Belly, correct Acrimony, are grateful to the Stomach, Lungs, and Liver, and mitigate a Cough.

Vitis alba, a Name for the *Bryonia alba,* or White Bryony.

Vitis Idæa. See *Vaccinia.*

Vitis marina, a Name for the *Fucus folliculaceus,* or Sea Lentils.

Ulmaria, Regina Prati, Offic. *Ulmaria, Barba Capri floribus compactis,* C. B. P. Meadow Sweet. It grows in moist Meadows, flowering in *July.* The Herb is used. It is antispasmodic, Antiepileptic, corroborative and astringent. Hence it is used by the Peasants for a Dysentery, *Diarrhœa,* and to repress Vomiting. It is of Service in regulating the disorderly Motions of the Heart, Blood, and Spirits; and wherever Condensation, Strengthing, and Astriction, are required, this Herb is of excellent Use. The Leaves are good for an Hæmoptoe; and the bruised Root is applied to Wounds, in order to stop the Blood, and consolidate the Part. A Decoction of the Root is proper in malignant Fevers. The Leaves have an herby, saltish and glutinous Taste; they give a faint red Colour to the blue Paper; the Root gives it a deep one; it is styptic, and a little bitter; its

Salt feems to refemble *Sal Ammoniac*; but it is united with a great deal of Sulphur, and a pretty deal of Earth. By the Chymical Analyfis it yields fome acid Liquors, and fome volatile concrete Salt, a good Quantity of Sulphur, and a pretty deal of Earth.

Ulmus, Offic. J. B. *Ulmus campeftris & Theophrafti,* C.B.P. Common Elm. It grows in Hedges, and the Bark and Leaves are ufed. The Bark is faid to have an agglutinating Virtue, to mitigate Arthritic and Ifchiadic Pains, to purge, and carry off Phlegm and Water. A Decoction of the internal Bark, is frequently us'd as a Gargarifm, in Quinfeys, and Afperities of the *Fauces.* The Leaves are aftringent.

Ulmus montana, Offic. C. B. P. *Ulmus latiore folio,* Park. Theat. The Wych Hafel. It grows frequently in Hedges. The Bark is ufed, which agrees in Virtues with the preceeding.

Umbilicus Veneris. This is already taken Notice of under the Article *Cotyledon.*

Urtica, Offic. *Urtica major vulgaris,* J. B. Common Stinging Nettle. It grows in Hedges, and among Rubbifh. The Nettle is furnifhed with fmall, flender Spines, of fo flexile a Nature at the Extremities, that when they enter the Skin they eafily bend; but when they penetrate the Flefh they cannot be drawn forth, but are there broken off as it were into Fragments, and excite an Inflammation and Veficles, which continue till the Pieces are expelled. The Decoction of the Leaves is aperitive, and commended againft the Gout. The greeneft and frefheft Stalks are ufed to whip the Limbs affected with the Gout or Palfy, in order to excite an Inflammation in the external Parts. This Plant is of Service in the Difeafes of the Kidneys and Bladder, Coughs, *Phthifis,* internal Hæmorrhages, *Hæmoptyfis,* Vomiting of Blood, an immoderate Flux of the Hæmorrhoids, and Bloody Urine. The Leaves bruifed and apply'd, refift a Gangrene, and a Decoction of them drank in the Manner of Tea, is an excellent Laxative. The Leaves of Nettles have an infipid, glutinous Tafte, and give no Tincture of red to the blue Paper; the Roots ftain it very little; they are infipid alfo, but a little ftyptic; from which we may conjecture, that the Nettles contain a Salt refembling that which is naturally in the Earth, that is to fay, compofed of *Sal Ammoniac,* Nitre, and Marine Salt; but in thefe Plants it is clogged with a great deal of glutinous Phlegm, and united with abundance of Sulphur and terreftrial Parts: For, by the Chymical Analyfis we obtain from Nettles fome volatile concrete Salt, a great deal of Sulphur and Earth, and feveral Liquors, which give a greater Indication of an acrid, than an acid Salt; fo that it is very probable, that the Phlegm of this Herb is thicken'd rather by the terreftrial Parts, than by the acid: But this thick Phlegm which is very confiderable, is entirely deftroyed by the Fire.

Urtica Romana, Offic. *Urtica Romana five mas cum globulis,* J. B. Roman Nettle. It grows in fandy Places, and the Seeds are ufed, which are recommended in Pulmonary Affections, the *Afthma,* ftubborn Coughs, Pleurify and Peripneumony.

Urtica mortua. A Name for the *Lamium album,* or white Archangel.

Ufnea Cranii Humani, Offic. *Mufcus ex Cranio Humano,* Ger. Emac. Mofs of a dead Man's Skull. This Species of Herb which adheres to the Sculls of Carcafes expofed to the Air, is by different Authors recommended as highly beneficial in various Difeafes. Thus it is extol'd as a Specific in Epilepfies, and all Diforders of the Head; in Hæmorrhages

pro-

produced by whatever Cause, and in Dysenteries. It is used internally, externally, alone, mixed with other Substances, and as an Amulet. In Hæmorrhages it produces its Effects, if only held in the Hand. Thus Boyle, in his Specifics, informs us, that he himself had an Hæmorrhage of the Nose stopt by using it in this Manner. Juncker whimsically informs us, that it renders the Body so impenetrable as not to be pierced with a Musket Bullet. Some affirm, that the Virtues of that Usnea are greater, which has been gathered from the Sculls, during a certain Position of the Stars; when for Instance, the Moon is in the Increase in the House of Venus, when she is in Pisces, Taurus, or Libra. Others affirm, that the Usnea gathered from the Heads of hang'd Persons is best. But Paracelsus asserts, that what is found on the Sculls of Persons broken on the Wheel is no less valuable. Grube in Arcan. Med. informs us, that those who greatly extol the Usnea in Medicine, suppose that the Vital and Animal Spirits of the deceased Person are collected in it, and by a certain Medicinal Force derived to any Part affected in a living Person. But as every one knows, that a Carcase has neither Vital nor Animal Spirits, those seem to be in the right who give no Credit to the peculiar Power of this Plant, or its specific Virtues in removing obstinate Disorders. But Juncker affirms, that the Virtues of this Plant are founded on Credulity, or some other Error. Besides, the Force of Imagination may be supposed to co-operate strongly with this Medicine, as Boyle thinks, when he informs us, that if a certain Person when Blood was taking from him, took Usnea in his Hand for the Sake of Curiosity, the Blood ceased to flow till he laid it aside again. Marx, a celebrated

Dealer in Aromatics in Nuremberg, does not hesitate to affirm, that the Usnea of the Human Cranium is of no other Use but to be preserved as a Rarity. And Boecler is of Opinion, that, as with the Bones of dead Bodies, so also with the Usnea many superstitious and impious Things are done. But Rieger is of Opinion, that in Hæmorrhages, where styptic Tents or Pessaries are expedient, the Usnea mixed with other proper Ingredients, may produce happy Effects. Besides where exsiccant and astringent Medicines are proper, its Powder, whether used externally or internally, must certainly produce some Effect; for it is of a drying and astringent Nature. Thus I agree (says Rieger) with Pauli, who speaks in this Manner: "Though the Usnea may produce good Effects in Spittings of "Blood, Hæmorrhages, and other "Fluxes; yet there is no Necessity "why a Physician should disgrace "his Profession by prescribing it, "since there are other Substances "equally astringent, and which no "Patient will refuse on account of "the Horror and Nausea they "produce." Etmuller informs us, that some supply the Place of the true Usnea with the Moss of a Tile, which in Hæmorrhages of the Nose they immerse in Vinegar, and apply to the Crown of the Head; whereas instead of the true Usnea, which is rare, others use one of the artificial Kind, which they obtain in the following Manner: They take the Moss of large Meadow Stones, gathered in the Month of April; this, when gently dried, they reduce to a gross Powder in a Glass Mortar, sprinkling it with Malmsey Wine, till it has acquired the Consistence of a thick Poultice. Then with a Knife they spread this Preparation very thin on the Cranium of a Carcase broken on the Wheel. As it becomes gradually dry, they fpread more of it on the *Cranium,* which in the open Air they expofe to the Rays of the Sun, removing it when Rains come on. This they repeat till the Plant begins to flourifh, and afterwards gather from it an *Ufnea* not inferior to that which grows fpontaneoufly from the Scull. *Ludovicus,* when treating of Vulneraries and Aftringents, fpeaks thus: " Mofs may be every-where " found ; and that obtained from " the Oak, and the common *E-* " *gyptian* Thorn, for Medicinal " Purpofes, in Peffaries ; for In- " ftance, Tents, and Ointments " are not inferior to the *Ufnea,* ga- " thered in the moft fuperftitious " Manner, or even that growing on " Human Sculls."

Uva crifpa, Goofe Berries. See *Groffularia.*

Uva Graina, Offic. *Vitis Idæa paluftris Virginiana, fruɛtu majore;* Raii Hift. Crane Berries. They are brought from *New England,* and are fuppofed to be excellent againft the Scurvy.

Uva marina, Sea Grape, or Shrub Horfe-tail. See *Ephedra.*

Uva $\begin{cases} paffa\ major. \\ paffa\ minor. \end{cases}$ See *Vitis.*

Uva Urfi. Spanifh Whortles. See *Vaccinia Urfi.*

Vulneraria. A Name for the *Anthyllis leguminofa,* or Kidney Vetch.

Uvularia. A Name for the *Biflingua,* or double Tongue.

Winteranus Cortex, Winters Cinnamon. See *Cortex Winteranus.*

Xanthium, Loufe Burr. This is already fpecify'd under the Article *Bardana.*

Xochinacaztlis, feu *Flos Auriculæ.* Hern. *Fruɛtus oblongus, cineraceus acidulus,* C. B. P. *Orejuelas, feu Orichelas,* Hughes. It grows in *New Spain,* and the Flowers enter the Compofition of Chocolate, in order to give it a fine Smell, and a plea-

fant Tafte. The Plant is hot and dry, difcuffes Flatulencies, attenuates Phlegm, and heats and ftrengthens a weak and cold Stomach.

Xylo-aloes. A Name for the *Agallochum,* or Aloes Wood.

Xylobalfamum. This is the Wood of the Tree, which produces the true Balfam, or *Balfamum è Mecha.*

Xylon. The Cotton Bufh. See *Goffipium.*

Xyris. A Name for the *Iris fætida,* or Stinking-Gladdon.

Yucca, Offic. *Yucca foliis Aloes,* C. B. P. Indian Bread. It grows fpontaneoufly in *America,* and is cultivated with us in Gardens. The Root is ufed, which affords a foft Pulp, which fome condemn as Poifon, others affirm to be efculent. The recent Root eaten is poifonous, but being bruifed, then dried in the Sun, it affords a Bread commonly eaten by the *Indians.* The Juice of the Root is fo poifonous, that they take Care to convey it deep under Ground, that it may not come to the Tafte of Animals, to which it would certainly prove mortal.

Zacintha, Cichoreum verrucarium, Offic. *Chondrilla verrucaria foliis Cichorei viridibus,* C. B. P. Wart Succory. It grows in Gardens, flowering in *June.* The Herb is ufed, which is diuretic, and edulcorating, and allays the immoderate Heat of the Blood. It is reported to be of furprifing Virtue in removing Warts.

Zea, Spelta, Offic. *Zea dicœcces vel Zea major,* C. B. P. Spelt Wheat. It grows in *Italy.* The Germans make Bread of Spelt, as white as that of Wheat, but lighter, and lefs nutritive ; while new it is fweet and eafy of Concoɛtion, but when ftale it is not fo grateful, and is befides difficult of Digeftion. Broth or Gruel made of the Flour of Spelt, is aftringent, and therefore adapted to the fame Purpofes, as if prepared

with

with Rice, being proper in an *Hæmop-tyfis,* Dyfentery, *Diarrhæa,* and the like, efpecially when boiled with Calve's Feet.

Zea verna, J. B. *Olyra,* Offic. *Zea Amylea five Olyra,* C.B.P. Sprat Corn. It is fown in *Germany,* and reaped late. The Seeds are ufed in the Kitchens of *Germany.* It agrees in Virtues with the preceeding, but is fomewhat lefs nutritive.

Zea monococcos. St Peter's Corn. See *Briza.*

Zedoaria. Zedoary. We have two Kinds of this Root, as the long and the round, but they are both the Roots of the fame Plant, the Body of which is round, and the Protuberances, or Ramifications long. The Plant they belong to is a Kind of *Colchicum,* defcrib'd by *Herman* in the *Paradifus Batavus.*

The firft is thus diftinguifh'd *Zedoaria longa,* Offic. C. B. P. *Gedwar aut Geidvar,* Ger. Emac. *Zedoaria Zeylanica Camphoram redolens,* Boerh. Ind. Alt. Long Zedoary. It is brought to us from the *Eaft-Indies.* It is reckon'd attenuant, detergent, emmenagogue, carminative, anthelmintic, cordial, alexipharmic, ftomachic, diuretic, heating and drying. It difcuffes Flatulences, and is principally ufed in Pains of the Colic, and of the Stomach : It cures the Bites of venomous Animals, ftops a Lientery, repreffes Vomiting, provokes the *Menfes,* and kills all manner of *Tineæ* infefting the Belly. The Dofe is from five Grains, to half a Dram in Subftance, and it may be ufed in Infufion like Tea. Some correct *Opium* with this Root.

The fecond is diftinguifh'd thus, *Zedoaria rotunda,* Offic. C. B. P. *Malankus,* Hort. Mal. Round Zedoary. This is alfo brought from the *Eaft-Indies,* and agrees in Virtues with the preceding, but is feldom to be met with in our Shops. This Species, cut into Slices, dry'd, and preferv'd in Sugar, is more excellent and commodious for Ufe than Ginger.

Another Species of Zedoary, is the *Zerumbet,* Offic. Garz. *Zinziber latifolium fylveftre,* Comm. Hort. Amft. *Kua,* Hort. Mal. *Walingbaru,* Herm. Muf. Zeyl. Zerumbeth. It grows fpontaneoufly in the Kingdom of *Malabar,* but is not to be met with in our Shops. It agrees in Virtues with the long Zedoary.

Zeopyrum. This is already fpecify'd under the Article *Triticum.*

Zingi, Anifum Indicum, Offic. *Anifum peregrinum,* C. B. P. Indian Anife. The Kernel of this Fruit, which is brought from the *Eaft Indies,* is good for the Colic.

Zingiber, Offic. C. B. P. *Zinziber,* Ger. Emac. Ginger. It is brought from *Calecut* in the *Eaft-Indies* principally, but it is now cultivated in *Jamaica* and *Barbadoes,* from whence we are fupply'd with it, either preferv'd or dry'd. It heats powerfully, opens, incides, and attenuates, and difcuffes Flatulencies in the *Primæ Viæ.* It is efteem'd beneficial to the Stomach, *Thorax,* and all the *Vifcera.* It excites an Appetite, and refifts Putrefaction and Malignity.

Zizyphus. The Jujube. See *Jujuba.*

VEGETABLES Omitted.

ABSINTHIUM Seriphium Gallicum, Offic. C. B. P. French Sea Wormwood. It grows about the Sea Shore of *France* and *England*. The Herb is used; which agrees in Virtues with the common Wormwood.

Absinthium Santonicum, Offic. *Absinthium Santonicum Gallicum,* C. B. French Worm Seed. This is brought from *Provence* in *France*. The Herb is used, which agrees in Virtues with the *Absinthium Seriphium.*

Absinthium Santonicum Judaicum, C. B. P. *Lumbricorum Semen Rauwolfio,* J. B. Arabian Wormseed. It is brought from *Judæa* to *Alexandria*, and is said by some, to be possess'd of the same Virtues with the common Wormwood.

Acer, Offic. *Acer campestre & minus,* C. B. P. The Maple. It grows in Hedges, flowering in *May*. The Root is used, which infused in Wine, is with great Success applied in Pains of the Liver.

Acer majus, Offic. *Acer montanum candidum,* C. B. P. The great Maple. It grows in Walks, and Churchyards, flowering in *May*, and the Fruit is ripe in *September*. The Juice that distils from the wounded Tree is used in Medicine, and is supposed to be beneficial in scorbutic Disorders. In the Beginning of *Spring*, when the new Buds swell with Juice, the Tree wounded in the Trunk, Branches, or Roots, yields a sweet and potable Liquor in Abundance, as the Birch does. Some use it for their ordinary Drink. The Inhabitants of *Canada* make a Sugar out of the Juice of this Tree.

Adianthum album, folio Filicis, J. B. *Dryopteris alba,* Park. The White Oak Fern. It grows in mountainous and rocky Places. The Herb is used, which agrees in Virtues with the common *Adianthum*, to which it is a *Succedaneum*.

Agnus Scythicus, Offic. *Agnus Scythicus Borometz,* J. B. *Frutex Tartaricus,* C. B. P. The Scythian, or Tartarian Lamb. This is brought from *China* and *Tartary*. The Down of this Plant, call'd *Poco Sempie,* Offic. Golden Moss, is used, which is recommended for spitting of Blood, in a Dose of six Grains; and three Doses are said to perform a Cure. The *Chinese* frequently apply it to recent Wounds, in order to stop the Bleeding. Many fabulous Stories are related of this Plant, as that it is a *Zoophyte*, and feeds upon Grass, and other Circumstances equally ridiculous; but the Truth is, that 'tis only a Kind of arborescent Fern, made artificially, so as to have some Resemblance to a Lamb, in order to amuse the Credulous, and surprize the Unwary.

Alcyonium. Bastard Spunge. This is a Sort of spungy Plant, which is found in the Sea, or upon the Shore, or rather a Froth of the Sea, which is hardened by the Heat of the Sun, and of different Shapes and Colours. What those Bodies are which the *Greeks* call *Alcyonia*, and whence they have their Original, has been a controverted

overted Point among the Botanists, and is not yet decided. *Pliny* writes that they are the Nests of some Sort of Bird, that build in the Sea. *Imperatus* would have them to be nothing but Bits of Straws and Hair, englobated into a Mass by the Agitation of the Waters. *Schroebius* affirms, they are produced by Reeds, and their Leaves, and that in several which he cut open, he found the very Plant, the Reed, rolled up and inclosed in the Middle.

Alcyonium durum, Offic. *Alcyonium spongiosum Officinarum*, J. B. Hard Bastard Spunge. The whole Plant is used, and is recommended for the *Eryfipelas*, the Ring Worms, the Itch, the Leprosy, and all other cutaneous Disorders, and to take away Freckles from the Face, being externally applied in Powder, or in Decoction.

Alcyonium stuppofum, Offic. *Alcyonium stuppofum Imperati*, J.B. Thready Bastard Spunge. The whole Plant is used, which is resolvent, and agrees in Virtues with the preceeding.

Alcyonium tuberofum, Offic. J. B. Tuberose Bastard Spunge. The whole Plant is used, which is proper to clean the Teeth, and if it is calcined with Salt, it makes a Depilatory, or Remedy to destroy Hair.

Alcyonium vermiculatum, Offic. J. B. *Alcyonium vermiculare Imperati*, C. B. P. Vermiculate Bastard Spunge. The whole Plant is used, which is esteemed good to excite Urine; to expel the Stone of the Kidneys and Bladder; to remove Obstructions of the Spleen, and for the Dropsy; it may be taken in Powder, or in Decoction. Being burnt it makes the Hair grow, if applied to the Part, mixed with a little Wine.

All the *Alcyonia* are deterfive and discuffive, and of an acrid Quality.

Alga, Offic. *Alga angustifolia vitrariorum*, J. B. Grass Wrack. It grows in several Places about the Sea Shore. The Herb is used, which is aperitive, refrigerating, deficcative, and vulnerary, and is esteemed good for the Gout, and Inflammations, and to kill Lice and Fleas.

Aloides, *Aloe palustris*, Offic. C. B. P. *Aloe five Aizoon palustre*, J. B. Water Aloes, or Fresh Water Soldier. It grows in moist Ditches, flowering in *June*. The Herb is used, which is esteemed vulnerary.

Ambrofia campestris, Offic. *Ambrofia campestris repens*, C. B. P. *Coronopus Ruellii, feu Nasturtium verrucofum*, J. B. Swine's Cresses. It grows among Rubbish, flowering in *June*. The Herb is used, which agrees in Virtues with the *Nasturtium*.

Anchufa lutea, Offic. *Anchufa lutea major*, C. B. P. Yellow Alkanet. It grows in *Germany* and *France*, flowering in *June*. The Root is used, but is seldom to be met with in our Shops. According to *Diofcorides*, it destroys flat Worms, if taken with Hyffop and Garden Cresses.

Angfana, Offic. *Draco Arbor Indica filiquofa, Populi-folio, Angfana fel Angfava Javanica*, Commel. Hort. Amft. It grows in the *East-Indies*. The Part used in Medicine is the Liquor which diftils from the wounded Tree, and condenfes into a red Tear, wrapt in thin, reedy Coverings, as fold in the Shops. The Gum of this Tree, as the very learned and ingenious *Commelin* says, is fold in the Shops for *Sanguis Draconis*. Hence I cannot but obferve, that either our Botanical Authors are at a great Lofs, and in much Confufion and Perplexity, about what Kind of Tree this fhould be, or elfe there are feveral Sorts of Trees which produce this Gum. It is efteem'd an Aftringent, and an excellent Remedy in *Aphthæ*.

Apium Pyrenaicum Thopfiæ facie, Tourn. Inft. *Seseli Pyrenaicum Thopfiæ folio*, Raii Hift. Mountain Parfley, or the second Baftard Turbith. It

It grows on the *Pyrenean* Mountains, and the Root is used, which serves the *Spaniards* instead of the Root Turbith, but it is of a noxious Quality.

Arbor Saponaria, Offic. *Saponaria sphærulæ arboris filici-foliæ,* J. B. *Nuculæ Saponariæ non edules,* C. B. P. *Baccæ Bermudenses,* Marl. Obs. Soap Berries. It grows in *Jamaica,* and other Parts of the *West Indies;* the Fruit is ripe in *October,* and when dry, is spherical, of a reddish Colour, and less than a Gall; of a large Eye, and a bitter Taste, but no Smell, containing one round black Stone. It is greatly recommended against the *Chlorosis,* and the Berries are reckon'd a singular and specific Remedy against that Distemper, working a perfect Cure, after an ineffectual Use of Chalybeates. The Spirit, Tincture, or Extract, are more proper to be used than the crude Berries.

Arbutus, Offic. *Arbutus Comarus Theophrasti,* J. B. The Strawberry Tree. It grows in Woods and Thickets. The Fruit is used, which is of a sharp, and austere Nature, hurtful to the Stomach, and causes Head-Achs. *Amatus Lusitanus* informs us, that they distil a Water from the Leaves and Flowers of this Tree, which is esteem'd a sacred Preservative and Antidote against the Plague and Poisons.

Arbutus folio non serrato, C. B. P. *Adrachne,* Offic. *Adrachne Theophrasti,* J. B. The Strawberry Bay. It grows in *Greece,* and the Fruit is used, which agrees in Virtues with the preceeding.

Aria, Offic. *Aria Theophrasti,* Ger. Emac. *Sorbus Alpina,* J. B. The White Boam Tree. It grows in Woods, and upon rocky Mountains, flowering in *April.* The Fruit, which is the Part used, is recommended for mitigating Coughs, and promoting Expectoration.

Arnica, Offic. *Doronicum Germanicum foliis semper ex adverso nascentibus villosis,* J. B. German Leopard's Bane. It grows in mountanous Places, flowering in Summer. The whole Plant is used, which is heating and drying, and of fine Parts. It is diuretic, sudorific, and sometimes a little emetic, and is found by frequent Experience to be a Discussive and Vulnerary, and is accounted the very best and only *Panacea,* for such as have hurt themselves by Falls from high Places. The Country People use it instead of Hellebore, for the Murrain in Cattle.

Atriplex sylvestris, Offic. J. B. *Chenopodium folio laciniato comâ purpurascente,* Tourn. Inst. Wild Orache. It grows upon Dunghills, flowering in the Summer. The Herb and Seeds are used, which are said to be emollient, and either raw or boil'd, are said to discuss Boils. The Seeds taken in *Hydromel,* cure the Jaundice.

Baccharis, Offic. *Conyza major Matthioli, Baccharis quibusdam,* J. B. Plowman's Spikenard. It grows in dry mountainous Places, flowering in *Autumn.* The Leaves and Root are used. The Leaves are astringent, and are good for the Headach, Erysipelas, and Inflammations of the Eyes, being made into a Cataplasm; the Smell of them provokes Sleep. The Root boiled in Water, is effectual in Convulsions, Ruptures, Falls, Difficulty of Breathing, old Coughs, and a Difficulty of Urine, it provokes the *Menses,* and given in Wine, is good against the Bites of venomous Creatures.

Bamia Moschata, Offic. *Alcea Ægyptiaca villosa,* C. B. P. *Mosch, id est Bamia Moschata,* Alpin. Exot. Mosch-Seed. It grows in *Egypt.* The Seeds are used, which are of a smutty Colour, Kidney like, and of

a very

a very fragrant Smell, like Musk. The *Egyptians* dry them slightly, and mix the Powder in their Coffee, to make it more effectual for the strengthning of the Head, Stomach and Heart. We use it in Fumigations.

Batatas, Offic. C. B. P. J. B. *Battatas Occidentalis India,* Park. Theat. Spanish Potatoes. They grow spontaneously in both the *Indies.* They are used either boiled, or roasted under Ashes, for loosening the Belly. They are of a fine Taste, and by some preferred to our Turneps. If they are taken new, and bruised and macerated with a little Water, they ferment of their own Accord, and produce a Drink used by the Inhabitants of *Brasil.*

Bifolium, Offic. *Bifolium majus, seu Ophris major quibusdam,* J. B. *Ophris bifolia,* C. B. P. Tway-blade. It grows in Woods and Thickets, flowering in *May* and *June.* The Herb is used, which is astringent and agglutinating, good to consolidate Ruptures, and heal Wounds, tho' it is seldom used.

Blattaria, Offic. *Blattaria lutea,* J. B. Moth Mullein. It grows by the Sides of Paths, flowering in *July.* The Herb is used, which agrees in Virtues with the *Verbescum,* or common Mullein.

Blitum album minus, C. B. P. *Blitum sylvestre spicatum,* Tourn. Inst. Small White Blite. It grows in Gardens, and the Herb is used, which is refrigerating, moistening, and emollient.

Brassica sylvestris, Offic. *Brassica maritima monospermos,* C. B. P. *Crambe maritima Brassicæ folio,* Tourn. Inst. Sea Cole wort. It grows in sandy Places about the Sea Shore, flowering in *July.* The Leaves are used, which are good to heal Wounds, and discuss inflammatory and other Tumors. This Colewort is used as an Aliment, like other

Cabbage, when very young, but is esteem'd more hot and dry.

Bunium, Offic. *Daucus Petroselini vel Coriandri folio,* C.B.P. Wild Parsley. It grows in stony and rocky Places, flowering in the Summer. The Herb is used, which is diuretic, heating, and brings away the After Birth: It is good for the Spleen, Kidneys and Bladder.

Cancamum, Offic. C. B. P. This is the Tear of an *Arabian* Tree, in some measure resembling Myrrh, of a very unsavoury Taste, and used in Suffumigations. At present we know not what the *Cancamum* was. Some take it for the *Lacca. Matthiolus* asserts the *Cancamum* of the *Greeks,* and the *Lacca* of the *Arabians,* to be the same Thing; in which, says the learned *Ray,* he is mistaken; for their Virtues are different. Others will have it to be the *Benzoin; Garcias* and *Amatus* affirm it to be the *Gum Anime,* so that, it seems none can be sure what it is. *Dioscorides* says it is endued with the Virtue of extenuating immoderately fat Bodies, if half a Dram of it be taken in Water, or *Oxymel,* every Day for a considerable Time. It is prescrib'd in Disorders of the Spleen, for the Epilepsy, and the *Asthma;* and, taken in *Hydromel,* it provokes the *Menses.* Macerated in Wine, it speedily exterges Cicatrices in the Eyes, and helps Dimness of Sight, and is as good a Remedy as any for putrid Gums, and the Tooth-ach.

Cardamindum majus, Rupp. Flor. Jen. *Acriviola maxima odorata,* Boerh. Ind. Alt. The great, or sweet Indian Cress. It is cultivated with us in Gardens, flowering in the Summer. It agrees in Virtues with the *Nasturtium Indicum.*

Carlina caulifera, J. B. *Carlina caulescens magno flore,* C. B P. Carline Thistle with a Stalk. It grows in Gardens. The Root is used, which

which agrees in Virtues with the *Carlina*, or common Carline Thistle.

Carlina sylvestris, Offic. *Carlina sylvestris quibusdam, aliis Atractylis,* J. B. *Cnicus sylvestris spinosior*, C. B. P. Common wild Carline Thistle. It grows in dry Pastures, flowering in *July* and *August*. The Herb is used, and is recommended by *Wedelius* for the Head-ach, and in other Respects agrees with the *Carlina*, or common Carline Thistle.

Caucalis, Offic. *Caucalis lato Apii folio*, C. B. P. *Lappula canaria latifolia five Caucalis*, J. B. Bastard Parsley. It grows in Fields, flowering in *June* and *July*. The Herb is used, and either eaten raw, or boil'd as a Pot Herb, is recommended by *Dioscorides* to provoke Urine.

Caucalis semine aspero, C. B. P. *Pseudo-Selinum*, Offic. *Anthriscus quorundam semine aspero hispido*, J. B. Hedge Parsley. It grows in Hedges and Thickets, flowering in *July* and *August*. The Seed is used, which provokes Urine and the *Menses*.

Cepa ascalonica, Offic. *Cepa sterilis*, C. B. P. Barren Onions, Eschalots. It is cultivated in Gardens for culinary Uses. The Root is used, which is heating, drying, inciding, aperient, and provocative. It excites an Appetite, and destroys Worms in the Intestines.

Cevadilla, Offic. *Cevadilla five Hordeolum causticum Americanum*, Park. Theat. *Hordeum causticum*, C. B. P. Indian caustic Barley. It is imported from *Mexico.* The Seeds of this Plant are so extremely burning and caustic, that they may be used in Gangrenes and putrid Ulcers, instead of the actual Cautery or Sublimate. The Seed powder'd, and sprinkled in Ulcers kills Worms, which sometimes breed therein, and cleanses them.

Chaerofolium, Offic. *Chaerophyllum sativum*, C. B. P. *Chaerophyllon*, J. B. Chervil. It grows in Gardens, flowering in *May*. The Leaves and Seeds are used. Chervil is diuretic, emmenagogue and lithontriptic, and is of fine Parts; it resolves coagulated Blood, and induces Sleep. It is used in Broths with good Effect, as a Promoter of Expectoration in an *Asthma*, and externally it is of great Use in the Colic, and in a Retention of Urine.

Chrysanthemum, Offic. *Chrysanthemum foliis Matricaria*, C. B. *Dioscorides's* Corn Marygold. It is cultivated, tho' but seldom, in Gardens, flowering in the Summer. The Flowers are used, and being bruised with Cerate, are said to discuss a *Steatoma*.

Chrysanthemum segetum, Ger. Emac. *Bellis lutea foliis profunde incisis majus*, C. B. P. Corn Marygold. It is frequently found among Corn. The Flowers are used, which are extoll'd by the *Germans*, as an extraordinary Remedy for the Yellow Jaundice.

Cicutaria vulgaris, Offic. *Cicutaria alba Lugdunensis*, Ger. Emac. *Myrrhis sylvestris seminibus laevibus*, C. B. P. Wild Cicely, Cow Weed. It grows frequently in Hedges, flowering in *May*. The Herb is used, *Tragus* being persuaded it was the *Myrrhis* of *Dioscorides*, advised the Use of it for the Suppression of the Terms; but *J. Bauhine* relates a melancholy Story of two Families, that had eaten the Roots of this Plant instead of those of Parsnips. They cause Difficulty of Breathing, Torpors, and Madness.

Cirsium, Offic. *Cirsium foliis non hirsutis*, Ger. Emac. Melancholy Thistle. It grows in several Places about *Montpelier*, flowering in *June*. The Root is used, which according to *Andreas* eases the Pains of *Varices*, if bound to the Part affected

Cistus

Cistus Hypocistidem ferens, Offic. Cistus mas folio oblongo, incano, C. B. P. Cistus with the Hippocistis. grows on Rocks, Hills, and in Woods, and flowers in the Summer. The Hypocistis, which adheres to the Tops of the Clods about the Root, used in Medicine. See Hypocistis.

Cistus fæmina, Offic. Cistus fæmina folio salviæ, C. B. P. Female Holly Rose. It is cultivated in Gardens, flowering in the Summer. The Leaves and Flowers are used, which agree in Virtues with the following.

Cistus mas, Offic. Cistus mas folio rotundo, hirsutissimo, C. B. P. Male Holly Rose. It grows spontaneously in Italy and Spain, but is cultivated with us in Gardens, flowering in the Summer. The Leaves, and Flowers are used. The Plant is of an astringent Quality; for which Reason, the Flowers bruised, and drank twice a Day in austere Wine, cure the Dysentery; made into a Cataplasm by themselves, they restrain Noma, or spreading Ulcers; and in a Cerate, they heal Ambustions, and old Ulcers of the Mouth.

Another Species of Cistus, is the Cistus, Ledon foliis Rosmarini ferruginis, C. B. P. Rosmarinus sylvestris quorundam, J. B. Bohemian Rosemary. It grows in Woods, flowering in July. The Herb is used, which is of an inebriating Quality; for which Reason, in many Places of Saxony, they boil it in their Beer, to make the Peasants drunk the sooner, whose Heads, when they have drank freely of this good Liquor, are affected with it for some Days afterwards: They lay it also among Cloaths to expel Moths.

Conyza, Offic. Germ. Conyza cærulea acris, C. B. Senecio sive Erigeron cæruleus, aliis Conyza cærulea, J. B. Blue Fleabane. It grows in barren Pastures, and flowers in July and August. The Herb is used, which is said to accelerate Suppuration.

Culithruvan, Mont. Exot. This is a hot aromatic Bark, and said to be found in New Guinea, but a Stranger in the European Shops. It is said to agree in Virtues with the Cortex Massoy.

Diospyrus, Offic. J. B. Mespilus Alni effigie, lanato folio minor, C. B. P. Vaccinia alba, Ger. Emac. White Whortles. They grow on Mountains, and on hilly Places. The Fruit is used, which agrees in Virtues with the Aria.

Heliochrysum, Offic. Heliochrysos quorundam, foliis Abrotani, J. B. Golden Cudweed. It is cultivated with us in Gardens, flowering in July. The Herb is used. It is recommended against the Bites of Serpents, and in Pains of the Hips, and Strangury. It is said to provoke the Menses, dissolve concreted Blood, and stop Catarrhs.

Helxine cissampelos, Offic. Helxine cissampelos multis, sive Convolvulus minor, J. B. Smilax lævis minor, Ger. Emac. Small Bindweed. It grows in Fields, flowering in June. The Herb is used, which being externally apply'd, is a good Vulnerary. The Juice of the Leaves, taken inwardly, is a good Cathartic.

Herba Vulneraria, seu Virga aurea vulgo Germanica, Offic. Conyzæ affinis Germanica, J. B. German Golden Rod. It grows on mountainous Places, flowering in July. The Herb is used, and agrees in Virtues with the Virga aurea; for which it is sold in the Shops of Germany.

Hordeum mundatum & perlatum, Offic. French, or Pearl Barley. What we call French Barley, because it is usually imported from France, is nothing but Barley decorticated in a Mill, adapted to that Purpose. What we call Pearl Barley, because it resembles Scots Pearls, is prepar'd after the same Manner; only is twice

twice or thrice subjected to the Mill, in Order to be ground, and made less. Both of them agree in Virtues with common Barley, only are more nutritive.

Jacobæa alpina, sive Achyllea, Cod. Med. *Chrysanthemum alpinum foliis Abrotani multifidis,* C. B. P. Five-leaved Mountain Rag-wort. It is cultivated with us in the Gardens of the Curious. The Leaves are used, which taken in Ptisan, or made into Tea, are recommended for an Asthma.

Iberis, Offic. J. B. *Iberis latiore folio,* C. B. P. Sciatica Cresses. They grow in Botanic Gardens, and resemble Garden Cresses in Smell, Taste, and Virtues, only they are less drying.

Laburnum, Offic. *Laburnum trifolium Anagyridi simile,* J. B. Bean Trefoil Tree. It grows upon Mountains, flowering in *June* and *July.* The Leaves and Seeds are used, which purge both upwards and downwards. The Leaves discuss Tumors; and the Decoction provokes Urine.

Libanotis altera, Offic. *Libanotis Fœniculi folio, semine foliaceo,* C. B. P. Candy All-heal. It grows in the Island of *Crete,* flowering in the Summer. The Root, Herb, and Seeds are used. The Herb, bruis'd and apply'd, stops the Bleeding of the *Hæmorrhoids,* mitigates Inflammations of the Parts about the *Anus,* and *Condylomas.* The Roots dried, cleanse Ulcers, and provoke Urine and the *Menses;* the Seeds drank, have the same Effects.

Lichen marinus, Offic. *Lactuca marina, sive Intybacea,* J. B. Oyster Green. This grows upon Oysters, and upon Rocks. The Herb is used, which agrees in Virtues with the *Alga.*

Ornithogalon, Offic. *Ornithogalum vulgare & verius,* J. B. Star of Bethlehem. It is cultivated in Gardens, flowering in *May.* The Roots and Seeds are used; the first of which are eaten either raw or boil'd, and the other is baked in Bread.

Pinguicula, Offic. *Pinguicula Gesneri,* J. B. Butter-wort. It grows in moist mountainous Places, flowering in *May.* The Herb is used, which is vulnerary, and good for *Hernias* in Children. A Syrup is prepar'd from it, which purges Phlegm very briskly.

CHAP. II.

Of ANIMALS.

ACCIPITER, Offic. *Accipiter Fringillarius,* Gefn. de Avib. The Sparrow Hawk. The whole Bird, its Fat, and Excrements are ufed. Oil wherein a Hawk has been boiled, is faid to cure Diftempers of the Eyes, if they are anointed with it. The fame Virtue is in the Fat. The fame Oil cures all Deformities of the Skin. The Excrements are of fo heating a Quality, that *Galen* will not admit them as Part of the *Materia Medica;* but there are fome who ufe them in Diforders of the Eyes; others however, advife them in Order to promote Delivery, taken inwardly, or by Way of Suffumigation. *Hippocrates* and *Pliny* refcribe them againft Barrennefs.

Acus, Ariftot. Aldrov. de Pifc. *etimbuaba,* Charlt. Pifc. The Tobacco Pipe Fifh. It is found in the *Adriatic* Sea, or Gulph of *Venice.* *Galen* recommends the Afhes of this Fifh, drank in fome convenient Vecle, for the Strangury.

Agnus. See *Ovis.*

Alauda criftata, Schrod. *Galeta,* Offic. *Alauda criftata major,* uii Synop. The Crefted Lark. The whole Bird, its Heart, and Blood, are ufed. The Heart and the Blood of Larks, are good for the windy Colic, and to extricate Gravel and Phlegm from the Kidneys and Bladder. The frefh Blood, taken in fharp Vinegar, or warm Wine, effectually relieves the Stone and Gravel. As the Lark ufes much Exercife, its volatile Salts muft be much exalted, and its Juices alcalefcent, efpecially as it feeds fometimes on Infects.

Alauda non criftata, Schrod. *Alauda,* Offic. Mer. Pin. The Sky Lark. The whole Bird, and its Blood are ufed, and agree in Virtues with the preceeding.

Album Græcum. See *Canis.*

Alce, Offic. Schrod. The Elk. The Parts ufed in Medicine, are the Hoofs, and the Nerves. The Hoof is efteemed a Specific againft the Epilepfy, apply'd either externally, or internally. Internally the Rafpings are taken. Externally a Bit of the Hoof is included in a Ring, and worn fuperftitioufly on the Finger, which is next to the little one, in fuch a Manner that the Portion of the Hoof may be next to the Palm. Sometimes the Hoof is held in the Hand, apply'd to the Pulfe; put into the left Ear, or fufpended about the Neck, in fuch a Manner, that it may touch the Skin. The Nerves are bound about thofe Limbs, which are moft fubject to Spafms. It feems the Elk is an Animal much fubject to epileptic Diforders, and it has been obferv'd, that it frequently fcratches its Head with the hind Feet, which was whimfically apprehended to be done, as a Remedy for the abovemention'd Diftemper. Hence the Hoof acquir'd its Reputation as a Medicine, but I am afraid no great Dependance can be had upon it.

K k

Ala

Alcedo, a Name for the *Ispida*, or King's Fisher.

Anas, Offic. *Anas domestica*, Aldrov. de Ornith. The Duck or Drake. The whole Duck alive, the Fat, Blood, and Dung, are used. A living Duck, stript Part of it bare of Feathers, and apply'd to the Belly, eases the Pain of the Colic. It is useful in external and internal Pains, as of the Sides, Joints, and in a cold Distemperature of the Nerves. The Blood is an Alexipharmic, and therefore sometimes used in Antidotes. The Dung is apply'd to the Bites of venomous Creatures.

Anas sylvestris, Offic. Schrod. *Boscas major*, Raii Ornith. The wild Duck, and Malard. The Fat, Blood, and Dung, are used, and agree in Virtues with the preceeding.

Anguilla, Offic. Aldrov. de Pisc. The Eel. The Fat is used, which is vulnerary, generates Hairs, is of Service in an *Alopecia*, cures Deafness, being put into the Ears, and mitigates the Hæmorrhoids.

Anguis. The Snake. See *Serpens.*

Anser, Offic. The Goose. The Fat, Blood, Dung, and Cuticle of the Feet is used in Medicine. The Fat is esteem'd to be more hot, subtle, penetrating, and resolvent, than that of the Swine, and is sometimes injected by Way of Clyster in Erofions of the Intestines; it cures Baldness of the Head; Fissures of the Lips, Ringings of the Ears, mollifies rigid Tendons, and relaxes the Belly, especially in Children. The Blood is alexipharmic. The Dung violently heats and dries, incides and opens, and powerfully provokes the *Menses*, and Urine, and expels the Secundines. It is much used in the Jaundice, Dropsy, and Scurvy. The Sportsmen are of Opinion, that when a Kennel is affected with Madness, the only Way to remedy this Evil is, to let a Flock of Geese lie in it every Night for a considerable Time, and I have some Reason to believe, that this Observation is not without Foundation. The Cuticle of the Feet dry'd and powder'd, is said to be astringent, and is sometimes used in immoderate Fluxes of the *Menses*, and is esteem'd a good Application for Chilblains.

Anser ferus, Offic. The wild Goose. It is found about the Sea Coasts, and agrees in Virtues with the preceeding.

Antilopus, Offic. *Capra strepsiceros*, Aldrov. de Quad. The Antelope. It is an *African* Beast like a Deer, and remarkable for its Swiftness. Its Hoofs and Horns are used, which are esteem'd anti-epileptic, and anti-hysteric.

Aper. The Boar. See *Porcus.*

Apes, Offic. Bees. The Bees themselves, their Honey, the Wax, and *Propolis*, or Bee Glue, are used in Medicine. The Salts of Bees are very volatile, and highly exalted; for this Reason, when dry'd, powder'd, and taken internally, they are diuretic, and diaphoretic. If this Powder is mixed in Unguents, with which the Head is anointed, it is said to cure the *Alopecia*, and to contribute to the Growth of Hair upon bald Places. Honey will taste of the Plant, from whence it is gather'd, as *Dioscorides* remarks with respect to the *Sardinian* Honey. And the Honey collected from the *Chamærododendros Pontica, maxima, Mespili folio, flore luteo*, which *Tournefort* takes to be the *Ægolethron* of *Pliny*, has been remark'd in all Ages to be poisonous. Honey is very penetrating and deterging, and is therefore good in all Obstructions, especially from viscid and tough Humours. In Infarctions and stuffing of the Breast, it is of great Efficacy, and wonderfully promotes Expectoration. In short, there is no Disorder from Phlegm, or any thing which

which is the Produce of a cold Constitution, in which it is not serviceable. But in thin and hot Habits it is not good. It was antiently used as Sugar is now; and great Pity it is, that it is not at present more used. It does great Service to such as are troubled in a Morning with thick tough Phlegm, with which they cannot be easy, until it is hawk'd up, tho' it gives much Difficulty and Straining to do it. For this Purpose it is very conveniently eat over Night upon a Toast, or dissolved in any warm Liquor. Some affirm it will destroy Worms, drank in Milk. It has been much used in Surgery to cleanse foul Ulcers, either by immediate Application, or washing them with Liquors in which it had been dissolved. It is remarkable that Honey was used by the Antients, in the Composition of their Antidotes and *Theriacas*, as in Mithridate, the *Theriaca Andromachi*; commonly called *Venice-Treacle*; and *Fracastorius* has follow'd their Example, in the Composition of his Confection, called *Diascordium*. Now, Honey, I apprehend to be a very proper Ingredient in such Compositions: For it opens the other Ingredients by fermenting; extracts, and in some Degree, alters their Virtues, and unites them in one common Efficacy. Besides, Opium, and other Narcotics, which are frequently directed in the Antidotes of the Ancients, are corrected by Honey; agreeable to which, is the Remark of *Dioscorides*, that Honey relieves the Disorders excited by taking the Juice of the Poppy. When, therefore, we make any of these Antidotes with *Diacodium*, a Medicine results from the Composition, of Virtues very different from those of one which is made with Honey. And this deserves the serious Consideration of Physicians who prescribe *Diascordium*, or any of the other Antidotes made with *Diacodi-*

um. With Respect to Honey, one farther Remark is to be made, which is, that there is a Peculiarity in some Constitutions, which renders them incapable of bearing the least Quantity of Honey, without excessive Gripes, Vomitings, and Uneasiness. And in others, it operates as a Poison; an Instance of which we find in the Philosophical Transactions Certain Balsams appear (says *Boerhaave*) in a very small Quantity, upon the Surface of the Leaves of some Plants, where they are inspissated by the Heat of the Sun, as seems manifestly to appear in Rosemary: There are also found in other Plants certain very minute Globules, rising from the open seminal Tufts in the main Part of the Flower. These can scarce be collected by any human Means; but I have sometimes found, upon frequently cohobating Spirit of Wine upon Rosemary Leaves, an unexpected and ungrateful Taste or Smell of Wax, fouling the Spirit, which before was good, and upon viewing these Leaves with a Microscope, I thought I discover'd little waxy Risings on the Surface; and upon handling them considerably, I evidently found Wax gradually sticking to my Fingers. Wax, therefore, appears to be a certain Species of Turpentine, which the fat Juices of Plants, when heated by the Sun, sweat out upon the Surface, or produce within the Cavities of the flowery Tufts. This the Bees collect, roll up into little Balls, and carry between their hind Feet to their Hives, where it is wrought into the Cells of their Combs; and from hence, after the Honey is separated from the drossy Parts, it is procur'd for human Uses. It is generally yellow, and not ungrateful either in Taste or Smell. It becomes hard, and almost brittle, in the Cold, but grows soft, and dissolves with Heat. Wax is heating, mollifying, and moderately inca-ning. It is mix'd in forbile Liquors, as an efficacious Remedy for a Dyfentery, and is recommended to prevent the Curdling of Milk in the Breafts of Nurfes. The white Wax is nothing but the yellow Wax, whiten'd by frequent Infolation. The *Propolis,* or Bee Glue, is a rude Wax-like, and thick Matter, or Glew, found in the Entrance of Bee Hives. It is gently heating, abftergent, and attracting: It foftens indurated Parts, alleviates Pains, and induces Cicatrices on Ulcers.

Apos, Offic. *Hirundo Apus,* Raii Ornith. The Black Martin, or Swift. It lives with us in *England* during the Summer. The whole Bird is ufed, which taken in Wine cures the Gripes.

Aquila, Offic. *Chryfeatos,* Aldrov. Ornith. The Eagle. The Gall and Dung are ufed. The Gall diftill'd with Oil of Violets, is recommended by *Avicenna* for Pains and Ringings in the Ears ; and the Dung againft Abortions.

Araneus, Offic. The Spider. Both the Spider and its Web are ufed. The Spider is faid to avert the Paroxyfms of Fevers, if it be apply'd to the Pulfe of the Wrift, or the Temples; but is peculiarly recommended againft a Quartan, being inclofed in the Shell of a Hazle Nut. The Web aftringes and conglutinates, and is therefore vulnerary, reftrains Bleeding, and prevents an Inflammation. The Country People have a Tradition, that a fmall Quantity of Spider's Web, given about an Hour before the Fit of an Ague, and repeated immediately before it, is effectual in curing that troublefome, and fometimes obftinate Diftemper. This Remedy is not confin'd to our own Country; for I am well inform'd, that the *Indians* about *North Carolina* have great Dependance on this Remedy for Agues, to which they are much fubject ; and I am acquainted with a Gentleman long refident in thofe Parts, who affures me he was himfelf cured by it of that Diftemper. And indeed Experience confirms the Efficacy of this Medicine in the Cure of Agues.

Araneus niger, Offic. The Black Spider. It is common in Woods, Thickets and Paftures. Among the approved Remedies of Sir *Matthew Lifter,* I find, that the diftill'd Water of Black Spiders is an excellent Cure for Wounds, and that this was one of the choice Secrets of Sir *Walter Raleigh.*

Ardea, Offic. The Heron. The Fat of this Bird is recommended to affwage the Pains of the Gout; for taking off Specks from the Eyes, and clearing the Sight ; and for curing Deafnefs, if put into the Ear. The young Herons are fometimes ufed as Food; but on Account of their Aliment, which is Fifh, their Salts muft be highly exalted, and their Flefh rank.

Ardea Stellaris, Raii Ornith. *Afterias,* Offic. The Bittern, or Mire Drum. The Skin and Feathers of this Bird, if burnt, are faid to ftop Hæmorrhages.

Aries. The Ram. See *Ovis.*

Afchia & Thymallus, Offic. The Grayling, or Umber. This Fifh refides in rapid, fhallow, and ftony Streams, and is efteem'd excellent Food. The Part ufed in Medicine is the Fat, which is faid to take away Specks and Pearls from the Eye: Melted in the Sun, and mixed with Honey, it takes away Freckles, and Marks left by the Small Pox.

Afelli. Wood Lice. See *Millepedes.*

Afellus, Offic. The Cod Fifh, or Keeling. Certain fmall Bones, found in the Head of this Fifh, called *Lapides Dentales* in the Shops, are ufed in Medicine. They are merely teftacious, and employ'd as fuch.

Afellus minor, Aldrov. de Pifc.

Oxij-

Oniscus, Offic. The Whiting. The Flesh and Gall are used. The Flesh is esteemed very wholesome Food, and the Gall is recommended in a *Phthisis*.

Asinus, Offic. The Ass. The Hoof, Blood, Milk, Urine and Dung are used in Medicine. The Hoof is recommended in an Epilepsy, like that of the Elk; and the Ashes of it, us'd externally, are esteem'd good for discussing strumous Swellings, and Imposthumations, for curing Chilblains, and Cracks of the Skin, for removing Films of the Eye, for expelling a dead *Fœtus*, and for rowzing Epileptic and Hysteric Patients out of their Fits. The Blood is said to be sudorific; and that of a young Ass to cure the Jaundice. Asses Milk is very nourishing, and abstergent, and is therefore esteem'd good in a Consumption, in Disorders of the Stomach, Abscesses of the Kidneys, the Stone in the Bladder, and Arthritic Pains. It is esteem'd gently cathartic, and was frequently directed by *Hippocrates* as a Purge in large Quantities. As a Topic, it makes the Gums firm, eases Arthritic Pains, and gives the Face an agreeable Whiteness, if wash'd with it. The Urine is said to be a powerful Remedy in Disorders of the Kidneys; cures the Itch, takes away Warts, and callous Excrescences; and relieves in Atrophies, and Palsies of the Limbs, and Pains of the Gout. The Dung is recommended to stop Hæmorrhages.

Aspredo. The Ruff. See *Cernua.*

Astacus, Offic. The Lobster. It is found in the Sea. The Shell of this Fish calcin'd, and drank in Wine, is said to break and carry off stony Concretions in the Kidneys; and it is likely enough to have some Effect in such Cases, because the Shells of Fish calcin'd are a Sort of Lime, and the Salts of Lime are the grand Dissolvents of stony Concretions.

Lobsters as a Food are highly alcalescent, and consequently must be very proper Food, when an acid Acrimony prevails in the Stomach, and general Habit; but the contrary, in case of a Tendency to an alcaline Putrefaction. They are esteem'd very nourishing, and good in a Consumption.

Astacus fluviatilis, Offic. The Crafish, or Crevis. They are found in Rivers, and the Parts of them used are, the Flesh, and what we call the *Lapilli*, or *Oculi Cancrorum*, known by the Name of Crab's Eyes. In their Head, according to some, or rather in their Stomach, are found two white Stones, as large as a Pea, of a Kind of lenticular or orbicular Form, but compress'd, and somewhat hollow on one Side; whereas the other is convex, and dispos'd in *Laminæ*. These Stones are of an earthy Taste. We frequently meet with a counterfeit Species of this Commodity, prepared of a whitish Earth, and made up in the same Form; but this factitious Kind is easily distinguish'd by breaking them, since they want those *Laminæ*, which are always found in the convex Part of natural and genuine Crab's Eyes. The Flesh of this Animal is cooling, moistening, and adapted to nourish such as labour under Atrophies The *Stones* or *Eyes* are cooling, drying, abstergent and discutient; they resolve tartareous Concretions, and coagulated Blood, and are possess'd of a lithontriptic Quality; for which Reason they are often prescribed in nephritic Pains, Pleurisies, Asthma's and Colics; they are also proper for cleansing the Teeth. The Shell is possess'd of the same Virtues with the Stones, and is besides of Service in curing such Itches in Children, as arise from saline Humours, and in carrying off the Paroxysms of Intermittent Fevers.

Attagen, Offic. The Gor Cock,

Moor Cock, or Red Game. It is found upon the highest Mountains. The Flesh and Gall are used. *Trallian* recommends this Bird in a *Phthisis*; *Galen* in nephritic Complaints; and *Avicenna* believed the Brains to increase the seminal Secretions. This Bird lives principally on Vegetables, and uses but little Exercise, scarcely ever being upon the Wing, unless to avoid Danger. Hence it does not abound with highly exalted Salts. It is a very agreeable and wholesome Food.

Balæna, Offic. The Whale. The Fat of the Whale is said by *Schroder* to be a good Topic for the Itch. The Oil is more used in Mechanics than Medicine, tho' it is by some recommended for the *Scabies*. It is called Train Oil.

Another Species of Whale, is the *Cetus*, or *Parmafitty* Whale. See *Sperma Ceti*.

Barbus, Offic. The Barbel. It is found in Rivers, and is greatly used in the Kitchen. The Spawn of this Fish, at some Seasons of the Year, is a most violent Vomit and Purge.

Bezoar. This is of two Sorts, either oriental or occidental. The oriental is found in the Stomach or *Omasum* of the *Capra five Gazella Bezoardica orientalis*, Offic. The Bezoar Goat. These Stones are of different Shapes and Sizes: Some of them are of the Form of a Kidney, or *French* Bean; others are round, oblong, and of an irregular Figure. Each Stone of this Kind is compos'd of several *Laminæ*, form'd of a greenish or Olive colour'd Substance, diversify'd with white Streaks, which run thro' the whole Body of the Stone. These *Laminæ* adhere so closely to one another, that breaking the Stone, we may observe several Layers of different Thicknesses, and even sometimes of different Colours. There are also found *Laminæ*, which upon breaking these Stones, disengage

and separate themselves very regularly from each other; which they also do, when a considerable Degree of Heat is apply'd to them. The Substance which possesses the Middle or Centre of these *Bezoars*, is usually hard, gravelly, and pretty smooth. The *Bezoardic* Layers, which cover this Substance, are easily broken between the Teeth, to which they adhere like a gently glutinous Substance, and tinge the *Saliva* a little. Authors advise us, to make Choice of Bezoar Stones which are of a moderate Bulk, of a brownish Colour, and which communicate a yellow Colour to Quicklime, a greenish one to Chalk, and which cannot be dissolv'd in Water. If prick'd with a hot Iron, no Bubbles ought to arise round the Iron, which is a Proof, that it is not adulterated with any Resins. The *Lamina* also must be fine, and dispose'd in *Strata*. The best Species of these Stones are taken from Animals that feed on large Mountains such as those of *Persia*. *Bezoar* is said to be alexipharmic, and a Promoter of Sweat; is good in Epilepsies, Palpitations of the Heart, Jaundice, Dysenteries, Stone, and Obstructions of the *Menses*; it cures Melancholy, and promotes Delivery; and in these important Intentions, *Schroder* assigns the Dose from three Grains to twelve. But we have no Instances from Experience to support any such Practice. It has neither Smell nor Taste; and upon taking into the Stomach, gives no Sensation, nor produces the least perceivable Effect, which is Ground enough to suspect it good for nothing, altho' our Physicians prescribe it in much larger Doses than what *Schroder* mentions, and others have ventured half a Dram, or a Dram at a time. Many Circumstances contribute to render the medicinal Virtues of *Bezoar* precarious, and not easy to be determin'd, as the Uncertainty of procuring that which is genuine, it being

being much adulterated, as is said, even in the *Indies*; not to mention the large Quantities that are made in *Europe*, in Imitation of the true: Again, the excessive Price it generally bears, makes it inconvenient to exhibit it in a great Number of Cases, and that in sufficient Quantities, and those long enough continued, to determine, whether the Virtues attributed to it are real or imaginary; and without this Test it is not possible to reason accurately and conclusively, with Respect to the Efficacy of any one Simple, tho' the Manner of its Production, and the *Analysis* are both taken into Consideration; neither does the Taste give us any surer Information. As to my own private Opinion, it is of no great Importance in the Case before us, because I have not very often directed it, and consequently am not a Judge of its real Effects: But I am informed from Physicians, who have industriously attempted to make the proper Experiments, that it has no Sort of medicinal Virtues, that they could perceive, which might give it the Preference to the testaceous Powders. I cannot, however forbear thinking, that if we had the genuine *Bezoar* Stone, we should find it endow'd with greater medicinal Virtues, than at present we have any Reason to believe it possessed of.

The *Occidental Bezoar* is produc'd by the *Cervus minor Americanus Bezoarticus*, the Lesser *American* Deer, being found in the Stomach of this Animal, and is easily known from the *Oriental*, from its being of a paler Colour: It is sometimes of a greyish white, and is form'd on Substances of the same Kind with the Oriental. Its *Laminæ*, are also sometimes thicker, and striated according to their Thickness. The Virtues ascrib'd to it, are much the same, as those ascrib'd to the *Oriental Bezoar*.

Blatta, Offic. The slow legg'd

Beetle. The Inside of this Insect, bruised or boiled in Oil, and dropp'd into the Ears, eases the Pains thereof.

Blatta Byzantina, Offic. *Blatta Byzantia, sive Unguis odoratus*, Park. Theat. The Constantinople Sweet Hoof. This exhibited internally, renders the Body soluble, softens the Spleen, and discusses peccant Humours. When used externally by way of Fumigation, it restores epileptic Patients, and Women under a Strangulation of the *Uterus*. In other Disorders its Effects are the same with those of the most tenacious Substances.

Bombyx, Offic. The Silk Worm. This Insect undergoes a strange and surprizing *Metamorphosis* in the several Periods of its Existence. This Animal, or Worm, is called *Bombyx*, in the Shops, and is produced from small Eggs, hatched by the genial Heat of the Sun, in the Spring of the Year. It feeds upon Mulberry Leaves, 'till it has arrived at a State of Maturity. After this they are usually put into a small Bag, where they wrap themselves up in a silken Case, which, coming from their Mouths, is without Interruption carry'd very often round them. This Case is sometimes of a palish Colour. In this Case, or Coat, it remains wrapt up, till it is transform'd into its *Chrysalis* or *Aurelia*, and appears dead: but at last, it sallies forth from its Coat in the Form of a Butterfly, with four Wings; and after a Copulation, which lasts for three Days, and proves immediately mortal to the Male, the Female lays a considerable Number of Eggs, and dies likewise. The whole Worm, and the silken Coat or Covering, are used in Medicine. Silk Worms dry'd, and reduc'd to a Powder, are by some apply'd to the Crown of the Head, for removing Vertigos and Convulsions. The Silk, and Case or Coat, are of a due Temperament between Heat and Cold, and corroborate and recruit the vital, natural, and animal Spirits. We muft take Care not to ufe the Coat, or Cafe, if it is either ftain'd with their Excrements, or if the *Aurelia,* or Worm remains dead in it.

Bos, Offic. This is a general Name for Black Cattle, as they are called, of which *Taurus* is the Male, or Bull, *Vacca* the Cow, *Vitulus* the Calf, tho' *Bos,* the Ox, is generally underftood of the Bull caftrated when young. The Horns, Gall, Liver, Spleen, Blood, Marrow, Suet, Oil of the Feet, Hoof, Urine, Dung, the Stones fometimes found in the Gall Bladder, the Milk, Butter, Cheefe, *Penis,* and the Balls found in the Stomach, are ufed in Medicine. The Rafpings of the Horn are fometimes ufed in an Epilepfy, and in Suffumigations, to purify contagious Air. The Gall is efteemed excellent in Ringings and Pains of the Ear, relaxes the Belly, and kills Worms. A Decoction of the Liver of a Calf, is ufed for Indurations of the Spleen, and a Suppreffion of the *Menfes;* and it is fometimes applied externally to the Region of the Spleen. The Milk is thick and nourifhing, and is good in Diforders of the Bladder, Diarrhæa, Dyfentery, Tenefmus, and Erofions of the Inteftines. The Butter is moderately heating, emollient, digeftive, lenient, refolvent, relaxing, and good for Dimnefs of the Sight. New foft Cheefe mitigates Pains of the Gout, and Heat of the Liver, and is reckon'd a good Application in an *Exomphalos* in Children: Old putrid Cheefe, is faid to promote the Solution of Aliment contained in the Stomach, and fuperior to the Powers of Digeftion. Old Leather made of the Hide, burnt or fing'd, is commended for the hyfteric Paffion. The Fat is of Service, wherever Emollients are required. The *Axun-*

gia, which is melted from the Hoofs, is more penetrating and emollient, becaufe of finer Parts; but the Marrow exerts its emollient Virtue wherever it is applied. The Bones calcin'd, and pulveris'd, are faid to ftrengthen the Bowels, to ftop a Loofenefs, and to be effectual againft Worms, and the Epilepfy, ufed either internally, or in Ointments, or Plaifters; but it muft be underftood of fuch Cafes where the Diforder proceeds from an Excefs of Humidity, or an Acid, and is to be fubdued by Driers and Abforbents. The Hoofs have an anti-epileptic Virtue: Being fried and fo taken, they may be of fome Service in a Dyfentery, where an alcaline, anti-acid, glutinous Faculty is required. The *Talus* of a Cow pulveriz'd, and drank in Wine, is commended by *Foreftus,* as a Specific againft Worms in the Inteftines. The *Membrum genitale,* or Pizzle of a Bull, pulveriz'd, or elfe in Decoction, is reported to create a Defire of Coition in Men, but an Abhorrence of the fame in Women; but Reafon does not comprehend thefe Contrarieties, nor Experience atteft them. There is a Stone fometimes found in the Gall Bladder of this Animal, which is called *Bezoar Bovinus,* and *Alcheron Lapis,* by the *Portuguefe, Mefang de Vaca,* and by the *Arabians, Haraczi;* which is faid by fome to have an alexipharmic and anti-epilepic Virtue. But this Stone is not to be confounded with the *Bulithum,* or Ball, which is fometimes found in the Stomach, and fometimes in the Inteftines of this Animal. Thefe are ufually called *Tophi Bovini,* and confift of Hairs, which it gets off by licking, from its Body, and fwallows, where by degrees they concrete into a Ball, which is commonly of the Colour of the Animal's Hair. Sir *Hans Sloane,* in his Hiftory of *Jamaica,* fays, that fome give half a Dram of it in Powder, er, as an Aftringent. Thefe Balls have fometimes a fhining Cruft over them, in which Refpect they imitate the true Bezoar Stone. The Spleen of an Ox is commended to provoke an Appetite, and diftill'd with Spirit of Wine, is recommended for all Infirmities of the Stomach; but the Virtue of this diftill'd Liquor, I fhould think, were owing to the Spirit of Wine, rather than any thing proceeding from the Spleen of the Ox. The Liver of an Ox dry'd and pulveriz'd, is commended as good in Fluxes of the Belly, and Hæmorrhages. If it be ferviceable in this Cafe, it acts as an abforbing, alcaline Powder; but then the Liver of other Animals will have the fame Effect. The Dung of an Ox is defervedly commended for its difcuffive Virtue in external Applications. Hence it is ufed recent, by way of Cataplafm, in Inflammations, paricularly the Gout, as an approved Anodyne. Some mix with it Earthworms, and apply it to the *Abdomen*, in order to cure the Colic, and difcufs Flatulencies; as alfo in the *Afcites*, to reprefs the Tumor, and difcufs the Water; for next to human Dung, that of an Ox is reckon'd the beft for this Purpofe. *Ettmuller* fays, it is very effectually applied to œdematous Tumors. It is alfo commended againft a Suppreffion of Urine, if applied to the *Pecten*, and the Region of the *Pubes*. The common People give the expreffed Juice in Pains of the Colic; and *Ettmuller* afferts, from certain Experience, that it is not only a prefent Remedy in the Colic, but alfo in the Pleurify; that of this Dung, in the fame Manner as of human Dung, by repeated Digeftion and Sublimation, may be prepared the *Zibethum Occidentale*, fo called by *Paracelfus*, becaufe it exhales a fweet Smell like Civet. *Diofcorides* fays, that the Dung of an Ox that grazes, apply'd

recent, mitigates the Inflammation of Wounds. It is wrapp'd, he fays, in Leaves, and heated in hot Afhes, and then apply'd to the Place; that a Fomentation of it affwages the Pain of the *Sciatica*; that it difcuffes Hardneffes, Pain, and *Strumæ*, being anointed with it, infufed in Vinegar; and that a Suffumigation of the Dung of the Male of this *Species* repreffes the falling down of the *Uterus*; and that the Smell of it, when kindled, drives away Gnats. On thefe Paffages *Mattbiolus* remarks, " We are to confider, that all Medi- " cines of this Kind are accommo- " dated to the hard Bodies of Ru- " ftics, fuch as Diggers, Mowers, " and fuch as are inur'd to Work " which requires bodily Strength; " to fuch as thefe, when affected " with fchirrhous Tumors, it is ap- " plied by way of Cataplafm with " Vinegar." *Valefcus de Taranta* affures us, that the Dung of an Ox, (or a Horfe) is of excellent Ufe in a Gangrene, to preferve the found Parts from Corruption: And, after him, *Sylvius* and *Barbette*, as they fay, made Ufe of the fame Remedy, which they kept as a great Secret. But it is really a fordid Medicine, hardly worthy of a Phyfician, and to be left to the poor Commonalty, rather than to be recommended to the rich and noble, according to *Heifter*. Cows Urine internally ufed, *Ettmuller* fays, cures the Gout, if it be taken in the Month of *May*, and the Feet are bathed a while in it, and, after that the *Norimberg* Plaifter is applied to them. *Diofcorides* fays, that the Urine of a Bull, with Myrrh, inftill'd into the Ears, cafes Pains thereof. *Helmont* propofes, as an approved Remedy for the Stone, the Liquor that ufually fills the Bladder of the *Fœtus* in a Cow, drank every Morning to the Quantity of about four Ounces, in a like Proportion of white Wine. The Blood

of

of a Bull fresh drawn, is reckoned poisonous, by causing a Difficulty of Breathing, and Suffocation ; but *Matthiolus* or *Dioscorides* observes, that except it be drank in great Quantities, and hot as it comes from the Veins, before it concretes, it does little or no Harm. This poisonous Quality, is not however confirm'd by later Experiments. But the Blood of Oxen and Bulls is commended, as internally used, for the Dysentery, an Excess of the *Menses*, and other internal Hæmorrhages; and for spitting of Blood, it is prescribed to be taken in Vinegar. Externally it is effectual in discussing and mollifying Tumours, and clearing the Face of Spots and Blemishes. *Ettmuller* says, the Blood is hardly used, but in Case of an Atrophy of the Limbs and Joints, after great Wounds receiv'd; and for Weakness and Pains in the Members and Joints, which, being thrust into the fresh Blood of an Ox, or a Dog newly kill'd, will be wonderfully refresh'd thereby, and render'd more pliable, and fit for Motion. The Blood of an Ox then, externally apply'd, has three Virtues in common with the Blood of other Animals; which Virtues are derived from its saponaceous Nature, whereby it is a Dissolvent and Aperient, its native Heat promoting its Operation. Internally taken, it is hurtful, by its natural Property, which causes it to concrete in the Stomach, and renders it insuperable by the vital Powers. *Helmont* says, that the Blood of a Bull is Poison, but not that of an Ox or a Cow; and assigns as a Cause the Fury of the Bull, dying with an eager Desire of Revenge, which impresses a Mark of Vengeance, and a powerful Signature, on the Blood. *Guainerius* says, that not only the Blood of a Bull, but that of an old Ox, is poisonous.

Botargum. The Salted Spawn of the Mullet. See *Mugil.*

Bubalus, Offic. The Buffal. The Parts used in Medicine, are the Horns, Hoofs, Tallow, and Dung, of which the Horns and Hoofs, are good against Convulsions; and the other Parts are reckon'd to be endu'd with the same Virtues as that of the Ox.

Buccinum, Offic. The Whelk. Whelks calcin'd, work the same Effects as the Purple Fish, but are of a more caustic Quality. Fill'd with Salt, and then burnt in a crude Earthen Pot, they make a good Dentifrice, and are applied with Success in Combustions, where it must be left alone to harden like a Shell; for, as soon as the burnt Place is brought to a Cicatrix, this Medicine falls off of itself. A Quicklime Lime is made of them. Whelks, are alcaline and absorbent, and by Calcination, are converted into Lime; and these Properties they possess in common with all other Shell Fish.

Bufo, Offic. *Bufo sive Rubeta*, Raii Synop. The Toad. *Ettmuller* informs us, that a live Toad bruised, proves an effectual Remedy for the Bite of the Viper, and other poisonous Serpents, when applied to the wounded Part. Some Authors, as *Helmont* informs us, order live Toads to be apply'd over both Kidneys, for removing the Dropsy, by a plentiful Discharge of Urine. *Paracelsus* affirms, that Toads are of excellent Service in the Cure of Pestilential Buboes in the Groin, and such as Women are afflicted with. *Franciscus Joel* affirms, that a Toad run thro' with a sharp Probe, dried in the Air, and moistened in Vinegar, if apply'd to pestilential Carbuncles, extracts all the Poison from the Body. *Helmont* also from the Toad, prepared an Amulet for the Plague; and others, as *Ettmuller* informs us, prepare Amulets for the same Purpose of the Bones of Toads,

or

whole Toads mixed up with L-g-glafs, which they fay extract Poifon, and prove a Prefervative, hung about the Neck. The a-re Author fays, that a dry'd Toad ng about the Neck, or in the Pit the Stomach, or applied to the m Pits, or even held in the Hand, ft effectually ftops and cures all nds of Hæmorrhages, and more ecially fuch as happen in malig-nt Fevers, Small Pox, and fome er Diforders of a like Nature. he Powder of dry'd Toads was celebrated Secret of *Kyperus*, for Cure of an *Afcites*. A dry'd ad inclofed in a filken Bag, with proper Quantity of the Mofs of e Sloe-Tree, if apply'd to the avel of a Woman afflicted with a mmorrhage of the *Uterus*, will p the Flux, as foon as it is warm the Part. It is by other Au-ors recommended to be put into a ken or linen Bag, and hung upon e Breaft for Incontinencies of U-ne, arifing from a Violence done any of the Parts. In the Cure a Cancer, fays *Etimuller*, and ore particularly unexulcerated Can-rs in the Breafts of Women, Toads e of fingular Service, either cal-n'd alone, or dry'd to fuch a De-ree, that they may be reduc'd to a owder. We are alfo told, that any Patients labouring under epi-emical Dyfenteries, have been hap-ily recover'd by the Ufe of this 'owder, which operates as a Sudo-ific. *D. Carlius* recommends the 'owder of calcin'd Toads, mixed vith the Powder of blue linen Cloth urnt, in Epilepfies of adult Perfons ttended with an Infpiffation of the Juices: He alfo informs us, that a Dofe, from ten or twenty Grains of he Powder of calcin'd Toads, ex-ibited internally, wonderfully mi-tigates arthritic Pains, and more e-fpecially thofe with which Wounds are attended. A Toad's Heart dry'd,

reduc'd to Powder, and exhibited an Hour before the Paroxyfm, has in fome Cafes cured Quartan Agues. A Toad dry'd, is by fome apply'd to the Soles of the Feet, by Way of an Epifpaftic in Fevers, and Difor-ders of the Head, and if apply'd to the Crown of the Head, is faid to cure Madnefs. The *Oleum Bufonum*, in the *Brandenburgh* Difpenfatory, is of great Service in Puftules of the Lips, and Cancers of the Breaft; and *Mufitanus* afferts, that it is a great Secret in curing the Falling off of the Hair. Others warmly recommend this Oil in Leprofies, and cutaneous Foulneffes. The *Em-plaftrum ex Bufonibus* of *Knoffelius*, when apply'd to the Throat, contri-butes to the Cure of fpurious Quinfeys.

Bupreftis, Offic. The Burn Cow. It feems to belong to the Kind of *Cantharides*, but it is more oblong in Body; and the cruftaceous Integu-ment of its Wings appears outwardly of a green, inclining to yellow, or rather is of a gold Colour; it has longer Legs, and fomewhat thicker. The Eyes are globulous and promi-nent, and from the Forehead, near the Eyes, proceed two oblong arti-culated Horns. The Head is but fmall, but the Mouth wide, hard, ftrong, forcipated, and armed with Teeth, with which it wounds and bites cruelly; the Belly is not round, but runs out in Length. It is of a feptic, exulcerating, and heating Quality; for which Reafon, it is mixed up with Medicines adapted to the Cure of a *Carcinoma*, *Lepra*, and malignant *Lichen*. Mix'd in emol-lient Peffaries, it provokes the *Men-fes*.

Buteo, Offic. The Buzzard. The Tefticles of this Animal is the only Part us'd in Medicine. A Decoction of them in Spring Water and Honey, is faid to prove a *Stimulus* to Ve-nory.

Cæcilia,

Cæcilia, Offic. The Blind Worm, or Sloe Worm. This is a Sort of Serpent, whose Bite has much the same Effects as that of the Viper; and is to be cur'd by much the same Methods. *Dale* from *Gesner*, gives an Account of a *Theriaca* being prepar'd of this Serpent, and Treacle-Water, for a Sudorific in the Plague.

Camelus, Offic. Camelus, Dromos, Gesn. de Quad. The Camel or Dromedary. It is found in *Asia* and *Africa*. The Parts used in Medicine, are the Blood, Gall, Dung, and Urine. The Blood helps the Dysentery, promotes Conception, and cures the Epilepsy; the Dung is recommended in Apoplexies; the Urine is thought to be effectual for cleansing and whitening the Teeth. Authors differ much about the Camel and the Dromedary. The Gentlemen of *Paris*, our *Ray*, and others, call by the Name of *Dromedary*, an Animal which has but one Bunch on his Back; but call a Camel, one which has two Bunches on that Part. But I have been told says *Dale*, by an ingenious Person, who very lately travelled into *Asia* and *Africa*, and agrees with *Johnson*, that the Camel is an Animal with only one Bunch on his Back, but the Dromedary has two; and that this latter was a very scarce Creature, and made use of by the Nobility only for its Swiftness; but the Camel was principally used for performing Journeys.

Cancellus, Aldrov. de Exang. The Wrong Heir. This Animal is brought from *America*; and the Oil distill'd from it, is esteem'd an excellent Remedy for the Rheumatism.

Cancer, Offic. The Sea Crab. The black Extremities of the Claws, and Shells, are principally used in Medicine, which are Absorbents, and esteem'd Sweetners of the Blood. *Schroder* says, they remove the Pa-

roxysms of Intermittents. The Crab consider'd as Food, has the Reputation of being good in a Consumption, and to cure the Strangury.

Cancer fluviatilis, Offic. The River Crab. Most Authors have blunder'd excessively, in speaking of this Animal, which they take for the Crawfish; whereas it is as different from the last mentioned, as the Sea Crab is from the Lobster. It is not found in the Rivers of *England, France* or *Germany*; but is frequent in those of *Greece, Crete, Sicily, Russia* and *Tartary*. Therefore, when *Galen* recommends the River Crab burnt, as a Specific against that Disorder, caus'd by the Bite of a mad Dog, Crawfish is not to be understood, but the true River Crab, the Subject of our present Enquiry. They are esteem'd refrigerating and moistening, and are said to ease Pain, and compose the Spirits. Hence they are used in Heat, and Pain of the Head, and Kidneys, a Quinsey, and Atrophy; and are said to be a good external Application in the *Ignis Persicus*, a Species of Carbuncle, and for Burns.

Canis, Offic. The Dog. The Head, the Fat, the Gall, the Blood, the Dung, called *Album Græcum*, the Urine, the Teeth, the Skin, and the Hairs are used in Medicine. Live Puppies laid upon the Belly, mitigate Colic Pains, and are serviceable to Paralytic Limbs; and there are many Instances in Authors, of inveterate Ulcers being cured, by being frequently lick'd by a Dog. The Head burnt, dries up Ulcers, cures Fissures of the *Anus*, and Tumors of the Testicles; internally it is of Service in a Jaundice. The Fat is esteem'd hotter than that of other Animals, and is given internally, in order to absterge and consolidate Wounds and Ulcers, in a Consumption, and to dissolve Blood coagulated by a Bruise. Externally it is used

:ed in Pains of the Ears, and Tor-
:res of the Gout, to kill Knits and
ice, for Deafnefs, and the Itch.
:he Gall of a black Puppy is e-
:eem'd a Specific in the Epilepfy;
:d externally applied, abfterges
:reckles on the Face, and cures
:pecks on the Eyes. The Blood
:ank is faid to be good againft the
:ite of the Animal, and Poifon. The
:ung dries, abfterges, difcuffes, o-
:ns, breaks Abfceffes, and deter-
:s Exulcerations; hence it is given
:ternally in a Dyfentery and Colic.
:xternally apply'd, it cures a Quin-
:y, and malignant Ulcers, mollifies
:rd Tumors. draws off the Waters
: Hydropic Patients, and cures
:arts. The Urine is apply'd to
:nning Ulcers, and Scurf of the
:ead, and to Warts. The Afhes
: the Teeth, facilitate the Denti-
:n of Children, and cure the Tooth-
:h. The Skin tann'd, cures
:e troublefome Itchings of the
:ands, and mollifies contracted Ten-
:ns. The Hair is faid to cure the
:ite of the Animal.

Canis Carcharias, Offic. The
:hite Shark. This Animal is found
:th in the *Mediterranean*, and main
:cean. The Teeth of the Serpent,
:d alfo of this Fifh, when petrified,
:e the *Gloffopetra* of the Shops. Its
:eeth are efteem'd good againft
:oifons. Women hang them about
:e Necks of Children, becaufe they
:e commonly thought to affift Den-
:ion, and prevent Frights. The
:*loffopetræ* are thought by fome to
: poffefs'd of an alexipharmic
:uality.

:*Cantharides*, Offic. Spanifh Flies.
:hefe are a Species of Infects too
:ell known to require a Defcription.
:hey are principally found in warm
:ountries, as *Spain, Italy,* and *France.*
:hey are extremely hot, corrofive,
:d diuretic, and are faid to be fome-
:hat emmenagogue; and they are
:markable for affecting the Bladder

and urinary Paffages with Inflammation, exceffive Pain, and Strangury,
either taken internally, or apply'd
externally; and fome have even affirm'd, that carrying a Quantity of
them in the Pocket for fome time,
has produc'd this Effect. Upon taking *Cantharides* internally, all the
Parts from the Mouth to the Bladder
feem to be corroded, the Breath
fmells like the Refin of Cedar; the
Præcordia, efpecially on the right
Side, are inflam'd; Urine is difcharg'd
with Difficulty and Pain; and at Intervals Blood is evacuated along with
it; the Stools are mucous and purulent, as in a Dyfentery; the Patient
loaths his Food; faints, is feiz'd
with a *Vertigo;* and at laft loofes the
Ufe of his Reafon. In order to mitigate thefe Symptoms, a Vomit muft
be exhibited, and copious Draughts
of diluting Liquors, with Emollient, oleous, and mucilaginous Subftances are to be given; but it is faid
that nothing is fo proper, as faline Acids, which refift Putrefaction,
drank in a proper Quantity, and apply'd externally. The beft for external Ufe is warm Wine Vinegar,
and in the Cafe of a Priapifm, the
Lees of generous Wine; but for internal Ufe, fimple Oxymel is faid to
be beft. Mean time, however, mucilaginous and cooling Clyfters are
frequently to be injected. Notwithftanding thefe Effects of *Cantharides,*
they are fometimes given internally
in Subftance, in nephritic Cafes particularly, and efpecially to Women,
well guarded with mucilaginous Subftances and Opiates; and *Groenvelt*
has wrote a Treatife, in order to
eftablifh their Ufe in this Manner.
Their Tincture, however, is frequently directed internally in nephritic Cafes, and as a Diuretic, when
the Conftitution abounds with Serum,
and the Urinary Paffages are obftructed; and fometimes they are exhibited in order to cleanfe, and deterge
                 the

the *Uterus*. The Use of *Cantharides* was known to *Hippocrates*, who mentions them frequently, but not with a View of exciting Blisters, for he directs them to be given internally as a Diuretic, for expelling the Secundines, and as an Emmenagogue; and he further advises them, as an Ingredient in Pessaries, in order to cleanse and deterge the *Uterus*. *Aretæus* was the first who order'd these Insects to be rubb'd on the Skin of the Head, in order to excite Vesicles. This Author recommends *Cantharides* in the Cure of an Epilepsy, and orders the Patient to use Milk for three Days before their Exhibition, to prevent the Injury the Bladder might otherwise sustain. The same Method of curing this Disease, and Palseys, was, according to *Aetius*, follow'd by *Archigenes*, whom we may reasonably suppose, to have been of the same Sect with *Aretæus*. *Galen* informs us, that Plaisters made of these Flies, may very properly be used for the Cure of Baldnesses, the Itch and Ring Worm; but according to *Le Clerc*, he either disregarded this Medicine in the Cure of most other Diseases, or, as appears from his own Writings, rarely used it, as being attended with dangerous Consequences. As the *Greeks* who came after *Galen* advanc'd very little new upon any Subject, so they have been no less indolent with Respect to this Particular. The *Arabians* also, are in vain consulted in this Affair, who, tho' strongly addicted to composing new Forms of Medicines, yet in this Particular, as in most others, follow'd the Footsteps of the *Greeks*. Among the *Latins*, *Cantharides* seem to have been in very little Repute; and *Celsus* himself, who deals very much in *Sinapisms*, makes no mention of them so far as we know, except when, in Imitation of *Mico*, he recommends them for deterging and removing Pimples. *Pliny* informs

us, that anointing the Parts affected with *Cantharides* is good against the Leprosy, the Ring Worm, and for extracting Darts. And *Scribonius Largus* is the only Author who extols them, when mixed with proper Cerates, for removing Scars. These are almost all the Cases in which the Antients apply'd *Cantharides* to the Skin; which was very rarely, and only when cold Humours were to be removed, and when the Disorder was become inveterate. Long after the Restoration of Learning, *Cantharides* were also as scantily used: For *Fernelius* only prescrib'd them in Blindness, and in Dropsies; but tells us at the same Time, that their Use requires the highest Caution and Prudence. *Hollerius*, a Cotemporary of *Fernelius*, an Author of a fine Taste, and a Man well acquainted with the Writings of the Antients, orders *Cantharides* to be mixed in stimulating Topics, for removing a Lethargy; tho' *Duretus*, who wrote the *Adversaria* to the Works of *Hollerius*, dissuades the Use of stimulating Topics in this Disorder, because it is accompanied with a Fever, in which Case hot Substances are highly improper. It is however, a memorable Cure, which *Paré* and *Hollerius* perform'd by *Cantharides*. They advised a certain Lady of Distinction, whose Face was all over deformed with burning Pimples, as if she had labour'd under an *Elephantiasis*, to apply a Vesicatory of *Cantharides* all over her Face, by which means she was afflicted with such racking Pains, and seized with a Fever so violent, that no hopes of her Life seem'd to be left: However, by the joint Care and Skill of these two, she was restored to Health, the Deformity of her Face disappear'd, and never created her any Trouble for the future. The same *Hollerius*, when speaking of Caustics, affirms, that sciatic and arthritic Pains, Hemicranias, and

Head-

ad-achs, are often relieved in con-
uence of the Blisters or Vesicles
sed by *Cantharides*. He also tells
that the *Viscera* are purg'd, the
dy entirely freed from recrementi-
us Sordes, and a large Number of
and obstinate Disorders cur'd, by
ans of *Cantharides*. But in our
ys, the external Use of *Cantha-
es* is very extensive, especially in
r own Country; and they are per-
nally apply'd in acute Distempers,
t I am afraid sometimes wantonly,
d without due Distinction; for as
e Salts of *Cantharides*, which ma-
estly get into the Blood thro' the
res, exert great Effects in the Bo-
, it is always worth while to con-
er, the Quantity proper to be ap-
ed, that their Degree of Action
ay be in some measure determin'd;
d 'tis farther worthy of Considera-
n, whether the Operation of these
lts is likely to be beneficial or o-
erwise, in the Distemper in which
ey are applied. For my own part,
imagine the great Use of *Cantha-
es* externally applied, is first in
isorders where *Serum* greatly a-
unds in the Blood, for the Discharge
xcited by the Skin, removes a Part
that which is redundant; and be-
les, the Salts acting in the Body,
en all the Glands and Emunctories,
d promote a farther Discharge of
rum, by the urinary Ducts, and very
kely by the salival Glands, and cu-
neous Pores. The external Ap-
lication of *Cantharides*, may be fur-
her very beneficial in most inflam-
atory Disorders, and all those
hich proceed from a Viscidity and
izinefs of the Blood and Juices, and
heir Tendency to Coagulation; for
he Salts of these Insects fuse the
Humours, render them more fluid,
nd not only prevent their Stagna-
on, but even farther exert great
Efficacy in reducing the Particles al-
eady coagulated and stagnating to a
due Fluidity, and thus removing Ob-

structions. And in all Distempers
whatever, particularly those which
affect the Head, the *Fauces*, or the
immediate Organs of Respiration,
Cantharides apply'd to distant Parts,
may by causing a Revulsion, and inviting the Humours to the Place
which they immediately affect, may
be very beneficial. Moreover in a
Langour of the Circulation, and *Stupor* of the nervous System, the external Application of *Cantharides*,
may be of very great Service by
their *Stimulus*. Upon the whole,
Cantharides appears to be adapted
particularly to cold Distempers, Constitutions, Climates, and Seasons; for
in those which are the Reverse of
these, they may over act their Part,
fuse the Blood, accelerate the Circulation, and stimulate too much,
and hence become greatly prejudicial;
and besides, their highly alcaline and
acrid Salts may incline the Juices to
Putrefaction, and hence become fatal. *Baglivi* made the following
Experiments, with a View to discover the Effects of *Cantharides*. At
Rome, says he, in the Month of *May*,
I open'd the right Jugular of a Ma-
stiff Dog fixed to a Table, and by
the Assistance of a Syringe, injected
two Ounces of the Tincture of *Cantharides*; and this Tincture consisted
of two Drams of *Cantharides* reduc'd to a Powder, and six Ounces
of the Water of *Carduus Benedictus*,
digested for three Days on hot Ashes.
After the first Injection, the Dog vomited an aqueous and viscid Substance, and discharged a viscid *Saliva* from his Mouth, till at last two
Ounces being injected, the Orifice
was stitch'd up, and calcin'd Vitriol
sprinkled in it. No sooner was this
Operation perform'd, than the Dog
dropt to the Ground, as if he had
been dead. He would eat no more
during the remaining Part of his
Life, but had a violent Drought,
for which Reason a Servant, prompt-
ed

ed by a Principle of Compaſſion, without my Knowledge, gave him about twelve Pints of Water, by drinking of which, he diſcharg'd a large Quantity of yellow Urine. In the mean time he howl'd, and his inſatiable Thirſt continued, but we gave him no more Water. Before his Death he was ſeiz'd with Convulſions, and on the fourth Night after the Injection was made, died howling in the moſt lamentable Manner. Upon opening his Body, we found that Part of his Neck, where the Injection had been made entirely ſphacelated and fetid. In the right Ventricle of the Heart, a large Quantity of very black Blood, little or not at all coagulated, fluctuated, and on the Surface of the Blood ſome ſmall Drops, as it were of Oil, floated. In the ſame Ventricle, we alſo found a ſmall *Polypus*, ſurrounded with ſome grumous Blood. In the left Ventricle of the Heart were found two long ſlender *Polypuſes*, and the Blood contained in it was highly black, and colliquated. The Lungs and other *Viſcera*, were entirely ſound; but that mucous Subſtance with which the Urinary Bladder is naturally lin'd, was entirely deſtroy'd, perhaps by the Acrimony of the *Cantharides*. The Bile in the Gall Bladder was become ſomewhat blackiſh. The Blood which flow'd from the open'd Veins or *Viſcera*, was highly black, but not at all coagulated, and had ſmall Drops as it were of Oil, floating on its Surface. At *Rome* in the Month of *July*, I injected two Ounces of the Tincture of *Cantharides* into the right Jugular of a young middle ſized Dog, fixed to a Table. After the Wound was ſtitched up, and dreſs'd, as in the former Caſe, the Dog forthwith vomited, and dropt down, as it were half dead. Two Hours after, he hung out his Tongue, with the greateſt Signs of an inſatiable Thirſt. He

would eat nothing, and notwithſtanding his Thirſt, I would allow him no Water. Six Hours after, he died howling in the moſt terrible Manner. Upon opening his Carcaſe, all his *Viſcera* were found to be ſound. His Blood, however, was highly black, and colliquated, and had, as in the former Caſe, as it were ſmall Drops of Oil floating on its Surface. This Dog was young, of a ſmall Size, and had drunk no Water; 'tis therefore no Wonder, if the Humours being ſuddenly diſſolv'd and colliquated by the Cauſtic Salt of the *Cantharides*, he ſhould die in ſix Hours after the Experiment was made. In both Dogs I obſerv'd, that after injecting the Tincture into the Jugular, no Part was ſo ſoon affected as the Head, which immediately nodded, and hung down; neither could the Animal ſtand with a ſtrait Neck. The Former of theſe Dogs immediately hung down his Head, and could ſcarce raiſe it up; but upon drinking twelve Pints of Water, he immediately ſtarted on his Feet, mov'd his Head freely, kept his Neck ſtrait, and became more briſk and chearful than before. But he had ſcarce ſooner diſcharg'd the Water by Urine than he dropt down to the Ground, raiſed his Head no more, but died on the fourth Night half ſtupid, and nodding his Head. Hence it may be inferr'd, that *Cantharides* are principally prejudicial to the Head, and conſequently highly improper in acute and inflammatory Diſorders of that Part. But this Aſſertion muſt rather be confirm'd by Experience, than eſtabliſh'd by Conjecture and *Hypotheſis*. At *Rome*, in the Month of *April*, I took eight Ounces of Blood newly taken from a certain Patient, this Blood divided into two Veſſels; immediately after Extraction I mixed a Scruple of powder'd *Cantharides* with the Blood contain'd

in

in one of the Veffels, and left that in the other without any Mixture at all. The Blood mixed with the *Cantharides*, coagulated before that left without any Mixture; but afterwards affumed a livid b'ackifh Colour, and a flender blackifh Pellicle appear'd on its Surface. At laft over the whole Surface of the Blood appear'd a large Number of Veficles, which, when broken, difcharg'd a blackifh Serum, and foon after the whole of the Blood was diffolv'd into a black, and fomewhat livid Serum. The Blood in the other Veffel, and which remain'd without the Addition of any thing, did not undergo the like Changes. In the fame Month, after taking Blood from a certain feverifh Patient, *Baglivi* feparated the *Serum* from the Blood, and mix'd with the former a Scruple of the Powder of *Cantharides*. A little after the Mixture he obferv'd; that the Powder was precipitated to the Bottom of the Veffel without communicating any Colour to the *Serum*, which only became more liquid, thin, and fcarce afterwards to be coagulated.

Caper, Offic. The Goat. The Parts in Ufe of this Animal are the Blood, the Marrow, the Suet, the Milk, the Whey, the Stones in the Stomach, the Dung, the Urine, the Bladder, the *Omentum*, the Skin, and the Gall. The Blood is accounted alexipharmic, deobftruent, proper in Dyfenteries, and calculated for refolving coagulated Blood, and diffolving the Stone. The Marrow is more acrid and dry, and confequently more efficacious, than that of other Animals. The Suet is a powerful Difcutient, relieves thofe afflicted with Arthritic Pains, removes Stranguries, and allays Hæmorrhoidal Pains. The Milk is of a nutritive and abftergent Quality, and efteem'd proper for hectic and phthifical Patients, and fuch as are confumptive or emaciated. The Whey is preferable to that obtain'd from the Milk of any other Animal, as it is aperient, abftergent, attenuating, and laxative; and for that Reafon ufed in Infufions for purging Melancholy. The Stones found in the Stomach and Gall Bladder, are faid to be poffefs'd of a refolvent and diaphoretic Quality. The Dung is of a heating, drying, abftergent, digerent, aperient, and acrid Nature; for which Reafon it is principally ufed in hard Tumors of the Spleen and other Parts, Swellings of the Parotid Glands, Bubocs, and for confolidating defperate Ulcers, as alfo in Dropfies, and fciatic Pains. When calcined, it makes a fine Powder, proper in all Cafes where the Ufe of Detergents is indicated, fuch as an *Alopecia* and Ring-worms. Internally it is properly exhibited in Diforders of the Spleen, Jaundice, Obftructions of the *Menfes*, and other Difeafes of a like Nature. The Urine is reconmended above that of all other Animals for diffolving the Stone, and promoting a Difcharge of Urine; for which Reafon it is proper in a Dropfy. The urinary Bladder dry'd and reduc'd to a Powder is faid to be a Medicine of peculiar Efficacy in an Incontinence of Urine. The *Omentum* apply'd hot, allays and checks turbulent Motions of the Spirits, for which Reafon it is very properly ufed in Colic Pains and a *Mania*. The Skin relieves *Diarrhæas*, ftops Hæmorrhages, and efpecially that of the Noftrils. The Gall is faid to cure Quotidian Fevers.

Capra Alpina, Offic. The Chamois or Gems. It is frequently met with among the *Alps*, belonging to *Switzerland*, and the Country of the *Grifons*, being a Sort of wild Goat, in Shape and Size refembling the tame one, with fhort Horns, the Extremities of which are hook'd.

The

The Parts used in Medicine, are the Blood, Fat, Liver, Gall, Dung, and the *Ægagropila,* or *German Bezoar,* which is a little Ball found in the Stomach of this Animal, which some have pretended to be formed by the *Doronicum,* or Leopards Bane, on which this Animal feeds; but it is now certain that it consists only of Hairs, which it swallows, and the like Balls are sometimes found in the Stomachs of Cows, Hogs, Boars, and other Animals. The fresh Blood of this Animal is a Cure for the *Vertigo;* the Fat is good for the *Phthisis,* and Exulceration of the Lungs; the Liver stops a Looseness, the Gall clears the Eye of an *Albugo,* and helps a *Nyctalops.* The Dung wastes and expels the Stone: And the *Ægagropila* besides its Virtues in almost all Manner of malignant Diseases, is thought to procure an easy Delivery.

Capra Bezoardica. The Bezoar Goat. See *Bezoar.*

Capreolus, Offic. The Roe Buck. It is found in *Scotland.* The Parts used in Medicine are the Rennet, Liver, Gall, and Dung. The Rennet is good for a *Diarrhæa* and Dysentery, the Liver is supposed to sharpen the Sight, and stops an Hæmorrhage, especially at the Nostrils; the Gall clears the Face of Spots, the Eyes of *Albugines,* Films, or other Defects, helps the Ringing in the Ears, and mitigates the Tooth Ach: The Dung cures the yellow Jaundice.

Carduelis, Offic. The Gold-Finch. The whole Bird is used, which if roasted, and eat, is said to be a good Remedy against Iliac and Colic Pains.

Carpio, Offic. The Carp. The Gall of the Carp is good for Dimness of Sight, and Clouds in the Eye. The Fat is of Service in hot Affections of the Nerves. The triangular Bones found in the Mouth called *Lapides Carpionum* are recommended in the Colic, Stone, and Epilepsy; and are said to extinguish Thirst in Fevers, and restrain Hæmorrhages of the Nose, if held in the Mouth.

Caseus, Cheese. See *Bos.*

Castor, Offic. The Beaver. There are two Sorts of *Castor,* the *Russian* and the *American,* but the *American* is esteem'd by *Geoffroy* of very little Value. The *Castor* or Beaver is an Animal which lives very much in the Water, and is furnish'd with two large Glands near the *Anus,* which separate an oily Liquor probably of the same Use, as the oleous Glands about the same Parts in Fowls, which supplies them with an unctuous Liquor, that they anoint their Feathers with, to preserve them from being too much affected by the Water. Hence it has been fabled that this Animal, sensible the Hunters pursue him for the Sake of his Testicles, sometimes stops and bites them off, and leaves them to his Pursuers in order to save his Life; for the Beaver, when hunted, and when just going into the Water, frequently stops, putting his Mouth towards the *Anus,* in order to furnish himself with the Oil these Glands contain, to anoint his Fur with, and preserve it from being injur'd by the Water. But the Animal which produces the *Russia Castor,* is said to be vastly different, from that whence the *American Castor* is produc'd. The Fat of the Beaver is said to be peculiarly adapted to Disorders of the Nerves and *Uterus,* and therefore to be good in Epilepsies, Palsies, Convulsions and Apoplexies. The Skin is recommended in the Gout and Palsies. The Glands abovemention'd, which are not the Testicles, are what we usually call *Castor,* which heats, dries, attenuates, opens, discusses Flatulences, corroborates the nervous System and Head, excites

xcites the Spirits when torpid, re-
ists Poisons, causes Sneezing, is A-
nodyne, and provokes the *Menses.*
Hence it is of Use in a Lethargy,
Apoplexy, Epilepsy, Palsy, Vertigo, Tremor of the Limbs, Defluxions on the Joints, Hysterics, and
Colic Pains, both externally and in-
ernally used. It has further the
Reputation of curing Ringing of the
Ears, Difficulty of Hearing, and
Pains of the Teeth, and of correct-
ng the Virulence of *Opium.* As
Castor consists of very minute and pe-
etrating Parts, and is possess'd of a
ertain Acrimony, it should seem to
e a tolerable Medicine, when the
ntention is to rouze and excite a languid Circulation.

Catulus. A Puppy. See *Canis.*

Catus & Felis, Offic. The Cat.
The Fat, Blood, Head, Dung, Skin,
nd Secundines are used in Medicine.
The Fat of a wild Cat heats, molli-
es, discusses, and is of great Ser-
ice in Affections of the Joints. The
lood cures a *Herpes.* The Head of a
lack Cat incinerated is said to be an
xcellent Medicine for Diseases of
he Eyes, as the *Unguis, Nubecula,
Albugo,* and other Disorders. The
Dung cures an *Alopecia,* and helps the
Gout. The Skin is worn to heat
he Stomach, and contracted Joints.
And the Secundine is hung about the
Neck, to preserve the Eyes from
Disorders.

Cera alba, & citrina, white and
ellow Wax. See *Apes.*

Cernua, Offic. *Aspredo fluviatilis,*
Gefn, de Aquat. The Ruff. This
Fish is common in many of our large
Rivers. *Gesner* recommends a Bone
ound in the Head of this Fish, for
he Stone in the Kidneys; and for
ungent Pains about the Ribs, and
n other Parts.

Cervus, Offic. The Stag. The
Parts used in Medicine of this Animal are, the Bone found in the Heart,
he *Penis,* the Testicles, the Blood,

the Tears, the Marrow, the Suet,
the *Astragalus,* or the Bone of the
Heel, the Stones found in the Stomach and the Horns. The Bone of
the Heart is recommended against
Poisons, and for procuring Longe-
vity, and is particularly adapted to
Disorders of the Heart; for which
Reason it is an Ingredient in Medicines of a cordial and comforting Nature. It is externally recommended
as an Amulet in Hæmorrhages, but
all these Virtues seem to be founded
on Superstition. The *Penis* is diuretic, stimulating to Venery, is good
for Dysenteries and Pains of the Colic, and for Hysteric Disorders. It
is further recommended for Ruptures, dry'd and taken in Powder.
Externally it is used for a Difficulty of
discharging the Urine; as also for
bloody Urine, the Plague, and for
promoting Deliveries. Exhibited in
Wine, it is said to be good against
the Bites of venomous Animals. The
Testicles are said to excite venereal
Inclinations, and Abilities.——The
Blood when dry'd and infus'd in Clysters, cures Ulcers of the Intestines, and
inveterate Fluxes; and when drank
in Wine is effectual against Poisons.
It is also commended against the
Gout, Sciatica and Pleurisy. The
Dose is from half a Scruple to a
Dram. The Tears of the Stag,
which are the *Sordes* collected in the
greater or anterior Angle of the Eye,
resembling indurated Wax, or rather
the indurated Wax of the Ears, and
which smell somewhat rank, like the
Sweat of the Animal, are recommended for their drying, corroborating, astringent, and diaphoretic Qualities. They are also said to be good
against Poisons, and contagious Diseases; and to be proper in difficult
Labours, and for expelling the dead
Fœtus. These Tears are by some
called the Stone, or *Bezoar* of the
Stag. The Marrow of the Stag is
by some thought preferable to the

Marrows of other Animals, for alleviating Pains, and healing malignant Ulcers. *Diofcorides* informs us, that thofe who are anointed with it are Proof againft Poifons. When this Marrow is old, it becomes rancid, acrid, inflammatory, corrofive, and of a cauftic Quality : But, when recent, it is of a mild and oleous Nature, and confequently proper for foftening indurated Parts, and moiftening fuch as are dry. Hence we know when its Ufe is proper, either externally, for anointing any Part affected, or when exhibited by way of Draught ; or when injected, by Way of Clyfter, in Gripes of the Inteftines. *Galen* recommends it for provoking the menftrual Difcharge. That the Suet banifhes Serpents from thofe who are anointed with it, as *Diofcorides* informs us, feems to be founded on the Perfuafion, that the Stag, and all its Parts, are poffeffed of a Quality, whereby they refift Poifon. This Suet is alfo faid to be good for foftening Tumors, conglutinating Wounds, curing Chilblains, and alleviating Pains, even thofe of the Gout. It is alfo faid to be good for *Hernias*, Excoriations of the *Perinæum*, and Freckles and Exulcerations of the Face. It is a proper Ingredient in Clyfters intended for the Cure of Fluxes and Dyfenteries. The Oil diftill'd from this Suet is faid greatly to alleviate Arthritic Pains, if the Part affected, is frequently anointed with it every Day. According to *Hoffman*, when laid upon a Linen Cloth, melted at the Fire, and apply'd to the Gums, it furprifingly alleviates the Tooth-Ach, and extracts the Worms which create the Pain. According to *Ettmuller*, " The Suet of the Stag is " an excellent confolidating Medi- " cine in fuperficial Excoriations. " In a falling down of the *Anus*, let " the Part be anointed with it warm, " and gently put up. It is alfo an " excellent Medicine for an *Inter-* " *trigo*, or Galling of the Skin ; " as alfo for Fiffures of the Hands " and Feet produc'd by Cold ; for it " is of a more penetrating and refol- " vent Nature than any other pin- " guious Subftances. Dr. *Neftor* " put one Drop of Stags Suet in " the Urine of any Patient who was " thought to be dangeroufly ill. If " this Drop fubfided in the Urine, " he pronounc'd the Cafe defperate ; " and, if it floated, he prognofti- " cated a Recovery." *Hippocrates*, in his Book *de Morb. Mul.* ordered melted Stags Suet, mix'd with Oil of Rofes, to be laid upon Wool, and put into the *Pudenda*, in Child-Bed-Women, when the *Lochia* were not difcharg'd. The fame Author recommends this Suet as a proper Ingredient in Peffaries againft Exulcerations of the *Uterus* ; and when, in order to provoke the menftrual Difcharge, acrid Peffaries have been us'd, he orders thefe to be laid afide, and the Suet of the Stag, melted in Wine, to be apply'd. As for the Ankle Bone of the Stag, or that fmall fquare Bone protuberating above the Hoof, the Powder of it is by fome highly commended againft Dyfenteries, Colics, and the Stone. *Johnfton* informs us, that *Rhafis* recommends the Brain of the Stag in Pains of the Hips and Sides ; as alfo for the Cure of Fractures. The Skin of the Stag is recommended againft Strangulations of the *Uterus*. When applied to the Loins, it is faid infallibly to promote the Expulfion of the *Fœtus*. *Burrhus* recommends Stockings of it againft the Gout. The Shavings of this Skin taken off with a Pumice Stone, and triturated with Vinegar, are faid to be proper for anointing an *Eryfipelas*. The fame put in Beds is faid to be a Remedy for an involuntary Difcharge of Urine. The Lungs of the Stag, if ufed as an Aliment, are faid to be of

eafe

easy Digestion, and *Pliny* informs us, that the Lungs and *Oesophagus* of this Animal, dry'd in the Smoak, beat with Honey, or daily taken in Wine, are good against a Cough and *Phthisis*. The Stones found in the Stomach of a Stag, is said to agree in Virtues with the *Bezoar*. But the Part of a Stag most celebrated in Medicine is the Horns, which when crude are said to resist Putrefaction, correct Malignity, and to preserve the Texture of the Blood. Hence it is used in the Small-Pox, Measles, and malignant and putrid Fevers, but in these Intentions as well as in all others where it is recommended, the Horns of the Buck are used promiscuously with those of the Stag, and must be equally effectual. Calcin'd Hartshorn is generally recommended against Putrefaction, for stopping Fluxes and Hæmorrhages, for killing Worms, and exciting a *Diaphoresis*. It is also recommended for provoking the *Menses*, for curing the Jaundice, Spittings of Blood, Ulcers, and Defluxions of the Eyes. It is also recommended for Dentifices, and against Pains of the Bladder, in Conjuction with Tragacanth. Some absolutely reject calcin'd Hartshorn, affirming that by the Calcination it is reduc'd to a dead Earth, and destitute of all Medicinal Virtue. *Ettmuller* tells us, " That it is a pure dead Earth, " which either as an Alexipharmic, " or Diaphoretic, produces no Effect at all; except, perhaps, in a " very remote and accidental Manner, by powerfully absorbing the " Acids of the *Primæ Viæ*; render-" ing them insipid, or changing " them, and, by that Means, pre-" venting their Action on the Parts " of the Body. But in *Diarrhæas*, " and a Laxity of the Intestines, by " absorbing the Humidity, it pro-" duces good Effects, and may,

" therefore, be properly exhibited " in acute Disorders, attended with " Fluxes, Hæmorrhages, Vomit-" ings, and a *Cholera*. Where an " Acid abounds in the Intestines, it " is also properly prescrib'd; for it " powerfully absorbs Acidities, and " various acrid Humours." It is also properly exhibited for expelling Worms of the Intestines, especially those of Children. Upon the whole calcin'd Hartshorn seems to act as an alcaline Absorbent only. Decoctions of the Shavings of Hartshorn uncalcin'd, in Water, may prove beneficial, where the Acrimony of the Humours is to be corrected, where the Constitution is dry, and wants to be moisten'd, and where Thirst is to be allay'd; but they are more proper in Disorders arising from Acidity, than in such as arise from an alcalescent State in the Juices. In some foreign Countries a Water is distill'd from the tender Horns of the Stag, which is esteem'd prodigious cordial, and is particularly celebrated, in the Disorders of Childbed Women, and for promoting the Expulsion of the *Fœtus*; but it is highly improbable, that it should be possessed of any more Virtues, than common distill'd Water.

Cervus minor Americanus. The lesser *American* Deer. See *Bezoar*.

Cetus. The Parmasitty Whale. See *Sperma Ceti*.

Chama, Offic. The Bastard Cockle. It is found in the *Mediterranean* Sea. *Dioscorides* says, that the Broth of this and other such Shell-Fish, made by boiling them in Water, is laxative, and keeps the Belly open: He adds, that it is usually taken with Wine.

Chamæleon, Offic. The Chamelion. The Gall, Heart, and the Animal itself are used in Medicine. The Gall removes Suffusions. *Pliny*

re-

recommends the Heart against Quartans, and *Trallian* recommends it against Epilepsies and the Gout.

Cicada, Offic. The Baulm Cricket. This Insect is common in *Italy*, but unknown in *England*. It is furnish'd with Wings, and is somewhat like a Cricket, very noisy, and living only on Dew. In the Kingdom of *Naples* innumerable Multitudes of these Insects are continually sucking and feeding upon the *round leav'd Ash-Tree*, from whose Wounds, by Exsudation, proceeds *Manna* as is said. These Insects are used, when dry'd, in Colics; and are recommended to be eaten roasted, in Disorders of the Bladder. The Ashes of these, burnt, are said to wear away the Stone.

Cicindela, Offic. The GlowWorm. The whole Insect is used, and is recommended by some against the Stone. *Cardan* ascribes an Anodyne Virtue to it.

Ciconia, Offic. The Stork. This Bird is seldom found in *England*. The Parts used in Medicine besides the whole Bird, are the Gall, Fat, Dung and Craw. The Stork is a remarkable Alexipharmic, being supposed a most excellent Remedy for all kinds of Poison, and especially the Pestilence; and also for Affections of the Nerves and Joints. The Gall is recommended for Diseases of the Eyes; the Fat is good to anoint gouty and trembling Joints; the Dung, drank in Water, is supposed to cure the Epilepsy, and other Diseases of the Head; and the Ventricle, or Craw, dry'd and pulveriz'd, is accounted an extraordinary Secret in Cases where Poison is concern'd.

Cimex, Offic. The Wall Louse, or Bugg. It is found in Beds, being a small Insect, of a Rhomboidal Figure, and a dark brown Colour, with six Feet, and a very tender Skin, so that it bursts with the least Compression, and emits a most offensive Smell. Given to the Number of seven, as Food, with Beans, they help those who are afflicted with a Quartan Ague, if they be eaten before the Accession of the Fit; swallowed alone without Beans, they are good against the Bite of an Asp; the Smell of them relieves under hysterical Suffocations; drank in Wine or Vinegar, they expel Leeches that have been swallow'd and pulveriz'd, and introduc'd into the urinary Passages, they cure a Difficulty of Urine.

Coccinilla, Cochineal. See *Cochinilla*.

Coccus Polonicus. This is a *Nidus* of an Insect found adhering to the Roots of the *Polygonum cocciferum*, or *Polonian Knawel*, and is used in dying Scarlet. The learned *Paulli* informs us, that the common People in *Silesia* swallow every Year three Grains of it, in order to prevent the Attack of Fevers; but he justly censures this as a superstitious Practice, as it is not attended with the proposed Success. The same Author also brands, with the odious Name of Superstition, the Practice of the credulous and giddy Multitude, who, about the Middle of the Day, on St. *John*'s Eve, dig up these Grains, in order to imprint on their Shirts and Breasts certain Characters, with the bloody Juice they yield upon being bruis'd, thinking, by this Means, to escape Falls, Contusions, Wounds, the Bites of mad Dogs, and a large Train of other Diseases. But tho' this learned Author affirms, that he has just Cause to detest and condemn the internal Use of them, yet I see, (says *Rieger*) no Reason why they should be rejected for medicinal Purposes, since the whimsical Uses, to which superstitious Fools apply any Medicine, can never rob it of its real and inherent Virtues. This he is the rather inclin'd to think, because the *Coccus Polo-*

Polonicus, is found from Experience, to have the same Efficacy in Medicines as the *Kermes,* and may be safely used as a *Succedaneum* to them. They are not, however, as yet received into the Shops. If in Cases of this Nature, Conjectures are pardonable, I am inclined to think, that the *Cocca Polonica,* if subjected to the same Chymical Analysis as the *Kermes,* would yield the same Principles, and discover themselves to be of a similar Nature.

Cochinilla, or *Coccinilla,* Offic. Cochineal. This is an Insect generated in, and feeding upon the *Ficus Indica major, Lævis, five non spinosa, Vermiculos, quos Cochinilla vocant, proferens,* Plukn. Phytog. which grows plentifully in *New Spain,* and *Mexico.* It is esteem'd greatly cardiac, sudorific and alexipharmic, and is said to cure all Fevers, however malignant; it is therefore often given in the Plague and petechial Fevers. *Geoffroy* says, that Cochineal is used in all the same Intentions with *Chermes.* I have no Reason to believe these Insects to be possess'd of any considerable Medicinal Virtues. They are principally employ'd in giving a red Colour to Tinctures.

Cochlea terrestris, Limax terrestris, Offic. *Cochlea testacea,* Schrod. The Snail. Snails are said to refrigerate, incrassate, consolidate, lenify, and to be agreeable to the Nerves and Lungs; hence they are used against Coughs, Consumptions, Spitting of Blood, and other Affections of the Lungs; against a hot Intemperature of the Liver, and a Colic. Externally they maturate, and break Carbuncles, consolidate Wounds, particularly of the nervous Parts, heal Ulcers, mitigate Inflammations, restrain Hæmorrhages, and make hydropical Tumours of the Belly and *Scrotum* to subside. The Shells act as Absorbents; but when calcin'd are a Sort of Lime.

Cochlea minor ex lutea & nigro variegata, Offic. The *Paris* Garden Snail. This is frequent in the Gardens at *Paris,* the Shell is used in *Collyria.*

Cochlea aquatica, Offic. The Water Snail, or Periwinkle. This agrees in Virtues with the common Snail.

Cochlea cælata, Aldrov. de Exang. This is a Species of Sea Snail, found in the *Mediterranean* Sea. Its *Operculum,* or Covering, is according to some, the *Umbilicus marinus* of the Shops, which is said to stimulate to Venery.

Columba, Offic. The Pigeon, or Dove. The Parts in Use are, the living Pigeon, the Blood, the Coat of the Stomach, and the Dung. The live Pigeon, dissected in the Middle, and applied to the Head, while the Blood is hot, mitigates the Violence of the Humours, and discusses Melancholy and Sadness; whence it is a very convenient Remedy in the Phrensy, Head-ach, Melancholy, and the Gout. The warm Blood, instill'd into the Eyes, helps Pain and Lippitude, discusses Cataracts and stagnated Blood, cures recent Wounds, has a peculiar Virtue in stopping an Hæmorrhage from the Membranes of the Brain, and mitigates the Pain of the Gout. The Coat of the Stomach, dry'd and pulveriz'd, is recommended in the Dysentery. The Dung is violently heating, on which Account it is a Caustic, and Discutient, and excites a Redness of the Skin, by attracting the Blood thither; whence it is of frequent Use in stimulating Plaisters, and Cataplasms. Triturated and sifted, and applied with the Seed of Cresses, it relieves under inveterate Disorders, as the Gout, *Hemicrania, Vertigo,* Head-ach, and others; internally it wastes the Stone, and provokes Urine.

Con-

Concha, Offic. Shell Fifh. This is a general Name comprehending a great many Sorts of Shell Fifh. The Shells of thefe Fifh in general, are drying, abforbent, correcting, and precipitating; for which Purpofes, thofe beat to a fine Powder are preferable to thofe levigated on a Marble with Water, which are commonly called *Concha Preparata.* What are ufually kept in the Shops, under this Title, are the Shells of Mufcles, and are recommended for exciting a *Diaphorefis* in Intermitting Fevers, if a Scruple, or half a Dram is exhibited, about an Hour before the Paroxyfm, in *Carduus* Water, or that of the leffer Centaury; ordering the Patient, at the fame time, to be kept warm, in order to encourage a *Diaphorefis.* But, when the Shells are calcined, they become Lime, and do not abforb and correct, but ftimulate and refolve, in Confequence of the Acrimony they have acquired by Calcination. In this Cafe they are fo far from correcting the Acrimony of the Juices, that they rather increafe the Heat of the Stomach and *Fauces. Olaus Wormius,* in his *Mufeum,* informs us, that the Afhes of Shell-fifh are poffefs'd of a cauftic Quality; that they are recommended againft Leprofies, Freckles, and Spots of the Skin; that when they are previoufly wafhed, like Lime, they cure Ulcers, and Eruptions on the Head; and that, in the *Netherlands,* they are ufed as a Cure for the Hæmorrhoids. *Pliny* defcribes their detergent Quality in the following Words: " The " Afhes of the Shells of Fifh, if " ufed by way of Ointment, with " Honey, remove Spots in the Faces " of Women in feven Days time, " render the Skin fmooth, and on " the eighth, the Part is to be a- " nointed with the Whites of Eggs." *Concha Venerea,* or *Veneris.* This

is what we call *Venus's* Shell. It is a Fifh, whofe Shell is univalve, wreath'd, and has a fmall longitudinal and denticulated Chink or Aperture in it. That this Species of Shell Fifh, was ufed by the Antients, as an Aliment, we read in *Seneca,* Epift. 95. *Mundius* afferts, that they prove a *Stimulus* to Venery, and provoke Urine. *Rondeletius* informs us, that they are good to remove Fluxes, and cure Ulcers of the *Uterus.* Excellent Dentrifices are prepared from this Species of Shell; which is alfo ufeful for curing Ulcers in the *Canthus* of the Eye, and the *Fiftula Lachrymalis.* It is remarkably drying, without exciting any Heat. *Wormius* informs us, that he has heard Spoons of thefe Shells highly commended for curing the Chin Cough in Children, if they fup Broths, or other proper Liquors with them. The Powder of thefe Shells is poffefs'd of an abforbent drying Quality, and is faid to be a Cure for the *Yaws.*

Coracinus, Offic. The Crow Fifh. This is a Fifh mentioned by *Galen Aldrovandus,* and *Bruyerinus.* It is found in Rivers, particularly in the *Nile* and the *Mediterranean* Sea. Certain Bones, found in the Head of this Fifh, are faid to be poffefs'd of fome Medicinal Virtues: They are called *Lapides Coracini,* and are recommended againft nephritical and colical Pains, and the Jaundice.

Cornix, Offic. The Carrion Crow. The Dung of this Bird is ufed, which taken in Wine, is recommended for the Cure of a Dyfentery.

Corvus, Offic. The Raven. Young Ravens, calcin'd to Afhes, are recommended againft the Epilepfy, Gout, and that Species of Leprofy called *Alphus.* The Brain is alfo taken Notice of among the Remedies for an Epilepfy. The Fat and Blood are faid to render the Hair black.

black. The Dung, fufpended about the Necks of Children, is reported to eafe their Coughs, and procure them an eafy Dentition.

Coturnix, Offic. The Quail. The Fat is faid to be good for Specks in the Eyes; and as this Bird is faid to feed upon Hellebore, the Dung is faid to be a Kind of a Specific in an Epilepfy.

Crabro, Offic. The Hornet. It is recommended in a Drench for that Diforder in a Horfe, which *Vegetius* calls *Scrofula*, meaning, I believe, what we call the Strangles. The Sting of the Hornet is very troublefome, making the Part affected to fwell very much, with an exceffive Pain. I fhould apprehend, that anointing it with Oil of Olives, would be the moft effectual Remedy.

Crangon, Offic. The Prawn. This fifh is efteemed extremely nourifhing, and therefore good in Confumpions.

Crocodilus, Offic. The Crocodile. This is found in the River *Ganges*, the *Nile*, and other large Rivers. The Blood and Fat of this Animal are ufed. The Blood is faid to clear the Sight; and the Fat is recommended for Wounds and Cancers.

Cuculus, Offic. The Cuckow. The whole Bird and its Dung, are ufed in Medicine. The Bird burnt whole, is recommended for the Gravel, Pains of the Stomach, and exceffive Humidity of the fame Part. It is given with good Succefs alfo in the Paroxyfms of Fevers. The Dung of the Cuckow drank, as is faid, cures the Bite of a Mad Dog.

Cuniculus, Offic. The Rabbit. The whole Animal, its Fat, and Brains are ufed A Rabbit calcin'd whole, is faid to cure a Quinfey, or Inflammations of the *Fauces*. The Fat is ufed for refolving the Indurations of the Tendons and Joints, and the Brains are faid to refift Poifons.

Cygnus, Offic. The Swan. The Fat of the Swan is ufed, which is efteem'd emollient, attenuating, and lenient, and is therefore faid to be good for the Piles, and Indurations of the *Uterus*. Mixed with Wine, it removes Freckles of the Skin, if thefe are anointed with it. The Skin of a Swan is fometimes directed to be applied to the Parts affected with a Rheumatifm. It is faid to fortify the Nerves and Stomach, to difpel Flatulencies, and to affift Digeftion, when applied to the Stomach.

Dama, Offic. The Fallow Deer. As this Animal lives entirely on Vegetables and Water, the Salts are not highly exalted; nor is it much inclined to alcaline Putrefaction, on account of its Aliment. But the habitual Exercife of the Animal exalts and volatilizes the Salts in fome Degree. The Venifon of a Deer, kill'd when cool, differs very much from that of one kill'd when heated with Exercife: The Fibres of the firft are more hard, the Flefh more tough, and confequently lefs eafily diffolvable in the Stomach. The fecond is more tender, more diffolvable, but has a greater Tendency to an alcaline Putrefaction, which however, may be, in a great Degree prevented, by fuffering the Deer to bleed plentifully when killed; as the *Jews* were directed to do with Refpect to all Sorts of Beafts and Fowls in *Leviticus*. The recent Blood of this Deer, drank immediately after being taken from the Vein, is faid to remove Dizzinefs of the Head. The Gall is faid to be deterfive, to cure Dimnefs of the Sight, and take away Films of the Eyes. The Liver is recommended againft a Diarrhœa, and the Horns agrees in Virtues with Hartfhorn.

Delphinus, Offic. The Dolphin. This is found in the *Britifh* Ocean, and in other Places. The Belly, Liver, Afhes, and Fat are ufed. The

The Belly dried, triturated, and exhibited in some proper Liquor, is said to cure splenetic Patients. It is said, that the Liver roasted, and used with Aliments, perfectly cures Tertian and Quartan Fevers; as also, that Species of nocturnal Fever known by the Name of *Typhus.* The Afhes, are by *Pliny,* enumerated among the Medicines which cure the Ringworm and Leprofies. According to the fame Author, the Fat melted, and drank with Wine, cures dropfical Patients.

Dentalium, Offic. The Dog-like Tooth Shell. This is a fmall Shell, or oblong conical Tube, of a white Colour, which inclofes a Sea Worm. It is found on the Coafts of *England,* and is alcaline, abforbent, cordial, and aftringent. There is another Kind of *Dentalium* found on the Coaft of *Normandy,* which is no more than a fmall Heap of Sand, in which a Worm hides itfelf. It is not much ufed in Medicine; but what Virtues it poffeffes, feem to be much the fame as other teftaceous Subftances.

Draco marinus, Offic. The Weaver. This Fifh is taken in the *Mediterranean* Sea. The Parts ufed, are the Head, newly burnt to Afhes, and the Bones. *Rondeletius* affirms, that the Afhes of the Head, newly burnt, are good againft all Poifons; and *Pliny* writes, that the Tooth-ach is eafed by fcarifying the Gums with the Bones of this Fifh.

Ebur. Ivory. See *Elephas.*

Echinus marinus, Offic. The Sea Hedge Hog. It is taken in the main Sea: It is friendly, and beneficial to the Stomach and Belly, and provokes Urine. The crude Shell, roafted, is a good Ingredient in Medicines for abfterging the *Pfora;* and the Afhes of it burnt, cleanfe foul Ulcers, and reprefs fungous Flefh.

Echinus ovarius, Offic. The great Sea Urchin. The Part ufed in Medicine is called the *Lapis Judaicus,* or *Jews* Stone of the Shops, which is thought to be the Spines or Prickles of this Animal petrified.

Echinus terreftris, Aldrov. de Quad. The Hedge Hog, or Urchin. This Animal is found in Thickets, and Hedges. What is ufeful in Medicine, are the whole Animal, the Liver, the Feet, and the Ventricle. The Hedge Hog boiled, or burnt to Afhes, helps an involuntary Difcharge of Urine, is grateful to the Stomach, and excites Excretions by Urine and Stool; externally it cures the *Alopecia,* being rubbed on the Part. The Liver, or the Body, dry'd, and taken in *Oxymel,* is effectual in nephritic Diforders, and cures a Cachexy, Dropfy, Convulfions, and *Elephantiafis,* and dries up Rheums in the *Vifcera.* The Fat is moft fuccefsfully ufed in a *Hernia.* The Membrane, or Coat of the Ventricle, is recommended for the Colic. The Decoction, or Broth of the Flefh, is very ferviceable in the Dropfy, by provoking Urine.

Elephas, Offic. The Elephant. The two large Teeth in the fuperior Jaw, are the Parts of the Elephant principally ufed in Medicine, as well as Mechanics. It is called *Ebur,* Offic. Ivory. It is a Refrigerant and Drier; is moderately aftringent, inciding, and a Strengthener of the *Vifcera:* It ftops uterine Hæmorrhages, affords Relief in the Jaundice, expels Worms, is good for inveterate Obftructions, cures Pains and Weaknefs of the Stomach, and the Epilepfy, preferves from Melancholy, and refifts Poifons and Putrefaction. *Ebur uftum,* Offic. *Spodium Arabum,* Burnt Ivory, is efteem'd an Aftringent.

Encraficholus, Offic. The Anchovy. Anchovies pickled with Salt, and kept in Barrels, and the whole Fifh, as well as its Pickle, are ufed in Medicine; the Fifh pickled is

appply'd like Herrings to the Soles of the Feet ; and both their Pickles serve for the same Purposes. It helps Digestion, and fortifies the stomach with its volatile and saline principles, which cause a gentle and moderate Heat in that Part, and disperse and attenuate the Aliments that are contained therein.

Entalium, Offic. The Entaglia. It is a Shell much longer and thicker than the *Dentalium.* It is imported from the *East Indies.* It is but little used in Medicine ; tho' probably, it may be serviceable for the same Purposes, and in the same Disorders, as other Substances of the testaceous Kind.

Equus, Offic. The Horse, or Mare. The Parts used in Medicine are the Blood, Rennet, Milk, Dung, Warts, *Lichen*) Testicles, Fat, Hoofs, Hairs, Saliva, Teeth, the Stone found in the Stomach or Intestines, which, for its Figure and Structure, consisting of *Laminæ,* is not unlike the *West-Indian* Bezoar. The Blood is mixed with Caustics and Septics : The Rennet, called *Hippace,* is particularly serviceable in the cœliac Passion, and the Dysentery. The Milk is thought to be good in the Epilepsy, *Phthisis,* Cough and Asthma. The Dung used externally, stops Hæmorrhages, and expels the dead Child and Secundines ; internally, it is exhibited in the Colic, Strangulation of the Uterus, Pleurisies, and also for the Expulsion of the dead Child, and After-Birth ; where that of a Stone Horse is most effectual. The Warts are particularly recommended in Hysterics, and for the Stone and Epilepsy. The Testicles are a present Remedy for expelling the Secundines, and are recommended in Colics. The Fat is used to good Purpose in anointing Luxations, and the Hairs repress an Hæmorrhage, the *Saliva,* or Spume of the Mouth, drank for three Days,

cures a Cough, and mitigates the violent Heat of the Fauces. The Teeth, when they first begin to appear, are said to facilitate Dentition in Infants. The Stone called the *Hippolithus,* is supposed to be endu'd with the same Virtues with the *West Indian* Bezoar.

Equus marinus, Offic. The Sea Horse. The Parts used in Medicine are, the Pizzle, which is a round, bony Substance, a Cubit, or more in Length, thick, ponderous, and solid, and much thicker and rounder at the End, near the Glans ; and the Teeth, which are great, long, thick, ponderous, hollow, and white. The Pizzle pulveriz'd, is used to expel the Stone ; the Teeth for Service and Value, are compared to Ivory, and are made into various Forms, as into Rings for the Cramp, and for other Purposes.

Erinaceus. The Hedge Hog. See *Echinus terrestris.*

Eruca, Offic. The Caterpiller. This is the *Fœtus* of a Sort of a Butterfly, and undergoes the same Metamorphosis as the Silk Worm, and at length passes into a Butterfly. There are many Species, but that which ought to be used in the Shops, is an Insect known to every body, that feeds upon Cabbage Leaves. Caterpillers bruised, or the Powder of them, raise a Blister like *Cantharides,* and take off the Skin. *Mouffet* says, they will cause the Teeth to fall out of their Sockets ; and *Hippocrates* writes, that they are good for a Quinsey.

Felis. The Cat. See *Catus.*

Ficedula, Offic. The black Cap. This Bird eaten as Food sharpens the Eyesight.

Formica, Offic. The Ant. This is a small, oblong, red, or blackish Insect, arm'd with a Sting, and living in Swarms ; the Male is wing'd, the Female destitute of Wings ; the Animal and its Eggs, are used in Medicine They are heating and drying, and incite to Venery; their acid Smell mightily refreshes the vital Spirits. They are said to cure the *Psora, Lepra,* and *Lentigo.* The Eggs are effectual against Deafness, and correct the Hairiness of the Cheeks in Children, being rub'd thereon.

Formica major, Offic. The Horse Ant. This Insect provokes to Venery, and the Oil thereof, by Infusion, is good for the Gout and Palsy.

Fulica, Offic. The Coot, or Bald-Coot. The Heart is recommended against Epilepsies; and the Flesh is said to be good for the Poison of Serpents.

Galbula, Offic. The Yellow Hammer. *Pliny* commends this Bird for the Jaundice.

Galerita. The crested Lark. See *Alauda criftata.*

Galeus. The Name of a Sea-Fish, called also *Muftelus Spinax,* Offic. The Hound-Fish, falfly called Seal. It is an Inhabitant of the cavernous Places of the Sea; and its rough Skin is of Use to Artificers in polishing Alabafter, Marble, and other things, the Flesh is highly alcalefcent, and confequently proper where Acidities abound.

Gallina aquatica, Offic. The common Water Hen, or Moor Hen. It is commonly found in Fish-Ponds. The Parts ufed in Medicine are, the Craw, the Feathers and their Afhes. The Craw is recommended in the *Afthma;* the Smoke of the Feathers is fuppos'd to be good for Hyfteric Fits, and their Afhes dry up old Ulcers and Fiftulas.

Gallina domeftica, Gallus, Offic. The Cock and Hen. The Parts ufed are, the whole Bird, the Brain, the Coats of the Ventricle or Craw, the Tefticles, the Gall, the Fat, the Throat, the Dung, and the Eggs. An Hen flit, and apply'd to the Head while the Blood is hot, is of good Effect in the Phrenfy, *Cephalalgia* and other Diforders of that Part: It is alfo faid to cure the Bites of venomous Animals, being ufed in the fame Manner. Laid on a Carbuncle, it draws out the Poifon; and, what deferves Obfervation, ftops an Hæmorrhage in recent Wounds, being apply'd thereto: The living Hen, ftript of its Feathers about the *Anus,* and apply'd, extracts the Poifon of *Buboes.* The Brain is of an incraffating Quality, and ftops Fluxes. The inner Coat of the Ventricle, extracted, dry'd, and pulveriz'd, has a Virtue of binding and ftrengthening the Stomach, and by that Means, of reftraining Vomiting and Fluxes of the Belly; and is, alfo, a Lithontriptic. The Tefticles of the Cock are faid to have a wonderful Effect in reftoring loft Strength in Difeafes, in fupplying prolific *Semen,* and venereal Vigour. The Gall deterges Spots in the Skin, being rub'd thereon, and is good for the Eyes. The Fat of Hens and Capons, heats, moiftens, mollifies, and is lenitive, and of a middle Nature between the Fats of a Swine and a Goofe, correcting Acrimony: It is of Ufe in Fiffures of the Lips, Pains of the Ears, and Puftules of the Eyes. The Throat of a Cock burnt, and not confum'd, but fcorch'd and dry'd, and given at Night before Supper, cures involuntary nocturnal Difcharges of Urine, by a fpecific Property. The Dung is faid to perform all the fame Effects as Pigeons Dung, tho' in an inferior Degree; but it is particularly ufeful in Pains of the *Colon* and *Uterus;* it is, alfo, efficacious in the Jaundice, Stone, and Suppreffion of Urine; the white Part of the Dung is obferv'd to be the beft. The Afhes dry up *Achors* of the Head, and other running Sores, being fprinkled thereon: The brown Part of the Dung confolidates an Exulceration

of

of the Bladder. The Eggs afford, for medicinal Uses, the Shells, Membranes, *Albumen*, and Yolk: The Shells are lithontriptic, and are endu'd with the Virtue of inciding a tartareous Mucilage: The Membranes have a diuretic Quality, used either inwardly or outwardly, and are apply'd to the Prepuce of Infants: The *Albumen* is refrigerating, astringent, and agglutinating, and is of frequent Use in Redness of the Eyes, and in Conglutination of Wounds (with the common Bole). In Fractures, and the like Cases, it is, also, of Service for *Anacollemas*. *Hippocrates* exhibited three or four Whites of Eggs to Persons in a Fever, as a Refrigerant and Expellent: The Yolk of an Egg has an anodyne, maturating, digesting, and relaxing Virtue; for which Reason, it is a very frequent Ingredient in Clysters, and mixt with a little Salt, is usually apply'd, in the Shell of a Walnut, to the Navel of Infants, to provoke Excretion of the *Faeces*. The white of a new laid Egg raw, pretty much resembles the *Serum* of the Blood, and is the Nutriment, from which all the solid Parts of the Chicken is form'd; hence 'tis perhaps, the very best Nutriment, where a Weakness of the digestive Organs prevails. The best Way of taking is, to beat it up with a little Sugar, and drink it with equal Parts of Milk and Water.

Gallinago, Offic. The Woodcock. The Ashes of this Bird, burnt, are said to be lithontriptic. The Woodcock consider'd as a Food, is said to be nourishing, strengthening, and restorative. The Salts of this Bird are highly exalted by their habitual Exercise, which renders it a very proper Aliment, where there is a Redundance of Acid.

The *Gallinago minor*, is the Snipe or Snite, which agrees with the preceeding in Virtues, except that it is

more easily digested, and esteem'd more delicate to the Taste.

Garum. The Pickle of the Anchovy, is so called. See *Encrasicholus*.

Gazella. The Bezoar Goat. See *Bezoar*.

Glis, Offic. The Rell or Rell Mouse. The Flesh if eaten, is said to cure the *Bulimia*; if the Soles of the Feet are anointed with the Fat, it is said to procure Sleep; the Excrements, drank in any convenient Vehicle, have the Reputation of dissolving the Stone; and mixed with Vinegar and May Dew, cure an *Alopecia*, the Part affected being anointed therewith; the Ashes clear the Sight.

Glossopetra. See *Canis Carcharias*.

Glottis, Offic. The Great Plover. This is found about watery Places, and the Gall is used, which is said to be good in Disorders of the Eyes. A Jelly made of the Flesh of this Bird, is by some esteem'd an Analeptic.

Gobius. The Gudgeon. This Fish affords good Nourishment, produces good Juice, is easy of Digestion, and provokes Urine. Several Authors affirm, that People recovering from Sickness may eat it. It contains much Oil and volatile Salt.

Gobius niger, Offic. The Sea Gudgeon, or Rock Fish. It is taken among the Rocks by the Sea Shore. Broil'd and eaten without Salt, it cures the Dysentery, Lientery and *Tenesmus*. It is said to be good for the Bites of Serpents and Dogs.

Graculus, Offic. The Cornish Chough. This Bird is found in *Cornwall*, and many other Places. Externally apply'd it is said to resolve Tumors, and to be good against scrophulous Swellings.

Grus; Offic The Crane. The whole of this Bird, its Fat, its Gall, its Head, its Eyes, its Stomach, and

the

the Marrow of its Legs, are ufed. The Bird itfelf, becaufe nervous, is faid to be highly beneficial to the nervous and membranous Parts; hence the Ufe of it is recommended in Colic Pains. Its Fat, if dropt into the Ears, leffens Deafnefs, foftens Hardnefs, and obftinate Tumors of the Spleen; it quickly relieves a Stiffnefs of the Neck, and is faid to be of the fame Nature with the Fat of a Goofe. The Gall is beneficial to the Eyes. The Head, Eyes, and Stomach, when reduc'd to a Powder, are fprinkled upon Fiftula's, Cancers, and varicofe Ulcers. An ophthalmic Ointment is prepar'd of the Marrow of the Legs.

Gryllus, Offic. The Cricket. This is an Infect with Wings, of a rufty Colour, an Inhabitant of the Fire, and highly officious with its fqueaking Notes. The Afhes of it exhibited, are faid to be diuretic; the exprefs'd Juice, dropt into the Eyes, is a Remedy for Weaknefs of the Sight, and alleviates Diforders of the Tonfils, if rub'd on them.

Halcedo. A Name for the *Ifpida,* or King's Fifher.

Halec, Offic. The Herring. The Parts of this Fifh, ufed in Medicine are the Veficles, called *Animæ,* and the entire Fifh. The *Animæ* are faid to excite Urine, taken internally. Salted Herrings are fometimes apply'd to the Soles of the Feet in Fevers, with an Intent to derive the Humours from the Head, and mitigate the febrile Heat. The Pickle of Herrings is ufed in Clyfters, for Pains in the Hips, and a Dropfy; externally apply'd, it mundifies fetid Ulcers, ftops the Progrefs of a Gangrene, and diffipates ftrumous Swellings. It is alfo, of Service in a Quinfey, if the Parts affected are anointed with this and Honey, mix'd together.

Hippocampus, Offic. The Sea Horfe. It is taken in the *Mediter-*ranean Sea. The Afhes of the burnt Fifh, mixed with Tar or Pix, or *Unguentum Amaracinum,* and the Part anointed, cures an *Alopecia.* It is a Remedy againft the Bite of a mad Dog.

Hippolithus. A Name for a Stone found in the Stomach, or Inteftines of a Horfe. See *Equus.*

Hippopotamus, Offic. The Sea Horfe, or rather River Horfe. The Teeth and Tefticles of this Animal are ufed in Medicine; the Tefticles dried and triturated, are drank againft the Bites of Serpents. The Teeth, made into Rings, are fuppofed to be of great Virtue againft the Cramp.

Hircus. The Goat. See *Caper.*

Hirudo, Sanguifuga, Offic. The Leech. There are two Sorts of Leeches, found in frefh ftagnating Waters. The fmaller of thefe are prefer'd for medicinal Purpofes, as making a lefs Wound, and confequently more eafy to be ftopt. They are only ufed for taking away Blood, and with this View they are apply'd to the Temples, under the Ears, to the *Anus,* Feet, Arms, and many other Parts.

Hirundo, Offic. The Swallow. The whole Bird, its Heart, Blood, Neft, and Dung, are ufed in Medicine. Swallows, with their Young, burnt to Afhes, are a Specific in the Epilepfy, and for Dulnefs of Sight, and Lippitude, if made into a *Litus* with Honey; they alfo cure the Quinfey, and Inflammations of the *Uvula.* The Heart alfo, is faid to be good againft the Epilepfy, and to ftrengthen the Memory; fome eat it againft a Quartan. The Blood is thought to be of fingular Benefit to the Eyes. The Neft helps the Quinfey, and cures Rednefs of the Eyes, and heals the Bite of a Viper, if apply'd to the Place. The Dung heats mightily, and difcuffes, being of an acrimonious Quality. It is of excellent Service againft the Bite of a

mad

d Dog, in the Colic, and nephri-
Diforders, and excites the Belly
Excretion. *Celfus* tells us that it
is commonly faid, " That whoever eats a young Swallow, fhall be
free from all Danger of a Quinfey for a whole Year."

Hirundo Indica, Offic. The *Indi-
Swallow.* It is found in the ma-
ime Places of *China.* Its Neft,
hich is the Part ufed in Medicine,
of an hemifpherical Figure, of the
ze of a Goofe's Egg, pellucid, and
Subftance refembling the *Ichthyo-
lla.* It ftimulates to Venery. In
hina thefe Nefts are efteem'd deli-
ous Food.

Hirundo riparia, Offic. Schrod.
he Sand Martin. The whole Bird
d its Blood are ufed in Medicine,
hich agree in Virtue with the com-
on Swallow.

Homo, Man, is not only the Sub-
t of Medicine, but contributes
th his Body to the *Mtteria Medi-*
. Officinal Simples, furnifh'd from
e Parts of the human Body, whilft
ive, are the Hairs, Nails, Saliva,
ar Wax, Sweat, Milk, Menfes,
cundines, Urine, Dung, *Semen*,
ood, the Stones of the Bladder,
hich are the *Bexoar Microcofmi*,
d the Membrane which covers the
ead of the *Fœtus.* The *Hair* is
mmended for the Production of
airs, for the Jaundice, Luxations,
d for ftopping an Hæmorrhage.
he *Nails* are faid to provoke Vo-
iting, and to be an Hydragogue
Dropfies. The *Saliva* of a Man
fting is recommended againft veno-
ous Bites, as thofe of Serpents, a
ad Dog, and the like. The *Ear-
ax* is faid to be a prefent Remedy
the Colic; outwardly ufed, it
ares the Stings of Scorpions, con-
lutinates Wounds, and Fiffures, and
uts in the Skin. The Sweat is
id to be effectual againft the *Scro-
bula*, if it be mixed with the Herb
and Root of Mullein, and wrapt up
in the Leaf, and fo applied to the
Place. The *Menftrual Blood*, of the
firft Flux, dried, is commended,
taken inwardly, for the Stone, and
the Epilepfy: Externally ufed, it
eafes the Pains of the Gout; it is
alfo faid to be of Service in the Peftilence, Abfceffes, and Carbuncles;
it cures the Eryfipelas, and cleanfes
the Face from Puftules. The *Secundine* are extol'd for removing ftrumous
Tumors in the Throat, againft the
Epilepfy, and for invalidating the
Effects of *Philtra*, or Love Potions;
for exterminating a Mole and a dead
Fœtus, and for deftroying noxious
Vermin. The *Urine* heats, dries, refolves, abfterges, difcuffes, cleanfes,
refifts Putrefactions; and is, therefore, of principal Service in Obftructions of the Liver, Spleen, Gall
Bladder, in the Dropfy, Jaundice
and as a Prefervative againft the
Plague. A Draught of the Hufband's
Urine, which the old Women call
Water of Caftor, is faid to facilitate
the Delivery of the Wife in hard Labour: Outwardly ufed, it dries the
Habit, diffolves Tumours, cleanfes
Wounds, even though poifon'd, prevents a Gangrene, loofens the Belly,
abfterges Scurf from the Head, mitigates the Paroxyfms of Fevers, cures
Exulcerations of the Ears, helps
Rednefs of the Eyes, removes Tremblings of the Limbs, difcuffes Tumors of the *Uvula*, and eafes Pains
of the Spleen: There is prepared of
it a *Sal Ammoniac*, which is an artificial ftriated Salt, made into Cakes,
of a white Colour, and of a bitterifh pungent Tafte; the Method of
Preparation is, by boiling together
Urine, Soot, and common Salt:
Chufe what is pure and white. There
feem to be fome Footfteps of a natural *Sal Ammoniac*, in *Diofcorides*,
Pliny, and other antient Authors,
who defcribe it, as found under the

Sands

Sands of *Lybia*; but no such thing is to be found in the Shops at present; nor is it known what it was. Human *Dung* is mollifying, maturating, and anodyne; whence it is very serviceable in mitigating Pains excited by Charms, for ripening pestilential Carbuncles, and for a Phlegmon, particularly of the Throat, as in a Quinsey; and to prevent an Inflammation in Wounds: Some even prescribe it inwardly for the Quinsey, to repress the Paroxysms of Fevers, and for the Epilepsy. The *Semen* or *Sperm*, is whimsically used by some for dissolving the malific Influence of Spells, causing Impotence; and of the same is prepared a magnetic Mummy, which serves for a Philtre. The *Blood*, drank recent and hot, is said to be effectual against the Epilepsy, if thePatient afterwards uses the vehement Motion of running till he sweats; it stops all Sorts of Hæmorrhages: Used outwardly, it also represses all Eruptions of Blood, and especially from the Nose. The *Stone* in the human Bladder dissolves the Stone, and all tartareous Matter in any Part, and expels the same; for which Reason, it frees from all Obstructions. The *Membrane*, which sometimes surrounds the Head of the *Fœtus*, is said to be of extraordinary Efficacy against the Pains of the Colic. Officinal Simples, taken from the human Carcase, are the *Mummy*, which is a resinous, harden'd, black shining Surface, of a somewhat acrid and bitterish Taste, and of a fragrant Smell. Under the Name of *Mummy* are comprehended, first, the *Mummy* of the *Arabians*, which is a Liquament, or concreted Liquor, obtain'd in Sepulchres, by Exudation from Carcases embalm'd with Aloes, Myrrh, and Balsam. If this *Mummy* could be procured right and genuine, it would be preferable to the other Sorts. The second Kind of *Mummy*

is the *Egyptian*, which is a Liquament of Carcases, season'd with *Pissasphaltus*. A third Substance, which goes by the Name of *Mummy*, is a Carcase torrified under the Sand, by the Heat of the Sun: but such a one is seldom to be met with in our Country. The other Parts useful in Medicine are, the Skin, Fat, Bones, Marrow, *Cranium*, and Heart. *Mummy* resolves coagulated Blood, and is said to be effectual in purging the Head, against pungent Pains of the Spleen, a Cough, Inflation of the Body, Obstructions of the *Menses*, and other uterine Affections: Outwardly, it is of Service for consolidating Wounds. The Skin is recommended in difficult Labours, and hysteric Affections, and for a Withering and Contraction of the Joints. The Fat strengthens, discusses, eases Pains, cures Contractions, mollifies the Hardness of Cicatrices, and fill up the Pitts left by the Measles. The *Bones* dried, discuss, astringe, stop all Sorts of Fluxes, and are therefore useful in a Catarrh, Flux of the *Menses*, Dysentery, and Lientery; and mitigate Pains of the Joints. The *Marrow* is highly commended for Contractions of the Limbs. The *Cranium* is found by Experience, to be good for Diseases of the Head, and particularly for the Epilepsy; for which Reason, it is an Ingredient in several anti-epileptic Compositions. The *Os triquetrum*, or triangular Bone of the Temple, is commended as a specific Remedy for the Epilepsy. The *Heart* also cures the same Distemper.

Hystrix, Offic. The Porcupine. It is found in the Province of *Caragu*, and is of the Size of a Pig eight Months old. The Parts used in Medicine, are the whole Animal, and the Stone, called *Pedro del Porco*, found in the Gall Bladder, called also, by the various Names of *Bezaar Hystricum, Lapis Hystricis, Lapis Malacensis*, *acenfis, Lapis Porcinus,* Mont. Exot. and *Lapis feu Pila Hyftricis,* Ind. Med. This Part is rather to be called an *Ægagropila,* than a Stone, as confifting of a woolly Kind of Fibres, and a reddifh, bitterifh, and friable Matter, with its Outfide cover'd in fome Parts, with a Kind of blackifh Scales, like Nails. It has neither *Laminæ* nor Membranes, and is neither ponderous nor fmooth, like the Bezoar, but light, and fomewhat like the *Ægagropila.* This Animal feems to be poffefs'd of the fame Virtues as the *Echinus terreftris.* Dr. *Tancred Robinfon* obferves, that it is efteem'd an excellent Alexipharmic.

Ibex, Offic. The Stone Buck. This Animal is found in the higheft Parts of the *Alps. Gefner* recommends the Blood taken in Wine, againft the Stone. The Dung is faid to be good in Arthritic and Ifchiadic Pains. And *Seraphinus* afcribes the fame Virtues to the *Coagulum,* or Runnet, as to that of the Hare.

Ichneumon, Offic. The Egyptian Rat. The Part of this Animal principally ufed in Medicine is the Dung, which, together with Muftard Seed, and Vinegar, is efteem'd a good Tonic in the Gout ; and is faid to be fudorific, to be good for the Colic, and venomous Bites, and to purify the Blood.

Ichthyocolla, Offic. The Ifinglafs Fifh. The Glue of this Fifh, commonly called *Ifinglafs,* is ufed, and is of a yellowifh Subftance, made up in a fpiral Form, of a glutinous Confiftence, and of no Smell. It is prepared of the Skin, Inteftines, Stomach, Fins and Tail of this Fifh, in the following Manner. Thefe Parts of the Fifh, when cut in fmall Pieces, are macerated in a fufficient Quantity of Water: Then they are boiled over a flow Fire, to the Confiftence of a Poultice ; after which they are to be moiften'd, and fpread into Pellicules, before they become

cold, and reduced to a hard Mafs. This Subftance, according to *Schroder,* is of a drying, incarning, and, in fome Meafure, of an emollient Quality ; it infpiffates the Blood, and is of an anodyne Nature : It is ufed in Exulcerations of the Lungs and *Fauces,* and in a *Fluor Albus* it is exhibited with Succefs : Some alfo prefcribe it in Dyfenteries. It is of a conglutinating Nature, when externally applied.

Ifpida, Offic. The King's Fifher. It is found about Rivers. The Heart is ufed, which dry'd, and hung about the Neck, prevents Epileptic Fits in Children.

Julius, Offic. The Rainbow Fifh. This Fifh is frequently found about *Genoa.* The Broth thereof loofens the Belly, and is diuretic, *Pliny* and *Orbafius* efteem'd this Fifh as good Food.

Julus, Offic. The Gally Worm. This is a terreftrial Infect, furnifhed with many *Annuli,* or Rings, and creeping on many Legs, and rolling itfelf up, when touched. It is common in Gardens. *Charlton* recommends it, taken in Wine, againft the Jaundice, and Difficulty of Urine.

Kermes, five Chermes, Ind. Med. *Grana Chermes & Coccus Baphica,* Offic. *Chermes, Grana Tinctorum, Coccus Baphica, Coccum infectorium,* Mont. Exot. Kermes Berries. This Grain is found adhering to the Branches, but rarely to the Leaves of the *Ilex aculeata cocciglandifera.* It is of a fpherical Figure, as large as a Pea, or Lentil, fmooth, fhining, and of a blackifh brown Colour. After the moft diligent Scrutinies of the Naturalifts into this Matter, 'tis now certain, that the Production of this Grain is owing to a certain Infect, or fmall Worm ; and that it is, in Reality, nothing but a certain *Nidus* or Follicle, fill'd with the numerous Progeny of that Animalcule. *Marfigli* affirms, that the Subftance of

Kermes Grains is richly impregnated with a volatile Salt, of an alcaline Nature. M. *Geoffroy* also, upon distilling *Kermes* Grains by the Retort, obtain'd urinous and volatile Liquors, which, when pour'd into the Tincture of Turn-sole, produc'd no Change, but tinged the Tinctures of Roses and Violets with a greenish Colour. From one Pound of *Kermes* he obtain'd half an Ounce of pure concreted volatile Salt, and about a Dram or two contaminated with a yellowish Oil. A large Quantity of fetid Oil was yielded, which was not black, but of a deep yellow Colour, and thick like Butter. Hence he concludes, that the Principles of the *Kermes* can be more properly compared to nothing, than to the Products yielded by crude Silk, when chymically examined. As for the Medicinal Virtues of the *Kermes*, *Dioscorides* describes them in the following Manner: This Substance is of an inspissating Quality; and when triturated with Vinegar, is highly proper for anointing Wounds, and cut Nerves. *Matthiolus*, from *Galen*, informs us, that the *Kermes* is possessed of an astringent, and, at the same time, of a bitter Quality, both of which dry without creating Pain; for which Reason it is proper in large Wounds, especially those of the Nerves; for which Purpose some triturate it with Vinegar, and others with *Oxymel*. *Pliny* informs us, that it is to be laid upon recent Wounds, triturated with Vinegar; upon the Eyes, when affected with Defluxions, triturated with Water; and to be dropt into inflamed Eyes. From these Passages it is obvious, that the Antients thought *Kermes* proper in Cases where the Use of astringent, and consequently of inspissating and repelling Medicines was indicated. The Moderns, with the *Arabians*, ascribe a highly corroborating and cordial Quality to the *Kermes*. The

Cloth dyed with these Grains, commonly called Crimson, or Scarlet Cloth, is also highly extoll'd, on account of these Qualities, and is, for that Reason, used not only for bringing forth the Measles, by wrapping the Patient in it, but also for corroborating the Heart, by the Application of Epithems, wrapt up in it, to the Region of that Organ. The Application of a Piece of this Cloth, is also thought good for curing Venereal Buboes. *Schroder* in his *Pharmacopœa*, informs us, that it is a common Practice to tie a silken Thread of this Colour, about the Parts affected with an *Erysipelas*, in order to remove that Distemper. *Simon Paulli*, in his *Quadripartitum Botanicum*, affirms, that the Eruption of the Measles is greatly promoted in Children, by wrapping them up in this Cloth; and that he has seen it successfully applied, by Men of Skill, to Venereal Buboes. For preventing Abortion, and strengthening the *Fœtus*, some Women use, as an infallible Remedy, a Belt of this Sort of Cloth next their Skins, all the Time of their Gestation. Others use the like Belt for suppressing an immoderate Flux of the *Menses* and Hæmorrhoids. *Ludovici* in his *Pharmacopœa*, insinuates, that these external Applications, are none of the best and most effectual. " To " add, says he, the Knap of Scarlet " Cloth to medicated Bags and Epi- " thems, is a Practice more osten- " tatious than useful: To tie up " bleeding Parts with a Scarlet " Thread, or to sollicit the Erup- " tion of the Measles, by wrapping " the Patient in Scarlet Cloth, seems " a Practice only worthy of ignorant " Women." And *Hoffman*, in his *Claro. Schrod.* informs us, that, when Scarlet Cloth is used for promoting the Eruption of the Measles, the Effect must rather be produc'd by the Force of the Patient's Imagination, than

than any expulsive Virtue lodged in the Cloth itself. Nor according to *Lanzanius*, does a Scarlet silken Thread, tied about the Part, remove the *Eryfipelas*. If we consider that the Principles which compose an Animal Body, have a Tendency to an alcalescent Disposition; if also we consider that the Animalcules of the *Kermes* Grain, as yet retain some Properties of the Substance by which they were nourish'd, especially the astringent Qualities peculiar to the Juice of the Shrub, we cannot deny that the *Kermes* Grains contain very considerable Virtues, which is indicated by their bitter and astringent Taste; in Consequence of which Quality it is corroborating, and calculated for removing the Laxity of the Fibres, and correcting the Peccancy of the acescent Humours. It is also obvious, that the saline alcaline Substances it yields in a chymical Distillation, are proper in Disorders, where an Acid is to be corrected and subdued. Hence 'tis evident, whether we use the alcaline Salts produced by the Fire, or the unchanged Substance of the Grains, that they are only to be commended as excellent Corroboratives, and Cordials, in particular Cases; but not in every Case indiscriminately, and without having a Regard to the predominant Fault in the Constitution. Hence the Reason is plain, why the Powder of *Kermes* Grains, in a poach'd Egg, with the Addition of a little Frank-incense, or Mastick, is successfully used by the *Italian* and *Portuguese* Women, for preventing a Miscarriage; and why, according to *Clusus*, the Powder of *Kermes* is properly exhibited to the Women of *Montpelier* in difficult Labours, and Loss of Strength; for by corroborating Medicines, Abortion is prevented, where the Fibres, in too lax a State, are to be braced, that they may not lose what ought to be retain'd. The

Expulsion of the *Fœtus*, on the other Hand, is promoted by increasing the contractile expulsive Force of the Parts, which depends on the Corroboration of their constituent Fibres. As for the Medicinal Virtues of Scarlet, or any other red Cloth, the deeper the Cloth is tinged with a strong and lively red, the more powerfully it reflects the Heat sent from the Part to which it is applied. Hence its medicinal Effects are owing to its heating Quality, since it neither absorbs nor dissipates, but powerfully reflects the Heat it receives. The same is applicable to the Scarlet Silk Threads.

Lacertus, Offic. The Lizard, or Eft. It lives in Caverns, and Ruins, and desolate Places. The large green Lizard is esteem'd above the rest; but, this being rarely found in these Countries, what we say is to be understood of the common Lizard. Being cut in Pieces, or bruised, especially the Head, and applied with Salt, it extracts Splinters, Pieces of Glasses, and the like, out of the Flesh. The Flesh, or the Ashes of it, burnt, made into a *Litus*, with Fat, cure an *Alopecia*: It is also good against the Sting of a Scorpion, and the Bite of other venomous Creatures.

Lacerta viridis, Aldrov. de Quad. Ovip. The green Lizard. It is larger than the common Lizard, and found in *Ireland*; the Animal itself is used, and agrees in Virtues with the preceeding.

Lacertus aquatilis, Offic. *Salamandra aquatica*, Raii Synop. The Water Eft. It is found in stagnant Waters. The Powder is good for facilitating the Extraction of Teeth.

Lampetra, Offic. The Lamprey, or Lamprey Eel. It is frequently found in large Rivers, and in the Sea. The Flesh is used, which is esteem'd very nourishing, and provocative to Venery.

M m 2 *Lanus,*

Larus, Offic. The Coddy Moddy. The Brain, Heart and Stomach, are used in Medicine. The Brain dried, cures an Epilepsy, according to *Cælius Aurelianus.* The Heart is said to facilitate Delivery; and the Stomach to help Digestion.

Leo, Offic. The Lion. The Fat only is in Use; which, washed and put into the Ears, eases the Pains thereof, and is successfully used to anoint Limbs benumbed with Cold: Some use it for scirrhous Tumours, and Chilblains.

Leopardus. The Leopard. See *Pardus.*

Lepus, Offic. The Hare. However delicious the Hare may be esteem'd among the modern *Britons,* our Ancestors thought it a Crime to taste it, as we learn from *Cæsar;* and in this they agreed with the *Jews.* Tho' the Hare lives on Vegetables and Water only; yet the habitual Exercise of this Animal exalts its Salts, and renders it somewhat alcalescent; and this Tendency is much increas'd, if it is killed immediately after being heated by strong Exercise: The Ashes, Head, Eyes, Blood, Lungs, Brain, Heart, Liver, Gall, Kidneys, Testicles, *Uterus, Congulum,* Fat, Dung, Hair, and the Bone called *Astragalus,* are used in Medicine. The Ashes of the entire Hare, burnt to a Blackness, or of the whole Skin, are recommended in the Stone, an *Alopecia,* and Chilblains, apply'd externally in the two last. The Head cures an *Alopecia,* and whitens the Teeth. The Eyes are esteem'd effectual for promoting Delivery, and for expelling the Secundines, and a Mole: The Blood cures Freckles and Pimples of the Face; and is said to be good in a Dysentery, the Cœliac Passion, and the Stone; the Lungs are good for an Asthma, Epilepsy, and for Chilblains; as a Topic, the Brain rubb'd on the Gums of Child-

ren, facilitates Dentition, and is good for Tremors of the Limbs; the Heart cures the Epilepsy, Pains of the *Uterus,* and a Quartan; the Liver moderates a *Diarrhæa,* and hepatic Flux; the Gall is good for an *Ophthalmia,* and the Tooth-ach. The Kidneys and Testicles are given for the Stone, to promote Conception, for Incontinence of Urine, and Disorders of the Bladder. The *Uterus* also promotes Conception; the *Coagulum* or Rennet, discusses concreted Blood, promotes Conception, and cures the Epilepsy. The *Astragalus* is recommended against the Gravel, Colic, Epilepsy, and for promoting Delivery. The Fat, especially if old, apply'd externally, is said to draw Thorns and Splinters out of the Flesh; to break Abscesses, and to cure Pains of the Teeth. The Dung is recommended for the Stone and Dysentery, and is esteem'd a good Application to Burns; and the Hairs stop Hæmorrhages.

Lepus marinus, Offic. The Sea-Hare. It is taken in the Sea, and according to the Description of *Dioscorides,* resembles a small *Loligo,* or Cuttle Fish. Bruised either by itself, or with the *Urtica marina,* (a sort of Shell Fish) and the Part anointed therewith, it extirpates the Hair.

Leuciscus, Offic. The Dace, or Dare. It is found in Rivers. The Flesh is used in the Kitchen, and the Fat and Gall in Medicine. The Fat is good for Pains of the Ears, and mix'd with the Gall, it is good for a Dimness of Sight.

Limax ater, Offic. The Black Snail. Bruised and applied to Ulcers, they have a lenient Effect in an extraordinary Measure, according to *Enxelius.*

Limax ruber, Offic. The red Snail. It is found in Fields. The Liquor of Snails, which is what is used in Medicine, is prepared by cutting

ing the Snails in small Pieces, then mixing them with an equal Quantity of Salt, and afterwards putting them into *Hippocrate*'s Sleeve, and leaving them in a Cellar, or cool Place, where they dissolve, and pass off in a Liquor. This Liquor is used to anoint the Parts affected with the Gout, and to extirpate Warts, being first scraped with a Penknife; it also cures a *Prolapsus*, or falling down of the *Anus*.

Limax terrestris. See *Cochlea.*

Linaria, Offic. The common Linnet. The Flesh of this Bird is recommended by some as an Analeptic, or Restorative; it also expels Stones from the Kidneys and Bladder.

Locusta, Offic. The Grashopper. It is a winged Insect, of a green Colour, living in open Fields. Locusts in a Suffumigation, relieve under a Dysury, especially such as is incident to the Female Sex. The *Locusta*, called *Asiratus*, or *Onos*, has no Wings, but large Members, while recent. This dried, and taken in Wine, is a very good Antidote against the Poison of the Scorpion.

Lucius, Offic. The Pike, or Pickerel. It is common in Rivers, and the Parts used are the Mandible, or lower Jaw, and the Fat: This latter is a common Remedy, and used to anoint the Soles of the Feet, and the Breasts of Infants, in order to make a Revulsion of a Catarrh, or to mitigate a Cough. The Mandible is drying and abstergent, for which Reason, it is prescribed as a Specific in a Pleurisy: It is of Service also, as well as the other Bones of the Head, in the Stone, the *Fluor Albus*, and difficult Child Birth. The Ashes, used outwardly, stop a Discharge of Ichor, cleanse old Wounds, and dry the Hæmorrhoids. A Water distill'd from the Gall, is esteem'd in Disorders of the Eyes. The Gall of a Pike is much recommended for cold Dis

orders, attended with an Inactivity of the Bile. It is also reckon'd good for Agues, if taken upon the Approach of the Fit; the Dose is seven or eight Drops in a proper Vehicle. It is likewise said, that the Heart produces the same Effect. Small Stones are found in a Pike's Head, which are looked upon as serviceable for purifying the Blood, forwarding the *Menses*, and provoking Urine; for expelling the Stone from the Kidneys and Bladder; and for the Falling Sickness. The Dose is from twenty five Grains to a Dram.

Lumbricus terrestris, Vermis terrestris, Offic. The Earth Worm. It is an Hermaphroditic, long Animal, without Legs, of the Thickness of a Goose-Quill, soft, carnous, and annulated, of a faint blood Colour, with a red Neck, living underGround, of an earthy Taste, and no Smell. Earth-Worms are remarkablely diuretic, diaphoretic, and anodyne; they discuss, mollify, open Obstructions, increase Milk, and conglutinate Wounds, and divided Nerves. They are principally used in Apoplexies, Convulsions, and other Affections of the Nerves and Muscles, in the Jaundice, Dropsy, and Colic, and have a specific Virtue against the scorbutic Gout: They mitigate Pains of the Gout, and their Ashes are said to cure the Tooth-ach. Earth-Worms are often used in Compositions for cooling and cleansing the *Viscera*. They are accounted much of the same Nature as Snails; but they seem to have more of an earthy or nitrous Salt, which makes them afford Parts more penetrating and detersive. They are good in Inflammations and Tubercles of the Lungs; and are particularly useful in Affections of the Kidneys, and urinary Passages, which they cool and cleanse very much. The compound Water, which has its Name from them in the Shops, is esteem'd a very good Medicine in the above-mentioned Cases.

Lupus, Offic. The Wolf. The Parts of this Animal used in Medicine are the Teeth, Heart, Liver, Intestines, Fat, Bones, Dung and Skin. The Teeth, set in Silver, are given to Infants, to rub their Gums, in order to make Way for the Eruption of their Teeth. The Heart is said to be good for the Epilepsy. The Liver corrects hepatic Disorders, and is, therefore, good for those who are hydropical, or emaciated, and for such as are molested with Coughs. The Intestines are exhibited as an extraordinary Remedy in the Pain of the Colic; which they are, also, said to cure, if only tied about the Patient: The same Effect is ascribed to the Skin. The Fat is of equal Virtue with that of the Dog; it heats, digests, cures Diseases of the Joints, and is good for sore Eyes. The Bones are effectual in the Pleurisy, and for Blows and Punctures. And the Dung is good for the Colic.

Lupus marinus, Schonf. Ichth. The Sea Wolf. It is found in the Sea, the *Dentes Molares* of this Fish, called the Toad-Stone in the Shops (*Lapis Bufonites*) are used, which are said to be excellent in the Plague, and against Poisons.

Luscinia, Offic. The Nightingale. The Flesh and the Gall are used, the former of which is effectual in a Cachexy, and comforts the Brain; and the Gall, made into a *Litus* with Honey, mightily sharpens the Sight.

Lutra, Offic. The Otter. It is found in large Rivers, and the Fat is used; which, being mixed, and boiled up with digestive Medicines, is very serviceable in removing Diseases of the Joints. The Liver, dried, powdered, and taken in the Quantity of a Scruple, or a Dram, is recommended for a Dysentery. The Testicles likewise, dried, pow-

der'd, and taken in the like Dose, are said to cure an Epilepsy.

Lynx, Offic. The Ounce. The Parts used, are the Fat, and the Claws; the Fat is proper for Resolutions, Strains and Luxations of the Joints; the Claw is set in Gold and Silver, and worn as an Amulet against the Epilepsy and Convulsions.

Mæna, Offic. The Cackerel. It is taken in the *Mediterranean* Sea. The Head, burnt to Ashes, and sprinkled on the Parts, cures callous Fissures of the *Anus*. The *Garum*, or Pickle prepared of the Fish is good to wash putrid Ulcers in the Mouth.

Manati, Offic. The Sea Cow. The Part of this Animal which is used in Medicine is the *Os Petrosum* of the Head, which is crustaceous, white, and like Ivory, of various Forms. It is much recommended for wearing away the Stone in the Kidneys and Bladder, and for easing Nephritic and Colic Pains. *Geoffroy* says, that it has the Reputation of preventing an Hæmorrhage, if worn about the Neck. *F. Hoffman* recommends it in the Epilepsy.

Mater Perlarum, Offic. Mother of Pearl. This is found in the *Mediterranean* Sea, and other Places. The Shell, besides the Virtues it possesses in common with the other *Testacea*, are said to have a cordial Quality, but I dont find this Assertion has any real Foundation from Experience. The Pearls found in these Shells are of two Sorts, *Oriental* and *Occidental*, the former of which are most esteem'd. They are a kind of *Bezoar*, bred in this, and sometimes in Oysters and Muscles; and accordingly they consist of several *Stratas* and are really stony Concretions. The best *Oriental* Pearls are found in the Island of *Ormus*, in the *Persian* Gulf: They are likewise gathered in the Gulf of *Mexico*, in the Province of *Costa Rica*, and in seve-

ral

al other Places of *America* ; but hese *Occidental* Pearls are lefs e-teemed than the former. SmallPearls, ommonly called Seed Pearls, are ikewife, found on the Coafts of *cotland.* Sometimes they are found rom two to feven in one Oyfter; vhich fhews how unjuftly they are ermed by fome *Uniones,* as if there vas only one in each Shell. *Valen-ini,* on the Credit of one *Kregger,* retends, they are the Eggs of thefe Animals; but this needs Confirma-ion. When thrown into the Fire, hey give an urinous Smell, in a mall Degree : They may fome-imes be whitened by taking off the uter *Stratum,* when yellowifh; but his diminifhes their Size. Pearls are very good Abforbent, being levi-ated on the Pophyry, like Crabs-Eyes; but they have, likewife, o-her Qualities, fince they yield a vo-atile Salt by the Retort, being, on hat account, Cordial and Depura-ory.

Melanurus, Offic. The blackTail. It is a Fifh taken in the *Mediterra-nean* Sea. Being eaten boil'd, it fharpens the Sight, and the Broth thereof cures the Colic, as we are affur'd by *Kyranides.*

Mileagris, Offic. The Turkey. The Flefh is efteemed analeptic, or reftorative, and ftimulative to Vene-ry. The Food of Turkeys is prin-cipally of Vegetable Subftances, and the habitual Exercife not very great, hence their Salts are not very much exalted. They are efteemed to be of eafy Digeftion, efpecially when young.

Mergus, Offic. The Goofander, or Dun Diver. This is a Fowl well known upon the Sea Coafts. The Liver of it, when ftale, taken with *Hydromel,* in the Quantity of two *Ligulæ,* is faid by *Diofcorides* to expel the Secundines. *Aetius* recommends the Liver roafted, and taken with Oil, and a little Salt, as an excellent Remedy againft the Confequences of the Bite of a mad Dog. The entire Bird, roafted, is efteem'd good for a Leprofy, and Diforders of the Spleen. The Blood is an Alexipharmic, and good againft venomous Bites ; and the Eggs are faid to be a Reme-dy for a Dyfentery, and Diforders of the Kidneys and Stomach.

Merops, Offic. The Bee-eater. It is frequently found in *Crete,* and *Ita-ly.* The entire Bird, and its Heart, are recommended in cardiac, icteri-cal, and ftomachic Diforders. The Gall, mixed with Honey, and the Juice of Rue, is faid to cure Suffu-fions of the Eyes.

Merula, Offic. The Black-Bird. *Pliny* informs us, that this Bird roafted with Myrtle Berries inclofed in it, cures the Dyfentery. The Dung, mix'd with Vinegar, takes off Freckles.

Merucla is alfo the Name of aFifh, called the Cook-fifh, which is found in the Ocean. *Trallian* recommends it in an hepatic Dyfentery from cold Intemperature, and Epilepfy. *Pliny* relates, that it is good in Diforders of the Liver, and Fevers.

Millepedes, Afelli, and *Onifci,* Of-fic. Wood-Lice, Sows, or Church-Bugs. They are fmall Infects, fcarce a Finger's Breadth in Length, and near half a Digit in Breadth, and of a livid blackifh Colour. They are found under Veffels that hold Wa-ter, and at a Touch with the Hand, roll themfelves up in a fpherical Fi-gure. They are of fine Parts ; di-geft, attenuate, abfterge, and open. Hence they are of fingular Efficacy in refolving a tartareous Mucilage, and reducing the Stone to a Muci-lage, in opening Obftructions of the *Vifcera,* and, confequently, for the Jaundice, nephritic Pains, Dyfury, Colic, *Afthma,* and the like. Out-wardly, the Powder of them is good for the Eyes, and Pains of the Ears ; and, made into a *Litus,* for the Quinsey; apply'd alive, they cure a *Phagedæna*. *Sennertus* commends them against the Stone in the Bladder; and *Riverius* gives Inftances of Wonders perform'd by them in inveterate *Strumas* and Ulcers.

Milvus, Offic. The Kite or Glead. The whole Bird burnt. the Head, Liver, Gall, Dung, and Fat are ufed in Medicine. The Afhes of the Bird burnt, are faid to be effectual in the Gout and Epilepfy, being taken inwardly; the fame is faid of the Head and Liver, being burnt; and the latter is, alfo, an Ingredient in ophthalmic Medicines. The Blood, mix'd with Nettles, and apply'd, is faid to give Relief under the Gout; the Gall enters the Compofition of *Collyria*, for the Eyes; and the Fat is ufed to anoint the Parts pained with the Gout.

Milvus is alfo the Name of a Fifh, called the Kite Fifh. It is taken in great Plenty in the *Ocean* and *Mediterranean*, and the Gall thereof is ufed to abfterge an *Albugo*, or whatever elfe may caufe a Dimnefs of Sight.

Monedula, Offic. The Jackdaw. The Flefh of this Bird externally apply'd, diffolves Tumors, and proves beneficial in fcrophulous Swellings.

Monoceros, *Unicornu*, Offic. The Unicorn. It is a Fifh taken in *Davis*'s Straights; and the Part in Ufe is the very large, white, round, ftriated turned Tooth, growing out on the left Side of the upper Jaw, almoft in the fame Manner as that of an Elephant; but that on the right Side foon falls off It is diftinguifhed from Ivory by the Finenefs of its Fibres: It is alfo, generally more folid and ponderous; in other Refpects it refembles Ivory. As to the Virtues, it is fudorific, alexipharmic, and cordial, whence it is commended againft Poifons, contagious Difeafes, and the like; it is, alfo, thought effectual in the Epilepfy of Infants. *Andreas Baccius* has written a whole

Book of this Animal, in which he directs Fragments of it to be fet in Rings, and worn upon the Fingers, or hung about the Neck inftead of an Amulet, fo as to touch the Skin. It has the fame Virtues as Hartfhorn, Ivory, and the like Subftances. The Fragments of Horns, which are fold under the Name of *Unicorn's Horn*, are no other, as we are affured by *Paulus Ammanus*, than Bones of the Whale, Sea-Horfe, or Teeth of the Elephant, which, as *Cardan* fays, may be made, by artificial Means, to refemble this Horn.

Mofchus. Mufk. This is produc'd from the *Animal Mofchiferum*, Offic. *Capra Mofchus*. Aldrov. de Quad. Biful. This Animal feems neither to be of the Goat, nor of the Hart kind. The only Part of it in Ufe is, Mufk, which is a grumous, pinguious, and unctuous Subftance, not unlike grumous Blood, of a blackifh rufty Colour, of a fomewhat acrid and bitter Tafte, of a fragrant grateful Smell, and found in Follicules, fituated near the Navel of the Animal. It is of an heating, drying, attenuating, difcutient, cordial, alexipharmic, and, confequently, cephalic Quality. It is principally ufed in Palpitations, and all other Diforders of the Heart, becaufe it cherifhes, roufes, and refrefhes the vital Spirits. For the fame Reafon it is, alfo, ufed in Diforders of the Head and Nerves, produced either by Cold or grofs Humours, as, alfo, in Colics. Externally it deterges Specks of the Eyes, dries up moift Defluxions. proves a *Stimulus* to Venery, and reftores the diminifhed Hearing Mufk has of late Years been found by Experience, an excellent Remedy in nervous Diforders, particularly Convulfions, and in Fevers it has been given with great Succefs, where Sleep has been wanting, and alfo in maniacal Cafes, as I have been informed; but in fuch Cafes, it is given in very large Quantities,

ies, for Example, thirty Grains, d repeated as Occasion requires.

is an Ingredient in the celebrated *mquin* Remedy, for the Bite of a ad Dog.

The Generation of Musk has laid Foundation for no small Disputes mong Authors; some affirming one, d some another Thing; for some aintain it to be a purulent and ex-crementitious Humour, concocted nd collected in the Follicule; near e Navel of the Animal: But, according to them, the Animal itself, which is of a salacious and lascivious disposition, by rubbing its Belly against tones and Trees, tears this Follicule, and, by that Means, discharges e Humour contained in it, which, eing coagulated by the Air and Sun, concreted into that Substance we all Musk. Others maintain, that e Musk is not evacuated by any Dilaceration of the Follicule, but ows spontaneously through an excretory Duct, allotted for that Purose. Others affirm, that Musk is nly the Follicule of the Animal, ut out after it is killed: And this Opinion is confirmed by our Merhants, who, for the most Part, buy he Musk contained in its natural ollicule. Others are of Opinion, hat Musk is Blood extravasated, and ollected into Apostems, by beating he Animal till Tumors and Abscesses re raised, which being, as it were, y a Ligature constricted into Follimules, are afterwards cut out, and fford the Musk. Others are of Opinion, that all the Parts of the Aninal afford Musk. In my Opinion, says *Dale*,) Musk seems to be an xcrementitious Blood, which has undergone various Concoctions and Alterations in its proper Follicule, and is either naturally secreted, nd collected by human Industry, or ontained in the Follicule of the Animal, when killed at a proper Season: But the crafty and fraudulent

Merchants add the Blood, Skins, and other Parts of the Animal to the Musk; and with this Mixture they stuff Bags, made of the Skin, and sell them for true and genuine Musk Follicules: But this Piece of Fraud is easily discover'd by the Skilful, and the cautious; for that Musk, which, when burned, evaporates, is thought to be genuine; but if, when burned, there remains something like a Coal, it is adulterated.

Motacilla, Offic. The Water Wagtail. This Bird is celebrated for its Virtue in wasting the Stone.

Mugil, Offic. The Mullet. It is taken in the Sea; the Flesh is used in the Kitchen, and the Part serviceable in Medicine, is the *Botargum*, or salted Spawn, which is prepar'd in the following Manner: They take out the Follicles of the Spawn entire, and cover them with rough bruised Salt for four or five Hours; after this they put them in a Press, between two wooden Planks or Boards, for a Day and a Night: Then they wash them, and afterwards dry them in the Sun for thirteen or fourteen Days together, taking them into the House at Night. Others say they hang them up in the Smoke, but far enough from the Flame, that they may not be injur'd by the Vehemence of the Heat. This excites a decay'd Appetite, and provoke Thirst, and give a Relish to Wine.

Mullus, Offic. The lesser Mullet. This Fish, frequently eaten, is thought to procure a Dimness of Sight; being cut open, and apply'd raw, it cures the bites of the Sea-Dragon, the Scorpion, and the Spider.

Mulus, Offic. The Mule. This is an Animal got by an Ass upon a Mare. The Hoof, Urine, and Dung, are used in Medicine. The Hoof, used as a Suffumigation, is said to check too profuse menstrual Discharges; burnt and taken internally, it is reported to cause Barrenness, and in an Ointment, to cure an *Alopecia.* The Urine, together with its Sediment, is recommended as a Cure for Corns. The Dung stops Hæmorrhages of the Womb, and is good for a Dysentery, and Pains of the Spleen.

Mamia, Mummy. This is already specify'd under the Article *Homo.*

Mus, Offic. The Mouse. The whole Animal, and its Dung, are used in Medicine. The Mouse, cut up alive, and apply'd, draws out Splinters, Darts, and Arrows, and cures the Bites of Scorpions, extracting the Poison; the Ashes cure the involuntary, or nocturnal Flux of Urine; the Dung purges Infants by Stool, is used in Clysters, cures an *Alopecia,* absterges Scurf from the Head, diminishes Stones in the Kidneys, or Bladder, and removes a *Condyloma, Verruca, Ficus, Marisca,* and the like Tumors affecting the *Anus.*

Mus alpinus, Offic. The Mountain Mouse. It lives in the highest Parts of the *Alps,* and the Fat is used, being recommended in nervous Affections, and for Stiffness and Contractions of the Joints.

Mus Araneus, Offic. The Erd Shrew, Hardy Shrew, or Shrew Mouse. It is an Inhabitant of the Fields, and has been found by Experience, as is said, to be peculiarly serviceable in Affections of the *Anus,* being burnt, and apply'd with the Fat of a Goose.

Mus major, Offic. The Rat. The Part used is the Dung; nine Pieces of Rat's Dung swallowed, are accounted, by some of our good Women, a singular Remedy for a Suppression of the *Menses.*

Musca, Offic. The Fly. There are various Species of Flies, but the common Sort are most generally used, and these prevent a Falling off of the Hairs.

Mustela, Offic. The Weasel. This Animal itself it used, when disemboweled, preserved in Salt, and dried in the Shade. Its Stomach, is, also used. Two Drams of the Animal, prepared in the Manner abovementioned, and drank in Wine, are said to be an instantaneous Remedy against the Venom of all Kinds of Serpents; and against Poisons, take internally. The Stomach, when filled with Coriander Seeds, and preserved for a due Time, if drank in some proper Liquor, is beneficial in Epilepsies, and Wounds inflicted by Serpents. This Animal, when burnt in an earthern Vessel, is serviceable in arthritic Pains. Strumous Swellings are lessened by being anointed with the Blood of this Animal, or its Ashes mixed with Vinegar. These are, also, beneficial in Epilepsies.

Mustela is also the Name of a Fish, called the Eel-Pout. This Fish is found in Rivers, and its Liver, Stomach, and Spine are used. The Liver, when suspended in a glass Vessel, and exposed to a due Degree of Heat, is colliquated into a yellow Liquor greatly beneficial in Specks of the Eyes, and Dimness of Sight. The Stomach is highly recommended against Disorders of the *Uterus;* but, when drank in some proper Liquor, is principally beneficial in expelling the Secundines, and removing Colics. The Spine, when reduced to a Powder, is said to cure the Epilepsy.

Mustelus-Spinax, A Name for the *Galeus,* or Hound Fish.

Mytulus, Offic. The Muscle. It is taken in our Seas. The Shell is useful in Medicine, and is an alcaline Substance, of the same Virtues with other Shells.

Noctua, Offic. The Barn or white Owl. The Flesh, Fat, and Gall, are e ufed. The Flefh cures the Palfy, and melancholy Perfons, and the like. The Afhes of the Bird, burnt intire with the Feathers, being induced into the Throat, have an admirable Effect in opening and breaking the Impofthume in a Quinfy. The Gall abfterges Specks in the Eye, and the Fat fharpens the fight.

Oculi Cancrorum, Crabs Eyes. See *Aftacus fluviatilis.*

Onifcus. The Whiting. See *Afellus minor.*

Oftreum, Offic. TheOyfter. Oyfter-fhells Powder, without Calcination, are abforbent and drying, and are faid to provoke Sweat and abfterge. Hence they are often ufed in thofe Sorts of Fevers which terminate by a *Diaphorefis.* Externally they are ufed in Dentifrices, and are applied to Excrefcenes about the *Anus.* But when Oyfter-fhells are calcin'd, they become Lime, and act in a quite different Manner; and then prudently manag'd, they are excellent in Flatulencies, the Stone, Gravel, and Infarctions of the urinary Paffages. Oyfters apply'd to peftilential Buboes are faid to extract all the Venom. They are efteem'd nourifhing, good in a *Phthifis,* and both the Shell and the Flefh, are faid to excite venereal Inclinations and Abilities.

Ovis, Offic. The Sheep. The Parts ufed in Medicine are the Brain, Gall, the *Oefypus,* the raw or unwafhed Wool (*Lana fuccida*) the Fat, Lungs, Cawl, Dung, Urine, Bladder, Head, Feet, incinerated Bone, and Rennet. The Brain of a Ram is faid to be effectual in preventing immoderate Sleep in epidemic Difeafes, and to facilitate Dentition. The Gall loofens the Belly; applied outwardly, cures a *Carcinoma,* and is of Service in a Purulency of the Ears. The Gall of a Lamb is prefcribed for the Epilepfy. The *Oefypus* is emollient, refolvent, heating, anodyne,

and proper in Luxations, Contufions, and the like. The Wool of a Lamb is good to mitigate and mollify Tumors in the Neck. The raw Wool of a Sheep is heating, emollient, lenient, and has the fame Virtues as the *Oefypus.* The Fat, given, in red Wine, ftops Hæmorrhages, and cures a *Diarrhæa,* Dyfentery, and Gripes. The Lungs, applied to the Head, mitigate the Pains, and immoderate Heat thereof, and compofe the difordered and tumultuous Spirits; whence it is of principal Service in Phrenfies, Want of Sleep, and the like Diforders. The Cawl applied hot, cures the Pain of the Colic. The Dung is refrigerating, drying, aperitive, and difcutient: Whence it is of very great Efficacy in the Jaundice, and other Diftempers; and, ufed externally, cures a Tumor of the Spleen, a *Thymus,* Corns, Warts, and other cutaneous Tumors; and is, alfo, very comfortable in Ambuftions. The Urine, drank, expels the Water in an *Anafarca.* The Bladder, burnt, and exhibited, relieves thofe who cannot retain their Urine. The Head and Feet of a Wether, well boiled in running Water, are ferviceable in *Atrophies* and Contractions. The Bones of a Lamb, incinerated, promote the Confolidation of Wounds, even of thofe which are moft difficult to be confolidated. The Rennet is good againft Poifons; to curdle Milk, and for venomous Bites.

Palumbus, Offic. The Ring Dove. It is an Inhabitant of the Woods; the Virtues are much the fame with thofe of the common Pidgeon, or Dove; the burnt Feathers are faid to cure the Jaundice, and to be good for the Stone and Dyfury.

Pardus, Offic. The Leopard. The Fat which is the Part ufed, is reckon'd one of the beft Cofmetics.

Parus, Offic. The Titmoufe. This Bird is celebrated for its Virtues againft gainst the Stone in the Kidneys, and Colic Pains, if eaten as Food, or burnt, and taken as a Medicine.

Passer troglodytes, Offic. The Wren. This Bird is very much commended for its Virtue in the Attrition and Expulsion of the Stone, whether it be taken whole, and eaten raw feason'd with Salt, or burnt to Ashes, and fo exhibited.

Passer vulgaris, Offic. The Houfe Sparrow. As this Bird is very falacious, it is recommended, efpecially the Brain of it, as a Strengthener and Incentive to Venery.

Pastinaca marina, Offic. The Poyfon-Fifh, Fire or Fierce-flaw. It is taken in the main Sea; the Parts of it ufed in Medicine are the L and the Priekle, which grows out of its Tail. The Liver is faid to be good for the Itch; and, boiled in Oil, deterges the Lichen and Leprofy; the Prickle, as *Dioscorides* fays, cures the Tooth-ach, by breaking and expelling the grieved Tooth.

Pavo, Offic. The Peacock. The whole Bird, the Fat, Gall, Dung, Feathers, and Eggs, are ufed in Medicine. The Broth of a Peacock, efpecially if it be fat, is faid to be a Specific againft the Pleurify; the *Fat*, with the Juice of Rue, and Honey, is an excellent Medicine for the Colic. The Gall cures Dimnefs of Sight, repreffes Defluxions of the Eyes, and cures the Afperities of the Eyelids. The *Dung*, dried and pulveriz'd, and the Weight of a Dram macerated at Night in Wine, and exhibited for many Days together, have a peculiar Virtue of curing the *Vertigo* and Epilepfy. The *Feathers* are ufed in Suffumigations, for Hyfterics; and the Eggs are prefcribed for the Cure of what they call the *Erratic Gout*.

Pectunculus, Offic. The Cockle. The Fifh is efteemed a delicious Food, either raw or boil'd. Of the Shells

calcin'd, and powder'd, excellent Dentifrices are prepar'd.

Pediculus, Offic. The Loufe. Lice are taken by the Country People, as a Remedy againft the Jaundice, and an Atrophy. *Schroder* takes Notice of a very whimfical Ufe of this Infect, which is, to put it into the Beginning of the *Urethra*, in order to excite Urine.

Pedro del Cobra. See *Serpens Indicus*.

Pedro del Porco. The Name of a Stone, found in the Gall Bladder of the Porcupine. See *Hystrix*.

Perca, Offic. The Pearch. This Fifh is frequently found in Rivers; and the only Part of it ufed in Medicine are the Bones found in the Head near the Beginning of the *Spina Dorfi*, and in the Shops called *Lapides Percarum*; which in Virtues agree with the other teftaceous Powders, and are ufed in diffolving the Stone, and cleanfing the Kidneys. Externally they are, alfo, ufed in Dentifrices, and for drying Wounds.

Perdix, Offic. The common Partridge. The Parts of this Animal, ufed in Medicine, are the Flefh, Marrow, Blood, Liver, Gall, and the Feathers. The Flefh, if eaten, augments the Quantity of *Semen* and Milk, and proves a *Stimulus* to Venery. The Marrow, as, alfo, the Brain, when drank in fome proper Liquor, are faid to afford Relief to thofe who labour under a Jaundice. The Gall is, by fome, highly extolled in Diforders of the Eyes. The Blood is ufed as an Ointment for the Eyes, when they are Blood fhot, and in recent Wounds of them. The Liver, dried before the Fire, and reduced to a Powder, ftops an Epilepfy; and is accounted an highly efficacious Medicine againft Fevers, if frequently exhibited in Yarrow-Water. The Feathers ufed by Way of Fumigation, and applied to the

Noftrils,

Noftrils, are beneficial in a Suffocation of the *Uterus*, as, alfo, for alleviating, mitigating, and removing Colics, and other Pains of a like Nature.

Perdix rufa, Aldrov. Ornith. The red Legg'd Partridge. It agrees in Virtues with the preceding.

Phoca, Offic. The Soile, or Sea Calf. The Flefh and the Fat of this Animal are ufed in Medicine. The Flefh is commended by *Avicenna* in the Epilepfy, and Suffocations of the *Uterus,* and the Fat is greatly recommended by *Hippocrates,* in the Diforders of Women.

Pica, Offic. The Magpy, or Pianet. This Bird is very much commended againft Dimnefs, Rednefs, and Pains of the Eyes, being eaten, or incinerated, and the Afhes put into the Eyes, or any other way apply'd. The Afhes are alfo exhibited in the *Mania,* Epilepfy and Melancholy.

Pila marina. This is a Species of *Alcyonium,* or a round fpherical Ball, found on the Sea Coaft, among Wrack. It is generally as large as a Perfon's Fift, but fometimes larger, and fometimes lefs. It is lanuginous, of a dark Colour, and formed by a Collection of Hairs, Sand, and other Impurities of the Sea, united by means of fome glutinous Liquor. It is faid to be proper for killing Worms, and preferving the Hairs, when applied externally. The *Pila marina* cannot be reduced to a Powder, till it is thoroughly calcin'd. Authors are of Opinion, that this Subftance is good againft fcrophulous and ftrumous Diforders, not only on Account of its drying Nature, but, alfo in Confequence of fome other latent Quality. Neither can I totally reject this Opinion, fince it is a Subftance, whofe faline Quaity is not deftroy'd by Calcination.

Porcus, Offic. The tame Swine, or Hog. The Parts of this Animal ufed in Medicine, are the Lard, the Gall, the Dung, the Lungs, the *A-*

ftragalus, and the Bladder. As the Lard is not of a very hot Quality, it is therefore made an Ingredient in refrigerating Ointments, and ufed for alleviating inveterate Pains of the Loins and Joints. *Diofcorides* informs us, that the Gall of this Animal is ufed with great Succefs againft Ulcers of the Ears, and of all other Parts. It is alfo, faid to prevent the Growth of the Hairs. The Excrements are of an emollient and difcutient Quality, and for that Reafon beneficial in Itchings, excanthematous Eruptions, Corns of the Feet, and other hard Tubercles; the Excrements, alfo, cure the Bites of venomous Animals, and ftop Hæmorrhages of the Nofe; the Lungs are highly beneficial, if apply'd to Abrafions of the Skin, contracted by the Shoes. The *Aftragalus* is recommended for Fractures of the Bones; as alfo for Pains of the Neck and Head. The Bladder is beneficial to thofe who difcharge their Urine involuntarily. It produces the fame Effects, when applied to the *Pubes,* and is faid to provoke Urine. There is faid to be found a triangular Bone, within the *Cranium* of a Swine, at the *Bafis* of the *Dura Mater,* which when properly applied is faid to be almoft a Specific in an Epilepfy, and to be much in Ufe among the Vulgar in *Germany* for that Diftemper.

Aper, Offic. The wild Swine, or Boar. The Lard, the Teeth, the *Penis,* the Gall, the Excrements, and the Urine are ufed in Medicine. The Lard is poffefs'd of the fame Qualities, tho' in a ftronger Degree, with that of the tame Swine. The Teeth are exhibited as a Specific in the Pleurify, and are faid to cure the Quinfey. The *Penis* and Tenicles are faid to remove Impotence and Barrennefs. The Gall difcuffes ftrumous Swellings. The Excrements when dried, are thought beneficial in ftopping Vomitings of Blood, and

H—

Hæmorrhages, when applied externally. The Urine is a Specific for resolving and expelling the Stone of the Bladder.

Proscarabæus, Offic. The Oil Beetle. It is found creeping by Path-sides, and in Woods, in the Months of *May* and *June,* and the Insect itself, and its yellowish Liquor are used in Medicine. It is much of the Nature of *Cantharides,* forces Urine and Blood, and is of extraordinary Efficacy against the Bite of a mad Dog. Taken in Powder, or preserved, it cures the wandering Gout. Its Liquor is by some esteemed of Efficacy in Wounds, it is an Ingredient also, in Plaisters for pestilential Buboes and Carbuncles, and in Antidotes; an Oil is prepared by Infusion of the living Animals in common Oil, which some use instead of Oil of Scorpions.

Propolis, or Bee Glue. This is already specify'd under the Article *Apes.*

Pulmo marinus, Offic. Sea Lungs. This Substance floats in the Sea; is of a pellucid bluish Colour, resembling in some measure, that of Crystal, and so tender, that it can hardly be taken out of the Sea entire. When recently triturated, and used by way of Ointment, it cures Gouts and Chilblains.

Purpura, Offic. The Purple Fish. This Fish is frequently found in the *Mediterranean* Sea. In the Shops no Part of it is used, except the Shell, which is strong, furrow'd, striated, and rough, with short Tubercles. In former Ages the *Sanies* of this Fish was used for dying: The Shell is of an alcaline Quality, and in Virtues agrees with other testaceous Medicines.

Raia, Offic. The Thornback. The Flesh, Liver, and Gall of this Fish, are used in Medicine. The Flesh is analeptic, and is said to in-

crease Venereal Vigour. The Gall is recommended against Dimness of Sight, and Exulcerations of the Eyes, and is a Remedy for the Itch.

Rana, Offic. The common Frog. The Animal itself, and its Spawn, are used in Medicine. The Frog itself is greatly recommended, as an Antidote for the Bites of all Kinds of Serpents, and for a Stiffness of the Tendons; apply'd to a pestilential Carbuncle, till it dies, it is said to extract the Poison. The Spawn refrigerates, constipates, incrassates, mitigates Pains, cures the Itch in the Hands, a Whitloe, and *Herpes;* is good in an Erysipelas, Burns, and Inflammations, and is a good Application for a red Face.

Rana viridis, Offic. The Tree Frog. The whole Frog, and its Blood, are used in Medicine. The Animal agrees in Virtues with the common Frog, and its Ashes sprinkled on Wounds, are said most effectually to restrain their Bleeding. The Blood is recommended as of peculiar Efficacy in a Philtre.

Rangifer, Offic. The Rain Deer. It is an Inhabitant of *Lapland,* and its Horns and Hoofs are of use in spasmodic Affections.

Remora, Offic. The sucking Fish. It is taken in the main Sea. As to its Virtues, it restrains Venery, prevents Abortion, and retains the *Fætus* till Maturity.

Rhinoceros, Offic. The Rhinoceros. The Part in Use is the black Fissile, pyramidal Horn, a Cubit in Length, of the Figure of a Buffalo's Horn, and perfectly solid, or without Cavity. This Horn is commended against contagious Poisons, and other Distempers which require Sudorifics, and therefore in such Cases, may supply the Want of the Unicorn's Horn. *Monti* writes that the Horn is alexipharmic, cardiac, stomachic, diaphoretic, and a Sweetner. Though there are various Kinds

Quadrupeds with one Horn deib'd by Authors, I take them all, s *Dale*, to be fictitious, except the *inoceros*, which is the only Uni-n, or one Horn'd Quadruped, d perhaps the very same with that the Antients, whose Horn *Ælian* irms to be black. And *Schroder*, well as others, ascribe the Virtues d to be in the Horn of the Uni-rn, to the Horn of the *Rhino-os*.

Ricinus, Offic. The Tick. It is nasty little Animal, of a livid Co-ur, with a blunt and roundish Tail, d full of Blood, and very much fects Cows, Swine, Goats, Sheep, d Dogs. The Blood of those icks which live about Dogs, as *liny* says, is a *Psilothrum*, or Me-cine to take off Hair, and mitigate n *Eryspelas*; and we are told by *matus*, that it is an admirable Re-edy for an obstinate and malignant *mpetigo*.

Rubecula, Offic. The Robin red reast, or Ruddock. This Bird when aten, is by some esteemed to excite Venereal Inclinations.

Rubicilla, Offic. The Bull-finch, Alp, or Nope. The Flesh of this Bird is recommended against the Co-ic.

Rutilus, Offic. The Roche. The Flesh of this Fish is said to promote Venereal Inclinations.

Salamandra, Offic. The Sala-mander, or Quench Fire. The Ashes of this Animal, are an excellent and effectual Cure for scrophulous Ulcers, being sprinkled on the Parts affected.

Sanguisugæ, Leeches. These are are already taken Notice of under the Article *Hirudo*.

Scarabæus cornutus, Offic. The Stag Fly. This Insect is, as I take it, what is usually called the Cock Chaffer. It is recommended as an Amulet for an Ague, or Pains and Contractions of the Tendon, if ap-

lied to the Part affected. *Schroder* reports, that if tied about the Necks of Children, it enables them to re-tain their Urine. An Oil is prepared by Infusion of these Insects, is re-commended by the same Author in Pains of the Ears, if drop'd into them.

Scarabæus pilularis, Schrod. The Powder of this Insect sprinkled upon a protuberating Eye, or prolapsed *Anus*, is said to afford singular Relief.

Scincus, Offic. The Scink. It is an aquatic Animal, cover'd with Ash colour'd Scales, and mark'd with a Sky colour'd List, which reaches from the Head to the Tail. It is an Alexipharmic, and Provoca-tive to Venery.

Scolopendra, Offic. The many Feet. It is a flat, slender Worm, three Digits in length, of a yellowish or reddish Colour, furnish'd on both Sides with a Multitude of Feet, two pretty long *Antennæ*, and a bifid Tail. Being boil'd in Wine, it is esteemed by some a Depilatory, or Medicine to take off Hair.

Scolopendra marina, Offic. The Sea many Feet. It is found in the Bottom of the Sea, according to *Gesner*, or in Oister Beds, as *Mouffet* says. Boiled in Oil, and the Parts anointed therewith, it takes off the Hair; but the Touch thereof ex-cites Itching.

Scolopax. A Name for the *Gal-linago*, or Woodcock.

Scomber, Offic. The Mackrel, or Macarel. It is commended for the Jaundice, and Obstructions of the Liver.

Scorpio, Offic. The Scorpion. It is an Animal with eight Feet, re-sembling a Crab, only less, and of a blackish, or sooty Sort of Colour. Burnt alive, and the Ashes exhibited, they provoke Urine, when obstructed by the Stone in the Kidneys or Blad-der; bruised and applied to the Place, they cure the Poison of their own Stings, others take it bruised

in

in Wine ; and others inftill Oil of Scorpions into the Wound. The Oil of Scorpions, is by fome recommended as effectual in a Suppreffion of U-rine, the Bladder being anointed with it hot, or before a Fire.

Scorpius marinus, Offic. The Scorpion-Fifh. It is taken in the *Mediterranean* Sea ; the Gall of it is good for Cataracts, an *Albugo,* or other Infirmities of the Eyes which darken the Sight.

Sepia, Offic. The Cuttle-Fifh. This Fifh is a Kind of *Polypus* ; it has a Bag in its Neck, containing a black Liquor, like Ink, which it e-mits to trouble the Water, when purfued by other Fifhes. The Parts ufed in Medicine, are the Bone, or Shell, the black Liquor or Humor, and the Eggs. The firft is a teftace-ous Subftance, white and fmooth, and tumid on each Side ; on the up-per Part it is fomewhat hard, fmooth and glabrous ; on the lower, fun-gous, foftifh, fomewhat rough, and friable. It grows on the Back of the Fifh, and taftes a little acrimoni-ous. This Subftance dries and ab-fterges ; cures Spots, Freckles and the tumid Itch ; is good for the Eyes, removes Swellings in the Gums, gives Relief in the Afthma, ftops a Gonorrhæa, expels the Stone, and provokes Urine. The black Hu-mour found in the Bladder within the Body, is faid to loofen the Belly, and the Eggs abfterge the Kidneys and Ureters, and provoke Urine and the *Menfes.*

Seps, Offic. The Serpent Seps. This is a very poifonous Serpent, a-bout three Foot long, and proporti-onably thick, faid to be found in *Syria, Croatia,* and many other Coun-tries. *Diofcorides* informs us, that taken in Wine, it cures its own Bite. The Poifon of its Bite acts like that of the Viper, and is cured by the fame Means.

Serpens, Offic. The Snake. The Fat, Slough, or caft Skin, and the Gall are ufed in Medicine. The Fat mollifies ftrumous Swellings, cures Rednefs of the Eyes, clears them from Specks, and fharpens the Sight ; it mitigates the Pains of the Gout. The Slough, boiled in Wine, and the Decoction inftilled into the Ears, eafes their Pains ; and, ufed as a Col-lution, helps the Tooth ach, cures an Impetigo, and makes the Hairs grow. The Gall applied to the Part affected, extracts the Poifon caus'd by the Bites of Serpents.

Serpens Indicus, Offic. The *Indian* Serpent. This is a very venomous Serpent. The Part of this Serpent in Ufe, is the Stone, or rather the Bone, of the Head, called *Pedro del Cobra.* This Stone of the Ser-pent, called in *Ind. Med.* by Miftake, *Piedra di Cabra,* is of an Oval Fi-gure, plain on one Side, and gib-bous on the other, of a brown Co-lour, Shining with Pores interfperfed. It expels all Sorts of Poifons, either taken inwardly, or outwardly applied. It refifts Putrefaction, promotes in-fenfible Perfpiration, raifes the vital Spirits, comforts the Heart, com-municates a new Fermentation to the Blood, and relieves Nature under all malignant Diftempers. Though this Stone be defcribed by *Garcias, Redi,* and others, yet the Learned among the Moderns differ about it principally in two Refpects, as, 1. Whether it be a Thing natural or fac-titious. *Kircher,* in his *China Illu-ftrata,* and *Thevenot,* in his Relati-on of Voyages and Travels, affirm thefe Stones to be found in the Head of a great *Chinefe* Serpent ; Mr. *Boyle,* in the Head of an *African* Serpent. Others on the contrary, as Father *Boccone,* in *Mufeo di Fifica,* fuppofe them to be artificial Subftan-ces, as calcined Bones, and other teftaceous Fragments ; and *Thevenot* the Younger will have them to con-fift of a Mixture of the Afhes of fome burnt

burnt Roots, and a Sort of Earth found near *Diu* in the *East Indies.* Another thing in which they differ, is about their Virtues. Father *Kircher* relates several Experiments of their Virtues in extracting the Poison infused by the Bite of a Viper, or another Serpent. Mr. *Boyle* in his Treatise of Specific Medicines, affirms the same from an Experiment made on a young Cat. And *Clayton,* in his Account of *Virginia* in the *Philosophical Transactions* writes, that he was present when the said Gentleman tried the Experiment on some Chickens, which all recover'd. Dr. *Havers* was an Eye-Witness, as he tells us, of the Salutary Effects of this Stone upon a Dog; and Dr. *Tyson,* in his Anatomy of the Rattle Snake, relates an Observation which he receiv'd from a celebrated Physician of *London,* who, by means hereof, cured a Man, who was bit by a Viper. *Baglivi* also performed the same Thing for one who was stung by a Scorpion. But tho' these Experiments succeeded well with all the Persons before mentioned, yet others, as *Redi* and *Charas,* made the same Tryals, with different Success. Having given this brief Account of the Opinions of the Learned on both Sides, my best Way, (says *Dale*) I think is, to endeavour to reconcile them. For this End, I shall only observe, that I have seen two Sorts of this Kind of Stone, one of which was like a Bone, porous, and had visible Marks of the File; the other was of a more compact Substance, and polished. This I suppose, (says *Dale*) to be the factitious Stone, and a Counterfeit of the former; and therefore conjectures, that the unsuccessful Experiments were made with those artificial Stones, and not with the true. The *Lapis colubrinus,* which formerly went at a high Price, is now sold very cheap at *Manila;* but what

is thus sold, is not taken from the *Coluber* (Snake) but is made of Hartshorn luted up in an Earthen Pot, where it is burnt to a Blackness; and afterwards polished. The *Moors* call this adulterated; but say, it is made of a strange Kind of Clay, like *Terra Sigillata.* The true *Lapis Colubrinus* cures the Bites of Serpents by Application. In a Fever, attended with Purple Spots, several of these Stones applied, relieve the Patient. In the Year 1681, I saved, says *Camellus,* from present Death, a Boy of three Years old at *Brana,* who had swallow'd Arsenic dissolv'd in Milk, by the repeated Application of this Stone. It is a Question, whether the Virtue of this Stone is to be ascribed to the Salt in the Hartshorn not being thoroughly burnt, or to its Pores, by which it attracts like a Cupping Glass.

Serpens marinus, Offic. The Sea Serpent. It is found in the *Mediterranean* Sea. The Flesh is said to cure Incontinence of Urine, if taken with Lily Root.

Silurus, Offic. The Shoar-fish. This Fish is found in the *Danube,* and its Flesh is nourishing when eaten fresh, and loosens the Belly; but seasoned with Salt, affords very little Nourishment, but clears the *Aspera Arteria,* and mends the Voice The salted Flesh applied draws out Splinters; and the Pickle cures a recent Dysentery, being used by Way of Fotus, by attracting the Flux of Humours to the Superficies; a Clyster of the same cures the *Sciatica.*

Simia, Offic. The Ape. The Parts in Use are the Stone, or *Bezoar Simiae,* which is sometimes found in the Stomach of this Animal, the Heart, and the Flesh. The Heart roasted, or boiled in *Hydromel,* sharpens the Sight. The Flesh is cold and dry, austere, of very bad Juice, and unfit to eat.

N n

Smaris, Offic. The white Cackerel. This is a Fish found in the *Mediterranean* Sea. The Head of this Fish salted and burnt, is said to reprefs the tumid Lips of Ulcers; to reftrain phagedenic Ulcers; and confume Corns, and thofe Excrefcences called *Thymi.* The falted Fifh is faid to be a good Application in Cafe of the Sting of a Scorpion, or the Bite of a mad Dog.

Sperma Ceti. This is agreed on all Hands to be the Product of the *Cetus,* Offic. or the Parma-fitty Whale. *Pomet* pofitively affirms that *Sperma Ceti* is the Brain of a Sort of Whale call'd *Byaris,* and, by the People of St. *John de Luz, Cachalot,* and he alfo affirms, that he has not only feen it prepar'd, but has often prepar'd it himfelf. This *Sperma Ceti* (fays *Pomet,*) is ufually prepar'd at *Bayonne,* and St. *John de Luz;* and this Work is fo rare in *France,* that there are not above two Perfons at the latter Place who know how to prepare it. Thofe who prepare it, take the Brain as aforefaid, and melt it over a gentle Fire; then they caft it into Moulds, like thofe wherein they refine Sugar; and after it is cold, and drain'd from the Oil, they take and melt it again, and proceed after the fame Manner, till fuch time as it be well purified, and very white; then with a Knife, made for the Purpofe, they cut it into Scales or Flakes, juft fo as it appears when brought to us. *Pomet* may poffibly be right, as to the Procefs generally ufed for making *Sperma Ceti;* but I have feen *Sperma Ceti* which has undergone no treatment at all, except being put into Paper Bags, fo that the Oil which adheres to it, may be abforb'd. The true *Sperma Ceti* is very white, and is in very fmall Flakes, not much larger than the Cryftals of Tartar: It diffolves by rubbing upon the Hand into a Sort of Oil; and does not adhere to the Palate when chew'd, as the common Sort will; which makes me fufpect, that it is mix'd with fome other Subftance, perhaps Wax, by thofe who make it for Sale. I can affirm with Certainty, that *Sperma Ceti* is neither the Oil, Brain, nor Sperm of the Whale, but a particular Subftance found principally in the Head of the Fifh; and flakes like boil'd Salmon, or Cod, when taken out. It is alfo found in other Parts of the Fifh, but not in fo large Quantities, or fo good, as in the Head. It is a noble Medicine in many Cafes, tho' principally ufed in Bruifes, inward Hurts, and after Delivery. It is an excellent Balfamic in many Diftempers of the Breaft; and gently deterges and heals. In Coughs, from fharp Rheums, Erofions, and Ulcerations, it is very fafe, pleafant, and effectual; as alfo in Pleuriffes, and inward Impofthumations. Where the *Mucus* of the Bowels has been abraded by Acrimony and Choler, as in *Diarrhæas,* and Dyfenteries, this is a very good Healer. In Ulcerations of the Kidneys, and bloody Urine, it is likewife a very fuitable Medicine; and, by foftening and relaxing the Fibres, it contributes frequently to the Expulfion of Gravel, by enlarging the Paffages. It is moft conveniently made up into the Form of Electuaries and Boles, with proper Conferves, and things of the like Kind: And in fuch Forms, if it be fkillfully mixed, it gives them an agreeable Smoothnefs, and is not difcoverable by the Patient. It is alfo very properly diffolv'd in a Draught, by the help of the Yolk of an Egg; or it is made into an Emulfion by the fame Management. The ufual Dofe is about half a Dram. It is emollient and healing, outwardly ufed; but its greateft Ufe that Way is in the Small Pox, melted with Oil of Almonds: With this the Puftules are juft kept moift,

moift, when they begin to harden; and it wonderfully prevents thofe fcars they are apt to leave, by foftning, and healing them up fmooth. Altho' this is but a modern Practice in this Diftemper, yet *Schroder* takes notice of its Ufe in his Time, in fmoothing and filling up the Fiffures, or Cavities, made by Blotches and Scabs. It is fometimes ufed as a Cofmetic, both in Paints, and in Paftes, to wafh the Hands with.

Spodium. Burnt Ivory. See *Elephas.*

Squatina, Offic. King-ftone, or Monk-fifh. It is taken in the *Brifh,* and other Seas. The Eggs, Skin, and Afhes, are ufed. The dry'd Eggs are found to be very ferviceable in ftopping a Loofenefs, by the Experience of the Fifhermen, who ufe it for all Manner of Fluxes. If the Skin is prepared an excellent *fmegma* for the *Pfora* and *Scabies;* and the Afhes are effectual againft the *Alopecia* and *Achors.*

Squilla, Offic. The Shrimp. It is taken in the Sea, and agrees in Virtues with the *Aftacus,* or Lobfter.

Struthio, Offic. The Oftrich. The Parts of this Animal ufed in Medicine are, the Coat of the Craw, the Fat, and the Eggs. The inner Coat of the Craw corroborates the Stomach, and diffolves Stones in a furprifing Manner. The Fat is agreeable to the nervous Parts, mollifies the Hardnefs of the Spleen, and mitigates nephritic Pains, the Parts being anointed therewith. The Eggs burnt and triturated in Vinegar cure the *Impetigo.*

Sturio, Offic. The Sturgeon. It is an Inhabitant of the Sea, but for the moft Part it is found in Rivers. The Parts ufed are the Bones, and the *Caviar,* which is a Mafs refembling green *Hamburgh* Soap, both in Colour and Subftance, and is exported in great Quantities from *Ruf-*

fia to *Italy* and other Countries. The Way of preparing it is thus related by *Gefner*. They take the Spawn of the Sturgeon, and firft cleanfing them from the Nerves which are therein, wafh them in Vinegar, or white Wine, and fpread them upon a Table to dry. This done, they put them into a Veffel, and cover them with Salt, then break them abroad with the Hand, not ufing an Inftrument, and afterwards put them into a Bag of a rare Texture, that the Humour may run through. When this is done they put it into a Pot with a Hole in the Bottom, by which the remaining Humour, if any, may be evacuated, and after well preffing and covering it clofe, fet it afide for Ufe. The Bones are commended for the wandering Gout, and are exhibited in the Pain of the Colic. The *Caviar* is nourifhing, increafes the *Semen,* and provokes to Venery.

Sturnus, Offic. The Stare or Starling. It makes its Neft about Towers, and the Tops of Houfes. Its Dung is efteemed a Cofmetic, and is faid by *Galen* to cure the *Alphi, Pani, Impetigo,* and Morphew.

Sus, Offic. The Sow. See *Porcus.*

Talpa, Offic. The Mole. It lies in Burrows under the Earth; and the Animal itfelf, the Heart, and the Blood, are ufed in Medicine. The Afhes of the burnt Mole, is good for the Leprofy, ftrumous Swellings and Fiftulas. Taken inwardly in Beer or Wine, it cures the wandering Gout, and *Scrophula.* The Heart cures an *Hernia,* and the recent Blood cures an *Alopecia,* being rubb'd on the Part.

Taxus, Offic. The Badger. The whole Animal incinerated, its Blood, and its Fat, are ufed in Medicine. The Afhes of the burnt Animal are exhibited with Succefs in Pulmonic Diforders, and an *Hæmoptoe.* The Blood dry'd and pulveriz'd, is faid to be good

for the Leprofy ; and the fame, diftilled, to be effectual againft the
Peftilence. The Fat, as it is a little
thicker, fo it is fomewhat hotter, and
more efficacious, than the Fat of the
Swine; It gives Relief under Pains
of the Kidneys proceeding from the
Stone, mitigates the Heat of Fevers,
and reftores Contractions and Weak-
neffes of the Joints and Nerves.

Tellina, Offic. The Limpin. Frefh
Limpins are good for the Belly, efpecially the Liquor of them : Salted
and burnt, then triturated, and inftilled
with Refin, they prevent the Hairs
of the Eye-Lids, which have been
pulled out, from ever growing again.

Teredo, Offic. The Wood-eater.
There is great Difpute among Authors about the *Teredo*, fome making
it one thing, fome another. *Aldrovandus* makes four Kinds of *Teredo* ;
one Kind is found in Wood, another
is called *Vermiculus*, a third *Thris*,
and a fourth *Coffus* ; to thefe *John-
fon*, from *Agricola*, adds a fifth,
which, from its Copper Colour, is
called *Kupfferworm*. But that Worm
with fix Legs, from which is produced the *Scarabæus minor arborum*,
commonly found in Trees, is fuppos'd to be the *Teredo* of the Shops.
The Parts of this Infect in Ufe are the
farinaceous Excrements, call'd *Powder of Poft* This Powder is drying,
whence it is fprinkled, with good
Succefs, on humid and watry Ulcers;
and for the fame Reafon, is in much
requeft among the good Women, for
drying up the Excoriations of Infants.

Teftudo marina, Offic. The Sea
Tortoife, or Turtle. The Legs, *Penis*, and Gall of this Animal are ufed
in Medicine. The Legs are fuperftitioufly worn as a moft approved
Amulet againft the Gout ; the Gall
is good for the Eyes, and the *Penis*
is recommended by fome in nephritic
Diforders. The Flefh is efteem'd
reftorative, and good for the venereal
Difeafe.

Teftudo paluftris, Offic. The Water Tortoife. The Blood and Gall
are ufed, which agree in Virtues with
the other Tortoifes.

Teftudo terreftris, Offic. The Land
Tortoife. The recent and crude
Blood of this Animal is prefcribed in
an hectic Fever ; and the fame dry'd,
is recommended for the Epilepfy.

Thunnus, Offic. The Tunney-fifh,
or *Spanifh* Mackarel. The pickled
Flefh of this Fifh cures thofe who
are bitten by the Viper called *Pra-
fter* ; but the Patient is to vomit
plentifully and frequently with large
Draughts of Wine ; it is of great
Efficacy, alfo, againft the Bite of a
Dog, being rubbed on the Wound.

Thymallus. The Grayling, or Umber. See *Afchia*.

Tigris. Offic. The Tiger. The Fat of
this Animal is ufed in Medicine, and
agrees in Virtues with the Fat of a Dog.

Tinca, Offic. The Tench. It is a
mucous Fifh, which delights in marfhy
and muddy Waters. As to its Ufes,
it is cut into Pieces, and apply'd to
the Wrifts, and Soles of the Feet, in
order to mitigate feverifh Heats, and
to divert the Venom of the Peftilence ; in like Manner it is apply'd
in Pains of the Head and Joints.
Live Tenches, apply'd one after
another to the Regions of the Navel
and Liver, and kept there till
they die, are faid to cure the Jaundice ; for they contract, it feems, a
yellow Colour. *Schroder* fays, that
he has feen an incinerated Tench ;
and efpecially its Tegument, exhibited with Succefs in the *Fluor Albus*.
The Broth of a Tench is fuperftitioufly recommended in a Jaundice.

Torpedo, Offic. The Cramp-fifh. It
is taken in the *Mediterranean* Sea. It
mitigates the Violence of the Pain in
an inveterate Head-ach, being apply'd to the Part ; and, alfo, prevents and reftrains the falling down
of the *Anus*, being in like Manner
apply'd.

Trutta,

Trutta, Offic. The Trout. The [fat] of this Fish is ufed in Medicine, [an]d is of a lenifying and diffolving [n]ature; good for the Piles, and o[th]er Diftempers of the *Anus*, Ulcers [in] the Breaft, and Fiffures in the Nip[pl]es.

Turdus, Offic. The Mavis, or [T]hrufh. This Bird, when ftuffed [w]ith Myrtle Berries, and roafted, is [fa]id to be exhibited with Succefs to [th]ofe who labour under Fluxes. In [th]e Time of the Plague, it is faid to [be] highly beneficial when macerated [in] Vinegar. The Powder of this [B]ird is, by *Guainarius* recommended [a]gainft the Effects of the *Napellus*, [or] Monks-hood.

Turdus, is alfo a Name for a Sort [o]f Fifh, called the *Wrafs*, or Old-Wife. This Fifh is found in the [m]ain Ocean, and in the *Mediterra-nean*, and is greatly recommended [b]y *Trallian* in the Epilepfy and Pleu-[ri]fy.

Turtur, Offic. The Turtle Dove. [T]his Bird, and its Fat, are ufed. It [a]grees in Virtues with the Pigeon, [e]fpecially in ftopping Dyfenteries, [a]nd immoderate Difcharges of the *Menfes*. The Fat collected when [th]e Animal is roafting, is, according [to] *Schroder*, properly ufed as an [O]intment in Diforders of the Kid-[n]eys, *Abdomen*, Breaft, and Groins.

Vacca, Offic. The Cow. This is [a]lready fpecified under the Article *Bos*.

Vanellus, Offic. The Lapwing, [o]r Baftard Plover. This Animal de-[l]ights in Marfhy Places, and its Afhes, [H]eart, and Skin, are ufed for Medi-[c]inal Purpofes. The Afhes drank [i]n Wine, are beneficial in Colics; [a]nd when applied by way of Cata-[p]lafm, cure the Bite of a mad Dog. The Heart alleviates Pains of the [L]oins, and the Skin is efteeem'd good [i]n *Cephalalgias*.

Vermis terreftris. The Worm. [S]ee *Lumbricus terreftris.*

Vefpa, Offic. The Wafp. The whole Infect is ufed, and is fuppofed to open Obftructions of the Kid-neys and Bladder, to break the Stone, and is thought by fome to agree in Virtues with the *Millepedes*.

Vefpertilio, Offic. The Bat, or Flitter Moufe. It appears in Sum-mer Evenings, but in the Winter lies hid in Rocks and Caverns. The Flefh and Blood of this Animal are ufed; the firft of which, being pre-pared, is good for a *Scirrhus*, and the Gout; and the Blood cures an *Alopecia*.

Vipera, Offic. The Viper. The Fat, rub'd well into the Part bit by a Viper, prevents the ill Confequen-ces of fuch a Wound. The Flefh of the Viper is efteem'd alexiphar-mic, and fudorific, and is ufed in-ternally in all peftilential and ma-lignant Difeafes, as the Plague, pe-techial Fevers, Leprofy, and the like. It is alfo ufed as a Reftora-tive in Confumptions, and the Ve-nereal Difeafe; and for this Pur-pofe the Flefh is to be eaten dreft; the Broth in which it is boil'd, is to be drank, and the Fat is to be rub'd into the Spine of the Back and Joints. Thefe are the Virtues afcrib'd to the Flefh of the Viper, but I am afraid without any real Foundation from Experience; for I have given the Flefh, Broth, and Salt of Vipers, in very large Quantities, without any greater Effects, than I have obferv'd upon the fame Occafions from the Broths or Flefh, of Fowls, Veal, or Mutton, given in the fame man-ner; and with Refpect to the Salt of Vipers, it does not appear from Experience, that they are poffefs'd of any other Virtues, than Salt of Hartfhorn, or any other Animal Salt. What is advertis'd and fold in *London* under the Name of *Effence of Vipers*, is only a Tincture of *Cantharides*, which as it ftimulates to Venery, without imparting any ad-

additional Strength to the Constitution, must be very prejudicial, especially when used habitually.

Vitulus. The Calf. See *Bos.*

Viverra, Offic. The Ferret. The Flesh and Gall of this Animal, are recommended in an Epilepsy, and the Gout, and are said to be good against Poisons.

Ulula, Offic. The Gray Owl. The Parts used in Medicine, are the Gall, Fat, and Flesh. The Gall is commended for the *Albugo,* Cataracts, and Films; the Fat for clearing the Sight: the Flesh boil'd in Oil, and that Oil mixed with Sheeps Butter and Honey, is good to heal Ulcers. It is esteem'd by some for the Gout.

Umbra, Offic. The Grunter, or Shadow Fish. It is taken in the *Mediterranean* Sea. The Parts used in Medicine are, the Bones found in the Head, and called in the Shops *Lapides Umbrarum:* These are commended superstitiously for the Colic, and in *France* are commonly set in Silver, and sold by the Goldsmiths under the Name of Colic Stones: For, they say, if it be only carried about one, or worn about the Neck, it not only removes the Pain of the Colic, but prevents its Return.

Unguis odoratus. The Constantinople Sweet Hoof. See *Blatta Byzantina.*

Unicornu. The Unicorn. See *Monoceros.*

Upupa, Offic. The Hoopo. It is a melancholy and unclean Bird, living on Worms found in Dung, Caterpillars, Beetles, and the like. The Parts in Use are the Flesh and Feathers. The Flesh, and its Decoction, according to *Avicenna,* have a specific Virtue against the Colic. And the Feathers applied, are said to mitigate Pains of the Head.

Uranoscopus, Offic. The Star Gazer. It is frequently taken in the *Mediterranean* Sea. The Gall is

used, which is esteem'd a present Remedy in Cataracts of the Eyes.

Ursus, Offic. The Bear. The Parts of this Animal used in Medicine are, the Fat and the Gall. The Fat is emollient and discussive, and is of principal Use in an *Alopecia;* it cures also Pains of the Gout, the *Parotides,* and other Tumors, and heals Ulcers in the Legs. The Gall is recommended to be taken inwardly for the Epilepsy, Asthma and Jaundice. Outwardly it is of Service in cancerous and spreading Ulcers, the Tooth-ach, Dimness of Sight, and other like Diseases. The Skin is good for a Person bit by a mad Dog to lie upon, and serves instead of a Rug to Travellers in the Winter-time.

Urtica marina, Offic. Sea Blubber. It swims on the Water, and is often cast by the Tide on the Shore, being a round, compressed, pellucid Substance, resembling a Jelly, with red Veins interspersed. It agrees in Virtues with the *Lepus marinus,* or Sea Hare.

Vulpanser, Offic. The Shell Drake, Burrough Duck, or Ber-Gander. It lives in maritime Places, and the Fat, which is the Part used in Medicine, is recommended by some, against the *Herpes,* and Tumors of the Face.

Vulpes, Offic. The Fox. The Fat, Lungs, Liver, Gall, Melt, Skin, Blood, the whole Animal, and its Dung are used in Medicine. The Fat is of Use in Convulsions, Contractions, Tremblings, and the like Disorders; also in Pains of the Ears, Wounds of the Head, and an *Alopecia.* The Lungs are consolidating and abstergent, and therefore of Efficacy in Diseases of the Lungs, and Straitness of the Breast. The Liver of a Fox is of Use in hepatic, and splenetic Cases; the Gall cures a *Pterygium* of the Eyes, the Spleen, removes a Hardness and Tumor

Tumor of that Part; the Skin, with the Hair on it, is fuccefsfully wrapt about fuch Limbs as are refrigerated or infefted with Arthritic Pains; the Blood dry'd and triturated, cures the Stone in the Kidneys and Bladder; for which Purpofe, it is faid to be more effectual if taken recent: The whole Fox, or its Flefh burnt, is commended for Diforders of the Breaft: The Animal boil'd in Water or Oil, is a Remedy for Affections of the Nerves, and therefore good in Contractions and Pains of the Joints; and the Dung, in the laft Place, clears the Skin from Afperities.

Vultur, Offic. The Vulture. The Flefh, Fat, Brain, Gall, and Dung, are ufed in Medicine. The Flefh is efteem'd effectual in Cephalic Affections, as the Epilepfy, *Hemicrania,* and the like: The Decoction of it is faid to be good for cutaneous Difeafes; and the Fat is proper for the Nerves: The Brain ftrengthens weak Heads; the Gall is faid to cure the Epilepfy, being taken in Wine; and the Dung, by its nidorous Smell, to haften the Birth.

Zibethum. Civet. This Subftance is produc'd from the *Animal Zibethicum,* Offic. *Catus Zibethicus,* Schrod. The Civet Cat. The Animal which yields Civet, is a Kind of Wild Cat, called by the Antients *Hyæna.* There are two Kinds of it, one that comes from *Holland,* and another that comes from *Guinea,* which is browner than the former. When Civet is mix'd with Mufk and Ambergreafe, or lower'd by a Mixture of any other Powders, it has a very fine Smell; but alone the Smell is difagreeable. It is very little ufed in Phyfic. Some rub Children's Navels with it to cure their Colics, and it was formerly apply'd to the *Pudenda* of Women in Hyfteric Fits; but this laft Practice is not only ufelefs, but hurtful. Civet is a fat and unctuous Subftance, of the Confiftence of Honey or Butter, and of a moft fragrant and grateful Smell. It is hot, moift and anodyne. Civet is not the Seed, nor Suet, nor Tefticles, nor *Scrotum* of the Animal called the *Civet Cat,* as fome would perfuade us, for thefe have no Smell; but it is a peculiar Excrement, fecreted by Nature, and collected in fome little Bags of a glandulous Subftance, which in the Male are feated between the *Penis* and *Tefticles,* in the Female between the *Uterus* and *Anus.* The beft is what comes from *America,* and is not adulterated with Butter; the black imported from the *Eaft-Indies* is not good.

C H A P. III.

Of M I N E R A L S.

ACHATES, Offic. The Agate. This is a precious Stone, reckon'd commonly between the opake and tranfparent, of different Colours, and mark'd with Spots or Specks, which are imagined to reprefent Trees, Fifhes, and other Things. The fineft comes from the *Eaft-Indies,* the common Sort from *Germany, Bohemia, &c.* Great Virtues have been attributed to this Stone,

Stone, both cardiac and alexipharmic; but they seem all to be imaginary.

Adamas, Offic. The Diamond. This Gem is generally mentioned in Catalogues of Drugs, and some Virtues are ascrib'd to it, which are absolutely fabulous.

Ærugo. Rust of any Metal, particularly Copper, called Verdigrease.

Æs, Cuprum, Offic. Copper. This is never used inwardly as a Medicine, unless in Tincture; and that but seldom, because this Metal, and especially its Rust, are reckon'd Poisons; and any Kind of Food, or even Water, that has stood long in Copper Vessels, is pernicious. The Symptoms produced by this Poison, are Pains in the Stomach and Intestines, excessive Vomitings, Irritations to Stool, Ulcers in the Intestines, sometimes Difficulty of Breathing, and spasmodic Contractions of the Limbs, and lastly Death itself, if the Quantity of Poison be great. The Remedies proper in such Cases, are first, to take a great Quantity of Milk, Oil, or melted fresh Butter; then to drink warm Water, till the Patient vomits plentifully. Clysters made of Oil, Butter, or fat Broths, are likewise proper; and lastly strengthening Cordials, and a Milk Diet. Various Recrements of Copper are employ'd in Medicine, as the *Ærugo,* Verdigrise; *Flos Æris, Æs Ustum, Squama Æris;* of which the *Flos, Squama,* and *Ærugo* are mention'd by *Hippocrates;* but the *Ærugo,* or Verdigrise, is the only Recrement now much in Use. It is a green Rust, raised on Copper-Plates; the Method of making it is thus: The Husks, Stones, &c. of Grapes, being first dried, and after dipped in some strong Wine, are laid for nine or ten Days in Wooden or Earthen Vessels, till they begin to ferment; then being squeez'd together with both Hands, they are form'd into Balls, which are put into

proper Earthen Pots, and Wine is poured upon them, till about half is cover'd; the Vessels have a Straw Lid thrown over them, and are set in a Wine Cellar, where the Balls are left in Maceration for twelve or fifteen Hours, being turned every four Hours, that the Wine may penetrate every Part of them. After this the Balls are raised about a Finger's Breath above the Surface of the Wine, and set upon wooden Bars; the Vessels are then shut again, and left in that State for ten or twelve Days more. After which Time, the Balls emit a strong and penetrating Scent, and are then fit for dissolving Copper. For this Purpose, they are broken and bruised with the Hand, that the outer Part of them, which is dryest, may be exactly mixed with the inner, which is still moist with Wine; then they are stratified with Copper-Plates in the same Vessels, upon wooden Bars; the Plates making always the lowest Stratum, and the Balls the uppermost. The Plates are four Inches long, and three broad; and, if the Copper be new, they must be previously buried for twenty four Hours in Verdigrise, and then heated a little in the Fire. The Vessels being filled in this Manner, and shut close, are left without any farther Management, till the Verdigrise is made, which happens sooner or later, according to the Nature of the Copper. Some Copper yields its Rust in six or seven Days; some requires twelve or fifteen Days. The Verdigrise thus compleatly extracted, the Plates cover'd therewith are taken out of the Vessels, and their Edges moisten'd with the strongest Wine; they are then wrapped up in Linen Cloths, dipped in the same, and laid in a Wine Cellar for three Weeks. By this, the Makers tell us, the Verdigrise is nourished, and then it is separated off from the Plates with Knives, and kept for Use. Verdigrise grife is ufed by Painters and other Artifts, but is feldom prefcribed inwardly by Phyficians. It is often ufed outwardly to deterge and dry Ulcers, and to eat away fungous and callous Flefh. It is the principal Ingredient in the *Unguentum Ægyptia-cum.*

Atites, Aquilæ Lapis, Offic. The Eagle Stone. This Stone is big, as it were, with another Stone rattling in its Womb, of a dark, Ruffet, or Afh-Colour, and commonly of an oval Figure. The oriental is accounted the beft. *Ætius* informs us, that if it is tied to the left Arm, it retains the *Fœtus* in thofe Women who are fubject to mifcarry. But in Time of Labour it muft be taken from the Arm, and tied to the Thigh, and the Woman will be delivered without Pain. Mixed with Bread, it finds out Thieves; for a Thief will never be able to fwallow it. *Dale* having quoted *Schroder* for the fame Virtues which *Ætius* above afcribes to this Stone in retaining the *Fœtus,* and facilitating Labour, with this Addition, that after Delivery the Stone muft immediately be removed from the Thigh, for fear it fhould draw the Womb to it, fubjoins the following Remarks from *Amman:* The natural Effects of the Eagle Stone are commonly magnified, on Account of the Traces of fome Signature, while it is believed to be of Service in time of hard Labour, and to facilitate Delivery. This *Dale* does not deny; but this natural Effect of the Stone, was by *Galen, Pliny,* and others, immediately blended and overlaid with Superftitions. For who will prove (1) that an *Ætites* tied to the Arm prevents Mifcarrying? Which too is an Effect contrary to the former. (2) That the *Ætites* has fuch an attracting Power, as to make the Womb fall out. *Wormius* and *Valeriola* produce their Obfervations as to this

laft. But in my Opinion, fays *Dale,* thefe Obfervations are not well grounded. For we know by Anatomy, that the *Uterus* is held faft in its Situation, by Ligaments formed by Nature for that very Purpofe. How then can this Stone work fuch an Effect? Indeed, unlefs a Power of relaxing, or breaking the Ligaments, be afcribed to it by the forementioned Authors, we cannot admit the Obfervation of *Valeriola,* which he makes on a Woman of *Valentia,* unlefs we fuppofe the *Uterus* to be drawn out of its Place, by the violent and unfkilful Hands of the Midwife, which has fometimes been the Cafe. And yet too many fuch Abfurdities are inferted among Anatomical Obfervations. (3) There is no Proof that ever this Stone difcovered if Poifon were mixed with any Thing, as is reported. (4) That it finds out Thieves, being pulveris'd and mixed in their Bread, by their Incapacity of fwallowing it, is a precarious Affertion, depending on a fallible Mark, for Deglutition may be hinder'd by other Caufes. (5) It neither procures Love, nor increafes Riches, which it is faid to do. (6) Therefore if we ought to fpeak the Truth, let us content ourfelves with allowing the *Ætites* the fame Virtues as the feal'd Earth, in malignant Diftempers, and againft Poifons.

Alabaftrum & Alabaftritis, Offic. Alabafter. This is a white Stone very well known, and is a Kind of Marble, but fofter. It is found in *Staffordfhire, Derbyfhire,* and other Places. The Stone applied with Rofin, or Pitch, difcuffes Hardnefs; with Cerate, eafes Pains in the Stomach, and faftens the Gums.

Alabaftrum citrinum, Mont. Exot. Yellow Alabafter. This agrees in Virtues with the preceeding.

Alumen. Alum. There are three Sorts of Alum principally ufed, as the *Alumen rupeum,* Offic. *Alumen rapcum five Chryftallinum,* Ind. Med. *Alumen factitium,* Mer. Pin. Common Alum. This, together with the Method of making it, from the calcin'd Stone, *Kali,* and Urine, are fo well known, that they require no farther Notice. It is efteem'd drying, aftringent, and incraffating. Alum melted with a due Proportion of Dragon's Blood, is the celebrated Styptic of *Helvetius,* which is extremely beneficial in uterine Hæ morrhages, and others, and in the *Fluor Albus.* A large Nutmeg with an equal Quantity of Alum, powder'd, and divided into three Dofes, if one is given every Morning, is faid to cure an Ague. Burnt Alum is ufed as an Efcharotic to eat down fungous Flefh.

The fecond Sort of Alum, is the *Alumen Rochi Gallis,* Offic. *Alumen Romanum five rubrum,* Ind. Med. Roch Alum. It is fomewhat like common Alum, exeept that it is of a palifh red. It is imported from *Italy* and *Smyrna,* and is faid to be made like other Alum, but without the Help of *Kali* and Urine. It agrees in Virtues with the preceeding.

Another Alum, is the *Alumen plumofum,* Offic. Plumofe, or Feather'd Alum. This is found in Quarries in the Ifland of *Melos,* according to *Tournefort,* where it is produc'd fpontaneoufly, without the Affiftance of Art, and differs from the other Species of Alum, only in its Form, confifting of tender foft Filaments, almoft like a Feather. Some have erroneoufly confounded this with the *Lapis Amiantus.*

Ambra grifea, Offic. Ambergrife. The Origin of Ambergrife is a Point that has been long debated among Phyficians and Naturalifts, fome maintaining it to be the Product of the Animal, others of the Vegetable Kingdom. Some affert that it is the Dung of fome oriental Bird, and as a demonftrative Proof of their Opinion, fhew the Claws and Fragments of the Beaks of Birds, that are often found inclofed within its Subftance, which, being committed to the Fire, emit the Odour of an empyreumatic volatile Salt, which Sort of Smell is almoft peculiar to Bodies that derive their Origin from the Animal Kingdom. Others, on the contrary, attempt to prove, that Ambergrife is a Kind of Honey, which is made by the Bees in the Rocks by the Sea-fide; and being afterwards attenuated and digefted by the Heat of the Sun, becomes a Subftance of that Fragrancy as we find it. But thefe Errors may be foon detected by plain chymical Experiments; for all Dung of Animals, and Honey too, admit of a Solution in aqueous Menftruums; but obftinately refift the moft highly rectified Spirit of Wine. Some of the Moderns have thought it to be a peculiar Kind of Refin, or Tear diftilled from fome Tree as yet unknown to us, in the *Eaftern* Parts of the World, and afterwards transferred to the Sea, where, acquiring a more perfect Digeftion by the Heat of the Sun, and by the Sea Salt, it conftitutes a refinous Body of that Nature. But, befides many other Reafons, what directly thwarts, and overthrows this Opinion, is, that all refinous Bodies of Vegetables will admit of an eafy Solution and Extraction in the highly rectified phlogiftic Spirit of Wine; whereas the contrary is true of Ambergrife, which is very difficult to be diffolved in fuch a Spirit: Befides, it is obferved, that inflammable Bodies produced from the Earth, as Amber, *Bitumen Judaicum,* and Sea Coal, are alfo difficult of Solution, and are by no Means readily united with a very fpirituous Liquor. Thefe Things confidered, we agree in Opinion with thofe who hold, that Ambergrife is to be reckoned among the Spieces of *Bitumens,*

Bitumens, and owes its Rise to the Earth, out of whose Bowels it is torn, and washed away by the Waves, and carried into the Sea; for it is found in greatest Quantities in the Sea about the Island of *Madagascar*, where the subterranean Parts are believed to be pregnant with that Kind of *Bitumen*. It is a solid, sebaceous, or fat Substance, not ponderous, of an Ash-Colour, variegated like Marble, and marked often with white Specks. There are two Kinds of Ambergrise, the Ash-Colour'd, and Black. The First is to be preferred, when cleared of all Filth, with a strong Smell, and light, and which, being pricked with a hot Needle, drops a fat odorous Juice. The Black is less esteemed, as being mixed with Earth or Mud, or adulterated, according to some. The Glebes of Ambergrise are sometimes found so big, as to weigh above two hundred Pounds. It is gathered in great Quantities about the *Molucca* Islands, in the *Indian* Sea, and is frequently found on the Shores, both in the *East-Indies*, and in *Africa*. Pieces of it are likewise met with on the Northern Coasts of *England*, *Scotland*, *Norway*, and *Ireland*, being thrown ashore by the Tide. Ambergrise melts by Fire into a gold colour'd or yellow Resin. In distilling Ambergrise, we get first an insipid, then an acid Liquor, or Spirit, and a yellow Oil of a most penetrating Smell, with a small Portion of acid volatile Salt, like Salt of Amber, a black, shining, bituminous Matter remaining in the Retort. From whence it is plain, that Ambergrise consists of fine volatile Parts, intangled in other thicker Parts, both saline and bituminous. This Drug is very much used by Confectioners, and is recommended by Physicians as proper to raise the drooping Spirits, to supply the Defect thereof, and to accelerate their Motions. Hence it is both a cephalic and cordial Medicine, enlivens the Senses, and is very effectual in Faintings, and all other Affections of the Head and Nerves. It is thought to be very instrumental in prolonging Life, and in producing such Effects, as are necessary for Generation. This Opinion prevails chiefly among the Eastern Nations. It is used both outwardly and inwardly. The Dose, in Substance, is from one to four Grains, taken in a poached Egg, or in a Glass of Wine with Sugar and Spices. Ambergrise is sometimes counterfeited by mixing a little Musk and Civet, with Storax, *Labdanum*, and Aloes Wood. And sometimes it is adulterated, by mixing with it some of the above mentioned Perfumes, and a great deal of Bull's Blood dried.

Amethystus, Offic. The Amytheft. This is a precious Stone, of a Violet Colour, which arises from a Mixture of Red and Azure. It is found in *India*, *Arabia*, and *Armenia*. It is good to stop a Looseness, and to absorb the acid Particles when too much abounding in the Stomach, which Virtue it has in common with other alcaline Substances. It is pretended, that it prevents Drunkenness, being worn on the Finger, or bruised, and drank in Powder, but this Virtue is only imaginary. Hence it receives its Name.

Amiantus, Offic. Earth-Flax. This is a kind of scissile Stone, consisting of Filaments, in such a Manner as to be capable of being wove into a sort of Cloth. It is remarkable for resisting the Force of Fire, so as not to be consum'd by it; it is seldom or never used in Medicine, that I know of; tho' Superstition has ascrib'd some Virtues to it, as that it resists Magic and Witchcraft; but as the Legislator has thought proper to abrogate all the Laws before in Force against Sorcery, upon a full Conviction, of there being no such Thing, I think we we may, with equal Reaſon, ſtrike the *Amiantus* out of the Catalogue of Simples.

Ampelitis Terra, Offic. Canal Coal. This is a foſſile, ſtony, friable and black Kind of *Bitumen*. It is eſteemed drying and digeſtive, and to be a good Application to malignant Ulcers. It is ſaid to kill thoſe Worms, which eat Vines, and hence has been applied to the *Abdomen*, in order to deſtroy Worms in the Inteſtines.

Antimonium, Offic. Antimony. This is a metallic, ſolid, ponderous and friable Subſtance, almoſt of the Colour of black Lead, conſiſting of long ſhining *Striæ*, or Needles. It is found in Mines, in many Parts of the World, of different Colours, but the *Hungarian* and *Tranſilvanian* Antimony, of which little or none comes to us, is eſteemed much the beſt for medicinal Uſes. What we are furniſhed with is not the pure Mineral, but that melted and caſt into a pyramidal Form. We are obliged to *Baſil Valentine* for diſcovering the medicinal Uſes of Antimony. It was this Chymiſt who firſt uſed Antimony internally, and enriched Medicine with many Preparations of this Mineral. It is ſaid, that having thrown away ſome Antimony, which he had uſed in the Fuſion of Metals, he obſerved ſome Swine, who had accidentally eaten it, to purge conſiderably; and that, very ſoon after this, they became ſleek and fat. This gave him the Hint of trying what it would do in human Bodies; with this View he made a Multitude of Experiments with it, as appears by his Treatiſe, intitled, *Currus Triumphalis Antimonii*, and determined its Efficacy. After him *Paracelſus, Matthiolus, Angelus Sala, Jacobus Launæus*, and many other learned Men, pleaded the Cauſe of Antimony, and held it in great Eſteem. There were, however, others who looked upon the internal

Uſe of Antimony as moſt pernicious, amongſt whom was *Jacobus Grevinus*, who in 1566, publiſhed a Treatiſe, in which he repreſents Antimony as a moſt dangerous Poiſon, and adviſes the Magiſtrates to prohibit the Sale of it, as they had done that of Quickſilver and Orpiment. His Council was taken, and the medicinal Uſe of Antimony was forbid the ſame Year, by a Decree of the Faculty of Phyſic at *Paris*, which was confirmed by one of the Parliament; and in 1609, *Paulmier*, a Phyſician of *Paris*, was expelled the Faculty for uſing it in his Practice. In the Year 1637, the ſame Faculty allowed its Uſe as a Cathartic; and in 1666, the free Uſe of it was permitted by the Parliament of *Paris*, in Conſequence of an Opinion of the Faculty of Phyſic given in its Favour. Antimony was eſteem'd by the Antients, aſtringent and refrigerating, was principally uſed externally, as in *Collyria*, againſt Fluxions and Exulcerations of the Eyes, and by way of Coſmetic to tinge the Eye-brows and Eye-laſhes of a black Colour. It is very aſtoniſhing that ſo many Phyſicians, and ſome of them Men of Learning ſhould ſo ſtrenuouſly oppoſe the Introduction of Antimony, into Medicine, and without any Manner of Evidence from Experience, treat it as a deleterious Poiſon; for it appears that Antimony reduced to a Powder is neither Emetic nor Cathartic, tho' if given in very large Quantities, it may perhaps by its *Stimulus* and Weight gently looſen the Belly; and ſo far is it from being deleterious, that it is an excellent Alterative in the *Scabies*, or Mange of Horſes, other Cattle, and Man, and thoſe who take it are obſerved to grow fat after it, and to enjoy a better State of Health than before; and it is a very great Error to imagine as ſome have done, that Antimony boiled or macerated in Water,

Water, both vomits and purges, for it does neither. But if Antimony is mixed with an equal Quantity of Nitre, and put gradually into a red hot Crucible, so as to melt, it then becomes violently emetic, and is called *Crocus Metallorum*; and it further communicates an emetic Quality to Wine, or almost in any other Liquor in which it has been infused; and this Proportion of Nitre with the Antimony is said to render the Preparation more emetic than any other; for if either more, or less, Nitre is us'd, it is proportionably less emetic. Antimony consists of a sulphureous, and reguline Part, which when united together operate as an Alterative only; but as soon as the Union is dissolved, the Sulphur becomes emetic and cathartic, and the reguline Part drastic and virulent. If Antimony in Powder is boiled in Water impregnated with an Acid, an Alcali, or any Thing oleous, this will in some Measure dissolve the Union betwixt the sulphureous and reguline Parts, and communicate to the Liquor, the Qualities of the Parts it dissolves; thus an Acid dissolving in the reguline and metallic Parts renders the Liquor extremely emetic and drastic; but an alcaline or oleous Liquor acting upon the Sulphur, renders the Liquor more mildly emetic, cathartic, and sometimes diaphoretic. Hence we may conceive the Reason why crude Antimony may sometimes by Accident operate in the *Primæ Viæ*, that is, if it meets with any Thing acid, alcaline, or oleous therein, capable of dissolving the Union betwixt the reguline and sulphureous Parts. *Hoffman* asserts, that he has seen very great and good Effects from crude Antimony mix'd with Sugar; in an Atrophy, and Pains of the Limbs; and crude Antimony alone powder'd, is said to be excellent in paralytic Disorders, and Diseases of the Breast. The ce-

lebrated *Kunckel*, was cur'd by the Advice of *Sennertus*, of violent Pains in his Arms, by taking crude Antimony in Powder; and he afterwards found great Relief in the Gout, by taking crude Antimony mix'd with Sugar. And the Remedy for the Gout so much advertis'd of late Years, under the Name of the Gout and Rheumatic Powder, consists of nothing but equal Parts of crude Antimony and Nitre, reduc'd to a fine Powder, till no Particles of the Antimony remain visible; the Dose is twenty-seven Grains of both together. Crude Antimony is also an excellent Remedy for the Rickets, Worms in Children, the *Fluor Albus*, and all Diseases from glandular Obstructions; but *Geoffroy* advises to begin with a very small Dose, and increase it gradually, to avoid at the Time of taking it all Acids, and to mix it with treble or four times the Quantity of some Absorbent, as the *Oculi Cancrorum*. We find in the *Brandenburgh* Dispensatory a Preparation under the Title of *Morsuli Restaurantes Kunckelii*, consisting of crude Antimony, mixed with some aromatic and oleous Ingredient, and Sugar: These are greatly celebrated in *Germany* for putrid Fevers, the Itch, and Ulcers thence arising, for carrying off the Relics of the Small Pox, and in a virulent *Gonorrhæa* of long standing; and two Parts of Antimony with one of the Peruvian Bark, given in the Quantity of two Drams for a Dose, is esteem'd excellent in an intermitting Fever, and is said even to cure one that is continual; but of this I have no Experience. It is further asserted, that crude Antimony mix'd with melted Wax, or as it is called *Cerated*, is an excellent Remedy in a *Diarrhæa* or Dysentery. I think it is generally agreed by Chymists, that the Sulphur of Antimony differs very little from common mineral Sulphur; but that it operates

operates in a different Manner, is owing to a Portion of the reguline Part, from which it is very difficult to free the Sulphur. Upon the Whole, Antimony may be esteem'd one of the *Herculean* Remedies, for conquering obstinate Distempers, and if us'd with Judgment and Discretion, it is as innocent as any other Medicine. It is therefore astonishing, that any Instances should occur of Patients labouring under obstinate Disorders, who have been deserted, or at least not cur'd, by Physicians, who have afterwards found a Remedy in Antimony, administer'd by the Hands of Quacks, who don't so much as pretend to any Degree of medicinal Knowledge.

Aquæ minerales. Mineral Waters. These differ extremely on Account of their Contents. Those which are cold, and impregnated with mineral and diuretic Particles, are called *Acidulæ,* but improperly; for *Hoffman* has demonstrated, that they are of an alcaline, not of an acid Nature. The Principal of these are, the Waters of *Tunbridge, Astrop, Knaresborough, Road, Ipswich, Spaw, Islington, Felsted, Oulton,* and *Cannock* in *Staffordshire:* The principal saline and cathartic Waters are, those of *Epsom, Acton, Kensington, Colchester, Richmond, Lambeth, Stretham, Dulwich, North-Hall, Scarborough, Woodham Ferrers, Holt,* and *Cheltenham.* The principal hot sulphureous Waters are, those of *Bath* and *Buxton* ; *Bristol* and *Matlock* Waters are also somewhat warm. All these act by their Contents; and perhaps the Water itself may exert very great Efficacy in the Cure of Distempers. There are such a vast Number of, and infinite Variety in mineral Waters, that it would require a whole Volume to explain this Subject ; I must therefore refer the Reader to what *F. Hoffman* has wrote upon this Subject.

Arena maris, Offic. Sea-Sand. This dries up the redundant Moisture in hydropic Constitutions, if the Patient lies cover'd with it as far as the Head. It is sometimes heated, and applied by Way of dry Fomentation instead of Salt or Millet.

Argentum, Offic. Silver. Some Preparations from this Metal are used in Medicine, tho' I don't know, that by itself it is possess'd of any Virtues, tho' some were formerly ascrib'd to it, as it should seem without any real Foundation. It was said to be peculiarly adapted to Disorders of the Head and Brain, and was therefore recommended in an Epilepsy, Apoplexy, Vertigo, Melancholy, Weakness of Memory, and Folly, if this last may be esteem'd a Distemper. *Tachenius* tells us of an illiterate Silversmith, of so happy a Memory, that he could repeat Word for Word, whatever he heard; and this it seems was ridiculously ascrib'd to his swallowing Silver, as he work'd it.

Argilla, Offic. Clay. Clays of all Sorts are esteem'd drying, astringent, and abstergent.

Arsenicum. Arsenic. Of this there are three Sorts. *Arsenicum Album,* Offic. White Arsenic, or Ratsbane. *Arsenicum Flavum,* Offic. Yellow Ratsbane. *Arsenicum Rubrum, Factitium,* Offic. Red Arsenic. Arsenic properly so called, is a Substance extracted from an Ore found in *Saxony* and *Bohemia,* named *Cobalt.* As this Original of Arsenic, and the Way of preparing it, are not commonly known, I shall here shew what is the Nature of Cobalt, and in what manner Arsenic, and the other Substances found with it in the Ore, are extracted, also what are the Kinds of factitious, or artificial Arsenic. The Cobalt of the Shops, *Cadmia Metallica* of *Agricola,* is a ponderous, hard, fossil

Substance

ibftance, almoft black, not unlike ntimony, or fome Kinds of Pyes, emitting a ftrong fulphureou nell when burnt, often mixed with opper, fometimes with Silver. It dug out of Mines in *Saxony*, near oflar; in *Bohemia*, in the Valley of achim; and in *England*, on the undip Hills, in great Quantities. has fo ftrong a corrofive Quality, fometimes to turn and ulcerate the lands and Feet of the Miners, and a deadly Poifon for all known A-imals. All the three Kinds of rfenic are extracted from it; and it kewife ferves to make *Zaffera*, ufed y Potters, in giving a blue Colour) their Veffels; and the *Encauftum æruleum*, or that Kind of Blue ometimes ufed by Painters, and often y Women to mix with their Starch, or whitening and ftiffening Linen. he Way of making all thefe, is ught by *Kunkel*, in his Art of mak-ig Glafs. To this Purpofe, they ut the Cobalt in a calcining Rever-eratory Furnace, made for that urpofe, in fuch a Manner, as that ie Flame may juft graze upon the)re, and fo fet it on Fire. The 'lame of the Ore is blue, accompa-ied with a copious Smoke, which is eceiv'd on the Cieling of the Fur-ace, and from thence convey'd out hrough a large Funnel, made of oards, and above an hundred Ells a Length; but the greateft Part of fticks to the Infide of the Funnel, n Form of a whitifh Soot; and eve-y fix Months the Labourers fweep he Funnel with Brooms, and care-ully preferve this Soot, which af-erwards ferves to make both vhite, yellow, and red Arfenic. vhite Arfenic is made only by ublimating the Soot in Iron Veffels, nto an opake Subftance, fometimes vhite and fhining like the *Encauftum álbum*, fometimes ftreak'd with red ind chryftalline Veins. Yellow Arfe-uc is made of the fame Soot fublim'd

with common Sulphur, in the Pro-portion of one Part of Sulphur to ten of Soot. The fublimed Mafs is of a yellow Colour, folid like Sul-phur, fhining, and not altogether opake, eafily broken, but not eafily friable, or eafily crumbled into Duft, and diftinguifhable from Orpiment, by not taking Fire when thrown up-on burning Coals, as Orpiment pre-fently does. Red Arfenic is made of the fame Soot and Sulphur, mix'd with a fmall Proportion of a metal-lic Subftance, called the *Spuma of Copper*. The fublimed Mafs is folid, of a cinnabarine Colour, and opake. The calcin'd Cobalt, after the Eva-poration of the Fumes or Smoke, is powder'd and calcin'd again, and this Operation is repeated till the Cal-cination is judged to be perfect. Then being very finely powder'd it is mix'd with two or three times the Quantity of powder'd Flint Stones, and moiften'd with a little Water in large Tubs, where in a very fhort time it becomes a folid firm Mafs, called *Zaffera*, as already faid, which is ufed by the Potters, Glafs-Men, and Enamellers. If two Parts of calcined Cobalt, one Part of Pot-afh, and three of common Sand, be melted together, a vitrious, opake, and bluifh Mafs is produced, which is ground in Mills to a very fine blue Powder, which is called *Smaltum*, or *Encauftum Cæruluem*, ufed by Painters, and in wafhing Linen. Arfe-nic confifts of an acid Salt, and a Kind of mercurial or metallic Sub-ftance, which difcovers itfelf when it is diftilled in a Retort, mixed with Soap, Suet, Oil, or any Fat, or oily Subftance; for with a ftrong Degree of Fire the Arfenic will be raifed in-to the Neck of the Retort in a me-tallic Form, like Antimony. The Sulphur contained in Arfenic is in fo fmall a Proportion, that it does not flame when caft on burning Coals, though Cobalt contains a great Quan-tity

tity of Sulphur, which consequently has been separated from the arsenical Parts in the Calcination and Deflagration, and so evaporated; but the Smell of Arsenic proves, that some Sulphur still remains in it. Arsenic is very volatile; for if any Quantity of it is put into a Crucible, and set over the Fire, it will presently evaporate in white Fumes, without leaving any Remainder. If melted, stratified, or cemented with Copper, it turns it of a silver Colour; but, as it impairs its Ductility, this Change of Colour is rendered of no Use. Arsenic is a powerful Corrosive, and reckoned among the strongest Poisons. When taken inwardly, it causes many bad Symptoms, of which some are common to it with other Poisons; such as Anxieties, Swoonings, Palpitations, a sudden Dejection, or Sinking of the Strength and Spirits, Stupors, Deliriums, convulsive Motions of the Limbs, Palsies, Heat and Corrosion of the *Fauces*, Thirst, Fevers, Vomiting, Pain in the Stomach, and cold Sweats. Other Symptoms are peculiar to this Poison, such as not only an Erosion of the Stomach, but an Extenuation of it, in such a Manner, as that all its Coats taken together, shall not be thicker than a Poppy Leaf in many Places; and at the same time, the small Intestines are found corroded and perforated; a sudden Swelling, and Sphacelation of the Parts of the Body; and, after Death, a more speedy Putrefaction than is observed in other Cases, especially in the Parts of Generation belonging to Men. If Death does not immediately follow, the Patient becomes afflicted with an hectic Fever, Marasmus, Palsy, Tremors, and sometimes Madness. Some recommend Rock Crystal reduced to an impalpable Powder, as an Antidote against Arsenic; but I should depend much more upon drinking large Quantities of Milk, Oil, or

fat Broths, while the Poison remains in the *Primæ Viæ*; but after it has got into the Blood, alexiterial Medicines are to be used, such as *Venice* Treacle, Mithridate, Bezoar, *Contrayerva* Root, and such like, and afterwards a Milk Diet. Though Arsenic be a quick Poison both for Men and Brutes, it is recommended by some in intermitting Fevers; but, let it be never so much prepared and corrected, its deleterious Qualities are only lessened, never wholly remov'd; and therefore, though it may be a good Remedy for the present, it will afterwards prove a Poison, and bring on very dismal Symptoms. After giving the above Account of the Opinion of *Geoffroy*, with Respect to the internal Use of Arsenic, I need not caution the young Practitioners in Physic to hold as suspected the Advice of *Pitcairn*, who directs Arsenic to be given internally in a Dysentery; and of *Zacutus Lusitanus*, who advises the Use of it in Clysters for the same Distemper.

Asphaltus & Bitumen Judaicum, Offic. Jews Pitch. The *Asphaltum* of *Dioscorides*, and *Bitumen Judaicum* of the Shops, called *Carabe* and *Gummi Funerum* by *Serapion*, and by others *Mumia*, is a solid, brittle, ponderous Substance, of a red, blackish, or dark Colour; easily inflammable, and of a strong bituminous Smell, especially when warm, and fusible by Fire. It is found in several Parts, but the best is that which comes from *Judæa*, where it is gathered in the Dead-Sea, called from thence the Lake *Asphaltites*. It is probable, that a great Quantity of this *Bitumen* rises from the Bottom of that Lake to the Surface of the Water. At first it is so soft, viscid, and glutinous, that it can with Difficulty be separated from any Part which it touches, but in Time it grows harder than Pitch; and from the Place where

where it is found, it is called *Carabe of Sodom*; *Carabe* being used often by the *Arabians* to denote any solid *Bitumen*, and the *Dead-Sea* being the Lake where *Sodom* stood. The Names of *Gummi Funerum* and *Mumia* were given it, because the common People, among the *Egyptians*, used it in embalming and preserving dead Bodies. The true *Bitumen Judaicum*, is seldom brought to us; for *Dioscorides* directs us to make Choice of that which shines like Purple, and to reject the black Kind as being foul, and of small Value; but all that we see of that Kind is black; though even that, when broken in Pieces, appears against the Light, to be of a Saffron Colour; and therefore it is possible this may be the same Kind recommended by *Dioscorides*, only boil'd to a hard Consistence in Brass Kettles before it is sent to us. It is of a discutient, emollient, and agglutinating Quality. It dissolves coagulated Blood, and promotes the menstrual Discharge.

Asteria Gemma, Offic. The Bastard Opal, or Star Gem. This Gem is transparent like Crystal, but of a harder Nature. 'Tis thought to be a Species of the *Opal*, but neither the one nor the other are now kept in the Shops. If carried about with one, 'tis thought to procure Sleep, and prevent frightful Dreams.

Astroites seu Stellaris Lapis, Offic. Star Stone. This Stone is porous, moderately hard, and white, and as big sometimes as a Man's Head. It is found in some Quarries in *England* and *Germany*. It is esteem'd antipestilential, and is said to destroy Worms in Children.

Auripigmentum, Offic. Orpiment. The Orpiment of the Shops, is an Arsenical Juice, in squamous or foliaceous Glebes, like the *Lapis Specularis*, the *Squamæ*, or *Strata*, being easily separated from each o-

ther. Orpiment is of three Kinds; one of a Gold Colour, the second of a deeper red, or Cinnabarine Colour, mix'd with yellow; and the third greenish and yellowish, mix'd with a large Proportion of Earth, and therefore the least valuable. These three Kinds are found in the Veins of Gold, Copper, and Silver Mines; but we know not what was the other Kind of Orpiment mention'd by *Dioscorides*. Orpiment is of an acrid Taste, soluble in Oil, and inflammable by Fire, emitting a thin Flame, with a great deal of Smoke, smelling strongly of Sulphur or Garlick. This Smoke, if collected, turns to yellowish Flowers like Sulphur, and a red, or Blood colour'd Mass remains behind, which, when cold, concretes into a hard solid *Regulus*, like Cinnabar, called by some, red Orpiment, or *Realgar*. If the Orpiment be kept in a subliming Vessel for a long Time on the Fire, the whole Mass is raised to the upper Part of the Vessel, and there concretes into a beautiful, red, pellucid Substance like a Ruby, only a small Quantity of metallic Earth remaining at the Bottom. The first Fumes which come from this *Regulus*, will turn Copper white and brittle. Orpiment therefore must consist of the same Parts as common Sulphur, with some Mineral Particles mixed with them; or it is composed of an acid Salt, entangled in Particles of Mercury, and a bituminous Substance. Its corrosive Quality arises from the acid *Spicula* stuck into the Particles of Mercury; but it has that Quality in a less Degree than corrosive Sublimate, because of its bituminous Part. It is less inflammable than Sulphur, because the Energy of the acid Salts contain'd in it is weaken'd by the Mineral Parts; and, from its corrosive Quality, it is deservedly reckon'd among Poisons. It was antiently

used

used by Physicians to eat away fungous Flesh, but is now laid aside in that Intention, Chymistry having furnish'd us with much better Catherretics. It is used sometimes by Barbers, with a Mixture of Quick Lime, as a Depilatory, to eradicate the Hairs of any Part of the Body; but if they let it lie on too long. it corrodes the Skin   Some Physicians recommend the internal Use of Orpiment, in Substance, in a purulent *Phthisis,* accompanied with Expectoration, and in Asthmas. The Fumes of it may likewise be received at the Mouth in the same Intentions, and the *Chinese* reckon it among the purgative Medicines.   However I cannot think (says *Geoffroy,*) the inward Use of this Medicine in any Respect allowable; for it is a strong Poison, destructive to the Nerves, and accordingly is found by Experience to bring on very terrible Symptoms, such as Spasms in the Hands and Feet, Stupors and Contractions, cold Sweats, Palpitations of the Heart, Faintings, Thirst, inward Burning, Vomiting, Belly-ach, Erosions, violent Pains, and Death itself, according to the different Doses of this Poison; and in the Bodies of such as die in this Manner, the *Oesophagus,* Stomach, and Intestines are found to be inflamed, corroded, and perforated in several Places. The Antidotes for Orpiment, and all other Arsenical Substances, are whatever is able to blunt the Acrimony of these corrosive Medicines; such as Milk and Oil, drank in great Quantities, fat Broths, the Juice of Mallows, or Marshmallows, Decoctions of Flea-wort, and Linseed, Marshmallow Roots, and such like. Orpiment or Arsenic, worn about the Neck like an Amulet, cannot be so hurtful as some imagine; neither do we believe it of any Virtue in preserving against the Plague, or pestilential Diseases.

Aurum, Offic. Gold. The Use of Gold in Physic was unknown to the antient *Greeks.* The *Arabians* first talked of its Medicinal Virtues, and mixed it in their Compositions, being previously reduced to thin Leaves, upon a Perswasion that it comforted the Heart, and exhilarated the Spirits; and that therefore it was proper in Palpitations of the Heart, and in Melancholies. The Chymists add further, that a most powerful fixed Sulphur is contained in Gold, which, if it be mixed with the Blood, preserves it from all Corruption, and restores and revivifies human Nature in the same Manner as the Sun, the great Original of this Sulphur, enlivens Nature. Many Authors are of a quite different Opinion, because the Effects of Gold, are found not to answer these great Pretensions; and it may be reasonably question'd, whether Gold be at all useful in Physic. The Virtues of the Chymical Preparations of Gold are equally dubious, because they seem to derive their Energy, not from the Gold, but from the Menstrua, and other Substances mixed with it.

Belemnites, & Lapis Lyncis, Offic. Thunder Bolts. The *Belemnites* is a round, oblong Stone, ending in an obtuse Point, sometimes white, sometimes of a Gold, and sometimes of a dark Colour. Some of these Stones are solid, others hollow, and it is distinguished by Lines drawn from the *Axis* to the Circumference. It is commonly about an Inch in Length and Thickness; though some have been found as large as a Man's Arm, and in every one of them there is a Fissure or Slit running thro' its whole Length. The Name *Belemnites* comes from a *Greek* Word, which signifies the Point of an Arrow: It is also called *Dactylus Idaeus,* from its Resemblance to a Finger, and its being found in Mount *Ida,* in the Island of *Crete;* but it is

dog

dug up likewife in the *Alps*, and in many Places of *France* and *Germany*. It is without Ground taken for the *Lapis Lyncurius* of the Antients, fince it is evident, that by that Word *Diofcorides* underftood Amber, which he tells us, was by fome taken to be the concreted and indurated Urine of the *Lynx*. The *Germans* fay, that this Stone is good againft the Night Mare, and the Stone in the Kidneys. It is given in Powder, from half a Dram to a Dram in any convenient Vehicle.

Beryllus, Offic. The Beryl. This is a precious, fhining, tranfparent Stone, the Colour of which is commonly a Sea green; but there are fome of the Colour of Oil, or of Garlick, or pale, or yellow, or of the Colour of Gold: They call this laft *Chryfoberillus*; that is to fay, gilded *Beryl*. It is found in feveral Parts of *India*. It is not likely that Gems fhould be poffefs'd of any Medicinal Virtues, but thofe afcrib'd to this are, that when powder'd, and given internally, it ftops Hæmorrhages, and is good for Diforders of the Liver, Eructations, and Difeafes of the Mouth, Face, and Throat.

Bifmuthum, Offic. Bifmuth, Marcafite of Silver, or Tin Glafs. *Bifmuth* is a metallic, fufible, but not ductile Subftance, very brittle and heavy, and diftinguifhable from Lead and Tin by its Colour, which is fometimes fhining like Silver, fometimes of a faint Purple, refembling the *Regulus* of Antimony, but confifting of broader *Laminæ*, and ftaining the Fingers. It is prepared by Artifts, by being firft torrefy'd, and then melted into a *Regulus*. It is often found in the Silver Mines; and wherever the Miners find *Bifmuth*, they conclude they fhall find Silver; and hence they call it the Proof of Silver. The Mines of *Bifmuth* are in *Bohemia* and *Mifnia*. Some pretend that it may be extracted from

Cobalt melted into a *Regulus*, by a particular Procefs; but this is not certain. *Bifmuth* feems to have been unknown both to the *Greeks* and *Arabians*; for the *Arabian Marcafite* was the *Lapis Pyrites*. It is very feldom ufed in Phyfic, tho' fome prepare Flowers from it, which they fay are diaphoretic, but moft Phyficians have been afraid to ufe it inwardly, becaufe of the Arfenical Parts contain'd in it. The Magiftery of *Bifmuth* is prepared by diffolving the Metal in Spirit of Nitre, then precipitating it with a Solution of Sea Salt in Water. This Precipitate, being edulcerated by frequent Lotions, becomes a very white Powder, much valued by the Ladies as a Cofmetic, and much ufed by Dealers in Hair, to improve the Colour of it when dark or red. Pewterers mix it with Tin to harden it, and give it a more fhining Colour.

Bitumen, Offic. *Piffafphaltos nativum*, Schrod. Common Foffile Pitch. The *Bitumen* is produc'd in *Apollonia*, near *Epidamnos*, and is carried down the *Ceraunian* Mountains by the Current of a River, and thrown upon the Shores, where it concretes into Maffes, and fmells like Pitch mixed with Brimftone. The *Piffafphaltos* of *Diofcorides*, and of the Shops, or Mineral Pitch, is a black or red Kind of *Bitumen*, of a fragrant and not unpleafant bituminous Smell, vifcid, or of a middle Confiftence, between *Petroleum*, and a folid *Bitumen*, not unlike the common Pitch, fufible by Fire, concrefcible by Cold, and eafily inflammable. It is compounded of two *Greek* Words, which fignify Pitch and *Bitumen*, and the Compound might be render'd a bituminous Pitch, or pitchy *Bitumen*, the Reafon of which Name is not that it confifts of an artificial Mixture of thefe two Subftances, but it fmells like fuch a Mixture. It diftils from

Rocks,

Rocks, or springs from the Earth in several Countries. In *Italy* they use that which is found in the *Campania di Roma,* about sixty Miles from the City, near a little Town called *Catho.* It ouzes thro' the Crannies of Rocks in the Summertime, of the Consistence of Honey, of a black Colour, and penetrating Smell. There is likewise a plentiful Spring of this *Bitumen* in *Auvergne* in *France,* which is soft and black like Pitch, and of a bituminous Smell. If it be kept a great while, it grows hard, retaining still something of its fatty Consistence, and never grows so dry or hard as the solid *Bitumens.* Fresh *Bitumen* is digestive, maturating, and resolvent. It is used in ripening Buboes, resolving Tumors, discussing sciatic Pains, and to strengthen luxated Parts after they have been reduced. A Mixture of this, and slimy or muddy Clay, is called *Maltha,* and was used as Mortar in building the Walls of *Babylon,* according to *Vitruvius.*

Bolus, Bole. There are many fat Earths used in Medicine, which go by the Name of *Boli,* Boles, as the

Bolus Armena, Offic. Bole Armoniac. It is an earthy Substance, of a pale yellowish Colour, inclining somewhat to red. It is ponderous, pinguious, easily friable, and of a styptic Taste. It is dig'd out of the Mines in *Turky,* and thence brought to us. It is, at present very rare with us; for what is found in the Shops, approaching to the Colour of red Oker, is imported from *Spain* and *Normandy,* and is thought to be little different from the *Rubrica Sinopica.* It is an Alexipharmic, and corrects those Acidities in the Blood which are prejudicial to Health. It is astringent in some Degree, and, for that Reason, used in Fluxions of Humours When apply'd externally, it is of a drying Quality, and induces Cicatrices on Wounds. *Fracastorius* says, that *Bole Armoniac* given to a Person almost in the Agonies of Death, from the Bite of a Spider, instantly cur'd him.

Bolus Armena alba, Mont. Exot. White Armenian Bole. This Bole is brought from *Armenia.* It agrees in Virtues with the preceeding, but is not to be met with in our Shops.

Bolus Armena lutea, Mont. Exot. Yellow Armenian Bole. This Bole adheres to the Tongue, is a strong Astringent, and said to be a powerful Resister of Malignity.

Bolus Bohemica, Offic. *German* Bole. It is an earthy Substance, of the same Colour with the Bole Armoniac, but somewhat fainter. It has some Veins of a yellowish Colour running thro' it, and is heavy, easily friable, and of an astringent Taste. It is dig'd from the Mines of *Bohemia,* and thence imported to us. It agrees in Virtues with the Bole Armoniac, and is sometimes kept in our Shops. *Aldrovandus* informs us, that it is a very efficacious Medicine in all exanthematous Fevers.

Bolus candidus, Offic. *Unicornu Minerale,* Schrod. White Bole. This Bole is dig'd from the Earth at *Gran* in *Hungary,* and at *Goltberg* in *Liege.* It relieves and mitigates Pains of the Head, strengthens the Brain, and is singularly efficacious in curing Dysenteries, and the *Fluor albus.*

Bolus rubra nostras, Ind. Med. French Bole. *Dale* confesses he knows nothing of this Bole. I take it to be the red *French* Bole, which is got in many Parts of *France.* *Pomet* gives the following Account of the *French* Boles. " The Bole which " we sell, says he, is found in seve- " ral Parts of *France,* about *Blois* " and *Saumur,* or *Bourgogne,* and " which is of various Colours, as grey, " red, and yellow. The Yellow is " the most valuable, because it pas- " ses the readiest for Bole of the *Le-*

" *vant*, and becaufe it fits the Gil-
" ders beft. As thefe Boles are the
" deareft, becaufe of the Charge of
" tranfporting them to *Paris* from
" *Blois* and *Saumur*, we prefer that
" of *Baville* and other Places about
" *Paris*, becaufe the Peafants bring
" it at a cheaper Rate, than we can
" buy the other. The beft is the
" cleaneft, fmootheft, and well co-
" lour'd, of a light yellowifh red,
" which being tafted, feems to melt,
" like Butter, in the Mouth. Its
" Thicknefs is known by fticking to
" the Tongue. The counterfeit or
" adulterate Bole is of a fad-deep
" red, fandy, and gritty, being not
" of a third Part of the Price of the
" True. It is very drying and a-
" ftringent, good againft Fluxes and
" Gleets. It thickens thin Humours,
" refifts Putrefaction, and expels
" poifonous Bodies. It is alfo ufed
" in Spitting of Blood, bleeding
" Wounds, and alfo to confolidate
" broken Bones, and ftrengthen
" weak Limbs."

Bolus Toccavienfis, Offic. Tran-
fylvanian Bole. This Bole has all
the Characteriftics of the true *Armenian* Bole, and melts in the Mouth
like Butter. It is digg'd from the
Earth in *Tranfylvania* near *Tokai*. It
is greatly celebrated as an efficacious
Medicine in Catarrhs and the Plague.
It was firft apply'd to medicinal Purpofes by *Crato*, who prefers it to the
Armenian Bole brought from *Turky*.
I cannot determine, fays *Dale*, whether it is really different from all the
preceeding or not.

Borax. A Kind of Salt ufed in
mechanic Arts and Medicine. It is
alfo called *Chryfocolla factitia*, *San-
terna Plinii*, & *Tincar*, Offic. *Nitrum factitium*, *Arabice Borax*.
Worm. Borace. *Borax* is a Salt,
whofe Compofition, whether natural
or artificial, is but little known. Natural Hiftory, as well ancient as modern, affords us but little Light or
Information concerning this ftrange
Salt, and from what we can learn of
it from thence, we are not fufficiently inftructed to conclude, that it is
the true *Chryfocolla* of the Ancients;
though the *Spaniards*, who work
in the Mines of *Chili*, the *Venetians*,
and other Moderns, ftill give it that
Name, which they found in ancient
natural Hiftory. *Pliny*, fpeaking of
the *Chryfocolla* of his Time, divides
it into two Kinds; the Native, which
was taken out of the Mines of Copper; and the factitious, which was
made by ftirring and beating the U-
rine of young Children in Mortars of
Copper. *Paul Herman* in his *Materia Medica* fays, that they make
Borax in the *Eaft-Indies* of a nitrous
Earth, which, after they have calcin'd, and reduced it to Powder,
they boil and make thereof a ftrong
Lixivium; this they afterwards expofe to the Air, in order to make it
run into Cryftals; that this Salt never comes to a greater Perfection in
that Country; and that it is in the
Places whither it is tranfported that
they purify it. By thefe two De-
fcriptions, and efpecially *Pliny*'s, it
appears, that we are at a Lofs for
the true *Borax* at prefent; for in the
Effays which *Geoffroy* fays he made
on the Solution of this Salt in Water
without Addition, he could never
find a fingle Atom of Copper, whereas there ought to have been a confiderable Quantity, had it been the
Chryfocolla of *Pliny*. Nor had I, fays
he, any more Reafon, from what I
could difcover, to think that it might
be made of a nitrous Earth, taken in
the Senfe and according to the Properties of our Nitre at prefent, becaufe it cryftallized in a differentMan-
ner, and fufed upon Coal. But if
M. *Herman*, by his *Indian* Nitre
means the Nitre of *Agra*, and fome
other Places in the *Eaft-Indies*, which
is a *Natrum*, and confequently a
ftrong Alcali, *Borax* would be an al-

caline Salt of much greater Penetration, and of a much more acrimonious Taste than we find it, unless they have a Way of making this Salt, by adding to the *Natron* some sweetening Substance to take off the Acrimony, and so making an imperfect *Sal Salsum,* in which the Alcali is predominant. *Geoffroy's* late Brother, in the Lectures which he read at the Royal College upon the *Materia Medica,* and after the Perusal of some Memoirs of a *German* Traveller called M. *Narglin,* a good Naturalist, who had made many Essays upon that Salt, both in the *Indies* and at *Venice,* where it was formerly purify'd, tells us, " That *Borax* was produc'd in " several Parts of the *East-Indies,* but " most plentifully in the Dominions " of the Great *Mogul,* and in *Persia,* " that, in several Places of those " two Countries, there flow'd gently " from different Mines, but princi- " pally from those of Copper, a salt " Water, muddy and greenish, which " was carefully preserv'd; that, af- " ter it was evaporated to a certain " Consistence, they poured it into " Pits sunk in the Earth, and lined " with a Paste composed of the Mud " deposited from the same mineral " Sources, and the Fat of Animals; " that they laid over these Pits a Co- " ver of a convenient Thickness, " made of the same Paste; that at " the End of some Months they o- " pen'd them, where they would " find the Water partly evaporated, " and the Salt of the *Borax* crystal- " lized; that they took these Cry- " stals out of that fat Mud, with " which they were still mix'd or co- " ver'd, and in that Condition they " were brought to us from the *In-* " *dies.*" Our Merchants import *Borax* also from *China,* where it costs little; which makes it probable, that this Kind of Salt is natural to that Country, or at least very easy to make. These differant *Boraxes* are at present refined in *Holland;* but the Way of doing it is not a Secret only to the *Dutch,* for there is a private Gentleman in the *Fauxbourg St. Antoine,* who did refine it, and deliver it to the Merchants as fine and as pure as that of *Holland.* In this State of perfect Purification it is transparent like Rock-Crystal. The Use of Borax in Medicine is that of an incisive and aperient Salt, by Virtue of which it is effectual against Diseases which proceed from an Inspissation of the Humours, and Obstructions thence arising, acting at the same Time against the Acid, without exciting any Motion. The Dose is an entire Dram. It is thought by some to have a specific emmenagogue, and expulsive Virtue, which may probably be derived from the aforesaid incisive, deobstruent, and aperitive Qualities. However, its *Stimulus* does not seem strong enough to be depended upon for present Relief in a difficult Birth, unless it be join'd with some other Ingredients, that are of more Efficacy by their volatile *Stimulus.* For this Reason *Borax* is commonly given in Powder mixed with Saffron, Myrrh, Oil of Cinnamon, Castor, the volatile salt of Amber, and other Powders of known Efficacy, in promoting the Birth, and facilitating Delivery. Some advise a few Grains of it to be taken in a poach'd Egg, as a Provocative to Venery, especially to those whom poach'd Eggs alone have a good Effect upon; *Borax* calcin'd is reckon'd of specific Virtue in Fluxes of the Belly, or the *Semen,* because it is a Sort of styptic Earth. The Dose is from a Scruple to half a Dram, in Conserve of Roses, either alone, or with other suitable Ingredients, for Instance, the Bone of a Cuttlefish, or toasted Nutmeg. Outwardly it is apply'd, though but seldom, to confume carnous and fpongy Excrefcencies, in fordid Ulcers; it is recommended alfo for the Itch, and in Cofmetics. The Ufefulnefs of *Borax* in fuch Cafes may reafonably be expected from its faline, incifive, and refolving Qualities, which caufe it to be received into the *Unguentum Citreum,* which is recommended for making the Skin fmooth, and free from Afperities. Its faponaceous, abfterfive Virtue, for the Purpofes aforefaid, may perhaps more juftly be expected from *Borax* in its crude State, as it is fold in *India;* tho' according to *Garçias,* it is feldom ufed by the *Indian* Phyficians, unlefs for the Itch.

Calaminaris Lapis, Offic. Calaminar Stone. The Foffile *Cadmia* of *Agricola,* ftony *Cadmia* of *Schroder, Lapis Calaminaris,* or Calamine of the Shops, is a foffil Subftance, of a middle Confiftence between Stone and Earth, of different Colours, fuch as a pale Colour inclining to white, yellowifh, and a blackifh red. This laft is full of fmall ferruginous Globules, like Grains of Pepper, and mark'd with white Veins, and is found in great Quantities about *Bourges* near *Saumur,* in *Anjou,* in *France,* and in many Parts of *England.* The others are dug in *Germany,* near *Aix la Chapelle;* and all Kinds of it feem to partake of au Iron-Ore, becaufe the greateft Part is attracted by the Load-ftone. This Species of *Cadmia* was probably unknown to the ancient *Greeks,* or at leaft was not ufed by them in Phyfic, fince it is not mention'd either by *Diofcorides,* or *Galen.* It is now prefcribed, by fome Phyficians, to dry running Ulcers, to heal the excoriated Parts of Children, either in a fine Powder by itfelf, or mix'd with Ointments. The *Lapis Calaminaris* is much ufed in cooling, and drying Cerates; and is, in Powder, frequently fprinkled up-

on Sores and Ulcers, with a View of drying them, and difpofing them to cicatrize. I have been told, that the Surgeons have lately obferved, that *Lapis Calaminaris,* reduced to a very fine Powder, operates as an Efcharotic; whereas in a more grofs Powder it acts as a Dryer.

Calx, Offic. Lime. Quick Lime, by the *Greeks* called κονία, or τιταν⊙- ασβιτ⊙-, or fimply ασβιτ⊙-, is no more than a calcarious Stone, burn'd into a Calx of a white cineritious Colour, of an acrid and pungent Tafte, and which, when it has not been too long expofed to the Air, produces an Efferveicence, Smoak, and a confiderable Degree of Heat, when Water is poured upon it; but when it is penetrated by the moift and humid Parts of the Air, it ceafes to produce an Effervefcence, and becomes a Kind of Powder. Quick-Lime may be prepar'd not only of the Stone commonly called Lime Stone, but alfo of Marble, and other Stones of a clofe Contexture, and hard Nature. In fome Parts of *France* it is prepar'd of a Sort of Flint, which is capable of being calcin'd. In *Holland,* and fome other Countries, where Lime-ftone is not to be found, they prepare it of the Sea Shells found on the Shore, which they calcine by the Affiftance of a ftrong and violent Fire. But this Species is lefs proper, both for the Purpofes of Architecture and Medicine, than that which is prepar'd of Stone. The *Americans,* according to *Labat,* prepare a Quicklime of Sub-marine Plants and Lithophytes; and in feveral Parts of *England,* where a proper Stone cannot be had, Lime is made of Chalkftones calcin'd.

Quick lime is fometimes ufed by Surgeons as an Efcharotic; but taken internally it is efteem'd a Poifon. That Species, however, which is made of Shells calcin'd, is frequently given as a Medicine. Quick-lime is used in making some Sorts of Caustics. Lime-water, and the *Lixivium* or Ley, lately so much celebrated for calculous Disorders; and 'tis very certain, that the Salts of Lime may exert very great Effects in the Body, if taken in such a Manner as not to do Injury by their Corrosiveness and Heat. Lime Water is esteem'd a Specific, for that Species of Scurvy, to which Sailors are so very subject; and Fluids impregnated with the Salts of Lime, should seem to be very effectual for dissolving those Obstructions in the Vessels, which are form'd of earthy Particles.

Carbo fossilis, Lithanthrax, Offic. Pit-Coal, or Scotch-Coal. *Hoffman* informs us, that Coals, distill'd from a Retort by an open Fire, yield first a Phlegm, then a somewhat acrid sulphureous Spirit, then a subtile Oil, then a grosser Oil, which subsides to the Bottom of the Receiver; and, lastly, by a brisker Degree of Fire, a certain acidulated Salt, resembling that of Amber. In the Retort, there is left a light black Earth, which, upon the Application of Fire, emits neither Flame nor Smoke. I shall here give a brief, but accurate Description of the several Experiments made by *Hoffman,* in Order to investigate the Nature of these Principles. The Spirit yielded in Distillation, is at first White, but afterwards appears ting'd with a reddish brown Colour; which Phenomenon may also be observed in the Spirits yielded by Woods, Tartar, Myrrh, and other Substances of a like Nature. Upon an Affusion of the Acid Spirit of Salt, a large Number of Bubbles immediately appear'd at the Bottom of the Vessel, which becoming gradually and successively more numerous, ascended to the Surface of the Liquor, but without any remarkable Perturbation of the Mixture. With Spirit of Nitre the Conflict was greater, and the Liquor was render'd more turbid. Upon a sufficient Quantity of quick Lime being thrown into this Spirit, a strong volatile Spirit immediately afflicted the Nose in a forcible Manner. Upon an Affusion of Spirit of Nitre to this Mixture, a thick white Fume was forthwith emitted; which we always observe to happen, when we add Spirit of Nitre to volatile Salts or Spirits. The fetid Oil, intimately united and incorporated with Salt of Tartar, also diffused a Smell like that of volatile Salt. Upon Distillation, this Mixture yielded an alcaline, volatile, and oleous Spirit, which immediately became green with Syrup of Violets, as all Alcalis do; but, when mix'd with an Acid, rais'd a sudden Effervescence, and immediately assum'd a perfectly red Colour. The gross empyreumatic Oil of these Coals, obtain'd in the first Distillation, emitted a sulphurous Smell. When put into a Silver Spoon, to which a gentle Heat was apply'd, it immediately ting'd it of an obscure blackish Colour; a sure Proof, that a true mineral Sulphur is dissolved in it; for common Sulphur, dissolved in Oil of Turpentine, tinges Silver Vessels with the same Colour. The acid Salt, upon an Admixture of Oil of Tartar *per Deliquium,* assumed a near Affinity to that obtain'd from Amber by Distillation. Spirit of *Sal Ammoniac* excited a large Number of very broad Bubbles, which collected themselves in the Bottom of the Glass: But immediately after, the Mixture, which was before limpid, assum'd a reddish Colour; and, upon the Affusion of an Acid, returned to its former Transparence. 'Tis rarely observ'd, that an Acid is thus ting'd by an Alcali. That I might, therefore, says our Author, trace the Cause of this Phenomenon more accurately, I mix'd dissolved volatile Salt of Amber, which I thought of a like Nature with the Salt of which we

now

v ſpeak, with Spirit of *Sal Am-*
niac; by which Means, after ſome
nﬂiﬁ, the Mixture in a little Time
imed a beautiful browniſh red Co-
r; and an excellent Medicine, of
rtues not inferior to ſuccinated
rit of Hartſhorn, was produced.
eſe are the principal Experiments
nade, in order to inveſtigate the
ture of foſſile Coals; from which,
nink, it is obvious, that no dele-
ious Principle, nothing offenſive to
Maſs of Blood, and the minuteſt
ts of the Body, in a Word, no
cious Mineral, no Quantity of
ſenic, are found in them. That a
neral Sulphur is not ſo fatal as is
nmonly believed, is ſufficiently ated by thoſe Men who prepare,
e, and boil the Sulphur of Goſlar
o are found and vigorous, in com-
iſon of other Metal-workers. Nor
here, in the *German* Coal, a very
ſiderable Quantity of this Sulphur,
erwiſe it might be eaſily obtain'd
r, and in the Form of Flowers, by
blimation; for theſe mineral Coals
porous and ſpongious Earth, rich
and intimately impregnated with
bituminous and ſubterraneous
ce. Bitumen is their conſtituent
inciple, without which they would
ither emit Flame nor Smoak: But
Bitumen they contain, like all
e other Species of Bitumens, of
iich Amber is one, conſiſts of ole-
s, ſulphureous, acid, and fine alca-
e Parts, as is obvious from the
chymical Analyſis of Amber,
tumen Judaicum, Naphtha, Petro-
m, and all other reſinous Bodies.
far then are theſe Principles from
oving prejudicial to the vital Juices,
at, by drying up the ſuperﬂuous
umidity, they rather defend the
aſs of Blood, and the Body, from
orruption and Putrefaﬁion; for,
cording to *Galen*, all Bitumens are
dowed with a balſamic Vertue.
ſides, that bituminous Bodies ſet
fire, correﬁ the bad State of the

Air, and diſſipate its ſuperﬂuous Humidity, are Points admitted by moſt
modern Phyſicians; and the Antients
uſed Sulphur and Aſphaltus, in order
to correﬁ and purify the Air, when
Plagues and contagious Diſeaſes raged.
Places in which the Atmoſphere is
very moiſt, and impregnated with
aqueous Exhalations, which weakens
its Force and Elaſticity, are not
wholeſome; becauſe, by that Means,
Perſpiration being obſtruﬁed, a Load
of recrementitious and ſaline Sordes
are retain'd in the Body, and communicate a depraved and ſcorbutic
Intemperature to the Blood and Humours, from which terrible chronical
Diſorders ariſe. 'Tis therefore obvious, that the ſulphureous Vapour
of foſſile Coals is of ſingular Service,
in Countries where the State of the
Air is moiſt and unaﬁive; as is evident from the City of *Halle*: An
immenſe Quantity of aqueous Exhalations, ariſing not only from the
River *Sale*, diffuſed into many Branches, but, alſo from the Salt Works,
whilſt each Day at leaſt ten thouſand
Pounds of Water are evaporated into
the Atmoſphere ſurrounding that City, muſt of Courſe beſet the Town
at Morning and Night, with Clouds,
which every one muſt perceive to be
prejudicial to Health, unleſs an Eaſt-
erly or northerly Wind diſpel them.
And, in Times paſt, no City was
more obnoxious to Scurvies, Conſumptions, purple and malignant Fevers, than *Halle*; but ſince about
twenty Years ago, they began to
burn foſſile Coals, for boiling the
Salt, the Atmoſphere is ſo purify'd,
that theſe Diſeaſes are ſcarce heard of
in that City. In former Times the
Phyſicians, who practiſed in it, complain'd that no Diſeaſe occur'd to
them, which was not accompany'd
with a ſcorbutic Taint. Numbers of
young Men were cut off by Conſumptions and Dyſenteries; and petechical and ſpotted ſcorbutic Fevers

raged

raged excessively; but now these Disorders happen rarely, and then only a few are affected with them. But I am well appriz'd, that it is by some objected, that the Exhalations of fossile Coal, are rather pernicious than advantageous to Health; because they prey upon Metals, especially the Iron and Lead of Windows, which they consume; and because in Gardens which are near them, and thick set, they render the Trees and Shrubs barren and sapless. 'Tis also objected, that in *England*, and especially *London*, a Consumption is produc'd, peculiar to that Country, by a preternatural Dryness of the Vesicles of the Lungs in Consequence of this Smoak, as also, that its Smell is fetid, and highly disagreeable. But to all these Objections we answer, that tho' the Smoak arising from the Mineral Sulphur, and from Vinegar, are possess'd of a powerful Virtue, by which they consume the lighter and more porous Metals, Iron and Lead, they are not for that Reason, less proper for purifying the Air, when a Plague rages, or dissipating its superfluous Moisture, so prejudicial to Health. Besides that this Smoak does not in the least injure the Health of those People who inhabit the Houses exposed to it, and in which the Leads of the Windows are corroded, is a Fact attested by daily Experience, since few of them labour under any Disorders of the Breast. That this Smoak, however, may prove prejudicial, when thick and dense, is a Fact of which I am firmly persuaded; for as a large Quantity of Exhalations from a Balsamic Gum, which is friendly to Nature, for Instance, from Mastick, Benjamin, or *Peruvian* Balsam, is ungrateful; so 'tis not to be doubted, but the dense Vapour of Bitumen, which is not very grateful, may create Disorders;

which, however, seems to be owing not so much to its Nature, as to the Excess of its Quantity. 'Tis not therefore, to be wonder'd at, if in *London*, where a gross State of the Air, Gluttony, and excessive Drinking, especially of spirituous Liquors, induce a morbid State of the Humours, an excessive Quantity of Smoak, arising from fossile Coal, should prove prejudicial, and produce a Dryness of the Lungs. As to that Objection of the Smoak being fetid, disagreeable, hurtful to the Nerves and membranous Parts, and prejudicial to those who labour under a Weakness of the Nerves and Head, we answer, that tho' the Smells of fetid Substances are not always grateful to the Delicate, yet they are not, for that Reason, prejudicial to Health; as is obvious in the Spirits of Soot, Worms, and Hartshorn, which are all highly fetid. But how much these Spirits contribute to repair the Strength, and to preserve and purge the Mass of Blood and Humours, is known to almost every one concern'd in Physic. It must also be observed, that the Smell, even of Perfumes, is ungrateful to many; as we observe in Women who have weak Nerves, and who, not only bear Fetids more chearfully, but receive a Kind of Relief from them.

Chalcedonius, Offic. The Chalcedony. This is a precious Stone. As to its Medicinal Uses it is by some thought serviceable against all Disorders arising from black Bile, such as Sadness, Melancholy, and the unaccountable Dread of Dæmons and Spirits. Those brought from the *East Indies*, which are moderately pellucid, and variegated with whitish milky Streaks, if hung about the Breast, are said to generate Abundance of Milk. Some Authors are so ridiculously superstitious and whimsical, as to promise Victory to the happy Combatant who wears

wears the Chalcedony Stone about him. Its true and genuine medicinal Virtues seem to consist in its absorbent Quality, when it is reduced to a fine Powder, and exhibited like the other earthy and absorbent Powders. But because the Apothecaries have other Substances of the same Virtues, and, at the same Time, far more easily prepar'd, it is rarely prescrib'd by the Moderns.

Chalcitis, Offic. As the *Misy,* Sory, Chalcites, and Melanteria, are generally found in the same Mines, Authors usually treat of them together, whose Examples I shall follow. The χαλκῖτις of the *Greeks* takes its Name from χαλκὸς, Brass, and is commonly described to be a metalline Recrement, of the Colour of Brass, diversify'd with oblong, shining Veins, and produced in the same Ores, which give Birth to the Sory and Misy. Betwixt these two Substances it holds a middle Rank, not only with Respect to its Bed, but also with Respect to its Consistence; for, according to some, the Sory is thinner, and the Misy thicker; and, according to others, the Sory is thicker, and the Misy thinner than the Chalcites. According to *Galen,* the undermost Bed is of a stony Texture, and consists of Sory: Over this lies the second Bed, which is Chalcitis, and resembles an Efflorescence; and the uppermost Bed is that of the Misy, which resembles Verdigrise; but in Process of Time, the *Chalcitis* is converted into *Misy,* and the *Sory* into *Chalcitis.* According to *Pliny,* " That Stone is called *Chal-* " *citis,* from which the Brass itself " is obtain'd. It differs from the " Cadmia in this, that the former " is cut from Rocks above the " Ground; whereas the latter is " only obtain'd from such as lie " conceal'd under it. The Chal- " citis also becomes immediately

" friable, and assumes a soft Tex- " ture, in Appearance like that of " concreted Down. There is also " another Distinction between the " Cadmia and Chalcitis, which is, " that the latter contains three Kinds " of Substances, Brass, Misy, and " Sory; for it has oblong Veins of " Brass. That is thought best, " whose Colour resembles that of " Honey, has slender Veins, is fri- " able, and not of a stony Nature. " That which is recent is also ac- " counted best, because when old, " it becomes Sory." And accord- ing to *Dioscorides,* " That Species of " Chalcitis is best which resembles " Brass, is friable, not stony, re- " cent, and variegated with oblong " and shining Veins. This Sub- " stance is of an abstersive heating " Nature, and cicatrizes Ulcers. It re- " moves the tough and viscid Matter " which sticks in the Eyes, and their " Corners. In a Word, It is among " the Number of the gently corroding " Medicines. It is an effectual Me- " dicine against an *Erysipelas* and " *Herpes.* In Conjunction with the " Juice of Leeks, it stops Hæmor- " rhages from the Womb and No- " strils. The Powder of it cures " Disorders of the Gums, spreading " Ulcers, and Tumors of the Ton- " sils. When calcin'd and triturated " with Honey, it proves an excel- " lent Medicine for Disorders of the " Eyes. It removes and destroys " Callosities and Roughness of the " Eye-lids. It cures Fistulas of the " Eyes, when put into them, by way " of Collyrium. Of the *Chalcitis* " is prepared a Medicine distin- " guish'd by the Epithet *Psoricon.* " For this Purpose we must take " two Parts of the Chalcitis, one " of the Cadmia, and triturate the " whole in Vinegar. But this Me- " dicine must be buried in Dung, " in an earthen Vessel, for forty " Days, during the Appearance of " the

" the Dog-Star, that it may become
" more acrid, which the *Chalcitis*
" itfelf alfo does by the fame Me-
" thod. Others prepare the fame
" Medicine, by triturating equal
" Portions of thefe two Subftances
" in Wine. The *Chalcitis* is to be
" calcin'd in a new earthen Veffel
" placed over live Coals. It is cu-
" ftomary to calcine the moifter
" Kinds of the *Chalcitis* till it does
" not rife in Bubbles, and is become
" perfectly dry; but the other Kinds
" may be taken off the Fire when
" they have affum'd a florid Colour,
" refembling that of Blood or Mi-
" nium. The Sordes appearing on
" the Surface muft be blown off;
" or it may be calcin'd upon Coals,
" blowing them all the Time, till it
" affumes a palifh Colour; or put-
" ting live Coals under the Veffel,
" it is to be ftirr'd about till it flames,
" and changes its Colour." 'Tis
obvious, that the Antients reckon'd
the *Chalcitis* among the abftergent,
drying, acrid, cauftic, or efcharotic
Medicines. The Variety of Compofitions, in which, according to
Scribonius Largus, they ufed this Ingredient, is a fufficient Proof of this.
That it was applied to the fame
Purpofes by their Farriers, we may
find in the twenty fixth Chapter
of the fecond Book of *Vegetius.*
Foreftus recommends the calcin'd
Chalcitis for drying Ulcers. At
prefent torrefy'd *Chalcitis* is an Ingredient in the *Theriaca Andromachi,*
and in the *Emplaftrum Diacthalciteos
Galeni,* which is alfo called *Diapalma.*
ma. But, becaufe the *Chalcitis* is
not generally known, the Moderns
for the moft Part ufe white Vitriol,
either calcin'd or crude, or the *Vitriolum martis* in its Stead; which
laft *Schulzius,* in his *Blancardi Lex-
icon Renovatum* prefers, for making
the *Theriaca.* Whether the *Chalcites* is a proper Ingredient in the
Theriaca, is much difputed; but it

fhould feem that, it is not neceffary
in that Compofition, as will appear
from confidering what Kind of Subftance it properly is. *Matthiolus*
feems to have been the firft who
hinted at its true Origin, in the following Words: " It is obvious, fays
" he, to every one, from common
" Experience, that all Vitriol of every
" Kind, in Procefs of Time, dege-
" nerates into *Chalcitis:*" For it is
a Species of metallic Recrement,
called *Atramentum Rubeum,* generated of the *Pyrites* foften'd in Water,
which has Iron either pure, or mix'd
with Brafs, affociated with it, and
which is continually more and more
diffolved and divided till it appears
friable. This Recrement confifts of
moift and aqueous Particles lefs temperate, and with a fmaller Portion of
Sulphur, or fulphureous Acid, than
Vitriol. In Confiftence and Colour
it differs from *Sory* and *Mify,* is of
of an acrid, acid, and aftringent
Tafte, of a penetrating naufeous
Smell, and diffufes an ungrateful
Odour. From it are often obtain'd
in the Smelting Houfes, Brafs, *Cadmia, Pompholyx, Spodium,* and *Diphryges.* That Species of *Chalcitis*
is by fome efteem'd the moft genuine, which confifts of beautiful Purple colour'd Pieces: But for Ufe, 'tis
no Matter of what Colour it is; for
what is imported into *France* for
Sale from St. *Chriftopher's,* is, according to *Pomet,* of a greenifh Colour, like that of imperfectly calcin'd Vitriol. According to the
learned *Henckelius,* we ought rather
to enquire, after the Elixiviation of
the Vitriol, of what Nature it is,
whether it partakes of Iron or Copper, that we may be the better able
to judge, for what Medicinal Purpofes it is moft proper. Hence
'tis obvious, that they are in the
right, who call *Chalcitis* the *Colcothar,* or *Caput Mortuum* of Vitriol; as alfo thofe who clafs

it

mong the vitriolic Minerals, or
le and impure Vitriols. Hence
Reafon is alfo obvious, why it is
ome accounted a Species of Vi-
, and why *Boerhaave* calls it
iolum rubrum, becaufe for In-
ce, it is a Compofition of the
d of Sulphur and Iron, in which
e is perhaps, a fmall Admixture
Brafs. But it is more properly
'd the *Colcothar* of Vitriol than
re and perfect Vitriol, becaufe it
ts a Cryftalline Form.

he choiceft *Mify* comes from *Cy-*
, refembles Gold, is of a hard
ftance, and when broken, glitters
: Gold, and fhines with a Star-
: Splendor. It is calcin'd in the
e Manner, and has the fame Vir-
, as *Chalcitis*, only *Mify* produ-
no *Pforicon*: As to their Quali-
, *Mify* and *Chalcitis* differ only
h refpect to Intenfenefs and Re-
fnefs. The *Egyptian Mify* is pre-
d for its Strength, but is far infe-
 to the *Cyprian* in its ophthal-
Virtues. *Geoffroy* fays it feems to
nothing but an Efflorefcence of
lcitis.

iome have miftaken the *Sory* for
lanteria; but they are of different
ids, tho' not much unlike: But
, is the ftronger fcented, and cre-
: a *Naufea*. It is produc'd in E-
t, and fome other Countries, as
ica, *Spain*, and *Cyprus*; but the
y which bears the higheft Price is
it comes from *Egypt*, and, when
ken, appears of a blacker Colour,
full of Perforations, of a fattifh
ftance, aftringent, of a ftrong
ell and Tafte, and fubverts the
mach. That *Sory* which does not
rkle like *Mify* when it is broken in
ces, is reckon'd of another Kind,
l of little Value. It is calcin'd,
l has the fame Virtues, as the *Mi-*
nd *Chalcitis*. Put into a hollow
oth, it eafes the Pain thereof;
 it faftens loofe Teeth. Infufed

in Wine, it helps the *Sciatica*; and
clears the Skin of Pimples, if rub'd
thereon with Water. It is an Ingredient alfo in Medicines which make
the Hair black. Generally fpeaking, this and almoft all other Drugs
are ftronger before they are calcin'd
than afterwards, except Salt, Lees
of Wine, Nitre, Quick-Lime, and
the like, which are of little Efficacy
when crude, but have their Virtues
much improv'd by Calcination. *Ge-*
offroy fays the *Sory* of the *Greeks* is a
foffile Subftance, thicker and more
compact than *Chalcitis*; which emits
Sparks by Attrition, and is of a fpongy Texture, black colour'd, aftringent, naufeous Tafte, and of a ftrong
hurtful Smell.

This Defcription agrees very well
with a Subftance which the *Turkifh*
Women make Ufe of to take off
Hairs from their Bodies, call'd by
them *Rufma*, which is defcrib'd by
Bellonius to be a Foffil, almoft like
Excrement in Appearance, but light-
er, and of a black burnt Colour,
like Pitch, found in the Mines of
Gallo-Græcia.

The *Melanteria* is fometimes found
in the Entrance of Copper Mines,
where it concretes like Salt. Another Sort, which has an earthy Quality, is gathered from the uppermoft
Surface of thefe Mines. There is
alfo a foffil Kind found in *Cilicia*,
and in fome other Countries. The
beft *Melanteria* is of the Colour of
Sulphur, fmooth, equable, pure,
and which touch'd with Water, immediately turns black. It has the
fame cauftic Quality as *Mify*.

All thefe foffil Subftances are now
rarely found in Apothecaries Shops,
being to be had nowhere elfe but in
Cyprus, *Afia minor*, or *Egypt*. They
are cauftic, and burn to an *Efchar*,
and are, in fome Degree, aftringent.
Chalcitis was ufed in the *Theriaca* in
Andromachus's Time, but, as it can

feldom

seldom now be had, *Colcothar*, or Vitriol calcin'd to a Redness, is substituted for it.

Chalybs. Steel. See *Mars.*

Chia Terra, Offic. Earth of *Chios*. This Sort of Earth is to be chose whitish, inclining to an Ash Colour, and like the Earth of *Samos*. It is crusty and white, but made up in Masses of different Forms, and has the same Virtues as the *Samian* Earth. It clears the Skin of Wrinkles, and is good for Ambustions. *Terra Samia*, or *Cimolia alba*, may be substituted in its stead.

Chrysocolla. The same as *Borax*, which see.

Chrysolithus, Offic. The Chrysolite. This is a green diaphanous Gem, of a glittering Splendor like Gold. It is found in *India*, and other Countries; and is superstitiously said to be endued with the Virtue of stopping Hæmorrhages, and of mitigating Bile, Anger, and Phrensies.

Chrysopasius & Topasius, Offic. The Topaz. It is a diaphanous and pellucid Stone, of the Colour of Gold, and is supposed to be of a solar Nature from its Signature; for which Reason it is believed to strengthen the Mind against nocturnal Fears, to diminish Melancholy, to prevent troublesome Dreams, and to work other such good Effects; but these Virtues are entirely superstitious.

Cimolia alba, Offic. Tobacco-Pipe-Clay. This was very famous among the Antients. It acquir'd its Name from *Cimolus*, an Island near *Crete*, now call'd *Sicandre*, where it was found in great Plenty. *Tournefort* describes the *Cimolia alba* as a white, heavy, insipid Chalk, abounding with small Grains of Sand, which he thinks the same as that got about *Paris*, except that the *Cimolia* is fattish, and saponaceous, whence it is called *Terra saponaria*. The Inhabitants

he says, make Use of no other Soap for washing their Linen than the *Cimolia*. I apprehend the *Cimolia alba* is different from the common Tobacco-Pipe-Clay; but *Dale* informs us, that in *Cornwall* a Sort of Clay is found, which he calls *Steatites*, and which is used as a Soap. In the Shops this Earth, with the Mark of a Seal upon it, is called *Terra Sigillata alba*. It is also sometimes sold for the *Terra Samia*. *Dale* farther informs us, that the *Cimolia alba*, which he seems to think the same as Tobacco-Pipe-Clay, is drying and astringent, either apply'd externally, or taken inwardly; and further that it is an excellent Medicine either in continual or intermittent Fevers; and that it was the grand Secret of Sir *Theodore Mayerne*, in curing these Disorders.

Cimolia purpurascens, Offic. Fuller's Earth. This is seldom or never used internally; but applied, as a Topic, it is drying and astringent.

Cinnabaris nativa, Offic. Native Cinnabar. This Cinnabar is a Fossil, metallic, heavy Substance, not very hard, found sometimes pure, and sometimes mix'd with Stones. Of the pure Cinnabar there are several Kinds; one of a purple Colour, inclining to red, but which, by grinding, turns to a very beautiful Red; another of a blackish or liver Colour, resembling the *Lapis Hæmatitis*; and a third of a yellowish Colour, which is commonly so rich in Quick-silver, that, when heated in the least Degree, the Metal drops spontaneously from it. The other Kind of native Cinnabar is found in a fossile Stone, form'd of *Laminæ*, of an Ash Colour. It has been likewise found in a white metalline Stone, and sometimes in Form of a Gold or Silver *Pyrites*, such as was dug up some Years ago in several Places of *Normandy*. Native Cinnabar is found in *Hungary*, *Bohemia*, *Italy*, *Spain*, and *France*,

nce, and every one knows of what
s it is compofed. Quick-filver
btain'd from it, by diftilling it
a Quick-lime, or Filings of Iron;
Sulphur may likewife be had, in
mall Quantity, by boiling it in
ng *Lixivia,* and then pouring di-
'd Vinegar into the Decoction,
Quick-filver being firft feparated.
e internal Ufe of it is recommend-
y fome Phyficians in the Epilep-
Vertigo, Madnefs, and all fpaf-
dic Affections. In thefe Cafes
y choofe that of *Hungary* or *Ca-*
thia, which is of a fparkling red
lour, and free from all heteroge-
us Particles; and reject the dark
yellowifh Kind, as being more im-
re. Sometimes, however, native
nabar, by Means of fome vitri-
c, or even arfenical Particles affo-
ted with it, happens to excite
ufeas, Vomitings, Anxieties, and
artburns, which I have myfelf
re than once, fays *Geoffroy,* been
Witnefs to, even after the Cinna-
r had been purged by frequent
aftings. Every Pound of good
nnabar, yields fourteen Ounces of
uick-filver.

Cos, Offic. The Whetftone. *Di-*
orides informs us, that the Grit
ich is worn off the Whetftone, by
arpening Iron, caufes Hair to grow
on the Parts affected with an *Alo-*
ria; that it reftrains the Growth of
e Breafts in Virgins; and that,
ank in Vinegar, it confumes the
leen, and is good for an Epilepfy.
here are three different Sorts of
Whetftones, the Stone, the Grit-
one, and the black Whetftone. It
not eafy to determine which is
eant by *Diofcorides.*

Creta, Offic. Chalk. This is
ll'd by the *Greeks* Κρητικὴ γῆ, Cre-
n Earth, becaufe the beft Sort was
rought from *Crete,* now *Candia.*
entman takes Notice of fifteen dif-
erent Sorts of Chalk. *Geoffroy* de-
nes Chalk, a denfe, brittle, earthy

Subftance, which readily ftains the
Fingers, and fticks to the Tongue,
without any Aftringency. Many
Kinds of Earth come under the Denomination of Chalk. Chalk is now
found in many Countries befides
Crete. It raifes an Effervefcence
with acid Liquors, and is therefore,
defervedly looked upon as an alcaline, or abforbent Earth. It is us'd
with Succefs to allay the too great
Acidity of the Juices of the Stomach, particularly in the Difeafe
commonly known by the Name of
the Heart-burn; and alfo in Coughs,
that arife from a fharp Phlegm. It
is likewife ferviceable in Hæmorrhages, and is faid to kill Worms. In
a Word, the Property of all alcaline
Earths, is not only to abforb Acids,
but to allay the Acrimony of the
Fluids, and efpecially to reftrain the
violent Motion of the Bile, by detaining the Salts and Sulphurs thereof
in their fixed Parts. White Chalk is
given alone, from fourteen Grains to
a Dram. Powder'd Chalk is alfo giv-
en with Milk, to prevent its turning
Acid in the Stomach; and externally, it is commended for drying
Wounds, Ulcers, and Fiffures in the
Nipples. Chalk, when calcin'd,
becomes a Lime, and differs extremely in Virtues from Chalk uncalcin'd.
Chalk in large Quantities, put into
Springs or Wells of hard Water, is
faid to render it foft. Dr. *Slare,*
from Experience affirms, that Chalk
abforbs Acids fooner, and more powerfully, than Crabs Eyes, calcin'd
Hartfhorn, or Coral; and he therefore judges it to be a better Remedy
than either of thefe for deftroying
Acids in the Stomach. It is externally apply'd to running Puftules,
Achors, and Excoriations, and is farther faid to be of Service, when apply'd to an *Eryfipelas,* or to Parts
affected with gouty Pains. Chalk,
however, if taken in confiderable
Quantities, and without proper Ca-

· thartics

thartics to carry it through the inteſtinal Tube, when it has exerted the Effects intended, is known by Experience, to be productive of great Miſchiefs, by plaiſtering as it were the Inteſtines, obſtructing the Lacteals, and the Orifices of the inteſtinal Glands, and thereby cauſing Cachexies, Indigeſtions, and various Diſorders.

Creta Selinuſia, Offic. Earth of *Selinuſia.* This Earth is in moſt Eſteem, when it is reſplendant, white, friable, and readily diluted with a Fluid. It is drying and aſtringent, and is recommended as a good Topic for Ulcers.

Cryſtallus, Offic. Cryſtal. *Frederic Hoffman,* in many Parts of his Works, recommends Cryſtal as a Medicine, under the Name of *Cryſtallus montana. Schroder* informs us, that Chryſtal is aſtringent, and good in a Dyſentery, Diarrhæa, the Cæliac Paſſion, Cholera, and uterine Fluxes, that it increaſes Milk, wears away the Stone in the urinary Paſſages, and is beneficial in the Gout. He further ſays, from *Boetius de Boodt,* that two Scruples, or a Dram of this, exhibited in Oil of ſweet Almonds, is good for thoſe who have taken Mercury. *Schroder* takes Notice of the Salt, Magiſtery, Oil, Elixir, and Eſſence of Cryſtal: But I believe theſe are never either made or uſed. Rock Cryſtal is a ſoft tranſparentGem,reſembling Ice, and its Figure is that of an hexagonal Pillar, pointed at both Extremities; or it may be ſaid to be compounded of two Pyramids, with ſuch a Pillar between them. A ſecond Kind is found in *Ireland,* and in ſome Parts of *France,* eſpecially about *Troyes* in *Champagne,* which ſeems to be made up of Cryſtalline Plates, and fiſſile in the Direction of all its plain Surfaces, and, when reduc'd to Powder, it ſtill retains a rhomboidal Figure, ſo that even the fineſt Powder, view'd

thro' a Microſcope, ſhews a Congeries of very ſmall rhomboidal Solids. Another Property of this Cryſtal is, that all Objects, ſeen thro' it, appear double; which ariſes from a double Refraction of the Rays of Light. A third Species of Cryſtal is that mention'd by Dr. *Liſter,* which is very ſmooth, pellucid, and glittering, coming near to a Diamond. Its Figure is ſpherical, oval, depreſſed, and ſometimes repreſenting an Hemiſphere, or Hemiſperoide, and in others roundiſh and irregular. It is very hard, and has an exquiſite natural Poliſh, and is dug up in Pieces of different Sizes in ſeveral Places of *England.*

Diphryges, Offic. Scurf. It is a Sort of Metallic Recrement, which ſubſides upon a particular Treatment of melting Braſs with Water. At preſent the Shops are unacquainted with it. It is of a mixed Quality, containing in itſelf ſomething moderately aſtringent, and moderately acrimonious; for which Reaſon it is a very good Remedy for all ſtubborn Ulcers.

Eretria terra, Offic. Eretrian Earth. There are two Sorts of *Terra Eretria;* the one white; the other Aſh-colour'd. What is moſt eſteem'd, approaches to an Aſh colour, and is very ſoft, and drawn over Copper-Plates, leaves a Line of a Violet Colour. According to *Diſcorides,* it has an aſtringent, and refrigerating, with ſomewhat of a mollifying Virtue, incarnates, and conglutinates recent Wounds.

Ferrum. Iron. See *Mars.*

Gagates, & Succinum nigrum, Offic. Jet. It is a Kind of black, ſtony, cruſty Earth, ſo full of *Bitumen,* that it ſmells ſtrongly of it, and being kindled, flames almoſt like Pitch, and emits a very black Smoke. It differs from the *Terra Ampelitis,* in that this latter ſends forth no Flame, unleſs excited by Bellows,

d has no bituminous Smell; where-
the *Gagates*, held to the Fire,
tches Flame, and emits a Smell
e *Bitumen*. It is mollifying and
fcutient, and is fuppofed to cure
e Colic, and other Diftempers. It
of great Efficacy in Hyfterics, and
e Epilepfy; and is alfo a Diure-
. The Oil thereof is good for
e Palfy. *Tournefort* commends it
hyfteric, epileptic, hypochondriac,
d paralytic Diforders; the Dofe
from fix Drops to twelve. *Wormius*
ikes the *Gagates* only a harder
ecies of *Ampelites*, and fays, that,
en it is polifh'd, it is called by
iny, the *Gumma Samothracica*; by
cander, *Lapis Thracius*, and, by
me, *Lapis Obfidianus*. Though
rricola, fays *Aldrovandus*, fuppofes
e *Lapis Obfidianus* to be a Species
Gagates, and *Lapis Thracius*, I
lieve it to be a Subftance very dif-
ent from both. *Diofcorides* fays,
at, ufed in Suffumigation, it cures
e Fit of an Epilepfy, and revives
e Patient under hyfteric Diforders;
d that the Fume thereof drives
vay Serpents: It is an Ingredient
antiarthritic Medicines, and in
copa. It is produced, he fays, at
e Mouth of a River in *Cilicia*, near
City called *Plagiopolis*; and the
ace, or River, where it is found is
lled *Gagas*.

Granatus, Offic. The Granate.
his is a pellucid Gem, of a yellow-
red Colour, almoft like that of
ttive Cinnabar; it is faid, if pre-
tred, and taken internally, to be
ying and ftrengthening; to cure
alpitations of the Heart, and to reft Melancholy and Poifon; and to
op Hæmorrhages. It is alfo be-
ev'd by fome, to have the fame
ffects, if fufpended about the Neck.

Gypfum, Offic. Tarras, Plaifter
f Paris. Authors difpute about the
ypfum, fome will have it to be the
alx of *Alabafter*, others that of
lum of *Scajola*, others make it the

Calx of *Mufcovy* Glafs; and fome
that of the Selenite Stone: But our
Gypfum is a Lime made of fome
whitifh Stones, and opake Bits of
Talk, flightly burnt till they fparkle.
The beft, according to Dr. *Merret*,
is in *Derbyfhire*, and ufed in Floor-
ing and Cieling of Houfes. The
learned Dr. *Lifter*, in his *Journey to Paris*, fays, there are Quarries
of this *Gypfum* at *Monmartre*, and
that they burn it in an open Fire, the
hardeft Part requiring no more than
three or four Hours burning. He
faw alfo a Quarry of it at *Clifford-
Moor* in *Yorkfhire*, where it is called
Hall-Plaifter. It is of a drying
Quality, ftops Bleeding, and abforbs
as an Alcali the Acrimony which
falls from the Gums in the Scurvy.

Halcyonium, *Spuma maris*, Offic.
The Froth, or Foam of the Sea.
This is a bituminous or oleous Sub-
ftance, found floating on the Sea.
It is much controverted, whether this
is the Excrement, Sperm, or Milk,
of fome Animal, or a Kind of
Zoophyte; or a Juice of fome Sea
Plant; or fomething of a bituminous
Mineral Exfudation from the Bottom
of the Sea, converted into a Foam
by the Agitation of the Waves.

Heliotropium, Offic. The Helio-
trope. This is an opake Gem, of a
green Colour, mark'd with bloody
Spots or Veins. It is faid to refift
Poifon, and to ftop Hæmorrhages.

Hyacinthus, Offic. The Hyacinth.
This is fo called, from its Refemblance to the Plant of that Name,
in its yellowifh Colour, of which
there being feveral Degrees, the different Kinds of it are taken from
thence: Some are of the Colour of
red Lead, or bilious Blood, fome
of Saffron, fome of yellow Amber,
which are the leaft efteem'd. Hyacinths are diftinguifhed into Oriental,
which are brought from the *Eaft-
Indies*; and Occidental, which comes
from *Silefia*, *Bohemia*, *Auvergne* in

P p *France*,

France, and other Places: Thefe Hyacinths feem to be different from that mention'd by the Antients, efpecially by *Pliny*, which was of a fhining Violet Colour, like the Amethyft, tho' not fo ftrong. Many fuperftitious Virtues have been afcribed to this Stone. They faid it was of a cold Nature; that it ftrengthens the Heart, is gently aftringent, and procures Sleep.

Jafpis, Offic. The Jafper. It is an opake Gem, of a green, and fometimes a Blood Colour. It is found in the *Eaft Indies*, and is faid to ftop all Sorts of Hæmorrhages, and to exhilarate the Spirits.

Judaicus Lapis, Offic. The Jew's Stone. This is an oblong, roundifh Stone, of the Figure of an Olive, marked with Streaks and Furrows, running from the *Bafis* to the *Apex*, according to its Length, at equal Diftances from each other. It is of a whitifh or Afh Colour, and fhining within. It parts obliquely into thin *Laminæ*, and is given in Powder, to the Quantity of a Dram, in any proper Vehicle. It was called *Lapis Judaicus*, or *Syriacus*, from the Countries where it is found. By others it is named *Euroius*, as being of a diuretic Virtue. This laft Virtue *Geoffroy* very much queftions; but fays it is plain from Experience, that this Stone, the *Lapis Lyncis*, Crab's Eyes, and feveral other Things, faid to have a Power of diffolving the Stone, are really diuretic. But it cannot be concluded, that, becaufe oftentimes Gravel comes away with the Urine, therefore they have any lithontriptic Quality; for the fixed earthy Parts of thefe Stones, being mixed and incorporated with the Salts of the Fluids in the Body, become thereby more fixed, and more unfit to pafs off thro' the Pores of the Skin, but find their Way more eafily thro' the Strainers of the Kidneys. Therefore the Se-

cretion, by infenfible Perfpiration, being leffened, they are excreted in greater Quantities by Urine; and thereby whatever *Saburra* they find there, they wafh away; and hence the Urine becomes turbid, and is fometimes mixed with Gravel, fome Particles of which may be of a confiderable Size, when the Paffage is wide enough to tranfmit them. In this Manner the diuretic Quality of thefe Stones may be accounted for; but neither Experience nor Reafon can give any Ground for attributing to them a lithontriptic Quality.

Lapis Armenus, Offic. The Armenian Stone. This Stone is opake, with green, blue, or blackifh Spots, fmooth, and marked like the Azure Stone, with Gold coloured Specks, and friable. There is indeed, but very little Difference between the two Stones, they being often found in the fame Glebe, and ufed indifferently for each other, as having the fame Virtues; only the *Armenian* Stone is more ftrongly purgative. It is given from fix Grains to a Scruple; and externally ufed, it is detergent, with fome Degree of Acrimony and Stypticity. It is very feldom ufed in Phyfic; but the Painters employ it in making a beautiful blue Colour, with a greenifh Caft.

Lapis Affius, Offic. *Sarcophagus, five Affius Lapis.* De L et. The Affian Stone. *Galen* informs us, that this Stone is fo called from *Affos*, a City of *Troas* in the leffer *Afia*. It is of a tophous, foft, friable, and loofe Subftance; fomething grows upon it like very fine Meal, fuch as we fee fticking upon the Walls of Mills; they call it the Flower of the *Affian* Rock: It is of fubtile Parts, and confumes Flefh that is too foft and fluid, by Colliquation, without Mordacity. The Stone on which it grows, has the fame Virtue, but weaker; for the Flower is not only colliquative, digeftive, and prefervative

tive like Salt, but performs all its without any remarkably corrove Quality. *Dioscorides* informs s, both the Stone and the Flower ave an astringent, and gently colliuative Virtue, and being mixed ith Resin of Turpentine or Tar, iscuss Tubercles ; but the Flower esteem'd most effectual, and is, ideed, when dry'd, an extraordiary Remedy for inveterate Ulcers, hich are difficult to be cicatrized, id represses carnous Excrescencies. fixed with Honey, it absterges foul nd virulent Ulcers ; it deterges lso, and incarns Ulcers which are ollow ; and mixed with Cerate, estrains the spreading Kind. It is iade into a Cataplasm with Beanseal for the Gout ; and for splenee Disorders, with Vinegar and quick-lime. The Flower made into n Eclegma with Honey, is good in Phthisis. Vessels are made of the tone, in which gouty Persons put heir Feet when they bathe, and nd Relief thereby. Coffins are iade of the same, for the speedy Consumption of dead Bodies ; and 'ersons of a very fleshy and gross labit are extenuated, by sprinkling he Flower instead of Nitre, in their baths.

Lapis Bononiensis, Phosphorus Bononiensis, Spongia Solis, Lapis Lucidus, Mont. Exot. Bononian Phosphorus, Light Carrier. This is a small, grey, soft, glossy, fibrous, sulphueous Stone, about the Bigness of a arge Walnut ; when broken, having a Kind of Crystal or sparry Talk within ; found in the Neighbourhood of *Bologna* or *Bononia*, in *Italy*, and when duly prepared, making a Species of *Phosphorus*. It is esteem'd caustic, escharotic, and emetic.

Lapis Bufonites, Offic. The Toad Stone. Some affirm, that these Stones are found in the Heads of old Toads which have lived in dry Places ; and that the Stone is far more valuable,

when taken from the Toad immediately killed, than when it has been dead for a great while. The common People affirm, that an old Toad, if laid upon a red Cloath, will vomit up this Stone. Others for obtaining the Stone, order a Toad to be exposed to the Heat of the Sun, till it be parched with Thirst ; upon which they maintain it will vomit its Stone, as too great a Burden to its Head. Others, in Order to procure the Stone, order a very large live Toad to be put into an earthen Vessel full of small Holes, and the Vessel, when close stopp'd, is to be buried among a large Collection of Ants, for the Space of a Month ; for then they affirm, that the Flesh of the Toad being destroy'd by the Ants, nothing remains but the Bones, and the Stone which was lodged in the Head. I cannot forbear looking upon these Accounts as so many Fables, too palpable and glaring to deserve our Attention, much less our Assent. Our learned Countryman, Mr. *Brown,* in his *Vulgar Errors,* thinks, that People have some Reason to seek for such Stones in the Heads of Toads, because stony Concretions are often formed in the Head of many other Animals, but more especially Fishes and Snails ; but he doubts whether such a Stone is really found in the Head of the Toad ; and, if it is really there, he thinks it is the Cranium indurated or petrify'd. Others have asserted, that this Stone was produced from the viscid Spume deposited upon the Head of a large Toad, by a Collection of Toads lodged in a Cave in the Winter Season. Hence *Christophorus Salveldensis* informs us, that in *France* and *Spain,* this Stone is only produced by a certain Species of horned Toad, called *Borax,* and mark'd with Saffron colour'd Spots, and blackish livid Streaks. *Lanzonius,*

nius, from *Alb. Seba,* informs 'us, that the Origin of the Toad-Stone is very uncertain, and involved in a Kind of impenetrable Obscurity; since, notwithstanding the large Number of Authors who have wrote concerning them, and endeavour'd by Examination to discover their Natures, not one has hitherto dar'd to assert, that he has, with his own Hands, extracted a Stone of this Kind from the Head of a Toad, or even pretended to shew one obtain'd in that Manner; for *Vallisneri,* after all the Pains he could take, could by no Means obtain any Stone from the Toad; from which Circumstance, he thinks, he has Reason to conclude, that this Stone being found in the Toad is a Story, which, like some other Pieces of Imposture, has met with a kindly Welcome from the Credulity of Mankind. *Merret,* affirms, that the Stones called Toad-Stones, and accounted Gems, are only certain Teeth called the Grinders, in the *Lupus Marinus,* or Sea-Wolf. *Schroder,* as *Dale,* informs us, recommends the Toad-Stone, as a most valuable Medicine against the Plague, and all Kinds of Poisons. Some affirm, that the *Bufonites,* or Toad-Stone, carried about any Person, preserves him against all Kinds of Poison, and changes its Colour upon coming near a poison'd Cup. But, as these Things are not found to hold in Fact, I think it enough just to have mention'd them; only I must observe with *Boccler,* that the *Bufonites,* in Consequence of its being an alcaline Substance, may absorb Acids, and contribute to the Cure of Fluxes.

Lapis Galactites, Offic. Milk-Stone. It grows out of a Lime-stone, which it very much resembles too in other Respects. It is of an Ash Colour, and, being rub'd on a Whetstone, yields a milky and sweet Juice; whence it takes its Name. It increases almost every Year, so as at last to be as big as a Child's Head. It is somewhat heating and abstersive; whence it is proper to anoint the Eyes with it in Defluxions and Ulcers. After bruising it in Water, it ought to be reposited in a leaden Box, because of the glutinous Quality which it retains. Triturated, and drank in Water, or sweet Wine, after Bathing, it generates Plenty of Milk in the Breasts of Women.

Lapis Geodes, Matth. *Geodes,* Offic. The bastard Eagle Stone. This Stone is of an astringent and drying Quality, deterges such Things as darken the Sight, and mitigates Inflammations of the Breasts and *Testes,* being rub'd on the affected Parts with Water.

Lapis Hæmatites, Offic. The Blood Stone. *Lapis Hæmatites,* λιθο αἱματίτης, of the *Greeks, Sedenegi,* and *Sadanegi* of the *Arabians,* is a ferrugineous, hard, glebous, ponderous, metallic Substance, of a dark red or yellowish Colour, and sometimes blackish, or of the Colour of Iron, and of an earthy astringent Taste; being broken, it shews fine, long, sharp Fibres, like those of Wood. It was called *Hæmatites,* in *Greek,* from its Colour; or because it is endued with the Virtue of stooping Blood. *Pliny* distinguishes five Kinds of Blood-stone, according to the Countries where they are found, and their differing Colour and Hardness. Others divide them according to their different outward Appearance. Some Stones have an uneven and angular Surface, as those that come from *Spain;* some are clustered on the Surface, like Bunches of Grapes, from whence they are termed *Hæmatites Botryodes,* as we see in those brought from the *Hercynian* Forest in *Germany.* Others are formed in various Convolutions, like Intestines, the outer Surface of the Brain; thefe Surfaces are very well de-ated by *Aldrovandus* and *Impe-*. In Iron Mines, the Blood-ftone ften found, in a diftinct Ore; where-ever it grows, there are ays red Stones, and red Earth, r it. It is likewife found fome-es in the fame Places with the d-ftone, and indeed there is a at Affinity between thefe two, being both reckoned Iron Ores. e Blood-ftone is dug up in many ces of *Germany*, in *Italy*, and *in*, and this laft is reckoned the t. That Blood-ftone is to be de Choice of, which is hardeft l fmootheft, without any Mix-e of Filth or Veins; and this ne is carefully to be diftinguifhed another, fomething like it in lour, but fofter, which Pinters l Joiners make Ufe of, called by ftake in fome Books *Hæmatites*, its true Name is *Rubrica Fabri-* or Ruddle. Blord-ftone is a nd of Iron-Ore, from which Iron y be extracted; and, in the lley of *Joachim* in *Bohemia*, the nes of thefe Stones are fo rich, it it is thought worth while to ex-ct the Iron from them, which is o excellent in its Kind, as *Agrico-* relates. This Stone is diffolved Acids, in the fame Manner as n, and, with the vitriolic Acid, turned into green Vitriol. Both *ofcorides* and *Galen* ufed Blood-ne in Roughneffes and Cicatrices the Eyelids; and for this Purpofe ey firft rubbed it upon a Whet-ne with Water, a Decoction of mugreek-feeds, or the White of Egg; and they commend it, when luted in Milk, in Suffufions of the yes. In all Ages it has been ufed a fine Powder, from one to four ruples, in any proper Vehicle, for l Kinds of Hæmorrhages, in Spit-g Blood, and in Ulcers of the ungs, which it dries and heals. In

the *Fluor albus*, *Cachexy*, and Sup-preffion of the Menfes, it is as ef-fectual as the *Crocus Martis aperiens*.

Lapis Hibernicus, Offic. *Irifh* Slate. It is a foffile Stone, of a black Co-lour, fomewhat inclining to an A-zure, and of an earthy Tafte; and found in Mines, as well in *England*, as in *Ireland*. This Stone is fre-quently ufed in Contufions; for it refolves coagulated Blood: Some fay it is effectual in quartan Fevers; but it is much us'd in all Kinds of Hæmorrhages, uterine Fluxes, and Spitting of Blood.

Lapis Lazuli, Offic. Azure ftone. This is a hard blue Stone, with Gold and Silver colour'd Specks and Veins; and is found of two Kinds, one that can bear the Fire, and the other that cannot. The firft is brought from *Afia* and *Africa*, and is called the Oriental Stone; the o-ther is found in fome Places in *Ger-many* and *Italy*, being dug out of Gold, Silver, and Copper Mines, and is fofter than the Oriental. The Oriental produces the ultramarine Blue, which never changes with Age. But the *German* Ultramarine is eafily affected by external Caufes, and in Time turns green. The beft *Lapis Lazuli* is of a deep blue Colour, marked with fome gold Specks, hard to break, and durable in the Fire. It purges upwards and downwards, and is recommended by Authors in melancholy Affections, quartan A-gues, Apoplexies, and Epilepfies. They attribute to it a corroding Quality, with fome Aftringency; the firft of which, *Diofcorides* and *Galen* fay, may be corrected by wafh-ing it in Water; but they are mi-ftaken, for both wafhed and un-wafhed, it vomits and purges, and what the Water carries off from it differs from what remains, only in the Finenefs of the Parts. The blue Colour of this Stone arifes, undoubtedly, from fome Parts of

Coppe

Copper mixed with it, from which, alfo, its purgative Quality proceeds; but it may very reafonably be afked, why an acrid and purgative Medicine of this Kind fhould be ufed in the *Confeftio Alkermes,* defigned for a ftrengthening Cordial? To anfwer this, it is to be confidered, that the antient Phyficians acknowledged two Virtues in this Stone, one Purgative, the other Styptic; which, though contrary to each other, were neverthelefs found in the fame Subject. The ftyptic Quality, by which it becomes a Strengthener, they counted natural to it, when it was found in gold Mines, mixed with fmall Particles of Gold; the cathartic Quality they confidered as merely accidental, arifing from the Mixture of heterogeneous Parts. Therefore, on Account of the ftrengthening Virtue of this Simple, they endeavoured by various Ways to correct the other, as by repeated Ablutions and Calcinations; but whether they have fucceeded or not, is with me, fays *Geoffroy,* ftill a Doubt, though, fays he, I muft own, that long Experience has fhewn, that no bad Accident ever happens from the *Confeftio Alkermes* rightly prepar'd. Whence it may be conjectured, that by Calcination the purgative Virtue of the Stone is very much leffened, or entirely deftroyed; but he cannot fay, that it contributes any thing to the cordial Virtues of the Confection. The Antients thought it purged off particularly the *Atra Bilis,* but, I am afraid, upon no good Grounds; for the black Colour of the Stools, after taking it, is not fo much owing to the Nature of the *Fæces,* as to the Tincture which all Steel and Copper Medicines communicate to them. As there are many Medicines of more certain Efficacy among us, we feldom ufe the *Lapis Lazuli,* all

the Magifteries, Tinctures, and Elixirs, which the Chymifts prepare from it, being laid afide. When *Geoffroy* mentions the *Lapis Lazuli* as an Ingredient in the *Confeftio Alkermes,* he means a Sort directed in foreign Difpenfatories; for in ours it has been long omitted. The Dofe, according to *Schroder,* is a Dram of the Stone reduced to a fine Powder.

Lapis Melitites, Offic. The Honey Stone. This Stone only differs in Colour and Sweetnefs from the *Lapis Galactites;* and the Effects produced by both are, according to *Diofcorides,* the fame. But, according to *Galen,* it is fomewhat more hot and abftergent than the *Galactites. Agricola* affirms, that the *Galactites* and *Melitites* are produced in the fame Lime-ftone Rock. *Wormius* diftinguifhes between the *Morocthus,* the *Galactites,* and the *Melitites,* in the following Manner: The *Morocthus* yields a milky Juice, which is deftitute of the Sweetnefs of Honey, and is neither of a white nor cineritious Colour; but the *Galactites* is of a white or cineritious Colour, and yields a milky Juice, without any Tafte of Honey; whereas the *Melitites* is of various Colours, and yields a milky Juice, as Sweet as Honey. But *Jo. de Laet* diftinguifhes between thefe three Stones in the following Manner: That which is of a cineritious or black Colour is the *Galactites;* that which is yellow, and in Colour refembling Honey, is juftly called the *Melitites;* whereas that which is greenifh is the *Morocthus,* which fhines like a Gem more than any of the others.

Lapis Memphites, Offic. Memphis-ftone. This is a Stone of a pinguious Subftance, parti-colour'd, of the Size of an ordinary Pebble, and found in *Egypt* near *Memphis.* They fay this Stone, levigated, and rubbed on the Parts which are to suffer cutting or burning, renders them insensible without Danger.

Lapis Morochthus, Offic. White Marking-stone. This Stone which some call *Galaxius,* or *Leucographis,* is produc'd in *Egypt,* and is used by the Fullers in whitening their Linen, as being of a soft Substance, and easily diluted. It is supposed to be of an emplastic Quality, and good for Spitting of Blood, the Cæliac Passion, and Pains of the Bladder, being taken in Water, as also for uterine Fluxes, being taken in like Manner, or applied in a Pessary. It is likewise an Ingredient in *Collyria,* or ophthalmic Medicines of a soft Consistence; for it fills up a *Cœloma,* and represses Defluxions: Made into a Cerate, it cicatrizes such foul Ulcers as happen in the tender and soft Parts of the Body.

Lapis Nephriticus, Offic. The Nephritic-stone. This is a Stone very much variegated with green and other Colours, as white, yellow, blue, and black, but still with a greenish Cast: It is imported from *America,* but is, also found, in some Parts of *Spain* and *Bohemia.* It is idly worn as an Amulet against Pains in the Stomach and Kidneys.

Lapis Phrygius, Offic. The Phrygian-stone. *Galen* informs us, that this Stone is found in *Cappadocia.* The best is pale, moderately ponderous, of no solid Contexture, and distinguished by white Lines. This Stone whether crude or burnt, is an efficacious Astringent. It moderately cleanses, also, and has an escharotic Virtue, and with Cerate cures Ambustions: It is good in Diseases of the Eyes, and for Ulcers, and other Purposes; but is not at present used in the *English* Shops.

Lapis Schistus, Offic. The Cleaving-stone. It is exported from *Germany.* The best is of a metallic Substance, and of the Colour of Saffron; the others, which are not so good, are blackish, and consist of thin, shining, and transparent Laminæ, which stick to one another. The Virtues are the same with those of the *Hæmatites,* only weaker in every Respect. *Boetius* thinks it a Species of Talc; and *Agricola* perceives no Difference between it and the *Hæmatites* except in the Figure. *Dioscorides* informs us, that it fills up a *Cœloma* of the Eyes, being diluted with Woman's Milk; and is, also, very effectual for a Rupture, or falling out of the same Part, for Thickness of the Eye-lids, and a *Staphyloma.*

Lapis Specularis, Offic. Muscovy Glass. This is a Fossile-stone resembling Crystal, transparent, and divisible into very thin *Laminæ.* It is erroneously supposed, says *P. Amman* to be the *Glacies Mariæ,* (the Virgin *Mary*'s Looking-glass) as it was formerly believed to be the *Aphroseline* or *Selenites:* For both Opinions are fabulous; the first, because, it is uncertain whether the Virgin *Mary* ever made Use of such a Glass; and the last, because it neither contains the Image of the Moon, nor increases or decreases as that Planet does. We have it imported from *Muscovy,* *Spain,* and other Parts; and it is of Use in Surgery, in the Cure of sordid Ulcers. It is of Service, also, in difficult Labour, and is an *Arcanum* against the Epilepsy; and is also reckoned among Cosmetics.

Lapis Spongiæ, Offic. Spunge-Stone. This is a Stone quite friable, concreted in a Spunge, and of a white or grey Colour. It is an Attenuant without any remarkable Heat, and is good to break the Stone in the Kidneys and Bladder, and also to discuss strumous Swellings. The Stones found in Spunges

ges being taken in Wine, are good to break the Stone in the Bladder.

Lapis Thyites, Offic. The Greenstone. This Stone is of a greenish Colour, resembling the Jasper; tho', when diluted, it renders the Liquor used for that Purpose of a milky Colour. It is produc'd in *Ethiopia,* is of an highly pungent Quality, and, according to *Dioscorides,* removes Specks and Dimness of the Eyes.

Lapis Variolatum, Offic. The Small-Pox Stone. This Stone is by some idly recommended to be worn about the Neck, by Way of Amulet, in order to promote the Eruption of the Small-Pox.

Lithargyrus, Offic. Litharge. This was of two Kinds among the *Greeks,* differing only in Colour. One was yellow; called *Chrysitis,* or *Lithargyrus Auri;* the other white, called *Argyritis,* or *Lithargyrus Argenti;* and the same Distinction is still kept up. It is commonly made in those Furnaces in which Lead is separated from Silver, or where Silver is refined by Lead from the other Metals mixed with it. When the Workmen design to separate Silver from the Lead or Copper contained in the same Ore with it, they first make a Kind of Trough of Bone-ashes, in which they melt a great Quantity of Lead; and into this melted Lead they throw the Silver Ore to be purified, and continue to blow with Bellows, till all the Lead, mixed with the Copper or Lead contained in the Silver, swims on the melting pure Silver like Oil. Then they gradually blow this Lead towards the Sides of the Trough, and afterwards, cutting the Sides, the vitrified Lead runs down to the Ground; and there becomes Litharge, sometimes of a Gold, and sometimes of a Silver Colour; whence the Dealers in those Commodities have given out, that the one was made from

Silver, the other from Gold; whereas the Difference consists only in having been more or less exposed to the Fire, or in having a greater or less Mixture of Copper. Litharge is therefore nothing but vitrified Lead, either alone, or mixed with Copper: It is frequently used in Physic in outward Applications, being mixed with oily Substances to make the Basis of most Plaisters, by Reason of the emplastic Consistence, which this and other Recrements of Lead acquire, by being mixed with and dissolved in Oils. It is of a drying, detergent, and gently astringent Quality; and for this Reason is used in incarning and cicatrizing Ulcers. It is prepared by being well levigated in a Mortar with clear Water, till all the Lead, which is not perfectly calcined, or other metallic Fœces, fall to the Bottom, leaving the finer Parts incorporated with the Water, which, subsiding by Rest, are separated from the Water, and dried.

Lithocolla, Offic. The Stone-Gluer. This is a Mixture of Marble, or Parian Stone, with Bull's Glue. It is of Service, being applied with a heated Probe, in laying hold of the Hairs which incommode the Eye.

Ludus Paracelsi, Offic. Waren Vein. It is a Stone of the Colour of yellow Amber, but more opake, of different Sizes, distinguished by transcurrent Lines of a dark Ashcolour like Veins. It is frequently found in Maritime rocky Places, and is recommended by *Paracelsus* for a Lithontriptic. Doctor *Grew* thinks it a good Diuretic, and that it may be of Use for expelling Gravel.

Magnes, Offic. The Loadstone. This is a ferruginous, dense, fossile Substance, of a blackish, bluish, or reddish Colour, attracting Iron, or another Magnet, or repelling them; and directing its Poles always to those of the World, when it is at Liberty to move. This Substance is not to be confounded with the _Magnes_ of _Theophrastus_, which he says, was white, and shining like Silver; not hard, but easily made into Vessels by the Turners Art; neither did it attract Iron. It was however, named from the same _Magnesia_ in _Lydia_. Another Name of the Load-Stone is _Lapis Lydius_, which is also applied to what we call the Touch-Stone, by which the Truth of Gold and Silver are tried. These two Significations of _Lapis Lydius_ are, therefore, carefully to be distinguished, because they are very different. The Load-Stone is found in many Parts of _Europe_, and for the most Part in Iron Mines; but the best are those which come from the _East Indies_ and _Ethiopia_. It is undoubtedly, a Kind of Iron Ore; and in some Places of _Germany_, they actually extract the Iron it contains: When exposed in the _Focus_ of a great Burning Glass, it likewise manifestly discovers Iron. The Virtues of the Magnet is attracting and repelling Iron, and in its turning its own Poles to those of the World, are very wonderful; and especially its being able to communicate these Virtues to the Iron which it touches. The Load-Stone is not used inwardly in Physic; tho' _Galen_ says it has the same Virtues as the Blood Stone; and also, mentions its purgative Virtues, and recommends it, on that Account in Dropsies. _Dioscorides_ proposes, that it be given in the Quantity of three _Oboli_, to evacuate gross melancholy Humours. Some think it possess'd of a deleterious Quality, which is denied by others; but _Geoffroy_ imagines the poisonous Quality is to be understood of that Kind of _Magnes_ mention'd by _Theophrastus_, which he takes to be a Kind of Native Litharge. The true Load Stone, externally used, is drying, astringent,

and consolidating. It stops Bleeding, and is recommended by _Hoffman_ for the Cure of _Hernias_. _Paracelsus_ makes it an Ingredient in a Plaister, not only for extracting the Head of an Arrow from the human Body, but all manner of Dirt and Filth whatever.

Magnes albus, Mont. Exot. The white Marking Stone. This Stone is called by the _Italians_, _Calamita alba_, and _Magnes carneus_; because, as the true Load Stone draws Iron, this is suppos'd to draw Flesh. It is a white Stone, marked with black Spots, which, if laid on the Tongue, sticks very closely to it; and is no other than a Kind of rocky Marl, found sometimes in the same Mines with the Load Stone. It is foolishly and fictitiously said to be of wonderful Efficacy in Love Affairs. According to _Monti_, it absterges with an Astringency, and is reckon'd among Antiarthritics, Antiscorbutics, and Aperitives.

Magnesia, Offic. _Manganese_, Mer. Pin. _Sapo Vitri_, Mer. Arf. Vit. Soap of Glass. This is a fossile, metallic, ferruginous Substance, resembling Antimony in its shining Colour, and very brittle. _Pomet_ mentions two Kinds of it, one Ash-colour'd, which is not easy to be got, and therefore little used; the other black, which is very common. It is used in making and purifying Glass; for by mixing a small Quantity of it with Glass, whilst in Fusion, it clears it from any green, or bluish Colours, and makes it more transparent and bright. On that Account _Merret_ term'd it _Sapo Vitri_. If too great a Quantity be put in, it gives the Glass a Purple Colour. It is used by Potters in colouring their Vessels black, as the _Zaffara_ is for blue. _Merret_ also, says, the best _Manganese_ is that which is hard, heavy, sparkling, and blackish, and which, being reduced to a Powder,

turns

turns Lead black. It is dug in *Germany, Italy, Piedmont,* and in *England* near the *Mendip* Hills in *Somersetshire* : And *Merret* tells us, that wherever the Miners find *Manganese* they conclude, that there is Lead Ore under it ; but whether it contains any Lead, or not, has not been discover'd.

Malachites, Offic. The Malachite. This may be taken for a Species of the Jasper, or *Prasius.* It is opake, and of a Mallow green, whence it has its Name μαλάχη *Malache* in *Greek,* signifying a Mallow. It is found in *Cyprus, Meissen,* and the Country of *Tirol,* and is exhibited as a Febrifuge.

Marga, Offic. Marle. This is not only of various Species, but also of different Colours, such as reddish brown, grey and yellow. It is of a pinguious and medullary Substance, found in some Stones and Rocks, when they are split. It is of a drying, constricting, consolidating, and narcotic Quality ; but resolves Tartar, and coagulated Blood. *Kentman* enumerates various Species of Marles, such as the white, the pinguious, the soft, the subcineritious, and the stony Marle, used by Artists for making Images ; the yellow and crustaceous Marle, which is found in sandy Grounds, and contains some Portion of Gold ; and the hard, yellow, and sandy Marle found in *Holland,* with which the Inhabitants, as in other Countries, manure the Land.

Marga candida, Offic. White Stone Marle. This is found in *Germany,* and is a fungous, white, and friable Substance. It is of an astringent and refrigerating Quality ; stops Hæmorrhages, and immoderate Discharges of the *Menses.* The Powder of it is by Surgeons sprinkled upon Ulcers, in order to dry and consolidate them. It is esteem'd

a powerful Cosmetic. *Anselmus Boetius,* when it is hard, refers it to the *Lapis Galactites* ; but, if soft, he makes it a Species of Marle ; for he is of Opinion, that the *Morochthus,* the *Galactites,* and the *Lapis Melitites,* are only indurated Marle.

Marga saxatilis cinerea, Offic. Ash-colour'd Marle. This Species of Marle is found in the Cavities and Fissures of Rocks, consists of thick Crusts, is of a cineritious Colour, and a somewhat acrid Taste. It is of an astringent, emplastic Quality, and stops Hæmorrhages, when externally apply'd, it agrees in Virtues with the *Samian* Earth.

Marga Saxatilis Incarnata, Offic. Reddish Marle. This Species is produced in the Mountains of *Bohemia* and *Liege :* It is a pinguious, lubricous, and ponderous Earth, of a Carnation Colour, adhering to the Tongue, and tinging the Fingers with a yellowish Hue. This Kind of Marle, is not only beneficial in Ruptures, Fractures, Defluxions, the Hæmorrhoids, and Dysenteries ; but also resists Poisons, and pestilential Disorders.

Marmor album, Offic. White Marble. This differs from Alabaster only in Hardness, and in Splendor, when polished. *Galen* tells us, that taken internally, it dissolves the Stone.

Mars. This is the Chymical Name for *Ferrum* Iron, and is sometimes called in Pharmacy, *Chalybs,* Steel. *Melampus* is the first upon Record, who exhibited Iron by way of Medicine ; for he is said to have directed *Iphiclus* to take the Rust of a Knife, and drink it in Wine, ten Days together, in order to procure him Children. Iron is the most useful Metals for human Life ; for, besides the innumerable Kinds of Instruments made of it, it furnishes excellent Remedies in many Diseases. The Medicinal Virtues of Iron, taken

'ken inwardly, were not unknown ' the Antients. *Dioscorides,* attributes to it an aftringent Virtue, and recommends it in uterine Hæmorages. He likewife, orders Wine, or Water, in which a red hot Iron as been quenched, in the Cæliac affion, Lientery, and Dyfentery, nd for reftoring weak Stomachs. hyficians now acknowledge a twofold Virtue in Iron, one aperient, the other aftringent ; for it is obferv'd to cure a Suppreffion of the *Menfes,* to open Obftructions of the Liver, and Spleen, and other *Vifcera,* to ftop Hæmorrhages and Diarhæas, and to ftrengthen the relaxed Fibres of the Inteftines. On thefe Accounts it is reckon'd the grand fpecific in Hypochondriacal Affecions, and all Kinds of *Chlorofis.* Some attribute an aperient Virtue to ome Preparations of Iron, and an aftringent Virtue to others ; but the Truth is, all thefe Preparations are both aftringent and aperient, tho' not in the fame Degree. For Medicinal Ufes, Iron is preferable to Steel ; and the Filings of Iron, reduced to an *Alcohol,* or impalpable Powder, are prefer'd by many, to all other Preparations, in promoting the Flux of the *Menfes,* and in removing Obftructions of the *Vifcera,* being given from twelve Grains to half a Dram, once or twice a Day, in any convenient Form. Filings of Iron, tied up in a Linen Bag, are alfo prefcribed to be infufed in aperient Apozems, and alterative Broths. *Sydenham* tells us, that he was inform'd, " That the crude Ore of " Iron, is more efficacious in curing " Difeafes, than Iron which has " been refined by Fufion ; but, for " the Truth of this, fays he, I had " only the Author's Word, not be- " ing affured of it by my own Ea- " perience." And I have feen a Kind of Iron Ore, called at the Iron Works, *Cumberland Ore,* which

very much refembles Bole, and which rub'd with Quickfilver, unites with it, forming a Kind of Cinnabar, which promifes very fair to be an excellent Deobftruent. There is a Stypticity in Iron, by which it braces up the Veffels and *Vifcera* when relaxed ; hence the Organs of Digeftion, when weak and relaxed, are ftrengthen'd and enabled to perform their Offices. Hence alfo, by a prudent Ufe of Iron, the contractile Force of the Arteries is increas'd, and in Confequence of this, the Circulation is accelerated, and Obftructions are removed. But for the fame Reafon that Iron or its Preparations are of Service in a Weaknefs of the Solids, and a Languor of the Circulation, it becomes prejudicial in a high Degree, when the Solids are too tenfe, the Circulation too brifk, and the Conftitution inclin'd to Inflammation. Prudent Practitioners alfo, will be very cautious of exhibiting Iron in a full Habit of Body, without previous Evacuations, becaufe otherwife by increafing the Velocity of the Blood, in fuch Habits, Hæmorrhages, Fevers, Apoplexies, Convulfions, all Kinds of Nervous Diforders, and Death, will not unfrequently be produced. And for the fame Reafon it is always prudent to adminifter Steel, as it is called, or Iron, after due Evacuations, gradually, and in fuch Dofes, as will not accelerate the Circulation too fuddenly. Steel properly fo called, is not fo good as Iron for Medicinal Ufes.

Melanteria. This is already fpecify'd under the Article *Chalcitis.*

Mercurius. Mercury, or Quickfilver. This is a fluid, metallic Subftance, cold to the Touch, of a fhining Silver Colour, very heavy, volatile, and which will unite with moft Metals, efpecially Gold, to which it joins itfelf very clofely. It is fometimes found in its fluid Form in in the Bowels of the Earth ; and in that Cafe, it is firſt well waſhed with Water, to clear it from the Earth ; then ſometimes with Vinegar and Salt, to carry off all other metallic Parts ; and laſtly, it is paſſed thro' Cotton, or dreſs'd Leather, and then has the Name of Virgin Mercury. It is alſo found in Glebes, or in Form of a red ſulphureous Mercurial Mineral, called Cinnabar, or of a ſtony Glebe, ſometimes red, ſometimes yellow, ſometimes dark, and ſometimes of a Lead Colour. It was by the Antients rank'd among Poiſons. *Dioſcorides* aſcribes pernicious Effects to it ; and from his Authority, doubtleſs it was, that *Galen* reckon'd it highly corroſive ; for he owns he never made any Trial of it himſelf. The Name of it is not found in *Hippocrates* ; whence it is probable, that it was not in Uſe in his Time. But before *Avicenna* it was uſed externally, though ſeldom internally, being ſtill reckon'd a Poiſon by moſt Phyſicians. *Actuarius* ranks it, however, among Medicines ; but *Meſue* applied it only for curing cutaneous Diſeaſes, though *Avicenna* obſerves, that many had drank it without any bad Effect, and that it paſſed through the *Anus* unchanged. About two hundred Years ago, though it was ſtill believed by ſome to be poiſonous, it began by many to be uſed inwardly ; they having obſerv'd, as *Fallopius* relates, that it was given in that manner by Shepherds to their Cattle, to kill Worms, without any bad Effect ; whence they concluded, that it might be ſafely given to Men alſo, and that therefore, crude Mercury was not to be reckon'd a Poiſon. Thus *Braſſavolus*, and *Carolus Muſitanus* tells us, they gave it to Children troubled with Worms, from two to twenty Grains, and always with ſome Succeſs ; and that ſeveral Midwives gave it to Women in difficult

Labours, though perhaps, not always with any viſible good Effects. *Matthiolus* relates, that ſome Women with Child drank each a Pound of Quickſilver to procure Abortion without any bad Conſequence ; and it is commonly known, that the Workers in Quickſilver take this Method to cheat their Maſters of conſiderable Quantities, by firſt ſwallowing it, and then voiding it with their *Fæces*, from which it is eaſily cleanſed by ſimple waſhing. It muſt, nevertheleſs be owned, that the Uſe of it, whether outwardly or inwardly, can never be long continued without Miſchief ; for the Miners, and others employ'd about it, though of the ſtrongeſt Conſtitutions imaginable, ſeldom remain four Years in that State, but are ſeiz'd with Tremblings and Palſies, and die miſerable. By an injudicious Uſe of it, whether outwardly applied, or inwardly taken the Nerves are likewiſe affected, weaken'd, corrupted, and contracted ; whence Tremblings, Spaſms, Palſies, and too great an Attenuation of the Fluids, which often brings on a fatal Salivation, Ulcers in the Mouth and Throat, and incurable Looſeneſſes. Quickſilver judiciouſly adminiſter'd, is, however, undoubtedly a moſt excellent Medicine ; it opens the Pores, ſmall Veſſels, and Ducts of the Glands ; reſolves obſtructed Humours, attenuates thoſe which are too thick, and viſcid, eſpecially the *Lymphæ*; and diſſipates Concretions, even in the remoteſt Parts of the Body. On all theſe Accounts it is found to be of ſingular Service in Tumours, ſwell'd Glands, a ſchirrhous Spleen, Meſentery, or Liver, Ganglions, *Strumæ*, and other ſuch Diſeaſes. It alſo blunts the Acrimony of the Fluids, and hence performs Wonders in Venereal Tumors, Buboes, and Ulcers, in cutaneous Puſtules, Scabs, and other Affections of the Skin ; univerſal Remedies of the he Preparatory, and especially of the evacuating Kind, having not only gone before the Use of Mercury, but being continued along with it. For as all these Diseases arise from a viscid *Serum* become caustic by a long Stagnation, if it be divided and reduced to a fluid State by Quickfilver, before a Passage is prepared for it out of the Body, it must either exert its Efficacy on the Part where it was first lodged, or, by removing to the more noble Parts of the Body, bring on Symptoms more dangerous than the first. Therefore before the Patient begins to take Mercury in any Form, his Body ought to be cautiously prepared by Bleeding, to lessen the Plenitude of the Vessels; by warm bathing, and the Use of diluting Medicines, that the Humours may become more fluid, and the solid Fibres softer; as also, by purging, that Way may be opened for the Passage of the dissolved Humours out of the Body. These Passages are also to be kept open during the Time that the Quickfilver is taken, least the Humours be intercepted in their Course, and be turned a more dangerous Way; and the Patient ought to be kept warm, least Cold should stop or diminish insensible Perspiration, which ought likewise to be encouraged by gentle Exercise. Quickfilver, not only taken inwardly, but also by Unction, evacuates the Humours by Stool, Sweat, and insensible Perspiration; but the most common Method of its Operation, is by the Evacuation of a mucous *Saliva*, whence it is termed a Salivation. This Way of Purging was entirely unknown to the Antients, and is thought the most effectual Remedy for Venereal Diseases; for the Cure of which it was first used by *Jacobus Carpensis*, a Physician of *Bologna*. That is to be esteem'd, which is most pure, of the most

shining white Colour, most fluid, and which being evaporated, leaves no Remainder behind it. That is to be rejected, which is of a livid or pale Colour, which does not run into Globules exactly spherical, but oblong, resembling little Worms or Tears, which are sure Signs, that it is adulterated with Lead, Bismuth, or some other Metal. Mercury is sometimes so adulterated, as to produce very terrible and uncommon Symptoms: Thus Mercury is commonly adulterated with Lead; and this Fraud is, I think, adverted to by *Quercetan*, for by the Intervention of *Bismuth*, Lead, if its Quantity is not too large, may be forced thro' Leather, and rendered so fluid and moveable, as to prevent all Suspicion of Fraud. Hence 'tis obvious, how insufficient and superficial the Depuration of Mercury must be by such an Expression alone. But what terrible Effects are produced by Lead internally taken, is sufficiently obvious to any one, who is but a little conversant in the Writings of practical Authors; and a small Quantity of it is absolutely deleterious, when treated in a Manner not unlike that used when Mercury is adulterated with it. Crude Mercury is given in Substance, to kill Worms, from a Scruple to three Drams; being first well rubbed with Sugar in a glass Mortar, till it is dissolved into invisible Parts, adding a Drop or two of Oil of sweet Almonds, to keep it from returning to its native Form. Decoctions of Quickfilver are likewise much used, being made by boiling a Pound of Mercury in six Pints of Water for an Hour. The clear Liquor is given both to Children and Adults for their common Drink. Quick-filver is a great Enemy to all Sorts of Vermin, as well as to Worms; and it suddenly kills, or banishes them, being applied in an

Oint-

Ointment to any Parts of the Body where they are found. Crude Mercury is likewise given in very large Quantities in the Iliac Paffion, even two or three Pounds; and it often fucceeds in removing the Obftructions: But if the Obftruction be very great, fo that the Mercury remains a great while in the Inteftines, it may do them an Injury, merely by its great Weight. To cure the Itch, Quick-filver Girdles are ufed with very good Succefs, when the Precautions abovementioned are duly obferved. The Quick-filver is to be beat up with the White of an Egg, till both are turn'd to a thick Froth, which is rubbed on a Cotton Girdle, and, when dry, is wore round the Loins. It is very well worth the Notice of every Practitioner, that Mercury, or its Preparations, apply'd either externally, or taken internally, is an almoft infallible Remedy, for that Diforder which is induc'd by the Bite of a mad Dog, and a certain Prefervative againft it, and it has of late Years been ufed with great Succefs in many Diftempers, which were before efteemed extremely obftinate, if not incurable. *Rotario* a *Veronefe* Phyfician, of great Reputation, has wrote a Volume in *Folio*, on the Virtues of this *Herculean* Remedy. He advifes to divide it with Goofe-Greafe, for external Application, and for internal Ufe to mix it with Conferve of Rofes. He recommends it extremely in the Gout, conformable to the Sentiments of *Frederic Hoffman* upon that Subject, in the Dropfy alfo, even an *Afcites*, an *Afthma*, and many other obftinate chronical Diftempers, he affures us from Experience, that he has found it of infinite Service. But he feems to think it of much greater Service, when exhibited without raifing a Salivation, than when it excites one, and in this he agrees with many others of the Moderns,

who have wrote upon the fame Subject.

Naphtha, Offic. This is of the Colour of the *Babylonian* Bitumen, of a liquid Confiftence, very fubject to take Fire, fometimes white, fometimes black; it is feldom or never to be met with in our Shops; and therefore *Petroleum* commonly fupplies its Place. It is a Liquor of an oily Subftance, like rectify'd Spirit, very thin, pellucid, very penetrating, and fubject to kindle in to a Flame: It agrees in Virtues with *Bitumen*. There are fome, who, as *Agricola* affures us, are perfuaded, that the *Camphora* of the Antients was prepared of *Naphtha* by Sublimation; others there are, who will have it, that *Naphtha* and *Petroleum* are one and the fame Subftance; but fince we are not as yet certain what *Naphtha* is, we fhall not venture to determine in the Cafe. As for *Naphtha*, tho' it has many, and thofe very confiderable, Virtues in Medicine, which *Diofcorides* infifts upon at large, yet, at prefent, we are told by *Kempfer*, that he never knew the *Perfians* apply it to any other Ufe, than to temper their Vernifh.

Natron. This is the Nitre of the Antients, but is very different from our Nitre. It is a native Foffile dug out of the Earth, not pure but got by Lixiviation from the Earth, and is of an alcaline and abfterfive Nature, fo that it might well ferve inftead of Pot-afhes, for the making of Glafs or Soap. It was produced in *Egypt*, and now, at prefent, they dig at *Smyrna*, an Earth that is purely alcaline, which comes to *Paris* in great Quantities, and is ufed inftead of Pot-afh. *Clufius* writes, that the Nitre of the Antients is fo common at *Cairo*, that ten Pounds of it will hardly yield a *Meyden* (three Halfpence.) They ufe it for feveral

Par-

poſes ; for they incruſt Veſſels
h it, and mixed with the Pods
Acacia, it ſerves to dry Leather.
lonius informs us, that the Nitre
the Antients is very rarely found
ongſt us ; and confidently aſſerts,
t there is not a Grain of that Ni-
in *Europe* ; but that in *Egypt*
re is nothing more cheap and
nmon. This Nitre was not con-
tible, and inflammable like ours,
l, conſequently of no Uſe in mak-
; Gun-powder. This Difference
ng ſuppoſed, it plainly follows,
t what we find in ancient Writings,
thoſe of *Hippocrates*, *Pliny*, *Dioſ-
ides*, *Galen*, and others, of Ni-
: and its Virtues, is not to be un-
rſtood of our common Nitre, but
a native alcaline Salt. But though
llonius denies that there is a Grain
this alcaline Salt, or Nitre of the
icients, to be found in *Europe*,
ffman is of Opinion, that though
: have not ſo great Quantities of
rous alcaline Salt in the Earth of
ropean Countries, as in that of
ypt; yet that a purely alcaline
ed Salt may be produced from the
owels of the Earth, with all the
operties of Pot-aſhes, or Salt of
artar, or Nitre of the Antients
hich is ſufficiently proved by me-
cinal Springs, Baths, and Waters.
or a very pure alcaline Salt is ex-
eſted out of many of them ; for
iſtance, the *Selteran* and *Antonias*
Vaters, and in *Bohemia* thoſe of
luckfouerling, and *Wildungen*, which
ield a very pure *Sal Alcali*, as do
ie *Caroline* and *Emſen* Baths ; as
ie Springs of *Schwalback* and *Egra*
roduce an Alcali, and with it a Salt
f a middle Kind. So that I think
: can no longer be doubted, but
iat our Earth contains a fixed alca-
ne Salt, which is imbibed and car-
ied off by the Waters. This Con-
ideration will, alſo, ſerve to con-
ute the vulgar Notion of our mo-
ern Chymiſts, that fixed *Sal Alcali*

was the mere Product of Art, and
obtained by Fire ; nor could be extracted otherwiſe than from the Vegetable Kingdom, by Way of reducing Vegetables to aſhes.

Nitrum, Offic. Nitre. This is
very different from the Nitre of the
Antients, for an Account of which
ſee *Natron*. Our Nitre is artificially
prepared of two Elements, or Principles, one of which is the highly
Simple, univerſal, Acid, and primogenial Salt contained in the Air,
and the other an alcaline, ſulphureous and pinguious Earth, which like
a Matrix, or Load-ſtone, attracts
the univerſal Acid lodg'd in the Air.
Nor are Earths of every Kind, when
expos'd to the free and open Air,
fit for generating Nitre, but only
ſuch as are of an alcaline Nature,
and contain a pinguious and ſulphureous Subſtance. Hence, we find,
that the Earths, left after the burning of Houſes, are of all others the
moſt proper for generating Nitre.
The ſame holds true of calcarious
Subſtances; when, for Inſtance, Mud,
Earth, or Clay, is mix'd with Lime,
and expoſed to the free Air, the Salt
of Nitre eaſily breaks thro' it like
Froth. Quick Lime alſo, the Aſhes
of Wood, or of Soap-Boilers, as yet
turgid with an alcaline Salt, greatly
contribute to the Production of Nitre, when mix'd with Earth. The
Earth proper for generating Nitre
muſt not only be alcaline, but, alſo,
pinguious and ſulphureous; nay, a
volatile alcaline Principle is neceſſary
for this Purpoſe. Hence all Putrefaction contributes to the Generation
of Nitre in Sands. For this Reaſon
nothing in Nature ſo powerfully promotes the Generation of Nitre, as
dunging the Land with the Excrements and Urine of Animals. Hence
thoſe who prepare Nitre, diligently
dig up and preſerve the old and
ſqualid Earth, in Sheep-folds, Sta-
bles, and other Places where Ani-

mal

mals are kept. They also, carefully collect the Earth dug up about Bog-Houses, which being impregnated with the Salt and Sulphur of the human Excrements, is, for that Reason, highly proper for producing Nitre. They also chuse pinguious Earths of Church-Yards, Ponds, Marshes, and Walls, built of a pinguious Earth, and putrified Straw, especially their Surfaces taken off for about the Depth of a Finger's length, because these, being long exposed to the Sun and Air, have conceived a nitrous Salt, discoverable by the acrid and bitterish Taste. Hence it follows, that the more Putrefaction and volatile sulphureous Salt can be convey'd to the Earth, the more proper they are for producing Nitre. Earths, in order to yield a large Quantity of Nitre, must be managed in the following Manner: They are to be made up in Heaps, which are to be frequently watered or sprinkled with the Urine of Animals; by which Means, and the free Passage of the Air thro' them, they soon contract a nitrous Salt. But 'tis to be observed, that neither a too intense Heat of the Sun, especially such as burns the Earths, nor too pinching a Cold, nor too moist an Atmosphere, and especially rainy Weather, but rather a temperate windy Air, accompany'd with serene Weather, especially in the Spring or Autumn, and in the Night time, favour the Production of Nitre. The Heat of the Sun, is indeed, serviceable in drying the Earths from which the Nitre has been before extracted, but does not at all contribute to its Generation. Nor is its Generation promoted by intense Cold, southerly or westerly Winds, but by Winds blowing from the easterly or northerly Quarters bring the promogenial ethereal Acid. The Elaboration of Nitre does by no Means succeed under excessive Rains, which wash it out of the Earths. 'Tis also, to be observed, that from Waters impregnated with a nitrous Salt, by Elixiviation, there cannot be obtained any true Nitre, which is inflammable, and forms itself into Crystals, without the Addition of Ashes, in which there is an alcaline Salt, an Admixture of Quick-Lime, or that Lixivium which in boiling remains after former Crystallizations; for if the Lixivium, drawn from nitrous Earths, is boiled by itself, a saline *Magma* is only obtain'd, which neither runs into dry, much less inflammable Crystals, nor is easily dried, but is readily dissolved in the Air, especially when moist and humid. Hence we may reasonably conclude, that the inflammable Salt of Nitre is compounded of an acid Salt, a fixed Alcali, and a sulphureous Principle. And as neutral Salts are easily formed into Crystals, so, on the contrary, neither acid nor alcaline Salts, nor sulphureous acid Substances, mix'd with alcaline Earth, of which Kind this Lixivium, extracted from nitrous Earths, seems to be, are disposed to Crystallization. But that there is in Nitre such a fixed Alcali, is sufficiently obvious, not only from its Generation already described, but, also, from this, that Powder of Charcoal alone, added to Nitre fus'd in a Crucible, converts it into a pure alcaline Salt, commonly called fixed Nitre, tho' it is not, in Reality, different from Salt of Tartar, or any other alcaline Salt; as also from this Circumstance, that if this alcaline Salt is again combined with acid Spirit of Nitre, or *Aqua Fortis*, the Nitre is forthwith regenerated. Earths impregnated with a nitrous Salt, of which Nitre is prepared, are not only to be found in *Europe*, but 'tis, also, certain, that an inflammable Nitre may be prepared every where, because the Matter, or *Matrix* of Nitre, which is Earth rendered alcaline and sulphureous by Putrefaction,

tion, may be had every where. Neither is it to be doubted, but that the primogenial and universal Acid, which is formed into a nitrous Salt with the alcaline sulphureous Earth, is contained in the Atmosphere, wherever it extends. And, 'tis certain, that not only in the *Indies*, which are hot, but also in *Muscovy*, which is a cold Climate, a large Quantity of Nitre is prepared, which is better than the *German* Nitre, and far more fit for preparing Gun-powder. The *Indian* Soil favours the Generation of Nitre, because for several Months, no Rains fall to wash and carry off the nitrous Salt from the Earth.

The essential Characters, and Properties, by which Nitre is distinguished from all other Salts, are these (I.) Nitre is, by the Force of Fire, easily fus'd in a Crucible without flaming; but as soon as an oleous sulphureous Substance, capable of flaming, is added to it, it takes Flame, and produces an Explosion; which Effect happens not only by the Addition of common Sulphur, of Antimony which abounds with Sulphur, of Charcoal, of Tartar which abounds with Oil, of some Parts of Animals, the Blood or Bones, for Instance, but, also, by the Addition of Metals impregnated with Sulphur, such as Tin, Iron, and Zink; as also, by an Addition of *Sal Ammoniac*, which from the Urine receives a certain oleous, and sulphureous Principle. (II.) Nitre, mix'd and distill'd with a vitriolic Salt, or the Acid of Vitriol, yields an highly volatile acid Spirit, of an ungrateful Smell, and yellowish Colour, as appears in the Preparation of *Hoffman's Spiritus Nitri Fumans*, or *Aqua Fortis*; and because all Clay contains some Quantity of a vitriolic Salt, hence if three Parts of Nitre are mix'd with one Part of Clay, form'd into small Balls, and dry'd, the Nitre by Distillation yields its acid Spirit in the Form of a red Vapour; and because the Acid of Alum is of the same Nature with that contain'd in Vitriol, hence in Conjunction with Alum, as well as with Vitriol, an acid Spirit, or *Aqua Fortis*, may be distill'd from Nitre. It must, also, be observ'd, that no other Acid, except one of the vitriolic Kind, can by any Means extract the Acid of Nitre, since a very fix'd and strong Acid, such as that contain'd in Vitriol and Alum, is requir'd for that Purpose. (III.) Nitre, fus'd in a Crucible, is almost totally converted into an alcaline Salt; and this Effect is particularly produc'd mixing equal Quantities of Tartar and Nitre, and putting them into an ignited Crucible; by which Means the *Black-Flux-Powder*, commonly used by Workers of Metals in separating their Metals from adventitious Mixtures, is produc'd. Nitre, is, also, converted into an highly pure *Alcali*, when it is mixed and detonated with Powder of Charcoal; and by a strong Calcination it becomes an highly caustic Salt, of a Sky Colour, and this is call'd fix'd Nitre. 'Tis also, worth our Observation, that the whole of Nitre may be converted into a caustic Alcali, of an highly acrid Taste, and which, by pouring Water upon it, becomes intensely hot, when mix'd with an equal Quantity of Regulus of Antimony, and melted together to a Mass, in a red hot Crucible. The same *Phenomenon* is said to be produced with Zink and Tin. (IV.) Nitre is a Salt of so singular a Quality, that there is none like it in Nature; for, it not only cools the Tongue, when applied to it; but also the whole Body, when taken internally; and, when put into Water, augments its Coldness. (V.) A Solution of Nitre, put into Blood coagulated, and become black after it is taken from the Veins, not only renders it more fluid, but, also,

also, procures it a florid and beautiful red Colour; an Effect not to be expected from any other neutral Salt. By this Experiment we may, in some Measure, account for its Operations, and refrigerating Effect, on the human Body; for Nitre is a Salt, which, by Means of its aereo-acid Principle, is of an elastic and expansive Quality, allays and stops the tumultuous and exorbitant Motion of the Sulphur in the Blood and Humours, which, when confin'd, becomes more violent: And to this aereo-acid Principle, we are to ascribe the Fluidity, and florid Colour, which Nitre communicates to the Blood. Nitre, also, by procuring a greater Fluidity to the Humours, removes Stagnations, and Obstructions, and opens the Pores of the Skin, thro' which the hot and fiery Particles are exhal'd: And as Nitre stimulates the Ducts and Glands to a more copious Secretion of Lymph, hence it moistens the Body, and relaxes and softens Parts spasmodically contricted. (VI.) Nitre, when detonated with Sulphur, or any other inflammable Substance, is totally carry'd off in Smoke; by which Means, the whole *Crasis*, and as it were, the Substance of Nitre, which consists of an acid and alcaline Salt, together with a pinguious and sulphureous Substance, is totally destroy'd; for *Gun-powder*, kindled in a tubulated Re ort, is neither transform'd into an acid Spirit, nor an alcaline Salt, but yields a somewhat acid Phlegm. (VII.) 'Tis also, a Property peculiar to Nitre, that, when put into a Crucible, exposed to a calcining Fire, with Regulus of Antimony, Zink, Bismuth, Arsenic, Regulus of Cobalt, Tin, and Lead, it converts them to a Calx; by which Means the purer Metals, such as Gold and Silver, are separated from them. For this Reason, the most expeditious Way of separating Gold dispers'd in Antimo-

ny, is to calcine and fuse it with Nitre; whereas 'tis a speedy and laborious Task to separate its reguline and antimonial Parts by the Force of intense Fire; and as these Minerals are, in a great Measure, virulent, so when calcined with Nitre, they not only lose their deleterious Qualities, but partly become salutary Medicines. (VIII.) 'Tis sufficiently known to Chymists, that *Aqua Fortis* dissolves Silver, but not Gold; but it has not as yet been adverted to, that *Aqua Fortis* distill'd by Abstraction from common Nitre, does not dissolve Silver, but converts it to a Calx; whereas it quickly attacks and dissolves Gold. This will perhaps seem strange to him, who considers that *Aqua Fortis* is the Offspring of Nitre, and in every Respect agrees with the acid Spirit of Nitre, but his Surprize will cease, when he reflects, that in undeporated Nitre there is a large Quantity of common Salt, which must be separated by Art; and considers, that *Aqua Fortis*, drawn off common Salt, becomes an *Aqua Regia*, capable of dissolving Gold; for, if *Aqua Fortis* is even ten times drawn off depurated Nitre, its Virtues will not be alter'd by common Salt; but, if common Salt is mixed with the Nitre, the *Aqua Fortis* attacks and disentangles it; by which Means an highly subtile Spirit of Salt ascends, and this Spirit, in Consequence of its highly penetrating Subtilty, enters the most minute Pores of Gold, and, by Means of the elastic Sulphur of the Nitre, destroys the Cohesion of its constituent Parts. (IX.) 'Tis also, to be observed, that if Spirit of Nitre, or *Aqua Fortis*, are in a due Proportion drawn off common Salt, there remains in the Bottom a Salt, which deflagrates like Nitre; for the Acid of Nitre intimately associates itself with the alcaline Earth of common Salt, and with it is converted into

into Nitre, from which it expels the Spirit of Salt. Tho' Subſtances highly volatile enter the Compoſition of Nitre, it is nevertheleſs of a very fix'd Nature. The Volatility of its Principles is ſufficiently obvious from the Account before given of its Generation, whilſt, on the other Hand, its fix'd Nature is evinc'd from this, that it remains fus'd over a Fire for ſome Hours, without any Diminution of either Weight or Bulk; neither is its Texture alter'd by Flame, tho' a Change is ſoon produc'd in it by the Addition of a ſmall Quantity of ignited ſulphureous Earth. Tho' an highly volatile and corroſive acid Spirit, as alſo a very cauſtic fix'd alcaline Salt, may be prepared from Nitre, yet it is poſſeſs'd of a ſingular Power of removing the Septic, and conſequently the virulent and corroſive Qualities of almoſt all Subſtances, and rendering them propitious, temperate, and ſalutary. The violent and emetic Virtues of Regulus and Sulphur of Antimony are ſufficiently known; and 'tis certain, that by the Addition of a due Quantity of Nitre, and the Aſſiſtance of Fire, both theſe may be converted into mild, temperate, and gently diaphoretic Medicines. That moſt of the Inſects, which, by Means of their highly acrid Salt, excite Bliſters, are excellently corrected by Powder of Nitre, intimately mix'd with them, is certain from Experience: Thus Cantharides, and other Subſtances of a like Nature, may be ſafely exhibited even in delicate Conſtitutions, in order to remove a Difficulty of Urine, provided due Regard be had to the Cauſes of the Diſorder, and a ſmall Quantity of Camphire, which powerfully reſiſts Inflammation, is added. Some Purgatives are ſo highly draſtic, that, when imprudently exhibited, they raiſe violent Commotions in the nervous Syſtem, and often excite an Inflammation in the Coats of the Stomach: Of this Kind are Gamboge, Scammony, Reſin of Jalap, Coloquintida, Elaterium, and Spurge; which two laſt excite Bliſters, when applied externally. Now the cauſtic Quality of all theſe is greatly impair'd, by being mixed with any nitrous Salt, and if there is any genuine and efficacious Corrector of Purgatives, which guards the tender Membranes againſt Heat, Spaſms, and Inflammations, 'tis certainly Nitre. Aloes, which is otherwiſe of a laxative and balſamic Quality, has by its ſubtile acrid Salt been frequently obſerv'd to excite Hæmorrhages; but it is render'd more benign and propitious, by a proper Admixture of Nitre. The Bile, in Conſequence of its deterſive and bitter Quality, is a balſamic and natural Medicine, without which no Animal can long remain ſound, and in a due State: Now, if the Bile is vitiated by a Congeſtion of acrid Sordes retain'd in the Humours, it acts like Poiſon by irritating the nervous Syſtem, and producing preternatural Heat, Anxiety, Inquietudes, enormous Evacuations, and intenſe Pains: Now, in order to correct this peccant State of the Bile, no Medicine is more efficacious than Nitre. As Nitre is a powerful Cooler, when internally exhibited, ſo there is no more effectual Antifebrile, no Medicine which either ſo ſoon, or ſo ſafely, corrects the febrile Heat, and removes the woeful Train of Symptoms produc'd by it. Accordingly Angelus Sola informs us, that in quotidian and chronical tertian Fevers, as alſo, in that Species of Fever call'd the Putrid Hemitritæus, Nitre is uſed with wonderful Succeſs; for when the Patients are properly purg-ed before, and kept in a moderately warm Place, the Exhibition of Nitre twice or thrice two or three Hours before the Paroxyſm, gives ſuch a Change to the State of the Diſorder, that Health soon succeeds : And as all other Refrigerants, the most considerable of which are Acid, inspissate and coagulate the human Juices, so, on the contrary, Nitre attenuates and renders the whole Mass of Humours more fluid : Hence we understand why it is highly efficacious in extinguishing the Heat of the Body, and why no Salt is more friendly to the Constitution than Nitre. Upon injecting various Liquors into the Veins of Animals, it has been found, that several of them have been kill'd both by acid and alcaline Injections, only with this Difference, that the Acids produced too great a Coagulation, and the Alcalies too great a Fluidity of the Humours. But *Malpighi* informs us, that he injected a Solution of six Ounces of Nitre into the jugular Veins of a strong Dog, without producing any other Change, than a preternaturally copious Discharge of Urine. Hence we may justly conclude, that Nitre is excellently suited, and highly friendly, to the *Crasis* of the Blood : For this Reason Lord *Bacon* affirms, that a Scruple of Nitre frequently exhibited for a Dose, contributes greatly to the Prolongation of Life. Besides, Nitre seems to have a Kind of formal Existence in the human Blood, which, when dried, reduc'd to a Powder, and thrown upon live Coals, produces a Kind of Ebullition like that of Nitre. Nitre, also, prevents Putrefaction in Substances subject to Corruption ; and tho' common Salt is highly efficacious for this Purpose, yet 'tis doubted, whether Nitre is not preferable to it in preserving Bodies. Thus Blood taken from the human Veins, may, by an Admixture of a Solution of Nitre, be for a long Time preserv'd fluid and beautiful, without any Putrefaction. Besides 'tis sufficiently known, that Flesh either by Means of Nitre alone, or Nitre mix'd with common

Salt, for a long Time retains a beautiful red Colour, even after boiling ; the Reason of which seems to be, that this Salt exalts the red and beautiful Colour of the Remainder of the Blood contain'd in the minute Vessels of such Flesh. Hence 'tis obvious, that Nitre resists the Putrefaction, which is often form'd in the *Primæ Viæ*, and diffuses itself thro' the whole Body ; and may for this Reason be exhibited with Success in putrid Fevers, and Disorders of Children arising from Worms. Nitre, taken internally, powerfully promotes the Excretions by Stool, Urine, and Sweat : One Ounce of depurated Nitre, dissolv'd in Water, renders the Body soluble, and procures some Stools, tho' it answers these Intentions better, when mixed with a proper Quantity of the laxative Decoctions of Tamarinds, Sena Leaves, and *Manna*. When the Fluids are to be deriv'd to the inferior Parts of the Body, especially in Fevers, Nitre is highly efficacious. Among all the Class of Diuretics, none are better calculated for quickly removing the Obstructions of the urinary Ducts, rendering the Discharge of the Urine free, and dissolving calculous Concretions, than Nitre. *Penotus* affirms, that if a proper Dose of Nitre is taken once every Fortnight, it never suffers the Generation of Sand in the Kidneys, either in Patients subject to calculous Concretions or Dysuries, whether adult or young, robust or delicate. *Timæus* informs us, that he heard of a certain Man's being perfectly cured of the Gravel, by a long protracted Use of prepared Nitre ; and *Gralingius* informs us, that the *Sal Prunella,* is not only an excellent Preservative against, but also, an efficacious Cure for a *Nephritis* ; and *Hoffman* tells us, he has found from Experience, that an Emulsion of various Seeds, invigorated with Ni-

tre

tre, is with great Succefs exhibited for alleviating nephritic Pains. A proper Exhibition of Nitre renders Perfpiration more free and liberal, in Patients afflicted with immoderate Watchings, Thirft, and intolerable Heat, becaufe it corrects the Heat of the Blood, and checks the hot inteftine Commotions of the Fluids; by which means every Thing in the Conftitution is render'd calm, the preternaturally conftricted Parts are relaxed, and confequently the Blood is freely convey'd to the Emunctories of the Skin. In Practice we daily obferve, that the precipitatieg nitrous Powders excellently promote Sweat, in all Inflammations; but in languid, cold, and cachetic Conftitutions, the moving Force of whofe Mufcles is impair'd, a *Diaphorefis* muft be excited by more hot and active Medicines. Nitre is alfo an excellent Carminative. The Diforders arifing from Flatulencies, ftagnating, and pent up in the Inteftines, fometimes fpafmodically conftricted, are fufficiently obvious to Practitioners; for which Reafon they ought to be diffipated and expell'd with all Expedition. For this Purpofe *Hoffman* afferts, that he has found no Medicine more effectual and fuccefsful than Nitre, either alone, or mix'd with Carminatives; fince by its means, a Difcharge of Wind by the *Anus* is procur'd, the Flatulencies difcover themfelves by their Fluctuation and Noife, and are happily eliminated with an Explofion, which is in *Hoffman's* Opinion, principally owing to a Solution and Relaxation of the conftricted inteftinal Fibres: For which Reafon it is juftly commended in fpafmodic Colics, efpecially that of the bilious Kind, on which the Antients beftow'd the Epithet *hot*. But above all other Medicines, Nitre affords the moft confiderable Relief to hypochondriac and hyfteric Patients, fince it is excellently calculated for removing the Spafms and Flatulencies, which are the Caufe of all the Symptoms incident to fuch Patients. But one of the moft confiderable and important Virtues of Nitre is that by which it refifts Inflammations; for no Diforder is more injurious to the Animal Oeconomy than Inflammations; which in very acute Difeafes generally deftroy the Patient; fince, when they feize the Stomach, they produce Anxieties and Inquietudes; when they affect the *Meninges*, a Pain of the Head, a *Phrenitis*, or Convulfions; and when the Lungs, a Danger of Suffocation: When an Inflammation happens in other Parts, a preternatural Heat of the internal, and an exceffive Coldnefs of the external Parts, is produc'd, whilft, in the mean Time, Inflammations of the fanguiferous *Vifcera* eafily degenerate into Abfceffes or Gangrenes. In order, therefore, to cure the inflam'd Part, Nitre, either alone, or mix'd with a little Camphire, and other Bezoardic Subftances, is, of all other Things, the moft efficacious; fo that, if falutary Effects are not produc'd by it, the Cure may be juftly defpair'd of. In Practice, *Hoffman* fays, he has long ufed fuch a Powder with uncommon Succefs, and found that in Pleurifies, a *Phrenitis*, a Peripneumony, an *Angina*, an Inflammation of the *Oefophagus*, and ftomach, and an *Eryfipelas*, a frequent Exhibition of it has, in a great Meafure, remov'd the Heat, the Pain, the Thirft and Watching, by exciting a gentle Moifture all over the Body, which was before dry and parched: When mix'd with other proper Ingredients, and applied exte-nally, it alfo affords Relief to inflam'd Parts: Thus camphorated Spirit of Wine fo dexteroufly prepar'd, as not to be precipitated by an Affufion of Water, when mix'd with a Solution of N tre and a due Quantity of diftill'd Vinegar, difcuffes an Eryfipelas, and removes an intenfe Head-ach. Befides, Nitre is one of the moft confiderable of thofe Medicines calculated for the Cure of Spafms and Conftrictions, the Misfortunes excited by which, in the nervous Parts of the human Body, are fufficiently apparent to thofe who know Difeafes, and their various Caufes. At leaft 'tis certain, that enormous Hæmorrhages fometimes arife from no other Caufe, than an Inequality of the Circulation of the Blood; fince the Veffels, which in fome Parts are fmaller than in others, being fpafmodically conftricted, the Blood is impetuoufly convey'd to the adjacent Veffels, and their Ramifications, by too much diftending which, and opening their Orifices, violent Hæmorrhages are often produc'd : By this Means, Spittings of Blood, Hæmorrhages of the Nofe, exceffive Evacuations from the Hæmorrhoidal Veins, bloody Urine, and immoderate Difcharges of Blood from the *Uterus,* are produc'd. In the Cure of thefe Diforders, the moft rational Method of proceeding is, to relax the fpafmodically conftricted Parts, and reftore a free and eafy Circulation of the Humours thro' the Veffels. This Intention, as we learn from Experience, is excellently anfwer'd by Nitre, which in thefe Diforders is highly extoll'd by the moft judicious practical Phyficians. Thus *Riverius* extols it in an immoderate Difcharge of the *Lochia* ; in an exceffive Evacuation of the *Menfes* ; in a Spitting of Blood; in Hæmorrhages attended with a malignant Fever ; and for fimilar Purpofes. And as Spafms are frequently the Caufes of a Suppreffion of the ufual Evacuations of Blood from the *Uterus* in Women, fince its conftricted Parts refift the Impulfe of the Blood to the Uterine

Veffels, hence 'tis obvious, that Nitre in fuch a Cafe affords fingular Relief ; for which Reafon *Riverius* recommends it in a Suppreffion of the *Lochia* ; and *Grulingius* in a Diminution of the menftrual Difcharge. As Pains are often the Off-fpring of Spafms, fo thofe terrible Pains, which generally accompany the Excretion of Stones which affect the Inteftines, and are taken for a colical Indifpofition, are happily remov'd by the Ufe of Nitre : And *Welfchius* informs us, that by Nitre alone, a large Number of Soldiers in the *Hungarian* Camp were freed from an epidemical *Cephalalgia.* Though thefe Things are obvious in Practice, and confirmed by Experience, it is, neverthelefs, an additional Satisfaction to the Mind, to know the Reafon why, and the Manner in which, Nitre produces thefe Effects in the human Body.

Ochra, Offic. Yellow Oker. It is an argillaceous Subftance, of a yellow or luteous Colour, and an aftringent Tafte. As to its Virtues; it is drying, aftringent, difcutient, and repreffes Excrefcences. It is very feldom ufed, and never but externally, and that principally in Marks by Blows or Stripes, and in Collifions, and for difcuffing hard Tumours.

Oleum Terræ, Offic. Oil of Earth. This Oil is of two Kinds, the red, and the black : The red is brought from the *Eaft Indies,* and is of a pellucid red Colour, and has a ftrong Smell like *Petroleum,* but more grateful, as *Schroder* fays ; but as to what we know of this Oil, it is either the fame with *Petroleum,* or elfe is unknown in our Shops. The *Indian* Oil of Earth, defcribed by *Nonbovius,* is fcarcely ever brought over to us, but ingroffed by the *Afian* Potentates ; but whether it be a Species of *Petroleum,* or *Naphtha,* is not yet determined. What is brought to us from the *Indies,* and fold for

Oil

)il of Earth, is prepared of expref-
ed Oil of the Cocoa Nut, mixed
with medicated Earths, as *Boerhaave*
fays, he has been informed by a Perfon very fkilfull in thefe Matters,
and therefore wholly belongs to the
Clafs of Vegetables.

Onyx, Offic. The Onyx-ftone.
It is an opake, or not very lucid
Gem, of the Likenefs, Colour, and
fplendor, of the human Nail, being,
at leaft, of two Colours, white and
black, which appear in two diftinct
Zones, and rather opake, than diaphanous. As to its Virtues, it is
idly fuppofed to induceTranquillity of
Mind by compofing the Paffions, and
to quicken the Senfes.

Opalus, Offic. The Opal. This
is a beautiful Gem, of almoft all Colours: According as the Rays of
Light are refracted thro' it, it appears blue, purple, green, yellow,
red, milky, and black; and hence
it has been, by fome called the Gem
of Gems. The beft Opals are found
in *India*, the more ordinary Sort in
Cyprus, *Egypt*, *Hungary*, and in fome
Danifh Iflands. They all grow in a
foft Stone, marked with black or
dark Lines. It is faid to agree in
the fuperftitious Virtues afcribed to
other Gems.

Ophites & Serpentinus, Offic. The
Spleen-ftone, or Ophite. It is a very hardSort of Marble like Porphyry,
of a deep green Colour, interfperfed
with fome fainter Spots of the fame.
But we are told by *Diofcorides*, that
one Species of this Stone is ponde-
ous and black, another Afh-colour-
ed and fpotted, and a third diftinguifhed by white Lines. All of
them worn as Amulets, are whimfically faid to be effectual againft the
Bites of Serpents, and the Head-ach;
that with the white Lines, in particular, is faid to cure the Lethargy,
and Pain of the Head.

Ofteocolla, Offic. The Bone-Binder.
This is a Subftance of a feemingly middle Nature between Earth and Stone,
white, friable, teftaceous, fabulous; in
Figure refembling a Bone, and growing out of fandy Places, and other
ftony Soils: It is highly commended
for the fpeedy Conglutination of
Bones, becaufe it quickly affords
Matter for a proper *Callus*; and
confequently haftens the Conglutination. It alfo ftops the *Fluor Albus*,
and removes intermittent Fevers.
But *Hildanus* juftly cautions us to be
very circumfpect in exhibiting it to
young Perfons furnifhed with a laudable Habit of the Body, becaufe it
generally leaves an unfeemly Scar;
for which Reafon he thinks it is only
to be ufed in old and extenuated Patients, whofe native Heat is weak
and languid. According to *Wormius*, they in fome Shops fell for the
Bone-binder, a Species of the *Galactites*, which is white, porous, fmooth,
foft, eafily diffoluble into a Liquor,
and of a faline Tafte.

Oftracites, Offic. Hobgoblings-
Claw. This is a Foffil, very much
refembling the under Shell of an Oyfter, petrify'd. It is faid to check
the *Menfes* when profufe; to relieve
Inflammations of the Breaft, and
render the Skin fmooth.

Petroleum, Offic. *Petroleum, Oleum de Saxo, Naphtha, Oleum Petræ,*
Mont. Exot. Oil of Peter, or Rock-
Oil. It is a fat liquid Subftance, of
a black Colour, and a ftrong Smell.
There are two Kinds of it; one native, which flows out of Rocks and
Stones; and the other artificial, which
is diftilled from Charcoal and Fof-
fils. Of the Native, they reckon at
Paris two Sorts;

Petroleum rubrum five Gabianum,
Ind. Med. *An Petroleum rufum Schro-
deri.*

Petroleum flavum feu Italicum. Iud.
Med.

The *Bitumen*, or *Petroleum Gabianum*, is efteemed an antihyfteric;
and alfo, good for the Tooth-ach:

It heats and dries, confifts of fine Parts, is a Digeftive and Refolvent, and beneficial to the nervous Syftem. The *Naphtha* of *Dioscorides*, or *Petroleum* of the Shops, is a fubtile, inflammable, mineral Oil, with a fragrant bituminous Smell, of different Colours, either white, yellow, red, or black. Different Names are given it by Authors: The *Babylonians* gave the Name of *Naphtha* to an Oil either black or white, which flowed from fome Fountains near *Babylon*. It was likewife called, *The Oil of Media*, becaufe fhe is faid to have burnt *Creon's Daughter* to Death, by anointing her with this Oil. It had the Name of *Petroleum* becaufe it diftils from Rocks. By *Myrepfus* It is termed *Allicola*; by others, *The Oil of St*. Barbarus *the Abbot, the Oil of St*. Catharine, or *The holy Oil*. The Word *Naphtha* is faid to come from a Word which fignifies, to light, or kindle. There are few Countries in which this Oil is not to be found. In the Ifland of *Sames* a Kind of it is gathered, called by the Inhabitants by a Name which fignifies *Oleum Terræ*, and it is in great Efteem among the *Indians*. In *Italy*, near *Medena*, the Oil is gathered from Springs and Wells; and indeed this whole Dutchy abounds with it, efpecially a Place called *Fraimetio*. The Inhabitants dig Wells to the Depth of thirty or forty Feet, till the oily Spring is found; and there it is always mixed with the Water. The Wells dug at the Foot of the Hill furnifh a large Quantity of very red Oil; thofe near the Top, a white Oil, but in fmaller Quantities. There is another Rock in the fame Country near the *Apennine* Hills, where there is a perpetual Spring of Water, on which this Oil fwims, of a yellow Colour, and in fo great Quantities, that twice a Week they gather fix Pounds at a Time. *Petroleum* is found alfo in *France*; and

particularly in *Britany*, near *Beriers* and red Oil, mixed with Water. flows from the Crannies of fome Rocks, which is collected with great Care, being no Way inferior to the reft in Virtue. There is another fuch Fountain near *Clermont*, in *Auvergne*. *Petroleum* eafily takes Fire; and it is the Cuftom in many Places, to burn it in Lamps, inftead of common Oil. It is plentifully ftored with fine volatile Parts, which eafily evaporate, and are fo greedy of Fire, that if a lighted Torch, or any other flaming Body, be held in the Wells or Fountains of *Petroleum*, the exhaling *Effluvia* very often take Fire. It is difficultly mixed with Spirit of Wine. By Diftillation, it yields an oily Liquor, fomething more pellucid than before; but it lofes a great deal of its native Smell, and gives a more languid and fuliginous Flame. A fmall Quantity of a yellowifh *Magma* remains at the Bottom of the Alembic; therefore it is evident, that *Petroleum* is not meliorated by Diftillation. The beft *Petroleum* is reckoned that which is frefh gathered, of a fubtile, bituminous Smell, white, and pellucid; next to that is the yellow, then the red; but the black is accounted the moft impure of all. *Dioscorides* commends it in Suffufions, and Dimnefs of the Eyes. The *Petroleum* of *Britany* is given, a few Drops at a time, with great Succefs, in what is called a Suffocation of the *Uterus*, and to kill Worms in Children. It is proper in a Suppreffion of the *Menfes*, taken in the Quantity of twenty five Drops, or the Region of the *Pubes* being anointed with it. In a Palfy, accompanied with cold Pains in the nervous Parts, the Part affected is anointed with it. *Lufitanius* commends the Ufe of it in ftopping the Progrefs of a *Scirrhus*.

Piffafphaltus. See *Bitumen.*

Piffelæum Indicum, Offic. Barbadoes Tar. This is a Sort of *Bitumen*, found

und floating upon the Surface of
Lake in *Barbadoes*, at the Bottom
which it probably tranfudes out
the Earth. It is of a blackifh
olour inclinable to red, of a ftrong
nell, and of the Confiftence of
mmon Tar. It is a very good
ectoral, Stomachic, and Sudorific,
d hence is good in Coughs; it is
fo fometimes apply'd to Burns,
alds, and Inflammations, and is
id to be a good Remedy for a Scald
ead, and it is fometimes apply'd
the Soles of the Feet, and the
rifts, in order to cure an Ague.
octor *Towne*, in his Treatife on the
ifeafes of the *Weft Indies* reprefents
arbadoes *Tar*, given in the Quantity
two Drams, three times a Day, as
excellent Medicine in the *Colica
Bonum*, or dry Belly-ach, after the
in has been fomewhat mitigated by
evious Evacuations; and he furer tells us, that upon the very firft
ppearance of a tingling Uneafinefs
ong the Spine; the Fore-runner of
Palfy, generally fucceeding this
iftemper, an Embrocation of this
ar, with double diftill'd Rum, well
b'd into the whole Length of the
ine, and into the Limbs, will pre-
nt the impending Palfy, if any
ing can.

Plumbago, Worm. *Molybdæna,*
Plumbago faÏitia, Offic. Plumb-
e. This is that Recrement, which,
the Purification of Gold and Sil-
r with Lead, being concreted and
lcin'd, adheres to the Furnace.
s fuperior Part refembles Litharge,
inferior Afhes, and its middle is
Subftance compounded of both.
agrees in Virtues with Litharge,
nd is fomewhat cold, tho' at the
me Time, not poffefs'd of an a-
ringent Quality.

Plumbum, Offic. *Plumbum Saturnus*, Mont. Exot. Lead. Both
its crude State, and in all its Pre-
arations, Lead feems to be cooling,
hickening, repelling, abforbing, and

contracting, fo as to retard the Circulation of the Blood, hinder all the
Secretions, and injure the Nerves, by
caufing Spafms, Convulfions, Tremblings, Difficulty of Breathing, and
Suffocation. Whence it appears unfit for internal Ufe in any large Dofe,
or even in any at all; and accordingly its Medicinal Ufes are principally external. A Plate of Lead is
efteem'd a very good Application to
Ganglions, a Species of Tumor, often
appearing about the Wrifts, and Backs
of the Hand; and in Cancers, Lead
and its Preparations, externally apply'd, are efteem'd excellent. I have
known great Mifchief done, by the
internal Ufe of Sugar of Lead.
Ceruffa, or *Sandix*, White Lead,
is prepared by fufpending Plates of
Lead, in fuch a Manner as to receive
the Vapour of Vinegar, till it is corroded. This is only ufed externally;
and agrees in Virtues with Litharge.

Plumbum nigrum, Offic. Black
Lead, Wadt, Kello. This is accounted refrigerating, drying, and
repellent; and is fometimes applied
to ftrumous and cold œdematous Tumours.

Pnigites, Offic. Black Earth. It
is a fat, denfe, foft, black, aftringent,
and very acrimonious Subftance, of
the Tafte of Vitriol. To thefe
Marks, *Diofcorides* adds, that its Colour fomewhat refembles the *Eretria
Terra*, is cold to the Touch, and fo
glutinous as to adhere to the Tongue.
The fame Author fays, that it has
the fame Virtues as the *Cimolia*, only
is weaker: Some, he fays, fell it for
Eretria Terra.

Pompholyx, *Nil Album*, Offic.
This is a Metallic Powder, of a white
Colour, and lighter than *Tutty*; for
as that, in the making of Brafs, adheres to the Sides of the Furnace;
this mounts up to the Top. It is
very much efteem'd for Diforders of
the Eyes, and in general agrees in
Virtues with *Tutty*.

Por-

Porphyrites, Offic. Porphyry, or red Marble. This is a Species of Marble highly hard, and of a red Colour, it is brought to us from the Confines of *Egypt*, the Red Sea, and *Ethiopia*. It is thought to be possess'd of a lithontriptic Quality, and to agree in Virtues with the *Ophites*.

Prasius, Offic. The Green Stone. It is green for the greatest Part of it, but is seldom without black, and sometimes white Spots. Many take it for the Mother of the Emerald, because this Gem is sometimes found in it. It agrees in Virtues with the Emerald, but in a lower Degree.

Pumex, Offic. The Pumice Stone. This is a porous and spongious Stone, full of small Cavities and Perforations, and found in *Germany*, whence it is transported to us. It is of a refrigerating, drying, and extenuating Quality. It gently cleanses Ulcers, and render Cicatrices full and seemly. In Mount *Vesuvius*, *Ætna*, and other burning Mountains, large Quantities of this Species of Stone are found with the Sulphur.

Pyrites, Offic. *Marchasita*. Fire Stones. They are found in almost all Mines, being the most fruitful Matrix of almost all Metals, Salts, and Sulphurs; for it is not purely a Stone, but seems to be the most fertile of all Minerals. There are great Varieties of it, with Respect to Colour, Figure, Mixture with Metals, Stones and other Fossils, for it enters in various Proportions the Composition of Iron, Lead, Tin, Silver, Copper, and Alum, and also that of black Flints, Pit-Coal, Lime-Stones, Chalk-Stones, and others. The *Pyrites*, whether crude or burnt, is of an heating and abstersive Quality. It deterges such Things as darken the Sight, and concocts and discusses Hardnesses. Made into a Plaister with Rosin, it represses Excrescencies of the Flesh, by some-

what of an heating, join'd with an astringent Quality.

Rubinus, *Carbunculus*, Offic. The Ruby. This is a glittering diaphonous Gem, of a red Colour, and Proof against the File; the most beautiful are found in the Island of *Ceylon*. As to its Virtues, it is said to be a Preservative against the Pestilence, expels Sadness, restrains lascivious and evil Thoughts, prevents frightful Dreams, exhilarates the Mind, and preserves the Body in Health; but all these Virtues are entirely superstitious.

Rubrica Fabrilis. Offic. Red Oker, Ruddle, Marking Stone. This is an earthy, ponderous, and intensly red Substance, found in many Parts of *England*, and is used in vulnerary and drying Plaisters.

Rubrica Sinopica, Offic. Earth of Sinope. This ought to be thick, heavy, and all of one Colour, resembling Liver, and when diluted with Water, it ought to diffuse itself therein. It is dug out of the Earth in *Cappadocia*, is esteemed drying, and is said to restrain a Diarrhœa.

Sal. Salt. Salt is defined by *Geoffroy*, to be a solid, friable, pellucid, and sapid Mineral Body, dissoluble in Water, fusible by Fire, and easily concrescible in Form of Crystals. This Definition agrees to alimentary Salt, Nitre, Vitriol, Alum, *Sal Ammoniac*, and Borax. But by Salt, common alimentary Salt is generally understood, which is of three Kinds, that is, first, fossile Salt, of which what is transparent, or pellucid like Crystal, is called *Sal Gem*. Secondly, Salt obtain'd by the Evaporation of Sea Water, which is brought about, either by the Heat of the Sun, or by means of Fire. Thirdly, Salt obtain'd by the Evaporation of the Water of Salt Springs by Fire. Fossile Salt is got in great Quantities, in many Parts of the World, particularly in the

Moun-

ountains of *Catalonia*, and at *Vi-
ke* and *Bochna* near *Crackow* in
land, where there are prodigious
ines of Salt. *Sal Gem* is princi-
lly ufed in Clyfters, and Suppofi-
ries, in order to ftimulate the In-
tines to a Difcharge of their Con-
nts. In *Britany* in *France*, the
anner of making Sea Salt, is to
g fhallow broad Trenches, which
e lined with Clay. Thefe being
led with Sea Water by the Tide,
e Heat of the Sun evaporates the
ater, and a large Proportion of
lt remains behind. In *Normandy*
ey make fmall Heaps of Sand upon
e Shore, which imbibe the Sea
ater, and the infipid Humidity
ing afterwards evaporated by the
eat of the Sun, the Salt remains
nong the Sand. To feparate it,
ey firft boil it in frefh Water, and
en having ftrain'd off the *Lixivium*,
ntaining now only a Solution of
lt in frefh Water, they boil it
ain with a gentle Heat in leaden
auldrons, to a certain Degree of
hicknefs; then putting out the
ire, the Salt cryftallizes. Salt is
ade from Salt Fountains alfo, by
iling the Water till the Humidity
hales; and whilft it is boiling.
ey mix with it either Gall, or
ullock's Blood, which makes the
lt form itfelf more eafily into larger
umps; for the Parts of the Gall
· Blood, invifcate or intangle the
ituminous or earthy Parts, which
inder the Concretion of the Salt,
d are altogether thrown up as a
cum, or at leaft remain in the
rainers. But at *Droit-Wych* in
befbire, they add nothing to the
lt Water, during Coction. Sea
lt prepared by the Heat of the
un, is preferable to both, for culi-
ary and officinal Ufes. The Tafte
f it is well known; the Colour is
reyifh, becaufe of the Particles of
arth mixed with it; but if it be
iffolved and cryftallized by a gentle

Heat, it is formed into very white
cubical Grains. Salt made by boiling is white, but the Grains thereof
are not exactly cubical, becaufe of
fome Mixture of different Salts. By
the *Analyfis* of Salt, it appears that
common Salt confifts of a pure infipid Earth, an acid Spirit extremely
volatile; and Water; and it is highly probable that this Earth, before
it was united to the acid volatile
Spirit, was of an alcaline Nature,
and perhaps exactly the fame with
the *Natron* of the Ancients. What
makes this the more likely is, that
if any fixed alcaline Salt is impregnated with the acid Spirit of common Salt, a Salt will be formed
very nearly the fame with common
Salt, which the Chymifts call regenerated Salt. Common Salt has
many very extraordinary Properties.
(1) The fmalleft Cryftals of common
Salt are always of a cubic Figure,
that is, the Figure of a Dye. (2)
Upon the Application of Fire to it,
it crackles. This Decrepitation or
Crackling of Salt, feems to proceed
from the Air contained in its Pores,
which being rarify'd by the Fire,
breaks its Prifon and makes its E-
fcape. (3) Spirit of Salt is the
only Thing in Nature that will diffolve Gold; but not without being
joined with the Spirit of Nitre. (4)
Salt preferves all Vegetable and A-
nimal Subftances from Putrefaction,
as alfo Water, and is itfelf incor-
ruptible. This Property it entirely
owes to the Acid it contains. (5) A
greater Quantity of common Salt
will be diffolved in a given Quantity
of Water, than of any other Salt
whatever; for fix Ounces of common Salt may be diffolved in fixteen
of Water, but it muft be obferved,
that warm Water will diffolve more
Salt than cold, and that in Proportion to the Heat of the Water. This
Water in that Degree of Heat which
makes it boil, diffolves more Salt
than

than in any less Degree of Heat, infomuch, that as it grows cool, it will every Moment let fall more and more of the Salt which was diffolved in it, which will appear at the Bottom of the containing Veffel undiffolved; and when the Water is fo cold as to freeze, it will expel almoft all the Salt, which will ftick to the Bottom of the Ice in a folid Form. (6) Salt diffolved in Water, in a Heat equal to that of the Atmofphere, renders the Water confiderably colder. And yet, (8) notwithftanding this Increafe of Coldnefs, the Salt will keep the Water from freezing, infomuch that Water, wherein Salt is diffolved fhall not freeze near fo foon as pure Water: And hence we may obferve, that Salt, when interpofed between the fmall Particles of Water, has the Power of preventing their Affociation, that is, their Concretion into Ice; otherwife Salt, by increafing Cold, would promote freezing. (8) If Spirit of Salt is poured upon Ice reduced to Powder, it will increafe the Coldnefs thereof to a furprifing Degree; to a Degree much greater than ever was produced naturally, and in which every Animal muft die. (9) Salt thrown upon burning Coals, greatly increafes their Heat. This proceeds from the Air, Water, and Acid contained in the Body of the Salt; for the Air being forced out of the Salt by Heat, acts upon the Fuel like a Pair of Bellows; and that this will increafe the Heat of the Fire is known to all Smiths, who, when they would make their Fires intenfely hot, frequently fprinkle Water upon the burning Coals, (10) Salt made extremely dry, attracts the Moifture of the Air confiderably, even in the dryeft Seafons, infomuch that it is a common Thing for People who deal in Salt, to buy it at the *Wyches* very dry, and fo fell it a great many Miles diftant, for

lefs *per* Hundred, than it coft them; yet are they confiderable Gainers, becaufe the fame Quantity of Salt that weighs a Hundred at the *Wyches*, will be much heavier, after having imbibed the Moifture of the Air. The Virtues of Alimentary Salt are many, for firft as it is an excellent Prefervative againft Putrefaction, whenever any Aliments of an alcalefcent or alcaline Nature, or inclin'd to Putrefaction, are taken into the Stomach, in Quantities difproportion'd to the Powers of Digeftion, Salt by preventing Putrefaction, will guard againft thofe Mifchiefs, which would arife from fuch a Putrefaction of the Aliments in the Stomach; that is, what is ufually called a Surfeit; and by its *Stimulus*, will contribute much towards the carrying off the offending Matter, by Stool. On the other Hand, as Salt remarkably checks too great Fermentation, it will have a very good Effect, when fermentable Subftances are taken into the Stomach in too large Quantities, and by their Fermentation excite Flatulencies, Spafms, and Diftentions, and at the fame time ftimulates the alimentary Tube, to a Difcharge of its Contents. It likewife calms the too great Ebullition of the Fluids of the Body; and, as it readily joins with volatile urinous Salts, and changes them into a *Sal Ammoniac*, it is fitted to foften the Acrimony of the Fluids, and promote the Depuration thereof by Urine. By its little Points it likewife ftimulates gently the folid Parts, and thereby increafes their ofcillatory Motion, by which Means all the Functions of the Body are better perform'd. On thefe Foundations are built all the Virtues afcribed to Sea Salt, of drying, heating, deterging, digefting, opening, attenuating, increafing the Appetite, exciting to Venery, and of refifting Poifons and Putrefaction.

It

order'd in an *Apepfia*, want of
eftion, in want of Appetite, in
ivenefs, and Obftructions of U-

It has been obferv'd, that thofe
live for any long Time upon
h or Fifh, harden'd by Salt,
: been extremely afflicted with the
vy, fo that Salt is univerfally
ight to caufe the Scurvy, but late
:rvations have taught us, that
is fo far from being concerned in
Generation of the Scurvy, that
on the contrary an excellent Pre-
ative againft, and Cure for it, if
n in very confiderable Quanti-

Hence I fhould rather afcribe
fcorbutic Complaints thofe are
:ct to, who live on falt Provi-
i, to the Hardnefs, and confe-
it Indigeftibility of falted Ali-
ts; for Salt hardens, for the very
: Reafon that it prevents Putre-
on. Befides, as no Flefh or Fifh
be fo perfectly falted, but that
: Particles of it will be putrid
ng kept, thefe putrid Particles,
n mix'd with the Blood and Juices,
have a great Influence in exciting
: Diforders, which we errone-
y afcribe to Salt.

ppbirus, Offic. The Sapphire.
: is called by fome the Gem of
is, and is a hard Stone of a blue
)ur, like that of the clear Sky. It
es neareft the Diamond in Splen-
Tranfparency, and Hardnefs,
is of two Kinds; one pale,
d the Female Sapphire; the o-
of a deeper blue, called the
e. There is a third Sort, like-
, which has no Colour at all,
is fometimes made to pafs for a
nond, but it is neither fo hard,
'o brilliant. Sapphires are brought
I different Parts of the *Eaft-In*-
and are thence called *Oriental*.
reft are found in *Silefia* and *Bo*-
a, called *Occidental*. The Co-
of Sapphire may be taken out
Fire, and then it looks like a
nond; for which Reafon *Geoffroy*

believes this Colour to come from a
fmall Mixture of fine Sulphur of
Copper. Many are the ineftimable
Qualities fuperftitioufly afcrib'd to
this Stone; but, befides thefe, we
are told that it raifes and exhilarates
the Spirits, refifts Poifon, and cures
Ulcers of the Inteftines. *Schroder*
informs us, that it is of a cold and
dry Quality, aftringent; confolidating, alexipharmic, cordial, and ophthalmic.

Sardus, *Sarda*, *Carneolus*, Offic.
Sardius Lapis, Schrod. The Cornelian. It is a precious Stone, half
tranfparent, and like the Wafhings
of Flefh, or bloody Flefh; it is found
in *Sardinia*. The Powder is prefcribed to be drank in all manner of
Hæmorrhages; being worn, it is fuperftitioufly faid to exhilarate the
Heart, expel Fear, confer Boldnefs, a-
vert Fafcination, defend the Body a-
gainft all manner of Poifons, and by a
peculiar Property, to ftop Bleeding in
any Part of the Body; and ty'd about
the Belly, to prevent Mifcarriage.

Selenites, Offic. *Cryftallus Calca-
ria*, Mont. Exot. The Selenite.
This is a rhomboidal, pellucid Foffil,
divifible into thin *Laminæ*. It is found
in many Places, particularly near
Epfom Wells in *Surry*. It is faid to
agree in Virtues with the *Teftacea*, to
be a Sweetner of the Blood, and to
reftrain Hæmorrhages. Externally
it is ufed as a Cofmetic.

Silex, Offic. The Flint. According to *Schroder* Flints may be
ufed internally for inciding tartarous
Mucilage, refolving the Stone, and
opening Obftructions. They are,
alfo us'd as Dentrifices.

Smaragdus, Offic. The Smaragd,
or Emerald. This is a green diaphanous, fhining Gem, very pleafant to the Sight, but exceffively
brittle, which has given Occafion to
many Stories. It is divided into
oriental and occidental. The oriental is the beft in all Refpects. The
other

Other which comes from *Peru*, is not near so bright, and besides has generally some foul Spots. There is a third Kind of Emerald, or *Pseudo Smaragdus*, found in the Mountains of *Switzerland* and *Auvergne*, which is extremely tender, and of the palest green. Fragments of Emerald thrown upon a clear Fire, emit a fine Flame, and totally lose their Colour. which is a Proof sufficient that this Gem contains some Sulphur of Copper. Besides the superstitious Uses ascrib'd to it, it is said to stop Fluxes of all Kinds.

Smyris & Smerillus, Offic. Emery. It is a ferruginous, heavy, metallic, Substance, of a Colour inclining to black, and so hard, that Lapidaries use it in cutting and polishing their Diamonds, and Smiths to polish their Iron and Steel. *Emery* is of three Kinds ; the common, which is blackish, and very much used, is found in many Parts of *Europe*, especially in an Island on the Coast of *Tuscany*; and in *Guernsey* in the *British* Channel. The second is a hard uneven Sort, of a reddish Colour, like Bloodstone or Oker, but does not stain the Hands. This is by some reckon'd among the Blood-stones. The third is of a blackish red Colour, streak'd with Gold colour'd Veins. It is found in the Gold Mines of *Peru*, and really contains Gold This Kind is thought by Chymists to be a Gold Ore, or rather a Sort of immature or imperfect Gold ; and therefore they esteem it very much, and extract a Tincture from it with Spirit of Sea Salt, with which they fix Mercury in an Instant, and give this Substance the Name of the miraculous Precipitate, because they fancy they shall at Length attain the true Art of making Gold, by means thereof. *Emery* is recommended by *Dioscorides* and *Galen* as a Dentrifice ; but it corrodes the Teeth too much, and insensibly wears them away.

Sory. This is already taken Notice of under the Article *Chalcitis.*

Spodium Græcorum, *Nihil Gryseum*, Offic. Putty. This is the Ashes, or rather the metallic Flour, collected in the Furnaces and Shops of Copper Smiths, and differs from the *Pompholyx* in being more heavy, and not so pure. This is never given inwardly, but was sometimes applied externally. It is said to agree in Virtues with the *Pompholyx.*

Stannum. Offic. Tin. It is seldom used in Medicine internally, tho' its Virtues are highly extolled by some, particularly in Diseases of the Head, the Lungs and *Uterus*, the Falling Sickness, and the Bite of a mad Dog. It has been taken in crude Filings, to the Quantity of twenty Grains, or more, for some time, without Harm. It is reckon'd a good Remedy for the Worms.

Succinum & Carabe, Offic. Amber. We learn from *Frederic Hofman*, that Amber is produced plentifully in *Prussia*, which is famous for being the proper and native Country of it. Tho' this Bitumen be generated in the Earth, there is Plenty of it found in the *Baltic* Sea, by the Shore of *Ludwic*, where it swims on the Water, and is carried along by the Waves, whence it is taken up in Nets. The Places most remarkable for Amber, are the Villages of *Fisch hausen*, *Gross-ducstein*, *Weruichen*, and *Palmoniet*. Nor even is this Amber produced from the Sea, but in tempestuous Agitations of the Waters, is washed out of the Bowels of the Earth by the Waves, and at last thrown towards the Shores. Very properly then may this bituminous Body be reckon'd in the Class of Minerals ; for it is a Product of the Earth, and is contained within its proper Veins, as well as Pit-Coal, or other Minerals. The Courses of these Veins were discovered some Years ago, by Order of King *Frederic*

, in the following Manner. In
ing they firſt met with Sand,
h being removed, the next Thing
offered, was a *Stratum* of white
; digging under this they open
ligneous *Stratum*, that ſeemed to
ompacted of old Wood, which,
ever, could be ſet on Flame.
ler the Bottom of this *Stratum* in
t Parts, they found Ore of Vitri-
which being expoſed to the open
, ſhot forth into Flowers of Vi-
l, free from the leaſt Tincture of
per, and like thoſe which proceed
n the *Heſſian* Iron Ore. At laſt
ing ſtill deeper, they came upon
tatum of Sand; out of which in
ral Places, with convenient In-
ments, they extracted Abundance
hoice Amber. For it is a Thing
rthy Obſervation, that Sand is u-
lly the *Matrix* of Amber; ſo
t where they find a great Bed of
d in the Boſom of the Earth,
y are not without Hopes of meet-
with Amber. After the ſame
nner do they get it out of the
rcaſite, near *Kuſtrin*; and in the
rritories of *Stolpen* and *Dantzic*,
is alſo found in Lumps. Hence
ears the Falſity of the old Fable,
ich would have us believe, that
aber is the Reſin of Trees, which
tils from their Bark into the Sea,
l is there digeſted by the Heat of
Sun into a Body of that Kind.
e Manner in which this Bitumen
generated, ſeems to be this: From
t bituminous foſſile Wood, which
juſt now mentioned, by the Action of the ſubterranean Heat,
re diſtils an Oil much like *Naph-*
a, or *Petroleum*, which in pene-
ting the ſubjacent *Strata*, paſſes
ro' the Vitriol Ores, where by
xing with its Acid, it is coagulat-
into a Subſtance of a reſinous
rm. The Reaſonableneſs of this
pinion will appear from the follow-
g Conſiderations: 1. That Amber
its firſt Growth was liquid, may

be proved from its being often ſeen
conglobated by Nature itſelf into a
round Form. 2. Sometimes Inſects
of various Kinds ſtick and are included in Pieces of Amber, which
they could never have been, if the
Matter in which they are circum-
volved, had not been liquid. 3. We
may conclude, that Amber is a Concretion of an Oil much like *Petrole-*
um, becauſe Oil of Amber comes
near to *Petroleum*, both in Smell
and Virtue, and both of them are
equally difficult to be diſſolved by
the moſt rectified Spirit. 4. *Charl-*
ton, a very ſagacious Obſerver of
Nature, affirms, that Pieces of this
Bitumen have been frequently found,
which hold *Naphtha* and *Petroleum*
included within them. 5. The a-
cid Salt of Amber is of a very fixed Nature, and not inferior in Virtue to the Acid of Vitriol. 6.
What will afford great Light in
this Affair, is that phyſical Experiment, in which it is obſerved, that
all diſtilled Oils, ſcarce one excepted, and amongſt them aromatic Oils,
being mixed with Oil of Vitriol,
or pretty ſtrong *Aqua fortis*, con-
denſe into a reſiniform Maſs, which,
held to the Fire, is readily ſet on
Flame. 7. Beſides foſſile Woods and
Coals, by Diſtillation and Rectification, yield an Oil, very like Oil of
Amber and *Petroleum*. 8. Laſtly,
The very Diſpoſition of the *Strata*,
which we have related, is a good
Proof in this Matter. The firſt of
theſe is ligneous, the ſecond vitriolic,
and the laſt compoſed of Sand, at the
Bottom of which lies the Amber,
ſcattered here and there in Bits.
There is moſt Plenty of Amber along
the Shore of the *Sudwic* Sea, eſpecially when a tempeſtuous North
Wind blows; for it ſeems probable,
that the Sea penetrating by ſome ſe-
cret Paſſages into thoſe ſubterranean
Places, where the Amber is nouriſh-
ed, by violent daſhing and breakin

againſt them, feparate from Time to Time Pieces of this Bitumen; and carry them away with it. Amber is of various Colours; the beſt is reckoned the pellucid, quite free from Spots, and which bears the higheſt Price. For this the *Chineſe* give its Weight in Gold, and make their Idols of it after an elegant and maſter-like Manner. I lately faw, fays *Hoffman,* a convex burning *Speculum,* made of this pellucid Amber, in the Manner of one made of Glaſs, which the *Landgrave* of *Heſſe* keeps in his Cabinet of Curioſities. Next to the Pellucid is the White, after that the Yellow, and laſtly, the Brown, which is the worſt Amber of all. No leſs various are the Prices; for the larger and purer, fo much the dearer are the Pieces; and the more pellucid they are, the more are they valued. They talk much of a black Sort of Amber, which yet is no where to be met with, and fo is only believed upon common Report. Inſtead of this, they fell a black and folid Foſſile, which is a kind of *Aſphaltum;* and dug out of the Coal-Mines in *England,* and made into feveral Utenfils for the Uſe of the Inhabitants. Many great Virtues are aſcribed to Amber, efpecially when taken inwardly, in a cold State of the Brain, and in Catarrhs, in the Head-Ach, fleepy and convulſive Diforders, in a Suppreſſion of the *Menſes,* hyſterical and hypochondriacal Affections, in a *Gonorrhæa, Fluor Albus,* and Hæmorrhages. The Doſe is from a Scruple to a Dram, in a poached Egg, or any other proper Vehicle externally. Amber is uſed as a Fumigation, in Cataplaſms, and *Cucuphæ,* in Diforders of the Head or Brain. The Fumes of it, received at the Mouth, are often found fucceſsful in beginning Quinſeys, a falling down of the *Uvula,* or Swelling of the Tonfils from a Catarrh.

Sulphur. The Sulphur of the Shops; called · Ѳ in *Greek,* becauſe uſed in all expiatory and other facred Rites, is a mineral, concreted Juice, folid, dry, friable, fufible by Fire, and very eaſily inflammable. The Flame it emits is blue, and the Smell of burning Sulphur is ſtrong, fubtile, acid, and very prejudicial to the Lungs. Sulphur is of various Kinds; it is in the firſt Place divided into ἀπυρον, or native Sulphur, which has never been expoſed to the Fire; and ἐμπυρόμενον, or factitious Sulphur, prepared by Fire. It is either of a yellow, yellowiſh Aſh, or light Colour, and either pure or impure in Subſtance. Native Sulphur is of two Kinds; one pellucid, and ſhining like Gold, and either of a citrine or greeniſh Colour. This is found about the Gold Mines in *Peru* in *Switzerland;* and many other Places. The other opake, found either in hard, folid, ſhining, greeniſh, or yellow Lumps, or in Form of a clayiſh Glebe, of a light Aſh Colour, or yellow. This Kind is dug near all the burning Mountains, near fome fulphureous Springs, and in feveral other Places of *Europe* and *America.* Factitious Sulphur is prepared in different Manners. In fome Places it is obtain'd by boiling of Water; and at *Buda* in *Hungary,* according to *Agricola,* it is evaporated with the Water of the Mineral Springs, and concretes in the Covering or Dome of theſe Fountains, like the Flower of Brimſtone, and is gather'd from thence, once every Year, with great Care. It is alfo extracted from a Sort of Aſh-colour'd argillaceous Earth. Thus in fome Places of *Italy,* there are Mines, out of which a fat, white, argillaceous Earth is dug, mixed with fome blackiſh Veins; and this Earth being put into very capacious Veſſels, and diſtill'd, the melted Sulphur runs out at the *Roſtrum* of the Alembic into a Receiver, where it foon concretes into large Lumps.

Aſ

After the Diſtillation is over, a red Earth remains, which is thrown away as uſeleſs. Sulphur is alſo, often extracted from a Kind of *Pyrites*, eſpecially near *Liege*, where there is a Kind of *Pyrites* like Lead Ore, which being dug up, is broken into ſmall Pieces, and then thrown into very large Crucibles, or rather earthen Cucurbits of a quadrilateral Figure, with a narrow Orifice; Theſe Veſſels are placed in proper Furnaces, or an inclined Poſition, where the Sulphur contained in theſe Stones, being melted by the Fire, runs into Leaden Veſſels filled to a certain Height with Water, where it conretes immediately, the Subſtance which remains in the Cucurbit containing a large Portion of Vitriol. If by this firſt Operation, the Sulphur be not ſufficiently pure and clean, is melted a ſecond Time in Iron Veſſels, and boiled with the Addition of a certain Quantity of Linſeed Oil; afterwards it is made up, either in large Lumps, or is thrown into hollow Cylinders of Iron, rubbed over with Oil on the Inſide, and ſo is formed into Rolls: Sulphur ſo prepared is called Brimſtone, or common Sulphur, and is of two Kinds, yellow, or greeniſh, which laſt is preferr'd for the Extraction of Oils of Sulphurs from other Bodies, as containing the greateſt Quantity of vitriolic Salt. *Dioſcorides* informs us, that Sulphur is good in Coughs, when mixed with an Egg; and *Hippocrates* uſed it in hyſterical Affections accompanied with Coughing, by way of Fumigation, ſometimes alone, and ſometimes mixed with other Subſtances. The internal Uſe of Sulphur is recommended by Phyſicians in Diſeaſes of the Lungs, of which it is, by way of Eminence, termed the Balſam; becauſe it promotes Expectoration, and clears and ſtrengthens that Organ, and is therefore very beneficial in a *Phthiſis*, *Aſthma*, and

Catarrh. It has in all Ages been a famous Medicine in cutaneous Diſeaſes, Scabs and *Pſoræ*, uſed inwardly, or outwardly. Externally apply'd it diſcuſſes hard Tumors, ripens and digeſts Buboes; but no Medicine prepared with Sulphur is thought to be agreeable to Women with Child, becauſe it is ſubject to cauſe Abortion. Inwardly taken it is laxative, and promotes inſenſible Perſpiration, as may be perceived by the ſulphureous Smell of ſuch Perſons as have taken it, and by the browniſh or black Colour which it gives to the Gold or Silver they carry about them. It is therefore very quickly and readily diffuſed through the whole Body, and by its balſamic Parts, it blunts and entangles the acrid Salts, with which the Fluids abound in theſe Diſeaſes; and by its native, mild, ſoft, and oily Qualities, it readily cures ſmall Ulcers in the Lungs and Skin. Though Sulphur may be given inwardly, even in a groſs Powder, yet it is ſeldom order'd without ſome Preparation. It may be purify'd different Ways; ſome put it into Water with melted Wax, which ſwims at the Top while the Sulphur falls to the Bottom; and by repeating this Mixture till the Sulphur begins to acquire a red Colour, it is then thought to be more defecated. Some boil it in Water for ſeveral Days, changing the Water every now and then, and afterwards they ſet it for two Hours in hot Smoke, that ſome Fumes may exhale, and the remaining pale yellowiſh Sulphur they judge to be very pure. Others make Milks and Magiſteries of Sulphur, which they think much preferable to common Sulphur; but all theſe Preparations either change the true Nature of Sulphur, or elſe are of no Effect at all. The beſt Way to purify it, is by Sublimation, or the Reduction of it to Flowers, by which common Me-

tho

thod it is freed from the earthy or metallic Parts that may have been mixed with it. If taken crude into the Body, by fmall Dofes frequently repeated, it wonderfully cleanfes the firft Paffages, at length purges ftrongly, and then effectually cures certain cutaneous Difeafes, and fuch as proceed from Worms, or Mercurial Fumes.

Talcum, Offic. Talc. This is a fhining fiffile Stone, eafily divifible into very thin pellucid *Laminæ,* a little flexible. In the Fire it does not melt, is not calcin'd, nor does it lofe its Colour. Some Talc is of a Silver Colour, called by the Chymifts *Argyrolithos;* fome yellow, called folar Talc; fome greenifh, and fome black. That which is brought from *Venice* is reputed the beft, and is of a light green Colour. This Stone is feldom ufed in Phyfic, but it is very much in Vogue as a Cofmetic, the Ladies being of Opinion, that it cleanfes and whitens the Skin. Some Chymifts have endeavour'd, by the the Oil of Talc, to fix Quickfilver, and afterwards convert it into Silver, but they never confider'd, that what they called Oil of Talc, was intirely the Product of the other Subftances mixed with it.

Terra Japonica, Offic. Japan Earth. This is a gummy, indurated Subftance of a reddifh Colour, inclining to black; of an aftringent and auftere Tafte at firft, but afterwards fweet and grateful, and void of Smell. There are two Sorts of it; one purer, which, flightly tafted, melts, as it were, on the Tongue; the other harder, and lefs pure, and confequently of but little Ufe; and this perhaps led *Schroder* into an Error to miftake it for an Earth. The Learned are not agreed about the exotic Drug called *Terra Japonica,* and *Catechu,* or *Caetchu:* Some, who take it for a true and genuine Species of Earth, as its Name imports,

rank it among Minerals; others will have it to be a compound Subftance, participating of a vitriolic Nature; and others there are, who, and indeed rightly, reckon it in the Clafs of Vegetable Subftances, and take it for an infpiffated Juice. This *Catechu* is eafily diffolved in Water, incorporates with it, and communicates to it a red Tincture, as do many other Vegetable infpiffated Juices and Extracts: Befides, it is not feparated by Filtration, as Earths ufually are; but paffes the Filtre with the Water, and is, moreover, by Calcination, perfectly converted into Afhes, which Earths are not. That it participates not of a vitriolic Nature, will abundantly appear from the following Experiments: The firft is, that no vitriolic Salt can be feparated from it. Secondly, The Mixture of an Alcali with it excites or produces not the leaft Effervefcence or Precipitation. And laftly, a Solution of the fame, with the Addition of any Kind of vitriolic Subftance becomes an Ink. *Garcias,* and others after him, will have the *Catechu* to be the *Lycium* of *Diofcorides;* but are contradicted by *Clufius* and *Veftingius,* becaufe the Trees which yield the *Lycium* and the *Catechu,* are different in the Shape and Size of their Leaves and Fruits. Some affert it to be the infpiffated Juice or Extract of the Fruit called *Anacardium Occidentalium,* becaufe of the feeming Affinity of the Names, that Fruit being called *Cajou,* and *Catxu.* *Cleyer* affirms it to be the Extract of the Oriental *Acacia,* a Plant much like the Tamarind. *Paulus Ammannus* fays, it is an artificial Compofition, prepared of an Extract of *Indian* Liquorice, *Indian Calamus Aromaticus,* and the Juice of the *Areca,* which gives it its purple Colour. And laft ly, *J. Otho Helbigius,* a Perfon very well fkill'd in the *Eaft Indian* Simples, informs us, that it is extracted from a

Kind

Kind of fmall, hard, refinous, aftringent Fruit, which hangs in a fort of Clufters. This Fruit, he fays, with the Leaves of Betel, and Lime, are ufed over all *India*, in chewing, for cleanfing the Mouth; and is no other than what the Inhabitants of *Java* call *Faufel*, and thofe of *Malaya Pynang*. *Dale* declares himfelf of this laft Opinion. It is aftringent, corroborates the Stomach; removes a *Naufea*, excites an Appetite; reprelles Vomiting, and ftops Fluxes of the Belly, of the *Menfes*, and Hæmorrhages. But its moft remarkable Efficacy confifts in mitigating and curing a Cough, for which it is very effectual, if fuffer'd to diffolve gradually in the Mouth, and fwallow'd with the *Saliva*.

Terra Lemnia, Offic. Earth of Lemnos. This is a fat, vifcid, flippery Clay, of a pale red Colour. It is brought to us in little Cakes or Troches, marked with different Characters, each weighing about four Drams. It has its Name from the Ifland of *Lemnos*, where it is dug; and it is not a little furprifing to find how much this Earth has been celebrated in all Ages. Even in the Time of *Homer* and *Herodotus*, a great many very folemn Rites were obferved in digging it. In the Days of *Diof-corides*, it was made up with the Blood of a She-Goat, newly killed; and the Priefts of *Venus* ftamped it with proper Images. In *Galen*'s Time the Goat's Blood was omitted, but many other fuperftitious Ceremonies ftill remained; which, when *Petrus Bellonius* was at *Lemnos*, were laid afide, and others fubftituted in their Place. It is dug, fays that Author, only on the fixth Day of *Auguft*; as much being then taken out, as is fuppofed to be fufficient for a whole Year. When the Vein is opened, the *Greek* Priefts rehearfe fome Forms of Prayer, at which all the confiderable Inhabitants of the Ifland,

both *Greeks* and *Turks*, are prefent. The Vein being afterwards clofed, and cover'd with common Earth, the Inhabitants are forbid, under the fevereft Penalties, to open it any more during that Year. The greateft Part of this Earth is fent to *Conftantinople* to the *Grand Signior*, with whofe Seal it is marked; the reft is fold to Merchants by the Governor of the Ifland, fometimes with, and fometimes without his Seal upon it. *Bellonius* remarks, that at *Conftantinople* they have the Art of Counterfeiting it fo dexteroufly, that the falfe Earth can hardly be diftinguifhed from the true. That *Lemnian* Earth is reckoned the beft, which, when bruifed between the Fingers, or held in the Mouth, appears moft like Fat, and contains leaft Sand. The Antients have faid much about the Vertues of this Earth, but there is fome Room to think, that the Reputation it had among them, was more owing to the fuperftitious Ceremonies obferved about it, than to its intrinfic Qualities. *Dioſcorides* recommends it as an Antidote againft Poifon and Dyfenteries. *Galen* fays, that, when outwardly applied, it heals all frefh Wounds; and *Fernelius* is of Opinion, that whether applied outwardly or taken inwardly, it ftops all Fluxes of Blood. Some have celebrated its alexipharmic Qualities in all peftilential and contagious Diftempers; but many of the Moderns think it to be a mere alcaline Earth, endued with no other Quality but that of abforbing Acids. This, however muft be a Miftake; becaufe no Earth of this Kind raifes an Efferveſcence with Acids; and it appears by its Analyfis not to be altogether deftitute of the Virtues attributed to it by the Antients. It yields a fmall Quantity of volatile urinous Salt, and of a bituminous Oil, and of a Salt not much different from Sea falt; whence we may conclude, that this Earth is im-

pregnated

pregnated with a Kind of Sal Ammoniac, mixed with a bituminous Oil, by which the Action of Acids upon it is prevented; and that its Virtues must be, in some Degree, alexipharmic, diaphoretic, detergent, and vulnerary. This scaled Earth needs no other Preparation than to be finely powdered, or dissolved in a proper Liquor. In Dysenteries, Ulcers of the Intestines, and Hæmorrhages; it may be administered in Draughts or Boluses. In external Applications, this Earth is often joined with Bole. The Inconveniencies that may arise from using this Earth too long, or in too great Quantities, are common to it, with all the other absorbent Earths. They load the Stomach, by adhering closely to, or plaistering its inner Surface, which causes a very disagreeable Sensation; and, by closing the Orifices of the Glands of the Stomach and Intestines, they hinder Digestion, and may occasion the Fluids, which ought to be excreted there, to be carried to other Parts of the Body; from which Causes many Disorders may follow. The Way to prevent Accidents of these Kinds is, to give these Absorbents in small Quantities, diluted with much Liquor, and diligently to observe the Effects they produce.

Terra Lemnia alba, Offic. White Earth of *Lemnos.* It is a little tenacious and lubricous from its Fatness; whence it adheres to the Tongue, but without Mordacity: It is digged in the Island of *Lemnos.* As to its Virtues, it stops an Hæmorrhage from the *Uterus,* and the menstrual Flux; resists Poisons, and malignant Diseases; and is good for the Bite of a mad Dog.

Terra Melitea, Offic. *Terra sigillata Sancti Pauli vulgo.* Earth of *Malta.* This is a cretaceous ponderous Substance, of a whitish Colour, and astringent Taste. It is brought from *Malta* in small Cakes, sealed

with the Effigies of St. *Paul,* with a Viper. It is said to agree in Virtues with Chalk. The Earth of *Malta* is said to have received a Benediction from St. *Paul,* when shipwrack'd upon that Island; and hence alexipharmic Virtues are attributed to it, which it is not likely to be possessed of on that Account.

Terra Noceriana, Mont. Exot. Earth of *Nocera.* It is a white Kind of Earth found about *Nocera,* of an alexipharmic Quality, and of great Efficacy in malignant Fevers, and Heat of Urine. It is an Astringent, and an Edulcorant, or Sweetner.

Terra Portugallica. Earth of *Portugal.* It is a redish Earth, inclining to a Rose Colour, and of a styptic and astringent Quality, so as to adhere to the Tongue; it is made up into little Cakes, with the Figure of a Rose stamp'd upon them This Earth is said to be good for Fluxes of the Belly.

Terra Samia, Offic. Earth of Samos. This is an argillaceous, sebaceous, pinguious, and ponderous Substance of a white or pale Colour, and astringent Taste. It was brought from the Island of *Samos,* and is recommended by *Dioscorides* for checking Fluxes. It agrees in Virtues with the *Lemnian* Earth.

Terra Sicula;. Bexoardicum minerale, Mont. Ind. Exot. *Lapis Bexoar fossilis,* Geoff. Prælect. Mineral Bezoar, or Sicilian Earth. This is a Native of the Island of *Sicily.* It is esteem'd Alexipharmic, Sweetning, and Opening; and is recommended by *Aldrovandus* in malignant Fevers.

Terra Sigillata alba & rubra magni Ducis, Mont. Exot. White and red sealed Earth of *Tuscany.* It is said to be an Astringent, and an Edulcorant, or Sweetner.

Terra sigillata Livonica, Offic. sealed Earth of *Livonia.* This Earth is redder than the *Terra Silesiaca,.*
and

nd is very aftringent; whence it is ecommended in Dyfenteries, *Diarhæas,* and other Kinds of Fluxes.

Terra Silefiaca, Offic. *Terra Sigilata vulgo, five Terra Strigenfis. Terra figillata Germanica lutea Strigenfis Flava,* Schrod. *Bolus Silefianus,* Calc. Muf. Sealed Earth of *Striga.* It s of a luteous Colour, inclining to a right yellow; fat, vifcous; and runs broad like Butter in Water, or in he Mouth. It is generated in the Gold Mines of *Mons Acutus,* or St. George, near *Striganium,* a Town in he Dutchy of *Swidnitz,* among very hard Rocks. Hence it is digged, nd prepared with the greateft Care, by Direction of the Magiftrates, and educed into little orbicular Maffes, vhich are impreffed with a Seal, haing the Figure of the different Prominences of the Mountain, two Crofs-Keys, a Buckler, and on the Right Star. Under the Mountains are he Words, *Terra figillata montis auti. Wormius* mentions this Earth under the Diftinction of red coloured Earth. It is effectual in an *Hæmopoe, Phthifis,* Ulcers of the Lungs, nd Hæmorrhages of all Kinds; and eprefles a Dyfentery, and all other Fluxes of the Belly.

Terra Tripolitana & Tripolis, Offic. Englifh Oker. This is an earthy Subftance, eafily friable, of a yelowifh Colour, and of an aftringent Tafte. It is efteemed drying. Its principal Ufe is to mix with Salts in Diftillation, in order to keep them from melting.

Terra Turcica, Offic. *Turkey* Earth. The Infide of the Mafs is all of an Afh Colour, the Outfide red, anfwering in no Refpect to the *Terra Lemnia,* tho' it is fuppofed to have the fame Virtues, and is commonly fold for *Terra Lemnia.*

Terra vitriolata Sigillanda. M. Hoffm. Flor. Altdorff. This Earth is taken out of a fubterraneous Place, called *Dak Seiklock,* in the Territory of *Welden.* It is like the *Terra Silefiaca,* and has been found by a Multitude of Experiments to be of the fame Virtue in malignant Fevers, as we are affured by *C. Hoffman.*

Turchefia, Aldrov. Muf. Metall. *Turchois,* Offic The Turquois. The Virtues of this Stone, are faid to be great in Falls; a memorable Inftance of which is related by *Boetius* concerning himfelf. *Scylla* would have it to be a Sort of Fifh's Tooth. *Woodward* is of Opinion, that the Stones which the Jewellers call Turquoife are only Fragments of Bones, ting'd with a blueifh Colour in the Veins of Copper Mines, where they are found.

Tutia, Offic. *Cadmia Fornacia,* Geoff. Prælect. Tutty. This is a Recrement of Calamine melted with Copper, and not of Copper alone, as was that of the Antients. The officinal Tutty therefore may be defined a Sublimation of the Calamine, from melting Copper to the upper Part or Roof of the Furnace, where it concretes round Iron Rods placed there, into a hard Cruft, which is afterwards beat off into Pieces, like the Bark of Trees of a yellowifh Colour, fmooth on the Infide, and fonorous, of a blueifh Afh Colour on the Outfide, and powder'd, as it were, with very fmall Grains of the fame Subftance. This is perhaps the fame with the Tutty of the *Arabians;* for *Serapion* defcribes a Kind of Tutty, which is produc'd and collected in the Furnaces in which Copper is turn'd to a yellow Colour. But it is not certain, whether they might not likewife mean the *Calamine* itfelf by that Word. Tutty is reckon'd among the principal ophthalmic Medicines. It deterges and dries without Acrimony, and is therefore prefcribed with Succefs in Ulcers of the *Cornea, Adnata,* and Eyelids; and likewife in Itchings of the Eyes, inveterate *Ophthalmias,*

and

and to stop an involuntary Flux of Tears, and fistulous Humours. It is seldom used without Preparation, which consists in heating it red hot, and then quenching it three or four Times in Rose Water, and afterwards levigating it according to Art on a Marble or Porphyry.

Vitriolum, Offic. Vitriol. Some derive the Name Vitriol from *Vitrum,* because it has the Colour and Transparency of Glass; in *Greek* it is named Χαλκανθὸν, as if it were an Efflorescence of Brass, and in *Latin, Atramentum Sutorium,* because it is used in blacking Leather. Vitriol is either natural or factitious. The former is found in Crystals, or *Striæ,* sticking to the Roofs of Mines; and the latter is made by boiling the vitriolic Veins of some mineral Ores in Water, and afterwards letting them stand in the Cold to crystalize; or by corrupting and fermenting the *Pyrites,* or Marcasite, and then mixing it with Water, from which Vitriol is afterwards obtained by Coction and Crystallization. This Way of making Vitriol seems to have been unknown to the *Greeks.* White Vitriol is brought from *Germany,* made up in Loaves, like Sugar, and is of a sweetish astringent Taste: They are mistaken who think that white Vitriol of *Goslar,* is only the Green, calcined by the greatest Degree of Fire, for it is found in proper Mines, like a downy Efflorescence, which being dissolved in Water, to a due Consistence, is afterwards boiled till it concretes into a white Mass, like Sugar. Sometimes little Pieces of it are found in the same Mines, transparent like Crystal. This Vitriol contains an imperfect Iron Ore, or perhaps, an Iron Ore mixed with Calamine or Lead. Blue Vitriol is dry to the Touch, and concreted into blue Crystals, like Sapphires, of a Rhomboidal Figure, flattened, and consisting of ten Sides. It is brought

from several Places, especially from *Hungary* and *Cyprus*; and its beautiful blue Colour is owing to the Copper which it contains. The Taste of it is very acrid and austere. Green Vitriol has different Names, from the different Places where it is found; as *Roman, Swedish, English,* and *French.* It contains a large Portion of Iron, from whence its green Colour is derived: It is kept in the Shops, either in large rhomboidal Crystals, or in Heaps of small crystal Grains, sometimes a little unctuous, and sticking to the Hands. It is of an acid styptic Taste; and indeed it cannot well be supposed to have any other, Vitriol being an acid Salt, which having corroded Iron or Brass coagulates with them, and concretes into a pellucid Mass, either of a green or blue Colour, according to the Metal which it has dissolved. Some Authors mention likewise red Vitriol; but *Geoffroy* says, he has not been able to learn what it is. Vitriol is obtained by various Arts from Waters, Earths, vitriolic Stones, and especially from the *Pyrites.* In *Galen*'s Time, blue Vitriol was made in *Cyprus,* by the Heat of the Sun exhaling the Humidity of a vitriolic Water. In some Places of *Hungary,* the same Vitriol is now made by boiling and evaporating a Water of the same Kind; and the green Vitriol is made by a Method not much different, in other Places of *Germany.* In some Places it is made by frequent Ablutions of an Ash-coloured Earth, marked with Spots of different Colours; some of which look like the Rust of Iron, others like Verdigrise, with a strong sulphureous Smell, and an unpleasant bitter Taste: This Vitriol is therefore composed of a Mixture of Iron and Copper; and accordingly its Colour is a Mixture of Blue and Green. In *England,* green Vitriol is made from the *Pyrites,* which are heavy dense Stones,

Stones, of a dark Colour on the Outside, but their inner Surface is radiated from the Centre to the Circumference, the Rays shining like *Bath* Metal. See *Pyrites.* A Solution of Vitriol turns the Tincture of *Heliotropium* into a faint purple Colour, coagulates Milk, turns Syrup of Violets to a greenish Colour, but does not change a Solution of Corrosive Sublimate. When it is mixed with a Solution of Salt of Tartar, or Lime Water, the Colour becomes a little yellowish, and it communicates a black, or dark-purple Tincture to the Infusion of Galls, which indeed is peculiar to Vitriol. By Distillation an acid Spirit is obtained from Vitriol, by a very great Degree of Fire, called by the Name of the *Spirit or Oil of Vitriol,* which turns the Tincture of *Heliotropium,* and Syrup of Violets, to the Colour of Fire, coagulates Milk and Blood, and raises a strong Fermentation and Heat with any alcaline Salt. The Oil of Vitriol, or that strong acid Liquor obtained from it by Distillation, when mixed with common Water, raises an intense Heat; with *Sal Ammoniac* it raises an Effervescence, but generates Cold, tho' the Fumes that arise feel hot. After this Distillation is over, a blackish or red Earth remains in the Retort, called *Colcothar,* and it is the *Calx* or *Crocus* of either Iron or Copper, according to the Nature of the Vitriol that hath been distilled. From this Process it is evident, that Vitriol is composed of an acid Salt, subdued by metallic Parts; which is, also, easily demonstrated from the artificial Ways of producing Vitriol. If Spirit of Vitriol be poured on the Filings of Iron, a very good Vitriol is obtained; and if Copper Plates, stratified with Sulphur, be calcined in a Crucible, the Water in which this *Calx* is made to boil for some Time, if evaporated, will leave behind a true

blue Vitriol. The Virtues ascribed by Chymists to Vitriol are past Belief; neither do we find the Event to answer their Promises. *Dioscorides* mentions an emetic Quality of it; and says, that dissolved in Water, it is good against Worms in the Intestines, and after eating poisonous *Fungi.* He tells us farther, that this Solution snuffed up the Nose, purges the Head, and reckons it among the astringent, heating, and caustic Medicines. *Pliny* commends it in Diseases of the Eyes, Fluxes of the Blood, and for the Cure of Ulcers, and *Galen* made Use of it in *Collyriums.* At present it is used as an Emetic, Vermifuge, Styptic, Detergent, and Antiphlogistic; but is seldom given inwardly without Preparation. Externally, white Vitriol is principally used in Collyriums, to allay an Inflammation of the Eyes, and stop their Running. Powder of blue Vitriol is applied to the Extremities of the bleeding Vessels in Wounds, and stops the Bleeding, by cauterizing the Vessels, and coagulating the Blood. Among the Preparations of Vitriol, the first is Purification, called *Gilla* of Vitriol, in which white Vitriol is mostly made use of, it is purified by Solutions, straining and drying, twice or thrice repeated; and then being taken, from a Scruple to a Dram at a Dose, in a proper Vehicle, it will excite Vomiting: This is recommended by *Paracelsus,* and other Chymists, as an excellent Emetic, as not only cleansing the Stomach by gentle vomiting, . but, also, strengthening both Stomach and Intestines afterward, by its Astringency: Whence it is given with Success in Diarrhœas and Dysenteries. This *Gilla* was very much in Use before antimonial Emetics were known, and the Use of *Ipecacuanha* was discovered, but it is now almost left off.

Unicornu fossile, Offic. *Lapis Arabicus,*

ticus, Cæsalp. The Unicorn-Stone. This is a ſtony Subſtance, reſembling in Colour, Smoothneſs, and Shape, the Horns, Teeth, and Bones of Animals. It is made up of an outer, hard Part, of an yellowiſh, blackiſh, or Aſh-Colour, and a ſoft, friable, compact medullary Part, without Pores, of an aſtringent and drying Quality, ſticking very cloſe to the Tongue, and ſometimes of an agreeable Smell. It is ſaid to agree in Virtues with the *Terra Lemnia,* and is recommended againſt malignant Diſtempers; it reſembles, alſo, a Unicorn's Horn, particularly in reſiſting Poiſon, and curing the convulſive Motions of Infants; and is often uſed in the Small-Pox, and Meaſles. Of this Subſtance calcined, is prepared the factitious Turquoiſe.

CHAP. IV.

Articles *not properly reducible under the former Claſſes.*

SAL *Ammoniacum.* Sal Ammoniac. It is not at preſent well known what the *Sal Ammoniac,* or *Sal Cyreniacus* of the Antients was. It is ſaid to have been generated in the Sands by the Urine of Camels; for when Camels or other Animals depoſite their Urine in the barren Sands of *Africa,* the Heat of the Sun during the Day, makes all the Humidity evaporate; in the Night, the Acid of the Air is attracted by the alcaline urinous Salt, till it is perfectly neutraliz'd, and forms the antient *Sal Ammoniac,* or *Sal Cyreniacus,* which would be waſted in Vegetation, if the Soil was not utterly barren. In Imitation of this, all the different Sorts of *Sal Ammoniac* are made, by uniting an urinous Salt with ſome Sort of Acid. The Matter of the *Sal Ammoniac* made in *Egypt* is pure Soot, and nothing elſe, but ſuch a Soot as is ſwept from Chimnies where they burn Turfs of the Dung of Animals fed with Straw, which is the common Fuel in this Country, where they have no Wood. Theſe Turfs, which are impregnated with alcaline and urinous Salts, communicate to the Soot certain Properties which it could not

be expected to receive from the Smoke of Wood and Coal, and yet are abſolutely neceſſary for the Production of *Sal Ammoniac.* The Veſſels which contain the Matter are exactly of the Figure of Bombs. They are great round glaſs Bottles, a Foot and a half in Diameter, with a Neck two Fingers in Height. They caſe over theſe Bottles with a fat Earth, and fill them with Soot to four Fingers ſhort of their Neck, which continues void and open. They contain each about forty Pounds of Soot, which at the End of the Operation yield ſix Pounds of *Sal Ammoniac.* Soot of an extraordinary Quality affords above ſix Pounds; what is worſt, affords leaſt. The Furnaces are built like our common Ovens, except that their Vaults open with four Clifts in a Row lengthwiſe; upon each Clift are four Bottles, which are placed in ſuch a Manner, that the Bottom of the Bottle being ſunk in, and expoſed to the Action of its Flame, only the Neck of the Bottle remains expoſed to the Air; the Reſt of the Clift is ſtopped up, and well cemented. Every Furnace contains ſixteen Bottles; and md every great Laboratory confifts of eight Furnaces, difpofed in two Rooms, fo that it employs at once a hundred and twenty-eight Bottles. In each Furnace, for three Days and Nights together, there is kept up a conftant Fire made of the Dung of Animals mixed with Straw. The firft Day the grofs Phlegm of the Soot exhales in a thick Fume by the open Neck of the Bottle. The fecond, the acid and alcaline Salts, being fublimed, affociate toward the Top of the Bottle, where they touch the Neck, and, uniting, coagulate. The third Day the Coagulation continues, depurates, and is perfected. In the mean Time the Mafter makes a little Hole in the Side of each Bottle, a little below the Neck, to fee if the Matter be bak'd enough, and if there be nothing more to be fublimed. After he has made his Obfervations, he ftops the Hole carefully with the fat Earth, and opens it from time to time. At laft, when the Work is brought to the Point at which it ought to ftand, he takes away the Fire, breaks the Bottles, fhakes off the Afhes from the Bottom, and takes the round, white, and tranfparent Mafs, of the Thicknefs of three or four Fingers, that adheres to the Neck, which is what they call *Sal Ammoniac.* In two Towns of *Delta*, near one another, a League from the City of *Munfoure*, there are twenty-five great Laboratories, and fome fmall Ones, which make every Year fifteen hundred or two thoufand Quintals [Hundreds] of Sal Ammoniac. In all *Egypt* befides there are but three Laboratories more, two of which are alfo at *Delta*, and one in *Grand Cairo*, which do not produce above twenty or thirty Quintals of this Salt. There is alfo a Sort of Sal Ammoniac made in the *Eaft-Indies*, and thence imported into *Europe*. This Sort is made in the Figure of a Sugar Loaf,

with the Top cut off; the largeft of thefe Loaves are nine Inches in Diameter at the Bafe, and three Inches and a quarter at the Top, and eleven Inches and an half in height. To make a Comparifon between the *Indian* and *Egyptian* Sal Ammoniac, it appears, that they are of the fame Compofition, and as to their Qualities, and the Ufes to which they are applied, there can be no great Difference between them. That of the *Indies* has the Advantage of being pretty clean from Impurities on the Surface, and having only its Top of worfe Alloy than the Reft; fo that upon the whole Mafs there muft be lefs Wafte than in the *Egyptian* Loaves, which are charged with more Impurities in proportion to their Bignefs. Thefe are the Accounts we have of the Origins of the different Species of Sal Ammoniac. But it is fcarcely credible, that fo prodigious a Quantity of Soot, as to make fifteen hundred or two thoufand Quintals a Year, can be furnifhed by one Country, efpecially *Egypt*, which is a very warm Country, and where they only ufe Fires for culinary Ufes and at their Bagnios. We muft therefore furely conclude, that the *Egyptians*, who make Sal Ammoniac, have had the Addrefs to keep their Method of doing it a Secret from the *Europeans*; and that they make Ufe of fome other Ingredients befides Soot. Very good Sal Ammoniac is certainly to be made without any Soot at all, for I am well informed, that at the Sal Ammoniac Works carried on fome Years ago at *Newcaftle*, the Rule for making it was thus: Take of the *Bittern*, that is, the Liquor which drains from common Salt whilft making, one Gallon, and of Urine, three Gallons; let them ftand together forty-eight Hours to effervefce, and fubfide; then draw off the clear Liquor, and evaporate in leaden Veffels to Cryftallization. Sublime thefe Cryftals,

Cryftals, when dry, in proper Veffels, and a very good Sal Ammoniac will be produced. I am farther informed, that from one hundred Weight of Salt made from the *Bittern*, commonly fold under the Name of *Epfom* Salt, and three Hogfheads of Urine, fifty-fix Pounds of Sal Ammoniac may be procured. But it muft be remarked, that Sal Ammoniac is a very different Subftance from moft of the Preparations made from it; for when alcaline Salts are mixed with the crude Sal Ammoniac, they abforb the Acid, which renders the Sal Ammoniac neutral; and then the volatile urinous Salts, fet free from the Acid rife in Diftillation. *Boerhaave's* Character of Sal Ammoniac is, that it preferves all animal Subftances from Putrefaction, and its Brine penetrates into the moft intimate Parts, and is the nobleft Aperient, Attenuant, Refolvent, Stimulant, Errhine, Sternutatory, Diaphoretic, Sudorific, Antifeptic, and Diuretic. Sal Ammoniac is not employed fo much in Medicine, as it deferves to be; for as it is abfolutely a neutral Salt, confifting of an acid and a volatile alcaline Salt, it is extremely penetrating and refolvent, ufed either externally, or internally, and is a noble Deobftruent, and Cooler, where fuch Medicines are required.

Sal Catharticum amarum. Epfom Salt, or bitter purging Salt. Mr. *Brown,* in the Philofophical Tranfactions, gives us the following Account of this Salt. This Salt, fays he, was firft made by Dr. *Grew,* by evaporating the *Epfom* Waters. Some Years after, feveral other bitter purging Springs were found in different Counties, and Salts in fmall Quantities were boiled up from them, but from no Place, nor all the Places put together, in fuch large Quantities, as from the Springs on one Side of *Shooter's Hill* in *Kent,* about the Year 1700, which were then in the Poffeffion of thofe two Chymifts, Mr. *George,* and Mr. *Francis Moult,* and where they made fuch a large *Apparatus* for evaporating the Water, that they fometimes boiled down 200 Barrels in a Week, from which in a dry Seafon, and when the Land Waters did not get into their Drains, they have obtained two hundred and twenty four Pounds of Salt. After thefe Works had gone on fome time, Dr. *Hoy* found out a more expeditious Way of making a purging Salt, fo nearly refembling that from the purging Springs, in all its Properties, that it foon paffed on the World for the other, and continued fo to do. The great Confumption of thefe Salts (which went then only by the Name of *Epfom* Salts) as well at Home as Abroad, engaged fome of our own Phyficians, many Years before *M. Boulduc* took Notice of it, to fufpect that even what was made at *Shooter's Hill* was fpurious, and receiv'd an Addition of fomething to increafe the Quantity. But thefe Sufpicions, fays he, I dare pofitively affirm, were entirely groundlefs, as to the Salts made there, and readily believe the fame of any other Places, where the Spring Waters were boiled down for Salt. But upon a Confideration, that there were greater Quantities of this Salt confumed than all the Places where the Waters were boiled could produce, which was the real Fact at that time of Day, there was fufficient Room to fufpect that fome of them were not genuine, as appeared to be true fome time after. For the Secret which was then in a few Hands, of making thefe Salts cheap, gave thofe who had it, an Opportunity of underfelling thofe who made it from the Waters, and in a Year or two, render'd them incapable of making it to any Advantage: So that the Work on *Shooter's Hill* was thrown up; and d I believe there has not been a ndred Pounds of Salt made from e Waters since that Time in any art of the Kingdom: Some time for this Work at *Shooter's Hill* as broke up, some Pains were taken discover the Secret those had, who ld the Salt so cheap; and upon camining the several Salts that were ld about Town, those disposed of y Mr. *G.* and *F. Moult*, were cerinly genuine, and were therefore a roper Standard to judge of the rest y. But from all Experiments then iade, there could no material Diference be found between the Salt iade from the Waters, and that iade by them who were in the Seret. There was indeed a Salt sold y some, which in the Course of iose Trials, was found to be a *Sal Mirabile*, made from the *Oleum Virioli* and common Salt, but shot into ich small Crystals, as not at first ight to be distinguished from the ther: Necessity being the Mother f Invention, it was not long before was discover'd, and the Experinent was tried at the Lady *Carringon's* Salt Works near *Portsmouth*; vhere it was found the same Thing ould be done, as at another Work iot far from it, and in which Dr. *Joy* had been concern'd. It was ome Years after this Salt had been nade at *Portsmouth*, before the Salt Vlakers at *Lemington* attempted, or ndeed knew the Method of making t, who are now the greatest Traders n it, and have sent several Ton in Year to *London*, besides what has een directly exported from thence. It was the Opinion of the Proprieors of the *Salterns* near *Portsmouth*, hat this Purging Salt could not be nade at any other Salt Works but heirs, and that the bitter Taste in he Salt was communicated from the Earth to the Sea Water, whilst it tood exposed in their Sun Pans. But Fime has proved this Opinion false;

for besides what has been said of its being made at *Lemington*, it was some Time ago begun to be made near *Newcastle*, where it is still continued to be made, and doubtless may be made at any salt Works, where the common Salt is made from Sea Water by Evaporation. Whether any Thing of this Kind has been attempted at any of our Inland Salt Springs, either in *Cheshire* or *Worcestershire*, I am not yet satisfied. There is some Difference in the making the common Salt in *Hampshire*, from that about *Newcastle*. At the first of these Places, in the Beginning of the Summer, at Spring Tides, or at New and Full Moon, the Sea Water is let into their feeding Ponds, which are their Reservoirs for their Summers working, and from hence is convey'd into small square Pans, and again, after some Time, from these it is convey'd into large Pans, or Beds, which they call Brine, or Sun Pans, all which are made of Sea-Mud and Earth. In these last Pans, or Beds it lies exposed to the Sun and Wind, in order to exhale the weakest Waters; and it is in these Beds, if the Weather prove very favourable, that they can make as good Bay Salt as any we have from *France*; and at such a Time they never bring their Brine to the Boilers. But if the Weather is not hot enough for that Purpose, their Brine is exposed so long in these Pans, till it becomes of such Strength as to support their Eggs made of Glass or Wax, to a certain Heighth above the Surface of the Brine, which from thence is conveyed into large Stone Cisterns, and then into boiling Pans made of Iron, where it is boiled down (after having been frequently scumm'd) to a Sea Salt. 'Tis observable, that whilst the Brine is boiling, there precipitates a hard crusty Matter, which is partly taken out by Vessels placed

in

In proper Parts of the Pan for that Purpose, and Part of it fixed on the Bottom of the Pan so hard, as to be afterwards dug off, and this the Workmen call *Scratch*, and is what Dr. *Collins,* concerning the Sea Water boiled at *Shields,* calls a Stone Powder. When the Operation for the Sea Salt is finished, it is taken out hot, and put into wooden Troughs, with Holes at the Bottom; through which runs the superfluous Liquor: Under these Troughs are set other Vessels with Sticks fixed in them in a perpendicular Posture, to receive what runs through. In these Vessels the Liquor is suffer'd to continue some Time, and according to the Quantity of the Sea Salt still left in it, will crystallize to the Sticks, something like Sugar Candy, but in much larger Shoots; and this they call *Cat-Salt,* or *Salt-Cats,* and it holds some Share of the bitter Salt. When this Salt is broken small, or rather powder'd, it is so white, that some Gentlemen choose it for their Tables; but the greatest Consumption of it is among the Cake Soap Boilers. The Liquor that will not shoot to these Sticks, is what, at these Works, they call the *Bittern,* fit for making the *Sal Catharticum.* Near *Newcastle,* their Method is to receive the Sea Water into their Reservoirs at High Water, at any Time of the Moon, if there be no Fresh in the River, occasioned by Rain in the higher Country, and from these Reservoirs, without exposing of it in Beds, as at *Lemington,* they pump it into their boiling Pans, where evaporating it almost to a Pellicle, they fill it up again eight or nine Times, and then waste it with a gentle Heat for the common or Sea Salt. The Liquor that runs from this Salt, when taken out, and put into proper Vessels, is what they call the *Bittern,* which, if it stands some Time in those Vessels, a Salt will shoot and crystallize to the Sides, in Taste pretty much like the Sea Salt, but with a Share of Bitterness, and seems to answer to the Cat Salt of the *Lemington* Works, and very probably would shoot after the same Manner, if they made use of the same *Apparatus.* I could not but mention this general and loose Account of making the common Salt, as necessary to introduce the Liquor *Bittern,* which, before Dr. *Hoy* found out an Use for it, was always flung away, being so different in its Properties from the Brine made use of to produce the Sea Salt, that it requires some Skill in the Operator, to determine the Time when to take out the Sea Salt from the Pans, before the *Bittern* incorporated with it, which would otherwise spoil the whole making. The *Bittern* at *Lemington* not shooting to the Sticks, is carried by Channels into Pits made light with Clay, where it stands for some Months, and there will shoot again. What Liquor remains is boiled down, till it is observed to be in a Disposition to crystallize, and then is convey'd into wooden Coolers lined with Lead. The Liquor which will not shoot there, is boiled down after the same Manner, in order for another Crystallization. By this Time the Liquor seems to have alter'd its Property, and becomes of a very pungent biting Taste, and, if boiled down, will not longer shoot into Crystals, as before, but precipitates, during the boiling, as small grain'd Salt; and if they should continue to boil down the Liquor, separated from this Salt, each Quantity of Salt thus produced will be still more pungent than the other. If you boil down the whole Quantity of this Liquor, it will produce a Salt, which, if exposed to the Air, will run *per Deliquium.* The Liquor that produces this Salt is always flung away, wherever the *Sal Catharticum* made. This is what at prefent I n give no other Name to, than a rd Salt produced from the Sea ater, differing in fome Refpects, much from the other two, as they fer from one another. To return the feveral Cryftallizations, fuch mentioned to be fhot from the ttern; thefe will be of different es, as to their Figures, and hold ne Share of the third Salt, but now en Notice of, which makes them ject to give and diffolve; nor is ir Tafte come yet to that fimple ter of the pure Salt. Thefe there- e are either feparately, or altoge- r, to be flung into a Copper, h as much common Water as is ficient to diffolve them, and allow gentle Evaporation, till they are un ready to be poured into the olers in order for Cryftallization. is generally proves to be the pure Catharticum, thoroughly freed m either a Sea Salt, or the third :. The Liquor decanted from Shooting may be boiled down in, in order for a fecond Shoot- , and after that a third; but the Liquors from thefe Shoot- s are boiled away more or lefs, fo will fooner or later meet with pungent Liquor, which contains third Salt, as you did in the ner Shootings from the *Bittern*, n which the pure *Sal Catharticum* neceffarily required to be freed rom the common Salt; a Proof which cannot be better determin- than by the following Experi- ts, *viz.* that with the *Oleum Vi- i*, which will certainly ferment this Salt, if the Sea Salt has been well feparated from it, or ftill holds fome of the third Salt. when any of the Cryftallizations not ftand the Teft of this Expe- nt, they ought to be diffolved- fhot again, as before, by which ns the pure Salt is to be obtained. not mention, fays *Brown*, this as a l made ufe of at the Salt Works,

but what I have by Experience found to be true. And the fame Experiment will ferve to diftinguifh a *Sal Mira-bile* made at thefe Works, from that made with Oil of Vitriol and com-mon Salt. The Account they give of it is this: They take any Quan-tity of coarfer grained Cryftals boil-ed from the *Bittern*, which, when diffolved and evaporated, more than they would otherwife do for making the *Sal Catharticum*, they throw it in-to a wooden Bowl, with fome Oil of Vitriol, where it ftands for ten Days, and fhoots into large Cryftals, tranf-parent, and like the *Sal Mirabile*. But as this Salt, by this Method, is not fufficiently fatiated with the Oil of Vitriol, if they ufe any, fo it is eafily difcovered by the Oil of Vi-triol, which will readily ferment with it; whereas it has no Effect on the other *Sal Mirabile* made as a-bove. This is the Salt now fold in the Shops by the Name of *Epfom* and *Glauber's* Salts, and is a pretty good diuretic Purge, where the *Pri-mæ Viæ* are intended to be unloaded. But it fhould be given with a confi-derable Quantity of fome diluting Fluid, as mineral Waters. Dr. *Grew* recommends his *Epfam* Salts to excite a decay'd Appetite, to ftop habitual Inclinations to vomit, for Pains in the Stomach, in hypochon-driacal and hyfterical Diforders dif-folved in chalybeate Waters, for the Colic, in Worms, nephritic Pains, the Jaundice, Head-ach, and wan-dering Gout. But he cautions a-gainft ufing it in Dropfies; in a continual Fever, in an Ague; the Green Sicknefs, fpitting of Blood, *Cholera Morbus*, and the Palfy. Nor are they to be allowed to Women with Child, without great Circum-fpection. They may alfo prove hurt-ful in a Suppreffion of Urine; which depends upon an Ulcer in the Blad-der, or a Stone too big to pafs; in either of which Cafes the Patient is to abftain from all Diuretics. But

otherwife

otherwise I have often, says he, given this Medicine successfully, in bringing away the Urine, and Stones with it not of the least Size. *Quincy* is very much enrag'd at this Cheat, as he calls it, and seems to disapprove of the factitious *Sal Catharticum* as a Medicine. I must confess I am not entirely of his Opinion, because of the vast Quantity of these Salts used in Medicine, I have known no bad Effects produced, but on the contrary a great many good ones. When, however, this Salt is sold instead of the *Glauber's* Salt, it may be esteemed a very great Fraud; and the excessive Price, that the *Sal Catharticum* is generally sold at, is certainly another, for it does not cost four Pence a Pound originally.

Sal Polychrestum de Seignette. This Salt, which has been used in Medicine for many Years, takes its Name from Mr. *Seignette*, a Physician of *Rochelle*, who invented it, and during his Life kept it a Secret, which he only transmitted to his Children, who in their Turn kept the Secret so inviolably, that no Chymist was, for a long Time, able certainly to discover the Mystery, some taking it for one, and some for another Thing. The great Reputation of this Medicine, induced Mr. *Boulduc* to attempt a Discovery of its Composition. In order to make this Salt, we take, says he, the best calcined, whitest, and hardest *Alicant Kali*, reduced to a Powder; of this we make a strong *Lixivium* by boiling in Water, and filtrate the *Lixivium*, which is very transparent. Then we take separately some Cream of Tartar in Powder, upon which we pour this *Lixivium*, when warm. This Mixture excites a Fermentation, which lasts for a considerable Time, and which even after it has ceased, is renewed at certain Intervals. In the Time of this Fermentation, the Cream of Tartar is resolved; after

which there is a copious Precipitation of a spongeous and light Earth, which is to be separated from the Liquor by Filtration. Then we evaporate this Mixture to the Consumption of about a third Part. Then it is to be left at rest in earthen Vessels, by which Means, after some Days, we find Crystals transparent like Crystal, which when disengaged, and not supported by the Vessels, are formed into Cylinders or Columns, which through all their Length have many flat Surfaces, above nine of which I have some times, says he, counted, tho' they are not generally found in so great a Number. It is impossible exactly to determine the precise Proportion of the Salt of *Kali*, and the Cream of Tartar, since some Kinds of *Kali* contain a larger Quantity of Salt than others. But the most natural Way of finding this Proposition is, to dissolve in the *Lixivium* as much Cream of Tartar as it will receive, that is, to the Point of Saturation. A *Lixivium* of six Pounds of *Kali* generally absorbs two Pounds and three or four Ounces of Cream of Tartar, and when the *Kali* is very white and richly impregnated with Salt, the *Lixivium* of six Pounds some times absorbs an equal Weight of Cream of Tartar. This Difference as we may easily conceive, can only depend upon the Quality of the *Kali*, according as it is more or less impregnated with alcaline Salt. But when, says he, I took the Salt which subsided in the Solution or *Lixivium* of *Kali*, and the Configuration of which nearly resembles that of *Glauber's* Salt, half a Pound of this Salt dissolved, easily received thirteen or fourteen Ounces of Cream of Tartar, and the Mixture precipitated scarcely any Earth. This is the justest Proportion that can be proposed for the Substances which enter the Composition of Mr.

Seignette's

ette's Sal Polychreftum. If we wait for a fhort Time, we have Cryftals of *Kali*, after which the ture is more equally made, and t fubject to the Precipitation of lifferent heterogeneous Subftances h the *Kali* communicates to the *vium.* In a Word, this Salt n formed into Cryftals, and com- d with that of Mr. *Seignette* alfo tallized, was found to be pre- y the fame in all Circumftances; hey are figured like each other, eafily diffolved in cold Water, n reduced to a Powder, have fame Tafte, and communicate a in Coldnefs to the Tongue. en put upon a live Coal, they me fufed and bubble, yield the ll of burnt Tartar, and are at reduced to a black and fponge- Coal, which yields Tartar. If r this Examination, we fhould bt of the Conformity of this Salt h Mr. *Seignette's*, we may be inced of it by an Experiment, ch makes a fpeedy Decompofiti- of it: For if we diffolve equal ntities of both Salts feparately in m Water, and pour into each a So- on of Oil of Vitriol, till its Action es, in Proportion as thefe Solu- s become cold, a faline Concre- is formed, which when examin- is found to be true Cream of Tar- in Cryftals regenerated or fepa- d from the *Alcali*, whilft the Oil Vitriol is united with it, and af- vards by Cryftallization, forms h it a *Glauber's* Salt, in the fame nner as if this Oil had been pour- upon the *Lixivium* of the *Kali*. e *Sal Polychreftum de Seignette* is refore a Cream of Tartar render- Soluble by the *Alcali* of *Kali*. the Compofition of this Salt, we y underftand its Virtues in Medi- e. As 'tis a neutral Salt, in Con- ence thereof, it muft be attenu- ng, aperient, refolvent, and pe- rating, and fhould feem to be ch preferable to the *Sal Cathar-*

ticum amarum, in all Intentions where that is ufed.

Sandiver, Axungia Vitri, or Salt of Glafs, is a Kind of Salt which feparates from the Metal of Glafs whilft in Fufion. It is of an acrimonious and biting Tafte. The Farriers ufe it for clearing the Eyes of Horfes. It is alfo ufed for cleaning the Teeth, and is fome- times applied to running Ulcers, a *Herpes*, or the Itch, by Way of De- ficcative.

Sapo. Soap. This, tho' a Com- pofition, may be confider'd in this Place as a Drug. There are many Kinds of Soap, but the principal ufed in Medicine are thofe of *Venice*, A- licant, and Caftile. The general Method of making Soaps are, ac- cording to *Boerhaave*, thus. They take the fix'd alcaline fiery Salt, prepared with Quick-Lime; this they diffolve in fuch a Proportion of hot Water, that the Lie may fup- port a new laid Egg; and this the Soap makers call their capital Lie. They afterwards dilute Part of it with more Water, till a frefh Egg will fink therein; and this they call the weaker Lie. They afterwards mix their Olive Oil with an equal Weight of this Lie, by ftirring them well together, till the whole becomes white, then boil the Mixture with a gentle Fire, keeping it continually ftirring, till the Water being exhaled, the Remainder begins to unite, at which time they throw in thrice the Weight of capital Lie, in Proportion to the Oil, and mix and boil till the Mafs becomes fo thick, that a little of it laid upon a cold Stone, ap- pears to be of a due folid Confi- ftence; and if now a Part of this cold Mafs is diffolved in Water, it mani- fefts no Signs of Oil, this fhews that the Oil is well united with the *Alcali*; but if any Oil ftill appears, the Ad- dition of a little more capital Lie is required, and the boiling muft then uniformly be continued, till the

Soap

Soap will perfectly dissolve in Water. At this Time the Soap is tasted, and if it proves sharp and alcaline, it is a Sign that the Alcali abounds too much therein. Therefore a little more Oil is added, and the boiling continued, till at length a Mass is obtained, so hard as to cut in the Cold, and that will perfectly dissolve in Water, and neither taste alcaline upon the Tongue, nor run spontaneously in the Air; and thus the Soap is perfected. Instead of Olive Oil any other fat Substance may be used, as the Fats of Animals, and the Oils of Fish; thus black Soap is made from Train Oil, or the boiled Blubber of Whales; but the purer the Alcali is, and more scentless, tasteless, and less ungrateful the Oil, the better the Soap, especially for Medicinal Use. Soap so produced, tho' the Tenacity of the Oil is abolished, yet the former Virtue of the lixivial Salt remains, whereby it deterges without Danger of corroding; for when mixed with Water, it makes a strong saponaceous Lye, which by Heat, Motion, and Trituration, dissolves Gums, Oils, Resins, and gross Fats, rendering them also saponaceous, or soluble in Water; and thus it has a scouring, detergent, opening, cleansing Property. Hence it renders coagulating Humours fluid, opens old Obstructions, and thereby restores the lost Use of the Parts. It also has great Effects upon Concretions consisting of gross Earth and Oil; it prevents Acids from coagulating the Chyle or Milk; and even resolves them after Coagulation. Whence it appears to be almost an universal Opener, Diluter, Resolver, and Thinner in the Body, in the abovemention'd Cases, being drank upon an empty Stomach, well diluted and at different Times, in a sufficiently large Quantity, and assisted by the Motion of the Body. It is

likewise wonderfully serviceable, being externally applied in sinuous and fistulous Ulcers. It may be ting'd and disguis'd, by giving it a grateful Colour with Saffron, Turmeric, Cochineal, or other Pigments; and if it still proves disagreeable, on account of the nauseous Smell acquired by the Oil in boiling, it may be corrected by a little Balsam of *Peru.* But its Use is highly pernicious in those Distempers, where Life is in Danger from a Putrefaction, that dissolves and corrupts the Humours, as has frequently appear'd in the Plague, and other putrid Distempers, according to the just Observation of *Diemerbroeck.* Soap effects what neither Water nor Oil could perform, does that with Safety which Alcalies do with Danger, and can perform what other Salts cannot.

Spiritus Vini. Spirit of Wine, or more properly *Vinous Spirit;* for what is usually called Spirit of Wine, is procur'd from the fermented Juices of many other Vegetables besides that of the Grape. What is called *Proof Spirit* is generally esteem'd the best, but for common Uses *Molasses Spirits* may serve, as we are inform'd by the Compilers of the last College Dispensatory. Rectify'd Spirit is the same, depriv'd of all, or a great Part, of its Water, and freed as much as possible from its disagreeable Smell. We meet with nothing like Spirit of Wine before the thirteenth Century, when *Thaddæus* takes Notice of it. And some little Time after, *Arnaldus de Villa Nova* mentions it in very high Terms, under the Title of *Aqua Vini.* Spirit of Wine brought to a great Degree of Perfection, or what is called *Alcohol,* is the lightest Fluid next to Air, perfectly transparent, very thin, most simple, totally inflammable, without producing any Smoke, or diffusing any disagreeable Smell whilst it is burning; and is exceedingly

exceedingly volatile, without leaving any Fœces; absolutely immutable in Distillation; extremely expansible by Heat; very easily disposed to Ebullition by Fire; of a very pleasant Smell, and of a particular grateful Taste. All the Humours of the human Body, that we are acquainted with, it coagulates in an Instant, except pure Water, and Urine, whilst it hardens all the solid Parts, and thus preserves both from Putrefaction, or spontaneous Colliquation: It preserves the Bodies of Insects, Fish, Birds, and other Animals that are put into it, from Corruption, or Alteration, for Ages, if closely stopped: With Water, Vinegar, any acid Liquors, Oils, and pure volatile alcaline Salts, it suffers itself to be mixed, and that nearly with an equable Mixture; and gummy and resinous Substances it dissolves. So that we are acquainted with no Liquid, produced either by Nature or the Art of Chymistry, that is capable of being united with more Bodies than Alcohol is; but in a particular Manner it proves an excellent Vehicle for the *Spiritus Rector* of Vegetables, which by uniting with it, may be extracted from its proper Body, retained, and applied to medicinal, and other Uses. The great Masters of Chymistry, distinguished by the Title of Adepts, are supposed, in their Description of the artificial Preparation of this perfect Alcohol, to have shadowed out the Preparation of the Philosopher's Stone: But it is certain, that this Alcohol owes its Origin to Fermentation alone, nor can be prepared in any other Manner whatever. In the human Body, by its Smell, Taste, and Vapour, it wonderfully quickens, gratefully affects, and invigorates the animal, natural, and vital Spirits, Nerves and Brain: Hence it exhilarates the Mind and Senses, makes a Person brisk and agile, and proceeding thro'

various Degrees, at last causes Drunkenness, which, as it here comes on very suddenly, so likewise it goes off in the same Manner. The Blood, its Serum, and other thin Juices it coagulates in an Instant, and hence being drank imprudently, it is said to have killed Persons on the Spot. Applied externally, it dries, and corroborates the Vessels, and coagulates the Fluids contained in them, where-ever it can penetrate. The Extremities of the Nerves where it can reach it instantly dries, contracts, and deprives of all Sense and Motion. Hence it appears, how imprudently, and often, how unhappily, Alcohol, either pure or impregnated with aromatic Spirits, Camphire, or the like, dissolved in it, and ordered to be applied hot, and inforced with Friction, is made Use of as a Fomentation in chirurgical Cases. I would advise, therefore, to be cautious upon these Occasions, left under a specious Pretence of Vivification, Califaction, Dissipation, and Restoration of Agility, you obtain no other Effects than what I just now ascribed to these Spirits. In Wounds, Ulcers, and other visible Disorders, pure Alcohol performs the very same thing, (viz.) Coagulates, dries, and burns the Nerves. It is true indeed, it takes from the Nerves all Sense of Pain; but then at the same time it destroys all their Use. And it has the same Effect, in mitigating Punctures or Dilacerations of the same Parts. It stops bleeding at once by contracting the Vessels, and coagulating the Blood, where it is applied, but with the concomitant Circumstances just mentioned. Hence, therefore, it is a very speedy, and often an excellent Remedy in those Cases, though always attended with some Inconveniences. From what has been said, then, we learn what Effect pure Alcohol has upon animal or vegetable

table Substances immersed in it. For it dissolves into itself, and extracts whatever is oily in them, whence they become attenuated, contracted, and often corrugated. In this Manner the Preparations of the Parts of Animals have often been observed to be changed : And aromatic Flowers, Leaves, and Fruits are thus affected from the same Cause. Small Birds in their Feathers, and other little Animals cover'd with hard Scales, immersed in hot Alcohol, are preserved in their full Beauty, because this Attenuation, though it really happens, is concealed under their Feathers, and Scales. These Animals being macerated for some Time in the purest Alcohol, till they are thoroughly penetrated by it, and then taken out, and dried in a hot, but not fervid Oven, and afterwards put into Glass Vessels, and intirely debarred from any Communication with the external Air, may be kept in their proper Form for Ages, to the very great Advantage both of natural and medicinal History, because they afford lively and certain Characters by which they may be known. Since there are infinite, and often times very inviting, Occasions in which Chymists and other Artificers stand in Need of the true and purest Alcohol, the least Remainder of Water rendering the Operation unsuccessful, it is absolutely necessary we should have some Marks by which we may be able to distinguish, whether our *Alcohol* be pure or not : The principal of these are, if the supposed *Alcohol* contains any Oil dissolved in it, and so equally distributed through it, that it is no ways perceptible, then upon the pouring of Water into it, the Mixture will grow white, and the Oil will separate from the *Alcohol*. If any thing of an Acid lies concealed in *Alcohol*, a little of it mixed with the alcaline Spirit of *Sal Ammoniac* will discover the Acid by an Effervescence, for other-

wise there would be only a simple Coagulation. If there be any thing of an Alcali intermixed, it will appear by the Effervescence excited by the Affusion of an Acid : And as for other Salts, they are seldom found in it. But it is a Matter of greater Difficulty to discover whether there be any Water intermixed with it; and therefore Chymists have contrived certain Methods, by which this may be also determined. The first was the repeated Labour of so many Distillations, which they thought sufficient Grounds for them to presume that they were in Possession of pure simple Spirits, without the Admixture of any Phlegm; but, it is difficult by this Method to obtain pure *Alcohol*; but it would to the last retain something of Phlegm. Secondly, they put some *Alcohol* into a very clean, dry Spoon, and, heating it, set it on fire in a Place where there was not the least Wind, and if after the *Alcohol* was burnt out, there was no Moisture left in the Spoon, they pronounced it pure *Alcohol*. Some more curious Persons, however, by other Experiments, discover'd, that by the Action of the Flame, the Water that lay concealed in the Alcohol, might be dispersed into the Air, and consequently that the Absence of Water in the Spoon, after the Consumption of the Alcohol, was no certain Proof, that there was none contained in it, before it was set on Fire. In the third Place, therefore, they took some of the best Gun-powder, and drying it very carefully put a little of it into a clean and very dry Spoon, and poured some Alcohol upon it, which being heated, they just stirred it in the very Surface, and letting it burn down in a very quiet Place, if the Powder continued dry enough to take Fire by the Flame when just spent, they concluded that the Alcohol was pure : But against this Experiment there lies the very same Objection as against the former. Thefe two laft Methods, therefore, when they fucceed, demonftrate, that the *Alcohol* is in a very great Degree, but not abfolutely free from Water. In the fourth and laft Place, therefore, there has been another Way difcovered, by which it may be certainly known whether *Alcohol* contains any Water or not, which is this: Take a chymical Vial, with a long narrow Neck, the Bulk of which will hold four, or fix Ounces of *Alcohol*. Fill this two-thirds full with the *Alcohol* you intend to examine, into which throw a Dram of the pureft and drieft Salt of Tartar, coming very hot out of the Fire: then mix them by fhaking them together, and fet them over the Fire till the *Alcohol* is juft ready to boil; being thus fhaken and heated, if the Salt of Tartar remains perfectly dry, without the leaft Sign of Moifture, we are fure that there is no Water in this *Alcohol*: Hence the fingular Nature of Alcohol is abundantly determined by its individual Properties; efpecially if to what has been faid you add this Obfervation, that fuch an Alcohol is not vifible whilft it diftills through the Alembic: For it neither forms dewy Drops like Water, nor runs down in Striæ like ftrong Spirit of Wine, but it is quite invifible; which Property was not unknown to the ancient Chymifts, as evidently appears by their Writings. As all vinous Liquors borrow their intoxicating Qualities, and all their Properties wherein they differ from other Fluids, from the Alcohol which refides in them, I fhall make fome Remarks, with refpect to the Ufes generally made of them in common Life. Firft, then, as vinous Liquors have Effects upon animal Bodies, nearly allied to thofe of the *Gas Sylveftre*, or incoercible Spirit, which flies off from fermenting Liquors. It feems near a Certainty, that fermented Liquors inebriate,

and produce all their deleterious Effects by a Portion of this *Gas Sylveveftre* refiding in them. Hence appears the Imprudence, I fhould rather fay Madnefs, of thofe who take into their Stomachs large Quantities of a Fluid ftrongly impregnated with the moft fubtile and penetrating Poifon known in Nature, and which we find by daily Experience never fails to diforder, and if perfifted in, to deftroy the animal Machine. The Frequency of this Practice is amazing, and would fcarcely be credible, if it was not common. I fhould think myfelf happy, if any thing I could fay would put the leaft Check to this beftial Crime, to which it is aftonifhing there fhould be any Temptation; for I am fatisfied, that this alone deftroys more Lives than the Accidents of War, added to all the Diftempers with which Providence has thought proper to afflict Mankind; and it is very remarkable, that befides the Diftempers produced by drinking fpirituous Liquors, an habitual Ufe of thefe renders all Difeafes from other Caufes more difficult to cure. It is certain, that fermented Liquors are deleterious, in Proportion to their Strength, that is, in Proportion to the poifonous Spirit or Gas they contain. However, though fmall fermented Liquors do not immediately manifeft their Effects, yet I think it is not to be doubted, but that an habitual Ufe even of thefe, muft in the End induce an Alteration in the Conftitution to its Difadvantage. I am fenfible, a Habit of drinking thefe Liquors renders them fomewhat neceffary, and makes it difficult to leave them off, and fometimes even dangerous. It is therefore a great Imprudence in People of Condition, to inure their Children to the Ufe of Wine, and other fermented Liquor, from their moft tender Years. If we confider *Alcohol* as acting upon the Stomach only,

and

and at the same Time reflect, that it dries and contracts the Nerves, and deprives them of all Sensation and Motion, we shall readily perceive, that if taken in the Stomach, when it is empty especially, they must necessarily, by their proper Action, take away that Sensation which we call Hunger, and destroy that Elasticity of the Fibres of the Stomach, which is absolutely necessary to the Digestion of the Aliment. To these Inconveniencies arising from the internal Use of *Alcohol* it may be added, that it coagulates the animal Juices, and consequently all the Fluids it finds in the Stomach, I mean those Fluids which are separated in the Glands of the Mouth, *Fauces*, and Stomach, and which are designed by Nature to promote the Solution of the Aliment; now when these are coagulated, and rendered viscid, they are utterly unfit to promote the above-mentioned Solution, but rather prevent it. Every one that has seen a Person, much habituated to drinking Drams, take a Vomit, must have observed him to discharge from his Stomach great Quantities of a viscid ropy Jelly. If we consider spirituous Liquors as a Solvent of the Aliment, we shall find it so far from being fit to promote this Solution, that it greatly contributes to prevent it, for it hardens animal and vegetable Substances, and hinders their Solution in the Stomach, for the very same Reasons, that it prevents their Putrefaction out of it. It would be well if spirituous Liquors had any Virtues to make amends for the Havock and Destruction they make in the World. And to do them Justice, I believe, that rough austere red Wines may be of Service for bracing up a relaxed Habit, and promoting Digestion vitiated by an accidental Laxity of the Organs subservient thereto; and that the more penetrating white Wines, well dilu-

ted, may be of Service as Medicines. But with Respect to any thing more spirituous than Wine, there is scarcely any Case wherein they can be of sufficient Service to compensate for the great Mischiefs they produce; Insomuch that every Person who drinks a Dram, seems to me guilty of a greater Indiscretion, than if he set Fire to his House; and for the same Reasons, cordial Waters are the most dangerous Furniture for a Closet, particularly as there is something like Fascination in them, which obliges the Possessor to make Use of them, to the Destruction both of Health and Intellects. On this Account, I cannot forbear admiring the great Wisdom of *Mahomet*, who has strictly forbid his Followers the Use of fermented Liquors, for better Reasons than are generally apprehended. However *Alcohol*, and fermented Spirits in general, are of good Service externally apply'd in many Cases. Thus Spirit of Wine, especially camphorated, is a very good Addition to Fomentations designed to resolve Inflammations, whether external or internal. Wine used as a *Fotus*, or applied externally, cools, and allays the Heat of the Parts, notwithstanding it warms taken internally. Spirit of Wine does the same. *Pliny* says, it is the Nature of Wine to warm the *Viscera* taken internally but to cool externally apply'd. *Hippocrates* says, that Ulcers should be washed with nothing but Wine. *Galen* says, Wine is the best Medicament for Ulcers. *Dioscorides* says, that Wine in *Lana Succida*, is a good Application for Wounds and Inflammations. Dr. *Harris* from his own Experience affirms, that linen Cloths dipped in warm Spirit of Wine, often cure Burns from scalding Water, melted Pitch, Fire, and Gun-powder, better and sooner than all other Applications. He gives an Instance of a Boy that was blinded by

Drop of Pitch falling into his Eye,
d of another blinded by Gun-pow-
r, who both recovered their Sight
e very next Day, by a *Fotus* of
arm Spirit of Wine. Dr. *Harris*
o affirms, that warm Wine is the
ft Application for Wounds, Ul-
rs, and Inflammations, especially
ofe of the most sensible Parts, that
e full of Nerves, Tendons, and
ood-Vessels, as the Fingers and
oes, where Incisions and Punctures
ten cause great Pain, and endan-
:r a Mortification. The *Turks*,
ho are ignorant generally of Sur-
:ry, unless perhaps some wander-
g *Jew* practises it amongst them,
ment their Wounds, and wash them
ith Wine successfully. Gangrenes
ill sometimes happen from unskil-
lly cutting Corns, or the Nails of
e Toes, especially if they are ex-
perated with Unguents and Plaist-
s. Spirit of Wine and *Theriaca*
e the best Topics in such Cases.
pirit of Wine used as a *Fotus* for a
fficient Time, and upon some Oc-
sions repeated, extinguishes the
feat of an Erysipelas, sooner than
iy other *Fotus* whatever, whether
ie Erysipelas is cutaneous, true,
id genuine, or spurious, more pro-
und, and deeper in the Flesh. E-
ysipelatous Pains in Wounds and
Ilcers are cured by a *Fotus* of Spi-
t of Wine. If Vesicatories cause
reat Pains, and endanger a Morti-
cation, a *Fotus* of Spirit of Wine
ill cure them. Inflammations
aufed by Vesicatories, which are
ttended with violent Pains, and a
lackish Colour, and which tend to a
iangrene, are easily cured by fo-
ienting them with a linnen Cloth
oubled, and dipped in hot Wine, or
pirits of Wine, and afterward ap-
lying such a Cloth wetted with
Vine, or Spirit of Wine upon the
'art, without Plaisters, or unctuous
Aedicines. There is a Species of
Colic, which Women are subject to,

which is extremely painful, and is
sometimes fixed on the right Side,
sometimes on the left, below the
Navel, without Vomiting. Dr.
Harris says this is cured in a Day's
Time, or on the same Day, by an
Application of doubled linen Cloth
dipped in very hot Spirits of Wine,
and continued a long Time, even
where Narcotics are useless, or sometimes noxious. This I have frequently found of great Efficacy, in
the Case the Doctor mentions. As
this Author was a Man of undoubted
Integrity, his Authority has the
greater Weight.

Tartarus, Offic. Tartar. Wines,
especially those prepared from Grapes,
or of an acid, and austere Taste,
usually afford a copious Tartar, but
not in Perfection, till they are once
thoroughly fermented; and they
afford the purest, when put up in a
clean Vessel. It is more plentifully
obtained from the Wine, when this
has rested sometime upon the Lees;
and, in some Measure, gently confumed it. The Tartar of fine white
Wine is white; whence *Rhenish*
Wine affords the best, which is
white; and collected in thick Pieces,
for medicinal Use, and the whiter,
heavier, more shining, and thick
the Pieces are, the better. That of
red Wine is red, more impure, less
firm, and the Pieces less solid, and
more unctuous: This stony Salt of
Wine is difficultly dissolved in Water, or Wine itself, but remains almost like a Stone therein. If boiled in a large Proportion of Water, it
dissolves in some Measure, and makes
a turbid Liquor, wherein numerous
shining Corpuscles are observed to
float; and thus, in the Boiling, it
constantly throws up a Skin to the
Surface; which, if taken off with a
Skimmer, and put into a wide Ves-
fel to be dried, is called by the Name
of *Cream of Tartar*: And thus, by
Degrees, the whole Quantity of

Tartar may be converted into a Kind of white acid Powder, excepting only a few feculent Parts, remaining at the Bottom. If pure white Tartar be boiled with twenty times its Quantity, or more, of Water, till the whole is perfectly diffolved therein, and the boiling Liquor be now immediately put into a Cafk, without admitting any *Fæces,* a Cruft will prefently begin to form in all the internal Parts of the Veffel touched by the Liquor, and this Cruft increafes, till, in a fhort Time, nearly all the Tartar fhoots into little fhining figured Lumps, called *Cryftals of Tartar ;* which, being collected, and gently dried, are thus to be preferved feparate. The remaining Water, when cold, retains but little of the Tartar. Thefe Operations fhew, that the Nature of the Salt, which is produced by vinous Fermentation, entirely differs, in thefe Properties, from any other known Salt. A new Solution alfo of the Cream or Cryftals of Tartar, may be made in frefh boiling Water, fo as to obtain them each time more pure and white ; but the Virtue of them both, fcarce appears greater for any chymical or medicinal Ufes, than that of Tartar itfelf. It is a great Corrector of thofe Bodies which abound in a fharp bilious putrid Matter, and hence becomes an approved Remedy in acute Difeafes ; it cleanfes the firft Paffages, without much difturbing the more internal Parts. With a corrupt acrimonious Matter it loofes its Acidity, changes into a very foluble Subftance, and hence becomes a good aperitive Remedy. As Tartar is a Thing of very great Importance in Medicine it may be worth while in this Place, to confider its *Analyfis,* which I fhall give in the Words of the celebrated *Boerhaave :* " Fill two- " thirds of a Glafs Retort, with " choice Pieces of the beft white " Tartar, and place it in a fand Fur-

" nace, apply a large Glafs Receiver, " or one that is of the greateft Size, " and lute the Juncture with a com- " mon Mixture of Linfeed-Meal. " Apply a gentle Fire for fome " confiderable Time, fcarce ex- " ceeding one hundred Degrees, " there will come out a fmall Quan- " tity of a limpid, thin, tartifh, " fomewhat fpirituous, bitterifh, " and lightly odorous Liquor, " which is fo penetrating, as eafily " to fweat thro' the Luting ; let this " be kept feparate, then the Fire " being raifed to the Heat of boil- " ing Water, a white Vapour comes " over and along with it a highly " penetrating Spirit which is won- " derfully flatulent and will pafsthro' " almoft any Luting, and if we endea- " vour to confine it by that call'd " the *Lutum Sapientiæ,* it burfts the " Glafs by its Elafticity, and it ufu- " ally breaks out with Force, or per- " fpires at Intervals, thro' the Lu- " ting, and along with this " flatulent Spirit, there comes over " a thin, and extremely fubtile Oil, " of a yellow Colour, a fomewhat " aromatic Tafte, bitter, heating, " and of no ungrateful Odour. This " furprifing Oil I have found fo in- " credibly penetrating, that when " the Neck of the Retort enter'd " five Inches into the Mouth of the " Receiver, and the Juncture was " clofely luted, yet this volatile " Oil always returned back, and " paffed thro' the Body of the Lu- " ting fo as partly to diftill in Drops, " into a Cup fet underneath, and " in Part to run down the external " Surface of the Receiver, nor could " I hitherto by any Means prevent " this Effect ; for if a Luting be ap- " plied, that the Oil cannot pafs " thro', the Veffel flies to Pieces. I " did not therefore wonder to find " *Paracelfus* and *Helmont,* fo highly " recommend this Oil in Diforders " of the Ligaments, Membranes, and " Ten-

" Tendons, which they upon Experi-
" ence have declared may be cured by
" it even tho' contracted. The for-
" mer Matters being collected fe-
" parate, let the Remainder be
" urged gradually to the utmost De-
" gree of Heat that Sand will give,
" and thus again a Spirit will come
" over, and an Oil as before, but
" at the fame time a grofs, black,
" fetid, ponderous, glutinous and
" bitter Oil, leaving the remaining
" Tartar, black, fharp, and in every
" refpect truely alcaline. If this
" Mafs be urged with the ftrongeft
" Fire of Suppreffion, it will ftill
" yield a very thick, black and pitchy
" Oil, along with a certain Smoak,
" and thefe will continue to rife,
" how violent foever the Fire be
" made, and how long foever the
" Operation is continued, and there
" will ftill remain an extremely black,
" fharp, alcaline and dry Mafs, at
" the Bottom which being expofed
" to the open Air by breaking the
" Glafs, grows hot upon Contact
" therewith, and readily diffolves
" into a Liquor, nor can it be kept
" dry without great Caution, where-
" as the Tartar from whence it was
" produced, would fcarce diffolve
" in Water; when this dry black
" Mafs is expofed to a naked Fire,
" in the open Air, it takes Flame,
" and after burning, leaves a copious
" white alcaline Salt behind, as
" ftrong, fiery and pure as can any
" way be prepared. It affords but
" little Earth, and readily diffolves
" fpontaneoufly; if long detained in
" a ftrong Fire, it grows blue, of a
" marble Colour, and fometimes
" brown, and thus always becomes
" ftronger and ftronger." From
hence we learn many Particulars,
and firft how wonderful a thing Fermentation is, which feparates all the
grofs Parts, and leaves a tranfparent,
fubtile, fluid Wine, which generates
an almoft ftony Body that does not
diffolve in cold Water, while the
Principles of this Body lay concealed
in fo thin a Liquor. This ftony
Mafs alfo contains Water, a Spirit
and different kinds of Oil, thick and
copious. It is hard to conceive how
this Oil could lie concealed in the
Wine, which feems to contain Alcohol indeed, but no fuch Oil; but
what is more furprifing, the entire
Mafs of Tartar is merely acid, and
makes an Effervefcence with Alcalies
and yet by the bare Action of no
violent Fire, in a clofe Veffel, without any confiderable Separation of an
Acid, the greateft Part of its whole
Bulk is changed from an Acid to true
Alcali, and this perhaps is the only
Example where a fixt alcaline Salt is
produced in a clofe Veffel, by a moderate Fire, without the free Admiffion of the Air, whilft in other
Cafes only a black infipid Coal is
thus produced. Who wou'd have
thus fufpected that a manifeft Acid
could, by this Means, have changed
to an Alcali? And if the acid Water,
the Spirit and the Oil be poured back
upon this alcaline Mafs, from whence
they were before extracted, and the
Diftillation, performed as before,
fcarce any Acid will come over and
little Oil, but nearly the whole Mafs
will be turned into Alcali; whence
we fee that a large Quantity of a
very acid Matter may be eafily
changed to an alcaline Subftance,
but, on the contrary, I am acquainted with no Inftance in Chymiftry,
of fuch a manifeft Change of a ftrong
Alcali into an Acid; Whence I cannot fufficiently admire the particular
Nature of this Tartar, as knowing
nothing like it. The firft diftilled
and highly penetrating Oil of Tartar
is recommended for difcuffing cold
Tumours, and for reftoring Motion
to the dried tendinous Parts in contracted Limbs, together with the
Affiftance of proper Baths, Fomentations, and Frictions. If thefe Oils

be

be rectified and rendered more fubtile and penetrating, they are recommended by Chymifts, even for refolving gouty Knots and Concretions. It is faid by many that rich Perfumes may be exalted by this Oil, but they alfo fay that decayed Mufks and Civet may have their Scents invigorated, by being fufpended in a Jakes. Salt of Tartar may be thus prepared in a greater Proportion to the Tartar employed than by any other known Method, and in greater Plenty the flower the Diftillation was performed. This is alfo the beft, fharpeft, moft penetrating and pure of all the fixt Alcalies, nor is there any other known Body in Nature that affords more of fuch faline alcaline Matter than Tartar. And if the black alcaline Matter, remaining after the moft violent Diftillation, be fet by in the Retort flightly covered with Paper, it wholly refolves into a Liquor, which being filtered, affords an admirable Oil of Tartar *per Deliquium*, extremely fit for numerous chymical Ufes and particular Operations. If the fame be firft ftrongly calcined in an open Fire, it thus alfo refolves in the Air and affords an Oil of Tartar *per Deliquium*, but of a more fharp and alcaline Nature than the former.

Vinum. Wine. The Principles, or Elements, of which Wine is compofed, are, firft, an inflammable Spirit: Secondly, a Phlegm: Thirdly, an acid tartareous Salt: And, fourthly, a certain fulphureous and oleous Subftance. Wines therefore, differ from each other, with Refpect to Tafte, Smell, and Virtues, according to the Mixture and Proportion of thefe Elements. Such Wines as contain a large Quantity of inflammable Spirit, foon intoxicate, and heat the Body; but Wines in which the phlegmatic or tartareous acidulated Parts predominate, are of a laxative and diuretic Quality; nor do they

eafily affect the Head. Wines which contain a great deal of an oleous and fulphureous Subftance, fuch as old Wines, are of a deep yellow Colour, of a ftrong Tafte and Smell; and as they are not eafily tranfpired, fo they remain long in the Blood, and dry the Body. There is, alfo, another effential Element, or Principle, in Wines, which is a certain fweet, oleous, temperate, and vifcid Subftance, difcoverable in Wines which are not fufficiently fermented, or gently boiled; and fuch a Principle is, particularly, obferved in ftrong Sack, Frontignac, and *Hungarian* Wine. This Principle not only renders Wine grateful to the Tafte, but, alfo, of a nutritive and demulcent Quality. Tho' all Wines may be refolved into their conftituent Principles, that is, a Spirit, an Oil, a Phlegm, a fweet Subftance, and an acid tartareous Part, yet they differ in this, that fome contain a fweet and fubtile Sulphur, whereas others have a coarfer Sulphur, which is not fo grateful to the Tafte. The Colours of Wines depend on the fulphureous oleous Principle, which, by the inteftine fermentative Motion, is intimately refolved and mixed with the Parts of the Wine: The deeper the Colour, therefore, of Wine is, the larger Quantity of Oil they contain. When, therefore, the Spirit is abftracted from the Wine, the fpirituous, aqueous, and acid Parts, are carried off, and there is left in the Veffel a thick Mafs, of a darkifh and very deep Colour; to which if a confiderable Quantity of Water is poured, it is immediately tinged with the fame Colour the Wine had in its natural State; which is a fure Proof that the Wine derived its Colour from the thick, fulphureous, and oleous Mafs, which remains in the Veffel after Diftillation. Red Wines receive their Colour from the red Pellicles of the Grapes, upon which they ftand long

infused; the Acid, therefore, which in Musts, also, extracts and exalts the Colour which is contained in these Pellicles; for which Reason, that Colour is purely adventitious. All red Wines are possessed of an astringent Taste and Virtue, because they stand long infused not only with the red Pellicles of the Grapes, but, also, with their small Stones, which are of a manifestly astringent Taste. Hence they extract the astringent Principle from these two Substances, and receive it into themselves. The Countries lying between the fortieth and fiftieth Degrees of Latitude, such as *Hungary, Spain, Portugal, Italy, France,* a great Part of *Germany, Austria, Transylvania,* and a great Part of *Greece,* produce the best Wines; because, in these Parts, the Influence of the Sun is great. It is, also, certain, from Experience, that mountainous steep Places, with Rivers at their Roots, produce the best Wines; for, besides the Influence of the Sun, the Goodness of Wines, in a great Measure, depends on the fine and subtile Nourishment of the Grapes. Now because the Mountains are exposed to the Night Dews, which abound about the Rivers, and contain a subtile Water, intermix'd with an etherial Principle, it is not to be wondered at, if Dew should be the best Nourishment for the finest Vines. But Dew alone is not sufficient for the Nourishment of Vines, which, also, requires Rains. The Nature of the Soil, also, contributes much to the Production of good Wine; for we observe, that the best Vines grow not in fat, clayey, gross, and black Soils; but rather in such as are stony, sandy, or chalky; which Kinds of Earths, though apparently barren, are yet very proper for Vines; because they long retain the solar Rays, which, by cherishing the Roots, make the Nourishment pass thro' all the Pores

of the Plant. Besides, the Waters, passing thro' such Earths, are attenuated and strained, and their grosser Parts separated, and retained; so that the nutritive Juice of the Plant must be more pure and subtil. The Causes of the different Tastes, Salubrity, and Insalubrity of Wines, are, without doubt, placed in the different Nature of the Soil; since Tracts of Ground, lying on the same Mountain, with equal Aspects to the Sun, and bearing Vines of the same Species, yet yield Wines greatly different, with Respect to Salubrity, Taste, and a penetrating Quality. The superior Virtues of the *Tokay* Wine, are, by the Inhabitants of that Part of the Country, ascribed to the Gold there produced, but more justly to the large Quantity of corroborating Sulphur contained in the Earth; since neither Gold, nor any other Metal, can contribute to the Fruitfulness of the Earth, much less to exalt the Juices of Vegetables, or render them more salutary. But the Reason why all the *Hungarian* Wines are more salutary than others, depends on the Subtilty and Fineness of the Nourishment with which the Vines are nourished, and the large Quantity of the aerial and etherial Principle, which is intimately mixed with their Juices, and which renders both Aliments and Medicines far more salubrious than they would otherwise be.

In malignant Fevers, according to *Hoffman,* nothing is more excellent than Wine. The Malignity of these Disorders is known from a Defect of Motion and Strength, and from a Want of a due spirituous Quality in the Blood, arising from a slow Circulation of the same; all which indicate a certain Disposition of the Fluids to Putrefaction. It is, therefore, expedient, in all these Disorders, to restore the Strength, rouse the Spirits, increase the Circulation of the Blood, and promote Perspiration. These are the Designs

signs of all Alexipharmics. But all these Intentions are answered by Wine, as is obvious, not only from the Authorities of practical Writers, but, also, from Experience : In those Disorders where the peccant Matter is to be expell'd to the Surface of the Body, such as the Measles, Small-Pox and *Petecchia*, where Nature is weak, and the Motion of the Heart is sufficient for the Expulsion, or when, through Weakness there is a Retrocession of the Eruptions, Wine is highly proper ; but we are to abstain from its Use, when these Disorders are accompanied with an excessive Heat, an Ebullition of the Humours, and a quick Pulse. In continual Fevers, *Hippocrates* recommends white Wine, both alone, and mix'd with Water. Numberless Practitioners are of the same Opinion. Thus *Forestus* recommends fine small Rhenish white Wine ; and *Helmont* tells us, that they who moderately use Wine in continual Fevers, easily recover, preserve their Strength, and sooner recover their former State and Condition. Wine is still more proper in Intermittents, which generally arise from Crudities, an Obstruction of the Evacuations, and especially a Suppression of Transpiration. This Liquor is to be exhibited pretty liberally, on the Days of Intermission ; but sparingly, or not at all, during the Paroxysm, unless in the Decline of the Disease, and when the Body is disposed to sweat. The Reason why Wine ought to be prohibited in almost all Fevers, is this : A Fever is an intense Commotion of Blood, excited in order to remove and expel what threatens the Destruction of the Body. Now, it is sufficiently obvious, that where this Motion is intense, and too strong, Wine is to be sparingly used ; but if this Motion is so weak and languid, that Nature seems ready to sink, it is to be quickened by a proper Dose of white Wine, in order to restore languid Nature. In *Syncopes*, and Loss of Strength, nothing is more excellent than Wine. *Galen* orders those afflicted with a *Syncope* to drink Wine which is thin, of a yellow Colour, and old, rather than such as is new, or of a middle Age : Because the first not only restores the Strength, and recruits the Spirits ; but, also, by its Smell, or when applied to the Heart and Wrists, far surpasses all other Cordials, and Analeptics. In Nauseas, Weakness, Indigestion, and Inflation of the Stomach, nothing is more beneficial than Wine. Hence St. *Paul*, as we see in 1 *Timothy* v. 23. advises *Timothy* to use Wine for a certain Disorder of his Stomach. *Galen* tells us, that the Wines which are yellow or white, fragrant and thin, are excellent Stomachics, especially if they are gently astringent ; and such are the *Rhenish* Wines, which, on Account of their subtil, acid, spirituous, and astringent Principle, are highly beneficial, in exciting the Appetite, strengthening the Stomach, and promoting the Digestion of the Aliments. In a *Fames Canina*, or preternatural Voracity, *Hippocrates* recommends the drinking of Wine ; and this Advice is founded on Reason : But that Author did not, in this Passage, mean every Wine, but only such as is generous, pure, and old. For the Cause of this Disorder is an acid corrosive Humour in the Stomach, which, by such Wine is excellently corrected, just as the corrosive Nature of Spirit of Nitre, or Vitriol, is corrected by the Admixture of Spirit of Wine ; or as the Acidity of Tartar, so long as it is in Conjunction with the Wine, is so corrected, as to prove grateful to the Palate. In order to allay Thirst, nothing is more effectual than Wine mixed with Water ; for, by this Means, it far sooner extinguishes Thirst, than if Water had

been

been exhibited alone, since Thirst arises from an Obstruction and Constriction of those Glands which discharge the *Saliva* into the *Fauces*, for moistening them, and the *Oesophagus*; but these Glands are better opened by Wine and Water, than by pure Water; for which Reason *Hippocrates*, in acute Fevers, was not afraid to prescribe a Mixture of Water and Wine. In Vomitings of the Idiopathic Kind, or such as accompany Fevers as a Symptom, thin Wine is preferable to all other Liquors. In Colics, especially those arising from Flatulencies, or viscid Crudities, nothing is more beneficial than old *Rhenish* Wine. For this Purpose, *Hippocrates* recommends rich Wines, because it renders crude Matter fit for Concoction, attenuates what is thick, and discusses Flatulencies. *Crato* also recommends *Rhenish* Wine in Colics, but forbids the Use of *Moravian* and *Austrian* Wines, as also, the *Malmsey* Wines, which are sweet, thick, and turbid. In *Diarrhoeas* and Dysenteries, which appear as the Symptoms of acute Distempers, small *Rhenish* Wine, either alone, or mixed with a Ptisan, produces excellent Effects, since it is possessed of a subastringent Quality, by which the Tone of the Intestines, and their relaxed glandular Coats, are greatly strengthened: And as, in these Disorders, it is highly expedient to move the Humours from the Centre to the Circumference, to augment Perspiration, and provoke Urine, hence Wine is excellent, because it produces such Effects. Red Wines, on Account of their greater Astringency, are generally recommended; and if they are good, they may be used for that Purpose. In Obstructions of the Liver and Spleen, in the Jaundice, and Cachexy, Wine produces excellent Effects. *Solenander* a celebrated Practitioner, recommends a Mixture of chalybeate Water with a Wine which is white, pure, ripe, not strong, but pellucid, such as the *Rhenish* and *Moselle* Wines, as highly grateful to the Liver; and asserts, that by their astringent Quality, they corroborate the *Viscera*. But sweet Wines, because they increase the Quantity of the Blood, are greatly condemned by *Hippocrates* and *Guarinonius*. In Dropsies, *Hippocrates* extols austere, and aqueous Wines. And *Epiphan. Ferdinand.* informs us, that Persons labouring under an *Ascites* have been cured by the Use of *Malmsey* Wine alone. It is justly to be doubted, whether Wine is proper in hypochondriac Disorders; for I have frequently (says *Hoffman*) observed in Practice, that the Symptoms were exasperated by acid Wines, especially of the rough Kind. The Reason why hypochondriac Patients cannot bear Wines inclining to Acidity, seems to be this: On Account of the slow peristaltic Motion of the Intestines, their Contents are not promoted, hypochondriac Patients being generally costive, but become stagnant, and, by their Continuance, contract an Acrimony. Hence Wine, in such Patients, is by the Stagnation of the *Faeces*, converted into a strong Vinegar, which stimulates the nervous Parts to Spasms. But since hypochondriac Patients require a Reinforcement of Strength, and call for additional Force and Heat in their Stomach, Wine is not to be absolutely denied them. Hence *Brunnerus*, in hypochondriac Patients, prefers old *Rhenish*, or good *Hungarian* Wines, moderately used at Meals. But those affected with Disorders of this Kind, ought to abstain from red, austere, and sweet Wines, and from the excessive Use of all. In a Scurvy, which generates a large Quantity of fixed tartareous Salts, *Rhenish* Wine is excellent, because it is diuretic. Hence *Sachsius*, informs us, that *Rhenish* Wines are highly beneficial

ficial in a Scurvy, becauſe they by Urine, evacuate the tartareous *Sordes*; and that, in ſcorbutic Patients, he has obſerved an Evacuation of thick Urine, abounding with Tartar, procured by *Rheniſh* Wines. *Reiſner* recommends ſtrong, generous, and unmixed Wines, for ſcorbutic Patients ; but orders them to be drank in a ſmall Quantity ; and, if the Patient's Heat is increaſed, to be diluted with Water mixed with Raiſins. In the Stone of the Kidneys, ſweet, generous, and oleous Wines are by *Crato* juſtly condemned, becauſe the Stone is generally formed by a Redundance of Blood obſtructing the abdominal *Viſcera* and Kidneys, and producing, firſt, an Inflammation, and then an Ulceration of the Kidneys, and then the Stone. But that a *Plethora* is augmented by ſweet Wines, we have already obſerved. The Stone is, alſo, generated in the Kidneys, by turbid and auſtere Wines, ſuch as thoſe of *Numbergen* in *Germany*. But *Rheniſh* Wines are good againſt the Stone, becauſe they are highly diuretic. *Schulzius* recommends the *Neccarine* Wines. *Unxerus* extols rich Wines, moderately drank, after due Evacuation of the Body. *Montanus*, greatly recommends pure, ripe, and rich Wines of a white Colour, in nephritic Diſorders. A Strangury, according to *Hippocrates*, is removed by drinking Wine; but this Aphoriſm is to be underſtood principally of generous Wine, becauſe the Diſorder treated of generally ariſes from a Suppreſſion of Tranſpiration, which is reſtored by Wine of this Kind. It is a Queſtion of great Moment, whether Wine is proper in arthritic and gouty Diſorders? It is a common Perſuaſion, that theſe Diſeaſes are produced by Wine, and that they are only to be cured by drinking Water, and abſtaining from Wine. It is certain, that theſe Diſorders ariſe from a ſub-

tile Tartar, which lacerates the Membranes. Hence Wines, which contain a large Quantity of Tartar, ſeem to be prejudicial in them. But theſe tartareous Diſeaſes proceed from an Obſtruction of the Emunctories, and a Viſcidity and Denſity of the Humours. But Wine excellently conveys the morbific Matter through the Kidneys, which are the proper Emunctories of the Tartar. Hence there is no Reaſon why Wines ſhould not be admitted, eſpecially ſince the Gout generally derives its Origin from a Weakneſs of the Stomach, a Defect of a ſpirituous Quality in the Blood; and a ſlow Circulation of the Humours. Hence, Wine exhibited with a proper *Regimen*, and by the Direction of a Phyſician, may prove a Preſervative againſt the Gout, if it is uſed out of the Paroxyſm. But as there are great Differences, not only between Wines, but, alſo, between Conſtitutions, ſo the Phyſician ought to be circumſpect. Generous Wines, that are not acid, ſuch as the *Hungarian* Wines, agree with ſome Patients. *Crato* orders gouty Patients to drink a little *Hungarian*, or *Malmſey* Wines at Meals. And *Solenander* recommends the moderate Uſe of Wine for gouty Patients, on Account of the Weakneſs of their Stomachs. The ſame Author ſpeaks in the following Manner: " We are to " obſerve what the State of the Stomach, and of the reſt of the Bo- " dy, can bear. Nor is abſolute " Abſtinence to be enjoined Patients of " every Temperament, Conſtitution, " Age, and Method of Life ; be- " cauſe there are great Varieties of " Patients. If Wine, eſpecially of " the gently aſtringent Kind, is " drank moderately, and at a proper " Time, its Uſe will be beneficial, " inſtead of hurtful. Thus we ſee, " that by the Exhibition of a little " Wine in the Decline of the Pa- " roxyſm, gouty Pains are allevia-
" ted,

ed, becaufe by the Heat and Spirits excited, the peccant Humour is difcuffed, only the Patient muft abftain from Wine in the Beginning of the Paroxyfm." Having is confidered the Efficacy of Wine the Cure of internal Diforders, we ll now treat of the Injuries arifing m its prepofterous Ufe in fome Difers. It is, therefore, certain from perience and Reafon, that in all forders, where a great Quantity Blood is congefted, as in Inflamtions, and moft Diforders of the ad, efpecially an Head-ach arif; from an hot Caufe, a *Phrenitis*, idnefs, Vertigo, Epilepfies, Lergies, and all drowfy Diforders, ines of every Kind are prejudicial; fince in thefe Diforders the Blood impetuoufly convey'd to the Part ected, and collected there, it muft culate flowly. Hence Wine, which its Spirit afcends to the Head, i produces a greater Rarefaction the Blood, which it forces more pioufly and impetuoufly from the eart, to the Part obftructed, muft duce an Exafperation of thefe forders. *Hippocrates*, alfo, in a inful Repletion of the Brain, ors Abftinence from Wine; and afts, that apoplectic Patients ought ally to abftain from Wines; and further tells us, that in a *Sphace-* of the Brain, and a Lethargy, Patient is totally to abftain from ine. A phrenitic Patient, fays he, uld be warmed with warming Liors, and Potions; but Wine muft t be ufed for this Purpofe. And alfo tells us, that mad Perfons ght not to drink Wine. Wine is o hurtful in a Cough and Phthifis, caufe the *Afpera Arteria* cannot ar its acrid ftimulating Quality. t fince fweet Wine affifts Expectotion, the moderate Ufe of it is not jurious, nor when the Cough is on

the Decline, is old *Rhenifh* Wine to be prohibited, but rather prefcribed. *Tirellus* tells us, that Wines fupport the Sound, recover the Sick, revive the Languid, and perform Miracles. Extracts, Quinteffences, Bolufes, and Pills, are to be defpifed in Comparifon of Wines, which are the Support of the innate Heat; and ought, therefore, to be celebrated with Praifes, proportioned to the Advantages Mankind reap from them. What I have faid above with Refpect to Wines, muft be underftood of thofe which are pure, and unadulterated, and not of the Wines commonly made ufe of among us, which as they are manufactured, muft be extremely prejudicial both in Sicknefs and in Health. Wine as a Prefervative of Health, has always been in high Efteem, but with what Juftice I will not take upon me to determine; but I muft remark, that the Antients drank their Wines in a manner very different from the Moderns; for the former mix'd at leaft four Parts of Water, but generally fix, with their Wine, which muft be attended with mnch more falutary Effects to the Conftitution, than when taken pure, and undiluted, in the manner now generally practifed. It is certain that Health, and an equable Circulation of the Blood and Humours through the Veffels, contribute greatly to the Improvement of the Imagination, Genius, and Courage. And Wine has been faid to do this, in fo great a Degree, that the Wit, Courage, and fuperior Learning of the *Greeks*, have been afcribed to the moderate Ufe of their generous Wines; all which they loft, and degenerated into a kind of brutal Stupidity, as foon as the *Turks* conquered their Country, and deftroyed their Vines.

THE

THE NEW

English Dispensatory.

BOOK IV.

GENERAL EXPRESSIONS *including several* SIMPLES *at once.*

The five opening Roots.

SMALLAGE.
Asparagus.
Fennel.
Parsley, and,
Butchers Broom.

The five emollient Herbs.

Marsh-mallows.
Mallows.
Mercury.
Pellitory of the Wall, and,
Violets.

The four cordial Flowers.

Borage Flowers.
Buglofs Flowers.
Roses, and
Violets.

The four greater hot Seeds.

Aniseed.
Carraway Seed.
Cumin Seed, and,
Fennel Seed.

The four lesser hot Seeds.

Those of Bishops Weed.
Smallage.
Stone-Parsley, and,
Wild Carrot.

The four greater cold Seeds.

Those of Cucumbers.
Gourds.
Melons, and,
Water Melons.

The

The four leſſer cold Seeds.

hoſe of Endive.
   Lettice.
   Purſlane, and,
   Succory.

f the Weights and Meaſures at preſent uſed in the Shops; together with the ſeveral Characters of Abbreviation, which occur in Preſcriptions.

THO' it is certainly a Thing of the laſt Importance to preſerve e due Proportions of the ſeveral Inodients of Medicines, yet an Error this Reſpect has hitherto prevailed uiverſally. This unlucky Overſight occaſioned by the Uſe of different ecies of Weight in ſelling different ommodities. Thus Gold and Silr are ſold by Troy-weight, and oſt other Things by what we call verdupoize-weight. The Pound roy is divided into twelve Ounces, e Pound Averdupoize into ſixteen. at in theſe Weights neither Pounds r Ounces are the ſame, the Pound roy being much leſs than the Pound verdupoize, tho' the Troy Ounce heavier than that of the other. As e medicinal Pound is divided into ve!ve Ounces, ſo the various Sub-viſions of the ſame into Drams, cruples, and Grains, which the potbecaries uſe, are adjuſted to e Troy Ounce. But as Druggiſts d wholeſale Dealers ſell by the verdupoize-weight, ſo the Apoiecaries do not generally uſe Troy Veight for Pounds and Ounces; hence it happens that when me Ingredients are preſcribed in ounds, and others in Ounces, they re not proportion'd to the Intion of the Preſcription; and when ny Ingredients are ordered in any ubdiviſion, their ſmall Weights beig adapted to a greater Ounce,

than the Averdupoize, theſe Ingredients muſt of Courſe be diſproportioned.

Another Error in proportioning the Ingredients of Medicines is the applying the Names of Weights to Meaſures, tho' the Liquors contained in thoſe Meaſures have not the Weight implied by theſe Names.

To prevent the future Inconveniencies which might ariſe from theſe and other ſimilar Errors, the Compilers of the laſt *London Diſpenſatory* have aſcertained their Weight, which is that of Troy, and their Meaſure, which is what we commonly call Wine Meaſure, in the following Manner.

	contains	
℔ A Pound,		Twelve Ounces
℥ An Ounce.		Eight Drams.
ʒ A Dram.		Three Scruples
℈ A Scruple.		Twenty Grains

The Meaſures moſt in Uſe with us are,

	contains	
A Pint		Sixteen Ounces.
An Ounce		Eight Drams.
A Gallon		Eight Pints.
A Spoonful		Half an Ounce.
A Cyathus		An Ounce and an half.

An Explanation of ſome abbreviated Characters.

Cong. A Gallon.
Cochl. A Spoonful. We muſt obſerve, that a Spoonful contains half an Ounce of Syrups, and but only three Drams of diſtilled Waters.
M. A Handful.
S. V. R. Spirit of Wine, rectified.
C. C. Hart's Horn.
S. a. According to Art.
ſs. The Half of any Thing.
F. Form into.
B. M. Water Bath.
P. A Pugil, the eighth Part of a Handful.

P. E. Equal Parts.

C. C. C. Burnt Harts Horn.

q. s. A sufficient Quantity.

ana : of each.

q. v. As much as you please.

B. A. A Sand Bath, or Heat.

B. V. A Vapour Bath.

CHAP. I.

GENERAL RULES *for the gathering of* SIMPLES.

LET the annual *Roots* be gathered before they shoot out their Stems or Flowers; the biennial principally in the *Autumn* of that Year, in which their Seeds are first sown; and the perennial when the Leaves begin to fall, and therefore generally in the *Autumn.* Having first wash'd away the Filth, and cleared them of their withered and corrupted Fibres, hang them up in a shady, airy Place, that they may dry moderately. Let the thicker be cut in Pieces, either lengthwise, or transversely; preserving the cortical Part, and rejecting the Pith. Those Roots which loose their Virtues by drying should be kept covered with dry Sand.

Let *Herbs* be gathered at the Time of their Vigour, when they have shot into perfect Leaves; but before the Flowers are opened. Of some it is best to take only their flowering Tops. Let them be dried, as is directed above with Respect to Roots.

Let *Flowers* be gathered when they are moderately expanded, upon a clear Day, before Noon; but Roses, for, Conserve, in the Bud, before they open.

Let *Seeds* be gathered when ripe, and beginning to dry, before they fall spontaneously: The same is to be observed of Fruits, unless they be ordered green.

Woods for medicinal Uses are best felled in the Winter; and this is the best Season for shaving off their Barks.

Animals, and *Minerals* should be chose in their utmost Perfection, unless required otherwise.

These are the Rules laid down by the Compilers of the *Edinburgh* Dispensatory, who seem to have consider'd the Subject with Attention, and directed with Judgment and Accuracy.

Preparation of Fats.

The Fat, being first purged of its Membranes, Blood Vessels, and Strings, is to be wash'd in fresh Parcels of Waters, till it will no longer tinge the same Red; then let it be melted, and strained, and preserved from the Injuries of the Air. E.

The Directions of the *London* Dispensatory are to melt the Fats, with the Addition of a little Water, to keep the Fat from burning, or turning black, which they would otherwise be subject to do if the Fire was too intense. But they are first to be chopt into small Pieces, and at last strained when melted. The Fat of a Viper requires only separating, from the Intestines with a gentle Heat, and then straining thro' a thin Cloth; no Water being here necessary.

Prepared

Prepared, or washed Aloes.

Diffolve the Aloes in a fufficient quantity of Spring-water, over a ntle Fire; then ftrain it, and rowing away the *Fæces*, evaporate to the Confiftence of Honey. But e pureft tranfparent *Aloes* requires rwafhing. E.

Prepared Gum Ammoniac.

Diffolve *Gum Ammoniac* in Vine-r, ftrain the Solution, and after-irds evaporate the Vinegar with a ntle Heat. E.

Preparation of Bees.

Put Bees into a proper Veffel, and y them with a very flow Heat. E.

Preparation of Bole Armoniac.

Diffolve powder'd Bole, in a fuf-ient Quantity of Spring-water; r them well together, and after-irds decant the Water, now fatu-ed with the fine Flower. Pour on fh Water till the Bole is entirely Tolved, and only the fmall Sand d Stones are left behind. Mix e feveral Parcels of turbid Water, gether, then fuffer them to reft, d the Bole will fubfide, which, er the Water is poured off, muft dry'd for Ufe. E.

This is an admirable Way of redu-rg hardSubftances to a fine Powder, d is applicable to many other Parts the *Materia Medica*, both thofewhich :, and thofe which are not capable Solution. But in the Preparation fome which Water will fpoil, Spi-ofWine fhould be fubftituted in its ad.

Preparation of Toads.

Put live Toads in an earthen Pot, d dry them in an Oven moderately ated to fuch a Degree as that they iy be pulverized. E.

Preparation of Calamine.

Make Calamine thrice red hot, and as often quench it in Rofe-wa-ter; then levigate it with the fame Water, upon a Porphyry, and after-wards form it into Balls. E.

Care fhould be taken to powder Calaminefiner, or coarfer, according to theUfes it is to be apply'd to, for I am inform'd, that the Surgeons have ob-ferv'd Calamine finely powder'd, to act as a Sort of Efcharotic whereas in a more grofs Powder, it operates only as a Dryer. For the latter ufe, fimple Levigation will be fufficient, but for the former it fhould be treated in the Manner above directed for *Bole Armoniac*. To fave the Trou-ble of calcining Calamine, the *Lon-don* Difpenfatory directs that to be procur'd, which is ready calcin'd for the Brafs Works.

The Preparation of terreftrious and fuch other Bodies, as will not dif-folve in Water, from the London Difpenfatory.

Thefe Bodies are firft to be pound-ed in a Mortar, then levigated with a little Water upon a hard and fmooth Marble into an impalpable Powder, afterwards dried upon a Chalk-ftone, and then fet by for a few Days in fome warm, or at leaft, very dryPlace.

After this Manner are to be redu-ced into Powder, Amber, Antimo-ny, Bezoar, which fhould be leviga-ted with Spirit of Wine inftead of Water; becaufe this heightens the greenColour, Blood-ftone, Chalk, Co-ral, Crabs-Claws, Crabs-Eyes, Egg-Shells, firft feparated from the Mem-brane adhering to them by boiling in Water, Oyfter fhells, firft cleanfed, Pearls, Verdegrife, Tutty. The *Spiculæ* of Antimony if not reduc'd to exceffive fine Powder, are fubject to wound theCoats of theStomach, Care muft therefore be taken to powder it very fine, and the fame Caution is requifite with Refpect to Tutty, which is principally ufed for that tender Organ the Eye.

T t   *Th*

The Calcination of Hartshorn.

Burn Pieces of Hartshorn in a Potter's Furnace, till they become perfectly white; then reduce them to Powder after the same Manner, as other terrestrious Substances. L.

Preparation of Galbanum.

This is prepared in the same Manner as *Gum Ammoniac.*

Preparation of Lapis Lazuli.

Levigate this upon a Porphyry, then wash it several times in Spring-water, and afterwards dry the Powder. E.

Preparation of Litharge.

Litharge is prepared as *Bole Armoniac.* E.

Preparation of Filings of Iron.

Take such Filings of Iron as have been cleans'd by the Magnet, and set them in a moist Place, that they may turn to Rust, which grind to impalpable Powder. They are likewise prepared with Vinegar. They are also prepar'd by exposing the Filings of Iron to the Air, and moistening them with Vinegar or Water, till they are converted into Rust, and then they may be treated, as directed under the Preparation of *Bole Armoniac.* The dry'd Powder is by some called *Alcohol Martis.*

The Despumation, or Clarification of Honey.

Liquify the Honey by a *Balneum* of Water; that is, by setting the Vessel containing the Honey into hot Water; and let the Scum, that rises, be taken off. L.

Preparation of Millepedes.

Let Millepedes be inclosed in a thin Canvas Cloth, and suspended within a covered Vessel over the Steam of hot Spirit of Wine; and they will soon be killed by the Vapour, and be rendered friable. L.

In the *Edinburgh* Dispensatory, they are directed to be dry'd in a proper Vessel, with a very slow Heat.

Strain'd Opium, or the Thebaic Extract.

Take of Opium cut into small Bits one pound Weight; dissolve it into a Pulp with one Pint or less of boiling Water, taking care to avoid burning; and while it remains quite hot, press it strongly through a linen Cloth from its Dregs; then reduce the strained Opium by a Water Balneum, or other small Heat to its first Consistence.

Opium softened in this small Quantity of Water, passes the Strainer unaltered in its Substance, and freed only from Dregs; but if it be dissolved in a large Quantity of Water, the gummy and resinous Parts will divide from each other. L.

After the same Manner the rest of the Gums may be purified, such as Gum Ammoniac, Asa Fœtida, Galbanum, and the like. But a greater Quantity of Water may be safely used. If the resinous Part subsides, let it be taken out, and added towards the Conclusion of the Inspissation, that it may unite with the rest into one uniform Mass. Any Gum, as Galbanum, which easily melts, may be purified by including the Gum in a Bullock's Bladder, and retaining it in warm Water, till the Gum becomes soft enough to be separated from its Dregs by pressing through a Canvas Strainer.

Preparation of Opoponax and Sagapenum, according to the Edinburgh Dispensatory.

Opoponax should be prepared as *Gum Ammoniac;* so likewise should *Sagapenum.*

The Extraction of Pulps.

Pulpy Fruits, that are unripe, and those

ofe which are ripe, if dry, are to
: boiled in a fmall Quantity of
Vater, till they become foft ; then
e Pulp is to be preffed through a
rongHair-fieve; and afterwards boil-
l over a gentle Fire, and continual-
ftirred to avoid burning, till it is
ought to a due Confiftence. L.

Caffia is alfo to be boiled out from
e Pod or Cane bruifed, and redu-
d afterwards to a juft Confiftence
y evaporating the Water. The
ulps of Fruits, which are both ripe
d frefh, are to be preffed out with-
at any previous Boiling. L.

he Torrefaction of Rhubarb and Nutmegs.

Roaft them with a gentle Heat,
ll they become eafily friable into
owder. L.

Preparation of Goat's Blood.

About the Beginning of Summer
pen fome proper Artery of a middle
ged Goat, and draw out a Quanti-
y of Blood ; which, being received
a a clean Veffel, is to be dried either
y the Heat of the Sun, or a flack
ven. E.

The Baking of Squills.

Inclofe the Squill in Pafte of
Wheat-flower, having firft feparated
he external Skin and the hard Part,
rom which the fibrous Roots grow ;
han bake the Squill in an Oven,
ill the Pafte is dry, and the Squill
s rendered foft and tender through-
ut. This Operation is intended to

mitigate the Acrimony of the Squills;
but is of very little Ufe, as it by no
Means improves their medicinal Vir-
tues, and only fits it for entering as an
Ingredient, into that very trifling
Compofition the *Venice* Treacle.

The Exficcation of Squills.

Cut the Squill, after the external
Skin has been taken off, tranfverfely
into thin Slices, and dry it with a
very gentle Heat. By this Method
the Squills are faid to be fooner dried,
than when the feveral Coats, which
compofe the Squill are feparated from
each other.

The Burning of Sponge.

Heat the Sponge in a covered Veffel, till it becomes black, and is eafily friable, then reduce it to Powder
in a Glafs or marble Mortar. By
this Method, the Oil and volatile
Salt of the Sponge, are preferv'd in
the Subject, provided too intenfe a
Heat is not employ'd: A Glafs or Marble Mortar, fhould be employ'd, for
reducing it to Powder, when thus
calcin'd ; for 'tis faid that a Brafs, or
Bell-metal-Mortar, will render the
calcin'd Sponge offenfive to the Stomach.

The Straining of Storax.

Boil Storax in Water, till it becomes foft, then prefs it out between
warm Iron Plates, and feparate the
Storax now cleared of its Dregs, from
the Water. L.

C H A P. II.

Of W A T E R S.

THE incomparable *Boerhaave*
having laid down fome in-
ftructive Rules, for the Diftillation
of Simple Waters, it will be proper
in this Place to take Notice of them,
for the Information of thofe, who

are lefs acquainted with Pharmacy, and of fuch as have not duly confi-der'd what medicinal Virtues are to be expected in diftill'd Waters. The moft commodious Operation for this Procefs, is that perform'd by a Still-head, clofely fitted into the Mouth of a Veffel, fo as to collect and con-denfe the Vapour arifing by a boiling Heat, and tranfmit it without Lofs into a Receiver. The Defign in Di-ftillation is to collect whatever flies off from a recent Plant, by the natu-ral Degree of the Summer's Heat, up to that of two hundred and fourteen Degrees. And for this Purpofe we are to make Choice of a fapid and odorous Plant, which contains an inflammable, oily, and a fixable fa-line Part, as alfo a faponaceous one, confifting of the two. The Plants defign'd for this Operation are to be gather'd when their Leaves are at full Growth, and a little before the Flowers appear, or before the Seed comes on, becaufe the Virtue of the Subject expected in thefe Waters, is often little, after the Seed or Fruit is form'd, at which Time Plants begin to languifh : The Morning is beft to gather them in, becaufe the volatile Parts are then condenfed by the Cold-nefs of the Night, and kept in by the Tenacity of the Dew, not yet exhaled by the Sun. This is under-ftood, when the Virtue of the diftill'd Water principally refides in the Leaves of the Plants, as it does in Mint, Marjoram, Penny-Royal, Rue, and many more; but the Cafe dif-fers, when the aromatic Virtue is only found in the Flowers, as in Rofes, Lillies of the Valley, &c. in which Cafe we choofe their flowery Parts, whilft they fmell the fweeteft, which fhould be gather'd before they are quite open'd, or begin to fhed, the Morning Dew ftill hanging upon them. In other Plants the Seeds are to be preferr'd, as in Anife, Cara-way, Cumin, &c. where the Herb

and the Flower are indolent, but the whole Virtue remains in the Seed alone, where it manifefts itfelf by its remarkable Fragrance and aromatic Tafte. We find Seeds chiefly pof-fefs'd of this Virtue when come to perfect Maturity. We muft not omit, that thefe defirable Properties are found only in the Roots of cer-tain Plants, as appears in Avens, and in Orpine, whofe Root fmells like a Rofe; and here the Roots fhould be gather'd, for the prefent Purpofe, at that Time when they are richeft in thefe Virtues, which is generally at that Seafon of the Year juft be-fore they begin to fprout, when they are to be dug up in a Morning. If the Virtue here requir'd be contain'd in the Barks or Woods of Vegeta-bles, then thefe Parts are to be cho-fen for the Purpofe.

The Subject being chofen, let it be bruifed or cut, if there be Occa-fion, and with it fill two Thirds of a Still, leaving a third Part of it empty, without fqueezing the Mat-ter clofe; then pour as much frefh Rain Water upon it as will fill the Still to the fame Height, that is, two Thirds, together with the Plant : Fit on the Head exactly to the Neck of the Still, fo that no Vapour may pafs through the Juncture. Let the Joining of the Nofe of the Still Head to the Worm, be luted with a ftiff Pafte, made of Linfeed Meal and Water. Obferve, that the Ca-vity of the Worm be always cleanf-ed by paffing fair boiling Water thro' it, left otherwife the diftill'd Water fhould be foul'd. Apply a Receiver to the Bottom of the Worm, that no Vapour may fly off in the Diftil-lation; but that all the Liquor, be-ing cool'd in the Worm-tub, fill'd with cold Water, may be collected, which is beft perform'd by keeping the Worm-tub continually fupplied with cold Water.

Things being in this State, digeft

eft for twenty-four Hours with a moderate Degree of Heat, of one hundred and fifty Degrees. Afterwards raife the Fire, fo as to make the Water and the Plant boil; which may be known by a certain iffing Noife, proceeding from the breaking Bubbles of the boiling Matter; as alfo by the Pipe of the ftill-head, or the upper End of the Worm becoming too hot to be handed; or the Smoaking of the Water in the Worm-tub, heated by the Top of the Worm; and laftly, by the following of one Drop immediately after another, from the Nofe of the Worm, fo as to make an almoft continual Stream. By all which Signs we know, that the requifite Heat is given, and if it be lefs than a gentle Degree of Ebullition, the Virtue here expected will not be rais'd. But when the Fire is too great, the Matter haftily rifes into the Still-head, and fouls the Worm and the diftill'd Liquor; and the Plant being alfo rais'd, it blocks up the Worm; for which Reafon, it is proper to place a Piece of fine Linen, artificially, at the End of the Still-head Pipe, that, in Cafe of this Accident, the Plant may be kept from ftopping up the Worm. But, even in this Cafe, if the Fire be too violent, it will throw up the Herbs into the Still-head Pipe; whence the Paffage being ftopt, the rifing Vapour will forcibly blow off the Head, and throw the Liquor and Steam about, fo as to do much Mifchief, or even to fuffocate the Operator, without a proper Caution; and the more oily, tenacious, gummy, or refinous the Subject is, and confequently the more frothy and explofive, the greater Danger there is, in Cafe of this Accident.

Let the due Degree of Heat therefore be carefully obferv'd, and equally kept up, fo long as the Water, diftilling into the Receiver, is white, thick, odorous, fapid, frothy, and turbid; for this Water fhould be kept carefully feparated from that which will follow it: Whence the Receiver muft be often chang'd, that the Operator may be certain, that nothing but this firft Water comes over; for there afterwards rifes a Water that is tranfparent, thin, and without the peculiar Tafte and Odour of the Plant, but generally fomewhat tartifh and limpid, tho' fomewhat obfcur'd and foul'd by white dreggy Matter: And if the Head of the Still be not tinn'd, the Acidity of this laft Water will caufe it to diffolve the Copper, fo as to become green, naufeous, emetic, and poifonous to thofe who ufe it, efpecially weak Perfons and young Children, as operating both upwards and downwards, with fevere Gripings. If fuch a Misfortune fhould happen, it is remedied by drinking plentifully of Milk, fweeten'd with Honey, or of the common emollient Decoction.

The firft Water above defcrib'd, principally contains the Oil and diftinguifhing Spirit of the Plant, and always fomewhat faline, which in moft Plants is acid, but in the more pungent Antifcorbutics a volatile Alcali; for the Fire by boiling the Subject, diffolves its Oil, and reduces it into fmall Particles, which are carried upwards by the Affiftance of the Water, along with thofe Parts of the Plant that become volatile with this Motion. And if the Veffels are exactly clofed, all thefe being united together, will be difcharged without Lofs, and without much Alteration, into the Receiver annex'd; for if we may truft our Senfes, thofe Waters are richly impregnated with the Odour, Tafte, and particular Virtues of the volatile Parts of Plants: Hence, if the Botanift juftly affigns the Virtues of any Plant, as they are contain'd in that

Part which is volatile by a boiling Heat, the Chymist can present those Virtues separated from the rest. I have expresly observed, that the first of these distilled Waters contains only the Virtues of the Plants, residing in that Part which is volatile with this Heat; because, in the whole mix'd Juice of the Plant, there is a certain Virtue depending upon a Mixture of this first Water, and the Liquor remaining after that is drawn off. The fresh express'd Juice of recent Mint has certainly many more distinct Properties than the distill'd Water thereof: Whence Physicians are to observe, that the Virtues of this Water, and of the native Juice, are not the same, but very different.

The Water of the second Running wants the volatile Part above describ'd, yet scarce brings over the more fix'd Part of the Plant, except what is somewhat acid and vapid: If when this is come off, fresh Rain Water be pour'd upon the remaining Plant, and boil'd therewith, or strongly distill'd, there rises a more acid Water, containing very little of the particular Virtue of the Plant; almost the same Kind of Acidity appearing to rise thus from them all at last. This, says *Boerhaave*, I may venture to affirm upon Experience, that the Virtue of destroying Worms, which many celebrated Physicians have justly attributed to certain distill'd Waters, depends upon this, that the Acid of the Water of the last Running dissolves the Copper, and thus acquires a Virtue not its own. This Operation however, shews, that Plants contain an acid Salt so volatile as to rise and separate from the Subject, with two hundred and fifteen Degrees of Heat. But Experience shews, that the Water of this second Running has scarce any other Virtue than that of Cooling; as may be safely tried

by using a Glass Still-head instead of a Copper one, by which Means the Inconvenience of its dissolving the Copper is prevented.

And this is the best Method of preparing the distill'd officinal Waters, provided the two Sorts be not mix'd together, for both of them would be spoiled by such a Mixture; and will seldom remain perfect a Year.

A slight Fermentation is sometimes necessary, in Order to open the Bodies of some Plants, so as to make them afford their medicinal Virtues in Distillation. For this Purpose,

Take any recent, odorous, and sapid Plant, cut and bruise it, if that seems necessary, put it into a large Oak Cask, leaving a Space empty at the Top four Inches deep; then take as much Water as will, when added, fill the Cask to the same Height, including the Plant, and mix therein about an eight Part of Honey if it be cold winter Weather, or a twelfth Part if it be warm; in the Summer the like Quantity of coarse unrefined Sugar might, to the same Purpose, be added instead of the Honey, or Half an Ounce of Yeast added for each Pint of Water will have the Effect, but *Boerhaave* prefers the Honey: let the proper Quantity therefore of Honey and Water be warmed, and poured upon the Plant in the Cask; let the Cask stand upright, and have its wide upper Orifice, or Bung-hole, loosely covered with a wooden Cover, then set it in a Heat of about eighty Degrees, which is afterwards to be constantly kept up by covering the Outside with Cloths, and a due Regulation of the Fire, which must therefore be greater, and more carefully attended in cold Weather, but in the Heat of Summer little or no Fire is required. On the second Day a hissing Noise will begin in the Liquor,

iquor, with Bubbles, Frothing, d a grateful Smell of the Plant, e Plant now rifing to the Surface. 7hen this Fermentation has conti- ned fo long, that the Plant which as on the Top begins to fubfide id fink to the Bottom, the Opera- on is continu'd long enough for our urpofe, fo that now the Veffel muft e cooled and clofely bunged down ; r if it fhould continue longer open the fame Warmth, the Spirit and il now render'd more volatile, ould fly off, and the Virtues re- uir'd be loft ; fo that the Matter ould be now directly diftill'd. Take erefore as much of this Plant and s fermented Liquor as may fill two hirds of a Still, and work carefully om the firft ; for the Liquor, con- ining much fermenting Spirit, ea- ly rarifies with the Fire, froths, wells, and hence becomes very fub- ct to boil over. And as all this appens much quicker in this Diftil- ation than in the Diftillation of an nfermented Plant, we ought here o work flower, efpecially at the firft. And thus there will come over firft limpid, unctuous, penetrating, odo- ous, fapid Liquor, all which is to e kept feparate ; there follows a nilky, opake, turbid Liquor, ftill ontaining fomething of the fame Tafte and Odour ; and at laft comes ne that is thin, acid, not fragrant nd fcarce having any Refemblance f the Plant. There remains in the Still an Extract, infipid with refpect to the Plant, and retaining moft of he Subftance of the Honey. And ll thefe Particulars hold, when the Fermentation is continu'd till the Plant fpontaneoufly falls to the Bot- tom of the Cafk ; which, with the above-mention'd Degrees of Heat, ufually happens in five or fix Days. This firft Water, or rather Spirit, may be kept for feveral Years, in a clofe Veffel, without changing or growing ropy. It alfo excellently

retains the Tafte and Odour of the Plant, though a little altered ; but if lefs Honey were added, lefs Heat employed, or the Fermentation con- tinu'd only two or three Days, then the diftilled Water of the firft Run- ning would be white, thick, opake, unctuous, frothy, and perfectly re- tain the Scent and Tafte of the Plant, or much lefs altered than in the preceding Cafe ; though the Water will not be fo fharp and pe- netrating. After this is drawn off, a tartifh, limpid, inodorous Liquor will rife. There is alfo in this Cafe, always found fome Oil in the firft Water, which was not in the former Spirit. Again, if the Fermentation were to continue only for a Day or a Day and a Half, the Water that firft comes over would abound largely with Oil. In other Refpects Matters are nearly the fame in both ; for it is conftantly found, that the longer the Fermentation is continu'd, the lefs Oil appears in the diftilled Water, and therefore what runs firft is al- ways clearer and ftronger ; but upon mixing with common Water, the whole immediately becomes milky ; whence thefe Waters greatly differ from one another, accordingly as they are differently prepar'd in the above-mentioned Refpects. When the Fermentation is perfectly per- form'd, the firft Water will be lim- pid, the fecond milky, and if the third be forced over by a ftrong boil- ing Heat long continued, it will prove acid and limpid, refembling diftilled Vinegar. The Extract in this Cafe will always be the lefs im- pregnated with the Virtue of the Plant employed, the longer the Fer- mentation was continued, or the more perfectly it was performed, and *vice verfa* ; the Oil alfo, which in the other Method of diftilling Water, floats upon the Surface of the Water, becomes fo attenuated when the Plant is perfectly fermented

before

before Distillation, as intirely to disappear and lye concealed in the distilled Liquor; which may therefore be called Spirit, rather than Water. That this is the Case appears from hence, that if a large Quantity of Water be added to the Spirit, it presently grows white; which shews that there was Oil concealed in it: And, frequently, little Drops of Oil thus regenerated, will float upon the Surface of the Water.

Hence we learn that this Fermentation, when perfectly finished in the proper Time required for that Purpose, with a large Proportion of Ferment, and if the whole fermented Matter be for some Time contained closely bunged down in a Cask, affords these Waters extremely limpid, hot, aromatic, odorous, sapid, and penetrating without any Sign of their containing an Oil: and according as these Properties appear more in the Water, the native Virtues of the Plant are more changed; so that at last they can scarce be known; but when the Fermentation is perfect, each losing its proper Character they all become nearly alike. The Water of *Carduus Benedictus*, so prepared, is highly recommended, where sweating and Perspiration are required.

Hence the Taste and Smell of Plants, communicated to their distilled Waters, principally depend upon their native Spirit respectively. But, as this Spirit is wrapped up in a tenacious Oil, when this Oil is mixed with the Waters, it renders them more odorous and sapid, in the larger Quantity it is so mixed. This Oil is gradually thin'd, made less tenacious, more spirituous, and easier to mix with Water, by Distillation, Digestion and Cohobation in close Vessels, but thus the Spirit also becomes more volatile and disentangled, so as easily to fly off, unless it is every Way very closely confined in

the Vessels during the Distillation, which being performed, highly efficacious Waters may be thus prepared. But as Fermentation requires a Length of Time, the Admission of the Air, and open Vessels, it attenuates Oils by its Motion, so as to mix them with Water, and in this Form make an inflammable Liquor, which cannot happen without a Dissipation of native Spirit. It however renders Oils miscible with the animal Juices, and fit to enter the finest Vessels, but always destroys the peculiar Virtue of the Plant; in the mean Time, it proves the Medium of conveying, stimulating and grateful Virtues to the Nerves, especially those of the Nose, Mouth, Jaws, Throat, Stomach and Intestines.

The *Edinburgh* Dispensatory, orders simple Waters to be distill'd from the following Vegetables,

Angelica.
Baum.
Black Cherries, with their Stones crack'd.
Camomile Flowers.
Carduus Benedictus.
Elder Flowers.
Fennel.
Hyssop.
Mint.
Mugwort.
Parsley.
Penny-royal.
Red-Poppy Flowers.
Rose Buds.
Rue.
Savine.
Common Wormwood.

Aqua Alexiteria.

Alexiterial Water.

Take of the fresh Leaves of *Carduus Benedictus*, Baum, and *Scordium*, each ten Ounces; those of common Wormwood and Mint, each six Ounces; and those of Angelica, three Ounces; add two Gallons of Spring Water, and distil according to the Rules of Art. But observe that the Water thus obtain'd will be the better, if the *Carduus*, Wormwood, and *Scordium* be first fermented. E.

In the *London* Dispensatory, this Water is different from the former, and is order'd to be prepar'd thus.

Take of the green Leaves of Spear Mint, a Pound and a Half; the Tops of Sea Wormwood also green, the green Leaves of Angelica, of each a Pound; of Water as much, as is sufficient to prevent burning. Distill off three Gallons.

These differ from the Alexiterial Milk Water of the former *London* Dispensatory, as much as they do from each other. But they are all so excessively insignificant, that it would be trifling to determine which is best. Neither can be depended upon for curing any one Distemper, or alleviating any one Symptom. And they can be only us'd judiciously, as Vehicles to Things of greater Consequence.

Aqua Castorei.
Water of Castor.

Take of *Russia* Castor, one Ounce; of Water as much, as is sufficient to prevent Burning. Distill off a Quart. L.

This Water will be pretty strong of the Castor, and may serve as a Vehicle to other Medicines, in Cases where Castor can be serviceable, as in those Distempers which are improperly and, I may say, unintelligibly call'd *nervous*; but in these Cases Castor answers much better Purposes,

given in Substance, and without any Inconvenience, which the Water has not equally.

Aqua Cinnamomi sine Vino.
Cinnamon Water without Spirit.

To a Pound of Cinnamon add twelve Pints of Spring Water, and let them steep together for two Days; then draw off the Water till it ceases to run milky. E.

We are inform'd, that the Shops have been us'd to substitute *Cassia* for *Cinnamon* in this Water, an unpardonable Imposition, in those who are so well paid for their Time and Labour, as those are who deal in it. This should seem to be the very best simple Water we have; and the Virtues thereof may be understood from those of Cinnamon. It is advis'd to add an Ounce of white Sugar Candy to every Pint of this Water, to prevent the Separation of the ponderous Oil; and by this Means it is said to keep longer.

Aqua Corticum Aurantiorum simplex.
The simple distill'd Water of Orange Peel.

Take of the outer yellow Rind of fresh *Seville* Oranges four Ounces, of Water as much, as is sufficient to prevent burning. Distill off a Gallon. L.

In the Plan for the *London* Dispensatory, a Water was directed to be distill'd in the same Manner from Lemon Peel, which was, I presume, left out, because it loses its Flavour sooner than that of Oranges. Both should seem to be good simple Waters, as being impregnated with the Virtues of the Simples, an Account of which see under the Article of Vegetables.

Aqua

Aqua Menthæ Piperitidis simplex.

Simple Pepper Mint Water.

Take of the Leaves of Pepper-Mint dried, a Pound and a Half; of Water as much as is sufficient to prevent Burning. Distill off a Gallon. L.

This has been long kept in the Shops, but was received in the last London Dispensatory for the first Time. It is a very fashionable Water, and may be us'd properly as a Carminative, in Case of Flatulences in the Stomach, or whenever this Organ is intended to be warm'd, being very hot and pungent. But I don't believe it capable of curing any Distemper, tho' it may relieve a Symptom.

Aqua Piperis Jamaicensis.
Water of *Jamaica* Pepper.

Take of *Jamaica* Pepper, Half a Pound; of Water as much, as is sufficient to prevent Burning. Distill off a Gallon. L.

The Virtues of this Water may be learn'd from those of the *Pimenta*, which see under the Article *Caryophyllus*, amongst the Vegetables.

Aqua Ranunculi pratensis.
Water of Meadow Crowfoot.

Take of the Leaves and Flowers of the *Ranunculus pratensis*, or Meadow Crowfoot. Let them be distill'd in a common Alembic, in the same Manner as common simple Waters, as long as any Pungency remains in the Liquor. The distill'd Water is very hot and pungent, and requires lowering with common Water, till it may be drank. The Method of taking it is, to fill the Stomach first with about a Quart of warm Water; then give an Ounce of the Liquor, which in a few Minutes brings up the Water without any Violence. This is to be repeated, till the Patient has vomited sufficiently. There is, or at least was very lately,

a Man in *Cheshire,* commonly call'd the Vomiting, or Straw Hat Doctor, who render'd himself famous for exhibiting a particular Sort of Emetic, which he kept as a Secret; but I am inform'd, that this is his Vomit; and my Authority for this is very good. This Vomit has the Reputation of operating very soon, with great Ease and good Effect.

Aqua Rosarum Damascenarum.

Damask Rose Water.

Take of fresh damask Roses six Pounds; of Water as much as is sufficient to prevent Burning. Distill off a Gallon. L.

Aqua Seminum Anethi.

Water of Dill Seed.

Take of Dill Seed one Pound; of Water as much as is sufficient to prevent Burning. Distill off a Gallon. L.

For the Virtues of this Water, see those of Dill-Seeds, under the Article *Anethum.*

To these may be added, tho' 'tis rather procured by Resolution than Distillation.

Aqua Spermatis Ranarum.

Frog Spawn Water.

Hang any Quantity of Frog Spawn, in a Bag, so that the Water may run from it, into a Vessel set underneath to receive it, and to every Pint of the Liquor, thus obtained, add a Dram of Roch Alum. E.

This seems intended as a Cooler; but does not promise any great Effects, except such as is communicated to it from the Alum.

The *Edinburgh* Dispensatory informs us, that the Waters of such Plants, which are obtainable to no good Purpose by Distillation, may be made by dissolving a proper Proportion of their essential Salt in Spring Water.

An other

Another Method may be contriv'd of supplying the Place of simple Waters, thus, Grind an Ounce of dry Loaf Sugar, to an impalpable Powder in a glass Mortar, with a glass Pestle, and by Degrees add thereto a Dram of an essential Oil, or Half a Dram, if the Oil be very tenacious, and continue rubbing them together, till all the Oil be thoroughly mixed, and drank into the Sugar; the Oil, in this Operation, usually diffuses a Fragrancy to a great Distance, whence the Operation should be performed quick, and the Mortar be covered with a Cloth surrounding the Pestle. If a little fresh Yolk of Egg be added in the Grinding, and mixed in with the Sugar and Oil, the Oil thus becomes more easily miscible, but the Mixture will not thus keep so long without turning rancid. If a due Proportion of such an Eleosaccharum be dissolv'd in Water, this Water will be impregnated with the Smell and Taste of the Plant from whence the Oil was distill'd; that is, with the distinguishing Spirit of the Plant, which communicates to the distill'd Water all its Virtues. But if such an *Eleosaccharum* be dissolv'd in the distill'd Water of the same Plant the Oil was procur'd from, and the spirituous Water and Syrup of the same be added to it, this Mixture would be more impregnated with the Virtues of the Plant. And thus if the Virtues of Vegetables were accurately determin'd, Medicines of considerable Effects might be prepar'd.

With Respect to Simple Waters, the *London* Dispensatory, directs to add to them, about a twentieth Part of Proof Spirit in order to make them keep the longer. And we are farther there told, that the Herbs, if they are of prime Goodness, are to be taken in the Weights directed for each. Where green are prescribed, such are to be used. But in some of the Waters dry Herbs are allowed, because they are to be had at all Times of the Year, though green Plants afford rather the more elegant Waters. But the Weights here directed should be varied by the Judgment of the Operator, not only when green are used instead of dry, but whenever the Plants by a less favourable Season are weaker in Flavour.

The general Rules laid down in the *Edinburgh* Dispensatory for the Distillation of Simple Waters are, To use the Plants from whence they are distill'd, fresh gather'd; then bruise them a little, and let thrice their own Quantity of Spring-water be pour'd thereon; but less will suffice in Case they are juicy, and if dry, they must have a greater Quantity; for every Pint of Water thus added, draw off half a Pint, by the Alembic, with its Refrigeratory; the Junctures being first luted. But black Cherries require no Water to be added to them. Those Plants which abound with an aromatic and fragrant Oil, should be immediately committed to Distillation: But those that contain a more fix'd Oil, or owe Part of their Virtues to a Kind of volatile Salt, such as Wormwood, *Carduus Benedictus*, Mugwort, Chamomile, and some others, ought first to undergo an imperfect Fermentation, with Yeast; that is, they should be distill'd in the Beginning of the Fermentation, without staying till it is finish'd. If any Drops of Oil float upon the Surface of the Water, they must be carefully taken off.

As to the black Cherry-water now left out of the *London* Dispensatory, tho' I esteem it so insignificant, as to be not worth commenting upon; yet I must remark, that according to the best Information I could procure from those who had made Experiments with it upon Animals, purposely to discover its Effects, it is absolutely innocent, and attended with no ill Consequences whatever.

With Respect to the medicinal Virtues

tues of Simple diftill'd Waters from Vegetables, I muft remark, that as they are at prefent ufed, the Patient would receive no Injury in his Health or Conftitution, if moft, or perhaps all of them, were omitted in the Difpenfatories; for they are generally employ'd as the Bafis of a *Julap*, or Draught, with an Addition of an equally infignificant compound Water, and fome Syrup or Sugar; and are given in fuch Dofes, as it is unreafonable to expect any Manner of Effect from, except that of making the Patient believe it may do him Service, becaufe it taftes more like Phyfic than common Water, or Wine and Water, tho' the laft is frequently a much better Medicine. The College have, therefore, very well anfwer'd the Truft repos'd in it by the Legiflature, in expunging many of the Simple Waters to be found in former Difpenfatories. And I think the End, if any End is propos'd, of all or moft of them as commonly ufed, will be better anfwer'd by an extemporaneous Infufion of the recent Plant in cold Water, or one of the dry'd Vegetables in warm Water in a clofe Veffel, like *Tea*; for thus the Water will be impregnated with the diftinguifhing Spirit of the Plant. And I know that a flight Infufion of recent Mint has been commonly fold for the diftill'd Water of that Plant, and been univerfally efteem'd better than any other. Notwithftanding what I have faid, I believe the diftill'd Water of Plants may exert very great Efficacy in the Body, and contribute to the Cure of many Diftempers, if exhibited properly, that is, in Quantities fufficient to anfwer the End propos'd, and unmix'd with other Ingredients which may interfere with their Operation.

But whatever Virtues diftill'd Waters may be poffefs'd of, they will be found in the greateft Perfection in the Water made by repeated Cohobations, thus:

Take the Plant and Liquor, remaining in the Still after the Diftillation of an unfermentedPlant, and prefs them ftrongly thro' a Strainer, that all the Decoction may be obtained, and with this mix all the Water before drawn over. Return this Mixturn into the Still, and add to it as much of the fame recent Plant as was employed before, and if neceffary, add likewife as much Water as may make up the former Proportion to the Plant. Now clofe the Veffels exactly and digeft the whole with a hundred and fifty Degrees of Heat for the Space of three Days and three Nights, that the Herb being fo long fteep'd in its own Liquor, may be opened, loofened, and difpofed the eafier to part with its Virtues. This Digeftion being fo long continued, is of great Service, but if protracted too long introduces a Change tending to Putrefaction. Let the Water be now diftilled off as the firft Time, only proceeding more cautioufly and fomewhat more flowly at firft; becaufe the Liquor in the Still being now thicker more impregnated with the Plant, and therefore more flatulent and fubject to fwell upon feeling the Fire, it eafily boils over; but after about one half of the expected Water is come off, the Fire may be prudently raifed, and the Diftillation be continued fo long as the white, thick, odorous, and fapid Water comes over, and then the Operation muft be immediately ftopped. The Water fo obtained will be whiter, thicker, more odorous, fapid, frothy and turbid than that of the firft Diftillation of the Plant.

This Water preferves its Virtues much longer, and contains it in greater Perfection than that from a fingle Diftillation of the Plant, which fhows us the Way of concentrating the peculiar Virtue of Plants, fo far as it refides in their volatile odorous Parts. So likewife the remaining Decoction

in

this Proceſs is much ſtronger than the firſt Diſtillation, and as the Operation may be repeated as often as one pleaſes, both the Water and Decoctions may by ſeveral Repetitions, at length may be made exremely rich, ſo that by this Means excellent Medicines are procurable. Thus in the Year 1730, *Boerhaave* ſays, he diſtilled Baum after this Manner fourteen times ſucceſſively and found the Water at laſt had a balſaic Taſte and the perfect Fragrance of the Plant, ſo as to prove highly refreſhing even when barely ſmelt to or taſted: And no wonder, ſince the Virtue of many large Baſkets of Baum were here concentrated and wrought within the Compaſs of a ſmall Glaſs, and the Remainder, alo, at the Bottom of the Still being inſpiſſated, fill'd but another Glaſs and proved grateful, auſtere, and ſtrengthing, ſo that by mixing the two together, the Virtues of the Plant, might be thus highly concentrated, or brought into a very little Room. This Proceſs therefore does not only afford excellent Waters, but admirable Extracts alſo, which when properly mixed together, yield Medicines of ſuch Efficacy as can ſcarce otherviſe be imitated; for the native Virtues of Vegetables are little changed in this Operation, certainly leſs than in others, tho' it muſt be allowed that ſome Alteration is produced by ſo long a Continuation of the Boiling. But both the Odour, Taſte, and Effects demonſtrate, that the Waters thus prepared retain in a high Degree, the ſpecific Virtues of the Plant. And hence it is certain, that the medicinal Virtue of truely aromatic Vegetables, reſides in that Part of them which riſes with the Heat of boiling Water, and that it is poſſible by Art, to concentrate theſe Virtues ſo that they ſhall prove much more effectual than in the State they are naturally afforded, nor is there any Limitation; for by continuing

the Operation, the Virtue of Plants may be thus exalted to any Degree the Artiſt ſhall think proper.

Paracelſus aſſures us he found by Experience, that Baum is poſſeſſed of ſo great a ſpecific Virtue, as by inſinuating into the Humours of the Body, to reſtore a new youthful Vigour to the Aged, and by this Means perfectly to cure the Gout, and *Iſaac Hollandus* avouches the ſame. Now if theſe Authors ſaid true, I judged, ſays *Boerhaave*, that I might by Means of the preſent Proceſs procure the united Virtues of the Plant in their utmoſt Strength; and indeed, I have, ſays he, in myſelf experienced extraordinary Effects of the Water ſo prepared, by taking it upon an empty Stomach, and certainly it has ſcarce its Equal in hypochondriacal and hyſterical Diſorders, a Chloroſis and Palpitation of the Heart, as often as theſe Diſeaſes proceed rather from a Diſorder of the Spirits, than any Collection of morbific Matter, tho' it is indeed expenſive. He tells us he has reduced dried Mint by three or four Cohobations, into a Balſamic penetrating Liquor, which becomes an incomparable and preſent Remedy for ſtrengthening a weak Stomach, curing Vomiting proceeding from a cold viſcous Phlegm lodged about the Mouth thereof, as alſo in Lienteries. The Water, he ſays, he has in this Manner prepared from Lemonpeel has, by its fragrance, its agreeable penetrating and highly aromatic Taſte and Virtue, immediately cured Flatulencies, Deliquiums, Faintings, and irregular Motions of the Heart, tho' taken in a very ſmall Doſe. The like Water prepared by repeated Cohobations from recent Wormwood, has ſucceſsfully ſupplied the Want of Bile in the Body, ſtimulated all the languid Veſſels that aſſiſt in forming the Chyle, and killed and expelled Worms. The like Water from the Leaves of Savine has given an almoſt incredible Motion to the whole

ner-

nervous System, so as to prove the most excellent of all Medicines for promoting the Exclusion of the Fœtus and Discharge of the Menses and Hæmorhoids. The cohobated Water of Rue can never be sufficiently recommended for the Cure of the Falling Sickness, the hysteric Passion, for expelling Poison and promoting Sweat and Perspiration. Not to mention the Waters made from the Berries of the Juniper Tree and the Leaves of the *Arbor Vitæ,* both of them successfully curing the Dropsy, as that from Camomile Flowers cures tertian Agues.

These are the Virtues ascrib'd by that excellent Chymist and Physician *Boerhaave,* to the cohobated Waters of some Vegetables ; and as he was too penetrating to deceive himself, and too honest to lead others into Errors in so material a Point, I am inclin'd to believe him. It is therefore, Pity that the Gentlemen who were concern'd in compiling the last *London Dispensatory,* did not direct Waters prepar'd in this Manner from Vegetables of known Efficacy, to be kept in the Shops. It must be confess'd these Waters would have been somewhat expensive, and might have diminish'd the Profit of the Vender, especially as the Repetition of the Doses need not have been so frequent nor so long continu'd. But this is no Objection to their Use in a Country where the Physician is so liberally paid for his Care, and the Compounder for his Trouble.

I shall conclude the present Article of simple Waters, with some admirable Rules for making them from the above quoted Author.

Let the aromatic, balsamic, oleaginous, resinous, gummo-resinous, and strong smelling Plants, which long retain their natural Fragrance ; such as *Arbor Vitæ,* Baum, Bay, Hyssop, Juniper, Marjoram, Mint, *Origanum,* Penny Royal, Rosemary, Sage, &c. be gently dried a

little in the Shade, then digest them in the Quantity of Water already mentioned for twenty-four Hours; in a close Vessel, with one hundred and fifty Degrees of Heat; and afterwards distill in the Method above delivered, and thus they will afford excellent Waters.

When Waters are to be drawn from Barks, Roots, Seeds, and Woods that are very dense; ponderous, tough, and resinous; let them be digested for three, four, or more Weeks with ninety-six Degrees of Heat, in Vessels perfectly closed with a proper Quantity of Salt and Water, to open and prepare them better for Distillation. A considerable Quantity of Sea Salt, is here added partly to open the Subject the more, but principally to prevent Putrefaction, which otherwise would certainly happen in so long a Time, and with such a Heat; as is necessary in this Case, and so destroy the Odour, Taste, and Virtues required. And thus for Example may Waters be prepared from Aloes, Box, Cedar, Guaiacum, Juniper, Rhodium, and the like Woods.

Those Plants which diffuse their Odour to some Distance from them, and thus soon lose it, should immediately be distilled after being gathered in a proper Season, without any previous Digestion ; thus Borage, Buglofs, Jessamin, White Lillies, Lillies of the Valley, Roses, &c. are hurt by Heat, Digestion, and lying in the Air. Some Woods are also injured in the same Manner ; thus the Shavings of Sassafras, by being boil'd in Water, soon lose their Virtue, Taste, and Smell.

The Astringent, nutrimental, healing, consolidating, emollient, farinaceous, gelatinous, cooling and styptic Virtues of Plants are never, by these Means, communicated to the distilled Waters, but are to be sought either in the whole Plant, or its most fixt Part. Whence Pharmacy

acy should be relieved from the unneceffary Trouble of preparing uch Waters, and on the other hand, hyficians are diligently to be adonifh'd to feek for fuch Virtues in the Infufions, Decoctions, and Extracts of fuch Plants. Would it not e ridiculous to expect any Thing utrimental in the indolent and vapid iftill'd Water of Barley, or minced apons Flefh? Can any Man expect find the excellent Virtues of Sorel in hot, lax, putrid and bilious Conftitutions, from the diftilled Water of this Plant? So again it were bfurd to attribute the inimitable Virtues of Plantain to its diftilled Water; fuch idle and childifh Trifles re therefore to be rejected in the ferious Arts of Chymiftry and Medine.

The Cafe is far otherwife in thofe Plants whofe real Virtue refides enirely in that Part which is separable by Heat not exceeding 214 Degrees; for the Waters carefully prepared from thefe will contain all the Virtues which is loft in their Decocions and Extracts. The celebrated Virtues of Lavender Flowers, Lillies of the Valley, and of Rue, againft hat Species of the Falling Sicknefs which proceeds from a Difturbance n the Motion of the nervous Fluid, efide in the diftilled Water; but re abfolutely wanting in the Decocions or Extracts; fo, on the other land, the antiepileptic Virtue of Piony remains in the Decoction, but s wanting in the Water.

There are fome medicinal Plants whofe Virtues refide in a Part which s volatile, with the aforefaid Degree of Heat, but fo, that after they are raifed by Diftillation, the remaining Plant and its Decoction continue poffeffed of other Virtues of great Medicinal Efficacy. Such Decoctions re not therefore to be thrown away, but to be infpiffated with a moderate Heat that they may be kept uncorrupted; for being afterwards mixed

with the diftilled Water, the Virtues of both are thus united, and afford the whole Efficacy of the Plants; and of this Kind are Chamomile, Carduus Benedictus, the leffer Centaury, Germander, Ground Pine, Mugwort, Rofemary, Sage, Scordium, Wormwood, &c. This Tribe of Herbs indeed are exalted by Fermentation, fo as to afford the better Waters; but when their Decoctions come afterwards to be infpiffated, they either have lefs, or a different Kind of Virtue from the natural.

Acid, bitter, auftere, fweet, and flat Taftes rarely afcend from Plants in Diftillation, but commonly remain in their Extracts, though they afcend from Chamomile, Wormwood, and a few more; but the Colour of the Plants is fcarce ever raifed by Diftillation, though we have a blue Colour in the Diftillation of Camomile, and a green one in that of Wormwood; but thefe Colours are rather in the Oils than in the Waters. The faponaceous Virtue confifting in the Union of the Salt and Oil never rifes, but remains in the Extracts; and therefore Plants endowed with this Virtue are not to be thus diftilled.

The following Vegetables fcarce afford any Thing of Ufe in their diftilled Waters, that is Barberry, Beet, common Cherries, Colewort, Currans, Elder Berries, Endive, ripe Grapes, Ladies Mantle, Lettice, the Juice of Citrons, Lemons, Oranges, Purflain, Scorzonera, Sorrel, Strawberries and Succory. There are alfo very contrary Virtues in the fame Plant; thus the diftilled Water of Cinnamon of the firft running is deobftruent, heating, enlivening, ftimulating and good in Vomiting; but that of the fecond Running, aftringent cooling and naufeous, whilft the Decoction remaining in the Still is of a dark red Colour, opake, thick, of an auftere Tafte, aftringent, coagulating, and ftrengthening.

CHAP

CHAP. III.

Of Compound or Spirituous WATERS.

COMPOUND or spirituous Waters in general are only Brandy impregnated with medicinal Ingredients which contain some Parts so volatile as to rise with the Spirit in Distillation, and come over into the Receiver, so as the distill'd Water may be impregnated therewith. As to their Uses in Medicine, they appear to me not very extensive. For there is scarcely one Ingredient in their Composition which may not be given in Substance to much greater Advantage. Besides, I have a capital Objection, against their principal Ingredient, Brandy, and am convinc'd, that if they are given in Quantities sufficient to answer any Intention, the Brandy will do more Injury than the other Ingredients can countervail; for Brandy is known to have a very bad Effect on the Stomach, and to coagulate the Blood: And if they are given in so small Quantities, or so much diluted as to do no Mischief, they can have no Effect at all, and are given to no End or Purpose. In Fevers and Inflammations, which make at least three Fourths of the Distempers which occur, all Sorts of Drams, for compound Waters are nothing more, must be attended with very bad Consequences, as they make the Heat contract more forcibly, and frequently, and render the Circulation more rapid, in consequence of which the Heat and Fever is increas'd; but at the same Time it must be confess'd, that they raise the Spirits, and are therefore pleasing to the Patient and Prescriber; and this is a Circumstance much in their Disfavour; for hence being tempted to regard the immediate Relief only,

without considering the Consequences, People imperceptibly acquire a Habit of recurring to Cordials, till at last they cannot subsist without them, and then the Constitution is on the Verge of being totally and irretrievably destroy'd. I am afraid, that the Practisers of Physic have inadvertently been instrumental, by giving compound Waters as Medicines, in introducing the execrable Custom of drinking Drams, which at present does not only prevail amongst the Vulgar, but has made no small Progress among People of Rank and Distinction; insomuch that if it increases for forty Years more, in Proportion as it has done for the last half Century, there will be no Occasion for a second Deluge or a Conflagration, to exterminate the whole human Species from the Face of the Earth. For those who are habituated to Drams in a certain Degree, cannot long subsist themselves, and are absolutely depriv'd of all Hopes of leaving behind them a tolerably healthful Progeny. I must not omit to take Notice, that most acute Distempers are terminated or much reliev'd, by spontaneous and critical Sweats: Now 'tis obvious to the Observation of almost every one, that Brandy prevents, or checks Sweating, probably by coagulating the Blood; and if so, it must be improper in acute Distempers, when Sweating may be expected to relieve. It may be said, that compound Waters are generally given so much diluted, as not to be capable of checking Sweats; but if they are exhibited so as to act at all, the Effects will be such as I have above-mention'd; but if they are taken so much diluted to exert no Manner of Efficacy, this Case they are absolutely insignificant, and of no Service to any one but the Compounder; and their Exhibition betrays the Want of true medicinal Knowledge in the Prescriber, or something worse. If Cordials are wanting in Distempers, Wine is the most natural, and infinitely the best; and no Case can happen where Cordials can be required stronger than some Sorts of Wine; but when Wine alone is too powerful, it may be diluted at Pleasure, with some proper Water, or Decoction. Add to this, that some Kinds of Wine, as *Rhenish* and *Moselle*, are admirable Medicines, when mix'd in due Proportion with some proper farinaceous Decoction, and exhibited frequently, and plentifully to the Patient, at the same Time that they answer all the good Purposes of Cordials. It must, however, be confess'd, that Cordial Waters may sometimes have their Uses, by removing a present Symptom, in Faintings and excessive Languors, without contributing in the least to the Cure of the Distemper which excites them. But for these Purposes the Gin-shops can furnish Medicines equally efficacious with those of the Apothecaries.

General Rules for distilling compound Waters.

I. The Plants, together with their Parts, should be moderately and newly dried; except in those Cases when they are order'd fresh and green.

II. After they have been duly macerated, such a Proportion of Spring Water should be added thereto, as may prevent any *Empyreuma*, or burnt Flavour from the Still, or somewhat more.

III. The Liquor that runs off first in Distillation, is sometimes kept separate, under the Title of *Spirit*;

and the succeeding Part artificially fined down or freed from its Milkiness: But the best Way is to mix the several Runnings together, without Clarification; so as that the Waters may contain the full Virtues of the respective Plants, without regarding their Cleanness or Beauty.

Dr. *Fuller* advises to have all compound Waters made with highly rectified Spirit of Wine, and pure Water; by which Means not only the Composition will be untainted with the nauseous and fetid Phlegm, constantly remaining in Brandies, and the common Spirits sold by Distillers; but also a certain Rule will be had for making the same Waters, at all Times and Seasons, of the same Degree of Strength, and that too at a cheaper Rate, than by trusting to what the Distillers call Proof Goods; since one Gallon of well rectified Spirit of Wine will give three of a compound Water, as the Doctor judges, sufficiently strong.

Aqua Absinthii composita.

Compound Wormwood Water.

Take of *Calamus Aromaticus* the fresh external Rind of Oranges, and Cinnamon, each four Ounces; the Leaves of *Roman* Wormwood, half a Pound; of Garden Mint three Ounces; the lesser Cardamoms and Mace, each one Ounce: Slice or cut those Ingredients that require it, bruise the others, and pour thereon two Gallons of *French* Brandy, let them macerate together for four Days, then draw off two Gallons. E.

This is intended as a Stomachic and Cardiac, that is a Cordial, and seems well contriv'd for that Purpose, so as to give Relief in Languors, Fainting and Flatulences. Many of the Gin shops are furnish'd

U u   with

with a Dram not much unlike this, which they sell very cheap, to the great Comfort of the Basket Women about *Covent-Garden.*

Aqua Alexiteria Spirituosa.
Spirituous Alexiterial Water.

Take of the green Leaves of Spear Mint, half a Pound, the green Leaves of Angelica, the green Tops of Sea Wormwood, of each four Ounces ; of Proof Spirit one Gallon, of Water as much, as is sufficient to prevent burning, distill off one Gallon. L.

This seems to be intended as a Cordial and Stomachic. The particular Virtues, if any, may be learn'd from those of the Ingredients which enter its Composition, and from what has been said of Cordial Waters in general.

Aqua Alexiteria Spirituosa cum Aceto.
Spirituous Alexiterial Water with Vinegar.

Take the green Leaves of Spear Mint, the green Leaves of Angelica, of each half a Pound ; of the green Tops of Sea Wormwood, four Ounces ; of Proof Spirit one Gallon ; of Water as much, as is sufficient to prevent burning. Distill off one Gallon, and then add one Pint of Vinegar.

This should seem to be a much better Water than the preceding, for the Vinegar will prevent the Spirit from doing so much Injury as it might do without it; and indeed with this Addition, it may possibly do some Service.

Aqua Anhaltina.
Anhalt Water.

Take of the best Turpentine half a Pound, of Olibanum one Ounce ; Wood of Aloes reduced to Powder three Drams ; Grains of Ma-

stich, Clove-gilly-flowers, or Rosemary-flowers, Nutmegs, Cubebs, or Galangals, and Cinnamon, each six Drams ; Saffron two Drams and an half ; Fennel-seeds, and Bayberries, each half a Dram. Reduce all to Powder, and digest in five Pints of Spirit of Wine for six Days, adding fifteen Grains of Musk tied up in a little Bag; then distill in a slow *Balneum Mariæ,* separate what is clear from what is turbid.

N. B. *'Tis better to put the Musk in the Beak of the Alembic.*

This Water warms, dries, discusses, increases the Strength of the Heart, Stomach, and other Viscera ; for this Reason it is thought good in Faintings and Deliquiums. But it is more frequently used externally, and said to be of great Service in Catarrhs and Pains arising from a cold Cause, in the wandering Gout, in Palsies, Epilepsies, Apoplexies, Vertigos, Tremors, and Lethargies, by rubbing the affected Part well with it. This Water often occurs in the Writings and Prescriptions of foreign Physicians, and is much esteem'd abroad as a Cordial.

Aqua Bryonia composita.
Compound Bryony Water.

Take of Bryony Roots, one Pound ; those of wild Valerian, four Ounces, the Leaves of Pennyroyal and Rue; of each half a Pound ; the Leaves of Mugwort, the Flowers of Feverfew, and of the Tops of Savine, each an Ounce ; the external Rinds of fresh Oranges, and the Seeds of Lovage, each two Ounces ; upon these Ingredients, when duly cut and bruis'd, pour two Gallons and a half of *French* Brandy ; then let them macerate together for four Days, and afterwards draw off two Gallons and a half. E.

This

This is intended as a nervous and
antihysteric Medicine, and is said to
promote the uterine Discharges, to
accelerate Delivery, and relieve
Convulsions in Children. But I
must confess I have never observ'd
any Effects either from this, or any
other of the Bryony Waters, of
consequence enough to make it much
garded. But I have known many
Hysterical Women taught to drink
Drams, and in consequence thereof
absolutely destroy'd, by taking Bry-
ny Water as a Medicine.

Aqua Cinnamomi cum Vino.
Cinnamon Water with Spirit.

Infuse a Pound of Cinnamon in a
Gallon of *French* Brandy, and di-
still off the Water as the *Aqua
Cinnamomi fine Vino.* E.

This should seem to be the very
best and most useful of the spirituous
Waters. The particular Virtues
may be learn'd from those of Cinnamon. It sometimes happens that
the Peruvian Bark will not stay on
the Stomach, but be discharg'd by
Vomit, or run off by Stool. In
such Cases, I have often known it
retain'd by taking it with strong
Cinnamon Water.

Aqua Corticum Aurantiorum spiri-
tuosa.

The spirituous Water of Orange
Peel.

Take of the outer yellow Rind of
fresh *Seville* Oranges, half a Pound;
of Proof Spirit a Gallon; of Water as much as is sufficient to prevent burning. Distil off a Gallon.
L.

The Virtues of this Water may be
learn'd from those of Orange Peel.
There is a Dram exactly resembling
this sold in the Gin-shops by the
Name of *Covent-Garden*, so cheap,
that I am inform'd a Pint of it may
purchas'd for Six-pence. It is
esteem'd by the Ladies of the Town,

who are too delicate to drink Gin,
a very comfortable Cordial, and to
give great Relief in Flatulencies
and Lowness of Spirits, and to be
an excellent Stomachic.

Aqua Epidemia.
Plague Water.

Take of the Roots of Masterwort
and Butter Burr, each four Ounces;
Virginia Snake Root and Zedoary
each two Ounces; the Seeds of
Angelica and Bay-berries, each
three Ounces; the Leaves of *Scordium*, six Ounces; bruise and cut
the Ingredients, and pour thereon
two Gallons of *French* Brandy;
and when they have stood to
macerate for four Days, draw two
Gallons. E.

This is said to be intended as a
highly carminative Cordial, in very
low and languid Cases, and to raise
the Spirits in the Plague and malignant Fevers. But in these Cases I
should suspect it of doing great Mischiefs, for the very same Reason that
it gives a temporary Relief.

Aqua Melissæ composita.
Compound Baum Water, commonly
called *Eau de Carmes.*

Take of the fresh Leaves of Baum,
four Ounces; of the fresh external
Rind of Lemons, two Ounces; of
Nutmegs and Coriander Seeds,
each an Ounce; of Aromatic
Cloves, Cinnamon, and the Root
of *Bohemian* Angelica, each half
an Ounce. Bruise the Leaves, and
pound the other Ingredients, and
put them in a Glass Cucurbit; then
pour upon them a Quart of Brandy;
stop the Mouth of the Cucurbit,
and leave them to digest two or
three Days in a warm Place; then
add a Pint of the best simple Baum
Water, shake them together; fix
a Head to the Cucurbit, and to
that a Receiver: Then distil in
Balneo Mariæ, with a Heat sufficient to make one Drop follow

U u 2

ano-

another, which continue till the Ingredients in the Cucurbit remain almoft dry. When the Veffels are cold, take the Water from the Receiver, and preferve it in Bottles well ftopt.

This Carmelite Water, has been long famous in *France*, and is now in moft Parts of *Europe*, for its extraordinary cordial Virtues. It is faid to be extremely reviving, to be good in all Sort of Fits, Apoplexies not excepted, and to relieve in the Gout when it attacks the Stomach. The *Carmelites* at *Paris*, who make a confiderable Advantage by vending this Water, have endeavour'd to keep the Preparation of it a Secret. But I am pretty well informed, that the foregoing Receipt for it is the genuine Prefcription, by which thefe Religious make it. This is, alfo, ufed externally by Way of Embrocation to the Temples, the Region of the Stomach, and other Parts.

Aqua Juniperi compofita.

Compound Juniper Water.

Take of Juniper Berries, one Pound; Carraway Seeds, fweet Fennel Seed, of each one Ounce and a half; of Proof Spirit a Gallon; of Water as much as is fufficient to prevent burning. Diftill off a Gallon. *L.*

This differs from *Geneva* only by the Addition of the Seeds of Caraway and Fennel, which I don't apprehend communicate to it any additional Virtues. Thofe which it acquires from the Juniper Berries, may be learned from the Article of *Juniper* in the *Materia Medica.*

Aqua Menthæ Piperitidis Spirituofa.

Spirituous Water of Pepper-Mint.

Take of the Leaves of Pepper-Mint dried, a Pound and a half; of Proof Spirit a Gallon; of Water

as much as is fufficient to prevent burning. Diftill off a Gallon. *L.*

This Water feems intended to difcufs Flatulencies in the Stomach, and to relieve Colic Pains; but I fufpect that it acquires no good Qualities from the Brandy.

Aqua Menthæ vulgaris fpirituofa.

Spirituous Spear-Mint-Water.

Take of the Leaves of Spear-Mint dried, a Pound and a half; of Proof Spirit a Gallon; of Water as much as is fufficient to prevent burning. Diftil off a Gallon. *L.*

The Virtues of this may be learn'd from thofe of Mint. But I am afraid the Brandy will do more Injury in moft Cafes, than the Mint can compenfate.

Aqua Mirabilis.

The wonderful Water.

Take of Cinnamon two Ounces; of the external Rind of Lemons one Ounce; of Angelica Seeds, the lefler Cardamoms, and Mace, each half an Ounce; Cubebs, two Drams; and of Balm Leaves, fix Ounces; bruife them together, digeft them with a Gallon of *French* Brandy, for four Days; and diftil off one Gallon. *E.*

This is intended as a warm ftomachic Cordial, and is well contrived for that Purpofe. But I think it deferves the Confideration of Diftillers, much more than that of Phyficians, as it can anfwer no Purpofe but what may be provided for by much lefs pernicious Medicines.

Aqua Nephritica.

Nephritic Water.

Take of the frefh Flowers of white Thorn four Pounds; of Nutmegs bruifed three Ounces; infufe them together in a clofe Veffel with two Gallons of generous white Wine; and

and draw off by Diftillation twelve Pounds.

The Flowers of the white Thorn being efteemed very good in the Stone and Gravel, this Water is faid to have been much prefcribed in fuch Cafes by Dr. *Radcliff*. I don't believe it is of any great Efficacy; but Julaps and Draughts muft be continued in Practice, I fhould chufe this for its Infignificancy, preferable to many others which are more pernicious.

Aqua Nucis Mofchatæ.
Nutmeg Water.

Take of Nutmeg two Ounces; of Proof Spirit a Gallon; of Water as much as is fufficient to prevent burning. Diftil off a Gallon. *L.*

The Virtues of this may be known by thofe of Nutmeg. I muft remark, that this Water, if taken in Quantities fufficient to have any Effect, will be very fubject to render the Patient coftive, which in moft Difeafes is a very bad Circumftance.

Aqua Pæoniæ compofita.
Compound Peiony Water.

Take of the Roots of Peiony, two Ounces; thofe of wild Valerian, an Ounce and half; white Dittany an Ounce; of Peiony Seeds, fix Drams; of the recent Flowers of Lillies of the Valley, four Ounces; of thofe of Lavender and Rofemary, each two Ounces; of the Tops of Betony, Marjoram, Rue, and Sage, each an Ounce: Slice and bruife the Ingredients, pour upon them a Gallon and half of *French* Brandy, and after they have macerated four Days, draw off a Gallon and a half. *E*

This is greatly recommended as a cordial, cephalic, and nervous Medicine, and is made in Imitation of the *Aqua Epileptica Langii*. But I have been fo unfortunate as never to

have feen any Effects from it, which might not have been expected from a Dram.

Aqua Petrofclini compofita.
Compound Parfley Water.

Take of Parfley Root, four Ounces; frefh Horfe Radifh Root, three Ounces, and Juniper-Berries, fix Ounces; the Tops of *St. John's* Wort, biting Arfmart and Elder Flowers, of each two Ounces; the Seeds of wild Carrot, fweet Fennel and Parfley, of each an Ounce and half; flice and bruife the Ingredients, and add thereto two Gallons of *French* Brandy: let them fteep together for four Days, and then draw off two Gallons by Diftillation. *E.*

This is defigned for a Diuretic, and Lithontriptic. It may act in the firft Intention, but in the fecond nothing can be expected from it.

Aqua Pulegii fpirituofa.
Spirituous Penny Royal Water.

Take of the Leaves of Penny Royal dried, a Pound and a half; of Proof Spirit a Gallon; of Water as much, as is fufficient to prevent burning. Diftil off a Gallon. *L.*

The Virtues of this may be understood by thofe of Penny Royal.

Aqua Raphani compofita.
Compound Horfe Radifh Water.

Take recent Horfe Radifh Root, two Pounds; the frefh Leaves of Garden Scurvy Grafs, and thofe of Water Creffes, each two Pound; the external Rinds of frefh Oranges, and Lemons, each three Ounces; *Canella alba* four Ounces; Nutmeg, one Ounce; cut and bruife thefe Ingredients; add to them three Gallons of *French* Brandy, let them macerate together for two Days, and then draw off three Gallons. *E.*

In the College Dispensatory this is directed to be prepared thus:

Take of the fresh Leaves of Garden Scurvy Grass, four Pounds; fresh Horse Radish Root, the outer yellow Rind of fresh *Seville* Oranges, of each two Pounds; of Nutmeg, nine Ounces; of Proof Spirit, two Gallons; of Water as much, as is sufficient to prevent burning. Distill off two Gallons.

These seem intended as Diuretics, an' Antiscorbutics, and are well contrived to answer the End proposed. But the Juices of these Vegetables, mixed with Aromatics, in order to make them sit easy on the Stomach, should seem to promise fairer for a Cure.

Aqua Reginæ Hungariæ.
Hungary Water.

To two Pounds of Rosemary Flowers, add two Quarts of rectified Spirit of Wine; and just as the Flowers are fresh gathered, let them be immediately distill'd in *Balneo Mariæ*. E.

I don't know that this Water is of any Use in Medicine, tho' the Perfumers sell a great deal of it, which is used to communicate an agreeable Smell to Linnen. But I have never yet seen any made in *England* that was tolerable, if compared with that prepared in *France*. That made in the Manner here directed, gives Linen a disagreeable Scent when dry, instead of a pleasant one, which it acquires from the *French* Hungary Water.

Aqua Sclopetaria, sive Vulneraria.
The vulnerary Water, commonly called *Eau d'Arquebusade*.

Take of the Leaves and Roots of Comfrey, of the Leaves of Sage, of Mugwort, and of Bugle, each four Handfuls; of the Leaves of Betony, Sanicle, Ox-eye, of Daisy, of the greater Figwort, of Plantain, of Agrimony, Vervain, Wormwood, and Fennel, each two Handfuls; of St. John's-wort, of Long Birthwort of Orpine, of Paul's Betony, of the Lesser Centaury, of Yarrow, of Tobacco, of Mouse-ear, of Mint, and of Hyssop, each one Handful: Cut all these, and bruise them sufficiently in a Mortar; then put them into a large earthen Vessel, and pour twenty Pints of white Wine upon them. Stir the Whole with a Stick. Stop the Vessel, and suffer it to digest in a warm Dunghil, or any other such Heat, for the Space of three Days; then pour it over into a large Copper Cucurbit, whose Inside is covered with Tin; and, having adapted its Head and Refrigeratory to it, draw off the Moisture into a Receiver, by a moderate Fire, in the ordinary Manner. Thus you will have the Vulnerary Water, or *Eau d'Arquebusade*, which must be preserved in a close-stopt Bottle.

It is good for Contusions and Dislocations, and is very proper for discussing Tumors; applied externally, it deterges Wounds, and old Ulcers. It incarns, corroborates, resists Putrefaction, stops Gangrenes, and is by some used against Vapours. This Water is extremely celebrated by many foreign Physicians and Surgeons, and occurs frequently in their Writings and Prescriptions. It may possibly be a very good Water for external Uses, for which it is principally intended.

Aqua Seminum Anisi composita.
Compound Aniseed Water.

Take Aniseeds, and Angelica Seeds, of each half a Pound; of Proof Spirit a Gallon; of Water as much as is sufficient to prevent burning. Distill off a Gallon. L.
The Virtues of this may be understood by those of Aniseeds.

Aqua

Aqua Seminum Cardamomi.

Water of Cardamom Seeds.

Take of the lesser Cardamom Seeds husked four Ounces; of Proof Spirit a Gallon; of Water as much as is sufficient to prevent burning. Distill off a Gallon. *L.* The Virtues of this may also be learned from those of Cardamoms, in the *Materia Medica.*

Aqua Seminum Carui.

Water of Carraway Seeds.

Take of Carraway Seeds, half a Pound; of Proof Spirit a Gallon; of Water, as much as is sufficient to prevent burning. Distill off a Gallon.

See the Article *Carum,* under Vegetables, for the Virtues of this Water.

Aqua Theriacalis.

Treacle Water.

Take of the Roots of Butter-bur, a Pound; those of Angelica and Master-wort, each half a Pound; of Zedoary, four Ounces; of the Leaves of Rue and *Scordium,* each six Ounces; *Venice* Treacle, a Pound; *French* Brandy, three Gallons: digest all together for four Days, and afterwards distill off two Gallons and half of Water; to which add two Quarts of distilled Vinegar. *E.*

This is intended as a Sudorific and Alexipharmic, and may do Good where such Sorts of Medicines can be serviceable, which very seldom happens. But as I have a very bad Opinion of the Composition from whence it takes its Name, I should have a worse of this Water, if it was not for the Vinegar, which may possibly prevent it from doing much Mischief.

As the Water distill'd from Hartshorn is taken no Notice of by the Compilers of our Dispensatories, but is a Medicine much used by the *French* Physicians, we shall here give the various Methods of preparing it, directed in some of the most celebrated Dispensatories. In the *Brandenburgh Dispensatory,* therefore, and the *Pharmacopœia Parisiensis,* it is prepar'd by Distillation from the young and tender Horns of the Stag. According to *Ettmuller,* " it " is an excellent Medicine against " Palpitations of the Heart; and a " good Vehicle for exhibiting to " Children, Infants, and Adults, " Alexipharmic Medicines in Fevers, " and other Disorders of a malignant " Nature. It is he says proper for " promoting the Eruption of the " small Pox and Measles; as also " for curing Epilepsies either by " itself, or mix'd with other proper " Medicines. This Water is used " with Success by Child bed Wo- " men, when seiz'd with the pur- " ple Fever; as also in immoderate " Fluxes of the Lochia, Dysente- " ries, and Scurvy." Others also recommend it for promoting the Expulsion of the Fœtus. But it is in reality possess'd of scarce any other Virtues than those of common Water; for these young and tender Horns, as also all other Parts of other Animals, as *Zwelfer* justly observes, only send forth in such Distillation an elementary Water or Moisture possess'd of very inconsiderable Virtues; and which, tho' impregnated with an empyreumatic Smell, cannot from that Circumstance, be thought to possess so very powerful Qualities. The *Aqua Cornu Cervi è tenellis cum Vino,* in the *Brandenburgh* Dispensatory, receives besides the tender Horns, stimulating and alexipharmic Medicines, entire Citrons, Astringents, and other Substances, which in Distillation, do not yield their Virtues: all these are distill'd with Wine, and Water of

Germander. It is said to be alexi-pharmic and Cordial, which Qualities it more justly claims than the preceeding Water, not on Account of Hartshorn, but of the aromatic, . . . s, and heating Ingredients.
. . . passes his Judgment upon both in the following Words; they are supported upon a ground-"less and implicit Opinion, the "worst of Foundations. Some fond "Abettors of Antiquity, however, "ascribe a great deal to Composi-"tions of this kind. As there is no "Necessity for envying these Men "their *Nostrums*, they may be at "Liberty to enlarge at Pleasure the "Class of Cordials and Alexiphar-"mics. Of the simple Water, a "few Ounces may be exhibited for "a Dose; and of that prepared with "Wine, one is sufficient." Both these Waters are now in Disuse, because better and more judicious, or at least as good, Compositions are to be had with more Ease. They may, indeed, be us'd as Vehicles for other Medicines, that the Apothecary may have no Reason to complain of sustaining a Loss on Account of their

being discarded. The *Aqua Typhorum Cervi*, in the *Pharmacopœia Argen-toratensis*, is distill'd with Wine alone. This Preparation is by some com-mended, as an Alexipharmic, and good against Burning and Malignant Fevers. A few Spoonfuls may be given for a Dose. What rises in the Alembic seems to be simple Spirit of Wine, as may be also known from its Virtues and Properties. The *Aqua Cornu Cervi Citrata Waldschmidii*, in the *Pharmacopœia Argentoratensis*, is pre-pared of the Shavings of Hartshorn, distill'd with entire Citrons, and some distill'd Waters of Vegetables, com-monly call'd alexipharmic or stimulat-ing, with an Addition of the Water of Sorrel. This Preparation is accounted analeptic, and proper for allaying preternatural Heats. It is also said to be alexipharmic. A Spoonful of it may be exhibited at a Time; or it may be mix'd with other proper Liquors. From what is before said, 'tis obvi-ous, that whatever Virtues these Wa-ters possess are owing to the Ingredients us'd in Distillation, and not to the Hartshorn. All these are therefore, justly disregarded in our Pharmacy.

CHAP. IV.

SPIRITS *by* DISTILLATION.

Spiritus Vini Rectificatus.
Rectified Spirit of Wine.

TAKE any Quantity of *French* Spirit of Wine, or Brandy; drawn off by Distillation, one half, by a very gentle Heat.

This Spirit digested for two Days, with a fourth Part of very dry Salt of Tartar in Powder, and then di-stilled from a Glass Cucurbit, with an extreme gentle Heat, is *Alco-hol*. E.

Spiritus Cochleariæ.
Spirit of Scurvy Grass.

Take of fresh Scurvy-grass bruis'd, ten Pounds; and rectified Spirit of Wine, five Pints; let them ma-cerate together for twelve Hours; and then draw off five Pints of the Liquor, in *Balneo Mariæ*. E.

This is intended as an Antiscor-butic, and is given in any conveni-ent Vehicle, from twenty to one hundred Drops, or more. It is vul-garly called plain or white Spirit of
a Com-

urvy-grafs, to diftinguifh it from Compound, red Sort, commonly ld by the Name of Golden, or irging Spirit of Scurvy-grafs; hich is made by diffolving an Ounce Rofin of Jalap, Scammony, or amboge in the former. The Dofe the latter is faid to be from venty to fixty Drops, but is never 'd thatI know of in regularPractice.

Spiritus Lavendulæ fimplex.

Simple Spirit of Lavender.

'ake of frefh Lavender Flowers, a Pound and a Half; of Proof Spirit a Gallon. Diftill off five Pints, in a Bath Heat. L.

Spiritus Lavendulæ Compofitus.

ompound Spirit of Lavender, or Palfy Drops.

As this celebrated Medicine is fteem'd of fome Importance in Phyc, I fhall in this Place give the vaious Methods of preparing it, from ll our Difpenfatories.

'ake Flowers of Lavender, one Gallon; pour upon them four Gallons of *French* Brandy, and add frefh Flowers of Sage, Rofemary, and Betony, of each one Handful; of Borage, Buglofs, Lillies of the Valley, and Cowslips, of each two Handfuls; of the Leaves of Baum, Feverfew, and of the Orange Tree frefh gather'd; of the Flowers of Stœchas, Oranges, and Bay Berries, of each an Ounce; digeft thefe together, and draw off in *Balneo Mariæ,* two Gallons and a Half; then add of the outer Rind of Citrons, and of yellow Sanders, of each fix Drams; of Cinnamon, Nutmegs, and Mace, of the leffer Cardamom Seeds, and Cubebs, of each Half an Ounce; of Aloés Wood, one Dram; digeft thefe for twenty-four Hours, and filtre the Spirit; then if it be

thought proper, add of Mufk, Ambergrife, and Saffron, of each Half a Scruple; red Rofes dried, and red Sanders, of each Half an Ounce; let the Species be tied up in a thin Bag, and fufpended in the Spirit.

In fome of the firft Editions of the *Edinburgh* Difpenfatory, compound Spirit of Lavender, was order'd to be thus prepar'd,

Take of the Flowers of Lavender, one Pound; thofe of Lilly of the Valley, frefh gathered, thofe of *Arabian* Stœchas, and thofe of Rofemary, each two Ounces; the Tops of Betony, Marjoram, Balm and Sage, each an Ounce and Half; Cinnamon, two Ounces; the yellow Part of the frefh Citron or Lemon Peel, an Ounce; Bay Berries, the leffer Cardamoms and Nutmeg, each fix Drams; Cloves, Cubebs and Mace, each Half an Ounce: Bruife them all together, and pour thereon two Gallons of *French* Brandy, digeft for four Days; then in *Balneo Mariæ* draw off the Spirit as long as it will run, wherein fufpend the following Ingredients, contain'd in a Piece of fine Linen; *viz.* red Sanders in Powder, Half an Ounce; Cochineal, and Saffron, of each two Drams: and if the Spirit be defired perfumed, one Scruple of Ambergrife, and ten Grains of Mufk.

In the laft Edition of the *Edinburgh* Difpenfatory it is order'd thus,

Take of *French* Brandy, three Gallons; inftil into it gradually, fometimes fhaking it of the diftill'd Oil of Lavender, an Ounce and a Half; Oil of Rofemary, an Ounce; Oil of Marjoram, fix Drams, Oil of Lemon Peel, Half an Ounce; Oil of Nutmegs, three Drams; Oil of Cloves, two Drams; and Oil of

Cinnamon

Cinnamon, one Dram; let Half of this Spirit, thus faturated with the Oils, be diftill'd in a Bath Heat to two Thirds: Sufpend in the diftill'd Spirit, of red Sanders powder'd, one Ounce; Cochineal, and *English* Saffron, each two Drams, included in a fine Linen Rag, and if it is required to be perfum'd, fufpend in the fame Rag, a Scruple of Amber-grife, and Half a Scruple of Mufk.

The laft *London* Difpenfory, orders it thus,

Take of the *Spiritus Lavendulæ fimplex*, three Pints; of Spirit of Rofemary, one Pint; Cinnamon, Nutmeg, of each Half an Ounce; of red Sanders, three Drams. Digeft them together, and then ftrain off the Spirit.

As I have feldom known any us'd, befides that firft prefcrib'd, I cannot determine from Experience, which is the moft effectual, but they all feem to be admirable Medicines, as reviving Cordials, Balfamics, and Cephalics, and infinitely preferable to any of the Compound Waters, in moft of the Intentions, where the latter can be of any Ufe. *Quincy* informs us, that Spirit of Lavender has long been celebrated in all nervous Cafes, and is now greatly ufed in the Shops. In the Decays of Age, and convulfive, and apopleCtic Shocks, fuch as bring on Palfies and Lofs of Memory, this is of very good Service, and has been fo much remark'd for fuch Efficacies, as almoft univerfally to obtain the Name of *Palfy-Drops*; it may be taken from twenty, to one hundred Drops at a Time; the beft way is upon Sugar, and letting it gradually diffolve in the Mouth, becaufe by that Means it foaks more immediately into the Nerves, and gives a more fudden Supply to the Spirits, than

when it is diluted by any Vehicle, and carried with it into the Stomach.

Spiritus Matricalis.
Antihyfteric Spirit.

Take of yellow Amber, two Ounces; Myrrh, one Ounce and a Half, of *Ruffia* Caftor, one Ounce; pulverize them fine, and add as much Oil of Tartar *per Deliquium* as will make it into a foft Pafte, to which afterwards add, when gently dried, half an Ounce of *English* Saffron, and two Quarts of rectified Spirit of Wine: Digeft for four Days and draw off three Pints of Spirit in a glafs Retort. E

This Compofition, or fomething very like it, is in many foreign Difpenfatories, and is much us'd by Phyficians abroad, as an Uterine, and Antihyfteric.

Spiritus Bezoarticus Buffii.
Bezoartic Spirit of Buffins.

Take Spirit of Ivory, faturated with a fubtile Oil and volatile Salt about two Ounces, Sal Ammoniac four Ounces; Pot-afh firft diffolved in Water, eleven Ounces, Amber finely pulverifed, half a Pound, genuine Oil of Cedar, or of Juniper, half an Ounce, rectified Spirit of Wine a Pint and half. All thefe Ingredients being exquifitely mixed, in a glafs Cucurbit, are to be diftilled in a fand Heat, by which we extract a Spirit endued with confiderable Virtues. A volatile Salt firft rifes in the Alembic, which is afterwards fucceffively diffolved by the Spirit.

It is here to be obferved, that *Peruvian* Balfam, or the frefh Peel of Lemons, or Oranges, or Juniper berries, or any other balfamic and aromatic Powders may be ufed inftead of the Ingredients before mentioned. In the Procefs a limpid Spirit, t, like Water, comes over, but the longer it is kept in a Veſſel expoſed to the Air, the more yellow it turns, till its Colour be heightned almoſt to a Redneſs. If a Glaſs be filled with this Spirit and cover'd with a Stopple, it will continue clear, and ſuffer no Alteration of Colour.

This Spirit abounds with an oily volatile Salt, for the more a volatile Salt is impregnated, and intimately mixed with an Oil, the more eaſily and readily it unites, with highly rectified Spirit of Wine, and that Salt may immediately be precipitated from this Spirit, by mixing a few Drops of Oil of Vitriol with it, which produce a Coagulation and Precipitation of the Salt to the Bottom, where it firmly adheres to the ſides of the Glaſs. It is worthy our Obſervation, that this volatile Spirit of *Buſſius* is endued with an almoſt incredible Virtue in ſubverting and expelling all Kinds of Acids, tho' never ſo ſtrong, and theſe Effects are attended with different Circumſtances and Events. Thus if one Part of the Spirit of Nitre or Aqua-fortis, be poured to three Parts of this Spirit, all the Acidity is ſoon taken off, without any remarkable Ebullition, and nothing is precipitated to the Bottom, the Mixture acquires a mild nitrous Taſte, and being put into a Silver Spoon, and evaporated by the Heat of a Candle, leaves a Salt of an exquiſitely nitrous Flavour. This Mixture alſo, on Account of the volatile Nitre which it contains, is endued with excellent medicinal Virtues; for in acute Diſtempers, where volatile Medicines are of no Effect, becauſe of the violent Motion and Effervescence of the Blood, this Spirit, mixed with Spirit of Nitre, and render'd more temperate, gives all the Relief that can be wiſhed, by gently carrying off the morbific Matter.

If this Spirit of *Buſſius*, be mixed with Spirit of Salt ſtrongly concentrated there ariſes a greater Ebullition than in the former Caſe, but all the Acid is, in like Manner, in a very ſhort Time ſubdued, and the Liquor turns Salt, which in Diſorders of the Stomach, where the Appetite is loſt, may be given with Succeſs, for diſſolving viſcid Crudities. When this Spirit is mixed with diſtilled Oil of Vitriol, there immediately ariſes an Effervescence, the Mixture becomes turbid, and all the volatile Salt is precipitated to the Bottom, the Taſte of the Mixture has nothing of Acidity, but has a grateful Smell. The Reaſon why there is a Concretion and Precipitation of the volatile Salt, at the Mixture of concentrated Oil of Vitriol, but not with other Acids, ſeems to be as follows. Oil of Vitriol, as being a very ſtrong Acid, unites with inflammable Spirit of Wine, which is an oily Subſtance; hence the volatile Salt which it contains, is precipitated; but from other acid Spirits, which are weaker, and incapable of ſo intimate a Combination with the inflammable Spirit of Wine, there follows no Precipitation. From theſe Experiments we may draw this Concluſion, which is very uſeful in Practice: That this Spirit which abounds with an oily volatile Salt, may be given in large Doſes, without Inconvenience, in Diſtempers, eſpecially chronical ones, where a ſtrong and copious Acid is lodged in the Sinuſes of the Stomach and Inteſtines, and creates Diſturbance in thoſe Parts, as it does more remarkably in hypochondriacal Affections.

This Spirit takes its Name from its Inventor, *Buſſius*, an eminent Phyſician of *Dreſden*, and the Medicine itſelf is of univerſal Uſe in *Saxony*, and well deſerves our Notice, for it is a powerful Sudorific and Diuretic, with due Management, and is an excellent Anti-ſpaſmodic. Beſides, it recommends itſelf, on Account of its

grateful

grateful Flavour, having nothing of a nauseous empyreumatic Smell. The Foundation of the Preparation confists in mixing the volatile, urinous, and oily Spirits of Animals with highly rectified Spirit of Wine, and with an Addition of balsamic Species, distilling them over a proper Fire, by which Means we obtain a Spirit well impregnated with volatile Salt, an empyreumatic Oil, and resinous, sulphureous, balsamic Particles, and of no unpleasant Smell and Taste.

This Medicine is described by *Frederic Hoffman*, and introduced with the preceding Character. It somewhat resembles our *Spirit of Sal Volatile*, and promises fair to be an elegant, effectual, and agreeable Medicine. *Quincy*'s Directions for preparing the Spirit of *Sal Volatile*, or, as it is usually called, *Sal Volatile*, are thus,

Sal Volatile Oleosum.

Take of Sal Ammoniac, and Salt of Tartar, of each half a Pound, powder them apart, and mix them; put the Mixture into a Retort; put also into the Retort, the Leaves of *Marum Syriacum* half an Ounce, and of tartarized Spirit of Wine, one Pound and an half, impregnated with the essential Oils of Cloves half an Ounce; Cinnamon, one Scruple; Nutmeg, two Scruples, of Marjoram, Lemons, and Oranges, of each one Ounce; put to them of clean Water, two Pounds; and set all in a Sand Furnace, lute on a Receiver; and give Fire of the first Degree for one Hour and a half, increase to the second; which continue, five or six Hours, or until the white Salt which first shot at the Top of the Receiver, begins to melt down: Then put out the Fire, and pour the Spirit, which will have a great

deal of loose Salt in it, into a Vail by itself for Use; and the Salt hardened upon the upper Part of the Receiver into another.

This Preparation, is greatly now in Use; and for its preferable Fragrancy has almost excluded the Use of Spirit of Hartshorn, and the plain Spirit of *Sal Ammoniac*. It is a most noble Cephalic and Cordial, either to smell to, or take inwardly. Its Dose is from ten Drops, to one hundred or upwards, in Wine, or any common Vehicle. It is much varied according to the different Humours of the Maker; so that there would be no End of giving all the Receipts followed. This is one of the best, and whosoever pleases, may omit any of these Aromatics, or put others in their Room, if it may better suit any particular Intention. A *Sal Volatile* thus made with *Marum Syriacum* alone, is wonderfully penetrating, grateful and serviceable to the Head; and diluted to a convenient Strength, is one of the best Sternutatories that can be invented. It is easy to impregnate this with Steel. The slower the Fire is, the more Salt crusts upon the Top and Neck of the Receiver; and therefore if Care be taken not to draw it too near, whereby that Salt is melted down, a great deal may be preserved, which is vastly preferable to all of this Kind; not only for Fragrancy of Scent in Smelling Bottles, but for Efficacy internally used in all Nervous Cases.

Spiritus Salinus Aromaticus.

The Saline Aromatic Spirit.

In making the Compound Spirit of Lavender, according to the *Edinburgh* Dispensatory, only one half of the Spirit is directed to be used. Take, therefore, the remaining half of that Spirit impregnated with the essential Oils, and add to it of volatile *Sal Ammoniac* eight Ounces. Distill off imme-

imediately in a Sand Heat, two
irds.

This ſeems to be intended by the
ompilers of the *Edinburgh* Diſpen-
tory, for the ſame Uſes as the preceding.

Spiritus Volatilis Aromaticus.

Aromatic Volatile Spirit.

ake Eſſence of Lemons, eſſential
Oil of Nutmegs, of each two
Drams; of eſſential Oil of Cloves
half a Dram; of dulcified Spirit
of *Sal Ammoniac* a Quart. Diſtil
with a very gentle Fire. L.

This ſeems intended for the ſame
Iſes as the preceding. I don't com-
rehend why the Compilers of the
dinburgh, and *London* Diſpenſatories
ave thought proper to change the
lames of theſe and ſome other Me-
icines; becauſe it cauſes Confuſion
nd Perplexity, without any one Ad-
antage to compenſate it; and there-
ore Terms univerſally received in
he Art, ſhould be adher'd to, unleſs
here is ſome very good Reaſon for
he Alteration.

Boerhaave has given us a Proceſs,
or making an extemporaneous *Sal
Volatile Oleoſum,* thus,

Take one Part of Salt of Tartar,
three Parts of *Sal Ammoniac,* twelve
Parts of Aromatics, reduced to
Powder, and twenty ſix Parts of
rectified Spirit of Wine; mix them
together, by long ſhaking in a Bolt
Head. The alkaline Salt will thus
immediately unite with the Alcohol that floats above, the Water,
being attracted into the Salts; at
the ſame Time the Salts and Spirits will attract the Oil out of the
Spices, and thus the Liquor that
floats above, will preſently become
the *Sal Volatile* required; as the
famous *Le Mort* has obſerved.

Theſe are the Methods generally
directed for making the *Sal Volatile*
Oleoſum, which are all a Kind of volatile Soap, form'd by the Union of
Alcohol of Wine, with the Spirit of
Sal Ammoniac, and impregnated with
the preſiding Spirit of Vegetables.
Medicines may be prepared in this
Manner, to anſwer almoſt any Intention whatever; for when we are
certain of the Virtues of any Vegetable, and that theſe Virtues reſide in
the Oil, we may by the Methods a-
bove deſcribed prepare a volatile oily
Salt, impregnated with the particular
Virtues of the Plant. Thus if a Cephalic is wanted we may uſe Lavender, Roſemary, or Marjoram; if a
Cardiac, the Peel of Orange, Lemon, Citron, Cinnamon, or Nutmeg; if an Emmenagogue, Juniper,
Rue, Savine, or *Arbor Vitæ,* or the
diſtil'd Oils of either, or any of them.

Baſil Valentine is ſaid to be the
firſt Contriver of this Kind of Medicine; but its general Uſe was introduced by *Sylvius De la Boe.* But
as is uſual in ſuch Caſes, the Followers of theſe Phyſicians, uſed it too
univerſally, and without Diſtinction.
Boerhaave ſays, that volatile oily
Salts thus prepared, by their Odour,
Taſte, Penetrability, Mobility, ſaponaceous Virtue, and the Power they
have of correcting what is acid and
auſtere, afford a Remedy of ſingular
Efficacy, in the Hands of a prudent
Phyſician. For they are excellent in
all watery, mucous, cold, acid, auſtere
Diſtempers, where the Efficacy of
the Bile is wanting, and in all ſlug-
giſh Diſorders unattended with Inflammation or Putrefaction, eſpecially when the Diſorders, or unequal
Motions of the Nerves and Spirits,
occaſion troubleſome hypochondriacal and hyſterical Fits, with the Flatulencies thence proceeding. Hence
it is at preſent accounted a noble Re-
ſtorative, ſtomachic, warming, ſudorific, diuretic, diaphoretic, anti-
ſpaſmodic, and anti-epileptic Medicine, where the Diſtemper proceeds
from

from the Caufes above mentioned. But in inflammatory Diftempers, where the Juices are diffolved and putrid, in the alcaline Scurvy, the Phthific, Confumptions, and other Cafes, where the Body is almoft diffolved down, they often prove highly pernicious, and fometimes deftructive. Phyficians, therefore, are to be ferioufly admonifhed againft permitting Men, and particularly Women of a weak Conftitution, the frequent Ufe of thefe Salts.

Spiritus Volatilis fœtidus.

Fetid Volatile Spirit.

Take of any fix'd alcaline Salt, a Pound and a half; of Sal Ammoniac, a Pound; of Affa fœtida, four Ounces; of Proof Spirit, three Quarts; diftill off, with a gentle Heat five Pints. *L.*

The medicinal Virtues of this may be underftood from thofe of *Affa Fœtida.* It promifes fair to be a good Antihyfteric, and nervous Medicine, and to be capable of affording Relief in fpafmodic Diforders.

Spiritus Mindereri.

Mindererus's Spirit.

Take any Quantity of diftill'd Vinegar, and add to it by Degrees, as much of the Spirit of Sal Ammoniac as will put a Stop to the Effervefcence. *E.*

When the Vinegar is faturated with the Spirit of Sal Ammoniac, and the Mixture is perfectly neutraliz'd, it makes a Medicine of Virtues very different from thofe of either the Vinegar, or Spirit of Sal Ammoniac. It is extremely refolvent and penetrating, and is often given in Fevers and febrile Diforders, in the Quantity of half an Ounce, made into a Draught with fome fimple Water and Syrup, and repeated frequently. And in fuch Cafes it is much more likely to do Service, than the common

Draughts compofed of fimple and compound Waters, and Syrups. It may be made by faturating diftilled Vinegar with Volatile Sal Ammoniac. I don't know why the Compilers of the *Edinburgh* Difpenfatory have thought proper to make this a Shop Medicine, for it is prepared very readily extemporaneoufly, and is not worfe for being recently made. The common Draughts made by mixing the Juice of Lemons, with Salt of Wormwood, to the Point of Saturation, is intended for the fame Ufes as this *Spiritus Mindereri*, but I think the latter much preferable, provided the Vinegar made ufe of is the true *French* Vinegar, and not that four Beer, which is generally amongft us fubftituted in its Room. In extemporaneous Prefcription, where an Alcali and an Acid are united, with an Intent to form a neutral Mixture, it is impoffible to fpecify exactly the Quantity of Alcali fufficient to faturate the Acid, becaufe the one or the other, may happen to be ftronger or weaker. It is therefore beft to direct the Alcali to be added till the Point of Saturation is obtained, of which the Compounder only can be a Judge.

As the Virtues of neutral Salts in Medicine are not commonly underftood, tho' often exhibited as it were accidentally, and without any Defign, I fhall in this Place endeavour to explain their Ufes in the Words of a very celebrated Phyfician. Among all the various Salts in Nature, none are more fafe and efficacious, than neutral Salts, which are alfo, poffeffed of a cathartic Quality. Neutral Salts are thofe compounded of an alcaline Salt, or Earth, and an acid Salt, in fuch a Manner as that the one does not predominate over the other: Now as alcaline and acid Salts, when feparate, are of fo ftrong a Tafte and Quality, as often to approach to a corrofive Nature, fo

when

when mixed in a due Proportion with each other, they are, by the mutual Illision and Conflict of their Parts, so corrected, as not only with Respect to Taste, but also all their other Qualities, to become a Salt of a middle Nature, highly innocent in itself, and friendly to the human Constitution. Perfectly neutral Salts, therefore, are such as produce no Degree of Effervescence; but are perfectly saturated, upon the Affusion of any acid or alcaline Liquor.

Neutral Salts are of great Efficacy in the Cure of Diseases; possessed of an aperient and detergent Quality, capable of promoting all the Excretions, and, when exhibited in large Doses, of a cathartic Quality. 'Tis, also, sufficiently obvious, that Salts of this Kind are, of all others, the most salutary, and so friendly to Nature, that the Physician can neither practise successfully without them, nor easily produce any bad Effects by using them. But many Objections may be made to this Doctrine, since both Experience, and accurate Observation convince us, that those Medicines which are highly acid, as, also, volatile, urinous, and fixed alcaline Remedies, are so far from being unsalutary and unfriendly to the Constitution, that they may be said to be the most safe of any. But to this I answer, that neither acid nor alcaline Medicines, whether of the fixed or volatile Kind, ever produce a salutary Effect, unless by the internal Disposition of the Humours, especially those lodged in the *Primæ Viæ*, they are converted into a neutral Salt, and by that Means rendered friendly to the solid as well as fluid Parts of the human Body.

For this Reason, when a large quantity of Bile, especially of an alcaline and oleous Kind, is collected and becomes stagnant, in the flexure of the Duodenum, strongly affects the nervous System; and by

that Means often produces bilious Vomitings, Nausea, Loss of Appetite, hectic Heats, Cephalalgias, and an insatiable Thirst, then acidulated Liquors, such as Julaps, Refrigerants, or other acid mineral Spirits edulcorated, are of singular Service. Besides, when an intense febrile Heat, arising from a violent intestine Motion of the sulphureous Parts of the Blood, by destroying its temperate and due Texture, exhausts the Body, and impairs the Strength, Acids are in such Cases more beneficial than neutral Salts, alcaline Substances, or any other Remedies, because they are capable of fixing and subduing the sulphureous Particles, by whose Motion the Heat is produced. In malignant Disorders arising from a Putrefaction of the Humours, more Relief is to be expected from Acids than from any other Remedies, because a Putrefaction not only generates an Alcali, but also proceeds from a large Quantity of it: And when this Alcali is corrected and subdued by an Acid, the Putrefaction is forthwith stopt. In inveterate Scurvies, and Arthritic Disorders, large Quantities of Salts are generated in the Mass of Blood, which approach more nearly to an alcaline and lixivious, than to a neutral Nature. Hence the Blood of such Persons, when taken from the Veins, appears thin and florid, and their Urine is, for the most part, highly red, saline, and lixivious. And Experience teaches us, that in such Cases, more happy Effects are often produc'd by temperate Acids, than by alcaline, urinous, and volatile Medicines, or those of an hot and spirituous Nature.

Those Medicines which abound with an alcaline Salt, whether of the fix'd or volatile Kind, are by no Means to be promiscuously and indiscriminately used, tho' they are of singular Service, when prudently exhi-

exhibited; for when a Redundance of acid Humours is lodged in the *Prima Viæ*, and excites violent Symptoms, as we observe in hypochondriac, hysteric, and melancholic Patients, such as Corrosions of the Stomach and Intestines, Anxieties, Inflations of the Stomach, attended with a *Cardialgia*, Coughs accompanied with Pains of the Stomach, Cephalalgias, excessive Costiveness, or preternatural Looseness, accompanied with a Tenesmus, in these Cases, certainly, earthy Alcalines, and especially Crab's Eyes, prepared Shells, or Oil of Tartar *per Deliquium*, will produce more happy Effects, than any other Medicines, because by absorbing the Acid they convert it into a neutral Salt, which is afterwards easily carried through the excretory Ducts, without exciting any violent Symptom. But if there is rather a Defect than a Redundance of the Acid in the *Prima Viæ*, and if these are full of viscid and tenacious Humours, alcaline earthy Substances, taken in large Quantities, are highly prejudicial; for since they are not dissolved, they rather, by uniting with the earthy and slimy Particles, augment the Quantity of the Phlegm, and by that means destroy the Appetite, load the Stomach, obstruct the Mouths of the lacteal Vessels, and render the Patient costive. Thus we see, that the true Uses of alcaline and acid Medicines are, to neutralize the Juices, which then not only become perfectly innocent and inoffensive, but farther form excellent Medicines within the Body.

C H A P. V.

WATERS, by INFUSION and VINEGAR.

Aqua Aluminosa.
Alum Water.

TAKE of corrosive Mercury sublimate, and Roch Alum, each two Drams; powder them in a Glass Mortar, and boil them in two Pints of Spring Water; to the Consumption of half: Let it subside and pour off the clear Liquor. E.

This is only intended for external Uses, and even for these requires much Dilution, that is, with twice, thrice, or even four times its Quantity of Water. It is said to be useful in obstinate Eruptions, and foul chronical Ulcers.

Aqua Aluminosa Batteana.
Bate's Alum Water.

Take Alum, white Vitriol, each half an Ounce; of Water a Quart. Dissolve the Salts by boiling them in Water, and when the Fæces have subsided, filtre the Liquor thro' Paper. *L.*

Aqua Calcis seu Benedicta.
Lime Water.

Take a Pound of Quick Lime, and a Gallon of hot Spring Water stir them well together; afterwa suffer the Lime to subside, as pour off the clear, which is to be kept in Vessels carefully stopt. It is made in the same Manner as calcin'd Oyster Shells. E.

The *London* Dispensatory orders a Gallon and a half of Water, to a Pound of Quick Lime. This is recommended as an extraordinary Medicine in many Cases of Obstinacy; and if three or four Ounces of it be drank three or four times a Day, is said to cure red pimpled Faces, Strumas, Dysenteries, the *Fluor Albus*, rheumatic Pains, and the Diabetes. It is certainly a powerful Dryer; and very proper to use in Decoctions of the Woods, and all Ingredients of that Intention: But tho' the making of it is easy enough, yet here in *London* it may be had at any Time, as *Quincy* informs us, from the Sugar Bakers, by the Name of Lime Water, as it happens to be wanted; because they use it much in refining their Sugars. This is also much used for cleansing and drying up foul Ulcers, both by its internal Use, and washing them frequently with it.

Boerhaave remarks, that Lime when assisted by Heat, and the vital Motion, presently generates those fiery Spirits, that prove destructive to the tender pappy Mass of the Brain and Nerves; and the hotter, more agitated the Body, or the more it is affected with inflammatory Disorders, the more destructive the Use hereof is. But when the Body abounds with acid Water or Phlegm, the prudent Application thereof may sometimes of Service. We must also consider that the Lixivium of Quick Lime has a great Force in corroding, and extricating the muriafixed Salts in the Blood, and fitting them to be easily discharged; hence it becomes an extraordinary Remedy in that Kind of Scurvy, which principally proceeds from the above mentioned Causes: But in that kind of Scurvy, which proceeds

from Putrefaction, and consists in a sharp Oil and Salt, it proves highly prejudicial. Whence, perhaps, we may in some Measure reconcile the Experiments of some eminent Physicians in *France*, which shew the Lixivium of Quick Lime to be pernicious in that Country; whereas in *Germany* it appears a very advantageous Medicine. But all this holds more true of the Quick Lime prepared from Stone, than of that from Shells.

Aqua calcis minus composita.
The lesser compound Lime Water.

Take of Liquorice one Pound, of Sassafras Bark half an Ounce, of simple Lime Water three Quarts. Infuse two Days without Heat, and then strain off the Liquor. L.

Aqua calcis magis composita.
The more compound Lime Water.

Take of the Raspings of Lignum Vitæ half a Pound, of Liquorice one Ounce, of Sassafras Bark half an Ounce, of Coriander Seed three Drams, of simple Lime Water three Quarts. Infuse as before, and then strain off. L.

The Virtues of these may be understood by comparing those of the Ingredients, with those of Lime-Water.

Aqua Ophthalmica.
Eye Water.

Take of unprepared Bole Armoniac, two Ounces; unprepared Tutty, an Ounce; and of white Vitriol, half an Ounce; of Camphire two Drams; reduce them to Powder, and pour thereon two Quarts of hot Spring Water; boil them together, and stir the Mixture frequently; and after due Time allow'd for it to settle, pour off the clear. E.

This is only intended for external

X x

Uses; it is said to be good against Inflammations, and particularly to check Rheums in the Eyes; and if too sharp it may be lower'd by the Addition of Water. *Quincy* recommends a Water much like this, which he calls *Aqua Camphorata*, for cleansing Ulcers, by washing them frequently with it warm, and he says it keeps the Gums clean, and firm to the Teeth, if they are frequently rubb'd with it. He farther recommends it as a safe and efficacious Topic in the Itch, if the Eruptions, and Parts affected are frequently washed with it; with much the same Intentions, the *London* Dispensatory directs a Water under the Title of,

Aqua Vitriolica Camphorata.

Camphorated Vitriolic Water.

Take of white Vitriol half an Ounce; of Camphire two Drams; of boiling Water a Quart. Mix them, that the Vitriol may be dissolved; and after the Fæces have subsided, filtre the Water thro' Paper. *L.*

Aqua Ophthalmica altera.

Another Eye Water.

Take white Vitriol, and Bay Salt, of each one Ounce; decrepitate them together, till the Detonation is over, than pour upon them in an earthen Pan, one Pound of boiling Water; stir them together, and let them stand some Hours: A various colour'd Skin will fix upon the Surface; which carefully take off, and put the rest in a Phial for Use.

Quincy says, this was communicated to him as a wonderful Secret; and indeed says he, I have found it, by Abundance of Trials, very safely to cool and repel those sharp Rheums which sometimes fall upon the Eyes; and to clear them of beginning Films and Specks. If it be too sharp, it may be diluted with a little Spring, or Rose Water. *Q.*

Aqua Phagedænica.

Phagedenic Water.

Take a Pint of Lime Water, and half a Dram of corrosive Mercury sublimate, and make a Solution thereof. *E.*

This is intended for external Application only, and even thus must be used with great Caution, and much Dilution, either with Water, or Spirit of Wine, and thus it is said to be a good Lotion for old eating Ulcers.

Aqua Sapphirina.

Sapphire coloured Water.

Take a Pint of fresh Lime Water, and two Drams of *Sal Armoniac*; make a Solution thereof, and put it into a Copper Vessel till it has from thence acquired a blue Colour. *E.*

The *London* Dispensatory orders but one Dram of *Sal Ammoniac.*

This Water is in much Use for taking away Specks, or Films, or curing Ulcers in the Eye, for which Purpose two or three Drops are to be put into it. The Lime Water is drying; the *Sal Ammoniac* is extremely resolvent; and the Tincture it acquires from the Copper, renders it very mildly corrosive.

Aqua Styptica.

Styptic Water.

Take of blue Vitriol and Roche Alum, each half a Pound; Spring Water, two Quarts; boil them together till the Salts are dissolved, and afterwards filtre the Liquor; to each Pint whereof add a Dram of Oil of Vitriol. *E.*

The Title of this Water explains its Uses. The *London* Dispensatory directs a Water with much the same Intention, under the Title of

Aqu

Aqua Vitriolica cærulea.

The blue Vitriolic Water.

ake of blue Vitriol three Ounces;
Alum, the ftrong Spirit or Oil of
Vitriol, of each two Ounces; of
Water a Pint and a half. Boil
the Salts in the Water, till they
are diffolved; then add the Oil of
Vitriol, and ftrain the Mixture
thro' Paper. *L.*

Tar Water.

our a Gallon of cold Water on a
Quart of Tar, and ftir and mix
them thoroughly with a Ladle, or
flat Stick for the Space of three or
four Minutes, after which the
Veffel muft ftand eight and forty
Hours, that the Tar may have
Time to fubfide, when the clear
Water is to be poured off, and
kept covered for Ufe, no more
being made from the fame Tar,
which may ftill ferve for common
Purpofes.

This is the Method of making Tar
Water, as directed by the Bifhop of
Joyne, and as it is now in almoft
niverfal Ufe, I thought it not amifs
o take Notice of it in this Place.
ts Ufes may be learn'd from what
have heretofore faid upon the Sub-
ect of Balfamics.

Lotio Saponacea.

The faponaceous Lotion.

Take of Damask Rofe Water three
quarters of a Pint; of Olive Oil,
a quarter of a Pint; of the Ley
of Tartar the Meafure of half an
Ounce. Rub the Ley of Tartar
and Oil together, till they are
mixed; then gradually add the
Water. *L.*

This feems intended as a Detergent
nd Refolvent, but I can fee no End
t anfwers, which may not be pro-
ided for by extemporaneous Pre-
cription. For a Solution of fome
f the finer Soaps in Water will

anfwer all good Purpofes as well,
and may be render'd more deterfive
if requifite, by the Addition of a
Solution of Salt of Tartar, or any
other alcaline Salt.

Acetum diftillatum feu Spiritus Aceti.

Diftill'd Vinegar, or Spirit of Vine-gar.

Take any Quantity of the beft Vinegar, put it into a glazed earthen
Pan, and by the gentle Heat of a
Balneum Mariæ exhale about one
fourth thereof, then diftill the
Remainder by the Alembic; the
Fire being gradually increafed in
the Operation, fo long as the Spirit comes off clear. *E.*

The *London* Difpenfatory orders it
thus,

Let Vinegar be diftilled with a gentle Heat, as long as the Drops
fall free from any Empyreuma. If
fome Part of what comes firft off
be thrown away, what is referved
will be ftronger.

This is more properly called *Acetum
diftillatum,* than *Spiritus Aceti,* becaufe in the Diftillation of Vinegar,
the Phlegm rifes firft, and comes
over, leaving the heavier Acid behind;
whereas in the Diftillation of Spirits, the Spirit firft comes over, and
leaves the Water behind. The Virtues of diftill'd Vinegar may be
learn'd from thofe of Vinegar. But
I muft remark that the Vinegars generally made ufe of in *England,* are
far inferior in Virtues and Efficacy
to the true *French* Vinegar, made of
ftrong Wines by a particular Procefs.

Acetum Lithargyrites.

Litharge Vinegar.

Take four Ounces of Litharge of
Gold, and one Pint of the beft
Vinegar: Digeft them in a Sand
Heat for four Days, often fhaking
the Glafs, then filtre the Liquor.
E.

Xx2　　　　　　　This

This seems only intended for external Uses as a Cooler.

Acetum Rosaceum.

Vinegar of Roses.

Take of red Roses clipp'd from their white Heels, one Pound; the best Vinegar, one Gallon; let them stand to infuse in the Sun, put up in a well closed Vessel, for forty Days; then strain off the Liquor. The Operation may be sooner perform'd by letting them boil in *Balneo Mariæ* for some Hours. *E.*

This, as *Quincy* informs us, is seldom used, except to embrocate the Head and Temples, in some Kinds of Head-Achs, in which it frequently does Service.

Vinegars may be prepar'd in the same Manner from Rue, Elder, and other Vegetables. That of Rue should seem to be most considerable with Respect to its Medicinal Virtues.

Acetum Scilliticum.

Vinegar of Squills.

Take of Squills, cut small, one Pound; best Vinegar, three Quarts; let them stand to infuse in the Sun, as was order'd of Vinegar of Roses, and afterwards press and strain off the Liquor. *E.*

The Proportion of the Squills to the Vinegar is the same here, as in the *London* Dispensatory, but in the latter, the Digestion is order'd to be made in a gentle Heat, then the Vinegar is order'd to be press'd out, and set by till the Dregs are subsided, and afterwards a twelfth Part of Proof Spirit, is to be added to the depurated Vinegar, in order to preserve it from contracting Dregs by Time. But I am far from believing this Addition of any Service to the Medicine, for the Spirit, so far as it acts at all, must impair its Virtues. Vinegar of Squills was a Medicine

very much celebrated amongst the Antients. It is said to be the Invention of *Pythagoras*, or that he learned the Use of it from *Epimenides*. He began at the fiftieth Year of his Age, to take some of this Vinegar every Day, and to this it was attributed that he lived in perfect Health to the Age of a hundred and seventeen. It is esteem'd to preserve the Hearing, and open the auditory Passage, used by way of Gargarism. *Dioscorides*, who orders this Medicine to be made by infusing in the Sun, informs it is good to consolidate the too lax and humid Gums, and fasten loose Teeth. It is excellent to heal putrid Ulcers in the Mouth, and for an offensive Breath. Drinking of it hardens the Throat and Jaws, and makes them callous; it helps the Voice, and renders it clear and sonorous. It is administer'd to such as labour under Infirmities of the Stomach, have weak Digestions, to epileptical, vertiginous, melancholy, and mad People. It is given also in hysteric Fits, in Disorders of the Spleen, and the Sciatica. It wonderfully clears and revives infirm Persons, renders the Body sound, and gives a good Colour. It quickens the Sight, and dropped or poured into the Ears, helps Thickness of Hearing. But he condemns the Use of it in internal Exulcerations.

Acetum Theriacale.

Treacle Vinegar.

Take of the Treacle of *Andromachus*, or that of the College of *Edinburgh*, one Pound; best Vinegar, two Quarts; digest them together with a gentle Heat, for three Days, and afterwards strain off the Liquor. *E.*

It is said, that this is very powerful in raising a Sweat, and therefore it must be a good Medicine where

Sweating

Sweating is of Service. But such great Mischiefs are daily done by extorting Sweats imprudently, that it should not be attempted without great Caution and Judgment; for nothing is more frequent than Fevers of the most malignant Kind, excited from very small Beginnings, a Cold for Example, or slight Fever, which would have terminated in a few Days without any Assistance from Medicine, by the imprudent Use of heating Medicines and Diaphoretics.

CHAP. VI.

Of TINCTURES.

General Rules *for extracting of* TINCTURES.

I. LET the Vegetables be such as were lately and moderately dried; unless they are order'd fresh gather'd: They ought likewise to be sliced and bruised before the *Menstruum* is put to them.

II. When Digestion is performed in a Bath Heat, the whole Work depends upon well regulating the Heat, which ought all along to be very gentle, unless where the Ingredients are of a hard Texture; in which Case, the Fire may at length be so far increased as to make them boil a little.

III. Very capacious circulating Vessels should be used for this Purpose; and ought to be heated before their Junctures are closed.

IV. The Vessel should be frequently shook during the Time the Digestion is in hand.

V. Let Tinctures be clarified by settling, before they pass the Filtre or Strainer.

VI. The *Edinburgh* Dispensatory farther very prudently advises, never to substitute Malt, Molosses, or any other Spirit, instead of a true rectify'd Spirit of Wine, in those Tinctures and Spirits destin'd for internal Uses.

Beerhaave informs us that Alcohol, when perfectly pure, scarce extracts any thing more from well dried compounded Vegetables, than the inflammable Parts, Spirit, Balsam, Oil, Colophony, Resin, and resinous Gum, and what is merely saponaceous; leaving a pure, dry Salt and Earth behind. If, therefore, the Artist knows that all the particular Virtue required resides in these Parts, then the Operation must be performed with pure Alcohol alone; but when the Virtues required lies in a Mixture of the, oily, resinous, saline, and saponaceous Parts together, it is better to use the common rectify'd Spirit than Alcohol; because that Spirit acts by its aqueous Part, upon what is saline and saponaceous, and by its Alcohol, upon what is balsamic, oily, and resinous; so that by this Means the united Virtues may be obtained in the Tincture. This is evident in the Roots of Hellebore, Hermodactyls, Jalap, Mechoacan, and Turbith; because the Tinctures drawn from them with a Spirit only once rectified, purge much better than those extracted by pure Alcohol. For if a resinous Tincture be drawn by Alcohol from Jalap, it purges less; whilst the Remainder being boiled in Water, communicates a purging Virtue there-

thereto. But if the Tincture be extracted with common Spirit, it proves highly purgative; and the Remains contain scarce any thing worth the extracting. Hence we learn, that a fixed alcaline Salt is not required in the making of many Tinctures, because it would either destroy, or change their particular Virtues; and that they are not always to be made with Alcohol: But we are first to confider what Spirit should be ufed. All the Tinctures, prepared with pure Alcohol, will burn entirely away, almost like pure Alcohol itself; whence it is manifest that this Menstruum extracts only the inflammable Part from the Compound, and leaves the rest behind. If, therefore, the Virtue of a Plant entirely refides in the faline, faponaceous Part, to boil it with Water is better than Alcohol. The Opium diffolved in Water is the best, the next is that diffolved in Wine, and the next in Spirit of Wine, but always the worfe, the better the Spirit.

Tinctura Amara.

The bitter Tincture.

Take of Gentian Root two Ounces, and of the outer yellow Rind of Seville Orange Peel dried, one Ounce, of the leffer Cardamom Seeds husk'd half an Ounce, of Proof Spirit a Quart. Digeft without Heat, and then ftrain. *L.*

This feems to be intended for a Stomachic, and to fupply the Place of thofe bitter Drops and Tinctures, which are commonly ufed in the Taverns by way of Whet. I am afraid that the Spirit in fuch Bitters, do more Prejudice to the Stomach than the Advantage receiv'd from the aromatic bitter Ingredients can compenfate, tho' they may excite a temporary Appetite.

Tinctura Antimonii.

Tincture of Antimony.

Take of Antimony and Nitre, each two Ounces; reduce them to Powder; and throw it by Degrees, into four Ounces of Salt of Tartar, contain'd in a Crucible, and made to flow by a violent Fire; let them continue in Fufion for half an Hour: then pour the Mixture into an Iron Mortar, made hot and dry to receive it: Pulverife the Mafs, fuffer it to cool, throw it into a Matrafs, and laftly, pour thereon a Quart of rectified Spirit of Wine: Digeft them together for eight Days with a gentle Heat of a *Balneum Mariæ*, and afterwards ftrain off the Tincture, *E.*

Another Tincture of Antimony, is directed in the *London* Dispenfatory to be prepared thus,

Take of any fixt alcaline Salt, a Pound, of Antimony half a Pound, of rectified Spirit of Wine, a Quart. Mix the Antimony reduced to Powder, with the Salt, and melt them together for an Hour in a ftrong Fire, then pour all out, and being pulverized, pour on the Spirit of Wine, digeft for three or four Days, and afterwards ftrain off. *L.*

Tinctura Antimonii acris fimplex.

The fimple acrid Tincture of Antimony.

This is directed to be made in the *Brandenburgh* Difpenfatory, by digefting the *Scoriæ* of the Martial Regulus of Antimony juft made, and hot, in highly rectify'd Spirit of Wine. Another acrid Tincture of Antimony, called the *Regalin Tincture*, is made by digesting equal Parts of the Martial *Regulus* of Antimony detonated with an equal Quantity of Nitre, in highly rectified Spirit of Wine.

It is said, that neither of these take up much from the Antimony, but that all their Virtues are borrowed from the Nitre render'd alcaline and acrid, by being fused with Antimony. These Tinctures, given in a proper Vehicle, and a . considerable Dose, are said to bring away the serous Humours of cachetic Patients. They are also esteem'd good Deobstruents in hypochondriac Medicines. *Stabl* calls that Tincture of Antimony, which is made by throwing diaphoretic Antimony, immediately after Dentonation, into Spirit of Wine, and digesting it. *Tinctura Antimonii alcalina acris.* The Doses of these Tinctures are from ten to sixty Drops.

Tinctura Antiphthisica.

Tincture against the Phthisic.

Take of the *Saccharum Saturni* one Ounce and an half; Vitriol of Iron, one Ounce; rectify'd Spirit of Wine, one Pint; and without Heat draw a Tincture. *E.*

This has been long in great Esteem both in *England* and abroad, as a kind of Specific in hectic Fevers, and is said to be good in relax'd Habits, as it braces powerfully. But as I am bound by no Authorities whatever, I think it my Duty to declare, that I esteem it a very dangerous Medicine, if given in Doses sufficient to answer any Purpose; and I have known it excite excessive Gripes, excessive Faintings, and Weakness; all which are the known Effects of Lead taken internally.

Tinctura Saturnina.

The Saturnine Tincture.

Take Sugar of Lead, green Vitriol, of each two Ounces, of rectify'd Spirit of Wine a Quart. Reduce the Salts separately to Powder, and put them into the Spirit, then digest without Heat, and filtre the Spirit thro' Paper. *L.*

In the Remarks on the Translation of the last *London* Dispensatory, we are told, that if Heat is used in the making of this Tincture, it will unawares loose its Colour, after it has begun to promise a good one.

Tinctura Aromatica.

Aromatic Tincture.

Take of Cinnamon six Drams, of the lesser Cardamom Seeds husk'd three Drams, long Pepper, and Ginger of each two Drams, of Proof Spirit a Quart. Digest without Heat, and strain the Spirit off. *L.*

This is directed to be made without Heat, because that would dissipate the volatile aromatic Parts, and injure the Medicine. The Virtues of this Tincture, may be understood by those of the Ingredients. It is used in making the *Elixir Vitrioli Acidum.*

Tinctura Balsamica.

Balsamic Tincture.

Take of Balsam of Capivi, one Ounce; *Peruvian* Balsam, three Drams; Balsam of *Tolu,* two Drams; Benjamin, half a Dram; *English* Saffron, one Scruple; and of rectify'd Spirit of Wine, one Pint: Digest them for four Days in *Balneo Mariæ*, and afterwards strain off the Tincture. *E.*

This is intended as a Balsamic as its Title imports, and as such is of very extensive Use in Medicine. But I don't comprehend the Reason why so many different Sorts of Balsams are made use of. For if Balsam of *Capivi* is better than that of *Tolu,* why should that of inferior Virtues be employ'd at all in this Medicine?

It would be coming nearer to the Point, to determine which is of moſt Efficacy, and uſe that, omitting the other.

Tinctura Cantharidum.

Tincture of Cantharides.

Take two Drams of Cantharides, a Pint and a half of rectify'd Spirit of Wine? Digeſt them with a very gentle Heat for two Days; and pour to the ſtrained Tincture one Ounce of Balſam *Capivi*, half an Ounce of the Reſin of *Guaiacum*, and half a Dram of Cochineal. Digeſt them in *Balneo Mariæ* for four or five Days, then ſtrain off the Tincture, to which add two Drams of Camphire, and one Dram of the diſtilled Oil of Juniper. **E.**

This ſeems to be the beſt Tincture of *Cantharides* I have met with, and is render'd more ſafe by the Addition of Camphire. The Tranſlator of the *Edinburgh* Diſpenſatory informs us, that it is a better Preparation than that troubleſome one ſo highly magnified by Dr. *Quincy*, and deſerves the ſame Character, eſpecially for Gleets and ſeminal Weakneſſes, when other Remedies fail. The Character referr'd to of *Quincy's* Tincture, is its being a moſt excellent Medicine, in many Caſes where we have not its *Succedaneum*, nor any thing tending that Way. It is a moſt ſtimulating Cordial, and cannot fail to excite conjugal Intercourſe, where a Conſtitution, by any Misfortune has fallen into a Coldneſs or Indifferency that way; for (if the Expreſſion may be allow'd) where there is Fuel, it will infallibly kindle it. The *Satyrion*, and all of that Tribe, are not to be compared to it. In many Caſes alſo, where ſloughy and cold Humours have clogg'd the Reins and Genital Parts, and thereby occaſion'd other Mis-

chiefs, beſides an Inability to Coition, this Medicine is of mighty Service; and will anſwer where the moſt efficacious Balſams and Turpentines fail. It may be given from ten to one hundred Drops, in a Glaſs of Canary, or any other Liquor which a Patient may like better. But notwithſtanding theſe Commendations of this Medicine, which indeed cannot be greater than it deſerves; yet none but the truly Skilful muſt dare to meddle with it: For by an injudicious Adminiſtration, it may occaſion Stranguries, Eroſions, Excoriations, and even Convulſions.

Tinctura Cantharidum.

Tincture of Cantharides.

Take of Cantharides bruiſed two Drams, of Cochineal half a Dram, of Proof Spirit a Pint and half. After Digeſtion filtre the Spirit thro' Paper. **L.**

The Balſam of *Capivi* in the preceding Tincture of the *Edinburgh* Diſpenſatory, renders it a much better Medicine for that Addition, as appears from what I have ſaid of Balſamics in general, under the Article of Balſamics.

Tinctura Cardamomi.

Tincture of Cardamom Seeds.

Take of the leſſer Cardamom Seeds freed from their Husks half a Pound, of Proof Spirit, a Quart. Digeſt without Heat, and ſtrain off the Spirit. **L.**

The Medicinal Virtues of this may be known from thoſe of the Cardamoms.

Tinctura Castorei.

Tincture of Castor.

Take of *Ruſſia* Caſtor, an Ounce and half; rectify'd Spirit of Wine a Pint; digeſt them together in a gentle Heat for four Days, and after

afterwards ſtrain off the Tincture.
E.

In the *London* Diſpenſatory, they
der two Ounces of the Caſtor, to
Quart of Proof Spirit, and to be
geſted for ten Days, without any
eat at all. And Proof Spirit has
een found a better Menſtruum to
tract the Virtues of the Caſtor.
he Medicinal Virtues may be un-
erſtood by thoſe of Caſtor.

Tinctura Cephalica.
Cephalic Tincture.

ake of Piony Root, two Ounces;
the Roots of *Caſſummuniar*, and
white Dittany, each ſix Drams;
wild Valerian Root and Miſletoe
of the Oak, each one Ounce;
Peacock's Dung, and Roſemary
Flowers, each half an Ounce;
and of *French* white Wine, ſix
Pints : Digeſt them for four Days,
and then ſtrain off the Tincture.
E.

This is intended as a Cephalic, as
s Title imports, and is calculated
or Diſorders of the Head, for which
ıe Ingredients which enter its Com-
oſition are very much recommended.

Tinctura Cephalica purgans.
Purging Cephalic Tincture.

his is made, by adding to the pre-
ceding Tincture, two Ounces of
Senna Leaves; one Ounce of black
Helkbore Root; and a Quart of
French white Wine. E.

This ſhould ſeem to be a very good
urge in Diſorders of the Head.

Tinctura Cinnamomi.
Tincture of Cinnamon.

ake of Cinnamon an Ounce and a
half, of Proof Spirit a Pint. Digeſt them without Heat, and ſtrain
the Spirit off. L.

The Virtues of this may be under-
ood by thoſe of Cinnamon.

Tinctura Corticis Peruviani ſimplex.
The ſimple Tincture of the Peru-
vian Bark.

Take of the Peruvian Bark four
Ounces, of Proof Spirit a Quart.
After Digeſtion ſtrain the Spirit
off. L.

We are told by the Author of the
the *Pharmacopœia Reformata,* that a
Tincture of the *Peruvian* Bark has
long been pretty much in Eſteem,
and uſually kept in the Shops; but
as the College have not ſet down any
Standard Form for making it in
their *Pharmacopœia,* this Tincture
has been variouſly prepared, at the
Diſcretion of the Apothecary or
Chymiſt. Some have employ'd a
highly rectify'd Spirit of Wine as a
Menſtruum, which they have taken
Care fully to ſaturate, by Digeſtion
on a large Quantity of Bark. Others
have thought to aſſiſt the Action of
the Spirit by the Addition of a fixed
alcaline Salt; and many have given
the Preference to a vitriolic Acid,
which has been ſuppoſed to improve
the Medicine, by adding to the
Roughneſs of the Bark, and by giving a greater Conſiſtence to the Spirit, which enabled it to ſuſtain more
than it could by itſelf. Theſe various
Preparations have their various
Uſes, and may to good Purpoſe be
applied by the Skill of the Phyſician. For general Uſe the Form
introduced here is a very convenient. A weak Spirit is well
adapted Menſtruum to extract the
whole Virtues of the Bark, as it e-
qually affects its reſinous and ſaline
Parts, and therefore makes as little
Alteration as poſſible in the Medicine itſelf.

Tinctura Corticis Peruviani volatilis.
Volatile Tincture of the Peruvian
Bark.

Take of the Peruvian Bark four
Ounces, of Spirit of *Sal Armoniac*

moniac a Quart. Digest without Heat in a close Vessel, and then strain the Spirit off. *L.*

The last quoted Author remarks, that the volatile Spirit of *Sal Armoniac* has but lately been applied to the Bark as a Menstruum, on which it without Dispute acts powerfully, but its acrimonious Pungency is so great as to make its Doses very small. It might perhaps therefore conveniently be lower'd by the Addition of an agreeable simple Water, which would effectually remedy this Inconvenience, and render it more palatable, and leave the Menstruum sufficiently strong for the Purpose it is designed.

Tinctura Croci.

Tincture of Saffron.

Take of *English* Saffron one Ounce; and *French* Brandy, a Pint: Digest them together for three Days, then strain off the Tincture. *E.*

This Tincture is also prepared with Canary Wine. The Virtues of this may be known from those of Saffron.

Tinctura Foetida.

The fetid Tincture.

Take of Asa Foetida four Ounces, of rectified Spirit of Wine a Quart. After Digestion strain the Spirit off. *L.*

The Author of the *Pharmacopœia Reformata* is of Opinion, that a highly rectify'd Spirit is not so proper a Menstruum as a low one, for extracting this Tincture. It is not worth disputing, because *Asa fœtida* in Substance promises greater Efficacy than its Tincture. The Compilers of the *London* Dispensatory however, have judged extremely well, in giving this Tincture, and many others, in the simple Manner here directed; for those which are more complex, are less to be depended upon, and more uncertain in their Effects, causing besides great Confusion and Perplexity to the Prescriber.

Tinctura Fuliginis.

Tincture of Soot.

Take of Wood Soot two Ounces, of *Asa fœtida* one Ounce, of Proof Spirit a Quart. After Digestion strain off the Spirit. *L.*

This is directed in the *Edinburgh* Dispensatory exactly in the same Proportion. It is esteem'd a very good Cephalic and nervous Medicine, and has lately been in much Repute for the Cure of Epilepsies and Convulsions.

Tinctura Guaiacina volatilis.

Volatile Tincture of Gum Guaiacum.

Take of Gum Guaiacum four Ounces, of *Spiritus volatilis aromaticus*, or aromatic volatile Spirit, a Pint and a half. Digest without Heat in a well closed Vessel, and then strain the Spirit off. *L.*

It has been for some time the Custom both amongst Empirics and Physicians, to give a strong Tincture of Gum Guaiacum for Rheumatic and Gouty Pains, and I have known it sometimes succeed, but more frequently not. This here directed seems to be the best I have met with; but they all excite too much Heat, a Circumstance attended with many Disadvantages, in Disorders attended with a Siziness of the Juices.

Tinctura Hellebori nigri.

Tincture of black Hellebore.

Take of black Hellebore four Ounces; Cochineal, half a Dram; bruise them, and pour thereon a Quart of *Spanish* white Wine; digest them together, in a very gentle Heat, for four Days; and afterwards strain off the Tincture. *E.*

In former Dispensatories, when the Tincture of Hellebore has been ordered to be extracted with a spirituous Menstruum, Salt of Tartar has been generally added, in order to open

en the Body of the Root; but in
s it is omitted as not neceſſary.
his is a very good Diuretic and
obſtruent; and is much uſed for
moting the menſtrual Diſcharge,
many Caſes where Steel acts too
cibly, and excites great Commons in the Conſtitution. For a
ther Knowledge of its Virtues, ſee
ſe of Hellebore.

The *London Diſpenſatory* directs a
ncture of black Hellebore under
: Title of *Tinctura Melampodii* in
ich the ſame Proportions, but in
s Proof Spirit is ordered inſtead of
niſh Wine as a Menſtruum.

Tinctura Jalappæ.

Tincture of Jalap.

ke three Ounces of Jalap Root,
reduced to a groſs Powder; pour
ppon it a Pint of rectified Spirit of
Wine; let them digeſt for eight
Days, in a gentle Heat; then
ſtrain off the Tincture. E.

a the *London Diſpenſatory*, they or-
: eight Ounces of Jalap, to a Quart
P:oof Spirit.
Boerhaave is of Opinion, that
ſof Spirit extracts the Tincture of
s Root, much better than one
ich is higher, becauſe it diſſolves
th what is ſaline and ſaponaceous,
l what is balſamic, oily, and reſi-
1s. This is a very pretty and con-
ient Medicine, and may very pro-
ly be added to cathartic Infuſions,
coctions, and Solutions in order to
icken their Operation, in the Quan-
· of a Dram or more. *Boerhaave*
s, that if half an Ounce of ſuch a
ncture, be mixed with an equal
antity of the Syrup of Buckthorn,
ſotion will thus be obtained, which
thout occaſioning much Diſorder,
ntifully purges Water; whence
are furniſhed with an excellent
dragogue in thoſe Diſtempers that
uire it.

Tinctura Jalappæ compoſita.

Compound Tincture of Jalap.

Take of Jalap Root, ſix Drams;
black Hellebore Root, three
Drams; Juniper. Berries and the
Shavings of *Guaiacum*, each half
an Ounce; and of *French* Brandy,
one Pint and an half; digeſt them
for three Days, and ſtrain off the
Tincture. E.

This is ordered in the *Edinburgh
Diſpenſatory*, but it ſeems here to be
of but little Uſe, for the Tincture of
Hellebore, and Juniper Water, may
be added extemporaneouſly to the
ſimple Tincture, if they ſhould be
thought neceſſary.

Tinctura Japonica.

Tincture of Japan Earth.

Take of Japan Earth three Ounces,
of Cinnamon two Ounces, of Proof
Spirit a Quart. After Digeſtion
ſtrain the Spirit off. L.

This Tincture as it is more ſimple,
is much preferable to any we have yet
had in the Diſpenſatories, and is
of Uſe in Caſes where the Drug from
whence it takes its Name, is proper,
and is particularly excellent in a
Cough; but I know of no Virtues
it is poſſeſſed of, but what the *Japan* Earth has alone in a greater Degree.

Tinctura Ipecacuanhæ.

Tincture of Ipecacuanha.

Take of Ipecacuanha, in Powder, an
Ounce; Chochineal, a Scruple;
Spaniſh white Wine a Pint; digeſt
for two Days and filtre. E.

Of late Years a Tincture of Ipecacuanha has been very much uſed as
an Emetic, becauſe not attended with
ſome Inconveniencies, which are ſaid
to happen from the powdered Root
in ſome Conſtitutions, wherein it
cauſes an Aſthma. It is therefore
proper to have ſome Standard in the
Shops,

Shops, becaufe when it is wanted on any fudden Occafion there is not Time to make it according to any extemporaneous Prefcription.

Vinum Ipecacuanhæ.

Wine with Ipecacuanha.

Take of the Root of Ipecacuanha, two Ounces; of the yellow Part of *Seville* Orange-peel, dried, half an Ounce; of Canary a Quart. Infufe without Heat, and ftrain. L.

If this is intended as an Emetic, it will not be at all the better for the Orange Peel, but if as an Alterative, for the Cure of a Diarrhæa, or Dyfentery it is more proper. The Author of the *Pharmacopæia Reformata* affirms, that for the Purpofe of an Emetic, the Ipecacuanha is beft prepared by infufing it in warm Water, as may be fairly deduced from its Analyfis, and which has been further confirmed by repeated Trials.

Tinctura Laccæ.

Tincture of Gum-Lac.

Take of Gum Lac, one Ounce; Myrrh half an Ounce; reduce them to Powder; then pour on as much Oil of Tartar *per Deliquium,* as will make the Whole into a foft Pafte; after which, dry it by a gentle Fire, and add thereto a Pint and half of Scurvy Grafs; digeft all in *Balneo Mariæ* for four Days; and then ftrain off the Tincture. E.

Boerhaave directs a more fimple Tincture of Gum Lac to be thus made:

Take of pure Gum Lac, reduce it to fine Powder; and moiften it with Oil of Tartar *per Deliquium,* fo as to make it into a foft Pafte, which being put into a Glafs Veffel, place it in a gentle Heat. Then take out the Glafs, and leave it in the open Air without Fire, where the Oil of

Tartar will again refolve; after which it is to be dried a fecond Time in a gentle Heat; and thus by repeating the Liquefaction, and the drying alternately, the glaffy Tenacity of the Gum will be broke, and refolved into a Liquor of an elegant purple Colour. Then let it again be gently dried, and carefully taken out of the Glafs, as being thus prepared for affording a Tincture with Alcohol. Put the Matter into a tall chymical Glafs, and pour upon it pure Alcohol, enough to float three or four Inches above it; ftop the Glafs with Paper, and fet it in a Furnace, that it may fimmer for two or three Hours, which may be done without Danger of lofing the Alcohol, by Reafon of the long and flender Neck of the Glafs. Let the Liquor cool, and pour off the clear Tincture, by a gentle Inclination of the Veffel, into another Glafs, that is to be kept well ftopped. The Remainder may be treated in the fame Manner with more Alcohol, and the Tincture poured to the former, till the Matter, by boiling, will no longer tinge the Alcohol; after which the Matter may be thrown away as exhaufted. The feveral Tinctures being put together, and purified from their Fæces by ftanding, are to be diftilled by a very gentle Fire, in a Glafs Body, till one half of the Alcohol is come over, whereby being thickened, the Remainder is to be kept for Ufe.

This Tincture is of great Virtue in curing the Diforders of the Gums, Mouth, and Teeth, in the Scurvy, being frequently ufed by rubbing it on the Parts; and taken externally, it has the fame Virtue, and fafely cures that Diforder, if not attended with too much Heat. It is alfo of great Ufe in the Gout, the Rheumatifm,

, and Scurvy, from a sluggiſh
ſe, as alſo in a Leucophlegma-
Dropſy, or the like. It may be
n three Times in a Day in *Spa*-
or *Canary* Wine, after the Sto-
h has been firſt cleanſed and emp-
. It has a grateful Odour and
:rneſs, with an agreeable Aſtrin-
:y, that ſhews its ſtrengthening
:ue, and is therefore greatly com-
ded in the Cure of the *Fluor Al*-

Tinctura Martis.

Tincture of Steel.

te Filings of Iron, without any
reparation, three Ounces; dulci-
ed Spirit of Salt, two Pints; di-
eſt in a gentle Sand Heat, for
hree Days, and filtre the Tinc-
ure. E.

he Compilers of the laſt Edition
the *Edinburgh Diſpenſatory* have
ſtituted this Tincture of Steel in
Room of two others in their for-
r Editions, that of *Ludovicus* and
t of *Mynſicht*. The *London* Di-
ſatory orders a Tincture of Steel
ler the Title of,

inctura Martis in Spiritu Salis.

mcture of Iron in Spirit of Salt.

ke of the Filings of Iron, half a
Pound, of *Glauber*'s Spirit of Sea-
Salt three Pounds, of rectified Spi-
·it of Wine three Pints. Digeſt the
Filings in the Spirit of Salt, with-
>ut Heat, as long as the Spirit
will work on them, then after the
Fæces have ſubſided, evaporate
the Liquor poured off clear, to one
Pound, and to this add the Spirit
of Wine. *L.*

here is another Tincture of Steel
ected in the *London* Diſpenſatory
der the Title of,

Tinctura Florum Martialium.

Tincture of Martial Flowers.

ke of Martial Flowers four Oun-

ces; of Proof Spirit a Pint. After Digeſtion ſtrain the Spirit off.
L.

The late Mr. *White* uſed to take
equal Parts of *Sal Ammoniac*, and
Iron Filings, and calcine them over
a gentle Fire, in a flat unglazed earthen Veſſel, keeping them ſtirring all
the Time, till they concreted together into Lumps; this powdered
gives almoſt immediately a Tincture
to the Spirit poured upon it. This
and the preceding are intended to i-
mitate *Mynſicht*'s Tincture of Steel,
and afford better Medicines, with
much leſs Trouble. This Preparation of Iron with Sal Ammoniac,
will diſſolve in the Air *per Deliquium*,
and this Oil or *Liquamen*, is a very
good Medicine where this Mineral is
proper, perhaps inferior to none.

Tinctura Martis Ludovici.

Ludovicus's Tincture of Steel.

Take one Part of the Vitriol of Iron,
not acid, but perfectly ſaturated;
four Parts of Cream of Tartar,
and twenty Parts of Rain Water;
boil them together in a Glaſs Veſſel, often ſtirring them with a
Stick, till the Maſs becomes grey,
thick, and almoſt conſiſtent; but
with Care to avoid even the leaſt
burning. Put the Maſs into a tall
Bolt Head, pour common Spirit of
Wine thereon, ſo as to float four
Inches above it; boil them together
for an Hour or two, and a red Liquor
will be obtained; when cold decant and filtre it. Treat the Remainder with freſh Spirit as before,
and continue to do this ſo long as
the Spirit acquires any Redneſs,
then put the ſeveral Parcels together, which thus make *Ludovicus*'s
medicated Tincture of Iron.

Phyſicians having obſerved, that the
excellent medicinal Virtues of Iron,
had their Effect ſo long as the Iron
continued diſſolved in a mild Acid,
but

but vanished, and were precipitated into an unctuous Calx, upon meeting with an Alcali; hence prudently joined the Salt of Iron with a vegetable Acid, in Expectation that it might thus pass and act upon all the Vessels of the Body, whilst it more permanently retained a saline Nature; and this was the Reason of joining the Salt of Iron with the vegetable oily Salt of Tartar, to prevent its being easily precipitated in the Body into a *Crocus*, or astringent Calx. This Tincture has the Virtue of opening, attenuating, strengthening, and gently evacuating by the Belly and Kidneys; and hence proves curative in leucophlegmatic, scorbutic, icteric, hypochondriacal, and hysterical Cases, or when the Body is relaxed, weak through the Sluggishness of the Parts, ricketty, or abounding with Worms. It is taken in a Morning fasting, in the Quantity of a Dram, diluted with six times its Weight of Water, repeating it thrice, and each Time drinking after it a Quarter of a Pint of thin Whey, walking gently upon it, so as not to sweat; this may be continued for nine Days, with great Advantage. A few Drops of it may be given to Children troubled with Rickets or Worms, mixed with Syrup or Honey.

Tinctura Menthæ.

Tincture of Mint.

Take of Mint Water, one Pint; of the dry'd Leaves of Mint, one Ounce; macerate them in a close Vessel for four Hours in a warm Place, and strain off the Tincture. E.

This is added in the last Edition of the *Edinburgh* Dispensatory, and may be very useful in Cases where Mint can be of Service, especially as a Stomachic.

Tinctura Myrrhæ.

Tincture of Myrrh.

Take of Myrrh three Ounces, of Proof Spirit a Quart. Digest them together, and then strain the Spirit off.

Helmont imagined, that if Myrrh could find Entrance into the innermost Recesses of the Body, it would have a great Efficacy in the prolonging of Life, so far as this might be expected from an uncorrupted State of the vital Balsam. This Tincture by its detergent, embalming, or balsamic Virtue, excellently heals any foul Ulcers of the Mouth, Nostrils, Gums, or other Parts of the Body, by their being touched or rubbed therewith. If the Bodies of dead Creatures be penetrated with this Liquor, they having been first warmed, and then dried, it preserves them uncorrupted. Given internally, it is an admirable Remedy in all languid Cases, proceeding from a simple Inactivity. It is principally serviceable in those Female Disorders which proceed from an aqueous, mucous, sluggish Indisposition of the Humours, and a Relaxation of the Solids; and therefore has extraordinary Effects in the *Fluor Albus*, and all the Diseases arising from the same Cause. See the Article *Myrrha*, in the *Materia Medica.*

Tinctura Myrrhæ & Aloes.

Tincture of Myrrh and Aloes.

Take of Myrrh reduced to Powder, two Ounces; rectified Spirit of Wine, a Quart; let them stand together in *Balneo Mariæ* for eight Days; then add of the Powder of *Hepatic* Aloes, one Ounce; and digest again for two Days; then strain off the Tincture. E.

The Aloes here is prudently order'd to be added, after the Tincture

Myrrh is extracted, because if both were put in together, the Aloes would only saturate the Menstruum, leaving the Myrrh untouch'd.

Tinctura Opii, seu Laudanum liquidum.

Tincture of Opium, or Liquid Laudanum.

Take of crude Opium, without any previous Preparation, two Ounces; *English* Saffron one Ounce; *Canary* Wine, and *French* Brandy, each ten Ounces : Let a Tincture Be extracted by a gentle Sand Heat, which is to be strain'd. E.

Tinctura Thebaica.
Thebaic Tincture.

Take of Opium strain'd two Ounces, Cinnamon, Cloves, of each a Dram, of white Wine a Pint. Infuse without Heat for a Week, and then strain off the Wine thro' Paper. L.

This differs very little from *Sydenham's* Liquid *Laudanum*, except in the Alteration of the Name. It would have been no great Disadvantage to the Medicine, if the Cinnamon and Cloves were also left out, for these add no one Virtue to the Medicine, and mend the Taste but very little. And to confess the Truth it would be no Misfortune to Practice if all the Tinctures of Opium and Laudanums were omitted; for crude Opium without any previous Preparation, answers all Intentions much better, and the Dose of this is more easily ascertain'd. *Boerhaave* asserts, that Opium dissolved in Water is the best, the next is that dissolved in Wine, and the next in Spirit of Wine; but always the worse, the higher the Spirit.

Tinctura Rhabarbari.
Tincture of Rhubarb.

Take of Rhubarb slic'd and bruis'd

one Ounce; Tartar of Vitriol half a Dram; Cochineal, a Scruple; Cinnamon Water prepared without Spirit, a Pint; digest them together in a warm Place one Night; and then strain off the Tincture. E.

This seems to be a much better Medicine, than the common Tinctures of Rhubarb made with Spirit, but I should prefer common Water, as a Menstruum preferable to the Cinnamon Water, because Cinnamon, if it does any thing, checks the Operation of the Rhubarb. I am sensible, that as Rhubarb is esteem'd a good Medicine to check a Diarrhæa, that the Cinnamon Water may be order'd to assist the Rhubarb in preventing too copious and frequent Stools, but it requires the greatest Judgment to determine when it is necessary and proper to stop Discharges of the Excrements by the Anus, which I should apprehend ought seldom to be done, whilst there remains any thing in the Intestinal Tube, that stimulates to Excretion, and offends them. This Caution I judge the more necessary, because I have frequently known fatal and shameful Mistakes made in this Respect, where the Patient has been nearly destroy'd by checking a critical Looseness, which would otherwise have cur'd the Distemper, and which even has done it, after being brought on again, and promoted.

Tinctura Rhei Amara.
Bitter Tincture of Rhubarb.

Take of Rhubarb, one Ounce; Gentian, one Dram and a half; *Virginia* Snake Root, one Dram; Cochineal, one Scruple, and of *French* Brandy, one Pint : Digest them for two Days, and then strain the Tincture. This may be likewise made with *Spanish* white Wine, E.

I should

I should much prefer the Wine to the Brandy.

Tinctura Rhei dulcis.

Sweet Tincture of Rhubarb.

Take of the best Rhubarb, and sliced Liquorice, each two Ounces; Raisins of the Sun stoned, one Ounce; *Winter's* Bark, the lesser Cardamoms, each two Drams: And of *French* Brandy, one Quart: Digest for two Days, add to the Tincture, when strained, three Ounces of white pulverized Sugar Candy, and digest again till the Sugar Candy is dissolved. E.

Tinctura Rhabarbari Vinosa.

Tincture of Rhubarb in Wine.

Take of Rhubarb two Ounces, of the lesser Cardamom Seeds husk'd half an Ounce, of Saffron two Drams, of white Wine a Quart. Infuse three Days without Heat, and strain. L.

Tinctura Rhabarbari spirituosa.

Tincture of Rhubarb in Spirit.

Take of Rhubarb two Ounces, of the lesser Cardamom Seeds freed from their Husks half an Ounce, of Saffron two Drams, of Proof Spirit a Quart. Digest without Heat, and strain the Spirit off. L.

With Respect to these Tinctures of Rhubarb, I know of no great Use they are of in Practice; for Rhubarb in Substance has better Effects. They may indeed, be more proper in Clysters; and may be more agreeable to those who chuse to take a Draught, rather than a Powder, or Bolus; but then I should prefer an Infusion in Water, or Wine, to one made with Brandy; because it answers the End of a Laxative better, and is not attended with the ill Effects of a Dram.

Tinctura Rosarum.

Tincture of Roses.

Take red Rose Buds, the white Heels being cut off, half an Ounce, of the strong Spirit of Vitriol, called the Oil, one Scruple, of boiling Water, two Pints and a half, of double refined Sugar one Ounce and half. First add the Spirit of Vitriol to the Water in a Vessel of Glass, or Earth glased, and then infuse the Roses, strain the Liquor when cold, and add the Sugar. L.

This is intended for an Astringent and Cooler, and is a very proper Medicine in Hæmorrhages, and excessive febrile Heats, and is very good in many Cases as a Gargarism.

Tinctura Sacra.

Tincture of Hiera Picra.

Take of Succotrine Aloes, in Powder, an Ounce, of the lesser Cardamoms, and *Virginian* Snake-Root, each one Dram; Cochineal, a Scruple; *Spanish* white Wine, a Pint and a half: Digest for two Days in a gentle Heat; and strain. E.

That in the preceding *London* Dispensatory is by many prefer'd to this. It is made by digesting an Ounce of the *Species Hiera Picra* (which see) in a Pint of white Wine. It is intended as a stomachic Purge, but it has much better Effects if given in extremely small Doses, and those frequently repeated by way of Alterative, one Spoonful for Example at Night going to Bed. Taken in this Manner, it is very effectual in mending the Appetite, and is of good Service in a *Chlorosis*, Cachexy, and Suppressions of the Menses.

In the last *London* Dispensatory it is thus directed.

Take of Succotrine Aloes eight Ounces, of *Winter's* Bark so called two Ounces, of white Wine two Quarts. Pulverize the Aloes and

rk separately, then mix them
d pour on the Wine, infuse for
Week or longer without Heat,
e Glass being often shook, and
lly strain the Wine off.

s convenient to mix some clean
Sand with the Powders, that
Aloes may not concrete into a
p. L.

e Compilers of the last College
ensatory gave us the following
arks upon this Medicine.

ra Picra is a very ancient Com-
ion; but as it was originally an
tuary, and now with us is more
in Tincture, its Ingredients de-
a particular Review, that so
ent a Medicine may be render'd
tle disagreeable in Taste and Fla-
as possible, a Circumstance much
worthy of Regard in its present,
in its antient Form. The origi-
species, besides the Aloes, were
amon, Spikenard, Xylobalsa-
, and often *Schœnanthus* also.
hese the *Xylobalsamum* is little
vn to us; nothing has been
ght into *Europe* under that Name,
dry Sticks without any Taste or
ll. Our *Pharmacopœia* has sup-
d this Defect, by substituting
e in its Room. But at the last
isal the Medicine was much more
'd on Account of the exception-
Flavour of some of the Ingre-
ts; and it has been now thought
er to take this Composition will
er into Examination. The prin-
l Part of the Medicine is the
es, and the Improvement under
sideration consists in chusing the
r Ingredients of such Aromatics,
may at least correct the ill Smell,
ot alleviate the intense Bitterness
this principal Ingredient. All
Ingredients which have made a
of the Composition, either in
present, or former *Pharmaco-*
a, have been found upon parti-

cular Examination to be insignificant,
or to increase the Offensiveness of the
Medicine, both in Flavour and Taste,
except Cinnamon and Cardamom
Seeds; and of these the Cinnamon is
not free from Objection in regard to
the Taste. After Trial made upon
many other Materials both simple
and compounded together, the simple Form of the Medicine here exhibited has appeared to exceed all
others.

I should not apprehend it possible, by
any Means whatever, to render this
Medicine agreeable in any Degree
to the Taste; and therefore the Improvements in this Medicine should
be consider'd with Respect to the Medicinal Virtues only; and Experience
alone must determine whether it is
better or worse than the *Tinctura sa-*
cra of former Dispensatories. But I
shou'd suspect that it is not better.

Tinctura Salutifera.
Healthful Tincture.

Take the Roots of Angelica, *Calamus*
Aromaticus, Galangal, Gentian,
and Zedoary, Bay Berries, the
lesser Cardamoms, Cinnamon, and
long Pepper, of each a Dram:
To these Ingredients, ready slic'd
and bruis'd, add a Quart of *French*
Brandy; let them digest for three
Days, and afterwards strain off the
Tincture. E.

This seems intended for nothing
more than a Cordial Dram, and is
better Furniture for a Distiller's than
an Apothecary's Shop.

Tinctura Serpentariæ.
Tincture of Snake Root.

Take of *Virginia* Snake Root three
Ounces, of Proof Spirit a Quart.
Digest without Heat, and strain off
the Spirit. L.

The Virtues of this may be understood from those of the Root. It is
here directed to be made with Proof

Y y

Spirit,

Spirit, as a better Menstruum for the Extraction of the Virtues of the Root, than one that is higher.

Tinctura Serpentariæ composita.

Compound Tincture of Snake Root.

Take of *Virginia* Snake Root, two Ounces ; Venice Treacle, an Ounce ; Cochineal a Dram ; and *Spanish* white Wine, a Quart ; let them stand to digest in a gentle Heat for four Days, then strain off the Tincture. E.

This is a high Cordial and Sudorific, but a very dangerous Medicine, if used without the greatest Judgment ; for if it does not immediately do Service, it is sure to do a great deal of Prejudice, and to increase the Fever irremediably, which it was intended to relieve.

Tinctura ad Stomachicos.

Stomachic Tincture.

Take the Roots of *Calamus Aromaticus*, Galangal, Gentian, and Zedoary, Orange Peel, and *Peruvian* Bark, of each two Ounces ; the Tops of common Wormwood, and the lesser Centaury, Chamomile Flowers, and the Seeds of *Carduus Benedictus*, of each an Ounce ; crude Filings of Iron, tied up in a Piece of Linen, six Ounces ; when these Ingredients have, as they require, been sliced and bruised, pour upon them two Gallons of *French* white Wine, and digest for four Days, then strain off the Tincture. This Tincture may also be made without Iron.

This Preparation nearly resembles that given by Dr. *Cheyne*, which he recommends as proper to brace up the Solids, after a due Course of Evacuants and Attenuants. It is a very good Stomachic, and Strengthener, and may very properly be used, after a Course of the Bark, in order to prevent the Return of an Inter-

mittent, in the Quantity of a few Spoonfuls for a Dose. I think Dr. *Cheyne* orders it to be taken an Hour before, and two Hours after Dinner.

Tinctura Stomachica.

Stomachic Tincture.

Take of stoned Raisins four Ounces, of Cinnamon half an Ounce, Caraway Seeds, the lesser Cardamoms freed from their Husks, Cochineal, of each two Drams, of Proof Spirit a Quart. Digest without Heat, and strain off the Spirit. L.

This is intended as a spicy Cordial, but should seem to be of very little Use in Practice.

Tinctura Styptica.

The Styptic Tincture.

Take of calcined green Vitriol one Dram, of *French* Brandy tinctured by the Cask a Quart. Mix them that the Spirit may turn black, and then strain it off. L.

The Compilers of the last *London* Dispensatory have substituted this, in the Room of the celebrated Styptic of *Helvetius*, and it is said to be a good Remedy for Hæmorrhages. *Helvetius*'s Styptic, as publish'd by himself, is thus made:

Take four Pounds of the Filings of Steel, and eight Pounds of Tartar, well powder'd, mix these well together, and put them in a new earthen Pot, and pour thereon as much *French* Brandy as will make it into a Poultice. Let this stand fermenting in a Cellar for four Days, and stir it between whiles. Then put it into a *Balneum Mariæ*, and distil it according to Art, with a moderate Fire, to draw off the Brandy. When you find that nothing but the Phlegm comes off, take it from the Fire, and take out the Mass, stamp it very fine, that not the least Lump may remain ; then mix it again, as before, with a fufficient Quantity of Brandy, and put it into the Cellar to ferment, as before, and then diftil it a fecond time. This Operation may be reiterated feven or eight times, but the laft Time mix your Mafs well upon a Marble, and form it into two Ounce Balls. One of thefe Balls is fteep'd in a Pint of good *French* Brandy, a little warmed, and hung only in it by a Wire, till the Brandy has received the Colour of the Ball. But if you are in great Hafte, then grate a fufficient Quantity of the Ball in fome Brandy, ftir it well, and you may ufe it that very Inftant.

This is faid to be the fame as the celebrated Styptic of Dr. *Eaton.*

Tinctura Salis Tartari.

Tincture of Salt of Tartar.

Take of the Salt of Tartar, one Pound; put it into a Crucible; place it in a melting Furnace; and let it ignite gradually, till it is of a white melting Heat; cover it well with Coals, and keep it in the moft extreme Degree of Fire for five or fix Hours: Then pour it into a warm Mortar, and, whilft warm, powder it, and put it into a Matrafs, heated upon warm Sand to prevent its Breaking with the hot Salt; then pour upon it of tartariz'd Spirit of Wine, two Pints, invert and lute well to it another Matrafs, to make it a double Veffel; make a gentle Fire, and let it fimmer fix or feven Hours, and in that Time it will acquire a good Tincture; which when cold, put into a Vial, and keep it well ftopt.

This operates both by Sweat and Urine, and is an excellent Aperitive, and good in all fcorbutic Habits, and in Cachexies, Jaundice, and Dropfes. Its Dofe is from ten to fifty or fixty Drops.

Tinctura Salis Tartari Harveiana.

Harvey's Tincture of Salt of Tartar.

Take the black alcaline Salt, remaining in the Retort, after the ftrongeft Diftillation of Tartar; reduce it to Powder, in a hot Iron Mortar, with a hot Peftle, and immediately put it into a tall Bolthead; pour the beft common Spirit thereon, fo as to rife four Inches above it; boil with a gentle Fire, for twenty Hours; and thus a black, thin, bitter, aromatic, lixivious Liquor will be obtained, which, being decanted pure, may long be preferv'd perfect in a clofe Glafs for Ufe.

The common Spirit, confifting of Water, Acid, and Alcohol united, coming to boil with the Alcali of Tartar, that ftill remains oily, makes a mild and fafe Lixivium; the Alcali being here temper'd by the Acid, Oil and Alcohol: Whence we have a noble Kind of Medicine and Menftruum, wherein if Vegetables be boiled or digefted, it diffolves them to good Advantage. In Surgery, it is an excellent Remedy for cleanfing, deterging, drying, and healing all weeping, purulent, putrid, fanious, and virulent Ulcers, as well the fiftulous as the finuous and burrowing; and alfo for taking down proud Flefh, efpecially if artificially mixed with a little Oil. It has fimilar Effects when ufed internally, in Diftempers where acid, auftere, aqueous, mucous, or terreftrial Matters, and Coagulations abound, provided they be not attended with a putrid Diffolution of the Humours; and hence it is commended in old Obftructions of the *Vifcera,* Collections of Water, dropfical Difpofitions, the Green Sicknefs, Jaundice, and cold Gout. It acts ftrongly as a Diuretic, a Diaphoretic, and fometimes as a Purgative; and may be fafely given in a large Dofe. Two or three Drams thereof being mollified with an Ounce of the Syrup of the five opening Roots, and diluted with Fennel Water, will have a very good Effect, being taken in the Morning fasting, and repeated three or four times at due Intervals, or a better than most other Remedies. Hence the famous Dr. *Harvey* deservedly recommends it.

Tinctura Succini.

Tincture of Amber.

Take two Ounces of the Powder of yellow Amber, and as much Oil of Tartar *per Deliquium*, as will make it into a Paste; on which, when gently dry'd, pour twenty Ounces of rectify'd Spirits of Wine: Digest in a gentle Heat for eight Days, and afterwards filtre the Tincture. E.

Tinctura Succini Hoffmanni.

Hoffman's Tincture of Amber.

Mix very exactly Salt of Tartar, with an equal Portion of choice Amber, reduc'd to a very fine Powder, and pour thereon a sufficient Quantity of Spirit, to the Height of about four Inches above it. After a previous Digestion, let a Distillation be made out of a Glass Cucurbit, with a Sand Heat; and there will be drawn off a Spirit impregnated with the most subtile and fragrant Oil of Amber, which, though it be in itself endued with an extraordinary strengthening Virtue, will yet serve to much better Purposes, by contributing towards furnishing us with an excellent Tincture. The transparent Amber is to be chosen before that which is brown, or dark colour'd, as consisting of a softer sulphureous Matter. Let this be bruised and levigated in a Mortar to a very fine Powder; into which, being placed on a Marble Stone, drop Oil of Tartar *per*

Deliquium, and mix them very carefully till they come to a Paste, which must be dry'd gently. This done, pour thereon a sufficient Quantity of the Spirit prepared as above, and then digest them in a Glass Vessel, or Vial close stopp'd with a gentle Heat.

By this means we obtain the most generous and efficacious Essence of Amber; a Remedy highly to be valu'd, were it only on Account of its most grateful Taste and Smell.

The most convenient Way of taking it is by instilling some Drops of it into Sugar, or Syrup of Pinks, or of the acid Juice of Citrons. The Morning is the usual Time when Persons take it, for corroborating the Stomach, Head, and a weak, nervous System, drinking afterwards some Cups of warm Liquor, as Coffee or Chocolate; it may also be taken at Dinner in sweet Wine. It provokes the Menses, but restrains the *Fluor Albus,* and is an excellent Medicine in Rheumatic Disorders.

It is remarkable, that this Essence, dropp'd into Water, is not precipitated like other Essences or Solutions of Oils and Resins; and that a few Drops of it, instill'd into a large Quantity of Water, impregnate the whole with the grateful Odour of Amber, which so amply diffuses itself through the least Corpuscles of Water, is of very fine Parts, and by Consequence can make its way into the very innermost Fluids and Solids of our Bodies; so that a small Dose may be expected to produce a considerable Effect.

Tincture of Amber has an incredible Efficacy in all those Distempers, which proceed from too great a Mobility of the immediate Instruments of the human Affections, Spirits, and nervous System, and particularly from a Relaxation of the Parts thro' Weakness. And hence proves of wonderful Service in ypochondriacal, hysterical, languid, old, watery Cases, and Concretions often proceeding from them. So hat Mr. *Boyle* and *Helmont* have or this Reason placed it among the nobleft Anti-spasmodics, and Anti-pileptics, when the Disorder proceeds from those Causes. The Dose s from ten to eighty Drops, three imes a Day, in *Spanish* or *Canary* Wine.

Tinctura Sudorifica.

The Sudorific Tincture.

Take of *Virginian* Snake Root, five Drams; Cochineal, half an Ounce; *Ruffian* Castor, one Dram; *English* Saffron, two Scruples; Opium one Scruple; *Mindererus*'s Spirit, a Pint. Digest for three Days in a Sand Heat, and strain. E.

This, as its Name imports, is a powerful Sudorific, but a very dangerous Medicine in Fevers. *Sydenham*'s Method of treating Fevers is used like Probity, *laudatur & alget*, prais'd, but seldom practis'd; whilst that of *Morton*, which consists in the Exhibition of fiery Sudorifics, is prefer'd to it, tho' the Theory on which it was founded has been long exploded. I have frequently known a Cold, or very slight Fever, exalted into one very dangerous and fatal by the Use of such Medicines. But I don't recollect a single Instance of a Fever cured by hot Sudorifics, which I had not Reason to believe would have terminated spontaneously without them. And I am very certain, that the Custom so prevalent among the Unwary, of exhibiting Sudorifics, or Sweats, as they are call'd, in the Beginning of Fevers, causes more Gain to the Practisers of Physic, than half the Distempers which would otherwise afflict Mankind. The Use of this Medicine, therefore, and others of the like Intention, requires the utmost Judg-

ment and Caution, and, even with these, are seldom of any great Service to the Patient, whatever they may be to the Prescriber, or Dispenser.

Tinctura Tolutana.

Tincture of Balsam of *Tolu.*

Take of the Balsam of *Tolu* an Ounce and half, rectify'd Spirit, a Pint. Digest in a Sand Heat till the Balsam is dissolv'd, and strain.

The Virtues of this may be learn'd from those of Balsam of *Tolu*, and what has been said of Balsamics. Book IV. Chap. vi.

Tinctura Valerianæ simplex.

The simple Tincture of Valerian.

Take of wild Valerian Root four Ounces, of Proof Spirit a Quart. After Digestion strain off the Spirit. L.

The Valerian here is to be finely powder'd, upon which depends the Strength of the Tincture, which is said to be a neat and elegant Medicine, and no doubt of considerable Efficacy. But as no Inconvenience attends the taking the Root, I don't see what curative End can be answer'd by this Tincture; for the Spirit by no Means adds any Virtue to the Valerian.

Tinctura Valerianæ volatilis.

Volatile Tincture of Valerian.

Take of the Root of wild Valerian four Ounces, of the volatile aromatic Spirit a Quart. Digest them together in a close Vessel without Heat, and then strain the Tincture off. L.

This should seem to be a very good Medicine in those Cases which are usually call'd nervous, and particularly in relax'd Constitutions, that abound with an Acid.

Tinctura

Tinctura Veratri.

Tincture of white Hellebore.

Take of the Root of white Hellebore eight Ounces, of Proof Spirit a Quart. After Digestion filtre thro' Paper. L.

I think this is the first Time we
have had a Tincture of white Hellebore in our Dispensatory. It is an
excellent Medicine to quicken Purges,
when we intend they should operate
briskly, and with Efficacy, as in
Maniacal Cases, or Apoplexies,
when a strong Stimulus is requir'd.
In the last Case *Celsus* recommends
the Use of white Hellebore.

Elixir Paregoricum.

The Paregoric Elixir.

Take Flowers of Benjamin, Opium
strained, of each a Dram, of
Camphire, two Scruples, of the
essential Oil of Anniseeds half a
Dram, of rectified Spirit of Wine
a Quart. After Digestion strain
off the Spirit. L.

This is much the same as the *Elixir
Asthmaticum*, in the *London* Dispensatory. And here the Name is alter'd for some Purpose; for the Epithet *Asthmaticum* would be subject to
make the Unattentive consider the
Medicine as only proper in Asthmatic Cases; whereas 'tis on all Occasions an excellent Paregoric. *Quincy*
says there is not any Composition of
our Shops to be compared to it in the
Intention it is ordered. It admirably
allays the Tickling which provokes
frequent Coughing, and yet opens
the Breast, and gives more Liberty of
Breathing; forasmuch as the Opium
takes off the uneasy Sensation occasion'd by acrimonious Humours, and
so tends to thicken them, by occasioning them to be less agitated in
Coughing: The Benjamin and all
the other Ingredients serve to deterge
and cleanse the small Glands, and

make Way for their Discharges. In
this Composition also it is so manag'd,
that the Opium is rather an Opener,
by relaxing the Fibres, and thereby
enlarging the Capacities of the Vessel; in which consists the Cure of an
Asthma; because thereby the Blood
flows easier through the Lungs, and
they have more Room to respire in:
Whereas in those Compositions where
Opium is not join'd with warm Detergents, but rather with Things
which agglutinate, as in the Storax
Pill, such Humours are suffer'd to
lodge till they thicken and fill the
Vessels with Grumes and Viscidities,
and so increase all the Symptoms, as
sometimes to stop all Motion, and
end in Death. The Truce therefore
which Opium gives in this Medicine,
is only to procure the better Opportunity to the other Ingredients to rarify and thin the viscid Cohesions in
the Vessels, and fit them for Circulation and Secretion: So that as
stopping a Cough, in some Cases and
by some Means, is of fatal Consequence, by this Management it is a
good Step towards a Cure of what
causes one. Its Dose is from twenty
to one hundred Drops to grown Persons, in Hyssop Water or Canary, at
Night going to Bed; and from five
to twenty Drops to Children: For
whom, in what is called the Chin
Cough, it is peculiarly excellent.

Elixir Proprietatis, with distill'd Vinegar.

Take choice Aloes, Saffron and
Myrrh, of each half an Ounce; cut
and bruise them, put them into a tall
Bolt Head, pour twenty times their
own Weight of the strongest distill'd Vinegar thereon, let them
simmer together for twelve Hours:
Then suffer the whole to rest, that
the Fæces may subside, and gently
strain off the pure Liquor thro' a
thin Linen. Put half the Quantity of distilled Vinegar to the Remainder,

mainder, boil, and proceed as before, and throw away the Fæces. Mix the two Tinctures together, and distil with a gentle Fire, till the whole is thicken'd to a third; keep the Vinegar that comes over for the same Use; and what remains behind is the *Elixir Proprietatis* with distill'd Vinegar.

Thus we obtain an acid, aromatic Medicine of great Use in the Practice of Physic: for when externally apply'd, it cleanses and heals putrid, sinuous, and fistulous old Ulcers, defends the Parts from Putrefaction, and preserves them by a true embalming Virtue: It also heals Ulcers, and cures Gangrenes in the Lips, Tongue, Palate, and Jaws. It has the same Effects in the first Passages, when used internally, as often as putrefy'd Matter, corrupted Bile, concreted Phlegm, Worms, and numberless Distempers proceeding from these four Causes, are lodg'd or seated therein. Again, it has nearly the same Effects in the Blood and Viscera, as may easily appear from knowing the Virtues of the three Ingredients, when dissolv'd in a subtile Vinegar. It is to be taken in a Morning upon an empty Stomach, at least twelve Hours after eating: It is given from a Dram to two or three for a Dose, in sweet Wine, Mead, or the like; walking after it, or having the Belly gently rubb'd. If taken in a larger Dose, and with a somewhat cooler Regimen, it always purges: if in a less Dose, and often repeated, it cleanses the Blood by secreting thick Urine, and generally performs both these Operations successfully. But, if taken plentifully, while the Patient is in Bed, and the Body well cover'd, it acts as an excellent Sudorific; and afterwards usually purges, and proves diuretic, and thus becomes every

way useful: Whence it is the best acid *Elixir Proprietatis*, good in numerous Cases, and at the same time safe. *Paracelsus* declared, that an Elixir made of Aloes, Saffron, and Myrrh, would prove a vivifying and preserving Balsam, able to continue Health and long Life to the utmost possible Limits; and hence he calls it by a lofty Title the *Elixir of Propriety* to Man; but concealed the Preparation, in which *Helmont* asserts the *Alcahest* is requir'd. *Crollius* formerly used the Oil of Sulphur made by the Bell, as a Menstruum in this Case, upon considering, according to the Doctrine of *Paracelsus*, that an hungry Acid was proper in Stomachic Remedies; but when this is used, the Aloes and Myrrh are scorched, and acquire a stony Hardness, so as not afterwards readily to dissolve in Alcohol: For this Use they require that the strong Acid of the Sulphur should be diluted. Hence, says *Boerhaave*, I conjectur'd, that a mild, oily, vegetable Acid would prove a commodious and proper Solvent in this Case for Medicinal Uses; and, upon adding an equal Quantity of Alcohol to the Elixir prepared in this Manner, it becomes more balsamic, mild, and effectual. It in every Respect resembles the *Pilulæ Rufi*, and may be successfully used in their Stead. This is the Character given by *Boerhaave* of his *Elixir Proprietatis* with Vinegar; but many other Methods have been taken of making this celebrated and excellent Medicine, tho' the Ingredients in all are Myrrh, Aloes, and Saffron: so that the Difference results principally from the Menstruum. Some direct it to be made with *Alcohol*, others with Wine, and again others with the Addition of an Acid. *Boerhaave* also directs an *Elixir Proprietatis* to be made by digesting the Myrrh, Aloes, and Saffron in three times

the

their Weight of the Liquor of tartariz'd Tartar, in a close Vessel, for three Days, in order to dissolve the Ingredients, then adding twenty times their Weight of *Alcohol*, and suffering them to boil gently for twelve Hours; then decanting off the clear Liquor, more Alcohol is to be added, and this is to be repeated till almost the whole Ingredients are taken up. Then all the Liquors are to be mixed, and inspissated to the Thickness of Oil. This Elixir, he informs us, being prepared with an extremely opening Salt, is possess'd of many excellent Virtues, so that it is admirable in old inveterate Obstructions, which it powerfully resolves, without offending by any acid or alcaline Property: For these compound Salts, along with what they dissolve, generally pass quick through the Vessels of the Body.

The same Author farther directs an *Elixir Proprietatis* to be prepar'd in much the same Manner, only using the Liquor of Regenerated Tartar, instead of the Liquor of Tartariz'd Tartar. And by this Means he tells us, the Ingredients are almost wholly dissolv'd, so as to become uniform and potable; whence he asserts, that he has found this Elixir to have an incomparable opening, and dissolving Virtue in most Chronical Diseases, where it mightily liquefies the Concretions in the Vessels, agreeably stimulates the nervous System, so as to throw off the Matters thus dissolved, and prevents Putrefaction; which in these Cases is so frequent and destructive. Hence it relieves the Viscera, restores their Actions impaired by an obstructing Matter, resolves the Humours, and thus cures numerous Distempers, scarce otherwise curable. All these Elixirs differ in Virtues, according to the Difference of the Menstruum used, and ought to be ready prepar'd with different Menstruums for different Purposes. They all of them preserve the Bodies of Animals from Putrefaction, if suspended therein, except that prepared with Water. They are all of them excellent in case of carious Bones, except those prepared with Acids; and hence they should always be ready at hand for Practice, as being almost general Medicines: And no Wonder, since Saffron is a true Exciter of the Animal Spirits; Aloes an excellent and innocent Purgative; and Myrrh the highest Preservative: But in those Distempers where the Blood is too much broke, in large Bleedings, or the Hæmorrhoids, or where the Humours are in too violent a Motion, they are by no means proper, but hurtful.

The *Edinburgh* Dispensatory directs this Medicine thus,.

Elixir Proprietatis.
Elixir of Propriety.

Take one Ounce of pulveriz'd Myrrh, and as much Oil of Tartar *per Deliquium*, as will make it into a soft Paste; with a gentle Heat evaporate the Moisture, and add of rectify'd Spirit two Pints, digest in a Sand Heat for four Days, then add of Succotrine Aloes in Powder, an Ounce and half; *English* Saffron, an Ounce; digest again for two Days, and pour off the Elixir, after it is depurated by subsiding.

In the same Dispensatory it is directed to be prepar'd with an Acid thus,

Elixir Proprietatis cum Acido.
Elixir of Propriety with an Acid.

Take of Myrrh in Powder an Ounce and half; Succotrine Aloes in Powder, an Ounce; *English* Saffron, half an Ounce; rectify'd Spirit, twenty four Ounces, that is, a Pint and half; dulcify'd Spirit of Vitriol, six Ounces. Digest in a Sand

Sand Heat for four Days, and pour off the Elixir, after it is depurated by subsiding.

n the *London* Dispensatory, the oziginal Name of this Medicine is ang'd; to which I have the same bjection as I have to other Alterains of this Kind, which is, that it uses Confusion without rendering e Medicine the better, and with it any one Advantage resulting ther to the Prescriber, Compound-, or Patient. The simple *Elixir oprietatis* is order'd under the Tiof

Elixir Aloes.

Elixir of Aloes.

ake of the Tincture of Myrrh a Quart, Saffron, Succotrine Aloes, of each three Ounces in Weight, after Digestion strain off the Spirit. L.

n Imitation of *Helmont's Elixir oprietatis,* we have the

Vinum Aloeticum Alkalinum.

Aloetic Alkaline Wine.

ake of fixt Alkaline Salt eight Qunces, Succotrine Aloes, Saffron, Myrrh, of each one Ounce, of purify'd Sal Ammoniac six Drams, of white Wine a Quart. Infuse them together without Heat for a Week or longer, then filtre the Wine thro' Paper. L.

Elixir Myrrhæ compositum.

The compound Elixir of Myrrh:

ake of the Extract of Savine one Ounce, of the Tincture of Castor a Pint, of the Tincture of Myrrh half a Pint. After Digestion strain off the Tincture. L.

his seems to be an excellent Mezine to promote the Uterine Diarges, and should seem to be very cing, for which Reason it should yer be given when there is any Suspicion of Pregnancy. It may also promote the Expulsion of the Foetus and Secundines, but with this View it must be exhibited with Caution, for Fear it should bring on a Flooding. It is farther said to be a good Antihysteric, and to cure Fits in Children. But for this last Purpose there are much better Medicines.

Elixir Pectorale.

Pectoral Elixir.

Take Balsam of *Tolu* two Ounces, Gum Benjamin an Ounce and half, *English* Saffron, half an Ounce, rectify'd Spirit of Wine a Quart, digest them in a Sand Heat for eight Days, and then filtre the Tincture.

The Title of this Medicine expresses its Virtues; it should seem to be an admirable Balsamic and Pectoral.

Elixir Polychrestum.

Elixir of many Virtues.

Take of Gum Guaiacum six Ounces, *Peruvian* Balsam, half an Ounce; rectify'd Spirit of Wine, a Quart; digest them in *Balneo Mariæ* for four Days, and strain. E.

The *London* Dispensatory directs this, under the Title of *Balsamum Guaiacinum,* Balsam of Guaiacum, to be made by digesting in two Pints and a half of rectify'd Spirit, a Pound of Gum Guaiacum, and three Ounces of Balsam of *Peru.*

Both this, and that directed by the *Edinburgh* Dispensatory above, differ very little from the celebrated *Balsamum Polychrestum* which *Quincy* introduces with this remarkable Character: It is, says he, an efficacious Medicine for many good Purposes, but particularly to warm and defend the Nerves from those Defluxions which prejudice their Motions, and, when they prove of a saline tartarous

rous Kind, make the Gout in the Joints; to preserve against this last Distemper, there is not a better Medicine, considering the Conveniences of making and taking it. It will likewise answer all the Ends that are aim'd at by the Wood Diet-drink; it dries up or dissipates by insensible Transpiration all superfluous Moistures, is good in all Venereal and Scrophulous Cases, and very certainly wears off an old Gleet, where the Virulence has been previously removed. It will change an aqueous Vehicle milky, but may conveniently enough be given in any Liquor; and it is usually taken from twenty to thirty Drops, two or three times in a Day. Thus *Quincy*. But I have been so unfortunate as to be greatly disappointed in my Expectations from this Medicine, having very seldom known it succeed in the Manner he promises. But it will answer very good Purposes when mix'd and taken with *Elixir Proprietatis*, in small Doses, as an Alterative.

Elixir Salutis.

Elixir of Health.

Take of Senna Leaves, cleared of their Stalks, four Ounces; of Guaiacum Shavings, of dry'd Elecampane Root, of the Seeds of Anise, Caraway, Coriander, and of Liquorice Root, of each two Ounces; of Raisins stoned, eight Ounces; of *French* Brandy three Quarts; steep them together cold for four Days, and then strain out the Tincture for Use.

Some add Rhubarb, Scammony, Jalap, or other purgative Ingredients, in order to make it operate more briskly; for, as here directed, the purgative Ingredient, which is the Senna only, bears so small a Proportion to the Quantity of Spirit in a Dose sufficient for a Purge, that it is too strong for most Persons who have not been accustomed to spirituous Liquors; it is therefore to be deem'd rather a Carminative than a Cathartic, and in some Colic Pains it gives great Relief. Something very like this is the celebrated *Daffy's Elixir*, by which an immense Sum of Money has been got by the Dealers in it. What has contributed to the Success of this Medicine is, the Propensity of great Numbers to Drams, which immediately afford some Relief in Lowness and Flatulences, whatever bad Effects they may afterwards have; and it must be confess'd, that the Cathartic Ingredients render it less prejudicial, than it would be without them. It may be consider'd as a purgative Usquebaugh. It is a proper Purge for Drunkards, and is a great Favourite of old Women habituated to Drams. But can answer no good End but what may be much better provided for by Means less pernicious. It is directed in the *London* Dispensatory thus, under the Name of

Tinctura Senæ.

Tincture of Sena.

Take of stoned Raisins sixteen Ounces, of the Leaves of Sena one Pound, of Caraway Seeds an Ounce and a half, of Cardamom Seeds husk'd half an Ounce, of Proof Spirit a Gallon. Digest without Heat, and strain off the Spirit. L.

This is much stronger of the Sena than that of the last Dispensatory, and consequently a better Purge.

The *Edinburgh* Dispensatory directs it thus, under the Title of

Elixir Salutis.

Elixir of Health.

Take of the Leaves of Sena, two Ounces; choice Rhubarb, Seeds of Fennel, Juniper Berries, Raspigs of Guaiacum, each an Ounce; *rench* Brandy three Pints: Di-eſt for four Days, and to the rain'd Liquor add, white Sugar-andy in Powder four Ounces. E.

Elixir Stomachium.

Stomachic Elixir.

:e of Gentian Root, and the eſh yellow Rind of Oranges, :ch two Ounces; Cochineal half Dram; ſlice and bruiſe the In-redients, pour thereon a Quart f *French* Brandy, let them di-eſt for three Days, then ſtrain ff the Elixir. E.

iis ſeems intended to imitate *ghton's* Elixir, and may be very per for the Bar of a Tavern, where fit only is confider'd. But, in the tary Art of Phyſic, Diſtempers be cur'd without laying in the ent's Way Temptations to do ſelf a Miſchief, or leading him a Habit, that will infallibly de-y him, if perfiſted in, that is, of tting in a Morning. Aqueous ers anſwer much better Pur-:s, than thoſe which are ſpiri-us.

Elixir Vitrioli.

Elixir of Vitriol.

ke of dulcify'd Spirit of Vitriol, wo Pounds; inſtil gradually into :, of the Chymical Oil of Mint, ialf an Ounce; that of Lemons nd Nutmegs, each two Drams; nix. E.

Elixir Vitrioli Mynſichti.

Mynſicht's Elixir of Vitriol.

ke of Cinnamon, Ginger, and Cloves, of each three Drams; Calamus Aromaticus, one Ounce; Galangal an Ounce and an half; Sage and Mint dried, of each ialf an Ounce; Cubebs and Nut-negs, of each two Drams; Wood of Aloes, Citron Peels, of each a

Dram: Powder them together, and add to them white Sugar-Candy, three Ounces; Spirit of Wine, a Pound and half; and Oil of Vitriol a Pound: Digeſt them together for twenty Days; and then pour off the Liquor, and filtre it for Uſe.

Quincy ſays, the Spirit had better be digeſted upon the Ingredients ſome time by itſelf; becauſe the Oil of Vitriol gives a Thickneſs to it, and diſables it from taking out the Vir-tues of the Spices; and when it is put in, it muſt be done very gradu-ally, becauſe it will elſe cauſe ſo ſudden a Heat, as to endanger burſt-ing the Veſſel. Many have got a Way of putting in *Jamaica* Pepper for all the Spices; but it is not ſo juſt to vary from the *Recipe*, when there is no Reaſon for it but Cheap-neſs, and the Medicine thereby be-comes the worſe; which it certainly does in this Inſtance, becauſe that is a more oily Spice than thoſe here order'd, and therefore cannot make ſo good a Stomachic. The ſame Author alſo informs us, that this is deſervedly a very good Medicine, for it mightily ſtrengthens the Sto-mach, and will do good Service ſometimes, where Bitters avail no-thing, eſpecially in Relaxations from Debauches and Over-feeding. This very well imitates the Virtues of the celebrated Bark, and is properly given in all Intentions where that is found to ſucceed; ſo that by its Help Intermittents, and many Diſ-orders from too lax a State of the Solids, may be removed with a much leſs Quantity of the Bark than they might otherwiſe require. It has an Influence alſo over many Diſtempers of the Head to Advantage, and pre-ſerves againſt Epilepſies, Apoplex-ies, Palſies, and Rheumy Defluxions. It may be given from ten to thirty or forty Drops in any ſuitable Vehicle once,

once, twice, or thrice a Day; observing to take it when the Stomach is most empty, as in the Morning fasting, a little before Dinner, and in the Afternoon. This is the very Medicine which Mr. *Fuller*, Author of the *Medicina Gymnastica*, gives an Account of in his *Appendix*, to have been order'd to him by a Physician now of the greatest Note, and by the sole Help of which he was recover'd from a most deplorable Decay of Constitution, particularly of the Stomach, and continual Reachings to vomit for some time; though from a Return afterwards into the same Irregularities, which was driving away the *Hippo* by spirituous Liquors, he relapsed and died. *Bates* recommends this as an excellent Medicine for the Stomach and Intestines, for exciting the Appetite, and preserving from the Epilepsy and Apoplexy; for purging the Brain, for relieving the Head, together with the whole Body, from phlegmatic catarrhous Humours, and defending it from Pain.

Elixir Vitrioli acidum.
Acid Elixir of Vitriol.

Take of the aromatic Tincture a Pint, of the strong Spirit or Oil of Vitriol, the Weight of four Ounces. Mix them gradually, and when the Fæces are subsided, filtre thro' Paper. L.

This is the Method directed by the College for making *Mynsicht's* Elixir of Vitriol. Experience must determine, whether the Medicine is improv'd with Respect to its Efficacy, the principal thing to be consider'd.

Elixir Vitrioli dulce.
Dulcify'd Elixir of Vitriol.

Take of the aromatic Tincture a Pint, of dulcify'd Spirit of Vitriol eight Ounces in Weight. Mix them. L.

The *London* Dispensatory orders *Vigani's* Elixir of Vitriol to be thus made. It is intended for Stomachs which cannot bear the Acidity of the other.

The Author of the *Pharmacopœia Reformata* informs us, that what has been sold for *Vigani's* Elixir of Vitriol, is no more than the sweet Spirit of Vitriol, digested upon a small Quantity of Mint, curiously dry'd, until it has acquired a due Colour. Great Care must be taken that the Spirit be well freed from its acid Parts, either by a very prudent Rectification, or by leisurely distilling it from a small Quantity of fixed Alcaline Salt, for on this Circumstance depends its greenish Colour, in which consists the Secret, that alone being the Characteristic of the Genuineness of the Preparation. The Mint for this Purpose is most commodiously suspended in the Spirit in a fine Linen Cloth, to prevent the Necessity of filtering it, during which, its most volatile Parts will exhale.

Vinum Amarum.
Bitter Wine.

Take Gentian Root, the yellow Part of fresh Lemon Peel, of each one Ounce, of long Pepper two Drams, of white Wine, a Quart. Infuse without Heat, and strain. L.

This is intended as a Stomachic.

Vinum Antimoniale.
Antimonial Wine.

Take of the Crocus of Antimony washed, one Ounce, of white Wine one Pint and a half. Infuse without Heat, and then strain the Wine off thro' Paper. L.

It is something very astonishing that the Crocus of Antimony, or *Crocus Metallorum*, should communicate inexhaustibly an Emetic Quality to the Liquor it is infus'd in, which it is found to do. The Compilers of he *London* Dispensatory have alter'd the Name *Vinum Benedictum* which was formerly known by, to *Vinum Antimoniale*, as it should seem without any Necessity. In the former College Dispensatory it was directed to be made by infusing an Ounce of the *Crocus Metallorum* in a Pint and half of *Canary*, for several Days. *Quincy* says, the Dose is from two Drams to an Ounce. This was the common Emetic before *Ipecacuanha* was introduc'd, and was that generally made use of by *Sydenham*. who I presume observ'd no ill Effects from its Use, because if he had, he would not have prescrib'd it; and I never knew it do any Injury, where judiciously administer'd; and with respect to its Virtues I have strong reason to believe it much more effectual than *Ipecacuanha*; in particular I have never observ'd the good Effects from *Ipecacuanha*, given in the Beginning of the Small Pox, which the honest *Sydenham* ascribes to the Emetic Wine.

Vinum Chalybeatum.

Chalybeate Wine.

ake of Filings of Steel unprepar'd, three Ounces, Cochineal, half a Dram; *Rhenish* Wine, a Quart; digest in a Sand Heat for ten Days, and filtre. E.

This is much the same as *Boerhaave*'s Chalybeate Wine, and scarce differs, except in the Difference of Cochineal, an Ingredient of no Importance to the Virtues of the Medicine; but he only orders the Digestion to be continued three or four Days. *Boerhaave* says, that the soluble Part of Iron, is a most noble Medicine, for promoting that Power in the Body by which the Blood is made, as often as it happens to be weaken'd, thro' a bare Debility of the over relax'd Solid, and an inherent, cold, aqueous Indisposition

of the Juices. If an excellent Medicinal Virtue may, by any Experiment, be gained from Metals, certainly it is this; for no Virtue of any Vegetable or Animal Substance, no Diet, nor Regimen, can effect that in this Case, which is effected by Iron: But it proves hurtful where the vital Powers are too strong, whether this proceeds from the Fluids or Solids. I have often thought, says *Boerhaave*, whether this was not the potable Sulphur of the Metal, that so powerfully resists the Debility of Nature; a Medicine infinitely superior to the boasted *Aurum Potabile*, and a Medicine that never proves pernicious when given where required. Hence we see that Iron has a Part not very remote from a Vegetable, and even an Animal Nature; and which is extremely easy to dissolve. If a Dram of this Chalybeate Wine be mixed with thrice its Weight of Sugar, boiled to a proper Consistence, and be prudently given in the proper Cases, it makes an incomparable Remedy for the Young of both Sexes.

Vinum Chalybeatum.

Chalybeate Wine.

Take of Filings of Iron four Ounces, Cinnamon and Mace, of each half an Ounce, of *Rhenish* Wine two Quarts. Infuse a Month without Heat, often stirring, then strain it off. L.

This differs but little from the preceding, except in the Addition of the Spices.

Vinum Croceum.

Saffron Wine.

Take of Saffron one Ounce, of Canary one Pint. Infuse without Heat, and strain. L.

The Virtues of this may be learn'd from those of Saffron.

Vinum

Vinum Millepedatum,

Wine of Millepedes.

Take of live Millepedes, two Ounces; bruife them a little, and pour thereon a Pint of white *Rhenifh* Wine; let them infufe for a Night, and afterwards prefs out the Wine. E.

The Medicinal Virtues of this may be underftood by thofe of the Millepedes.

Vinum Viperinum.

Viper Wine.

Take of dried Vipers two Ounces, of white Wine three Pints. Infufe with a gentle Heat for a Week, and then ftrain the Wine off. L.

There has been fome Difpute whether living or dry'd Vipers are beft for Viper Wine, or whether a cold or a hot Infufion is preferable. The College has here preferr'd dry'd Vipers, and a warm Infufion; but the Medicine is not of Confequence enough to be worth difputing about, for I believe the Virtues it is poffefs'd of are very inconfiderable. A Medicine has been advertis'd in Town, under the Name of Viper Wine, which is faid to have had very extraordinary Effects, fuch as might be expected from a Tincture of Cantharides, which upon Examination I find it really to be.

Spiritus Vini camphoratus.

Spirit of Wine, with Camphire.

Take of Camphire, an Ounce; and rectify'd Spirit of Wine, a Pint; mix them fo as to make a Solution. E.

Julaps, Mixtures, &c.

Julepum e Camphora.

The Camphorated Julep.

Take of Camphire one Dram, of double refin'd Sugar half an Ounce, of boiling Water a Pint. Firft, grind the Camphire with a little rectify'd Spirit of Wine, till it is foftened, then with the Sugar till it is perfectly united; laftly add the Water by Degrees, and when the Mixture has ftood in a cover'd Veffel till it is cold, ftrain it off. L.

This is fubftituted by the College for the *Julapium Camphoratum,* or Camphorated Julep, which is thus prepar'd,

Take Camphire, two Drams, fet it on Fire, and extinguifh it in a Pint of Water; then light it again, and extinguifh it, which repeat till all the Camphire is confum'd.

This is an admirable Antihyfteric, and is excellent in Cafe of Flatulencies. I don't know whether the Burning of the Camphire may not make it a better Medicine. For I have feen better Effects from this, than from any fimple Solutions of Camphire.

Julepum e Creta.

The Chalk Julep.

Take of the whiteft Chalk prepared, one Ounce, of double refin'd Sugar fix Drams, of Gum Arabic two Drams, of Water a Quart. Mix all together. L.

This is an Abforbent, and feems intended for the Heart Burn, or Gripes in Children.

Julepum e Mofcho.

The Mufk Julep.

Take of Damafk Rofe Water the Meafure of fix Ounces, of Mufk twelve Grains, of double refined Sugar one Dram. Grind the Mufk and Sugar together, and gradually add the Rofe Water. L.

The Mufk in this Medicine is the only Ingredient to be depended upon, and

and this is given with much greater Effect in Substance. *Bates* has a Medicine not unlike this, under the Title of *Julapium Hystericum Moschatum*, with Orange Flower Water, which is a better Vehicle than Rose Water, and Dragon's Blood. This he orders to be taken at two Doses in Hysteric Fits. And *Fuller* has a *Julapium Moschatum*, which he recommends very much as a Cordial, and says it is excellent in a Hiccough attending a Fever; and indeed Musk is in this last Case very excellent, if given in Substance from ten to thirty Grains.

Lac Ammoniaci.

Milk of Gum Ammoniac.

Take of Gum Ammoniac two Drams, of simple Penny Royal Water half a Pint. Rub the Gum in a Mortar with the Water, till it is dissolved. L.

This is the common Method of dissolving *Gum Ammoniacum*, but it is so soon and readily done *extempore*, that it should not seem necessary to make it an officinal Medicine. The Virtues may be learn'd from those of Gum Ammoniac in the *Materia Medica*.

Of Decoctions, Infusions, &c.

What are usually called Infusions in the Shops, are made by pouring boiling Water, or Water very near boiling, to the Ingredients to be infus'd: If these contain any volatile aromatic Parts, which it is necessary to retain in the Medicine, the Vessel must be immediately accurately cover'd, which Circumstance is otherwise not so necessary. If the Ingredients are boiled in the Water, the Medicine hence resulting is called a Decoction, or Apozem. In Decoction the denser the Plant is, and the more resinous, the more oily Froth is thrown to its Surface;

and the less of that resinous, or oleaginous Virtue is communicated to the Water, because it is not dissolved therein; and therefore for preparing a Decoction of this Kind, a long previous Digestion, or the Addition of a fixed Alcaline Salt, and afterwards a longer Boiling, are required. But even in such resinous Vegetables, if boiled when they are fresh, green, and succulent, their native saponaceous Virtue still keeps their Resin soluble, which, running together when dry, becomes more difficult of Solution. This has been observed by those, who, in *America*, have boiled the Chips of Guaiacum in Water, whereby they soon obtained a very penetrating Liquor which cures the Venereal Disease; whilst the Wood that has been long kept, being now less soluble in Water, has a less Effect. And as Plants lose by Boiling all that which goes off in the Form of Vapour, with two hundred and twelve Degrees of Heat; all those Plants are unfit for this Operation, whose Virtue required is volatile with this Degree of Heat. But those whose Virtue resides in a more fixed Matter than can be separated by this Heat, are fit for Decoction. Let it, however, be carefully observed, that the peculiar Virtue of a Plant, which commonly resides in its presiding Spirit, does not always shew itself by some remarkable Odour, Fragrance, or aromatic Taste: On the contrary it may happen, that the Spirit shall be extremely active, without remarkably affecting the Senses; as appears in the black Hellebore Root, the *Cicuta aquatica Gesneri*, the *Solanum maniacum*, &c. whence all these Particulars are very cautiously to be consider'd, before any general Rule is laid down.

These Preparations may pass thro' the Lacteal and Mesenteric Vessels, and mix with the venous Blood of the

the *Vena Cava*, and thus by the vital Motion be mixed with the Humours of the Body, received into all the larger Kinds of Vessels, reach to the Viscera, and all the other Parts of the Body; for they are saponaceous, penetrating, and miscible with every Humour. And here they may act by their own peculiar Force remaining in the Liquor of the Infusion or Decoction; which Faculty of Action is then greatly increased by the Force of the vital Motion, and thus produces sudden Effects. But they want that Efficacy which remains in the distilled Water, tho' the Infusion contains more of it than the Decoction. But in the Decoction, however, this Want is supplied by a great Efficacy, which the boiling Heat communicates thereto, by enabling it to dissolve, and intimately mix the Virtues of the Plant with the Water by long Boiling. Whence, if the Operation were performed in a Still with its Alembic Head, and the exhaling Water returned to the remaining Decoctions, then these Decoctions would become exceedingly rich in the Virtues of the Plant; for such a Liquor will contain nearly all the Powers of the Subject. It must be well consider'd, that the Medicinal Virtues of Infusions and Decoctions, depend as much upon the Efficacy and Quantity of the hot Water received, as upon the Virtue of the Plant. This is known to Physicians. It is an Error, in condemning the Use of Tea, to attribute the Mischief wholly to the Leaves, when the larger Part is hot Water: And again, when we attribute the Virtue of enlivening the Spirits to the Drinking of Tea, the diluting Virtue of hot Water is not to be omitted. But we must remark, that some of the peculiar Virtues of Plants are alter'd by the Boiling. *Arum* grows milder by Decoction; the crude

Juice or Infusion of *Asarabacca* proves strongly Emetic; but this Virtue, by long continued Decoction, is changed to another, that is diuretic and aperient. For the Method of clarifying Decoctions, See Book I. Chap. ix.

Decoctum Album.
White Decoction.

Take calcin'd Hartshorn, an Ounce; Spring Water, three Pints; boil them together till only a Quart remains behind; to which without straining add, an Ounce of Cinnamon Water, made without Spirit, and two Drams of white Sugar; and mix them together. E.

The *Decoctum Album* of the *London* Dispensatory is thus directed:

Take of burnt Hartshorn prepared, two Ounces; of Gum Arabic, two Drams; of Water, three Pints; boil the Water away to a Quart, and strain it off.

Decoctum Album compositum.
Compound white Decoction.

Take of burnt Hartshorn, six Drams; Crab's Eyes, three Drams; Roots of the greater Comfrey and Tormentil, of each two Drams; Spring Water, three Pints; boil them together, so that there may remain a Quart of Liquor, when strained thick; to which add an Ounce of Cinnamon Water, made without Spirit; and half an Ounce of *Diacodium*; and mix them all together. E.

These Decoctions are generally us'd in Diarrhœas and Dysenteries, but often very imprudently, and with very bad Effect; for to check Stools which are critical, and meant by Nature to relieve some Disorder, either in the Bowels or whole Habit, which is generally the Case, is destructive to the Patient, as it confines the morbid Matter, and thereby excites a worfe Diftemper than is intended to cure, I have fre-ently known exceffive Gripes, and ngerous Fevers caus'd by ftopping ools injudicioufly. It is, there-re, feldom proper to ftop Fluxes, ithout previoufly carrying off the fending Matter by due Purging. has been obferv'd by all Phyficians ice *Hippocrates*, that a copious æmorrhage from the Nofe ter-inates a Fever, fometimes in its fancy; but that a flight Hæmor-iage is a fatal Symptom, becaufe it ews that Nature is making an in-fectual Effort for her Relief. Some-ing of the fame Kind happens ith Refpect to Diarrhœas, which ry frequently anticipate or cure a ever, if copious and profufe; but flight and infufficient for the Pur-ofe, they are to be efteem'd per-lcious, and of bad Prefage, and ught to be promoted rather than op'd. Thefe white Decoctions, owever, may fometimes be proper check the Exorbitance of Fluxes, no' feldom to ftop them. But their fe requires great Judgment.

Decoctum Amarum.

Bitter Decoction.

ake of Gentian Root, a Scruple; Tops of the leffer Centaury, Cha-momile Flowers, and the Seeds of *Carduus Benedictus*, each a Dram; Spring Water, fix Ounces; boil them together a little, then ftrain off the Decoction. *E.*

This was in the firft Edition of the *Edinburgh* Difpenfatory, but is o-nitted in the laft. It is intended as Stomachic.

Decoctum Amarum cum Senna.

Bitter Decoction with Senna.

n the former bitter Decoction, while hot, infufe, for a Night, one Dram of the Leaves of Senna; and ftrain off the Liquor. It is like-wife prepared with a double and triple Quantity of Senna. *E.*

This was, alfo, in the former Edi-tion of the *Edinburgh* Difpenfatory, but is omitted in the laft. It renders the preceding Decoction laxative.

Decoctum commune pro Clyftere.

Common Decoction for Clyfters.

Take of the Leaves of Mallows, of the Herb Mercury, and Chamo-mile Flowers, each half an Ounce; Fennel Seed, and Linfeed, of each two Drams; Spring Water, a Pint and half; boil them together till a third Part of the Liquor is exhaled, then ftrain off the Re-mainder. *E.*

The *London* Difpenfatory directs it thus:

Take of Mallow Leaves dry, one Ounce; dried Chamomile Flow-ers, fweet Fennel Seeds, of each half an Ounce; of Water, one Pint, after Boiling ftrain it off. *L.*

Thefe Decoctions are only us'd in Clyfters, as Vehicles for things of greater Confequence. In the for-mer College Difpenfatory it was thus directed; but the Differences are not very material.

Take of Leaves of Mallows, Vio-lets, Pellitory of the Wall, Beets, and Mercury, of each one Hand-ful; of Chamomile Flowers two Pugils; of fweet Fennel Seed, half an Ounce; of Linfeed, two Drams; and boil them in a fuffi-cient Quantity of common Wa-ter, to yield a Pint when ftrain'd.

Decoctum Diafcordii.

Decoction of Diafcordium.

Take of Diafcordium, an Ounce; *Japan* Earth, two Drams; Spring Water, a Pint and a half; boil them fo as to leave a Pint of Li-quor, when ftrain'd thick; to

Z z   which

which add of Cinnamon Water, made with Spirit, and the Syrup of *Diacodium,* each an Ounce; and mix them together. E.

This is an Astringent, and seems intended principally to check Fluxes, and may be taken by Way of Draught, or in Clysters. But it is a Medicine to be us'd with the utmost Caution. See the preceding Remarks on the *Decoctum Album.*

Decoctum emolliens pro fotu.

The emollient Decoction for Fomentations.

Take of the Leaves of Mallows, one Ounce; Flowers of Chamomile, Melilot, and Elder, of each half an Ounce; Seeds of Foenugreek, one Ounce; boil them in two Quarts of Spring Water.

It is also made without the Seeds of Foenugreek. The Title expresses the Uses.

Decoctum ad Ictericos.

Decoction for the Jaundice.

Take the Roots together with the Leaves of the greater Celandine, the Roots of Turmeric, and Madder, of each an Ounce; Spring Water, three Pints: Boil them together till there remains a Quart of the strain'd Liquor; to which, when cold, add the Juice of two hundred Millepedes, and two Ounces of the Syrup of the five opening Roots, and mix them together. E.

This seems very well contriv'd to answer the Design its Title expresses. But it must be taken in large Quantities, in order to answer any good Purpose.

Decoctum Lignorum.
Decoction of the Woods.

Take three Ounces of the Shavings of Guaiacum Wood; two Oun-

ces of ston'd Raisins of the Sun; a Gallon of Spring Water; boil them together over a gentle Fire to two Quarts; towards the End of the Operation, add one Ounce of the Shavings of Sassafras Wood, and half an Ounce of sliced Liquorice; then pour off the Decoction when settled. E.

Experience convinces us, that there is a very great Difference betwixt a Decoction of the fresh Chips, or Raspings of Guaiacum, and one of those which are old and dry, which is what are commonly used with us. The Reason of this should seem to be, that the naive saponaceous Virtue in the green Plant preserves the Resin soluble, the Parts of which cohere together when dry, and become more difficult to dissolve. See the Article *Guaiacum* in the *Materia Medica.*

Decoctum ad Nephriticos.

Nephritic Decoction.

Take of the Roots of Marsh-mallows, Liquorice, and Rest Harrow, each half an Ounce; Linseed, and wild Carrot Seed, of each three Drams; Pellitory of the Wall, an Ounce; four ripe Figs; ston'd Raisins of the Sun, two Ounces; Spring Water, three Quarts; boil them together, so as to make two Quarts of Liquor when strain'd. E.

As this Decoction is emollient, in Nephritic Paroxysms it may contribute much to the Relaxation of the urinary Passages, and consequently to the easy Passage of the Stone or Gravel. It will be a much better Medicine, if exhibited with an Addition of Nitre, and some Syrup of Marsh-mallows. It should be drank very plentifully.

Decoctum

Decoctum Nitrosum.
Decoction of Salt-Petre.

Take of well purified Nitre, half an Ounce; white Sugar, two Ounces; Cochineal, a Scruple; Spring-water, five half Pints: Boil them together to a Quart; then pour off the Decoction, after it is clarify'd by standing. *E.*

The Nitre renders this an admirable Medicine in Fevers, and febrile Distempers. But as Nitre is so really given in Substance, or dissolved in any diluting Fluid, this does not seem altogether necessary as a Shop-Medicine. If the Cochineal is intended for any thing more than to disguise the Medicine, it is very trifling; otherwise very unfair, and too much mysterious.

Decoctum Pectorale.
Pectoral Decoction,

Take of Raisins of the Sun stoned, and Barley, each an Ounce; four fat Figs; Spring-water, six Pints: Boil to four Pints, at the End of the Decoction adding of the Root of *Florentine* Orrice and Liquorice, each half an Ounce; of the Leaves of Harts-tongue and Colts-foot, each an Ounce: Strain off the Liquor. *E.*

The *London* Dispensatory directs the Pectoral Decoction thus:

Take common Barley, Raisins stoned, Figs, of each two Ounces; of Liquorice-root, half an Ounce; of Water, two Quarts. Boil the Water first with the Barley; then add the Raisins; and afterwards, towards the latter End of the Decoction, the Figs and Liquorice; the Decoction will then be fully compleated, when one Quart only of the Liquor will be left after Straining. *L.*

In the former College Dispensatory it was thus directed:

Take of stoned Raisins, one Ounce; of Dactyls, No. six; of fat Figs No. eight; of Barley cleansed, one Ounce; boil these in three Pints of Spring Water to the Consumption of a third Part, towards the End putting in of Liquorice-root, half an Ounce; of the Leaves of Maiden-Hair, Ground-Ivy, Scabious and Coltsfoot, of each one Handful. Let them stand in Infusion a quarter of an Hour, and then strain off the Liquor.

It would be very trifling to dispute which of these Pectoral Decoctions is best. It is of more Consequence to remark, that an Infusion of the Pectoral Ingredients in hot Water makes a Medicine much more agreeable to the Stomach, and not less efficacious. These Decoctions and Infusions must be taken in very large Quantities, in order to produce any considerable Effect; and indeed no great Dependance is to be had on them, without the Addition of something more efficacious.

Decoctum Tamarindorum cum Senna.
Decoction of Tamarinds with Senna.

Take of Tamarinds, six Drams; Crystals of Tartar, two Drams; Spring Water, a Pint and a half; boil them in an earthen Vessel to one Pint; in this, whilst hot, infuse, for a Night, one Dram of Senna Leaves, and to the strain'd Liquor add one Ounce of Syrup of Violets. This is also sometimes made with a double, or triple Quantity of Senna.

This is an admirable cooling Medicine in febrile Disorders, especially in Case of Costiveness.

Infusum amarum.
The bitter Infusion.

Take of the Root of Gentian, half a Dram; the Tops of the lesser Centaury, one Dram; pour upon

Z z 2

them four Ounces of boiling Spring Water: Infuse for four Hours and filtre it. *E.*

This, in the last Edition of the *Edinburgh* Dispensatory, is substituted for the *Decoctum amarum* of the former Editions, and seems to be a better Medicine.

Infusum amarum cum Senna.

The bitter Infusion with Senna.

To the preceding Infusion, add of the Leaves of Senna, one Dram; the Seeds of Fennel, half a Dram. *E.*

It is sometimes made with double or treble the Quantity of Senna.

The *London* Dispensatory orders a bitter Infusion, thus,

Infusum amarum simplex.

The simple bitter Infusion.

Take Gentian Root, the yellow Rind of Lemon-peel fresh, carefully separated from the inner white Part, of each half an Ounce; of the yellow Rind of *Seville* Orange-peel, also carefully separated from its inner white Part, but dried, a Dram and a half; of boiling Water, three quarters of a Pint: After infusing for an Hour or two, strain it, either through Paper or a Cloth, without any pressing out. *L.*

This is intended as a Stomachic Bitter, and seems very well adapted to that Intention.

Infusum amarum purgans.

The purging bitter Infusion.

Take the Leaves of Sena, the yellow Rind of fresh Lemon-peel, of each three Drams; Gentian Root, the yellow Part of *Seville* Orange-peel dried, the lesser Cardamom Seeds husked, of each half a Dram; of boiling Water, five Ounces: After infusing it till the Liquor is cold, strain it off. *L.*

This should seem to be a very good Stomachic Laxative; to which may be added at Discretion any proper Cathartic Ingredient, in order to render it more Cathartic.

Infusi Sennæ Unciæ quatuor.

A Four-Ounce Infusion of Senna.

Take of the Leaves of Senna, three Drams; and of the great Water Fig-wort, two Drams; bruised Ginger, and Salt of Tartar, of each ten Grains; boiling Water, four Ounces: Infuse them together for four Hours, then strain off the Liquor. *E.*

A Decoction or Infusion of Senna is the common Basis of Cathartic Potions; but is seldom given without the Addition of something to render the Operation brisker.

Infusum Senæ commune.

The common Infusion of Sena.

Take Leaves of Sena, one Ounce and a half; of Crystals of Tartar, three Drams; of the lesser Cardamom Seeds husk'd, two Drams; of Water, one Pint. Boil the Crystals of Tartar in Water till they are dissolved; then pour the Water, while boiling-hot, upon the Sena and the rest. When the Liquor is cold, strain it off. *L.*

In this the Crystals of Tartar seem to be judiciously substituted for the Salt of Tartar in the former College Dispensatory. It is, like the preceding, used for the Basis of Cathartic Potions.

Infusum Senæ Limoniatum.

The Infusion of Sena with Lemon.

Take of the Leaves of Sena, one Ounce and a half; of the Yellow of fresh Lemon-peel, an Ounce in Weight; of Lemon-juice, an Ounce in Measure; of boiling Water,
one

one Pint. Infuse till cold, and then strain. *L.*

In the Narrative prefix'd to the College Dispensatory, we are told that this Method of adding an Acid in the Infusion of Senna, whether of Tartar or Lemon-juice, is contrary to that in our present *Pharmacopœia*, where an Alcaline Salt is made an Ingredient. In Theory Acids weaken watry Tinctures from Vegetables; and Alcalies rather increase the Quantity extracted; but Experience has sufficiently shewn, that these Infusions as here directed, do not fail in their Intention; and, in a Medicine very nauseous to many, it is of principal Consequence to prepare it so, that the lightest and least disgustful Parts may be extracted.

Emulsio Communis.
Common Emulsion.

Take of the four greater cold Seeds, an Ounce; and blanch'd sweet Almonds, half an Ounce: Beat them very well in a Marble-mortar, then pour on by degrees a Quart of Spring-water. Mix them well, and, when strain'd, add an Ounce of Cinnamon-water, without Spirit, and two Drams of white Sugar. *E.*

Emulsio Arabica.
Arabic Emulsion.

This Emulsion is made after the same Manner as the preceding; first boiling in the Water, till perfectly dissolved, three Drams of bruised Gum Arabic. *E.*

The *London* Dispensatory orders the *Emulsio Communis*, or common Emulsion, thus:

Take of sweet Almonds blanch'd, one Ounce; of Gum Arabic, half an Ounce; of double refined Sugar, six Drams; of Barley-water, one Quart. Dissolve the Gum in the Barley-water hot, and, when the Water is quite cold, pour it gradually upon the Almonds pounded with the Sugar, rubbing them together, that the Liquor may grow milky; then strain it off. *L.*

Boerhaave remarks, with respect to Emulsions in general, that the Liquor thus prepared, resembles in many Respects the Chyle of Animals, which is itself prepared from Vegetables in their Bodies by Chewing, Ruminating, and the Action of the Stomach, before it is mixed with the Bile in the Duodenum. The Thing appears plain from the white Colour, the mild Odour, the sweet Taste, the thick Unctuousness, and the great Disposition they both have to turn sour. So likewise, if the Liquor thus prepared stands some Time in a tall cylindrical Vessel, it spontaneously separates into a white, thick and almost totally oily Part, which floats at the Top, and into a thinner, transparent, bluish Liquor, that remains below; wherein it perfectly resembles Milk, as dividing itself into Cream, and thin Milk. Again, if this Liquor be kept for some Time in a warm Air, it turns sour, and afterwards considerably sharp, tho' without acquiring the proper Rancidness of an express'd Oil; in which Respect also it perfectly agrees with Milk, which acquires the like Acidity in such an Air, without becoming rancid like pure Oil: Whence this farther Remark should be made, that in acute Distempers Emulsions may be given with greater Safety than express'd Oils. But I could never, says *Boerhaave*, by any Art of Coagulation obtain such a Curd from this Liquor as Milk affords; whence there is this Difference betwixt the Milk of Vegetables and Animals. The Reason of the Difference between an ex-

press'd

press'd Oil, and an Emulsion, seems principally this, that, the mealy Part in the Grinding being constantly in fine Particles interposed betwixt the pure Oil, the Parts of this Oil are so broke and separated from one another, that, its Tenacity being chang'd, it becomes miscible with Water, and thence appears in the Form of Milk, which also consists of a fat Substance dissolved in Water; whereas when a pure Oil is obtained by Expression, the Parts thereof, being in Contract with each other, do not admit of Water, nor suffer it to be mixed among them. Again, the large Quantity of Meal, intermix'd amongst the Oil in the Emulsion, causes it to turn sour, not rancid; and hence appears the Reason why the Liquor is white; for Whiteness always ensues as often as Oil is intimately divided and mix'd with Water. If Oil be pour'd upon a Glass of Water, the two Liquors will remain separate and transparent; but if shook briskly together, they will unite in some measure, and during that Union the Mixture will appear perfectly white; but if now suffer'd to rest, the Oil collects at the Top, the Water sinks to the Bottom, and the Whiteness immediately vanishes; and the same Thing frequently happens in Animal Milk, distill'd Oleaginous Waters, and these Emulsions. It is also certain, that the Whiteness becomes greater the larger the Quantity of Oil, and in this Case the Liquor sooner grows rancid; but the less the Oil, the less white the Liquor, and the sooner it turns sour. In the Summer, Emulsions will scarce keep above ten Hours, but in the Winter longer. To conclude, this Method of making Emulsions gives Light to the Action of Mastication; for, all the Foods prepared from Corn abounding with a latent Oil, and being ground by the Teeth in chewing, and mix'd with the Saliva, the

longer they are thus acted upon in the Mouth, the nearer they approach to these Emulsions, and at length always turn white, when the Saliva, Salt, and Oil are well ground together. The Operation thus begun in the Mouth is carried on in the Stomach, and more perfected in the Intestines, where the Matter still retains the same Nature, except that new Juices are perpetually mixing themselves therewith, and communicating their Properties; whereas in our Pharmaceutical Operation there is no Addition but of Water alone; and hence we may understand the artificial Distinction between the first Chyle, and the Milk of Animals.

Emulsions are so readily made *ex tempore*, and are so very soon spoil'd, that they are not fit for Officinal Medicines, but may be vary'd occasionally according to the Intention of the Prescriber. They are used when any considerable Acrimony abounds, and particularly when the Urine is discharged with Pain and Difficulty, from any Cause whatever.

Aqua Hordeata.

Barley-Water.

Take of Pearl-Barley, two Ounces; of Water, two Quarts: Wash the Barley first well with some cold Water; then, pouring on about half a Pint of Water, boil it a little while; and this Water, which will be coloured, being thrown away, put the Barley into the Quantity of Water above directed, first made boiling hot, and boil away to half. *L.*

This is the common Liquor used for cooling, moistening, and diluting in febrile Disorders. But as the Method of making it is universally known, as it is soon made, and will not keep, it was less necessary to describe it in a Dispensatory.

Four

Fotus Communis.

The Common Fomentation.

'ake the Leaves of Southernwood, or of Lavender-Cotton dry, the Tops of Sea-wormwood also dry, Chamomile-flowers, of each one Ounce; of Bay-leaves dry, half an Ounce; of Water, three Quarts. After a slight Boiling, strain the Water off. *L.*

This seems a convenient Basis for a 'omentation, to which Spirit of Vine, or whatever the Prescriber idges proper, may be added. The medicinal Virtues may be learned 'om those of the Ingredients which nter its Composition.

Jus Viperinum.

Viper Broth.

Take a Viper of a middle Size, without the Skin, Head, or Entrails; of Water, a Quart: Boil to about a Pint and half. Remove all from the Fire, and when the Water is cold, if the Viper be not a dried one, take away the congeal'd Fat; then take a Chicken of a middle Size, drawn, and the Skin, with all the Fat taken off, and put it whole into this Decoction while cold. Set it upon the Fire till it boils; then remove it from the Fire; take out the Chicken, and cut the Flesh of it into small Pieces, which put again into the Water, and set it over the Fire; but, as soon as it begins to boil up, pour it off, first having taken away whatever Scum may have risen. *L.*

It would be ridiculous to make Remarks upon this Culinary Preparation, because every Cook-maid in *England* is qualify'd to do it better han *Hippocrates* or *Boerhaave*, if they were now alive. I shall only observe, that the last-mentioned Author was of Opinion, that Broths taken frequently, and in a small Quantity at a Time, are most excellent Restoratives, and highly efficacious in relax'd Habits; and Chicken Broth may perhaps be as good as any other. On this Account the *Jus Viperinum* may be a good Restorative; but I esteem the Chicken the principal Ingredient to be depended on; for the Flesh of one Viper, let the Virtues of the Animal be never so great, cannot be sufficient to answer any Intention; and besides, so far as I have been able to learn from Experience, Vipers have no one Virtue to recommend them, that can in the least be depended upon; but it is very usual to overlook the Efficacy of Things we are daily conversant with, and ascribe their good Effects to others that are not so common, tho' less to be depended upon. And I am pretty certain, that whoever experiences Chicken Broth with and without the Viper, will find as much Service from the latter as from the former.

Mucilago Seminum Cydoniorum.

Mucilage of Quince-Seed.

Take of Quince-Seed, a Dram; of Water, six Ounces: Boil it with a gentle Fire till the Water grows roapy, resembling the White of an Egg; then strain it through a Linnen Cloth. *L.*

This and the Mucilage of Gum Tragacanth seem to be pretty equal with respect to their Virtues. They are principally used, mixed with other Ingredients, to hold in the Mouth, and be swallow'd gradually. Sometimes they are made a Vehicle for heavy Substances, which will not so readily be suspended in any thing that is perfectly fluid.

Serum Aluminosum.

Alum Whey.

Take of Cows-milk, one Pint; of Alum in Powder, two Drams;

Boil

Boil till a Whey is formed, which is to be well separated from the Curd. *L.*

The Virtues of this may be learn'd from those of Alum.

Serum Scorbuticum.
Scorbutic Whey. *

Take of Cows-milk, one Pint; of the Scorbutic Juices a Quarter of a Pint: Boil till a Whey is form'd, which is to be well separated from the Curd. *L.*

The Title expresses the Virtues.

CHAP. VII.
Of SYRUPS.

General Rules for making of Syrups.

I. THE Sugar, employ'd for Syrups made without Coction, should first be boil'd with Water to a Candy Consistence, observing to clarify it with the White of Eggs, and by Despumation.

II. Tho' a double Weight of Sugar, in Proportion to the Liquor, may be required in making such Syrups, yet a less Proportion will generally suffice. First, therefore, dissolve only an equal Quantity of Sugar; then, by degrees, add a little more in Powder till it remain undissolved at the Bottom; to be afterwards incorporated by the gentle Heat of a Water-bath.

III. Acid Syrups, or those made with the Juices of Fruits, should not be put into Copper Vessels, unless such as are tinn'd.

IV. The Vegetables used either for Decoctions or Infusions are to be moderately dried, unless where they are expressly required fresh-gather'd.

V. Syrups made by Coction are to be clarify'd with the White of Eggs, except *Diacodium*, which therefore requires the purest Sugar.

VI. The Solutive and Purging Syrups ought rather to be made of brown Sugar.

Syrupus ex Allio.
Syrup of Garlick.

Take of the Roots of Garlick sliced, one Pound; of boiling Water, a Quart. Steep the Garlick in the Water twelve Hours in a close Vessel, and in the Liquor strain'd dissolve a sufficient Quantity of Sugar, so as to make the Syrup. *L.*

The Virtues of this may be learn'd from those of Garlick. It seems principally intended as a Pectoral.

Syrupus de Althæa.
Syrup of Marshmallows.

Take of the Root of Marshmallow, three Ounces; candy'd Eryngo-Root, one Ounce; Liquorice, half an Ounce; Maidenhair, or *Trichomanes*, and Pellitory of the Wall, each one Ounce; Spring-water, six Pints: Boil to the Consumption of one Third. To the strain'd Liquor, depurated by subsiding, add white Sugar, four Pounds. Boil gently, continually stirring, till a Syrup is form'd. *E.*

In the *London* Dispensatory the *Syrupus ex Althæa* is thus prepar'd:

Take of the fresh Roots of Marshmallows, a Pound; of double refin'd Sugar, four Pounds; of Water, one Gallon. Boil the Water with the Roots till it is half wasted. After it is quite cold pour

our it off, and prefs it out. Let he Liquor ftand by for a Night, hat its Fæces may fubfide. In he Morning pour off the Clear, nd, adding the Sugar, boil all lown to the Weight of fix Pounds.

o great Efficacy can be expected n any Quantity of this Syrup t can be taken for a Dofe. It is I however, not improperly, to eten Emollient Decoctions or In- ons, principally thofe intended nake Gravel or a Stone to pafs with Eafe.

Syrupus Artemifiæ.
Syrup of Mugwort.

e of the Root of Madder, two unces; thofe of round Birth- orth and Turmeric, of each an unce; Spring-water, a Gallon. oil them together till a fourth art be wafted; and add, towards e End of the Operation, Leaves f Mugwort, an Ounce; thofe of alamint, Dittany of *Crete,* Fe- rfew with the Flowers, Origa- m, common Penny-royal, Rue, d Savine, of each half an Ounce; e Seeds of *Daucus* of *Crete* (or wild Carrot) and thofe of Lo- ge, of each three Drams. To e ftrain'd Liquor put fix Pounds white Sugar, and make it into Syrup, according to the Rules Art, by boiling it over a gentle re. *E.*

is Syrup is omitted in the laft on of the *Edinburgh* Difpenfa- ; but I have given it a Place becaufe it feems as well con- l, and to be of as great Efficacy ny of the other Syrups. It is lated principally for promoting Jterine Difcharges.

rupus è Cortice Aurantiorum.
Syrup of Orange-Peel.

of the external Rind of frefh anges, fix Ounces; boiling ring-water, three Pints. Infufe em in a clofe Veffel, with a

gentle Heat in *Balneo Mariæ,* for the Space of fix Hours; then ftrain off the Liquor, and add to it twice its own Weight of white Sugar; and thus make it into a Syrup, without Boiling. *E.*

A Syrup very like this is order'd in the *London* Difpenfatory, under the Title of

Syrupus è Corticibus Aurantiorum.
Syrup of Orange-Peel.

Take of the outer yellow Rind of frefh *Seville* Orange-Peel, eight Ounces; of boiling Water, five Pints. Steep the Peel in the Wa- ter for a Night in a clofe Veffel, and in the Morning diffolve in the Liquor ftrain'd, of double refin'd Sugar beaten to Powder, as much as is fufficient to make a Syrup. *L.* The Virtues of thefe two Syrups may be learn'd from thofe of Orange-Peel. They fhould feem to be grateful and beneficial to the Stomach.

Syrupus è Succo Aurantiorum.
Syrup of Orange-Juice.

Take of the clarified Juice of Oranges, a Pint; white Sugar, two Pounds; and make a Syrup thereof, without Boiling, accord- ing to the Rules of Art. *E.*

Syrupus Balfamicus.
Balfamic Syrup.

Take of the Syrup of Sugar, two Pounds, frefh made. Remove it from the Fire, and, when almoft cold, mix gradually with it of the *Tinctura Tolutana,* an Ounce, and let them be mix'd by Agitation. Then let the Syrup ftand in a Bath-heat till the Spirit is all ex- haled. *E.*

The Method of making the Bal- famic Spirit, directed in the *London* Difpenfatory, is thus:

Take of Balfam of *Tolu,* eight Ounces; of Water, three Pints. Boil the Balfam in the Water in a circulatory

circulatory Veffel, or at leaft in a Matras with a tall Neck, and the Orifice lightly cover'd, for two or three Hours. When the Water is cold, and ftrain'd off, add double refin'd Sugar to make it into a Syrup. *L.*

The Virtues of both thefe may be learn'd from thofe of Balfam of *Tolu.*

Syrupus Capilli Veneris.
Syrup of Maidenhair.

Take of the Herb Maidenhair, half a Pound ; fhaved Liquorice, two Ounces ; boiling Spring-water, three Quarts: Let them ftand together for a Night, then boil them a little, and ftrain out the Liquor by Expreffion; whereto add its own Weight of white Sugar, and boil it to the Confiftence of a Syrup. *E.*

This Syrup is omitted in the laft Edition of the *Edinburgh* Difpenfatory. As it is a very trifling Medicine, I have only given it a Place here for the Satisfaction of fome who have an Opinion of it. The Syrup of *Capillaire,* fold in the Coffeehoufes, ought to be made of the *Canada* Maidenhair and Orangeflower Water. The *London* Difpenfatory directs a Syrup of Maidenhair under the Title of *Syrupus Pectoralis,* which fee.

Syrupus Caryophyllorum.
Syrup of Clove-July-Flower.

Take of frefh gather'd Clove-Julyflowers, clipt clear from their white Heels, a Pound ; boiling Spring-water, three Pints : Let them ftand together one Night, then ftrain off the Liquor, and add thereto twice its own Weight of white Sugar, and thus make it into Syrup, without Boiling, according to the Rules of Art. *E.*

In the *London* Difpenfatory they order three Pounds of the Clove-Julyflowers to five Pints of boiling Water.

I think this Syrup is only valued for its Colour and Flavour, but is of no great Ufe in Medicine.

Syrupus de Cichoreo cum Rheo.
Syrup of Succory with Rhubarb.

Take of Rhubarb fliced and bruifed, fix Ounces ; boiling Spring-water, two Quarts : Let them infufe, in a gentle Heat, for two Days ; and, after a very little Boiling, ftrain off the Liquor ; to which add, of the clarified Juice of Succory, two Quarts ; and of white Sugar, fix Pounds : Then boil them up to a Syrup, in which, whilft it is yet warm, mix a Scruple of the diftill'd Oil of Cinnamon, firft received upon a little Sugar. This may alfo be made with the Decoction of Succory. *E.*

This is omitted in the laft Edition of the *Edinburgh* Difpenfatory. I have given it a Place here, becaufe it is a pretty Purge for Children, and much ufed.

Syrupus Croci.
Syrup of Saffron.

Take of Saffron-wine, a Pint ; of double refined Sugar, twenty-five Ounces ; which diffolve in the Wine fo as to make a Syrup. *L.*

This is a Cordial, and a very agreeable Syrup, and of Ufe in Medicine, as a fufficient Dofe of the Saffron to anfwer fome good Purpofe, may be thus given at once.

Syrupus Cydoniorum.
Syrup of Quinces.

Take of depurated Juice of Quinces, three Pints ; of Cinnamon, one Dram ; Cloves and Ginger, of each half a Dram ; of Red Wine, one Pint ; of double refined Sugar,

nine

nine Pounds. Digest the Juice with the Aromatics six Hours in a Heat of Ashes; then add the Wine, and strain the Liquor off; and lastly, add the Sugar to make a Syrup. *L.*

This is a very agreeable Syrup, and proper to sweeten Astringent Medicines, or take off the disagreeable flavour of others.

Syrupus Kermesinus.

Syrup of Kermes.

Take of the Juice of Kermes-berries, a Pound; white Sugar, two Pounds; and make them into a Syrup without Fire.

That is the best esteem'd which comes to us ready prepared from the Southern Part of *France*, especially no Fire be used in the making. *E.* The Virtues of this may be learn'd from those of the Kermes.

Syrupus è Succo Limonum.

Syrup of Lemon-Juice.

This is made of the Juice of Lemons after the same Manner as the Syrup of Orange-Juice. *E.*

In the *London* Dispensatory it is ordered thus:

Take of Lemon-juice, after it has stood till its Fæces are subsided, and it has been strain'd off, a Quart; of double refined Sugar, fifty Ounces. Dissolve the Sugar in the Juice, so as to make the Syrup. After the same Manner are made the Syrups of Mulberries, and of Raspberries. *L.*

The Virtues of these may be learn'd from those of the Ingredients.

Syrupus Myrtinus.

Syrup of Myrtle.

Take of Myrtle Berries, two Ounces; Tormentil Root, red Roses, red Sanders, Pomegranate Bark, Balaustines, and the Seeds of Su-

mach, each an Ounce; cut and bruise the Ingredients; then boil them in a Gallon of Spring Water, till only one half remains behind; to which, when strain'd, add four Pounds of white Sugar, and boil them together into a Syrup. *E.*

This is omitted in the last Edition of the *Edinburgh* Dispensatory; it is intended as an Astringent.

Syrupus Papaveris albi, seu de Meconio, vulgo Diacodium.

Syrup of white Poppies, or *Diacodium*.

Take of the Heads of the white Poppy, in a mild Degree of Maturity, and moderately dried, fourteen Ounces; boiling Spring Water, a Gallon : Let them infuse for a Night; then boil to the Consumption of one Half of the Liquor; strongly press out the Remainder, and add thereto four Pounds of white Sugar; and boil them up to a Syrup. *E.*

The *London* Dispensatory directs this to be thus made, under the Title of,

Syrupus è Meconio sive Diacodion.

Diacodion.

Take of the Heads of dried white Poppies without their Seeds, three Pounds and a half; of Water six Gallons. Slice the Heads, and boil them in the Water, often stirring them, that they may not burn, till about a Third only of the Liquor is left, which will be almost all imbibed by the Poppy Heads; then take all from the Fire, and press the Liquor strongly out from the Heads; in the next Place boil the Liquor by itself to about two Quarts, and strain it while hot, first thro' a Sieve, and then thro' a thin Flannel; set it by for a Night, that what Fæces may have passed the Strainers, may subside;

next

next Morning pour off the clear Liquor, and boil it with ſix Pounds of double refined Sugar, till the Whole comes to the Weight of nine Pounds, or a little more, that it may become a Syrup of a juſt Conſiſtence. *L.*

As this Syrup is of very great Importance in Medicine, I ſhall here obſerve, what has been ſaid of it by the principal Pharmaceutical Writers. Firſt, *Quincy* remarks, that this Syrup will not bear the uſual Way of Clarification, without loſing much of its Strength, as an Opiate. And ſuch Difference will happen on one Account or other, tho' made with the utmoſt Care, as renders it difficult to be found always of the ſame Strength. The Author of the *Pharmacopœia Reformata* judiciouſly remarks, that, notwithſtanding all the Care which the Committee have taken about this Syrup, it will ſtill greatly differ in its Strength; for in ſome Seaſons the Poppy Heads will contain more Opium in Proportion to their Weight than in others, nor will the different Skill of the Operator, and certain Circumſtances, in the Operation itſelf, contribute a little to render this Syrup unequal in Strength, tho' the utmoſt Care be taken. The Writers of the *Edinburgh* Diſpenſatory ſeem to have well weighed the Inconveniences which attend the uſual Methods of preparing this Syrup, and accordingly have ordered the Decoction of the Poppy Heads in a Manner which ſufficiently ſhews their Skill in Pharmacy. But perhaps all the Pains hitherto taken in the Preparation of this Medicine, are as unneceſſary as defective; for if an Opiate be really wanted in the Form of a Syrup, and if it be abſolutely neceſſary to determine, in a very exact Manner, the Strength of the Syrup, with Regard to the Opium, it would be more to the Purpoſe to diſſolve a certain Quantity of purified Opium, well ſepa-

rated from its reſinous Parts, in a certain Quantity of the white Syrup, or rather in ſome Water to be boiled down to a certain Pitch, and then made into a Syrup with a ſufficient Quantity of Sugar, without any farther Boiling. In my own Opinion this Syrup and all others of the ſame Kind, are of very little Uſe in Medicine; becauſe all the Ends it can anſwer, are much better provided for by crude Opium. The *Syrupus è Meconis,* or *Diacodium,* is, indeed, more readily taken by Children; but to theſe it is very ſeldom proper to give it; and beſides, this Circumſtance tempts Nurſes to exhibit it frequently to Children in order to compoſe them, to their utter Deſtruction.

Syrupus Papaveris Erratici.
Syrup of wild Poppies.

Take of the freſh Flowers of wild Poppy, four Pounds; of boiling Water, four Pints and a half. Set the Water poured on the Flowers over the Fire, and ſtir the Flowers in, till they are all thoroughly wet; and, as ſoon as the Flowers are ſunk, let them ſteep for a Night; next Day pour off, and preſs out the Liquor, ſetting it by for another Night, that its Fæces may ſubſide; then with a proper Addition of double refined Sugar make the Syrup. *L.*

This is alſo an Opiate. The particular Virtues may be learn'd from thoſe of the *Papaver Rubrum, ſive Erraticum.*

The Proportion of the Poppyflowers in this Syrup is greater to the Water than in that of the *Edinburgh* Diſpenſatory, which is thus directed under the Title of

Syrupus Papaveris Rhœados.
Syrup of Red Poppies.

Take of the freſh red Poppy-flowers, a Pound; boiling Spring-water, three Pints: Let them ſtand together

ther one Night, then strain the Liquor, add to it two Pounds of white Sugar, and boil it up to a Syrup. *E.*

Syrupus Pectoralis.
The Pectoral Syrup.

ke of the Roots of *Florentine* Orris, and of Elicampane, each an Ounce and a half; of Liquorice, two Ounces; of the Flowers of Coltsfoot, the Herb Maidenhair, or in Defect of that *Trichomanes*, of the Leaves of Groundivy, each an Ounce; of fat Figs, twelve in Number; Spring-water, eight Pints. Boil to the Consumption of one Fourth, and to the strain'd Liquor add six Pounds of white Sugar. Boil to the Consistence of a Syrup. *E.*

his, as it should seem, deserves : Name of a Pectoral Syrup much :ter than the following, and appears to be a very good Medicine in Cough and Hoarseness.

Syrupus Pectoralis.
Pectoral Syrup.

ke of the Leaves of *English* Maidenhair dried, five Ounces; of Liquorice, four Ounces; of boiling Water, five Pints. Steep the Ingredients for some Hours, and, when the Liquor is strain'd off, dissolve in it a proper Quantity of double refined Sugar to make a Syrup. *L.*

ee *Syrupus Capilli Veneris.*

Syrupus è Floribus Persicæ.
Syrup of Peach-Blossoms.

his is made with the Infusion of fresh Peach-Blossoms, in the same Manner as the *Syrupus Papaveris Rheados. E.*

t is said to be a pretty Puke for ildren, and opens a little downards; for which Purpose it is much in Use. Its Dose is from two Drams to one Ounce.

Syrupus è Peto, sive Nicotiana.
Syrup of Tobacco.

Take two Drams of the Leaves of *Virginia* Tobacco; half an Ounce of shaved Liquorice; and six Ounces of boiling Spring-water: Let them infuse warm for a Night; then strain off the Liquor, put to it an equal Weight of Honey, and boil it into a Syrup. *E.*

This is omitted in the last Edition of the *Edinburgh* Dispensatory, and very prudently; for I know of no Use it is of, except for a Vomit, and we have much better and safer Emetics.

Syrupus Pæoniæ.
Syrup of Piony.

This is made with an Infusion of fresh Piony-flowers, after the same Manner as the *Syrupus Papaveris Rheados. E.*

The Virtues of this may be learn'd from those of Piony,

Syrupus Pulegii.
Syrup of Pennyroyal.

Take of the Leaves of common Pennyroyal, six Ounces; boiling Spring-water, three Pints: Let them infuse warm in a close Vessel for one Night; then strain off the Liquor, clarify it, and add thereto twice its own Weight of white Sugar, so as to make it into a Syrup without Boiling. *E.*

If the Physician who prescribes this Syrup has any Intention in so doing, it may be much better answer'd by an Infusion of the Herb, like Tea.

Syrupus Quinque Radicum.
Syrup of the five opening Roots.

Take of the five opening Roots, each two Ounces; Spring-water, three Quarts;

Quarts: Boil them together till a 3d Part of the Liquor be evaporated; then press out the Remainder, and with four Pounds of white Sugar boil it up to a Syrup. *E.*

The former *London* Dispensatory directs eight Ounces of Vinegar to be added to it at the latter End. This, with the Vinegar, makes a very grateful Syrup, and is frequently prescribed amongst Pectorals and Aperients.

Syrupus Rosarum Pallidarum.
Syrup of Damask-Roses.

This is made with a double Infusion of fresh Damask-Roses, after the Manner of the *Syrupus Papaveris Rheados. E.*

This is esteem'd gently laxative.

Syrupus Rosarum Solutivus.
Solutive Syrup of Roses.

Take the Decoction left after the Distillation of six Pounds of Damask-Roses, and five Pounds of double refined Sugar: Boil down the Decoction press'd out to three Pints, and set it by for a Night, that its Fæces may subside: Next Morning pour off the clear Liquor, and, adding the Sugar, make it into a Syrup, by boiling it away to the Weight of seven Pounds and a half. *L.*

This makes a tolerable good Purge for Children and weak People, and is often added in Prescriptions to Cathartic Decoctions and Infusions.

Syrupus de Rosis siccis.
Syrup of dried Roses.

Take of red Roses, half a Pound; and of boiling Spring-water, two Quarts: Let them steep together for a Night; then, after a little Boiling, strain off the Liquor, add thereto four Pounds of white Sugar, and boil it up to a Syrup. *E.*

Syrupus Sacchari.
Syrup of Sugar.

Take of white Sugar and Spring-water, each an equal Quantity; and boil them up to the Consistence of a Syrup. *E.*

This Syrup seems to be as good as most of the Alterative Syrups; that is, for nothing at all, for any medicinal Purpose of Consequence.

This is directed in the *London* Dispensatory under the Title of *Syrupus simplex.*

Syrupus Scilliticus.
Syrup of Squills.

Take of Vinegar of Squills, a Pint and a half; Cinnamon, Ginger, of each an Ounce; of double refined Sugar, three Pounds and a half. Steep the Spices for three Days in the Vinegar, and, when strained, make the Syrup by adding the Sugar. *L.*

In the *Edinburgh* Dispensatory the *Syrupus Scilliticus* is thus order'd:

Take of Vinegar of Squills, two Pints; of white Sugar, four Pounds. Make into a Syrup without Coction. *E.*

These seem to be intended to promote Expectoration, and assist in bringing up viscid Phlegm.

Syrupus è Spina Cervina.
Syrup of Buckthorn.

Take of the Juice of Buckthornberries ripe and fresh, one Gallon; Cinnamon, Ginger, Nutmegs, of each one Ounce; of double refined Sugar, seven Pounds. Set the Juice by a few Days, that its Fæces may separate; then strain it, and, in a small Quantity of it, infuse the Spices. Boil down the rest, towards the End adding that wherein the Spices have been infused, but strain'd from them, that the

he Whole may be reduced to two
Quarts; then add the Sugar, and
make the Syrup. *L.*

his is, in the *Edinburgh* Dispensa-
y, order'd to be made somewhat
erently under the Title of

*upus de Spina Cervina, seu Rham-
no Cathartico.*

Syrup of Buckthorn.

ke of the clarify'd Juice of ripe
Buckthorn-berries, three Quarts;
brown Sugar, four Pounds; and
boil them over a gentle Fire to a
Syrup; and, whilst it is warm,
mix therewith a Dram of the dif-
ill'd Oil of Cloves, received upon
a little Sugar. *E.*

et Syrup of Buckthorn be made
whatever Manner, it will always
e a very disagreeable Taste; so
t it is no great Matter whether
rse or fine Sugar is used. It is a
fk Cathartic, and is particularly
em'd for purging off the Water
a Dropsy; and is often added to
ative Decoctions, Infusions, and
lutions, in order to quicken their
eration. The Dose is an Ounce,
more, if given alone.

Syrupus à Symphyto.
Syrup of Comfrey.

ke the fresh Roots of the greater
Comfrey, and the fresh Leaves of
Plantain, of each half a Pound:
Bruise them together, and strongly press out their Juice: Upon the
Pressing pour a Quart of Spring-
water, and boil it to the Consumption of one Half; then strain off
the Liquor, and mix it with the
express'd Juice: Add thereto an
equal Weight of white Sugar, and
boil them to the Consistence of a
Syrup. *E.*

'his Syrup is intended as a gentle
kingent and Vulnerary.

Syrupus Violarum.
Syrup of Violets.

Take of Violets, fresh and well colour'd, two Pounds; of boiling
Water, five Pints. Steep the Flowers a whole Day in a Glass or
earthen Vessel glazed; then pour
off the Liquor, and strain it thro'
a fine Linnen Cloth, with Caution
not to press at all the Flowers.
Afterwards with a proper Quantity of double refined Sugar make
it into a Syrup. *L.*

This Syrup is of very little Consequence in Medicine, and therefore it
is not much Matter how it is made,
tho' it is much recommended by
some. See the Article *Viola* in the
Materia Medica.

Syrupus Zingiberis.
Syrup of Ginger.

Take of Ginger sliced thin, four
Ounces; of boiling Water, three
Pints. Let the Ginger steep some
Hours, and strain off the Liquor;
to which add the proper Quantity
of double refined Sugar to make
a Syrup. *L.*

This is a very agreeable Syrup.
The Virtues may be learn'd from
those of Ginger.

Of Honies, Jellies, *and* Juices.

Mel Ægyptiacum.
Ægyptian Honey.

Take of Verdigris powder'd very
fine, five Ounces; of Honey, the
Weight of fourteen Ounces; of
Vinegar, the Measure of seven
Ounces. Boil all together over a
gentle Fire, till the Mixture acquire a proper Consistence and
reddish Colour. After a Time a
grosser Part will subside from this
Mixture, the upper and more liquid

quid Part of which is call'd the *Ægyptian* Honey. *L.*

The Uses of this are entirely external. It serves to cleanse and deterge Ulcers, and keep down fungous Flesh.

The *Unguentum Ægyptiacum* of the *Edinburgh* Dispensatory is much the same as this.

Mel Elatines.

Honey of Fluellin.

Take of the depurated Juice of Female Fluellin, four Pints; of clarified Honey, four Pounds. Boil them together to a proper Consistence. *L.*

I have never known this used in any Intention whatever. The Virtues may be learn'd from those of the *Veronica Fæmina.*

Mel Helleboratum.

Honey of Hellebore.

Take of the Roots of white Hellebore dried and sliced, one Pound; of clarified Honey, three Pounds; of Water, four Pints. After steeping the Roots three Days in the Water, boil them a little while; then boil the Liquor, well press'd out and strain'd, with the Honey to a due Consistence. *L.*

This partakes pretty strongly of the Virtues of the white Hellebore, and may be given in Maniacal Cases. I have known it excite very violent Efforts to vomit, when added to Clysters, in which it may sometimes be a proper Ingredient.

Mel Mercuriale.

Honey of Mercury.

Take of the Juice of Mercury and Honey, each three Pounds; and boil them together, clearing away the Scum as it rises, to the Consistence of a Honey. *E.*

This is principally used as an Emollient in Clysters.

Mel Rosaceum.

Honey of Roses.

Take of red Rose-buds quick dried, and their Heels cut off, four Ounces; of boiling Water, three Pints; of clarified Honey, five Pounds. Steep the Roses some Hours in Water; then to the strain'd Liquor add the Honey, and boil to a proper Consistence. *L.*

The *Mel Rosatum* of the *Edinburgh* Dispensatory differs very little from this. It is esteem'd a Detergent, and is principally used in Gargarisms for Ulcers and Inflammations of the Mouth and Fauces.

Mel Solutivum.

Solutive Honey.

Take the Decoction remaining after the Distillation of six Pounds of Damask Roses: Take also of Cumin-seed a little bruised, an Ounce; of coarse Sugar, four Pounds; of Honey, two Pounds. Boil the Decoction, press'd out, to three Pints; adding, towards the End, the Seeds tied up in a Cloth; then gently boil it, with the Sugar and Honey, into the Consistence of a liquid Honey. *L.*

This seems principally intended for Clysters, and is proper as an Addition to Decoctions for that Purpose.

Oxymel ex Allio.

Oxymel with Garlick.

Take of Garlick sliced, one Ounce and a half; Caraway-seeds, Sweet Fennel-seeds, of each two Drams; of clarified Honey, ten Ounces; of Vinegar, half a Pint. Boil the Vinegar a little while in a glazed earthen Vessel, with the Seeds bruised; then add the Garlick, and cover the Vessel. After all is cold, press out the Liquor, and with the Heat of a *Balneum* dissolve in it the Honey. *L.*

This

This is intended as a Pectoral and expectorant, and may do Service in Redundance of viscid Phlegm.

Oxymel Pectorale.
Pectoral Oxymel.

ake of the Roots of Elecampane, and *Florentine* Orrice, each Half an Ounce: Slice, bruise, and boil them in a Quart of Spring-Water, till it comes to a Pint and a Half: To the strain'd Liquor add of unprepar'd Gum Ammoniac, an Ounce, dissolved in four Ounces of Vinegar; add also eight Ounces of Honey; then boil them together, scum the Matter and strain it. *E.*

This promises fair to be an excellent Pectoral and Expectorant; and must therefore be very good in Asthmas and Coughs, and wherever viscid Phlegm abounds.

Oxymel Scilliticum.
Oxymel of Squills.

ake of Honey, three Pounds; and of Vinegar of Squills, a Quart: Boil them together to a Syrup; observing to scum it during the Operation. *E.*

This is directed exactly in the same Manner, in the *London* Dispensary.

This is an Emetic, if exhibited in large Dose, and is a very good expectorant. But it is more frequently given in small Doses, two or three Drams, for Example; and corrected with strong Cinnamon Water, and some Pectoral Syrup, in order to prevent the *Nausea* which would otherwise excite.

Oxymel Simplex.
Simple Oxymel.

ake of Honey, two Pounds; Vinegar, a Pint; and boil them toge-

ther according to the Rules of Art.

This is exactly the same in the *London* Dispensatory. It is of considerable Use as a Pectoral and Expectorant, and is very properly added to resolvent Cataplasms, when the Intention is to discuss inflammatory Tumors.

Of JELLIES.

Gelatina Berberorum.
Jelly of Barberries.

Take of Barberries with their Stalks pick'd off, white Sugar, each a Pound. Boil with a gentle Heat to a due Consistence, and pass it thro' *Hippocrates*'s Sleeve. *E.*

This is a very agreeable cooling Acid, and very proper to moisten the Mouth and Fauces, in febrile Diseases; or to be drank, dissolv'd in warm Water.

Gelatina Cornu Cervi.
Jelly of Hartshorn.

Take of the Shavings of Hartshorn, half a Pound; Spring Water, three Quarts: Boil them over a gentle Fire, in a glaz'd earthen Vessel, till one Half is wasted; then strain off the Liquor, and add thereto six Ounces of white Sugar-Candy in Powder; four Ounces of *Spanish* White Wine, and an Ounce of Orange or Lemon Juice; after which, with a gentle Fire, boil all together to a thin Jelly. *E.*

This relates more to Cookery than Physic. The Uses may be learn'd from those of Hartshorn.

Gelatina seu Miva Cydoniorum.

Jelly of Quinces, or Quince Marmalade.

Take of the clarify'd Juice of Quince, three Pints; white Sugar

gar, a Pound; and boil them up to a Jelly, according to Art. *E.*

This is an Astringent, and is sometimes given in Diarrhœas and Dysenteries. But is more frequently employ'd in giving Consistence to a Bolus.

Gelatina Ribesiorum.
Jelly of Currants.

This is made of the Juice of Currants, in the same Manner as the Jelly of Barberries. *E.*

This is very cooling and agreeable, and of more Consequence in Medicine than is generally imagin'd. It is frequently given in febrile Heats, without any farther View than to cool the Mouth and Fauces. But dissolv'd in warm Water, or Ptisan, it is an admirable saponaceous and resolvent Medicine. And, farther, many Chronical Distempers may be cur'd by a copious and long continu'd Use of Jelly of Currants; for after a long Use it will excite a *Diarrhœa* of so salutary a Kind, that the Distemper will be reliev'd eminently, or totally cur'd. *Boerhaave* remarks that it acts just like the saponaceous Juices of the Spring Grass, which in some Time will purge a surfeited Horse, after it has resolv'd the Obstructions which cause the Distemper. And then the Horse grows fat, sleek, and healthful.

Of JUICES.

Succus Glycyrrhizæ.

Take any Quantity of Liquorice Root; bruise it, and pour thereon as much boiling Spring Water as will float three Inches above it: Digest for three Days; and, after a little Boiling, press out the Liquor, and evaporate it, with a gentle Heat, to a proper Consistence. *E.*

The Virtues of this may be known from those of Liquorice.

Succus Pruniorum sylvestrium, seu Acacia Germanica.

The Juice of Sloes, or the *German* Acacia.

Take any Quantity of the Juice of unripe Sloes, and exhale it to a due Consistence, over a gentle Fire. *E.*

This, as it is an Astringent, may be properly us'd, whenever the whole Habit, or any particular Part, is too much relax'd. The Dose is, according to *Boerhaave*, from six Grains to a Dram and Half.

Succi Antiscorbutici.

Juices against the Scurvy.

Take of the Juice of Garden Scurvy Grass, that of Brook-lime, that of Water Cresses, and that of *Seville* Oranges, each a Pint; and of white Sugar, ten Ounces: Mix them together, and clarify them, according to the Rules of Art, and then add of compound Horse Radish Water, half a Pint.

In the *London* Dispensatory it is thus directed:

Take of the Juice of Garden Scurvy Grass, a Quart; the Juice of Brook-lime and of Water Cresses, each a Pint; of the Juice of *Seville* Oranges, a Pint and a Quarter. These being mix'd, let them stand till the Dregs subside; then let the Juice be pour'd off clear and strain'd.

The Title expresses the Uses. If given to any Purpose, they should be taken twice or thrice a Day in large Quantities, and be long continu'd.

Rob Baccarum Sambuci.
Rob of Elder-Berries.

Let the depurated Juice of Elder-Berries be inspissated with a gentle Heat to a proper Consistence. *L.*

The

The *Edinburgh* Dispensatory directs this to be made by evaporating our Pounds of the Juice of ripe Eller Berries, with Half a Pound of Sugar; but it is esteem'd better without the Sugar. This is not so much attended to in regular Practice as it deserves to be. There is not a better Medicine in a common Cold; if a Spoonful is taken at Bed-time dissolv'd in Half a Pint of Water. What has been said of Jelly of Currants is also applicable to this; but this is of much greater Efficacy, and more extensive Use; being highly saponaceous, resolvent, and antiseptic.

Elaterium.

Slit ripe wild Cucumbers, and pass the Juice, very gently pressed out, through a very fine hair Sieve into a glazed Vessel; set it by some Hours, till its thicker Part shall have subsided: Then pour off as much of the thin Part of the Juice, as can conveniently be done, by inclining the Vessel, and draw away the rest by the Filtre: Let the thicker Part, which remains, be covered over with a linen Cloth, and dried either in the Sun or by a gentle Fire. *L.*

This is an excessively violent Cathartic and Hydrogogue, and is but seldom prescrib'd, because it operates so very powerfully. I have never known above five Grains given for a Dose, tho' some Authors mention a much larger. Its Use should be principally confin'd to Apoplexies and Lethargies, arising from a Redundance of Serum, and where milder Cathartics will not operate with Effect. It is a Medicine of very great Antiquity, for *Theophrastus* relates that he saw some two hundred Years old in the Possession of a Physician. Mr. *Boulduc* made a kind of *Elaterium*, which should seem to be preferable to this, and

milder, by drying the wild Cucumber very well, and reducing it, together with its Seeds, to a Powder, which he found a very good Hydragogue.

PRESERVES, CONSERVES, *and* SUGARS.

From the *Edinburgh* Dispensatory.

Preserved Angelica.

Take any Quantity of fresh Angelica Root, cut it to Pieces, take out the Pith, and steep it, for two Days, in proper Parcels of Spring Water, which are to be once or twice renewed. After this, let them boil a little; then pour off the Water; and add as much Syrup of Sugar as will rise two Inches above them. In a Day or two, boil them again gently, if there be Occasion, to exhale the superfluous Moisture; so as that the Syrup may remain of its due Consistence.

And after the same, or a similar Manner, the following Simples may be preserved, *viz.* the Roots of Eryngo, Elecampane, *Satyrion, Scorzonera,* and the greater Consound; as also the Peels of Oranges, Citrons, and Lemons.

Nutmegs and Ginger are brought to us ready preserved from *India.*

All Kinds of Fruit, Flowers, and Seeds are likewise preserved, either by means of a Syrup, or crusting them over with Sugar: But the Confectioner's Art can hardly be admitted a Part of Pharmacy.

Iron also is a Subject of this Operation.

Mars Saccharatus.

Candied Iron.

Take any Quantity of clean Filings of Iron, unprepared; throw them into a brass Kettle, hung over a very gentle Fire; and, by Degrees, pour to them twice their own

Weight of Sugar, boil'd to the Confistence of Candy: Keep the Kettle in constant Motion, so as that the Filings may be crusted over with the Sugar; Care being had to prevent their Running into Lumps.

Conserves of the Leaves of *Roman* Wormwood.

Garden Scurvy Grass,
Wood Sorrel.
Mint.
Rue.
of the Flowers of Rosemary.
Mallows.
Betony.
Red Roses.
of the yellow Part of Orange Peel.
of Hips.

Conserves may be made of any of these Subjects, according to the Rules of Art; they being just clear'd of their Stalks, Fibres, or the like, and bruised to a Pulp; then adding, by Degrees, during the Operation, thrice their own Quantity of white Sugar. But for the more juicy Simples, twice their Quantity of Sugar will suffice: And the Pulp of Hipps requires a much less Proportion.

From the *London* Dispensatory.

Conserves of the Leaves of Garden Scurvy Grass.

Spear-Mint.
Rue,
Wood-Sorrel.
Of the Tops of Sea Wormwood.
Of the Flowers of Lavender,
Mallows,
Rosemary,
Red Roses, while in Bud.
Of the external yellow Part of *Seville* Orange Peel.

The Leaves are to be plucked from their Stalks, and the Flowers from their Calix's; the external Rind of the Orange Peel should be scraped off with a Rasp, or Grater; every one of them, when thus prepared, is to be pounded in a Mortar with a wooden Pestle, first by itself, and then with the Addition of three times its Weight of double refined Sugar, till they are well incorporated together. *L.*

Conserve of Hips.

Take of the Pulp of ripe Hips, one Pound; of double refined Sugar, twenty Ounces; and mix them into a Conserve. *L.*

The principal Use of this is to give a Confistence to an Electuary, or Bolus.

Conserve of Sloes.

Scald the Sloes in Water to soften them, taking Care, their Skins are not broken; then take them out, and express their Pulp, which mix with thrice its Weight of double refined Sugar. *L.*

The Virtues of this may be learn'd from those of Sloes.

Candied Eryngo-Root.

Boil the Roots, till the Rind will easily peel off: When peel'd, slit them through the Middle, and the Pith being taken out, wash them three or four times in cold Water. Then take, for every Pound of Roots so prepared, two Pounds of double refined Sugar; dissolve the Sugar in Water, set it over a Fire, and, as soon as it begins to boil, put in the Roots, and continue the Boiling, till they become soft.

In the same Manner Angelica Stalks are candied.

Candied Orange Peel.

Soke the fresh Peels of *Seville* Oranges in Water, and change it often, till the Peels lose all Bitterness; then boil them with double refined Sugar, dissolved in Water, till they become soft and transparent.

Lemon-peel is likewise to be candied in the same Manner.

The

The Virtues of these may be learn'd from those of Orange and Lemon Peel. They are of very little Use medicinally.

SUGARS.

Saccharum Hordeatum, seu Penidiatum,
Barley Sugar.

This is made of white Sugar, boiled with Barley Water, till it acquires such a ductile Consistence, as that it may be drawn out, and fashioned with the Hands, into twisted Sticks, like Ropes. *E.*

This comes more properly under the Cognizance of the Confectioner than the Physician; and is too trifling to deserve any farther Remark.

Saccharum Rosarum Rubrum,
Red Sugar of Roses.

Take of white Sugar, a Pound; and of the Juice of red Roses, four Ounces; boil them together, over a gentle Fire, till the Juice is almost totally exhaled; then throw in an Ounce of the fine Powder of dried red Roses; and after this pour the whole upon a Marble, and form it into Lozenges, according to Art. *E.*

This is directed in a different Manner in the *London* Dispensatory, under the Title of

Saccharum Rosaceum.
Sugar of Roses.

Take of red Rose Buds, quick dried, and their white Heels cut off, one Ounce; of double refined Sugar, one Pound. Reduce the Roses and Sugar to Powder separately, then mix them, and with a little Water form Lozenges, to be dried with a gentle Heat.

These Preparations are somewhat astringent, but of too little Consequence to deserve farther Notice.

Tabella Diatragacanthi.
Lozenges of the Powder of Gum Tragacanth.

Take of white Sugar, a Pound; and of Rose Water, four Ounces; make a Solution over a gentle Fire; then add of the compound Powder of Gum Tragacanth, three Ounces; after which throw the whole upon a Marble, and fashion it into Lozenges. *E.*

The Virtues of this may be learn'd from those of Gum Tragacanth, if it has any worth Notice.

CHAP. VIII.

Of POWDERS.

GENERAL RULES *for making of* POWDERS.

I. PArticular Care must be had, that nothing rotten, decay'd, or impure, be mixed along with Powders; besides which, the Stalks and all the corrupted Parts of Plants are to be first pick'd out, and thrown away.

II. When dry Spices are powder'd, they should be sprinkled with a few Drops of some proper Water.

III. The moister Aromatics should be dried with a very gentle Heat, before they are reduced to Powder.

IV. Gums, and the other Things that grind with Difficulty, are to be mixed with the drier Ingredients; so as to pass the Sieve together.

V. Powders should be made only in small Quantities; and ought to be kept in well stopt Glasses.

Pulvis Antiepilepticus, de Gutteta dictus.

Powder against the Falling-Sickness.

Take of the Roots of white Dittany, Piony, wild Valerian, and Misletoe, each equal Parts. Mix and make a Powder. *E.*

A a a 3   This

This is so readily made *extempore,* that it should not seem necessary to make it a Shop Medicine; particularly because it is best when fresh made. It is, however, well enough calculated for the Intention its Title expresses.

The *Pulvis ad Guttetam* in the former *London* Dispensatory stood thus:

Take of white Dittany, Misletoe of the Oak, Contrayerva, *Virginia* Snake Root, and Male Piony-Roots; of the Male Piony-Seeds, of burnt Hartshorn, and Elk's-Hoof, of each two Drams; of wild Valerian Root, an Ounce; of red Coral, and human Skull, of each three Drams; of Jacinth Stone, a Dram; of Occidental Bezoar, a Dram and a half; of the Oriental, a Scruple; mix them into a Powder; to which may be added, at Pleasure, of Musk five Grains, and of the Leaves of beaten Gold, thirty.

Pulvis Epilepticus niger.

The black epileptic Powder.

Take of the *Talus,* or Ankle Bone of a Hare, and of Ivory, both calcin'd to Blackness, each five Drams; of the Roots of Swallow-Wort, Piony, and Valerian; of Hartshorn calcin'd without Fire, red Coral prepar'd, Elk's Hoof, Amber prepar'd, *Muscovy* Glass calcin'd, each a Dram and half; of the Shells of Oisters prepar'd without Fire, two Drams; of the Herb *Carduus Benedictus,* and the Seeds of Columbine, each a Dram; Extract of wild Poppies, a Dram and half; depurated Salt of Amber, and Salt of Hartshorn, each a Scruple; the Oils of Mace and Chamomile, each fifteen Grains. Mix and make a fine Powder.

This Medicine is much esteem'd in *Germany* for the Epilepsy, and all

Spasmodic, Hysteric, and Hypochondriac Disorders; the Colic from Flatulencies, Gripings, and the internal or blind Piles; and, farther, in the Worms, and Crudities in the intestinal Tubes of Children. It should be always given fresh prepar'd, because the principal Part of its Efficacy depends upon the black, empyreumatical Oil, contain'd in the Ingredients thus prepared, which loses its Virtue with Keeping. Dr. *Linden,* in a Pamphlet wrote upon the Subject of this Powder, recommends, as a great Improvement, the Substitution of certain Bones found within the Cranium of a Hog, calcin'd in such a Manner as to preserve the black Oil. See the Article *Porcus,* in the *Materia Medica.*

I have a very great Objection to these Medicines calculated against an Epilepsy, on Account of the Number of their Ingredients, and indeed against all others which are much compounded. For if one Ingredient is better than another, why should the Efficacy of that be impair'd, by adding one more insignificant. Thus in the *Pulvis Epilepticus* of the *Edinburgh* Dispensatory, if the Valerian is better than the Dittany, Piony, or Misletoe, I see no Reason why that should not be used alone without the others. The full Dose is said to be a Scruple; which should seem to be too little to answer any good Purpose.

Pulvis Antilyssus.

Powder against the Bite of a mad Dog.

Take of Ash-colour'd ground Liver Wort, two Ounces; of black Pepper, one Ounce. Beat them together into a Powder. *L.*

This is the celebrated Remedy for the Bite of a mad Dog, and has the Reputation of preventing its Effects. I have never yet known it experienc'd in Man, except where other Methods

Methods have been try'd at the same Time; so that it was not possible to know to what to ascribe the Cure. But I have frequently known it given to Dogs, and not often with Success. I have also been well inform'd, that a Man near *Smithfield*, another at *Northampton*, and another at *Bury St. Edmunds*, all took this Medicine from the first, with the utmost Caution and Regularity, and yet all dy'd mad. It was originally taken Notice of by *Dampier*, the celebrated Traveller, and was publish'd many Years ago by Sir *Hans Sloane* in the Philosophical Transactions.

Pulvis Ari compositus.

Compound Powder of Cuckowpint.

Take of the Root of Cuckowpint, fresh dried, two Ounces; the Root of the yellow Water Flag, the Root of burnt Saxifrage, of each one Ounce; prepared Crabs Eyes, Cinnamon, of each half an Ounce, of Salt of Wormwood, two Drams. Let all be beat into a Powder, which must be kept in a very close Vessel. *L.*

It is best to give this Medicine fresh made, because the *Arum* or Cuckowpint Root spoils by Keeping. It is esteem'd good in the cold Scurvy. But Practitioners should be very cautious in the Use of hot Antiscorbutics; because a continu'd Use of them will dry the Liver, so as to render it almost friable; and hence Jaundice, Dropsy, and Death; which are often ascrib'd to the Distemper, tho' more generally the Effects of the Medicines thus injudiciously taken.

Pulvis Bezoardicus.

Bezoardic Powder.

Take of the compound Powder of Crabs Claws, a Pound; of Oriental Bezoar prepared, an Ounce. Make them altogether into a Powder. *L.*

In former Dispensatories, the *Bezoar* was an Ingredient in the *Gascoign's Powder*, or *Pulvis è Chelis Cancrorum compositus*. But in the last Dispensatory the College have directed it without Bezoar, and have order'd this for those who have an Opinion of the *Bezoar*. This was once a Medicine much in Use, and given in almost every Fever; but is at present pretty much out of Fashion, for so I must call it, because nothing but Fashion could support the Credit of so insignificant and trifling a Medicine, in which the Bezoar is of little Consequence as any of the other Ingredients. It is, however, of some Service to the Compounder, because, when used, it is generally repeated every three or four Hours. The Medicine which seems to bid fair for succeeding this in Practice, is *Raleigh's* Cordial, which tho' it answers the End of the Compounder as well, or perhaps better, is I am afraid not so innocent with Respect to the Patient.

Pulvis è Bolo compositus sine Opio.

Compound Powder of Bole without Opium.

Take of *Armenian* Bole, or of *French* Bole, half a Pound; of Cinnamon, four Ounces, Tormentil Root, Gum Arabic. of each three Ounces; of long Pepper, half an Ounce. Make them into a Powder. *L.*

This is intended as an Astringent.

Pulvis è Bolo compositus cum Opio.

Compound Powder of Bole with Opium.

Take of Opium strain'd three Drams, then let it be a little dried, that it may be commodiously reduced to Powder; and add it to the Species of the preceding Composition, before they are pulveriz'd, that they may be all beat together into a Powder. *L.*

This is like the preceding, an Astringent, and more powerful for restraining Fluxes of all Kinds, on Account of the *Opium.* I don't know what Service the long Pepper can be of, in either.

Pulvis Cephalicus.

Cephalic Powder.

Take of the Leaves of Asarabacca, Betony, and Marjoram, each equal Quantities. Mix and make a Powder. *E.*

A Powder much like this is directed in the *London* Dispensatory, under the Title of

Pulvis Sternutatorius.

Sneezing Powder.

Take the dried Leaves of Asarabacca, of Marjoram, of *Syrian* Mastick, Thyme dried, Lavender Flowers, of each an equal Weight, and rub all into a Powder. *L.*

Both these are intended as Errhines, to clear the *Membrana Pituitaria*, and by the convulsive Motion of Sneezing, and the subsequent Discharge, to relieve the Head.

Pulvis è Cerussa compositus.

Compound Powder of Cerusse.

Take of Cerusse five Ounces, of Sarcocol an Ounce and a half, of Gum Tragacanth half an Ounce. Make all into a Powder. *L.*

This is substituted for the *Trochisci Albi Rhasis.* It is entirely for external Use. It is said to be good in Inflammations, and to repel hot corrosive Humours; and it is us'd in Collyrias, Injections, and Lotions.

Pulvis è Chelis Cancrorum compositus.

Compound Powder of Crabs Claws.

Take of the Tips of Crabs Claws prepared, one Pound; prepared Pearls, red Coral prepared, of each three Ounces. Mix all together. *L.*

See the Remarks on the *Pulvis Bezoardicus,* above.

In the *Edinburgh* Dispensatory it is thus directed:

Take of Crabs Eyes, and red Coral, of each an Ounce; the black Tips of Crabs Claws, two Ounces. Mix and make a Powder.

I think both these not at all improv'd by leaving out the Amber; but even with that they are too trifling to deserve a serious Remark. They can only act as Absorbents, which most of the Testacea singly will do as well.

Pulvis Contrayervae compositus.

Compound Powder of Contrayerva.

Take of the compound Powder of Crabs Claws, a Pound and a half; of Contrayerva Root, five Ounces. Make them into a Powder. *L.*

I am far from thinking this Medicine any Improvement on the *Pulvis è Chelis Cancrorum compositus.* The best Character that can be given of the last is, that 'tis innocent; but the Contrayerva, in this, renders it dangerous, and in many Cases of fatal Consequence; because it increases Heat, when there was before too much; and may excite a symptomatical Sweat, which is always prejudicial, instead of one that is critical and salutary. It may, however, be of some Use, to continue or promote a critical *Diaphoresis*, when Nature has shewn the Necessity for it, by exciting it spontaneously. But in all Cases we should be ascertain'd that the Sweat is critical, before we attempt to increase or continue it; and then there is seldom any Occasion for such Helps. This Medicine may be of Service in relax'd Habits, abounding with an Acid in the *Primae Viae.* But, whenever there is any extraordinary Heat, it should be used with Caution.

on. It anſwers very well the luxative Views of the Compounder, ecauſe 'tis generally very frequently peated.

In the *Edinburgh* Diſpenſatory, the ulvis Contrayervæ compoſitus ſtands us:

ake of Contrayerva Root, half an Ounce ; of *Virginian* Snake Root, a Dram and half ; Cochineal, one Dram ; *Engliſh* Saffron, half a Dram ; of *Armenian* Bole, three Drams ; of the compound Powder of Crabs Claws, ſeven Drams. Make a Powder.

Pulvis Cornachini.

Cornachine Powder.

ake of Diaphoretic Antimony, Cream of Tartar, and Scammony, each a like Quantity ; and make thereof a Powder. *E.*

This and the *Pulvis Comitis War-ʒicenſis* only differ in the Proporon of the Ingredients to each other. he latter is directed with two unces of ſulphurated Scammony, ne Ounce of Diaphoretic Antiony, and half an Ounce of the ryſtals of Tartar. In other Diſenſatories, alſo, the Proportion of le Ingredients in the *Pulvis Corna-hini* differs from that in this. I ſteem it one of the beſt Shop Ca-artics we have. But the Preſcriber lay extemporaneouſly alter the Proortion of the Ingredients, accord-g to the different Intentions he as in View. Thus, if he intends ſhould act principally upon the tomach and Inteſtines, the Proporon of the Scammony ſhould be rge. 'Tis very probable that the ryſtals or Cream of Tartar may pen the Scammony, be impregnated ith ſome of its Virtues, convey lem into the Blood, and thus make lem operate in the Urinary Paſſages. Vhen, therefore, the Preſcriber inʒnds that the Medicine ſhould act

in this Manner, he will do well to increaſe the Proportion of the Cream or Cryſtals of Tartar. Experience has taught me, that Diaphoretic Antimony is not the inert Calx it is now faſhionable to repreſent it. On the contrary, it will operate powerfully, and with great Effect, if judiciouſly adminiſter'd. In the preſent Caſe, 'tis not unlikely, that the Diaphoretic Antimony may open the Scammony more than the Cryſtals of Tartar could do, and lead it thus open'd into the moſt remote Series of Veſſels and Glands, where it may do more Service than in the inteſtinal Tube. But, Reaſoning apart, I know for certain, that not only this Medicine, but many other Cathartics, operate very differently, and with very different Effects, when mix'd with Diaphoretic Antimony, from what they do without it.

Pulvis è Scammonio compoſitus.

Compound Powder of Scammony.

Take of Scammony, five Ounces ; of burnt Hartſhorn prepared, three Ounces. Grind them carefully together into a Powder. *L.*

This is ſubſtituted in the Room of the *Pulvis Cornachini*. But I apprehend the Omiſſion of the Cream or Cryſtals of Tartar, and Diaphoretic Antimony, to be no Advantage to the Medicine, for Reaſons given in the Notes to the *Pulvis Cornachini*.

Pulvis Diaromatum.

The Powder of Aromatics.

Take of Canella Alba, or wild Cinnamon ; of the Leſſer Cardamoms, Mace, and Ginger, each equal Parts. Mix and make a Powder.

This is added in the laſt Edition of the *Edinburgh* Diſpenſatory, where it ſeems to be ſubſtituted for the *Species Diambræ*, or *Pulvis Diambræ.*

bra. It seems a very good aromatic, cordial, stomachic Powder.

In the *London* Dispensatory it is thus directed under the Title of

Species Aromatica.

Aromatic Species.

Take of Cinnamon, two Ounces; the Lesser Cardamom-seeds, freed from their Husks, Ginger, Long Pepper, of each one Ounce. Make all into a Powder, by beating them together. *L.*

Pulvis Diasennæ.

Compound Powder of Senna.

Take of the Leaves of Senna, and Cream of Tartar, each two Ounces; of Scammony and Ginger, each half an Ounce: Make them into a Powder. *E.*

This is a Cathartic; but not very necessary for a Shop Medicine, as something of the same Kind may be easily prescrib'd extemporaneously. In the *London* Dispensatory it is thus directed, under the Title of

Pulvis è Sena compositus.

Compound Powder of Sena.

Take Leaves of Sena, Crystals of Tartar, of each two Ounces; of Scammony, half an Ounce; Cloves, Cinnamon, Ginger, of each two Drams. Powder the Scammony by itself, the rest altogether, and then mix them. *L.*

Pulvis Diatessaron.

Powder of four Ingredients.

Take of the Roots of Round Birthwort and Gentian, of Bay-berries and Myrrh, each two Ounces: Make them into a Powder; whereof, by the Addition of two Ounces of Ivory Shavings, is made the

Pulvis Diapente; or,

Powder of five Ingredients. *E.*

Vegetius, in his *Mulomedicina*, pre-scribes this as a Medicine of Consequence in the Diseases of Cattle. I never knew it used for Man.

Pulvis Diatragacanthi frigidus.

The compound, cooling Powder of Gum Tragacanth.

Take of Gum Tragacanth, an Ounce; Gum Arabic, five Drams; Starch, Liquorice, white Poppy-seed, of each two Drams; and the Root of Marshmallow, half an Ounce: Make them into a Powder. *E.*

This is a cooling and agglutinating Medicine, and is given when there is a considerable Acrimony of the Humours, in Stranguries, Coughs, and sometimes in Hectics; but is a Composition of no great Consequence.

In the *London* Dispensatory it stands thus, under the Title of

Pulvis è Tragacantha compositus.

Compound Powder of Gum Dragant.

Take of Gum Tragacanth, Gum Arabic, Marshmallow Roots, of each an Ounce and a half; Starch, Liquorice, of each half an Ounce; of double refined Sugar, three Ounces. Reduce all together into a Powder. *L.*

The Difference betwixt these two is not of Consequence enough to deserve a Remark.

Pulvis Hieræ Picræ.

Powder of Hiera Picra.

Take of *Succotrine* Aloes, four Ounces; the Lesser Cardamoms, and *Virginia* Snake-root, of each half an Ounce: Mix them, and make into a Powder.

When the *Hiera Picra* is made for the Sake of the Tincture, the Aloes only need be pulverized, and the other Ingredients well bruised. *E.*

he former *London* Dispensatory
od thus, under the Title of

Species Hiera Picra.

of Cinnamon, Zedoary, Afa-
n, the Lesser Cardamom-Seeds,
d Saffron, of each six Drams;
chineal, a Scruple; of the best
oes, twelve Ounces; and let
m all be made into a Powder
gether.

Hiera Picra.

Hiera Picra.

of the Gum extracted from
ccotrine Aloes, one Pound; of
ld-Cinnamon-bark, three Ounces.
wder them separately, and then
x them. *L.*

erience alone must determine
her this is better than the *Spe-
liera Picra* of the last *London
nsatory*; or whether the Com-
of the present have been more
us of Elegance and Taste than
ficacy, in this Composition.

Pulvis è Myrrha compositus.

mpound Powder of Myrrh.

of the dried Leaves of Rue,
ttany of *Crete*, Myrrh, of each
Ounce and a half; Afa Fœtida,
gapenum, *Russia* Castor, Opo-
nax, of each an Ounce. Beat
together into a Powder. *L.*

s is substituted for the *Trochisci
yrrha*, and is excellent for pro-
g the Uterine Discharges, and
xpulsion of the Fœtus.

Pulvis ad Partum.

wder to promote Delivery.

of Borax, half an Ounce;
ftor and Saffron, of each a
am and a half: Mix them, and
ke a Powder; to which add of
a distill'd Oil of Cinnamon, eight
ops; and of the distill'd Oil of
nber, six Drops; and mix all
gether. *E.*

s is excellent for promoting De-

livery, where forcing Medicines are
proper, and no Hæmorrhage is apprehended.

Pulvis Stypticus.

Styptic Powder.

Take of Roche Alum, half an Ounce;
and of Dragon's Blood, two Drams.
Mix them into a Powder. *E.*

This is said to be invented by *Helvetius*. It is a most excellent Styptic, and inferior to nothing in checking too copious Discharges of the
Menses, or other Hæmorrhages. It
may properly enough be taken with
Tincture of Roses.

Pulvis è Succino compositus.

Compound Powder of Amber.

Take prepared Amber, Gum Arabic,
of each ten Drams; Juice of the
Rape of Cistus, Balaustines, *Japan*
Earth, of each five Drams; of
Olibanum, half an Ounce; of
strain'd Opium, a Dram. Reduce
all into a Powder. *L.*

This is substituted for the *Trochisci
de Carabe* of former Dispensatories,
and seems intended for an Astringent, principally to check Fluxes;
but is of no great Use.

Pulvis Vermifugus.

Worm-Powder.

Take of the Leaves of the Female
Southernwood, of the Flowers of
Tansey, and of Worm-seed and
Coralline, each half an Ounce:
Mix and make them into a Pow-
der; whereto add of the distill'd
Oils of Rue and Savin, received
upon a little Sugar; each twenty
Drops; and mix all together. *E.*

The Title of this Medicine expresses its Uses.

Species è Scordio sine Opio.

Species of Scordium, or Water Germander, without Opium.

Take of Bole Armenic, or of *French*
Bole, four Ounces; of Scordium,
or

or Water-Germander, two Ounces; of Cinnamon, an Ounce and a half; Storax ftrain'd, Roots of Tormentil, Biftort, Gentian, Leaves of Dittany of *Crete*, Galbanum ftrain'd, Gum Arabic, Red Rofes, of each one Ounce; Long Pepper, Ginger, of each half an Ounce. Beat all into a Powder. *L.*

This is fubftituted for the *Species* for the *Confectio Fracaftorii,* the Opium being omitted, as the whole Compofition might have been, without any Difadvantage to the Practice of Phyfic. For it was originally, and ftill continues to be, a very unimportant Medicine, capable of anfwering no one Intention, which might not be provided for much better by extemporaneous Prefcription. It is intended as a Reftringent,

Species è Scordio cum Opio.

Species of Scordium, or Water-Germander with Opium.

Take of ftrain'd Opium, three Drams;

and add this to the former Species while they are pounding together; it being firft a little dried, that it may the more commodiously be beaten to Powder. *L.*

This is fubftituted for the *Diafcordium,* or *Confectio Fracaftorii.* I have never yet known this ufed. But with Refpect to the *Diafcordium,* a Medicine very much in Practice, I have never yet feen any good Effect from it, but what might have been expected from the Opium alone; and I think Opium a much better Medicine without any Addition. I muft confefs, that this feems to be a better Medicine than the *Diafcordium;* but nothing can be a more melancholy Proof of the wretched and uncertain State of Phyfic, than not only to fee fuch infignificant and unmeaning Compofitions in all the *European* Difpenfatories, but alfo to hear them mentioned with fome Degree of Veneration.

CHAP. IX.

Of Electuaries, Confections, Antidotes, &c.

GENERAL RULES *for making* **ELECTUARIES.**

I. THE Rules, laid down for making Decoctions and Powders, muft alfo be underftood to regard the Decoctions and Powders of Electuaries.

II. The Gums, infpiffated Juices, and other Ingredients that are not pulverifable, muft be diffolved in the Liquor prefcribed; the Powders being put in by Degrees, and the Whole briskly ftirr'd together, fo as to make a fmooth and uniform Mixture.

III. Aftringent Electuaries, and thofe wherein the Pulp of Fruits is an Ingredient, are to be made up in fmall Quantities; the fuperfluous Moifture of fuch Pulps being exhaled over a gentle Fire, before they are mix'd in with the reft.

Confectio Alkermes.

Confection of Alkermes.

Take of the Syrup of Kermes, three Pounds; and evaporate it, with a gentle Heat, to the Confiftence of Honey; then add to it the following Ingredients, reduced to very fine Powder;

owder; Cinnamon, and Yellow aunders, each six Drams; Cochieal, three Drams; Saffron, a Dram and a half; and mix them together. *E.*

his is directed in a different Manin the *London* Dispensatory, s:

ke of the Juice of Kermes, varm'd and strain'd, three Pounds; of Damask Rose-water, six Ounces n Measure; of Oil of Cinnamon, half a Scruple; of double refin'd Sugar, one Pound. Melt the Sugar, by a Bath-heat, into a Syrup with the Rose-water; then add the Kermes-juice, and, after it is cold, the Oil of Cinnamon. *L.*

his is a very agreeable and reing Cordial, and will answer much ter Purposes than Cardiac Was, without any of their bad Conuences. It is principally used in king up Boles; but may be emy'd for much better Purposes.

Confectio Cardiaca.
The Cordial Confection.

ke fresh Rosemary-tops, Juniperberries, of each a Pound; the LesserCardamom-seeds, freed from their Husks, Zedoary, Saffron, of each half a Pound: Draw a Tincture with about a Gallon and a half of Proof Spirit. Reduce, by a gentle Heat, this Tincture strain'd nearly to the Weight of two Pounds and a half; then finish the Electuary by adding the following Species, very finely powder'd, *viz.* of the compound Powder of Crabsclaws, sixteen Ounces; Cinnamon, Nutmeg, of each two Ounces; of Cloves, an Ounce; of double refined Sugar, two Pounds. *L.*

his is substituted for the celebrated nfection of Sir *Walter Raleigh*, or her is this Confection reduced rer the original Receipt of the thor. It is at present a Medicine ch in Vogue as a Cordial, and is nded with much less Inconve-

nience than Drams. But I must confess I have not been so fortunate as ever to have seen any Effects from it, sufficient to make it worth Preparing, or even Mentioning, unless it be to give some Cautions with respect to its Use. In debauch'd Constitutions, those vitiated by Spirituous Liquors, or relax'd by Accident or Chronical Diseases, and abounding with Acidities and Flatulences, it may be of Service, as a cordial warming Balsamic. But where-ever the Fibres are too rigid, the Heat too intense, and the Humours are inclined to an alcaline Putrefaction, all which happens in most acute Diseases, this Medicine must be extremely prejudicial, as it increases the Heat, Rigidity, and Tendency to Putrefaction; however, it may give a little present Relief, by raising the Spirits and warming the Stomach; and if it raises a Sweat, before the offending Humours are, in the Phrase of *Hippocrates*, concocted, or, in other Words, sufficiently attenuated, and disposed to pass thro' the cutaneous Pores, it must do Mischief in Proportion to the Degree of Sweat it excites, and the Quantity of the fine diluting Lymph it expels. And, when this Attenuation or Concoction is brought about, such Helps as this Medicine will afford are not wanting to compleat a Cure. *Hippocrates*, the Prince of Physicians, never advises the Use of heating Medicines in the Cure of acute Distempers. *Sydenham*, the modern *Hippocrates*, learn'd from Observation the bad Effects of such Remedies; and *Boerhaave* absolutely rejected them in such Cases. But, had they all approved them, I could not have so far distrusted my own Senses as to submit to their Opinion; for I have met with Cases where Patients have, in all Appearance, been much relieved by Evacuations; but upon the Repetition of a few Doses of this very Medicine, or something of the same Nature, the Heat has been

been violently increased, the Tongue has grown black, and a Delirium has come on, succeeded by Death, whilst the Patient has all the Time sweated profusely at every Pore. I am sensible that heating Medicines were originally brought into Practice by the Chymical Physicians, and a false Theory; but I am inclined to believe that Artifice has had a great Share in their Introduction, and Custom and Inattention have continued them; for their Use undoubtedly renders more Medicines, and more Attendance necessary than any other Method, and protracts a Fever, which would, in all Probability, terminate in a few Days, to almost as many Weeks. If Men were Statues, such Treatment would be only wicked; but when rational Creatures, endued with Sensibility, are designedly tortured by such a Prostitution of Science, Language is too barren to represent such Conduct in its proper Colours.

Confectio Paulina.

The Confection called Paulina.

Take Costus, or in its stead Zedoary, Cinnamon, Long Pepper, Black Pepper, strain'd Galbanum, strain'd Opium, Russia Castor, of each two Ounces; of the simple Syrup, boiled to the Confistence of Honey, an equal Weight to thrice the Species. Mix carefully the Opium, first dissolved in Wine, with the Syrup warm'd; then to the Storax and Galbanum, melted together, add by Degrees the Syrup, while it remains warm: Afterwards sprinkle in the other Species reduced to Powder. *L.*

This Medicine is the *Confectio Archigenis*, brought back nearly to the Form it is found in, and the Name it is call'd by, *Galen.* It is a very warm Opiate, but should seem to be

a very trifling Composition, of but little Use in Practice.

Electuarium Antidysentericum.

Electuary against a Dysentery.

Take of Dioscordium, two Ounces; of the Balsam of *Lucatellus*, one Ounce. Mix into an Electuary.

As there are many better Medicines for a Dysentery, this does not seem of much Consequence. It may, however, be of some Service when it is proper to check a Diarrhœa, or Dysentery, which requires great Judgment to determine. These Distempers are of great Emolument to the Venders of Medicines; for when stopp'd, without removing the Cause, they will certainly return at Intervals for Years, and perhaps for ever, and require more Medicines at every Return, without End.

Electuarium è Baccis Lauri.

The Electuary of Bay-berries.

Take of the Conserve of Rue, two Ounces; preserved Ginger, one Ounce; Bay-berries, half an Ounce; Zedoary, two Drams; Russian Castor, one Dram; Chymical Oil of Fennel, ten Drops; Syrup of Orange-peel, a sufficient Quantity to make an Electuary. *E.*

This is principally used as a Carminative in Clysters, in order to expel Flatulencies.

In the *London* Dispensatory it stands thus:

Electuarium è Baccis Lauri.

Electuary of Bay-berries.

Take the Leaves of Rue dried, Caraway-seeds, Common Parsley-seeds, Bay-berries, of each an Ounce; of Sagapenum, half an Ounce; Black Pepper, Russia Castor, of each two Drams; of clarified Honey, thrice the Weight of the Species, when powder'd. Mix

x the Species with the Honey
s an Electuary. *L.*

Electuarium Cardiacum.
The Cordial Electuary.

of the Conserve of Rosemary,
d of red Roses, each an Ounce
d a half; candied Orange-peel,
d Nutmeg, of each an Ounce;
eserved Ginger, six Drams;
infection of Alkermes, half an
nce; the distill'd Oil of Cinna-
on, twenty Drops; and Syrup
Cloves, enough to make the
hole into an Electuary, accord-
g to the Rules of Art. *E.*

e Remarks made upon the *Con-*
Cardiaca are equally proper
respect to this Composition;
this seems preferable to that ce-
ted Medicine.

Electuarium è Casia.
Electuary of Casia.

e the solutive Syrup of Roses,
e Pulp of Casia fresh extracted,
f each half a Pound; of Manna
ve Ounces; of the Pulp of Ta-
arinds, one Ounce. Rub the
Manna in a Mortar, and with a
entle Heat dissolve it in the Sy-
up; then add the Pulps, and, the
eat being continued, reduce the
Whole to a proper Consistence. *L.*

e *Edinburgh* Dispensatory has a
mposition not unlike this, under
Title of

Diacassia.

te of *Casia Fistularis*, twelve
Ounces; of Tamarinds, six Oun-
es; of *Calabrian* Manna, eight
Ounces; Syrup of pale Roses, one
Pound. Dissolve the Manna in
ot Water, and strain it; then
vaporate it together with the Sy-
up, to the Consistence of Honey,
nd afterwards mix in the Pulps,
nd make an Electuary.

th these are gentle Purges, but
y unmeaning Compositions, and

what might be very well omitted,
because the Ingredients are so readily
mix'd extemporaneously.

Diascordium.

Take the Leaves of Scordium, red
Roses, Cinnamon, Bole Armoniac, and *Japan* Earth, of each
an Ounce; the Roots of Bistort,
Gentian, and Tormentil; the
Leaves of *Cretan* Dittany, Gum
Arabic, *Storax Calamita*, and
Galbanum, of each half an Ounce;
long Pepper and Ginger, of each
two Drams; Opium, a Dram and
a half; Syrup of Diacodium,
boil'd to the Consistence of Honey, thrice the Weight of all the
Powders; Canary Wine, half a
Pint; Mix them together, so as
to make an Electuary according
to the Rules of Art. *E.*

This is directed thus in the *London*
Dispensatory, under the Title of

Electuarium è Scordio.
Electary of Scordium, or Water
Germander.

Take any Quantity of the Species of
Scordium, or Water Germander
with Opium, and thrice their
Weight of Diacodium, boiled to
the Thickness of Honey. Mix
the Species with the Syrup into an
Electuary. *L.*

See the Remarks upon the *Species è*
Scordio. With Respect to the Change
of *Diacodium* instead of Honey, it
may be much doubted whether this
is an Improvement or not. Honey
by its Fermentation induces a great
Alteration in the Ingredients of this
Composition, and probably renders
the Opium a better Medicine. It is
a Detergent, and possess'd of very
considerable Virtues, to those who
can bear it, which some cannot. I
have long esteem'd the *Diascordium,*
as 'tis generally us'd, a very pernicious, and often dangerous Medicine.

cine. But 'tis lefs fo with the Honey than with *Diacodium.* For Honey renders it lefs narcotic and aftringent, and fomewhat detergent; whereas *Diacodium* makes it more narcotic and aftringent. Upon the Whole, this Compofition feems very infignificant; for if it is meant as an Aftringent, lefs complex and more efficacious Medicines may be contrived extemporaneoufly; if as an Opiate, crude Opium without any Addition will anfwer better Pupofes, under the Management of the Judicious, and is lefs naufeous to the Patient. But a falfe Theory, and Inattention to Experience, has fupported the Character of this, as well as many other Medicines equally trifling.

Electuarium Lenitivum.

Lenitive Electuary.

Take of dried Figs one Pound; and of the Leaves of Sena eight Ounces; the Pulps of Tamarinds, of Cafia, and of *French* Prunes, of each half a Pound; of Coriander Seeds, four Ounces; of Liquorice three Ounces; of double refin'd Sugar, two Pounds and a half. Reduce the Sena with the Coriander Seed to Powder, and feparate by the Sieve ten Ounces; boil the reft with the Figs and Liquorice in two Quarts of Water, till it is boiled half away, then ftrain and prefs it out; let the ftrained Liquor be evaporated, to the Weight of a Pound and a half, or a little lefs; afterwards add the Sugar to make a Syrup; this Sugar mix gradually with the Pulps; and laftly ftir in the Powder before feparated by the Sieve. *L.*

In the *Edinburgh* Difpenfatory it ftands thus, under the Title of

Electuarium Lenitivum pro Clyftere.

Lenitive Electuary for Clyfters.

Take of the Root of Polypody of the Oak, two Ounces; the Leaves

of Mercury, Fœnugreek Seed, and Linfeed, of each an Ounce; Spring Water three Quarts: Boil them together till one half is exhaled; adding, towards the End of the Operation, two Ounces of Senna Leaves, and half an Ounce of Coriander Seed; then prefs out the Liquor, and put to it two Pounds of Honey; boil it to the Confiftence of a thick Syrup; and add thereto a Pound of the Pulp of *Damafcus* Prunes; and half a Pound of the Pulp of *Caffia fiftularis*; and make all together into an Electuary. *E.*

Thefe purge very gently, and are convenient enough to add in Clyfters. Internally they are more proper to prevent Coftivenefs, than to be exhibited as regular Purges. But I don't know any End they can ferve, which Manna alone will not anfwer. The College have thought fit to change the commonly receiv'd Name of *Electuarium* for that of *Electarium*, for Reafons too trifling with Refpect to the Practice of Phyfic, to enquire into.

Mithridatium five Confectio Damocratis.

Mithridate, or *Damocrates*'s Confection.

Take of Cinnamon fourteen Drams, of Myrrh eleven Drams, Agaric, Spikenard, Ginger, Saffron, Seeds of Treacle Muftard, or of *Mithridate* Muftard, Frankincenfe, *Chio* Turpentine, of each ten Drams; Camels Hay, Coftus, or in its Stead Zedoary, *Indian Leaf*, or in its Stead Mace, *French* Lavender, long Pepper, Seeds of Hartwort, Juice of the Rape of Ciftus, ftrained Storax, Opponax, ftrained Galbanum, Balfam of *Gilead*, or in its Stead, exprefled Oil of Nutmegs, *Ruffia* Caftor, of each an Ounce, Poley Mountain, Water Germander, the Fruit of the

he Balſam Tree, or in its Stead
ubebs, white Pepper, Seeds of
he *Daucus* of *Crete*, Bdellium
rained, of each ſeven Drams;
eltic Nard, Gentian Root, Leaves
f Dittany of *Crete*, red Roſes,
eeds of *Macedonian* Parſley, the
ſſer Cardamom Seeds, freed from
heir Huſks, ſweet Fennel, Gum
rabic, Opium ſtrained, of each
ve Drams; Root of the ſweet
lag, Root of wild Valerian, A-
iſeed, Sagapenum ſtrained, of
ach three Drams; Spignel, Saint
ohn's Wort, Juice of *Acacia*, or
i its Stead *Japon* Earth, the Bel-
es of Scinks, of each two Drams
nd a half; of clarified Honey thrice
he Weight of all the reſt. Diſſolve
he Opium firſt in a littleWine, and
hen mix it with the Honey made
ot; in the mean Time, melt to-
ether, in another Veſſel, the
albanum, Storax, Turpentine,
nd the Balſam of *Gilead*, or the
xpreſſed Oil of Nutmeg, conti-
ually ſtirring them round that
hey may not burn, and as ſoon as
heſe are melted, add to them the
ot Honey, firſt by Spoonfuls,
nd afterwards more freely; laſtly
hen this Mixture is near cold
dd by Degrees the reſt of the
pecies reduced to Powder. L.

is celebrated Medicine ſtands thus
ted in the *Edinburgh* Diſpenſa-
, under the Title of

Mithridatium Damocratis.

Mithridate of *Damocrates.*

e of Myrrh, Saffron, Agaric,
inger, Cinnamon, Spikenard,
ale Frankincenſe, and the Seeds
f Treacle Muſtard, each ten
rams; thoſe of Hartwort, Opo-
alſamum (or Blſam of *Peru*)
quinanth, Flowers of *Arabian*
tœchas, Coſtus (or Zedoary)
albanum, *Cyprus* Turpentine,
ng Pepper, Caſtor, Hypo-

ciſtis; *Storax Calamita;* Opoponax, and *Indian* Leaf, of each
an Ounce; *Caſſia Lignea*, Poley
Mountain, white Pepper, Leaves
of Scordium, Seeds of *Cretan*
Daucus, Carpobalſamum (or Cubebs) Troches of *Cyperus*, and
Bdellium, of each ſeven Drams;
Celtic Spikenard, Gum Arabic,
Macedonian Parſley Seed, Opium,
the leſſer Cardamoms, Fennel
Seed, Gentian Root, red Roſes,
and Dittany of *Crete*, of each five
Drams; Aniſeed, the Roots of
Aſarabacca, *Acorus verus*, Phu,
(or wild Valerian) and Sagapenum,
of each three Drams; the Root
of Spignel, true Acacia (or the
the *German*) the Belly Part of
Scinks, and the Seed of St. *John's*
Wort, of each two Drams and a
a half; of clarified Honey, thrice
the Weight of all the Powders;
and *Canary* Wine, enough to diſſolve the Gums and Juices: Mix
all together, and make an Electuary, according to the Rules of
Art. *E.*

I only inſert theſe out of Deference
to the Compilers of the *London* and
Edinburgh Diſpenſatories. But could
have wiſh'd that they had been left
out of both; for it is a Reproach to
Phyſic, to ſee ſuch unmeaning and
random Compoſitions in Diſpenſatories, which have the Sanction of
public Authority, after all the boaſt-
ed Improvements in Anatomy, and
the Theory and Practice of Medicine.
Such Remedies, if it were proper to
call them ſo, can anſwer no one Intention, which may not be better provided for by a more ſcientific Combination of ſome few of their Ingredients; and this would render the
Art of healing leſs ridiculous to Men
of Senſe and Knowledge, tho' leſs
myſterious to the Ignorant and Unattentive.

The

Theriaca Andromachi.

Venice Treacle.

Take of the Troches of Squills half a Pound; long Pepper, Opium strained, dried Vipers, of each three Ounces ; Cinnamon, Balsam of *Gilead,* or in its Stead expressed Oil of Nutmegs, of each two Ounces ; Agaric, the Roots of *Florentine* Orrice , Water Germander, red Roses, Seeds of Navew, Extract of Liquorice, of each an Ounce and a half; Spikenard, Saffron, Amomum, Myrrh, Costus, or in its stead Zedoary, Camels Hay, of each an Ounce ; the Root of Cinquefoil, Rhubarb, Ginger, *Indian* Leaf, or in its stead Mace, Leaves of Dittany of *Crete,* of Horehound, and of Calamint, *French* Lavender, black Pepper , Seeds of *Macedonian* Parsley, Olibanum, *Chio* Turpentine, Root of wild Valerian, of each six Drams ; Gentian Root, *Celtic* Nard, Spignel, Leaves of Poley Mountain, of St. *John*'s Wort, of Ground Pine, Tops of creeping Germander, with the the Seed, the Fruit of the Balsam Tree, or in its stead Cubebs, Aniseed, sweet Fennel Seed, the lesser Cardamom Seeds freed from their Husks, Seed of Bishops Weed, of Hartwort, of Treacle Mustard, or *Mithridate* Mustard, Juice of the Rape of Cistus, Acacia, or in its stead *Japon* Earth, Gum Arabic, Storax strained, Sagapenum strained, Lemnian Earth, or in its stead Bole Armenic, or *French* Bole, green Vitriol calcin'd, of each half an Ounce ; Root of creeping Birthwort, Tops of the lesser Centaury, Seeds of the *Daucus* of *Crete,* Opoponax, Galbanum strained, *Russia* Castor, *Jews* Pitch, or in its stead white Amber prepared Root of the sweet Flag,

of each two Drams ; of clarified Honey, thrice the Weight of all the rest. The Ingredients are to be mixed in the same Manner as in the *Mithridate.* L.

In the *Edinburgh* Dispensatory it stands thus :

Take of the Troches of Squills, six Ounces ; those of Vipers , the Mass *Hedychroon,* long Pepper, and Opium, of each three Ounces ; *Sclavonian* (or *Florentine*) Orrice Root, red Roses, the Leaves of Scordium, Agaric, *Opobalsamum,* (or Balsam of *Peru*) Juice of Liquorice, the Seeds of Navew, and Cinnamon, of each an Ounce and half; Myrrh, Saffron, Ginger, Rapontic (or Tormentil Root) Cinquefoil Root, the Leaves of Calamint, Horehound , *Cretan* Dittany, the Flowers of *Arabian* Stœchas, Squinanth, *Macedonian* Parsley Seed, Costus (or Zedoary) *Cyprus* Turpentine, Male Frankincense, white Pepper, black Pepper , *Cassia Lignea* , and *Indian* Spikenard, of each six Drams ; *Cretan* Poley Mountain ; Seeds of the Hartwort of *Marseilles* (or the common) those of Anise, of Bishops Weed, of *Amomum,* (or Cloves) of the lesser Cardamoms, of Fennel, and of Treacle Mustard ; the Roots of Gentian, of Spignel, of *Pontic* Phu (or wild Valerian) and of sweet Flag ; the Leaves of Germander , Ground Pine, and St. *John*'s Wort ; tree Acacia, or the *German,* Carpobalsamum, or Cubebs, *Lemnian* Earth, or Bole Armeniac, calcined Brass Stone, or *Roman* Vitriol, *Storax Calamita,* Gum Arabic, the Juice of *Hypocistis,* *Celtic* Spikenard, and *Indian* Leaf, of each half an Ounce; Tops of the lesser Centaury, the Seed of *Cretan* Daucus, small, or long, Birth-wort Root ; *Jews* Pitch, or Amber, Galbanum,

Opo-

Opoponax, Sagapenum, and Castor, of each two Drams; of clarified Honey, thrice the Weight of the Powders; and as much *Canary* Wine as will serve to diffolve the Gums and Juices: Mix all together, and make an Electuary thereof, according to the Rules of Art. *E*.

Quincey is very diffuse in his Remarks upon this *capital Medicine* of the Shops. The principal Effects I have ever seen from its Use, have been such as any one might reasonably have expected, from an Opiate united with heating Ingredients, and exhibited where they were sure to do Mischief, that is, to convert a Cold, or flight febrile Diforder, into a dangerous Inflammation. *Quincey* would, therefore, have been highly ungrateful, if he had not spoke well of a Medicine, which brings in its Consequences yearly to the Apothecaries many thousand Pounds, and something to the Physicians, who are usually called in when the Case is irrecoverable, and are complimented with a few Guineas, and the Reproach of the Miscarriage. What I have said with respect to *Mithridate* will hold equally true of this Composition. *Raleigh*'s Cordial at present seems to have supplanted *Venice* Treacle; and it must be confess'd it is less prejudicial, as having no Opium in it.

Theriaca Edinenfis.
The *Edinburgh* Treacle.

Take of the Roots of *Virginian* Snake Root, six Ounces; the Root of wild Valerian, and Contrayerva, each four Ounces; of the *Pulvis Diaromaton*, three Ounces; Rosin of Guaiacum, *Ruffian* Castor and Myrrh, each two Ounces; *English* Saffron, and Opium, each an Ounce; of clarify'd Honey, thrice the Weight

of the Powders, and as much *Canary* Wine, as will serve to diffolve the Opium: Mix all together, and make an Electuary thereof according to the Rules of Art. *E*.

Camphire may be occasionally added.

This is better calculated to answer the End of an Alexipharmic, than the *Venice* Treacle. But, perhaps, is not for that Reason a less dangerous Medicine.

Electuarium Pectorale.
Pectoral Electuary.

Take of the Conserve of Roses, two Ounces; of the compound Powder of Gum Tragacanth, half an Ounce; Flowers of Benjamin a Dram; balsamic Syrup a sufficient Quantity, to make an Electuary.

The Title of this Medicine expresses its Uses.

Electarium è Scammonio.
Electary of Scammony.

Take of Scammony an Ounce and a half; Cloves, Ginger, of each six Drams; of the essential Oil of Caraway Seeds, half a Dram; of Honey, half a Pound. Reduce the Scammony to Powder by itself, mix the Aromatics, fresh pounded together, with the Honey, then add the Scammony, and in the last Place the Oil. *L*.

This is substituted for the *Caryocostinum* of former Dispensatories, and is so contriv'd, that a Dram and half of this contains as much Scammony, as half an Ounce of the former, which renders it more commodious for taking. It is a brisk Purge, and may be taken either by the Mouth, or in Clyfters. The particular Virtues may be learn'd from those of *Scammony*.

Philonium Lond &c.

The *London* Philonium.

Take white Pepper, Ginger, Caraway Seeds, of each two Ounces; of Opium strained, six Drams; of Diacodion boiled to the Consistence of Honey, thrice the the Weight of all the rest. Mix carefully the Opium dissolved first in Wine, with the Syrup warmed, and then add the other Species reduced to Powder. *L.*

This is a very warm Opiate; but I am persuaded it will in very few Cases answer better than crude Opium.

N. B. All Electuaries, if they grow dry, should be reduced again to their Consistence with a small Quantity of *Canary*, and not with Syrup, or Honey: By this Means the Dose will be rendered the least uncertain; which is especially necessary in those, that are made up with Syrup, and contain a large Quantity of Opium, such as the Philonium, and the *Confectio Paulina.* The Reason for this Caution is, that the Quantity of the fresh Syrup, or Honey, will be so great, as to vary the Proportion of the whole to the original Ingredients, and make the Effect of the Medicine precarious.

L O H O C H S.

Lohoch ex Amylo.

Lohoch of Starch.

Take of Starch two Drams; *Japan* Earth one Dram; Syrup of Comfrey, and the White of Eggs, beat to a Liquor, of each an Ounce: Mix them together, and make a Lohoch. *E.*

This is intended as a gentle Astringent; and may be of Service in some Sorts of Coughs and Asperities of the Fauces. But a Lohoch is not a very convenient Form for Medicines, and is almost out of Use. And besides, I apprehend, that all Medicines, which can readily be made extemporaneously, are not proper for Shop Compositions; because they may, by the Judicious, be better suited to any Case that occurs, by Prescription; and Directing them, in officinal Dispensatories, serves only to indulge the Laziness of some, and Ignorance of others.

Lohoch commune.

The common Lohoch.

Take of fresh Oil of sweet Almonds, and of Pectoral or Balsamic Syrup, each an Ounce; white Sugar two Drams: Mix and make a Lohoch. *E.*

This may possibly mitigate a Cough, but cannot be much depended on.

Lohoch Diatragacanthi.

Lohoch, with the compound Powder of Gum Dragon.

Take of the compound Powder of Gum Tragacanth two Drams; of *Japan* Earth one Dram; of the White of Eggs, beat up, an Ounce; Syrup of Diacodium, two Ounces: Mix them together into a Lohoch. *E.*

This is also of some Use in a Cough, when excited by a Discharge of thin Rheum.

Lohoch de Lino.

Lohoch of Linseed Oil.

Take of fresh Linseed Oil, and of Balsamic Syrup, each an Ounce; Flowers of Sulphur, a Dram; white Sugar, two Drams; mix them together so as to make a Lohoch. *E.*

This seems to be the best of these Lohochs; but I believe the fresh drawn Linseed Oil would do as well by itself.

Lo-

Lohoch de Manna.

Lohoch of Manna.

:e of *Calabrian* Manna, of frefh
rawn Oil of Almonds, and of
yrup of Violets, each a like
Quantity: Mix, and make a Lo-
och. *E.*

Lohoch Saponaceum.

Lohoch of Soap.

:e of *Alicant* Soap, a Dram: Oil
f Almonds, an Ounce; of Pecto-
l or Balfamic Syrup, an Ounce,
nd a half; and make thereof a
ohoch, according to Art. *E.*

Lohoch è Spermate Ceti.

Lohoch Sperma Ceti.

Take of Sperma Ceti, two Drams:
Rub it with a fufficient Quantity
of the Yolk of an Egg; and add
of recent Oil of fweet Almonds,
half an Ounce; of Balfamic Syrup,
an Ounce. Mix, and make a Lohoch.

This and the two preceding do not
feem of any great Confequence;
for all the Simples which enter their
Compofition may be given more
agreeably, and with better Effect.

CHAP. X.

Of PILLS.

IERAL RULES *for making of*
PILLS.

THE three firft Rules, laid
down for the making of
'ders, are to be carefully ob-
ed in the making of Pills.

I. The Gums and infpiffated
es muft be firft foftened by means
he Liquor prefcribed; then the
'ders are to be added gradually;
laftly, a perfect Mixture is to be
le of the Whole, by repeated
ting in a Mortar.

II. All Maffes of Pills fhould be
t in Bladders oiled, or moiftened
he Liquor the Mafs is made up
1.

Pilulæ Æthiopicæ.

Æthiopic Pills.

:e of pure Quickfilver, the golden
Sulphur of Antimony, and Refin
f Guaiacum, each half an Ounce:
Rub them together in a glafs Mor-
ar till the Mercury is perfectly

extinguifhed; and then add of
Alicant Soap, half an Ounce; of
Balfamic Syrup, a fufficient Quan-
tity to make a Mafs for Pills. *E.*

I muft confefs I have not often
known this ufed; but am certain it
muft be a moft excellent Remedy for
many Chronical Diftempers. I fhould
expect it to have very great Effects
in the Rheumatifm, to do confiderable Service in the Gout, and to
exert great Efficacy in the Cure of
cutaneous Difeafes, from the Itch to
the Leprofy; and I fcarcely know a
better Medicine than this promifes
to be in venereal Diforders. 'Tis thro'
a Neglect of the Ufe of fuch Medicines, that Phyficians frequently fail
of curing obftinate Diftempers, and
thus bring Quackery into Vogue;
for the World is wife enough to
judge by Succefs; and if Quacks
perform a Cure where Phyficians
mifcarry, the general Application
will be to the latter. It is trifling
to infinuate, that fuch Remedies are
unfafe; for, in the Hands of the Ju-

dicious, they are attended with as little Danger as more unmeaning and less efficacious Medicines.

Pilulæ Mercuriales.
Pills of Mercury.

Take of Quickfilver, five Drams; of *Strasbourg* Turpentine, two Drams; of the Cathartic Extract, four Scruples; of Rhubarb, in Powder, one Dram. First grind the Quickfilver with the Turpentine, till it appear no longer; then beat them up with the rest into a Mass. If the Turpentine chance to be too thick, it is to be thin'd with a little Olive Oil. *L.*

This seems directed in Imitation of *Belloste*'s Pill, and is, like the preceding, capable of doing great Service in Chronical Cases. In this Manner an almost infinite Number of Compositions may be contrived extemporaneously to suit any particular Case or Constitution, by combining Quickfilver, properly divided, with cathartic Ingredients. Having seen some Pills which were sold under the Name of *Belloste*, I was of Opinion, from their Appearance and Efficacy, that they were not the same as those originally sent over, and which have been so much celebrated in *Europe*. But having since examined the Pills sold at the *Blue Flower-Pot* in *Broad-street* near *Golden-square*, by a Relation of Dr. *Belloste*'s, I have Reason to believe them the Genuine, and the same as those originally sold by that Author.

In the *Edinburgh* Difpensatory the *Pilulæ Mercuriales* are thus directed.

Take of pure Quickfilver, an Ounce; Honey, a fufficient Quantity: Rub them in a Glass Mortar till the Globules of Mercury difappear; then add of Gum Ammoniac, two Ounces; and make into a Mass for Pills.

This seems to be a very good Mercurial Alterative, and as such may be of confiderable Use in Practice.

Pilulæ Mercuriales laxantes.
Laxative Mercurial Pills.

Take of pure Quickfilver, an Ounce of Honey, a fufficient Quantity; Rub them together till the Mercury is perfectly divided; and then add of Gum Ammoniac, the Extract of black Hellebore, and choice Rhubarb, each half an Ounce. *E.*

Quickfilver thus divided, without fome Cathartic Ingredient, will be fubject to affect the Mouth; this, therefore, feems well contrived to prevent it, and may be ufed with very good Effect in Chronical Diftempers.

Pilulæ Aromaticæ.
Aromatic Pills.

Take of Succotrine Aloes, an Ounce and a half; of Gum Guaiacum, an Ounce; the Aromatic Species, Balfam of *Peru*, of each half an Ounce: Let the Aloes and Gum Guaiacum be powder'd feparately; then mix'd with the reft, and form into a Mass with the Syrup of Orange-peel. *L.*

These are made in Imitation of the *Pilulæ Diambræ*, and *Pilulæ Alephanginæ*. It is a warm Cathartic, and may agree very well with debauch'd Stomachs.

Pilulæ Cocciæ.
Pills called Cocciæ.

Take of *Succotrine* Aloes, Colocynth, and of Scammony, each an Ounce; of vitriolated Tartar, two Drams; of the diftill'd Oil of Cloves, a Dram; and with Syrup of Buckthorn, enough for that Purpofe, bring them into a Mass for Pills. *E.*

In former Difpenfatories there were two

two Sorts of thefe Pills, the *Pilulæ Cochiæ majores*, and *Pilulæ Cochiæ minores*. Thefe are the *Cochiæ minores*, with the Addition of vitriolated Tartar, to keep them from exciting Gripes. They are of very little Ufe, and work pretty roughly. When Purging brifkly is intended, Jalap-root, or fome more brifk Cathartic, will anfwer better than this.

In the *London* Difpenfatory they ftand thus, under the Title of

Pilulæ ex Colocynthide cum Aloe.

Pills of Coloquintida, with Aloes.

Take Succotrine Aloes, and Scam-mony, of each two Ounces; of the Pith of Coloquintida, one Ounce; of Oil of Cloves, two Drams: Let the dry Species be reduced to Powder feparately, the Oil mix'd among them, and the Whole form'd into a Mafs, with Syrup of Buckthorn. *L.*

Pilulæ de Duobus.

Pills of two Ingredients.

Take of Colocynth, and Scammo-ny, each an Ounce; of vitriolated Tartar, two Drams; of the dif-till'd Oil of Cloves, a Dram; and with a fuitable Quantity of Syrup of Buckthorn bring them into a Mafs for Pills, according to the Rules of Art. *E.*

This was much the fame in the preceding *London* Difpenfatory, ex-cept that the Oil of Cloves was only in the Quantity of half a Dram; and in this the vitriolated Tartar is added, to keep the Cathartic Ingre-dients from adhering to the Inteftines, and exciting Gripes. In the laft *London* Difpenfatory the Name of this Compofition is changed, and ftands thus, under the Title of

Pilulæ ex Colocynthide fimpliciores.

The more fimple Pills of Colo-quintida.

Take the Pith of Coloquintida,

Scammony, of each two Ounces; of Oil of Cloves, two Drams: Let the dry Species be reduced to Powder feparately, the Oil be mixed with them, and the Whole be formed into a Mafs with Syrup of Buckthorn. *L.*

I believe this Name now given this Compofition, is neither better nor worfe than the preceding; fo that it deferves no Notice. It is of more Confequence to remark, that the *Pilulæ ex Duobus* have been very much in Ufe as a ftrong Cathartic, and frequently employ'd in the Cure of a virulent Gonorrhæa; but they operate too roughly, and frequently bring on a *Hernia Humoralis*, or Swelling of the Tefticles; or leave an incurable Gleet, to the great Pre-judice of the Patient's Virility. Ma-ny young Gentlemen have alfo been brought into a Confumption by the too frequent Ufe of thefe Pills, for the Cure of a Venereal Diforder: And upon the Whole, as there are much better and fafer Purges, I think this might very well be omit-ted, efpecially as extemporaneous Prefcriptions may better anfwer any End that can be propofed.

Pilulæ Ecphracticæ.

Deobftruent Pills.

Take of the *Aromatic Pill*, three Ounces; Rhubarb, Extract of Gentian, Salt of Iron, of each one Ounce; of Salt of Worm-wood, half an Ounce. With the folutive Syrup of Rofes, beat them diligently into a Mafs. *L.*

This, as its Title imports, is a De-obftruent, and is ufeful in a *Chlorofis*, a Suppreffion of the Menfes, fome Kinds of Cachexies, and many Chro-nical Difeafes.

Pilulæ Ecphracticæ cum Aculeo.

Stimulating Deobftruent Pills.

Take of Succotrine Aloes, the Ex-tract

tract of black Hellebore, and Scammony, each an Ounce; of Gum Ammoniac, and Resin of Guaiacum, each half an Ounce; of vitriolated Tartar, two Drams; Chymical Oil of Juniper, a Dram; Syrup of Buckthorn, a sufficient Quantity to make a Mass for Pills. E.

Pilulæ Ecphractica Chalybeatæ.

Deobstruent Pills, with Steel.

Take of the *Pillulæ communes,* or *Rufus's* Pills, an Ounce and a half; Gum Ammoniac, and Resin of Guaiacum, each half an Ounce; Salt of Iron, five Drams; Elixir Proprietatis, a sufficient Quantity to make a Mass for Pills. E.

These are very well contrived for Deobstruents; but exert their Effects as such best, if taken in small Doses, as Alteratives.

Pilulæ Fœtidæ.

Fœtid Pills.

Take of Assa Fœtida, a Dram and a half; *Russian* Castor, a Dram; Camphire, half a Dram; distill'd Oil of Hartshorn, a sufficient Quantity: Beat them together into a Mass for Pills.

This is intended as an Antihysteric.

Pilulæ de Gambogia.

Pills of Gamboge.

Take of Succotrine Aloes, Extract of black Hellebore, Gamboge, and Calomel, each two Drams; Chymical Oil of Juniper, half a Dram; Syrup of Buckthorn, enough to make a Mass for Pills. E.

I never knew this Medicine used; but it appears to me too rough, tho' corrected by the Oil of Juniper; and for that Reason of no great Use.

Pilulæ Gummosæ.

Gum Pills.

Take Galbanum, Opoponax, Myrrh, Sagapenum, of each an Ounce; of Assa Fœtida, half an Ounce: With the Syrup of Saffron make them into a Mass. L.

The *Pilulæ Gummosæ* of the *Edinburgh* Dispensatory are differently directed thus:

Take of Gum Ammoniac, and Sagapenum, each half an Ounce, *Russia* Castor and Myrrh, each three Drams; Assa Fœtida and Galbanum, each two Drams; distill'd Oil of Amber, half a Dram; and with a sufficient Quantity of *Elixir Proprietatis,* bring them by Art into a Mass. E.

Both these are intended as Antihysterics and Emmenagogues.

Pilulæ Pectorales.

Pectoral Pills.

Take of Gum Ammoniac, half an Ounce; Benjamin, three Drams; Myrrh, two Drams; *English* Saffron, one Dram; and with a sufficient Quantity of Balsam of Sulphur, made with Oil of Anniseeds, bring them into a Mass, according to Art. E.

The Title expresses the Design of this Pill.

Extractum Catharticum.

The Cathartic Extract.

Take of Succotrine Aloes, an Ounce and a half; of the Pith of Coloquintida, six Drams; Scammony, the lesser Cardamom-seeds husk'd, of each half an Ounce: of Proof Spirit, a Pint. The Spirit being poured upon the Coloquintida, cut small, and the Seeds bruised, draw a Tincture with a gentle Heat continued four Days; then to the Tincture, pressed out, add the Aloes and Scammony, first sepaeparately reduced to Powder; nd thefe being diffolved, draw off he Spirit, and reduce the Mafs to he Confiftence of a Pill. *L.*

his is fubftituted for the *Pilulæ lii*, which are thus directed in the nburgh Difpenfatory.

Pilulæ, feu Extractum Rudii.

Pills, or Extract of *Rudius*.

ke of the Roots of black Helle- ore and Colocynth, each two)unces: Bruife them well, and dd thereto two Quarts of Spring- vater: Boil them to the Con- umption of one Half; then prefs ut the Liquor, and exhale it to he Confiftence of Honey; after- vards put to it the following In- redients, reduced to a very fine owder, *viz.* of *Succotrine* Aloes, wo Ounces; and of Scammony, n Ounce; laftly, having remov'd he Mafs from the Fire, mix with a Dram of the diftill'd Oil of Cloves. *E.*

his Pill is a very good brifk Cath- c, and much in Ufe.

Pilulæ Rufi.

Rufus's Pills.

ke of *Succotrine* Aloes, two Oun- es; Myrrh and Saffron, of each ne Ounce: Make them into a Aafs, with Syrup of Saffron. *L.*

his is directed in the *Edinburgh* penfatory, under the Title of *Pi- communes,* with only half an ace of Saffron, and to be made with Syrup of Orange-peel. It moft excellent Cathartic, and moft ufeful of any in the Shops, aken in the Quantity of half a m; but it anfwers much better pofes to take it at Night, or ht and Morning, as an Altera- , in lefs than one Fourth of the Dofe: For thus it improves the etite and Digeftion, and, I am

pretty certain, exerts very confider- able Virtues in the Blood and Juices.

Riverius directs a Pill, of which this is the Bafis, under the Title of *Pilulæ contra Morbos deploratos,* and which I fhall call

Pilulæ Riverii.

Riverius's Pills.

Take of Pill *Rufi,* two Drams; of Gum Guaiacum, and Diaphoretic Antimony, each one Dram; Elixir Proprietatis, a fufficient Quantity to make them into Pills.

Riverius extols thefe Pills very highly, and indeed they deferve con- fiderable Encomiums. If twelve Pills are made of every Dram, and three are exhibited every Night and Morning, or at Night only, if they operate too much, they will do great Service in a Cachexy, Chlorofis, a Cough, Flatulences, and many Chro- nical Diforders. There is not a bet- ter Medicine for Women at the grand Period of Life, when the Catamenia begin to be irregular, or intirely ceafe, if duely perfifted in.

Pilulæ Matthæi.

Matthews's Pills.

Take of the Extract of Opium, black Hellebore, Liquorice, and the Soap of Tartar, each four Ounces. Let the Hellebore and Liquorice be made into a fubtile Powder: Beat and mix thefe four Ingre- dients very well; then, with two or three Ounces of this Mafs, mix an Ounce of *Englifh* Saffron, cut into fmall Pieces, and beat them well together, till the Saf- fron is perfectly incorporated with the Mafs, fo that no Part of it be difcernible from the reft; then beat and mix that with the reft of the Mafs as well. If this Mafs be too dry, you may mix it with fome of the Oil which comes from the Soap, which it fpues out when

it

it ſtands a long time by; or in its ſtead, ſo much rectified Oil of Turpentine as is ſufficient to make a Maſs fit to form into Pills; then put it into a wide-mouth'd Glaſs, or Gally-pot, tied over with a Bladder or Leather.

Quincy remarks, that there are many Ways of making this Medicine: *Bates* puts in white Hellebore. But how much ſoever it may be imagined to ſtand corrected here, it is much ſafer left out; and the Medicine will be ſtill left efficacious enough to all the Intentions it is ordered for. The Saffron in this is not ordered by *Bates*, but much improves the Medicine. In many Caſes it is an admirable and ſafe Opiate, and promotes the Diſcharges both by Sweat and Urine; and the Soap of *Tartar* is ſo aperient, that it makes it ſafe even in Aſthmas, when no other Preparations of Opium dare be ventur'd upon. It may be given from three to ten Grains. When it grows dry with keeping, it muſt be again moiſtened with freſh Oil of Turpentine; but the oftener it has had thoſe Amendments, its Doſe may be enlarged; for the Turpentine will not dry away ſo much, as not to leave enough behind to give ſome Augmentation to its Bulk. So far *Quincy*. And this Medicine is really very well contrived for an aperient Opiate. I like the Soap of Tartar, the black Hellebore, and Saffron, and have many Reaſons, reduced from Practice, to believe the Medicine much the better for them; tho', in general, Additions to Opium are either inſignificant or prejudicial. This Medicine is ſeldom omitted in Nephritic Caſes; and in many other Caſes it may be given with good Effect, where other Preparations of Opium, or Opium itſelf, are not ſo ſafe.

Pilulæ Starkei.

Starkey's Pills.

Take Extract of Opium, four Ounces; Nutmegs, and Mineral Bezoar, each two Ounces; Saffron and *Virginia* Snake-root, each one Ounce: Beat the Nutmegs and Saffron together into a Paſte, ſo that they cannot be diſtinguiſhed from one another. Let all the Mineral Bezoar and Snake-root be in impalpable Powder; then mix all together, with half a Pound of the Soap of Tartar; of Oil of Saſſafras, half an Ounce; and two Ounces of the Tincture of Antimony: Let them be all well incorporated, by beating in a Mortar; then keep them in a Glaſs, or Gally-pot, tied over with a Bladder and Leather, for Uſe.

This Mr. *George Wilſon* ſays he had from Dr. *Starkey*'s own Mouth, in the Year 1665, a little before his Death; who then told him, he gave *Matthews* the former for a little Money; but that was what he ſucceſsfully made uſe of himſelf. It is both more diaphoretic and more anodyne than the former; and they who have made Uſe of it in their Practice, affirm it to be the beſt Laudanum they ever met with; and yet this is not the Sort which is kept in the Shops, and it is not by much ſo conſtant Preſcription as the former. Indeed there are hardly any of the Shops that prepare this; ſo that a Phyſician may write for it in vain, while the other is ſo ready for a Succedaneum.

This may be given in a good handſome Doſe, and is not ſo hazardous in its Effects as common Opium, or any other of its Preparations.

Thus far *Quincy*: But I don't know that I ever either knew it made or uſed. It promiſes fair to be a very good Opiate. I don't think it the better

etter for the warm Alexipharics.

The *Edinburgh* Dispensatory directs *Matthews*'s Pills thus, under the Title of

Pilulæ Pacificæ, vulgo Matthæi.

Anodyne Pills, commonly called *Matthews*'s Pills.

Take of *Russian* Castor, two Ounces; *English* Saffron, and Opium, each an Ounce; Soap of Tartar, three Ounces; Balsam of Capivi, a sufficient Quantity. Make a Mass for Pills.

I don't think the Addition of Castor, or the Omission of the Helleore, any Improvement in this Medicine.

Pilulæ Saponaceæ.

Soap Pills.

Take of Almond Soap, four Ounces; of strain'd Opium, half an Ounce; of Essence of Lemons, a Dram: Beat the Opium, softened with a little Wine, along with the rest, till they are perfectly mix'd. *L.*

In the *London* Dispensatory this seems substituted for *Matthews*'s Pill. Experience must determine whether it is better or worse; but I strongly suspect it is not better.

Pilulæ Scilliticæ.

Pills of Squills.

Take of *Alicant* Soap, one Ounce; Gum Ammoniac, prepared Millepedes, and fresh Squills, each half an Ounce; and as much Balsam of Capivi as will make them into Pills, according to the Rules of Art. *E.*

This seems intended as a Deobstruent and Diuretic, and to be a good Medicine in a Jaundice, Dropsy, and Cachexy.

Pilulæ Stomachicæ.

Stomach Pills.

Take of *Succotrine* Aloes, an Ounce; of Rhubarb, six Drams; of Gum Ammoniac, three Drams; of Myrrh, and Extract of Gentian, each two Drams; of Saffron and vitriolated Tartar, each one Dram; Chymical Oil of Mint, half a Dram; and, with a sufficient Quantity of Syrup of Sena and Rhubarb, make them into a Mass for Pills. *E.*

The Title of this expresses the Intention.

Pilulæ è Styrace.

Storax Pills.

Take of strain'd Storax, two Ounces; of Saffron, one Ounce; of strain'd Opium, five Drams: Beat them diligently together, till they are perfectly mixed. *L.*

This is intended as a Pectoral Opiate, and is often given in a Cough, frequently mix'd with a gentle Cathartic.

In the *Edinburgh* Dispensatory it is thus directed:

Take of *Storax Calamita*, five Drams; of Gum Tragacanth, one Ounce; Olibanum, and Opium, each half an Ounce; and, with a sufficient Quantity of *Diacodium*, make them into a Mass, according to the Rules of Art. *E.*

CHAP. XI.

Of Troches.

GENERAL RULES *for preparing* TROCHES.

I. THE three preceding Rules, laid down for the making of Powders, must be likewise understood of the preparing Powders for Troches.

II. When the Mass is so glutinous as to stick to the Fingers, whilst the Troches are forming, let the Hands be rubb'd with sweet Oil, or any other of the Aromatic Tribe, or the Powder of Starch or Liquorice.

III. In order to the well-drying of them, let them be laid upon an inverted Sieve in a shady, but open airy Place, and keep them frequently turning.

IV. Let them be kept for Use in Vessels of Glass, or of glazed Earth.

Trochisci albi Rhasis, seu Sief album.

The white Troches of *Rhases.*

Take of Ceruse, ten Drams; Sarcocol, three Drams; Starch, and Gum Tragacanth, of each two Drams; Camphire, half a Dram; and a proper Quantity of Rosewater; in which dissolve the Gum Arabic and Gum Tragacanth, so as to make a Mucilage; and, the other Ingredients being reduced to Powder, make Troches of the Whole, according to the Rules of Art. *E.*

The *London* Dispensatory substitutes the *Pulvis è Cerussa compositus* for this. 'Tis only for external Use, and is esteem'd an Antiphlogistic and Repellent.

Trochisci Bechici albi.

White Pectoral Troches.

Take of double refined Sugar, one Pound and a half; of Starch, an Ounce and a half; of Liquorice, six Drams; of *Florentine* Orris, half an Ounce. All the Ingredients being reduced to Powder, with the Mucilage of Gum Tragacanth, form Troches. *L.*

These Troches are intended for a Cough: They must be held in the Mouth, and suffer'd to dissolve gradually. In the *Edinburgh* Dispensatory they are thus directed:

Take of white Sugar-candy, a Pound and a half; *Florentine* Orriceroot, an Ounce and a half; Liquorice-root, an Ounce; Starch, half an Ounce; Mucilage of Gum Tragacanth made with Rosewater, as much as will serve to form the Whole into Lozenges. *E.*

Trochisci Bechici nigri.

Black Pectoral Troches.

Take Extract of Liquorice, double refined Sugar, of each ten Ounces; of Gum Tragacanth, half a Pound. By moistening with Water, make Troches. *L.*

These are also intended for a Cough, but are of no great Consequence. In the *Edinburgh* Dispensatory they are thus order'd:

Take of the Juice of Liquorice, two Ounces; Balsam of *Tolu*, a Dram; of Gum Tragacanth, half an Ounce; of white Sugar, four Ounces;

unces; Hyffop-water, a fuffic-
ent Quantity to form Troches.

chifci *Cypheos, pro Mithridatio.*

ches of *Cyphis,* for Mithridate.

e of the Pulp of ftoned Raifins
f the Sun, and *Cyprus* Turpen-
ne, each three Ounces; Myrrh
d Squinanth, of each an Ounce
nd a half; Cinnamon, half an
unce; Saffron, a Dram; Bdel-
um, Spikenard, *Caffia Lignea,*
und or (long) Cyperus-root, and
uniper-berries, of each three
rams; of *Rhodium,* (or Yellow
anders) two Drams and a half;
f *Calamus Aromaticus,* nine Drams;
little *Canary* Wine, and a fuffi-
ient Quantity of clarify'd Honey.
et the Bdellium and Myrrh be
round with the Wine to the Con-
ftence of Honey; then add, by
egrees, the Pulp of Raifins, the
urpentine, the Honey, and, laft-
y, the other Ingredients reduced
o a very fine Powder; and fo
nake them into Troches, accord-
ng to the Rules of Art. *E.*

his is one of thofe infignificant
npofitions that deferves no No-

chifci *dicti Magma Hedychroi, pro
Theriaca Andromachi.*

ches, call'd the Mafs *Hedychroon,*
for the Theriaca.

ke of the Leaves of Marum and
Marjoram, of *Rhodium* (or Yellow
anders) and of the Root of Afa-
abacca, of each two Drams; of
quinanth, *Calamus Aromaticus,*
ontic Phu (or the Root of wild
Valerian) Xylobalfamum (or A-
oes Wood) Opobalfamum (or Balam of *Peru)* Coftus (or Zedoa-
y) and Cinnamon, each three
Drams; of Myrrh, *Indian* Leaf
or Bay-leaves) *Indian* Spikenard,
Caffia Lignea, and of Saffron, each

fix Drams; of Amomum (or
Cloves) an Ounce and a half;
of Maftich, a Dram; and, with a
requifite Proportion of *Canary*
Wine, make them up into Troches
according to Art. *E.*

This is a Compofition of very little
Confequence, and deferves no farther Remark.

Trochifci de Minio.
Troches of red Lead.

Take of red Lead, half an Ounce;
corrofive Mercury Sublimate, an
Ounce; Crums of white Bread,
four Ounces; with a fufficient
Quantity of Rofe-water, form oblong Troches. *E.*

Thefe are intended for an Efcharotic; but muft be ufed with great
Caution.

Trochifci de Myrrha.
Troches of Myrrh.

Take of Myrrh, half an Ounce; of
Madder-root, the Leaves of common Pennyroyal, *Ruffian* Caftor,
each three Drams; the Seeds of
Cumin, Affa Fœtida, and Galbanum, each two Drams; the diftill'd Oils of Rue and Savine, of
each twenty Drops; and a fufficient Quantity of *Elixir Proprietatis:* Let the Gums, by means
of the Elixir, be reduced to a Mafs
of the Confiftence of Honey: Afterwards add the Oils and Powders, fo as that Troches may be
artificially formed thereof. *E.*

This is intended for an Antihyfteric, an Exciter of the Menfes, and
the Lochia. In the *London* Difpenfatory the *Pulvis è Myrrha compofitus* is fubftituted in the Room of
thefe Troches.

Trochifci è Nitro.
Troches of Nitre.

Take of purified Nitre, four Ounces;
of double refined Sugar, a Pound.
Make

Make them into Troches with the Mucilage of Gum Trogacanth. *L.*

The Nitre here is a very good Ingredient; but this is not the beft Form for its Exhibition.

Trochifci è Scilla.
Troches of Squills.

Take of baked Squills half a Pound, of Wheat Flower four Ounces. Pound them together, and form them into Troches, to be dried with a gentle Heat. *L.*

This is of no Ufe that I know of except for the *Venice* Treacle.

In the *Edinburgh* Difpenfatory, the Troches of Squills are thus ordered under the Title of

Trochifci Scillitici, pro Theriaca Andromachi.

Troches of Squills, for the Treacle of Andromachus.

Take an entire Squill, after the Leaves and Stalks are dry, and, having pull'd off its outfide, include it in a Pafte made of Wheat Flower, and bake it in an Oven till the Cruft becomes hard: Then take three Ounces of the Squill thus baked tender, and grind it in a Mortar, adding thereto two Ounces of the Meal of the white Vetch, fo as to make a Pafte; whereof Troches being form'd, let them be dried in the Shade. *E.*

The mere Pulp of the Squill is juftly preferred to thefe Troches.

Trochifci è Sulphure.
Troches of Sulphur.

Take wafhed Flowers of Sulphur, two Ounces; of double refined Sugar, four Ounces. Beat them together, and by gradually adding the Mucilage of Quince Seeds form Troches. *L.*

In the *Edinburgh* Difpenfatory, fomething of the fame Intention are directed under the Title of

Trochifci Diafulphuris.
Troches of Sulphur.

Take of the Flowers of Sulphur, an Ounce; the Flowers of Benjamin, a Dram; of white Sugar, four Ounces; and a fufficient Quantity of the Mucilage of Gum Tragacanth; mix them all together, and make Troches thereof according to Art. *E.*

I don't fee any Advantage in thefe, more than in Sulphur alone, unlefs any one fhould like to take them better in this Manner. But the Difference cannot be great.

Trochifci de Terra Japonica.
Troches of Japan Earth.

Take of Japan Earth, two Ounces; of Gum Tragacanth, half an Ounce; of white Sugar a Pound; and a proper Quantity of Rofe Water to make Troches, with this Beat up the Troches. *E.*

Thefe are by much the beft Troches that I have met with for a Cough, which they relieve very eminently, if fuffer'd to diffolve gradually in the Mouth. But the *Japan* Earth alone is much better, us'd in the fame Manner, for thofe who can bear the Tafte.

In the *London* Difpenfatory they are thus directed:

Take *Japan* Earth and Gum Arabic, of each two Ounces; of Sugar of Rofes, fixteen Ounces: Beat them together, and with a little Water make Troches. *L.*

In both thefe the Proportion of Sugar is too large. They will have a much better Effect with lefs than half the Sugar, tho' they are then not quite fo agreeable.

Trochifci Viperini, pro Theriaca Andromachi.

Troches of Vipers, for *Venice* Treacle

Take half a Pound of Viper's Flefh feparated from the Skins, and the
Entrails

ntrails, the Fat, the Heads, and he Tails, and boiled till it grows oft in Spring Water, feafoned with a little Dil and Salt, and afterwards cleared of the Back-bone; f Bifket Bread, ground and feared, two Ounces; beat them up ogether, with a proper Quantity of the Broth, remaining after the Vipers were boiled, into a Mafs, o be formed into Troches, according to Art. *E.*

hefe Troches are brought to us n other Parts, ready prepared; the dried Flefh of the Viper is h Juftice preferred thereto.

Tabellæ Cardialgicæ
Cardialgic Lozenges.

ke of prepared Chalk, four Ounces; of prepared Crabs-claws, two

Ounces; of Bole Armenic, or French Bole, half an Ounce; of Nutmegs, a Scruple; of double refined Sugar, three Ounces. Make all into a Powder, and then with a little Water form it into Lozenges. *L.*

Thefe are very powerful againft that Diforder improperly called the Heart-Burn.

Trochifci Cardialgici.
Troches for the Heart-Burn.

Take of Oifter-Shells, and Chalk, powder'd, each two Ounces; Gum Arabic, half an Ounce; Nutmegs, half a Dram; fine Sugar, ten Ounces; Baum Water, enough to make Troches. *E.*

Thefe are of the fame Ufe as the preceding.

C H A P. XII.

Of O I L S in General.

THERE is a certain Part in Plants, which being either ontaneoufly fluid, or eafily made by a gentle Heat, is called their il. This Oil may become thick by ng ftanding, as we fee in the Oil of urpentine, which, tho' extremely, id at firft, manifeftly thickens by egrees. It may, alfo, grow thick ith Cold, and thus appear knotty ce Fifh-fpawn; and may become lid, as we fee in Wax; but by hat Means foever it thus becomes ard, it flows again upon being aplied to the Fire. This Oil, therebre, whenever it becomes liquid, at the fame Time unctuous, or exeeding foft and flippery to the ouch; tho' it has at the fame Time rtain Tenacity or Vifcofity in its arts, not found in Waters and Spits. Again, thefe Oils are always

inflammable, and feed both Fire and Flame, being themfelves difpofed to go into the Flame; a Property not found in Air, Water, or Earth: Laftly, Oil will not intimately mix with Water; but when fhook therein, repels the Water from it, collects together, and feparates into a diftinct Liquor; in which Refpect it differs from Spirits. Vegetable Oil, therefore, is an unctuous inflammable Liquor, that does not mix with Water.

This Oil is found of many different Kinds in Plants; the volatile Sort, which is produced in the Diftillation of the Waters from unctuous Vegetables, lodges the prefiding Spirit, which contains the Tafte and Smell of the Plant; whence in this Oil the particular fenfible Properties of the Plant manifeftly refide, which, being

iAg

ing once separated, robs the Plant of its Nature. Thus, if all this Oil were totally extracted from Cinnamon, Mace, Cloves, or Nutmegs, these Bodies would remain of their pristine Form, so as to be perfectly distinguishable, tho' they retain nothing of their peculiar Properties: For when all this Oil is taken away, those Spices can no longer be distinguished by the Smell or Taste; tho' the Body of the Oil receives not its Smell and Taste from itself, but intirely from that Spirit, which, when present, distinguishes these Oils, and when absent leaves them scarce distinguishable, and almost of one and the same Nature.

Sometimes in certain Plants, and particular Parts thereof, this Oil is collected pure, in little peculiar Cells or Receptacles: At other Times oily Particles are mixed with the Juices of Plants, and so dispersed therein as scarce to appear in the Form of Oil, but lie concealed in that of Soap. But when these latent oily Particles associate, or separate from the rest, they immediately appear in the Form of Oil. Thus the Juices of a Plant being extracted with Water, inspissated, made saponaceous, and dried, it is manifest they contain Oil by their Burning. On the other Hand, a pure Oil distils from Incisions made in the Fir, the Pine, and the Larch-Tree. A transverse Section being made into the Root of Masterwort, newly dug up in the Winter, we may, by the Help of a Microscope, perceive little Drops of Gold-coloured Oil ouzing out from certain Vessels on the Surface: And the same holds true of a Nutmeg, or Almond, cut with a warm Knife. But we find this Oil no where more plentiful than in the Cotyledons, or seminal Lobes of Plants, where it defends the tender Embryo from the pernicious Effects of unseasonable Water, or too great Cold; for

Freezing might probably prove destructive to so fine a Structure. This Oil also is, in the Winter-time, found driven towards the Bark by the preceding Summer; and being there more drained from its watery Moisture, is collected in great Abundance, especially in the Ever-greens. The Oil of Vegetables, therefore, chiefly abounds in their more dureable Parts, in order to defend the other natural and more necessary ones, and is therefore found in such Parts as are farthest removed from the absorbing Vessels of the Roots, and the nutrimental Juice drawn in from the Earth; and thus more Oil is found in ripe Linseed, than perhaps in all the other Parts of the Plant together. Sometimes also this Oil is collected in such Quantity, as spontaneously to appear in its proper Form, burst its Cells, and run out; whence the Barks of Trees and Fruits principally afford it, as we see in Pine-apples, Juniper-berries, &c. especially in the Ever-greens, where the outward Bark is often cased over with this Oil. The Trees in the Northern Regions, which grow upon the high Mountains, exposed to the freezing Cold, more particularly afford it; whence it should seem, that this Oil is highly requisite to defend the Life of Vegetables against the freezing Cold of Winter. We likewise observe, that these fat Oils chiefly grow and collect in full-grown Plants, that soon after seem, as it were, to sleep or become aged; for both Herbs and Trees contain little Oil in their young growing State, but are distended with a dilute, thin, watery Juice. Thus Flax, soon after it is first sown, rises in the Form of Grass, and is merely aqueous; but, when come to Maturity, it loses its Greenness, grows yellow, and now affords a copious Oil, especially in its Seed: And the same holds true of a young Pine, e, compared with one that is -grown. It is also observed, that shrubby Plants, which have live-Roots, gradually contract themres upon the Approach of Winter, with-hold their Juices, perspire little, receive but little Nourishment from the Earth, nor throw much off into the Air; and thus they continue to do in a higher Degree, as the Winter comes on, till length they in a manner rest. On other Hand, as the Spring approaches, all begins to move again; y take in Nourishment, and perre. If these Autumnal or Winter tions may be call'd Times of ep, and the Summer and Vernal riods Times of Waking, in Plants, will generally appear that the Oils Vegetables are increased in their eping, but the Water in their aking. Thus the Root of Maswort, being perfectly leafless in Winter, and lying hid and unive in the Earth, may be called rmant; but if now dug up, and amined, it will be found rich in l; but if again dug up in *May*, it pears aqueous, saline, and by no ans so oily as before; and the ne is observed in Trees. Lastly, see that old Trees are oppressed th their own Oil, and thence suffated, thro' the Abundance of Fat, the Pine, the Fir, *&c.* where this I appears in the Form of a Gum; t in others, under that of Rosin, l, or Balsam. And hence it is, at Gardeners so frequently comain of the Death of Trees, obacted in their Bark, which thus , as Animals do, when choaked th their own Fat.

he Chymist, therefore, who would tract the Oils of Vegetables, should t learn from Botany, that there certain Seasons wherein Plants ound with Water and Salt, and m but little with Oil; and again, t there are other Seasons where-

in they principally abound with Oil, and but little with Water and Salt: For whilst new Leaves, Flowers, and Fruit are forming in Plants, the Motion of the aqueous Juices, pregnant with Salt, is promoted, and the sluggish Oils excluded; but when the Leaves begin to wither and fall off, the Flowers to shed, or the Fruit to ripen, or spontaneously fall off, when perfect, then the oily Parts gradually collect together, and preside, the more subtile ones being dissipated by the Summer's Heat: Whence Builders fell their Timber in the Midst of Winter, that it may be durable, and Proof against Moisture and Rottenness; for all the hardest, most ponderous, and lasting Woods, are found to abound with a ponderous Oil: Thus Cedar and Lignum Vitæ contain an exceeding heavy, compact, and copious Oil. Chymists, therefore, must chuse their Subjects for Salt at a certain Season, and for Oil at a very different one.

Oils *obtained by Expression.*

Oleum Amygdalarum dulcium.
Oil of sweet Almonds.

Take any Quantity of sweet Almonds, fresh dried and blanched; bruise them in a Marble Mortar, put them into an Hempen Bag, and gradually force out the Oil by Means of a Press, with the Assistance of Fire.

In the same Manner are procured the Oils of bitter Almonds, Walnuts, Mace, Nutmegs, Lin seed, and Mustard-seed, the Iron Plates of the Press being first moderately warm'd.

Both ripe and unripe Olive Oil, as also Oil of Bays, are brought to us from foreign Parts. *E.*

In the *London* Dispensatory the Oil is ordered to be press'd out without the Assistance of Fire.

C c c

Oil

Oil of fweet Almonds contains very little Salt, tho' evidently much of the particular Nature of the Plant, as our Senfes inform us; but, whilft frefh, it fheaths, blunts, and mollifies what is acrimonious in the Humours; relaxes the Fibres, Membranes, Veffels, and Vifcera, when applied thereto; foftens the Hardnefs of the Flefh, and cures its Crifpature. It mollifies and moiftens dead and dry Efcars, and renders them feparable from the found Flefh by the vital Actions. It defends the naked Parts in Wounds, and prevents the dry Air from hurting them by Deficcation. It alfo prevents the thin Humours from exhaling too much thro' the open Mouths of the Veffels in Wounds, and thus fpoiling the extreme Veffels; and hence it becomes an excellent Remedy for expeditioufly healing recent Flefh Wounds. It is alfo accounted a great Anodyne, both as it is emollient and relaxing. But thefe Oils have one ftrange Property, whereby, with the Heat only of feventy Degrees, they prefently degenerate, without any foreign Body being mixed with them, and thus become thin, fharp, bitter, rancid, yellow, corrofive, and inflammatory; whereas they were before thick, mild, fweet, almoft infipid, white, anodyne, and relaxing; and thefe furprizing Changes happen in a few Days in the Summer's Heat. Frefh drawn Oil of Almonds will prove healing and fuppling to the parch'd rough Mouth and Jaws in the Quinfey; and the fame Oil, in a few Days afterwards, fuddenly inflames the Jaws of a Perfon in Health; and the fweeter it was when frefh, the fharper it proves when old and rancid. Hence Almonds, Walnuts, and Piftachoes become exceedingly naufeous when rancid, and fubject to occafion a fudden Quinfey in the Throat, and excite a Fever, thro'

the burning Effect they have upon the Mouth, Throat, Stomach, and Inteftines. Phyficians, therefore, fhould be cautious when they order Oil of Almonds in acute Diftempers, that it be frefh drawn, from Almonds that were not rancid, and, in the Heat of Summer, not kept above twenty-four Hours. The fame thing is alfo found in Butter, Animal Fat, Marrow, and the more perfect Oils hereof: All which, though innocent when frefh, become highly naufeous by ftanding unfalted in a hot Air, where they turn yellow, blue, or green, become rank, corrofive, and very poifonous in the Plague. Thus a great Acrimony is fometimes found in Cheefe that has been long kept, whereby the whole Mouth is fometimes violently inflamed; whence we may eafily conceive, what Effects it might have upon the Vifcera. It is an obvious Experiment, that Oil by Boiling, will foon turn yellow, red, black, bitter, fharp, and unwholfome. And this fhews us how Oils may, in fix Hours time, become extremely bitter in the Stomach; and when vomited up, be erroneoufly taken for the Bile; for this Matter takes Flame at the Fire.

OILS *made by Infufion and Decoction.*

Oleum Abfinthites.
Oil of Wormwood.

Take a Pound of the bruifed Tops of frefh common Wormwood; and three Pints of ripe Olive Oil; Boil them gently till the Herb becomes crifp, and then ftrain off the Oil with Preffure.

In the fame Manner are made

Oleum *Anethinum,* Oil of Dill, from the Leaves of the Plant.

—— *Chamæmelinum,* Oil of Chamomile, from the Flowers.

Ole

um Hyperici, Oil of St. John's-
vort, from the Tops.

— *Liliorum alborum*, Oil of White
lillies from the Flowers.

— *Rosarum rubrarum*, Oil of red
Roses, from the Flowers.

— *Rutaceum*, Oil of Rue, from
he Leaves. *E.*

Oleum Hyperici.

Oil of St. John's-wort.

te of the Flowers of St. John's-
vort, full blown, fresh, and care-
ully picked from their Calyxes,
our Ounces; of Olive Oil, a
Quart. The Oil being pour'd on
he Flowers, let them stand to-
ether till the Oil is sufficiently
inged. *L.*

his is intended for external Use.
: Virtues may be learned from
e of *Hypericum* in the *Materia*
ica.

Oleum Lumbricorum.

Oil of Earth-worms.

e of Earth-worms, well wash'd,
alf a Pound; of ripe Olive Oil,
Quart; of white Wine, half a
int; and boil them together in
alneo Mariæ till the Wine is
onsumed; after which strain out
e Oil by Expression. *E.*

Oleum Mucilaginum.

Oil of Mucilages.

e of the recent Roots of Marsh-
allows (or of white Lillies)
uised, four Ounces; of fresh
quills bruised, two Ounces; Seeds
Fœnugrec, and Lin-feed, each
Ounce and a half: Let these
: macerated in a sufficient Quan-
y of Spring-water; then let
em boil till they form a thick
d viscous Mucilage; which be-
g strongly press'd out, add of
live Oil, four Pints. Boil with
gentle Heat, or in a Bath-heat,
all the aqueous Moisture is

consumed, continually stirring it,
to prevent Burning.

In the *London* Dispensatory it is
thus directed, under the Title of

Oleum è Mucilaginibus.

Oil of Mucilages.

Take of the Root of Marshmallows,
fresh, half a Pound; Lin-feed,
Fenugreek-feeds, of each three
Ounces; of Water, a Quart; of
Olive Oil, two Quarts. Boil gently the Roots and Seeds bruised,
in the Water for half an Hour.
Afterwards add the Oil, and renew the Boiling till the Water is
quite wasted; then pour the Oil
cautiously off. *L.*

Oleum Sambucinum.

Oil of Elder.

Take of Elder-flowers, one Pound;
of Olive Oil, a Quart. Boil the
Flowers in the Oil till they are
almost crisp; then press out the
Oil, and set it by, that the Fæces
may subside. *L.*

The Virtues of this, as a Topic,
may be learn'd from those of Elder-
flowers.

Oleum viride.

Green Oil.

Take Bay-leaves, Leaves of Rue,
of Marjoram, of Sea Wormwood,
and of Chamomile, of each three
Ounces; of Olive Oil, a Quart.
The Herbs being bruised, boil
them slightly in the Oil till they
are become crisp; then press out
the Oil, and, after the Fæces have
subsided, pour it off. *L.*

The Ingredients of this Composition are very warm, and consequently the Ointment must be good in the
same Intentions as the *Unguentum*
Nervinum.

Ccc 2

Of

CHAP. XIII.

Of Artificial Balsams.

Balsamum Anodynum, vulgò Guidonis.

Guido's Anodyne Balsam.

Take of Galbanum and Tacamahac, each half a Pound; *Venice* Turpentine, one Pound: Put them into a Retort, so as they may fill one Third of its Capacity, and distil, gradually increasing the Fire. Let the red Oil, or Balsam, be separated from the other Liquor. *E.*

This Balsam should seem to be extremely penetrating and resolvent.

Balsamum ad Apoplecticos.

Apoplectic Balsam.

Take of the Oil of Nutmegs obtained by Expression, an Ounce: Melt it in a Silver Vessel, and, being removed from the Fire, add thereto, of the distill'd Oils of Cloves, of Lavender, of Rosemary, each half a Dram; of the Oil of Amber, half a Scruple; of Balsam of *Peru,* a Dram; and mix them together according to Art. *E.*

This is made in Imitation of the *Balsamum Apoplecticum.* As it warms and enlivens, it is very proper to excite Sensation in the Nerves, by being smell'd to, or rub'd on the Temples, or on Paralytic Parts. A few Drops may also be exhibited internally, in any convenient Form.

Balsamum Locatelli.

Locatelli's Balsam.

Take of Olive Oil, a Pint; *Strasburg* Turpentine, yellow Wax, of each half a Pound; of red Saunders, six Drams. Melt the Wax, with some Part of the Oil, over a gentle Fire; then add the rest of the Oil, and the Turpentine: In the last Place, mix in the Saunders, and stir the Whole well together, till it is nearly cold. *L.*

The Compilers of the *London* Dispensatory have very prudently continued the red Saunders in this celebrated Composition, as being a much more suitable Ingredient than Dragon's Blood, tho' the latter may perhaps give it a better Colour; a Circumstance not to be put in Competition with the Efficacy of a Medicine. It has been the Fashion to laugh at this Balsam as an injudicious Composition, and of little or no Efficacy. But whoever considers attentively the Ingredients, will be inclined to think it a very good Medicine, as an internal Balsamic and Vulnerary; but its greatest Excellence should seem to be in a Dysentery, and Erosions of the Intestines. People often speak and write of Medicines, upon Theory, without consulting Experience, which is only capable of determining the Character of any Remedy. And this has been the Case with respect to *Locatelli's* Balsam. As to its external Use, there are much better Medicines for any Purpose that can occur.

In the *Edinburgh* Dispensatory it is thus directed:

Take of yellow Wax, a Pound: Melt it by a gentle Heat, in a Pint and a half of Olive Oil: then add of *Venice* Turpentine, a Pound and a half; and, when it is removed from the Fire, add of *Peruvian* Balsam, two Ounces; Dragon's Blood, one Ounce; stirring it continually till cold.

The

e red Saunders is a better Ingre-
t than the Dragon's Blood.

*famum Saponaceum, vulgo Opo-
deldoc.*

: faponaceous Balfam, commonly
call'd *Opodeldoc*.

:e of rectify'd Spirit of Wine,
ur Pints; *Alicant* Soap, one
ound; digeft in a gentle Heat,
ll the Soap is diffolv'd; then
ld of Camphire two Ounces;
ıymical Oil of Rofemary, and
f Origanum, each half an Ounce,
ıd let thefe be mix'd well in by
irring, or fhaking. *E.*

lon't know why the Oil of Ori-
ım is here added.

ıis is the celebrated *Opodeldoc*,
:h is greatly recommended, and
without Reafon, for refolving
rulated Blood and Juices, when
ıating and exciting Pains; as in
fes, Strains, and Rheumatic Pains.
a much better Medicine for thefe
pofes is thus prepar'd, by the Ti-
ıf

— In the *London* Difpenfatory,
Linimemtum Saponaceum is fubfti-
d for this.

Balfamum Vitæ.

Balfam of Life.

:e of the beft Spirit of Turpen-
ne, two Ounces; and diffolve
ı it of Camphire, fix Drams.
ake alfo, of the beft Spirit of
al *Ammoniac*, an Ounce and half,
nd diffolve in it half an Ounce
f *Spanifh* Soap. Mix thefe gra-
ually together, and, if the In-
redients are very good, they will
oagulate, and form a Kind of
oap.

ıave met with nothing that more
verfully refolves ftagnating Juices;
more effectually removes fix'd
rumatic Pains, after the Ufe of
Evacuations, and Attenuants.

But fome Caution is requir'd in its
Ufe, for it is not always proper to
remove fix'd Pains in the external
Parts, left they fhould fix on the
Vifcera, where they may do more
Prejudice. If a due Proportion of
Opium, or its Tincture, is added,
it becomes an excellent and fafe
Anodyne, for external Ufe; and
may be given internally, either with,
or without the Opium, as a faponaceous and extremely penetrating Refolvent, where there is no Excefs of
Heat, and no Tendency to an alcaline Putrefaction.

Balfamum Anodynum Bateanum.

Bates's Anodyne Balfam.

To the *Balfamum Saponaceum* above
defcrib'd, add of the Tincture of
Opium a fufficient Quantity, more
or lefs, as it is intended to be more
or lefs Anodyne. *E.*

The Anodyne Balfam is thus directed in the *Edinburgh* Difpenfatory.
It is certainly an extremely penetrating and refolvent Anodyne, both
for internal and external Ufe. *Quincy*
recommends it ftrongly for a nervous
Colic, the Jaundice, and as a Topic
in Arthritic Pains; but in this laft
Cafe I fhould not be very forward
to ufe it. Its great Excellence fhould
feem to be in Nephritic Pains, after
due Evacuations; for the Soap acting, as it were, under the Conduct
of the Opium, is capable of affording great Relief. If the Chymical
Oils were left out of the *Balfamum
Saponaceum*, I fhould efteem it a
better Medicine. And if the Saffron, formerly order'd in it, was continu'd, I fhould think it not the
worfe.

Offa Helmontiana.

Helmont's Soap.

Take of the alcaline Spirit of Sal
Ammoniac, fo ftrong as to leave
much of its Salt undiffolved at

the Bottom ; put it into a cold and dry cylindrical Glafs with a narrow Mouth, fo as to fill about one half thereof ; pour to it gradually, a Quantity of pure cold *Alcohol*, fo as to run gently down the Sides of the Veffel, till it be full ; a white Coagulation will be made upon the Surface, where the lighter *Alcohol* refts upon the alcaline Spirit. If the Glafs be now inverted, there will inftantly appear a white opake Coagulation, where the *Alcohol* and alcaline Spirit mix ; and when they are both well fhaken together, the whole becomes a white opake confiftent Mafs, concreted like Stone, fo that not a Drop will fall out of the Glafs, while inverted. Stop the Veffel clofe, and fet it by ; Thus the Mixture will foon refolve into a Fluid, that floats at Top, and a denfe, faline Concretion, that falls to the Bottom ; fo that, in a Year's time, the Salt will almoft become folid below, with a Liquor floating above it. If the whole Mafs, thus produc'd, be diftill'd with a gentle Fire, an alcaline, balfamic, oily, folid Salt will fublime. The colder the Seafon, and the Place, in which the Experiment is made, the better it will fucceed.

This is one of the moft difficult Experiments in Chymiftry, as it requires both the Liquors to be perfect, and the Obfervance of feveral Circumftances, any one of which being neglected, will caufe it to mifcarry ; but, if they all be obferved, it will fucceed. Here we fee, that a pure volatile alcaline Salt will clofely attract to itfelf the moft fubtile Oil that is known, that is, an *Alcohol* ; whence the Soap, fo produced, is the moft fubtile and penetrating of all Soaps, confifting of an exceedingly fubtile and volatile *Al-*

cali and Oil, wonderfully united together in an Inftant. If this Medicine be diluted with *Canary*, and taken upon an empty Stomach, it paffes perhaps, thro' all the Veffels of the Body, refolves Concretions, opens Obftructions, excites the vital Powers, and thus fuccefsfully cures many dangerous Diftempers, proceeding from an obftructing Matter, capable of being refolved by it. But its Virtue vanifhes too foon, as being fo extremely volatile, and therefore becomes unequal to the more ftubborn Diftempers. It is highly commended in the Jaundice, unattended with an acute Inflammation ; it does not diffolve the Stone, or prevent the Concretion or Increafe thereof ; it diffolves in a gentle Heat, like Ice, and returns to a folid Form in the Cold. If pure *Alcohol* be thus mixed with one third of dry volatile *Alcali*, it makes a much more folid Soap, as being without Water, which is always double the Quantity in the ftrongeft alcaline Spirit, with refpect to the pure Salt.

Linimentum Saponaceum.
Saponaceous Liniment.

Take of the Spirit of Rofemary, a Pint ; of hard *Spanifh* Soap, three Ounces ; of Camphire, one Ounce. Digeft the Soap with the Spirit of Rofemary till it is diffolved, then add the Camphire. *L.*

This is contriv'd for much the fame Ufes as the *Balfamum Saponaceum*, for which it is fubftituted.

Balfamum Traumaticum.
Vulnerary Balfam.

Take of powder'd Benjamin, two Ounces ; *Peruvian* Balfam, an Ounce and half ; hepatic Aloes, half an Ounce ; of rectify'd Spirit of Wine, a Quart ; digeft then in a Sand Heat for four Days, and ftrain. *E.*

In the *London* Difpenfatory this Medicine is thus directed :

Take of Benjamin, three Ounces ; of ftrain'd Storax, two Ounces ; of Balfam of *Tolu*, one Ounce ; of Succotrine Aloes, half an Ounce ; of rectify'd Spirit of Wine, a Quart. Digeft them together till as much as may be of the Gums are diffolved, then ftrain the Spirit off. *L.*

Both thefe are made in Imitation of a Medicine, which has been of confiderable Ufe in private Families, call'd the *Jefuit*'s Drops, or *Fryer*'s Balfam. There are, I believe, at leaft twenty People in *London*, who get a comfortable Subfiftance by felling it as an Arcanum, under various Names and Titles. And one has had the Impudence to obtain a Patent for it, tho', in order to this, he muft have been obliged to fwear it is own Invention, in Defiance of Confcience and the Pillory, notwithftanding that *Pomet* publifh'd the Receipt, in his Hiftory of Drugs, many Years ago. It is much celebrated Abroad, under the Name of *Baume de Commandeur de Berne*, or

Balfamum Commendatoris.

The Commander's Balfam.

The Receipt ftands thus :

Take dry Balfam of *Peru*, one Ounce ; Storax in Tears, two Ounces ; Benjamin in Tears, three Ounces ; Aloes Succotrine, the beft Myrrh, Olibanum in Tears, Roots of *Bohemian* Angelica , Flowers of St. *John*'s Wort , of each half an Ounce ; Spirit of Wine, one Quart ; beat all together , and put them into a Bottle well ftopt, which hang in the Sun during the Dog-days ; at the End of which Time, the whole muft be paffed thro' a Li-

nen Cloth, and ufed for the Purpofes under fpecified :

All Gunfhot Wounds, and fuch as are made with fharp Inftruments, if they are not mortal, are cured in the Space of eight Days, by the Application of this Balfam, either with a Feather, Cotton, or by way of Injection, provided the Wound has been firft of all drefs'd with it, and no other Medicines have been ufed ; for when the Wound is at firft dreffed with it, no Pus will afterwards be formed; whereas the Generation of Pus is always the Effect of dreffing with the ordinary Medicines. There is no Occafion either for Tents or Plaifters when this Balfam is apply'd, efpecially at the firft Dreffings. Upon its firft Application to the Wound, it creates an intolerable Pain ; but that foon goes off, and is no more felt. This Balfam is fo admirable a Remedy for the Colic, that if four or five Drops of it are intimately mixed with a Glafs of Wine, and drank, the Patient's Indifpofition is foon after removed. It is alfo a fovereign Remedy for the Gout, when apply'd to the Part affected with a Feather or Cotton. In a Tooth-ach it is of fingular Service, when Cotton, foak'd in it, is apply'd to the Tooth affected. All Sorts of Ulcers, as alfo Cancers and Chancres, are cured by it. It is effectual againft the Bites of venomous Animals, thofe of mad Dogs not excepted. It prevents Pitting by the Small-pox, if the Puftules are anointed with it as foon as they appear on the Face ; for it dries them before Pus is form'd in them, upon which Circumftance the Pitting depends. It proves an excellent Remedy for the Hæmorrhoids, if they are rubb'd with it when the Patient goes to Bed. It is excellent for Defluxions and Bruifes, if the Parts affected are anointed with it.

Five

Five or fix Drops of it, exhibited internally, in four or five Spoonfuls of Broth, prove an excellent Remedy for the Purple Fever. It is alfo good for fore Eyes, when put into them with a Feather. It is alfo excellent for Pains in the Stomach, in which Cafe, if the Patient is feverifh, he muft take it in Broth, and, if not, in Wine. It cleanfes the Stomach, and procures an Appetite. It muft never be warm'd, but always be apply'd cold, and it becomes dry as foon as it is apply'd to the Part affected. Five or fix Drops of it, taken in Wine or Broth, are very proper for provoking the *Menfes*, when defective ; and giving a Check to them, when too luxuriant. When we pour out any Quantity of this Balfam, we muft ftop the Phial immediately after, to prevent its Evaporation. If any Wound has been previoufly dreffed with other Medicines, it muft be wafhed with warm Wine before the Application of this Balfam, which will cure it effectual-

ly, tho' not fo fpeedily as if th Balfam had been ufed at firft. I cures Fiftulas, however old, and in whatever Parts of the Body. Five or fix Drops of it, exhibited in white Wine, or in three or four Spoonfuls of Broth, are an excellent Remedy for Fluxes and Hæmorrhages. It is good for the Pricking of Horfes, when fhoed ; by pouring a Drop or two into the Hole from which the Nail is drawn, it is cured immediately.

Balfamum Viride.

The green Balfam.

Take of Linfeed Oil, and Oil of Turpentine, each a Pound ; of Verdigrife reduc'd to Powder, three Drams ; and boil them together, keeping the Mixture ftirring, fo as to diffolve the Verdigrife. *E.*

This fhould feem a very good Medicine to cleanfe and deterge foul Ulcers, and keep down fungous Flefh.

CHAP. XIV.

Of OINTMENTS and PLAISTERS.

GENERAL RULES *for making* OINTMENTS *and* PLAISTERS.

I. SUCH *Ointments* and *Plaifters* as have Plants in their Compofitions, are to be boiled till the Herb becomes almoft crifp, with Care to avoid their turning black ; then after ftraining, they are again to be fet over the Fire, to evaporate all their Moifture, let the Plants be frefh gather'd, fucculent, and well bruifed, unlefs they are order'd dry.

II The *Metalline Powders* are to be firft boiled with the oily or fat Ingredients, till they are thoroughly

incorporated : But Plaifters require to be mixed with Spring Water, till they become of the proper Confiftence. *Gums* which are readily diffolvible, as alfo *Powders* and *Turpentine*, are to be added towards the End of the Operation.

III. *Ointments* as well as *Plaifters* are not all to be made of the fame Confiftence, the fofter *Plaifters* come under the Name of *Cerates*, and ought to be kept in Gallipots or Bladders ; as thofe of a more folid Nature are formed into Rolls. But the Compofition of both is fo various, that at particular Rules are generally ded to direct the Artift.

OINTMENTS.

Unguentum Ægyptiacum.

Egyptian Ointment.

ake of Verdigrife, reduced to fine Powder, five Ounces; of Honey, fourteen Ounces; of Vinegar, feven Ounces; boil them together over a gentle Fire, to the Confiftence of an Ointment. *E.*

This is of confiderable Ufe in Surery, to keep down fungous Flefh, nd cleanfe fordid Ulcers.

Unguentum album.

The white Ointment.

ake of Oil of unripe Olives, three Pints; of Cerufe, a Pound; of white Wax, nine Ounces; and mix them together, according to Art, fo as to make an Ointment. *E.*

This is intended principally as a :ooler.

Unguentum album Camphoratum.

White Ointment with Camphire.

This is made by adding to the preceding white Ointment, when remov'd from the Fire; an Ounce of Camphire, rubb'd with a few Drops of Oil of Almonds, and mixing them together. *E.*

The *Unguentum album* of the Lonon Difpenfatory is thus directed:

ake of Olive Oil, one Pint; of white Wax, four Ounces; of Sperma Ceti, three Ounces. Melt all together with a gentle Heat, and ftir them very brifkly without ceafing, till they are fully cold. *L.*

This feems well contriv'd for a :ooling Ointment, and muft be proer enough for flight Excoriations. he Cerufe is left out, becaufe, as we

are told, it may be dangerous when apply'd to the tender Bodies of young Children; but there feems to be no Foundation for this Apprehenfion.

If a Dram and half of Camphire, beat with a few Drops of Oil of Almonds, be added to this, it is then call'd *Unguentum album Camphoratum.*

Unguentum Antipforicum.

Ointment for the Itch.

Take of Elecampane Root, and the Root of fharp-pointed Dock, each three Ounces; flice and bruife them; then pour thereon three Pints of Spring Water, and a Pint of Vinegar; boil them to a half, and ftrongly prefs out the remaining Liquor; to which add, eight Ounces of the Leaves of frefh Water Creffes well bruis'd, and add four Pounds of Hogs-Lard; then boil all together, till the aqueous Moifture is exhaled, and prefs out the Ointment, whereto put four Ounces of the Oil of Bays, and the fame Quantity of yellow Wax; afterwards mix the whole together. Sulphur may be hereto added occafionally. *E.*

The Title expreffes the Ufes.

Unguentum Antipforicum, cum Mercurio.

Ointment for the Itch, with Mercury.

This is made of the preceding Ointment, by adding thereto four Ounces of Quickfilver, kill'd by being ground with a proper Quantity of *Venice* Turpentine, and mixing them together according to the Rules of Art, fo as to make an Unguent. *E.*

Some Care and Caution is neceffary in the Ufe of this; otherwife it will raife a Salivation.

Unguentum, seu, Linimentum Arcai.

The Ointment, or Liniment of *Arcaus.*

Take of Hogs-Lard, a Pound; of Goats Suet, two Pounds; of Gum Elemi, and *Venetian* Turpentine, each a Pound and half; melt them together, then strain the whole, and make thereof an Unguent according to Art. *E.*

Arcaus, the Author of this Composition affirms, that it ripens, digests, deterges, and incarns.

In the *London* Dispensatory it is thus directed under the Title of

Unguentum è Gummi Elemi.

Ointment of Gum Elemi.

Take of tried Mutton Suet fresh, two Pounds; of Gum Elemi, one Pound; of common Turpentine, ten Ounces. Melt the Gum with the Suet, and all being removed from the Fire, add forthwith the Turpentine, and, while the Mixture is fluid, strain it. *L.*

This is intended as a Digestive, and an Incarnant, for which it is pretty much in Esteem.

Unguentum Basilicon.

The Ointment Basilicon.

Take of yellow Wax, Goats Suet, white Rosin, dry Pitch, and *Venice* Turpentine, each half a Pound; of Olive Oil, two Pounds and a half: Dissolve the other Ingredients in the Oil, stir them well together, then strain the whole for an Ointment. *E.*

This is us'd as a Digestive and Incarnant.

Unguentum Basilicum flavum.

Yellow Basilicum.

Take of Olive Oil, a Pint; yellow Wax, yellow Rosin, *Burgundy* Pitch, of each a Pound; of common Turpentine, three Ounces.

Melt the Wax, Rosin, and Pitch with the Oil, over a gentle Fire, then take them off, add the Turpentine, and strain the Mixture while it remains hot. *L.*

This is intended for the same Uses as the preceding.

Unguentum Basilicum nigrum vel tetrapharmacum.

Black Basilicum.

Take of Olive Oil, a Pint; yellow Wax, yellow Rosin, common Pitch, of each nine Ounces. Mix all together, and strain the Mixture off while hot. *L.*

This is not much in use; and is said to be subject to generate fungous Flesh in Ulcers.

Unguentum Basilicum viride.

Green Basilicum.

Take of yellow Basilicum, eight Ounces in Weight; of Olive Oil, three Ounces in Measure; of prepared Verdigrise, one Ounce. Mix all into an Ointment. *L.*

This is considerably detergent, and proper in order to keep down fungous Flesh in Ulcers.

Unguentum è Lapide Calaminari.

Ointment of *Lapis Calaminaris.*

Take of yellow Wax, eighteen Ounces; melt it in Oil of Olives, two Pints; then gradually sift into it, of powder'd *Lapis Calaminaris,* ten Ounces and a half. *E.*

This is made in Imitation of the celebrated Cerate of *Turner,* which he thus directs,

Ceratum de Lapide Calaminari.

Cerate of *Lapis Calaminaris,* commonly call'd *Turner's Cerate.*

Take of fresh-made unsalted *May* Butter, and of the best yellow Wax, sufficiently defecated, each three Pounds and an half; of pure

pure and newly prepared Oil of Olives, four Pounds ; and of the best Calamine Stone, sufficiently triturated, and pass'd thro a Sierce, two Pounds and ten Ounces : Let the Wax and Butter be put into a proper Vessel, with the Oil, and melted over a gentle Fire ; then strain them thro' a Linen Cloth into another Vessel, and immediately sprinkle the Powder of the Calamine Stone into it by Degrees, continually agitating the Mixture, and stirring from the Bottom of the Vessel, till it begins to cool, and becomes so thick, that the Powder, in consequence of its Weight, can no longer subside to the Bottom of the Vessel.

Turner gives the following Encomium of this Cerate:

As I have had, says he, ample Experience of this Cerate, I may be allow'd, I hope, to judge of its singular Properties, and good Effects, in all cutaneous Ulcerations and Excoriations, either from Scalding, Burning, or Fretting of the said Parts, by means of salt, acrid, or sharp Humours ; upon which Accounts, not straining a Tittle beyond its deserved Eulogy, I am bold to affirm, it will do more in all these superficial Hurts of the Body, than either *Unguentum Tutiæ, Diapompholyx, Nutritum, Desiccativum Rubrum, Rosatum*, or all the Epulotic Medicines now in Use ; and for which Cause I can, for the public Benefit, sincerely recommend it to all the Professors of the Art ; and do wish, that the Apothecaries would keep it made up in their Shops, to deliver, at a suitable Price, to indigent, or poor People, instead of their ridiculous *Lucatellus's* Balsam, and other improper Medicines, which they call for, ignorantly, to heal their Skin-keep Maladies. I know the Medicine

has been imitated by several ; and I have seen somewhat like it in some Gentlemen's Salvatories ; but I know not more than two Persons I ever communicated it to, as I was wont to prepare it for my own Use. The Medicine, thus prepared, is of a good Consistence, and a true Cerate, serving both for Pledget and Plaister, neither sticking troublesomely, nor running off, or about, by the Heat of the Parts ; but keeping its Body, and performing Things incredible. Whoever thinks fit to take it into Practice, will never repent it, nor perhaps (when he has experienced it as I have done) think I have said too much in its Commendation. This is the Medicine I have so often taken Notice of, under the Name of *Ceratum de Lapide Calaminari*, which, that I might contribute my Mite to the Surgeon's Treasure of Medicine, I here have publish'd, and leave it to take its Fate.

Unguentum Cæruleum fortius.

The stronger blue Ointment.

Take of tried Hogs - Lard, two Pounds ; of Quicksilver, one Pound ; of the simple Balsam of Sulphur, an Ounce. Rub the Quicksilver with the Balsam of Sulphur, till the Quicksilver no longer appears ; then add by Degrees the Lard warmed, and diligently mix them. *L.*

Perhaps the Balsam of Sulphur, here directed, may be a little Check upon the Quicksilver, and prevent its rising to the Mouth so readily as it would do otherwise. It is also said to divide the Mercury sooner and better than Turpentine.

Unguentum Cærulcum mitius.

The weaker blue Ointment.

Take of tried Hogs Lard, four Pounds ; of Quicksilver, one Pound ; of common Turpentine,

an

an Ounce. Rub the Quickfilver in a Mortar with the Turpentine, till the Quickfilver appears no longer, then add, by Degrees, the Lard warmed, and mix them diligently. *L.*

Unguentum Mercuriale.

Mercurial Ointment.

Take of Hogs Lard, two Ounces; Quickfilver, half an Ounce; rub them in a Mortar, till the Globules of Quickfilver no longer appear.

This may be made with only a double, or triple Quantity of Hogs Lard, to the Quickfilver. *E.*

In all thefe the Axungia is in too great a Proportion to the Quickfilver, which renders it more troublefome to rub in.

Unguentum Citrinum,

The yellow Ointment.

Take an Ounce of Quickfilver, and two Ounces of Spirit of Nitre; diffolve them in a Sand Heat, and, while very hot, mix therewith a Pound of melted Hogs Lard; before the Lard is cold, ftir them briſkly together in a Marble Mortar, ſo as to make an Ointment. *E.*

An Ounce of ftrong Spirit of Nitre, or *Aqua fortis duplex*, will readily diffolve an equal Weight of Quickfilver; and this, I think, ſhould be the Proportion for this Ointment. It is an Efcharotic, and is fometimes apply'd to Chancres, or us'd for eating down the Callofities of Ulcers.

Unguentum deficcativum rubrum.

The red drying Ointment.

Take of Olive Oil, a Pound and half; and of white Wax half a Pound; melt them together, and, when remov'd from the Fire, fift in the following Ingredients reduc'd to Powder, *viz.* of Calamine, fix Ounces; of Litharge of Gold and BoleArmoniac, each four Ounces; and of Camphire, firft rubb'd with a little Oil of Almonds, three Drams; then ſtir them briſkly together into an Ointment. *E.*

This, as its Title expreffes, is intended as a Deficcative.

Unguentum Dialthææ.

Ointment of Marfhmallows.

Take of the Oil of Mucilages, two Pounds; of yellow Wax, half a Pound; of white Rofin, three Ounces; and of *Venice* Turpentine, an Ounce and half; mix them together, and make an Ointment according to Art. *E.*

This is prepar'd fomewhat different in the *London* Difpenfatory, under the Title of *Unguentum ex Althæa,* thus:

Unguentum ex Althæa.

Ointment of Marfhmallows.

Take of the Oil of Mucilages, three Pints; of yellow Wax, one Pound; of yellow Rofin, half a Pound; of common Turpentine, two Ounces. Melt the Rofin and Wax with the Oil, then, thefe being taken off of the Fire, add the Turpentine, and ftrain the Mixture while it is hot. *L.*

This is much us'd as an Emollient and Relaxer.

Unguentum Diapompholygos.

Ointment of Pompholyx.

Take of Oil of unripe Olives, twenty Ounces; of the Juice of common

mon Nightſhade Berries, or of the *Solanum lethale,* eight Ounces; boil them together over a gentle Fire, till the Juice is exhaled; then, towards the End of the Operation, diſſolve five Ounces of white Wax in the Oil, and, removing it from the Fire, add thereto, whilſt it yet remains hot, the following Ingredients reduced to Powder, four Ounces of Ceruſe; of calcin'd Lead and Pompholyx, each two Ounces; and of clean Frankincenſe, an Ounce. Mix all together into an Ointment. *E.*

It is intended for hot, inflam'd, and corroſiveUlcers, which diſcharge a ſaline, acrimonious, and corroſive Matter. But I don't know that it is much in Uſe.

Unguentum Epiſpaſticum.
Bliſtering Ointment.

Take of Hogs Lard and *Venice* Turpentine, each three Ounces; of yellow Wax, one Ounce; of Cantharides, three Drams: Melt the Lard and Wax together, then add the Cantharides in Powder; laſtly, the Turpentine; and mix all together into an Ointment. *E.*

This, as the Title imports, is deſign'd for a Veſicatory; and intended for dreſſing of Bliſters, to keep them running, or rendering them perpetual, as they are call'd.

Unguentum ad Veſicatoria.
Ointment for Bliſters.

Take of tried Hogs Lard, and of the bliſtering Plaiſter, equal Weights. Melt them together with a very gentle Heat, and ſtir them well, till fully cold. *L.*

This is deſign'd for the ſame Uſes as the preceding.

Unguentum è Mercurio præcipitato.
Ointment with precipitated Mercury.

Take of the ſimple Ointment, an Ounce and a half; of precipitated Sulphur, two Drams; of white precipitated Mercury, two Scruples. Mix all together, and moiſten them with the Ley of Tartar, to bring the whole to the Conſiſtence of an Ointment. *L.*

Boerhaave ſtrongly recommends an Ointment made of an Ounce of *Pomatum,* or Ointment of Roſes, and a Dram of the white Precipitate of Mercury, for all cutaneous Diſorders, in which Caſes it is really very excellent. This Ointment is an Imitation of his. But the white Precipitate ſeems to be in too ſmall a Proportion. I don't know from Experience, whether the Sulphur imparts to it any Virtues, but I ſhould ſuſpect that it does not.

Unguentum Nervinum.
Nerve Ointment.

Take of the Leaves of Male Southernwood, Marjoram, or *Origanum,* Mint, Penyroyal, Rue, and Roſemary, each ſix Ounces; let the Herbs be freſh gather'd, well bruis'd, and boil'd till their aqueous Part is evaporated, in five Pints of Neat's Foot Oil, and three Pounds of Beef Suet, then preſs out all that will run; add thereto half a Pound of Oil of Bays, and mix them together into an Ointment. *E.*

This is a warm invigorating Topic, and may be us'd with good Effect, to excite the Nerves to Action, when too languid.

Unguentum viride.
Green Ointment.

Take of the green Oil, three Pounds; of yellow Wax, ten Ounces. Melt the Wax with the Oil over a gentle Fire, continually ſtirring till the Mixture is cold. *L.*

This

This feems calculated for the fame Purpofes as the preceding.

Unguentum Nutritum.

The Ointment called Nutritum.

Take of Litharge of Gold, and of Vinegar, each half a Pound; of Oil of unripe Olives, a Pound and a half: Rub them well together in a Mortar, pouring in at one time a little Oil, and at another a little Vinegar, till the latter no longer appears difunited, but the whole Mixture becomes a white Unguent. *E.*

This is a great Deficcative, or Dryer.

Unguentum Tripharmacum.

Ointment of three Ingredients.

Take of the common Plafter, four Ounces in Weight; of Olive Oil, two Ounces in Meafure; of Vinegar, one Ounce in Meafure. Set them together over a gentle Fire, continually ftirring them, till they are brought to the Confiftence of an Ointment. *L.*

This is fubftituted for the preceding, in the laft *London* Difpenfatory.

Unguentum Ophthalmicum.

Ointment for the Eyes.

Take of the Ointment of Tutty, an Ounce and a half; of the Ointment of Lead, two Scruples; of Camphire, half a Scruple: Mix them together, and make thereof an Ointment by the Rules of Art. It may alfo be made with a double or triple Proportion of Camphire.

This is defigned as a drying and aftringent Topic, to be ufed in Rheums, and Defluxions of the Eyes.

Unguentum Ophthalmicum Sloanei.

Sir *Hans Sloane's* Ophthalmic Ointment.

Take of prepared Tutty, one Ounce; of *Lapis Hæmatitis* prepared, two Scruples; of the beft Aloes prepar'd, twelve Grains; of prepar'd Pearl, four Grains. Put them into a Porphyry, or Marble Mortar, and rub them with a Peftle of the fame Stone very carefully, with a fufficient Quantity of Vipers Greafe or Fat to make a Liniment: To be ufed daily, Morning or Evening, or both, as hereafter directed.

Sir *Hans Sloane* informs us, that this Remedy was communicated to Sir *Theodore Mayerne* by Sir *Matthew Lifter,* and that Sir *Theodore* probably communicated it to Dr. *Thomas Rugeley,* Father to Dr. *Luke Rugeley,* who ufed it with extraordinary Succefs in the Cure of fore Eyes. He farther informs us, that for a pecuniary Reward he procured the genuine Receipt, in the Doctor's own Hand-writing, from a Perfon whom Dr. *Rugeley* employ'd in making it; and that he, Sir *Hans,* reform'd, improv'd, and us'd it, for many Years, in the Form above fpecify'd. The principal Improvement Sir *Hans* takes Notice of, is, the Subftitution of Vipers Fat for Hogs Lard, which was directed in the original Receipt.

Sir *Hans* informs us, that the Method which has beft fucceeded in facilitating the efficacious Ufe of this Liniment, is to bleed and blifter in the Neck and behind the Ears, in order to draw off the Humours from the Eyes; and afterwards, according to the Degree of the Inflammation, or Acrimony of the Juices, to make a Drain by Iffues between the Shoulders, or a perpetual Blifter: And, for r wathing the Eyes, he generally :commends Spring-water, which he inks preferable to any fpirituous otion, whether fimple or compound. And the beft inward Medines he has experienced to be Conrve of Rofemary-flowers, Antipileptic Powders, fuch as *Pulvis ad uttetum*, Betony, Sage, Rofemary, yebright, wild *Valerian*-root, Caf-or, *&c.* wafhed down with a Tea ade with fome of the fame Ingreients; as alfo Drops of *Spiritus lavendulæ compofitus*, and *Sal Volat. leof.* If the Inflammation returns, rawing about fix Ounces of Blood rom the Temples by Leaches, or upping on the Shoulders, is very roper. The Liniment is to be ap-fied with a fmall Hair Pencil, the ye winking, or a little opened. n profecuting the Cure of fore yes, he has been fometimes fur-rized at Want of Succefs, till at ngth he found that the Caufe was lurking intermitting Fever, every 'it of which affected the Eyes, and endered their Diforder obftinate; herefore, upon taking off the Fe-er by a proper Ufe of the Bark, he Cure has been effectually per-ormed.

This Medicine has cured many, hofe Eyes were covered with opake ilms, and Cicatrices left by Inflamnations and Apoftems of the Cor-ea; which though they happen to 'erfons of all Conditions, yet are nore common among the poorer ort of People; many of whom were totally deprived of Sight, as to e under a Neceffity of being led; nd, after fome Time, could per-ctly well find their Way without a 3uide. And it is not only very be-eficial in fuch Cafes, but alfo where here is an exceffive Pain in the Eyes, hooting thence up into the Head, as e particularly remembers in a great ady, who had fuch Pains in her re Eyes, and Head, that fhe had,

when he firft faw her, taken about fifty Drops of Laudanum thrice in twenty-four Hours; of which Complaints fhe and many others have been relieved by this Medicine, without the Help of any Opiate.

He fays, it is to be obferved (contrary to the common Practice, and to the Opinion which he himfelf en-tertained in his earlier Days, and communicated to the Public in the Introduction to his *Natural Hiftory of Jamaica*) that Cathartics, efpe-cially with the Addition of Mercury, are prejudicial in Difeafes of the Eyes, which are cured by this Medicine.

It is, fays he, alfo worthy of Re-mark, that People afflicted with weak Eyes are over-fond of Hood-winking, or covering them from the Light, which fometimes retards the Cure, by keeping their Eyes too warm; and, therefore, he has con-ftantly advifed them to throw away thefe Coverings, as foon as they could poffibly bear the Light.

Unguentum è Pice.
Ointment of Tar.

Take of Tar, of tried Mutton Suet, equal Weights. Melt them together, and ftrain while hot. L.

Unguentum Populeon.
Ointment of Poplar.

Take a Pound of the frefh gather'd Buds of the black Poplar, bruife them, and mix them well with four Pounds of frefh Hog's Lard, to be kept in this State, put up in a clofe glaz'd Veffel, till the following Herbs are in Seafon: Then take of the Leaves of Hemlock, black Henbane, Garden Poppy, and common Nightfhade, each fix Ounces: Bruife them all, and put them to the Lard, mix'd with the Poplar-buds: Now boil them over a gentle Fire till the aqueous Moifture is confumed; then ftrain

and

and strongly press out the Ointment, in which dissolve four Ounces of yellow Wax. *E.*

This is intended for a cooling Topic, but is not much in Use.

Unguentum Rosaceum, vulgò Pomatum.

Rose Ointment, commonly called Pomatum.

Take any Quantity of Hog's Lard, cut it into small Pieces, put it into a glazed earthen Vessel, and pour thereon as much Spring-water as will float some Inches above it: Let them stand together for ten Days, the Water being shifted once a Day; then melt the Lard with a very soft Heat, and throw it into a sufficient Quantity of Rose-water, wherein let it be well work'd; then pouring the Water off from it, add a few Drops of Oil of Rhodium. *E.*

Unguentum simplex.

The simple Ointment.

Take of tried Hog's Lard, two Pounds; of Rose-water, three Ounces. Pound the Lard with the Rose-water, till they are well mix'd; then melt the Lard with a very gentle Fire, and set it by a little while, that the Water may subside: Afterwards pour out the Lard, and leave the Water; then stir and beat the Lard, without ceasing, while it is growing cold, that it may be broke into as light and yielding a Mass as may be; and then add as much Essence of Lemons as shall be requisite to give it an agreeable Scent. *L.*

These two are substituted for the *Unguentum Pomatum* of former Dispensatories.

Unguentum Sambucinum.

Ointment of Elder.

Take of Elder-flowers, full blown,

four Pounds; of tried Mutton Suet, three Pounds; of Olive Oil, one Pound. Boil the Flowers, till they become almost crisp, in the Suet and Oil first melted together: Then press them out. *L.*

In the *Edinburgh* Dispensatory the *Unguentum Sambucinum* is thus directed:

Take of the internal fresh Bark of Elder, and of fresh Elder-flowers, each four Ounces: Bruise them well, and boil them in two Pints of Linseed Oil to the Consumption of the Moisture; then press out the Oil, and melt in it, of white Wax, six Ounces. Mix into an Ointment.

The particular Virtues of these may be learn'd from those of Elder. In general, it seems intended for a relaxing, anodyne Topic, and as a proper and safe Application to an *Erysipelas.*

Unguentum Saturninum, vulgò Balsamum Universale.

Ointment of Lead, commonly called the Universal Balsam.

Take of Litharge of Gold, and red Lead, each a Pound; of Vinegar, four Pints; and boil them together till one Half of the Liquor is wasted; then strain off the other: To the Remainder add the same Quantity of Vinegar, and proceed to boil and strain as before, till the Operation shall have been performed six several Times: Then mix all the Parcels of strain'd Liquor together in a glaz'd earthen Vessel, and exhale them to the Consistence of an Extract. Take of this Extract, and of white Wax, each three Ounces; of Olive Oil, a Pound; and mix them together, according to the Rules of Art, so as to make an Ointment. *E.*

This

This is very much used as a Desic-
tive, and Cicatrizer, and in all In-
ntions where Lead can be of Ser-
ce. But in the last Edition of the
Edinburgh Dispensatory it is thus
rected:

ake of the Sugar of Lead, two
Ounces; of white Wax, three
Ounces; of Olive Oil, one Pint.
Let the Wax be melted in the
Oil, and then gradually add the
Sugar of Lead, stirring it in per-
petually, till the Ointment grows
stiff by Cold.

n the *London* Dispensatory it is
us ordered:

ake of Olive Oil, half a Pint; of
white Wax, an Ounce and a half;
of Sugar of Lead, two Drams.
Rub the Sugar of Lead, first
brought to a very subtile Powder,
with some Part of the Oil; then
add this to the Wax, melted with
the rest of the Oil, and stir the
Mixture till it is fully cold: *L.*

n this the Proportion of Sugar of
ead is much less than in the pre-
ding.

Unguentum è Sulphure.
Ointment of Sulphur.

ake of simple Ointment, half a
Pound; of Flowers of Sulphur
unwashed, two Ounces; of Essence
of Lemons, a Scruple. Mix all
together. *L.*

This seems intended for the Itch;
it the common black Brimstone is
d to be more effectual than the
owers of Sulphur. This Oint-
ent may be improved by an Addi-
in of Salt of Tartar; and, in some
stinate cutaneous Cases, Pepper is
ded with good Effect.

Unguentum Tutiæ.
Ointment of Tutty.

akd any Quantity of prepared
Tutty, and mix it with as much

purified Vipers Fat as is requisite
to bring it to the Consistence of a
soft Ointment. *L.*

This seems intended for a Desiccative, principally for sore Eyes. I
suppose the Vipers Fat is here of-
dered, on Account of the Character
given of it by Sir *Hans Sloane*, for
Disorders of the Eyes, in treating of
the *Unguentum Ophthalmicum* above
described.

In the *Edinburgh* Dispensatory the
Unguentum Tutiæ is thus directed:

Take of white Wax, three Ounces:
Melt it over a gentle Fire, in ten
Ounces of the best Oil of Olives;
then gradually sift into it, of Tutty, two Ounces; of Calamine, one
Ounce; continually stirring it till
the Ointment grows cold.

This may be also made *extempore*,
by mixing these Powders with four
times the Quantity of unsalted Butter.

Unguentum Vermifugum.
Ointment against Worms.

Take of the Leaves of Female
Southernwood, common Wormwood, Rue, Savine, and Tansey,
each two Ounces: Bruise and boil
them, with a Pound and a half of
Olive Oil, and a Pound of Hogs
Lard, till the aqueous Moisture is
consumed; then strain and press
out all that will run; in which
melt three Ounces of yellow Wax:
Afterwards add of the Gall of an
Ox, and of *Succotrine* Aloes, each
an Ounce and a half; of Colocynth, and Worm-seed, each an
Ounce: Boil them all together,
keeping them continually stirring,
so as to make an Ointment. But
observe that the Aloes, the Colocynth, and the Wormwood, are
first to be reduced to very fine
Powder. *E.*

This seems to bid the fairest of any
Composition I have seen, or heard

of, to destroy Worms by external Application.

Linimentum album.

White Liniment.

Take of Olive Oil, three Ounces in Measure; of Sperma Ceti, the Weight of six Drams; of white Wax, two Drams: Melt all together with a gentle Fire, briskly stirring, without Intermission, till the Mixture is become quite cold. *L.*

This differs from the *Unguentum album* only in the Proportion of the Ingredients, so contrived as to render this softer.

Linimentum Tripharmacum.

Liniment of three Ingredients.

Take of the common Plaister, four Ounces in Weight; of Olive Oil, four Ounces in Measure; of Vinegar, the Measure of one Ounce: Set them over a gentle Fire, continually stirring, till the Liniment has acquired its due Consistence. *L.*

This differs only in Consistence from the *Unguentum Tripharmacum.*

Linimentum volatile.

Volatile Liniment.

Take of Oil of Almonds, one Ounce in Measure; of the Spirit of Sal Ammoniac, the Weight of two Drams. Shake them together in a wide-mouth'd Vial, till they perfectly unite. *L.*

This is ordered to be made with Spirit of Sal Ammoniac, with an alcaline Salt; not that made with Quick Lime. This is so readily made extemporaneously, that it does not seem proper for a Shop Medicine.

PLAISTERS.

Emplastrum adhæsivum.

Sticking Plaister.

Take of simple Diachylon, two Pounds; of *Burgundy* Pitch, a Pound; and melt them together, so as to make a Plaister. *E.*

The Title of this Plaister expresses the Uses, which are generally only to preserve Dressings on the Part. The *London* Dispensatory directs an adhæsive Plaister, under the Title of

Emplastrum commune adhæsivum.

The common sticking Plaister.

Take of the common Plaister, three Pounds; of yellow Rosin, half a Pound: Throw the Rosin, first reduced to Powder that it may the sooner melt, into the common Plaister, melted with a very gentle Heat, and stir them well together. Otherwise,

While the Oil and Litharge are boiling together, add the Rosin a little before the Plaister is finished, and then boil all together to the proper Consistence. *L.*

Emplastrum ex Ammoniaco cum Mercurio.

The Ammoniac Plaister, with Quickfilver.

Take of Gum Ammoniac strained, a Pound; of Quickfilver, three Ounces; of the simple Balsam of Sulphur, a Dram. Rub the Quickfilver with the Balsam of Sulphur, till it no longer appear; then add by degrees the Gum Ammoniac melted, a little before it is cold, and mix them carefully. *L.*

This seems a very well contrived Mercurial Plaister. It is a high Resolvent, and proper to be apply'd to indurated Parts, a Scirrhus, Tophs, and Nodes. But where this can be

Service, perhaps a well contrived rcurial Ointment would have a ter Effect.

ith the same View the *Edinburgh* pensatory directs the following ister:

Emplastrum Mercuriale.

Mercurial Plaister.

ke of Diachylon with the Gums, Pound and a half: Melt it; hen add eight Ounces of Quick-ilver, an Ounce of *Venice* Tur-)entine, and an Ounce and a half)f liquid Storax; which are to be irst thoroughly mixed together in a Mortar, till the Quicksilver re-nains no longer discernible. E.

nplastrum commune, cum Mercurio.

e common Plaister, with Quick-silver.

ke of the common Plaister, one Pound; of Quicksilver, three Ounces; of the simple Balsam of Sulphur, a Dram: Mix them to-gether, after the same Manner as n the Ammoniac Plaister, with Quicksilver. L.

Emplastrum Anodynum.

Anodyne Plaister.

ke of white Resin, eight Ounces; of Tacamahac powder'd, and Gal-banum, each four Ounces: When they are melted, add Cumin-seeds in Powder, three Ounces; black Soap, four Ounces: Make into a Plaister, according to Art. E.

This is a Discutient and Resol-nt.

Emplastrum Antihystericum.

Antihysteric Plaister.

ake of Galbanum, twelve Ounces; of Tacamahac, and yellow Wax, each six Ounces; of *Assa Fœtida*, four Ounces; of the Seeds of Cummin and *Venice* Turpentine, each four Ounces. Mix them to-

gether, and make a Plaister ac-cording to Art. E.

This may be apply'd to the Navel, or whole Abdomen, with very good Effect, in Hysteric Cases.

Emplastrum è Meliloto.

Melilot Plaister.

Take of the fresh Herb Melilot, six Pounds; bruise it well, put it into three Pounds of melted Beef-suet; boil them together till the Herb becomes almost crisp; then strong-ly press out the Suet, and add thereto eight Pounds of white Resin, and four Pounds of yellow Wax, boiling them a little toge-ther, so as to make a Plaister. E.

This is principally used for dressing Blisters.

Emplastrum attrahens.

Drawing Plaister.

Take yellow Rosin, yellow Wax, of each three Pounds; of tried Mut-ton-suet, one Pound: Melt all to-gether, and strain the Mixture, while it remains fluid. L.

This is substituted for the Melilot Plaister.

Emplastrum Cephalicum.

Cephalic Plaister.

Take of *Burgundy* Pitch, two Pounds; of soft Labdanum, one Pound; yellow Rosin, yellow Wax, of each four Ounces; of that called the expressed Oil of Mace, one Ounce. The Pitch, Rosin, and Wax being melted together, add first the Labdanum, and then the Oil of Mace. L.

In the *Edinburgh* Dispensatory the Cephalic Plaister is thus directed:

Take of yellow Wax, three Ounces; white Resin, Tacamahac, each two Ounces; Myrrh and Castor, each two Drams; *Venice* Turpen-

tine

tine, three Ounces; Chymical Oil of Lavender, and Oil of Amber, each a Dram. Mix, and make a Plaister, according to Art; but the Oils of Lavender and Amber are to be mix'd in, when the reft are taken from the Fire.

This feems a much better Plaister for the Purpofes the Title expreffes, than the preceding.

Emplaftrum de Cicuta, cum Ammoniaco.

Plaifter of Hemlock, with Gum Ammoniac.

Take of Gum Ammoniae, half a Pound; and diffolve it in a fufficient Quantity of Vinegar of Squills: Add to the Solution four Ounces of the Juice of the Leaves of Hemlock, ftrain the Whole, and boil it into a Plaifter. *E.*

This is intended as a Difcutient, and as fuch is ufed fuccefsfully.

Emplaftrum è Cymino.

The Cummin Plaifter.

Take of *Burgundy* Pitch, three Pounds; yellow Wax, Cumminfeeds, Caraway-feeds, Bay-berries, of each three Ounces. The Pitch and Wax being melted together, fprinkle into them the reft reduced to Powder, and ftir all well together. *L.*

This is much recommended as a Difcutient of Flatulences.

Emplaftrum Defenfivum.

Defenfive Plaifter.

Take of the Juice of Shepherd's-purfe, Knot-grafs, Horfe-tail, Yarrow, Plantain, the greater Houfeleek, common Nightfhade, and the greater Comfrey, each half a Pint; of Olive Oil, three Pints; of Hog's Lard, two Pounds; of Litharge of Gold, two Pounds

and a half; and of red Lead, half a Pound: Boil them up together almoft to the Confiftence of a Plaifter, and diffolve therein of yellow Wax and white Rofin, each four Ounces; then add of Olibanum and *Venice* Turpentine, each four Ounces; as alfo the following Ingredients reduced to Powder, *viz.* of Bole *Armeniac*, a Pound; of the greater Comfreyroot, Pomegranate-bark, Balauftins, Maftich, Dragon's-blood, and red Saunders, each two Ounces: Mix them, and make thereof a Plaifter according to the Rules of Art. The Plaifter may alfo be made without the Juices. *E.*

This is an Aftringent.

Emplaftrum Diachylon fimplex.

Simple Diachylon.

Take of the Oil of Mucilages, four Pounds; of Litharge of Gold, a Pound and a half; and boil them up to a Plaifter. *E.*

This is efteem'd an Emollient, Digeftive, Maturant, and Refolvent.

Emplaftrum commune.

The common Plaifter.

Take of Olive Oil, one Gallon; of Litharge, finely powder'd, five Pounds: Boil them together with about a Quart of Water, over a gentle Fire, continually ftirring, till the Oil and Litharge are united, and they acquire the due Confiftence of a Plaifter; and if the Water is wafted, before the Operation is over, more Water muft be poured on hot. *L.*

This is fubftituted for the *Diachylon fimplex.*

Emplaftrum Diachylon cum Gummi.

Diachylon with Gums.

Take of the Oil of Mucilages, four Pounds; of Litharge of Gold, two Pounds; and boil them in the he Confiftence of a Plaifter, then add thereto of Gum Ammoniac, Galbanum, *Venice* Turpentine, and yellow Wax, each half a Pound, and boil them into a Plaifter according to Art. *E.*

his very powerfully digefts, matues, and refolves.

Emplaftrum commune cum Gummi.

he common Plaifter, with Gums.

ke of the common Plaifter, three Pounds; of Galbanum ftrained, eight Ounces; common Turpentine, Frankincenfe, of each three Ounces. To the Galbanum and Turpentine melted together with a gentle Heat, fprinkle in the Frankincenfe reduced to Powder, and then gradually add to them the Plaifter firft melted, likewife with a very gentle Heat. Otherwife, tead of the common Plaifter finifhed, make Ufe of the Oil boiled with Litharge, as foon as they are joined, and not yet brought to the Confiftence of a Plaifter. *L.*

his is fubftituted for the *Diachy-*
1 cum Gummi.

Emplaftrum Diapalmæ dictum.

Diapalma.

ke of Litharge of Gold, and of Olive Oil, each three Pounds; of Hogs Lard, two Pounds, and boil them together, keeping them continually ftirring, till they become a Plaifter. To which, if there be added four Ounces of burnt *Chalcitis*, or calcined white Vitriol, it becomes the *Emplaftrum Diachalciteos*, or Vitriol Plaifter. *E.*

Emplaftrum Epifpafticum.

Bliftering Plaifter.

ke of Melilot Plaifter, and *Burgundy* Pitch, each eight Ounces; of *Venice* Turpentine, three Ounces; Cantharides, five Ounces. Mix them together, and make

them into a Plaifter, according to Art; but obferve to reduce the Cantharides to a very fine Powder, and add them to the other Ingredients, firft melted together. *E.*

Emplaftrum Epifpafticum.

The compound bliftering Plaifter.

Take of *Grecian* Pitch, ten Ounces; yellow Wax, four Ounces; white Refin, two Ounces; melt them together, and add, of *Venice* Turpentine, eighteen Ounces. Melt all together, and whilft hot, fift in the following Ingredients, firft reduced to a fine Powder, and mix'd together, continually ftirring them in, *viz.* Muftard Seed, and black Pepper, each an Ounce. Verdigrife, two Ounces; Cantharides, twelve Ounces. Make a Plaifter. Both this and the preceding, are to be kept in Bladders, anointed with Oil.

Emplaftrum Veficatorium.

Bliftering Plaifter.

Take of the drawing Plaifter, two Pounds; of Cantharides, one Pound; of Vinegar, half a Pint. The Plaifter being melted, a little before it hardens, fprinkle in, and mix the Cantharides, reduced to a very fine Powder; then add the Vinegar, and beat all well together. *L.*

The three laft Plaifters are intended to raife Blifters only; and either will anfwer that Purpofe very well. But I muft remark, that when Applications are made to the Feet, with an Intent to ftimulate ftrongly, excite Pain therein, and relieve the Head, Cataplafms compofed of equal Parts of fcrap'd Horfe Radifh, and powder'd Muftard Seed, moiften'd with old Yeaft, and very fharp Vinegar, will anfwer the Defign more expeditioufly, ftrongly, and with much better Effect, than any Application in which Cantharides is an Ingredient.

Emplaftrum de Minio fimplex.

Simple red Lead Plaifter.

Take of red Lead, a Pound; of Olive Oil, a Pound and a half; and of Vinegar, half a Pint; and boil them together over a flow Fire, fo as to make a Plaifter. *E.*

Emplaftrum è Minio.

Red Lead Plaifter.

Take of Olive Oil, two Quarts; of red Lead finely powder'd, two Pounds and a half. With thefe the Plaifter is to be prepared in the fame Manner as the common Plaifter, only here more Water is required, and more Caution, that the Plaifter may not be burnt, and turn black. *L.*

Thefe are faid to be good for drying and cicatrizing.

Emplaftrum de Minio cum Sapone.

Red Lead Plaifter, with Soap.

This is made by adding to the fimple red Lead Plaifter, when taken off the Fire, whilft it yet remains hot, after the Exhalation of the Moifture, half a Pound of *Venice* Soap, thin fliced, and ftirring them forcibly together, fo as to diffolve the Soap, and make a Plaifter according to Art. *E.*

The Soap in this Plaifter renders it very refolvent. It is apply'd fometimes to Arthritic Tumors and Strains.

Emplaftrum è Sapone.

Soap Plaifter.

Take of the common Plaifter, three Pounds; of hard Soap, half a Pound. To the common Plaifter liquefied, add the Soap, then melt all to the Confiftence of a Plaifter, and take particular Care that it

does not grow too cold before it is formed into Rolls. *L.*

Emplaftrum è Mucilaginibus.

Plaifter of Mucilages.

Take of yellow Wax, fourteen Ounces; of the Oil of Mucibges, eight Ounces in Meafure; of Gum Ammoniac ftrained, half a Pound; of common Turpentine, two Ounces. The Gum Ammoniac being melted with the Turpentine, add to them gradually the Wax melted with the Oil in another Veffel. *L.*

The *Emplaftrum è Mucilaginibus*, is principally us'd as a Suppurative. But I am inclin'd to believe the Mucilages mix'd with fomething oily to keep them from drying, will have a better Effect.

Emplaftrum Oxycroceum.

Oxycroceum.

Take of yellow Wax, one Pound; common Pitch, and Galbanum, each half a Pound; melt then over a gentle Fire, and add of Myrrh, Olibanum, and Venice Turpentine, each two Ounces. Mix all together, and make a Plaifter according to Art. *E.*

It is efteem'd a Refolvent, and is faid to fortify the Nerves and Mufcle, and to relieve Pain.

Emplaftrum Roborans.

Strengthening Plaifter.

Take of the common Plaifter, two Pounds; of Frankincenfe, half a Pound: of Dragon's Blood, three Ounces. To the common Plaifter melted, add the reft reduced to Powder. *L.*

The Title expreffes the Intention of this Plaifter.

Emplastrum Stomachicum.

Stomach Plaister.

Take of yellow Wax, eight Ounces; Tacamahac powder'd, four Ounces. When melted together add the following Ingredients reduced to Powder, *viz. Venice* Turpentine, six Ounces; of Bay Berries, powder'd, two Ounces; of Cubebs powder'd, an Ounce; expressed Oil of Mace, an Ounce and half; chymical Oil of Mint, two Drams. Mix them, and make thereof a Plaister according to Art. *E.*

This is prepar'd in a different Manner, in the *London* Dispensatory, thus:

Take of soft Labdanum, three Ounces; of Frankincense, one Ounce; Cinnamon, expressed Oil of Mace, so called, of each half an Ounce; of essential Oil of Mint, one Dram. Add to the Frankincense melted, first the Labdanum, a little heated till it is become soft, and then the Oil of Mace, afterwards mix in the Cinnamon with the Oil of Mint, and beat them together in a warm Mortar into a Mass, which is to be kept in a Vessel well closed, *L.*

Both these are intended as warm and cordial Applications to the Stomach; and exert very considerable Effects, when such Things are wanted.

Emplastrum Volatile.

Volatile Plaister.

Take of *Venice* Turpentine, an Ounce; grind it in a Mortar, gradually pouring thereto an Ounce of Spirit of Sal Ammoniac, and when they are thoroughly incorporated, add to them, by Degrees, half an Ounce of Tacamahac in Powder, and mix them together. *E.*

This seems intended as a very stimulating Resolvent.

CERATES.

Ceratum album.

White Cerate.

Take of Olive Oil, four Ounces in Measure; of white Wax, four Ounces in Weight; of Sperma Ceti, half an Ounce in Weight. Melt all together, and stir them well till the Cerate is quite cold. *L.*

This differs from the white Ointment, and Liniment, only in Consistence.

Ceratum citrinum.

Yellow Cerate.

Take of yellow Basilicum, half a Pound; of yellow Wax, an Ounce. Melt them together. *L.*

This differs from the yellow Basilicon only in Consistence.

Ceratum Epuloticum.

Cicatrizing Cerate.

Take of Olive Oil, a Pound; yellow Wax, prepared Calamy, of each half a Pound. Melt the Wax with the Oil, and as soon as the Mixture begins to congeal, sprinkle in the Calamy, and stir all well, till the Cerate is quite cold. *L.*

This seems to be intended to imitate *Turner*'s Cerate.

Ceratum Mercuriale.

Mercurial Cerate.

Take yellow Wax, tried Hogs Lard, of each half a Pound; of Quicksilver, three Ounces; of the simple Balsam of Sulphur, a Dram. Melt the Wax with the Lard, then add them gradually to the

Quick-

Quickfilver, firft well divided by the Balfam of Sulphur.

The Ufes of this may be known from thofe of the Quickfilver, which enters its Compofition.

EPITHEMS.

Epithema Veficatorium.

Bliftering Epithem.

Take of Cantharides reduced to a very fine Powder, and of Wheat Flower, equal Weights. With a fufficient Quantity of Vinegar, make them into a Pafte. *L.*

Epithema volatile.

Volatile Epithem.

Take equal Weights of common Turpentine, and of Spirit of Sal Ammoniac. Stir the Turpentine in a Mortar, and gradually drop in the Spirit, till the whole is reduced to a white Mafs. *L.*

This fhould feem to be a ftrong ftimulating Refolvent.

Cataplafma è Cymino.

Cummin Cataplafm.

Take of Cummin Seeds, half a Pound; Bay-berries, the Leaves of Water Germander dried, *Virginia* Snake Root, of each three Ounces; of Cloves, one Ounce, with Honey equal to thrice the Weight of the fpecies powder'd, make a Cataplafm. *L.*

This is fubftituted for the *Theriaca Londinenfis,* and is a very warm Topic, of confiderable Ufe, when Heat is to be excited in any Part.

Cataplafma difcutiens.

The difcutient Cataplafm.

Take of Bryony Root, two Ounces; the Root of common Flower de Luce, one Ounce; the Flowers of Chamomile and Elder, each half

an Ounce; Spring Water, a fufficient Quantity; boil them till they are tender, then bruife them well, and add, of Gum Ammoniac, diffolv'd in Vinegar, half an Ounce; crude Sal Ammoniac, two Drams; camphorated Spirit of Wine, one Ounce. Mix into a Cataplafm. *E.*

This feems an excellent Cataplafm for the Purpofes exprefs'd in the Title.

Cataplafma maturans.

Maturating Cataplafm.

Take of dried Figs, four Ounces; of yellow Bafilicum, one Ounce; of ftrained Galbanum, half an Ounce. Beat well the Figs with a little Wine or ftrong ftale Beer; then carefully mix in the Ointment, firft melted with the Galbanum. *L.*

The Title exprefles the Ufes.

Cataplafma fuppurans.

The fuppurating Cataplafm.

Take of white Lilly Roots (or thofe of Marfh Mallows) four Ounces; of fat Figs, one Ounce. Boil in a fufficient Quantity of Spring Water, till they are tender, bruife them well, and add, of crude Onions bruis'd, fix Drams; Galbanum, diffolv'd in the Yolk of an Egg, half an Ounce; of the *Unguentum Bafilicon,* and Oil of Chamomile, each an Ounce; the Meal of Linfeed, a fufficient Quantity. Mix and make a Cataplafm.

The Title exprefles the Intention, for which it feems excellently calculated.

Sinapifmus fimplex.

The fimple Sinapifm.

Take of Muftard Seed bruis'd, and the Crumb of Bread, each equal Parts; of the fharpeft Vinegar, a fufficient Quantity. Mix, and make a Cataplafm.

Sina-

Sinapifmus compofitus.

Take of Muftard Seed bruis'd, and the Crums of Bread, each two Ounces; bruis'd Garlic, half an Ounce; black Soap, one Ounce; the beft Vinegar, enough to make a Cataplafm.

Both thefe ftimulate very powerfully. See the Notes to the *Emaftrum Veficatorium.*

Coagulum Aluminofum.

Alum Curd.

Take of the White of an Egg at Pleafure, and ftir it in a Pewter Veffel, with a fufficient Lump of Alum, till it is coagulated. *L.*

This is a very good aftringent Epithem. I have known it apply'd to inflam'd, or over moift Eyes with very good Effect, receiv'd upon a little Tow. But it will fometimes excite Pains; and in this Cafe it muft be difcontinued; for nothing is more prejudicial to the Eyes, than Applications which give Pain.

A NEW

A NEW
English Difpenfatory.
BOOK V.
CHYMICAL MEDICINES.

CHAP. I.

CHYMICAL PREPARATIONS *of* VEGETABLES.

Diftill'd OILS.

Oleum Abfinthii.

Oil of Wormwood.

TAKE any Quantity of the Plant of Wormwood, moderately dried in the Shade, and cut to pieces; as much Spring Water as will commodiously keep it a-float, and a proper Quantity of Sea Salt to give the Liquor a tolerable Sharpnefs; let them ſteep together for for eight Days, then diftil them by the Alembic, with a ſomewhat ſmarter Fire, than what is uſual in the Diftillation of Waters, and afterwards ſeparate the Oil from the Water, according to the Rules of Art. *E.*

In the ſame Manner are diftill'd,

Oleum Hyſſopi.	Oil of Hyſſop.
Majorana.	Marjoram.
Mentha.	Mint.
Origani.	Origany.
Pulegii.	Penny-royal.
Roris Marini.	Roſemary.
Ruta, &c.	Rue, *&c.*
Florum Chama-	Flowers of
meli.	Chamomile.
Lavendula, &c.	Lavender,*&c.*
Seminum Aniſi.	Seeds of Aniſe.
Carui.	Caraway.
Cumini.	Cummin.

Oleum Fæniculi, &c.	Fennel, *&c.*
Corticis Limonum.	Lemon Peel.
Caryophillorum.	Cloves.
Cinnamomi.	Cinnamon.
Macis.	Mace.
Nucis Moſchata.	Nutmeg.
Ligni Saſſafras.	Saſſafras Wood.

But obſerve that all the *Seeds* and *Spices* ought to be bruiſed, before they are ſet to ſteep. *E.*

All Manner of unctuous *Vegetables* will afford their Oil by this Treatment, provided the Time of Digeſtion be ſuited to the Strength and Texture of the Subject. The tendereſt Plants ſcarce require any Maceration at all, thoſe of a ſoft and yielding Nature require one, two or three Days; and the viſcous ones of as many Weeks. The longer the Maceration is continued, the larger Quantity of Sea Salt is to be added; inſtead whereof may be uſed *Nitre* or any *fixed acid Spirit*; the Water ſeparated may be employed to Advantage in future Diftillations. *E.*

Diftilled and *Eſſential Oils*, are ordered to be prepared in the *Latin* Difpenfatory

From the Root of Saſſafras;
From the Leaves of Sweet-Marjoram

Wild-Marjoram,
Pepper-Mint,
Spear-Mint,
Penny-Royal,
Rosemary,
Rue,
Savine,
Wormwood;
From the Flowers of Chamomile,
Lavender;
From the Seeds of Anise,
Caraway,
Cummin,
Dill;
From Juniper-Berries,
From the Spices,
Cloves,
Nutmeg, and others.
These Oils are obtained by Distillation, with an Alembic and large Refrigeratory. Water must be added to the Materials in sufficient Quantity to prevent their Burning, and the Subject must be macerated in that Water a little Time before the Distillation. The Oil comes over with the Water, and either swims on the Top, or sinks to the Bottom, according as it is heavier or lighter. The Virtues of all these Oils may be learn'd from those of the Vegetables from whence they are distill'd.

Oleum Baccarum Juniperi.
Oil of Juniper.

Take any Quantity of bruised Juniper-berries, half their Weight of Spring Water, and a small Proportion of Yeast. Let them stand together for some Days to ferment, but not too long, and then add a sufficient Quantity of Spring Water, and distil the whole by the Alembic, separating the Oil, according to Art from the Water.

After the same Manner are distilled the Oils of Bayberries, and other Berries of that Kind; the Oils of Savin, and other Plants of that Nature; and indeed all the Oils of viscous Subjects, or those of a close Texture. E.

Boerhaave tells us, that essential aromatic Oils have almost an inimitable Virtue, intirely depending upon the Spirit, which is sharp, inflammatory, grateful, refreshing, heating, attenuating, and stimulating to the animal Spirits, and nervous Fibres; and by these Properties the Oils proves serviceable in cold, aged, watery, and phlegmatic Constitutions; and again, in cold Intermittents, moist and cold hypochondriacal and hysterical Cases, or other Diseases proceeding from cold, acid, or aqueous Flatulences in the Intestines; and, when prudently used in these Cases, they prove generally powerful and safe Medicines; but, when indiscreetly applied in Distempers attended with violent Heat, Motion or Inflammation, they prove poisonous. The Chymists have prudently observed, that these Oils act by Means of their Spirits, which, as lodged in the Oil, come to be applied to the Parts of the Body, so as there to produce their proper Actions, which would otherwise easily be lost thro' their extreme Volatility; and, when both the Oil and the Spirit act together, the Effect is more gentle, but more lasting. These Spirits, therefore, have, and communicate to the Oil, a certain Acrimony, which gives the Sensation of Fire to the Tongue, and presently occasions Pain; and the like Effect it shews when applied to the naked Nerves: When applied to the external Skin, they soon occasion the whole Series of an Inflammation, and end in a gangrenous Eschar. If applied to the Lips, or the internal Parts of the Nose or Palate, where the Nerves lie bare, it occasions the same, with great Violence, and presently brings on dangerous Inflammations. Whence we easily see, what Effects they may produce upon the Mouth, Throat, Stomach, and Intestines, when imprudently exhibited. Hence these
Oils

Oils may juftly be called inflammatory; tho' 'tis obferved, there is no better Remedy for immediately raifing the Spirits, by their grateful and extraordinary Virtue, which can fcarce be explained, for want of general Principles, otherwife than by direct Experiment. They have not only this refrefhing, but alfo an heating Virtue ; for if externally applied, or internally taken, they immediately begin to heat the Parts of the Body, and prefently increafe this Heat thus once begun ; but the colder and more languid the Body, the lefs they heat it, and *vice verfa* ; fo that, when rubb'd upon a dead Carcafs, they produce no Heat at all: Whence it is highly dangerous to give them in a burning Fever. They alfo increafe the Motion of the Nerves by Irritation, propelling the Spirits, and, perhaps, agreeably warming them both ; and whilft they perform all this, they attenuate and diffolve Vifcidities, fo far as can be done by increafing the Motion of Circulation. They have, however, befides thefe, other Virtues no lefs confiderable, and peculiar to each. Thus the Oils of the *Arbor Vitæ,* and of Savine, are powerful Emmenagogues, where the Stoppage of the menftrual Difcharge arifes from a languid Circulation. The effential Oil of Rue is of Service in the Epilepfy, from a cold relaxed State of the Nerves; and, alfo, in hyfterical Diforders from a cold Caufe ; that of Juniper Berries, in the cold Scurvy, and the Pains and Heavinefs thence proceeding; and, alfo, in nephritic Complaints, from cold Obftructions : That of Mint, in an almoft paralytic Weaknefs of the Stomach ; that of Lavender in the Palfy, Vertigo, Lethargy, and other cold Diforders of the Head: The fragrant un-inflammatory Oil of Rofes, is a noble Reviver of the languid Spirits ; that of Cinnamon,

very advantageous in a Deficience of Spirits without Inflammation, either during the Periods of Pregnancy, Delivery, or immediately afterwards, if at the fame Time there be no Rupture of the Veffels : Thofe of Wormwood, *Carduus Benedictus,* the leffer Centaury, Chamomile, and Tanfey, are ufeful againft Worms ; for which Purpofe they may be formed into Pills with Crums of Bread, and given in a fufficient Dofe upon an empty Stomach, the Patient refraining from all Kind of Aliment for two Hours afterwards: Thofe of Baum and Lemon peel, in Palpitations of the Heart, from cold phlegmatic Humours ; and thofe of Marjoram, Rofemary, and Sage, in Obftructions and mucous Difcharges of the Uterus, from a cold Caufe.

If thefe Oils be ftrongly ground for a confiderable Time, with thrice their own Weight of pure and dry Sea Salt, fo as to divide them well, and then again diftilled with Water, they become clean, pure, and limpid, or freed from their mucilaginous, or gummy Part, and fitter for keeping, if put up into Glafs Veffels having clofe Necks well fitted with ground Glafs Stoppels, and fet in a dry cold Place: But they lofe of their Quantity by this Rectification, much grofs Matter remaining behind in the Still, unable to afcend by Reafon of its Tenacity. Their Virtues, alfo, are leffened, which depend upon their Spirits, becaufe thefe remain in the Water ufed in the Diftillation, and are alfo diffipated in the Water which comes over. This Mr. *Homberg* fhews, by a laborious and inftructive, tho' dear Experiment ; for, upon diftilling fuch an Oil, with frefh Water every Time, fix and twenty times over, he at length obtained a fourth Part thereof ; the other three Fourths becoming an infipid, tenacious Subftance, whilft the Water, four and

twenty

enty times cohobated with the Oil, is rendered exceeding sharp, aromatic, saline, or spirituous.

When these pure Oils are, without addition, distilled in a Glass Retort, with a Fire gradually increased, they always exhale some Water, and afterwards become more clear, liquid, penetrating, and light; leaving at the bottom of the Retort, after the Distillation is performed by a strong Heat, a black, fixed, spongy terrestrial Matter: And if the Operation be thus several Times repeated, the greatest Part of the Oil will be converted into what the Chymists call *Caput Mortuum*. The excellent Mr. *Boyle*, by this Means, reduced a Pound of essential Oil almost wholly into Earth.

They who have distilled these Oils from pure Chalk, in clean Vessels, have found that by cohobating five Ounces of Oil eight Times upon fifteen Ounces of Chalk, it afforded only two Ounces and one Dram of Oil, two Drams and forty-five Grains of Salt, and half an Ounce of a strongly saline Water, containing the volatile Salt of the Oil, according to the Observation of Mr. *Bourdelin*.

Again, these Oils distilled from Lime slacked in the Air, and afterwards made exceedingly dry, are so changed, that a Pound of Oil being six times distilled, in the Way of Cohobation, upon fresh Quantities of Lime, with an extreme Degree of Fire, there came over fifteen Ounces and a half of Water, and one Ounce of Oil, according to the Observation of Mr. *Homberg*. Hence these Oils are found to consist chiefly of elementary Water and Earth, a little Oil, Spirit and Salt, and therefore new from the Union of those different Principles by the Action of the Fire: Whence Oil is not a simple elementary Body, but a Compound of several others. But whether this be really the Case, or whether

Experiments may shew, that these Oils are rather transmutable, I do not take upon me to determine.

This may be said with greater Certainty, that the more excellent of these Oils being dissolved in high rectified Spirit of Wine, digested and distilled with a gentle Fire of one hundred Degrees, give out their native Spirit to the Spirit of Wine, leaving a tenacious oily Matter behind; which being again treated in the same Manner with fresh Spirit of Wine, affords more; and thus, at last, remains an indolent, scentless, insipid, thick, and tenacious Body of Oil, perfectly deprived of all its Spirit: And if even pure Water be long shook with these Oils, it takes to itself their Spirit, becomes rich therewith, and thus robs the Oil of its Virtue; so that if the Operation be often repeated, it at length leaves the like indolent Remainder as the Spirit of Wine! And hence we are furnished with excellent Preparations; and learn, that these Oils are separable into Spirit and Oil, a little Salt, much Water, and much Earth; at least, that these are producible from them by Distillation. But nothing here seems stranger than that Water should remain so tenaciously mixed with these Oils, as not to be separated from them by Distillation twenty times repeated.

Hence it is confirmed by this, that the peculiar Taste and Odour of Plants wholly reside in their native Spirit: That the Taste and Odour of distilled aromatic Waters are solely owing to this Spirit, as peculiar to each Plant: That essential Oils, also, have their respective Characteristics from these Spirits alone: That the volatile Oil of Plants chiefly serves for detaining these Spirits, and the fixed Oil for connecting the solid Parts together; whence the Difference of these two Oils is very great: That both the expressed and distilled Oils

Oils are natural in the Plants themselves. And, that the Difference of Oils is principally owing to their Spirits.

Frederic Hoffman's Remarks on Essential Oils.

It frequently happens that Oils in Distillation, are yielded either too acrid, or of too deep a Colour, especially if they are urged by too strong a Fire ; and this is principally to be observed, when those Herbs, which abound with a large Quantity of acrid Salt, such as Thyme, Savory, Marjoram, and *Cretan* Origanum, are subjected to Distillation ; for if the Distillation is accelerated by too brisk a Fire, the Oils not only lose their grateful Smell, but also acquire a brownish or reddish Colour, which by no Means happens, if the Distillation is carried on by a moderate Fire.

Hence we learn, that excessive Heat is of great Efficacy in changing the Texture of Oils : And this Observation is applicable to the human Body, since we see, that by the intense Heat in Fevers, the temperate and sulphureous Parts of the Blood and Humours are surprizingly agitated ; so that it is not to be wondered at, if the oleous and temperate Principle of the Blood is converted into an highly saline sulphureous Matter, which being discharged by Stool and Urine, renders the Fæces bilious and yellow, and the Urine intensely red.

It is not to be doubted, but if right Measures are taken, those Oils which by too intense an Heat in Distillation, have in a great Measure, lost their grateful Taste, their Fragrance, and their Colour, may, by Rectification, be reduced to a due Degree of Perfection : But if the Rectification is attempted by putting the Oils in a Glass Retort, and carrying on the Distillation by a Sand

Heat, we find ourselves deceived, since, by this Means, these Oils have an ungrateful empyreumatic Smell, and are so far from acquiring their due and grateful Sweetness, that they are rather rendered more acrid. The Rectification is therefore to be made in another Manner : Those Oils, for Instance, are to be mixed with common Salt, with which they are to be strongly triturated, taking three Parts of Salt to one of Oil : Then adding a sufficient Quantity of Water, the Rectification is to be made from an Alembic, by which Means there is yielded an Oil far clearer, and of a more grateful Colour ; and what is surprizing is, that in the Bottom of the Alembic there is found a thick black Mass, which firmly adheres to the Hands, and the Quantity of which is the greater, the thicker and deeper colour'd the Oils are : I have often observed, that Oil of Marjoram contained more of this resinous Substance than other Oils, since an Ounce of it generally affords a Dram of such a Substance : The Oils of Mint, Spike, and Lavender, thus treated, do not leave so great a Quantity of Resin ; but the Oils of Thyme and Savory afford a large Quantity of it : We also find that such Oils as are of a gross Consistence, yield a large Quantity of this Resin.

This Experiment sufficiently evinces, that Oils are nothing but subtile and liquid Resins, closely united with Phlegm, and some ethereal Spirit ; as also that those Oils are hottest which contain the largest Quantity of Resin : For which Reason such Oils should always be cautiously prescrib'd internally by the Physician, because all subtile oleous Substances induce an intense and long-continuing Heat on the Humours of the human Body.

It is also to be observed, that Oils rendered more limpid by this Rectification, are not so soon dissolved by
rectified

&ctified Spirit of Wine as they were afore; but for this Purpose they require highly rectified Spirit of Wine, since they are formed into small Globules, and with great Difficulty incorporated with common Spirit.

It is also certain from Experience, that ethereal, limpid, and fragrant Oils become thicker by Age, and lose a great deal of their Fragrance; and, if we want to restore this Fragrance, we must infuse them with recent Herbs and Leaves, and reiterate the Distillation from an Alembic; by which means they are again impregnated with that subtile, sweet, and spirituous Principle, which they had oft by excessive Age.

From this Experiment we learn, that, besides a sulphureous, saline, earthy, or aqueous Principle, there is also another in Oils, which the Antients called Spirits, which is highly active, of a thin, ethereal Substance; and necessary to preserve the natural Crasis and Texture of the Oil.

This Spirit is principally disposed to Evaporation, by the Heat of the Air; and when this Spirit is lost, we find that the Oil is greatly changed in its Consistence, Smell, Taste, and Virtues. If, therefore, we intend to preserve Oils, we must not only carefully stop the Vessels which contain them, but also deposite them in cold Places, so that the Spirit being pent up in them, their Texture may remain entire.

Because the Air, especially when hot, induces a greater Change on the Nature of Oils, and the Quality of the oleous Mixture, than any thing else, whilst by long acting upon them, it deprives them of their grateful Taste and Smell, and inspissates them; the express'd Oils tending to a rancid State; and those distill'd to a terebinthinaceous Nature; the Colour also being in some greatly changed. Hence Oils are carefully

to be preserved from the free Access of an hot Air, which may be done by filling the Vessels in which they are kept, allowing only a small Space for Rarefaction, lest, upon the Approach of Heat, they should burst. They are also to be carefully stopt, and put into cold and dry Places.

Some, in order to preserve Oils, add some Water; such, for Instance, as distill'd Rose-water; which is of excellent Service, when there is not Oil enough to fill the whole Glass; since the Water, by its Exhalation, keeps the Consistence of the Oil thin, and hinders it from being inspissated.

It is also certain, from Experience, that Oils can never be intimately united and incorporated with Water; but these Substances, naturally immiscible, may by Art be so mixed, as not to be separated from each other. This is most commodiously done by pouring a few Drops of any aromatic Oil on Sugar, then putting it into Water, and shaking it; by which means the whole Oil, in a Moment, enters the Pores of the Water. Thus we may, in an extemporaneous Manner, prepare the Waters of Cinnamon, Cedar, Nutmeg, Mint, Baum, and Hyssop, which are otherwise to be only obtained with considerable Labour by Distillation. Besides, by the Addition of a small Quantity of Spirit of Wine, these Waters become spirituous.

It is an opprobrious, tho' true Assertion, that the true and genuine Oils of Plants are rarely to be had in the Shops; since, in order to increase their Quantity, it is customary, in distilling them, to mix them with some pinguious or other Substances of little Value. As for the dear Aromatic Oils it is certain, from Experience, that they are almost all adulterated, as is obvious in the Oils of Cinnamon, Cloves, Nutmegs, and Mace. But in these the Fraud is easily

sily

fily detected by pouring *Alcahol* of Wine, or highly rectified Spirit of Wine, upon them; for this Liquor immediately resolves, and imbibes the Particles of the purer Oil, leaving in the Bottom a large Quantity of expressed Oil, either of Almonds, or Ben-nuts. But the more skilful of the Chymists have an artful Method of concealing this Piece of Fraud; for they dissolve pure Oil of Cinnamon, or Cloves, by adding an equal Quantity of highly rectified Spirit of Wine, which may be so prepared, that one Part of the Spirit may absorb one Part of the Oil, whilst the Taste remains, and the Smell continues sufficiently strong and penetrating; so that the Imposition is with Difficulty discovered. But this Piece of Fraud is also quickly discovered, if these Oils are poured into common Water; for then the Water immediately becomes milky, which Effect is not produced by pure Oil, when put into cold Water, and left to itself. There is still another Method of adulterating the Oils of Plants, by mixing Oil of Turpentine, or Pine, with the Herbs to be distill'd; and this Piece of Fraud is most commonly committed in preparing Cephalic Oils from Plants, which abound with a balsamic Resin, such as Mint, Origanum, Sage, Rosemary, Marjoram, Savory, Thyme, Mother of Thyme, and the Flowers of Spike and Lavender; from which, by the Addition of these Oils, they obtain a large Quantity of Oil, tho' of a bad Kind, and inconsiderable Virtues; but such Oils, if the Plants are recent, retain their specific and distinguishing Taste and Smell. But this Piece of Fraud is easily detected; for if such Oils are kept for some time, they lose their grateful Smell, and the disagreeable Odour of the Turpentine remains. But there is still a more expeditious Method of discovering this Fraud; for if a Piece of Cloth, macerated in such Oil, is put in a warm Place, or exposed to an hot Furnace, the subtile Fragrance is immediately exhaled, and the Smell of Turpentine discovers itself.

Besides, the Cephalic Oils, adulterated with Turpentine, or Oil of Pine, are more limpid than the genuine Oils, which are of a deeper Colour. There is also another Method of detecting this Fraud; which is, when the Letters of the Signature, put upon the Mouth of the Glass, become successively pale, which does not happen with the genuine Oils; for the Effluvia of the Turpentine contain a subtile Acid, which in Process of Time, destroys the Colour of the Ink. Some, in the Distillation of these Oils, instead of Turpentine, add Seeds, which contain a large Quantity of pinguious Juice; such as those of Poppies; and by this means that thick Oil, which at other Times is generally express'd, with Difficulty passes the Helm, is raised and distilled in Conjunction with a Portion of subtile and æthereal Oil; and this is the usual Method of adulterating the Oil of Rue; for tho' Rue is of a strong Taste, and penetrating Smell, yet there is hardly any Plant which affords a smaller Quantity of Oil: But pure Oil of Rue is easily distinguished from that which is adulterated; since, when genuine, it does not become thick and coagulated, when exposed to the Cold; but is inspissated, when it is adulterated with any express'd Oil. The Oils of Chamomile, and the Tops of Yarrow, when pure and recent, are of a beautiful bluish Colour, which is afterwards changed into that of brown: but if this bluish Colour of the Oil of Chamomile-flowers remain above a Year, it is a sure Sign that it is actul-

erated; for it is cuſtomary to
with it Oil of Turpentine, which
a deep-bluiſh Colour, on Ac-
t of the Tincture it receives
the Copper of the Veſſel. It
great Importance to the Phyſi-
to be able to diſtinguiſh ge-
from adulterated Oils; for
balſamic and cephalic Oils not
loſe much of their Efficacy, but
acquire a foreign Quality, by
g adulterated; and it is ſuffi-
ıy known, that all terebinthi-
ous Subſtances violently exagi-
the Maſs of Blood and Humours,
create an intenſe Heat in the
y.

Oleum Terebinthinæ.

Oil of Turpentine.

e of any Quantity of Turpen-
ne, melted over a gentle Fire,
ıd pour it into a Glaſs Retort,
as to fill one Half thereof;
en, fitting on the Receiver, diſtil
a Sand-heat, and with a gentle
ıre: There will come over an
cid Spirit; then, the Fire being
radually increaſed, a limpid Oil,
ommonly call'd Æthereal Spirit;
ıd at length a yellow Oil, leaving
ıe Colophony at the Bottom;
hich, being urged with the laſt
Degree of Fire, will alſo afford a
ed and duſky-red Oil, that falls
ır j' the other Liquors to the
ottom of the Receiver. *E.*

ıe Gums Ammoniac,
    Caranna,
    Elemi,
    Galbanum,
    Sagapenum,
    Storax,
    Tacamahac, &c.
ill'd in the ſame Manner, afford
acid Liquor and an empyreuma-
Oil.

urpentine, diſtill'd by the Alem-
, with four times its own Quan-
of Water, yields a limpid Oil,

leaving the Colophony behind, after
the Evaporation of all the Water,
which may be kept for Uſe; or may
be diſtill'd by the Retort, by which
means it affords a yellow, a red, and
a duſky-red Oil. *E.*

In the *London* Diſpenſatory the Diſtillation of Turpentine is directed
much as before; thus,

Turpentine is to be diſtill'd with
Water in a Copper Still, like the
eſſential Oils of Vegetables. *L.*

After the Diſtillation, the yellow
Roſin remains in the Still.

This Oil is often, tho' improperly,
called Spirit of Turpentine.

Oleum Terebinthinæ Æthereum, &

Balſamum.

The Æthereal Oil, and the Balſam
of Turpentine.

Let the Oil of Turpentine be diſtill'd
in a Retort, with a very gentle
Heat, till what remains is become
of the Conſiſtence of a Balſam.

Balſam of Turpentine may alſo be
diſtill'd from yellow Roſin; whence
after a Portion of Oil, which muſt
be removed in time, will come a
thick Balſam; a blackiſh Roſin remaining in the Retort, which is called Colophony. *L*

The Æthereal Oil of Turpentine
has of late Years been much recommended for a Sciatica, taken in large
Doſes in Honey, or any other convenient Vehicle.

Oleum Guaiaci.

Oil of Guaiacum.

Take any Quantity of Guaiacum-
Chips, put them into a Retort of
Earth or Glaſs, and gradually diſtil them in a naked Fire, or a
Sand-Furnace: An acid Liquor
will firſt aſcend, then a light-red
Oil; and at length, with the utmoſt Degree of Heat, a thick
black Oil, that ſinks thro' the

other Liquors to the Bottom of the Retort.

In like manner Oils are diftill'd from any Kind of Wood. *E.*

This acid Water of *Guaiacum* is highly penetrating, aperitive, atte-nuating, healing, detergent, and fa-ponaceous, fo as to prove antifcor-butic, diuretic, diaphoretic, and fu-dorific, efpecially after being well purified and rectified.

Oleum Capaivæ compofitum.

Compound Oil of Balfam of Ca-paiva.

Take Balfam of Capaiva, two Pounds; of Gum Guaiacum, four Ounces: Diftil them together in a Retort. *L.*

It is doubted whether the Guaia-cum adds any Virtues to the Ca-paiva. This Oil is an excellent Balfamic, and is likely to do Good in all thofe Cafes where Tar-water can be of Service; but fhould feem to be a much better Medicine than the latter.

Oleum Buxi.

Oil of Box.

Diftil Pieces of Box in a Retort, with a Fire gradually raifed: The Oil will come over with an acid Spirit, from which the Oil is to be feparated by a Funnel. *L.*

See the Article *Buxus,* in the *Ma-teria Medica.*

Flores Benzoini.

Flowers of Benjamin.

Take any Quantity of powder'd Benjamin, and put it into a glazed Pot, and fit a Cone of Paper to the Brim thereof; then adminifter a flow Fire, that the Flowers may fublime; and repeat the Operation till the Paper becomes foul with the afcending Oil. *E.*

Thefe are faid to be a wonderful Pectoral, and particularly excellent in Afthmas; for they gently atte-nuate, and open the vifcous Obftruc-tions, and cleanfe the Bronchia. They are convenient almoft in any Form, and give a very grateful Scent to any Compofition. The Dofe is from three to ten or twelve Grains.

In the *London* Difpenfatory we find the following Directions, with re-fpect to the Flowers of Benjamin:

Put powder'd Benjamin into an earthen Pot placed in Sand, and, with a fmall Heat the Flowers will rife, and may be caught by a Paper Cone placed over the Pot. Or elfe,

The Benjamin may be put into a Retort, and the Flowers will af-cend into and faften themfelves about its Neck. *L.*

The Flowers, if tinged yellow, are to be mix'd with Tobacco-pipe Clay, and fublimed again.

Oleum Lateritium.

Oil of Bricks.

Let Bricks, heated red-hot, be plung'd into Olive Oil, till the whole Oil is imbibed; then the Bricks being fufficiently broke, are to be put into a Retort; and by a Sand-heat the Oil will afcend with a Spirit, which is to be feparated from the Oil. *L.*

The Author of the *Pharmacopæia Reformata* tells us, that this Prepa-ration has had a Place in moft Di-fpenfatories, under the pompous Names of Oleum Philofophorum, Oleum Sanctum, Divinum, Bene-dictum; but whatfoever Opinion fome may have of this Preparation, it is a very indifferent, as well as difagreeable one, and is rarely ufed for medicinal Purpofes; and it is pro-bable, that, for thefe Reafons, the *Edinburgh* Difpenfatory has rejected

The Liquor which comes over along with this Oil in Distillation, is very improperly called Spirit, being really no more than Phlegm, or Water tainted with the empyreumatical Taste of the Oil.

Oleum Picis Barbadenfis.

Oil of *Barbadoes* Tar.

Let *Barbadoes* Tar be distill'd in a Sand-heat, and an Oil will ascend with a Spirit. *L.*

See the Article *Piffaleon*, in the *Materia Medica*, among the Minerals.

Extracts *and* Refins.

Extractum Plantaginis.

Extract of Plantain.

Take any Quantity of Plantain-Juice; clarify it either by Yeast, the Filtre, or the White of Eggs; and afterwards evaporate it to the Confiftence of Honey. *E.*

In the fame Manner are prepared Extracts of all acid, cold, fucculent, and ftyptic Plants.

Extractum Abfinthii.

Extract of Wormwood.

Take any Quantity of dried Wormwood, and a fuitable Proportion of Spring-water; boil them together, pouring on frefh Water, till the Water has extracted all the Virtue of the Plants; then filtre the Decoction, and evaporate it over a flow Fire to the Confiftence of Honey. *E.*

The Extracts of Gentian-root, black Hellebore-root, &c. of the Herb Centaury and Chamomile-flowers, are prepared in the fame Manner; so likewife are the Extracts of all fixed Aromatics. *E.*

Extracts of the Roots of Elecampane, Gentian, black Hellebore; and

Extracts of the Leaves of Rue and Savine.

Boil them in Water; ftrain and prefs out the Decoction, and fet it by till its Dregs are fubfided; then boil it to the Confiftence of a Pill, with Care, toward the End, to avoid Burning. *L.*

The Virtues of all thefe Extracts may be learn'd from thofe of the refpective Vegetables whence they are drawn.

Extractum Glycyrrhizae.

Extract of Liquorice.

Boil the Roots of Liquorice lightly in Water; ftrain and prefs out the Decoction: Then, after its Dregs have fubfided, boil it away, till it will not ftick to the Fingers, ufing due Care, toward the End, to avoid Burning. *L.*

See the Virtues of Liquorice in the *Materia Medica.*

Extractum Jalapii.

Extract of Jalap.

Pour upon Jalap-root powder'd, rectified Spirit of Wine; and, with a due Heat, draw a Tincture, and boil the Refidue feveral times in Water: After Straining, draw off the Spirit from the firft Tincture till it begins to thicken. Infpiffate alfo the ftrain'd Decoctions; then mix the two Extracts, and with a gentle Fire reduce them to the Confiftence of a Pill. *L.*

In the *Edinburgh* Difpenfatory it is directed much in the fame Manner, only Salt of Tartar is added to the Jalap-root, after the Tincture is extracted by the Spirit. This is contrived to get the faline as well as refinous Part of the Jalap; and it may poffibly be almoft of as much Ufe

E e e 2 in

in Practice as the simple Root, without any Preparation.

Extractum Corticis Peruviani, molle & durum.

Extract of *Peruvian* Bark, both soft and hard.

Take of *Peruvian* Bark, reduced to Powder, one Pound; of Water, ten or twelve Pints: Boil for an Hour or two, and pour off the Liquor, which will be red and transparent; but as soon as it grows cold, becomes yellow and turbid: Boil the Bark again in the same Quantity of fresh Water as before, repeating these Boilings till the Liquor remains transparent, when cold; then evaporate all these Decoctions strain'd and mix'd together, to the proper Consistence, over a very gentle Fire, with due Care to avoid Burning. This Extract is to be prepared under a double Form, one of the Consistence of a Pill, the other hard enough to be reduced to Powder. *L.*

The medicinal Virtues of this Extract may be learn'd from those of the *Peruvian* Bark. We are inform'd in the Narrative of the Committee, that it is design'd for those whose Stomachs are so tender, as not to be able to bear the Bark in Substance in the Quantity requisite. But these Stomachs do not often occur in Practice; and in all others, the Bark in Substance is a better Medicine.

Extractum Ligni Campechensis.

Extract of Logwood.

Take of Logwood in Powder, one Pound: Boil it four times, or oftener, in a Gallon of Water, to a Half; then boil all the Liquors, mixt together and strain'd, to a just Consistence. *L.*

This seems intended to fortify the Bowels, when weaken'd by a Diar-rhœa or Dysentery; but should not be used till due Evacuations are made.

Extractum Ligni Guajaci, molle & durum.

Extract of Guaiacum-wood, soft and hard.

Take of the Shavings of Lignum Vitæ, one Pound: Boil it four times, or oftener, in a Gallon of Water, to half; then inspissate the Liquors, after they have been strained; but when the Water is near all dried away, add a small Portion of rectified Spirit, by which the Extract shall be brought to a uniform and tenacious Mass.

This Extract is also to be prepared under two Forms, one softer, and the other harder. *L.*

For the Virtues of this Extract, see the Article *Guaiacum* in the *Materia Medica.* I should apprehend, that a Decoction of Guaiacum will be much more likely to enter the Lacteals, and impregnate the Blood with the Virtues of the Wood.

Boerhaave takes Notice of a Kind of Extracts, which he calls *Essential Extracts,* of which he gives an Example in the

Extractum Croci.

Extract of Saffron.

Nature has prepared, in particular Parts of certain Vegetables, a determined kind of Body, so different from all others as scarce to be referred to any other known Kind; and has at the same time endowed it with Virtues, otherwise inimitable. We have an Example of this in the Chives of Saffron, which the principal Chymists have esteem'd so much as to call it the *Philosopher's Spice,* and to denote it by the initial Letters *Aroph,* which stand for *Aroma Philosophorum.* It is incredible how rich this Saffron is in Colour, Taste, Odour, and Virtue; how small the

Bulk

is that possesses all these rich ...ities; and how tender and easi...orruptible the Thing itself is; therefore requires a peculiar Me...of Operation.

...e, therefore, two Ounces of the ...oicest fresh *English* Saffron dried, ...d either cut small, or remaining ...hole; put it into a clean Bolt...ead, with a long and slender ...leck; pour upon it so much of ...e purest Alcohol as may float ...ur or six Inches above it: Then ...op the Glass slightly with a ...Vreath of Paper. Put it into a ...urnace, so that it may be exposed ...) a Heat of only a hundred De...rees. Leave it thus in Digestion ...hree Days, the Vessel being often ...ook: Let it afterwards rest for ...wenty-four Hours in a cold quiet ...lace; then carefully strain off all ...he tinged Liquor, thro' a Piece of ...lean Linnen, placed in a Funnel ...et in a clean Glass, and keep it ...losely stopt. It will be of a ...right-red Colour; the Saffron re...maining at the Bottom of the Glass ...vill be found paler than before. ...To this pour the like Quantity of ...resh *Alcohol*, and proceed as be...fore; and mix the Tincture thus ...acquired, with the former. Let ...these Tinctures be distill'd in a Glass Body, fitted with its Head, and perfectly well closed, with a Fire of a hundred Degrees, till about an Ounce remains behind; which, when cold, is to be pour'd into a Glass Vessel, to be kept carefully stopt. It will prove of an exceeding red Colour, a highly fragrant Odour, and a bitter, aromatic, penetrating Taste, and have the Consistence of thin Oil. Let it be kept under the Title of the *Essential Extract of Saffron*. The Spirit that comes over in the Distillation will be limpid, and colourless; but retains the grateful and aromatic Smell and Taste of Saffron. This is to be reserved for the same Use, and thus every time becomes the richer.

This surprising Experiment shews us a new Species of Matter, which we can neither call Oil, Spirit, Gum, Rosin, resinous Gum, Wax, or Balsam; but it is something perfectly singular, and of a spirituous oily Nature. This Extract mixes with Water, Spirit, and Oil, and has such exhilarating Virtues, that, being used too freely, it occasions an almost perpetual and indecent Laughter; but, used moderately, it becomes properly exhilarating. It tinges the Urine red, and is particularly said to destroy the petrifying Power thereof in the Kidnies, and therefore to be an extraordinary Remedy against the Stone. It is the true *Aroph* of *Paracelsus*. There is no Occasion previously to digest the Saffron with Bread in the Heat of Horse-dung, in order to procure its Tincture, which is thus render'd rather worse than better; for in our present Preparation, all that is efficacious is brought together without Loss, or impairing its peculiar Virtues, or any sensible Change. And these Preparations being miscible with any Liquor, and of a very penetrating subtile Nature, easily enter the finest Vessels of the Body; and, by their extraordinary Mobility, diffuse their Virtue thro' the Whole, and chiefly excite the Animal Spirits. Lastly, they have that admirable Virtue, which the Author of Nature has planted in them, and which can never be explained upon any Principle, and can only be known in itself from its Effects.

The like Extracts may be obtain'd from Ambergrise, Musk, Civet, Balm of *Gilead*, liquid Amber, liquid Storax, Cloves, Mace, Nutmeg, Angelica, Galangal, Orrice, and other

Barks,

Barks, and Flowers of a subtile Fragrance: Whence it is plain, that these Spirits of particular Bodies may be extracted and collected by *Alcohol*; and hence their sudden Action seems to proceed; because the most spirituous *Alcohol*, uniting with these active Spirits, makes a Medicine that immediately diffuses its Virtues every Way, and carries it thro' the Body; and when a similar Remedy is prepared from several such Ingredients mixed together, it easily appears, that thus an admirable Remedy may be compounded, rich in united Virtues, according to the Intention of the Artist; so that nothing of this Kind can be invented more effectual. These Extracts are best taken in *Canary*, or the like rich unctuous *Spanish* Wine.

Gummi & Resina Aloes.

The Gum and Resin of Aloes.

Take of *Succotrine* Aloes, four Ounces; of Water, a Quart: Boil the Aloes till it is dissolved as much as may be, and set all by for a Night: The Resin will be precipitated to the Bottom of the Vessel. The Liquor, pour'd off or strain'd, being evaporated, will leave the Gum. *L.*

We are told, that the Intention of the Separation of the Resin from the Gum, in this Preparation, is, to procure in the Gum a Medicine less purgative, and more agreeable to the Stomach. But I have never had any Reason, from Experience, to think that Aloes, on any Account, wants such Treatment.

Resina Jalappæ.

Resin of Jalap.

Take any Quantity of well-bruised Jalap-roots, and pour thereon as much rectified Spirit of Wine as will rise four Inches above it: Digest them together in *Balneo*

Mariæ, so as to extract the T... ture; which being filter'd, p... into a Glass Cucurbit, and ... off one Half by a Sand-heat: ... the Remainder pour a suffic... Quantity of Spring-water, and ... Resin will precipitate to the ... tom, which is afterwards to ... dried with a very gentle He... *E.*

Thus likewise are prepared ... Resins of Guaiacum, *Peruvian* B... and Scammony, &c. But the R... of Guaiacum is more commodi... made from the Gum than ... Wood.

The Resin of Jalap is not by ... so good a Medicine as the R... without any Preparation; of w... those who have much used bot... their Practice, must be abund... sensible; tho' in comatose Disor... and violent Affections of the H... perhaps the Resin may be prefer... because it stimulates and gripes ... than the Root.

Salts *both essential and fixed,* with the Preparations of Tart...

Sal Essentiale Acetosæ.

Essential Salt of Sorrel.

Take any Quantity of the Juice ... Sorrel, clarified by standing; ev... porate two thirds of it away, st... the remainder thro' a Flannel b... and again exhale it to a Pellic... then put it into a Glass Ves... and pour a little Olive Oil up... the Top; set the Vessel in a Ce... lar, till numerous Crystals app... therein, which are to be first ge... washed with Spring Water, ... then dried. *E.*

The essential Salts of the Le... Centaury, Succory, Eyebright, ... matory, Plantain, Oak, &c. ... obtained in the same Manner, ... also the Salts of all acid, a...

ngent and bitter Plants, that con-
but very little Oil.

eerbaave remarks, that Salts may
rocured in this Manner from the
e of any other succulent Vege-
e; but a different Salt will be
ys produced according to the
rent Nature of the Plant em-
ed. If the Juices were either
ifestly and purely acid, or acid
some Degree of Austerity, the
will resemble the Tartar of acid
re Wines. If a perfectly suc-
nt Plant were chose, and neither
or oily, as many medicinal ones
the Salt will be of another par-
lar Nature, perhaps resembling
re. Such a Salt is afforded by
oklime, Endive, Fumitory, Dwarf-
r, Grafs, Knot-grafs, Plantain,
-heal, Succory, Water-cresses,
ter-lillies, &c. Whence the Juices
hese Plants are greatly medicinal,
bounding with this Kind of ni-
s Salt, so as to open inveterate
structions, resolve the black bili-
Juice, and cure chronical Dis-
s. But when the viscous Juices
Vegetables are used in this Pro-
, as those of Purflain, Comfrey,
he like, their Salt cannot be ob-
ed without a previous Fermenta-
, to dissolve their Tenacity. In
Manner, all the Juices abound-
with Oil are unfit for this Pur-
e; for tho' they contain a Salt,
it is so entangled with the tena-
s Oil, as to prevent its uniting
h the Particles of its own Nature,
forming Cryftals; for Oil al-
s prevents the Cryftallization of
s; and again, Plenty of Oil oc-
ons a Lofs of Salt, and *vice verfa*,
vell in Animals as Vegetables; on
ich Account those Salts are not
ly obtained from such aromatic
nts as abound in Oil and Balfam.

Sal Abfinthii.
Salt of Wormwood.

the   of Wormwood be put

into an Iron Pot, and kept red-hot
for some Hours by a ftrong Fire,
often ftirring them, that all Remains of Oil may be burnt out;
then boil them in Water, ftrain
the Water, which will be impregnated with the Salt, thro' Paper,
and evaporate it to Drynefs.

In this Manner is to be prepared the
fixt alcaline Salt of any Plant, whose
Ashes will yield that Kind of Salt. L.

When the Oil is sufficiently burnt
out, may be judged of, as the Ashes
are ftirred up from time to time;
for while the Oil remains in them,
they will take Fire and sparkle, upon their being turned up to the Air.
And this turning up the Ashes, which
lie at the Bottom, to the Air, is neceffary, that the Oil may be effectually consumed.

The Method of making fixed Salts
directed in the *Edinburgh* Difpenfatory, differs from this very little, except in the Circumftance of keeping
the Ashes red-hot for some Hours,
which is there omitted; and in the
repeated Solutions, Filtrations, and
Coagulations there directed, in order
to render the Salt pure and white; but
the whiter and purer the Salt is, it becomes in Proportion the worfe for
medicinal Ufes, becaufe it is then
deprived of moft or all of the Oil
of the Vegetable, which I think of
great Confequence. See Book I.
Chap. vi. where the Medicinal Ufes
of thefe Salts are explain'd.

After the same Manner are obtain'd
the fix'd Salts of Bean Stalks, Broom,
and many other Vegetables.

The Spirit, Oil, and fix'd Salt of Tartar.

Fill two thirds of a Glafs Retort, with
choice Pieces of the beft white
Tartar, and place it in a Sand
Furnace; apply a large Glafs Receiver, or one that is of the great-

E e e 4   eft

est Size, and lute the Juncture with a common Mixture of Linseed Meal. Apply a gentle Fire for some considerable Time, scarce exceeding a hundred Degrees; there will come over a small Quantity of a limpid, thin, tartish, somewhat spirituous, bitterish, and lightly odorous Liquor, which is so penetrating, as easily to sweat thro' the Luting. Let this be kept separate; then the Fire being raised to the Heat of boiling Water, a white Vapour comes over, and along with it a highly penetrating Spirit, which is wonderfully flatulent. and will pass thro' almost any Luting; and, if we endeavour to confine it by that called the *Lutum Sapientiæ*, it bursts the Glass by its Elasticity; and it usually breaks out with Force, or perspires at Intervals, thro' the Luting; and, along with this flatulent Spirit, there comes over a thin, and extremely subtile Oil, of a yellow Colour, a somewhat aromatic Taste, bitter, heating, and of no ungrateful Odour.

Paracelsus and *Helmont* highly recommend this Oil in Diseases of the Ligaments, Membranes, and Tendons, which they, upon Experience, have declared may be cured by it, even tho' contracted.

The former Substances being collected separate, let the Remainder be urged gradually, to the utmost Degree of Heat that Sand will give; and thus again a Spirit will come over, and an Oil, as before; but at the same Time a gross, black, fetid, ponderous, glutinous, and bitter Oil, leaving the remaining Tartar black, sharp, and in every Respect truly alcaline. If this Mass be urged with the strongest Fire of Suppression, it will still yield a very thick, black, and pitchy Oil, along with a certain Smoke. And these will continue to

rise, how violent soever the Fire be made, and how long soever the Operation is continued; and there will still remain an extremely black, sharp, alcaline, and dry Mass at the Bottom; which being exposed to the open Air, by breaking the Glass, grows hot upon Contact therewith, and readily dissolves into a Liquor: Nor can it be kept dry, without great Caution; whereas the Tartar, from whence it was produced, would scarce dissolve in Water.

When this black dry Mass is exposed to a naked Fire in the open Air, it takes Flame; and after Burning, leaves a copious white alcaline Salt behind, as strong, fiery, and pure, as can any way be prepared. It affords but little Earth, and readily dissolves of itself; if long detained in a strong Fire, it grows blue, of a Marble Colour, and sometimes brown; and thus always becomes stronger.

The first distilled and highly penetrating Oil of Tartar is recommended for discussing cold Tumours, and for restoring Motion to the dried tendinous Parts in contracted Limbs, together with the Assistance of proper Baths, Fomentations, and Frictions. If these Oils be rectified, and render'd more subtile and penetrating, they are recommended by Chymists, even for resolving gouty Knots and Concretions. It is said by many, that rich Perfumes may be exalted by this Oil. Salt of Tartar may be thus prepared in a greater Proportion to the Tartar employed, than by any other known Method, and in greater Plenty the slower the Distillation was performed. This, also, is the best, sharpest, most penetrating, and pure of all the fixed Alcalies; nor is there any other known Body in Nature, that affords more of such a saline alcaline Matter, than Tartar. And if the black alcaline Matter, remaining after the most violent Distillation,

ion, be set by in the Retort, slight-covered with Paper, it wholly re-lves into a Liquor, which, being tered, affords an admirable Oil of artar *per Deliquium*, extremely fit r numerous Chymical Uses, and rticular Operations. If the same lt be first strongly calcined in an en Fire, it thus also resolves in the ir, and affords an Oil of Tartar r *Deliquium*, but of a more sharp d alcaline Nature than the former.

n the *Edinburgh* Dispensatory, Salt Tartar is thus order'd to be made:

Sal Tartari.

Salt of Tartar.

ake any Quantity of white Tartar, wrap it up in moisten'd Cap-paper, and calcine it in a reverberating Furnace, till it becomes very white; then dissolve it in hot Water, filtre the Solution, and exhale it in a clean Glass Vessel, till it becomes as white as Snow, and perfectly dry, keeping it continually stirring with an Iron Ladle towards the End of the Operation, to prevent its sticking to the Bottom of the Vessel. If the Salt of Tartar be required stronger, let the white Salt be fused with a very violent Fire, in a Crucible, and rever-berated for some Hours, till it turns of a greenish or blue Colour. *E.*

n the *London* Dispensatory it is di-ted in much the same Manner. e the Article of *Alcali*. Chap. vi. ok I.

quamen Salis Tartari, vulgo Oleum per Deliquium dictum.

quor of Tartar, commonly called Oil of Tartar *per Deliquium*.

ake any Quantity of Salt of Tar-tar, put it into a flat glass Vessel, and expose it to the Air of a moist Place for some Days, so as that it may dissolve into a Liquor, which

is either to be filtred, or freed from from its Fæces, by inclining the Vessel. The higher this Salt is calcined, the easier it resolves. *E.*

In the *London* Dispensatory it is thus directed under the Title of

Lixivium Tartari.

Ley of Tartar.

When the Tartar is calcined white, let it be put in a damp Place, that it may liquefy by the Moisture of the Air. *L.*

In this Process the Liquor is rather more pure, than if the calcined Tar-tar were dissolved directly in Water.

Nitrum fixatum.

Fix'd Nitre.

Fill a strong and large Crucible with very dry powder'd Nitre, laid lightly in; set the Crucible firm in the Furnace, and surround it with burning Coals at a Distance; then gradually bring them nearer, that the Crucible, with the Nitre it contains, may be thus heated equal-ly, to prevent Bursting. When all is now thoroughly hot, apply as strong a Fire as is necessary to make the Nitre run like Water; then take a little Piece of Wood-coal, thoroughly ignited, and put it gently into the melted Nitre, now at rest. The Coal (not the Nitre) will thus instantly take Flame with a hissing Noise, and move over the whole Surface of the melted Nitre with a brisk Mo-tion, till it is consumed, and the Flame extinguished, so as to leave the Nitre melted, as before it was thrown in. Now throw in another Bit of live Coal as before, and the same Phænomena ensue. Con-tinue repeating the Operation, till at length the Nitre remains fixed with the same Degree of Fire, so as to flow no longer, nor give

give Flame to the Coal thrown in, which at length will always prove the Case. This State may be known to approach, when the Nitre begins to lose its Fluidity, and the Coal leaps briskly about, and sometimes flies out of the Crucible: At this Time, therefore, the Fire should be a little increased. And when the Coal ceases to flame any longer, let all cool, and there will remain in the Crucible a Mass, with an hollow Part on its Top, where the last burning Coal had rested: This Mass is solid, ponderous, of a Colour betwixt white and green, fiery, alcaline, and presently runs in the Air; therefore, whilst yet very hot, let it be presently taken out by breaking the Crucible, and put into a clean Glass, to be carefully stopped.

The Alcali, thus produced, is very difficult to keep dry; but presently relents in the Air, and runs into a strong fiery alcaline Liquor, leaving a large Quantity of Ashes behind.

Tartarus Regeneratus.
Regenerated Tartar.

To a Quantity of sharp, pure, and dried fixed Alcali, contained in a large Glass with a narrow Neck, pour strong distilled Vinegar, till it almost covers the Salt; scarce any sensible Effervescence will appear: Shake them strongly together and then some small, but not lasting Ebullition appears. Pour on more distilled Vinegar, and then a greater Ebullition will arise, and appear sufficiently manifest: After shaking the Glass, add a third Quantity, and then a violent Ebullition, Frothing, and Hissing will be found; and proves the stronger, the more the Glass is shook; and this continues a long while: so that the Vinegar poured

on, makes the stronger Effervescence, the nearer the Operation approaches to the Point of Saturation with the Alcali; which Point is generally obtained, when about fourteen Times the Weight of strong distilled Vinegar is added to the Alcali. Now towards the End, let the Mixture be well heated, and long and strongly stirred, that no more Acid may be poured on, than is exactly required to obtain the Point of Saturation; which will at length be hit, by continuing to add a little of the distilled Vinegar by Degrees, and well agitating the Mixture, till the Addition, and Shaking in of a little more, no longer causes an Effervescence, even in the Heat. Then let the Mixture stand warm for twenty-four Hours; and, if upon shaking, it makes no Ebullition, again drop in a little Vinegar, and shake the Vessel; and if now no Effervescence arises, then the exact Point of Saturation is hit. During the Operation, the violent Effervescence throws off a very elastic Vapour, which bursts out of the Glass with a hissing Noise, after having been confined, by pressing the Hand against the Mouth of the Glass, whilst it was shook, and then suddenly taking it away: And if the Orifice should be closely and strongly shut up during the Effervescence, the Glass would be burst to pieces. The Liquor, thus prepared, is transparent, of a particular Odour, and not acid, and of a Taste neither acid nor alcaline, but particularly saline, and almost without Acrimony. It has a mild and innocent Virtue, tho' powerfully attenuating and resolving; being purgative, diuretic, and sudorific; whence it proves an admirable Remedy in chronical Diseases, attended with a tenacious

ous Matter, being given in a proper Dose at proper Seasons.

The Liquor being decanted clear from its Fæces, and diſtilled in a Glaſs Alembic, affords a pure ſimple Water; whilſt the Liquor remaining behind, becomes of a brown blackiſh Colour; and, at length, perfectly black, fat, thick, of an extremely penetrating Taſte, which diſcovers it to be of a ſaponaceous, penetrating, and reſolving Virtue. Take a little of this Liquor, and mix it with a little Vinegar; if it makes an Efferveſcence, this ſhews, that the Alcali ſtill predominates; and, therefore, the whole muſt be again ſaturated, by the careful Addition of diſtilled Vinegar; and as this uſually happens to be the Caſe, the Point of Saturation is to be carefully and anxiouſly ſecured.

When at length this is happily obtained, let the Liquor be ſeparated by Reſt from its Fæces, and then all the Water be drawn off by a gentle Fire, till a ſaline Maſs remains at the Bottom, of a black, reddiſh Colour, and a highly penetrating, but very particular ſaponaceous Taſte. This Maſs will have attracted, and retained all the Acid of the Vinegar, and given out all the Water. Mr. Homberg has laboriouſly ſhewn, that the Weight of the fixed Alcali is here increaſed nine Twentieths, in reſpect of the Alcali, by the Acid of the Vinegar ſo attracted; and that his Acid, with reſpect to the Vinegar, was in the Vinegar about a thirty-ſeventh Part of the whole, the other thirty-ſix Parts being pure Water. And thus the Salt is procured, which the Chymiſts call *Regenerated Tartar*.

If the Salt, thus laboriouſly prepared, be urged with a ſtrong Fire, it becomes volatile, and flies off in the Air. When carefully dried with a very gentle Fire, it appears like a Maſs that had ſtrangely concreted in the Cold, by the Appoſition of little thin Plates like Talc. It preſently runs with Heat, into a Kind of thick Oil, but again appears leafy in the Cold; and hence it has been called *Terra foliata*: And *Tachenius* pretending it to be diſſolved Talc, is taken to task for it by *Zwelfer*, in his apologetic Diſcourſe againſt *Tachenius*.

There is not, in all Chymiſtry, a more inſtructing Operation than this; it ſhews us a new, unexpected, and particular Appearance of Alcali and Acid, in the making of an Efferveſcence. We here ſee all the Degrees of Colour, from the tranſparent Whiteneſs of Water, up to Blackneſs; we ſee that a fat inflammable Oil is regenerated from Alcali, calcined by a violent Fire, and a thin, hungry Spirit of Vinegar; for this dry Salt takes Flame in the Fire, and, when diſtilled with a ſtrong Heat, affords a true Oil. Hence we learn, that Salts produced by a Mixture of Acid and Alcali, are not barely made up of the Acid and Alcali, as they are again ſeparable, but that a new Thing is produced, of which no Sign appeared before. We are taught what Proportion of Acid, and what Proportion of Water, is contained in an acid Liquor; what Proportion of Acid is required exactly to ſaturate an Alcali; and the true Manner of converting fiery, fixed Alcali, into a mild compound, volatile, ſaponaceous, oily Salt. This Salt, when properly prepared, is a moſt admirable Menſtruum, converting its Subject, by Mixture and Digeſtion, into an uniform ſoluble Maſs, that will readily paſs thro' the Body, and remain rich in its own Virtues: It is the greateſt Reſolvent in the Body hitherto known, and therefore highly valuable, as it is not hurtful in hot Caſes, yet ſerviceable in cold ones, and almoſt ſuited to every

Patient: *Boerhaave* thinks this, *Helmont*'s volatile Salt of Tartar, which he so highly recommends, and substitutes for the *Alcahest* itself. It seems certainly to be the *Acetum radicatum* of the ancient Chymists, as, in its Preparation, Vinegar returns, and is joined with its own Matrix of calcined Tartar; but whoever shall over carefully endeavour to dissolve, purify, filtre, inspissate, or calcine this Salt, in order to make it white, he will find it fly off into the Air, and be lost; and may thus, indeed, be convinced of its Volatility, with the Loss of his Labour and Cost. And this Admonition *Boerhaave* tells us he gives, because *Senertus* recommends a scrupulous Diligence in purifying this Salt; which is not only a lost, but an impoverishing Labour.

.I have given this Preparation from *Boerhaave*, as he seems to have been the most exact and particular; and must remark, that the Medicine is not at all the better for its Whiteness; nor the worse for its wanting the foliated Appearance.

In the *Edinburgh* Dispensatory it is thus directed:

Take any Quantity of dry pulveriz'd Tartar, put it into a large Glass Vessel, and pour on gradually as much Spirit of Vinegar as will saturate it; evaporate the filtrated Liquor over a very gentle Fire, till it becomes dry, but take Care it does not attract an Empyreuma; pour again upon the remaining Salt as much Spirit of Vinegar as will saturate it, then carefully evaporate the depurated Liquor to a Salt. *E.*

In the *London* Dispensatory it is thus order'd under the Title of
Sal Diureticus.

Diuretic Salt.

Take of any alcaline fixt Salt, one Pound; and boil it in four or five Pints of distilled Vinegar, with a very gentle Heat; when the Fermentation ceases, add more distilled Vinegar, and when the Fermentation arising from the Addition is over, pour on another Quantity of the like Vinegar, and proceed thus till the Vinegar, being near all evaporated, fresh Vinegar will not excite any Fermentation, which will generally happen by the Time about ten Quarts of Vinegar shall have been used; then gently evaporate to Dryness. The Salt left will be impure, which is to be melted for a time, but not too long, with a gentle Heat, afterwards dissolved in Water, and transcolated thro' Paper. If the Melting has been rightly performed; the strained Liquor will be limpid and colourless, like Water, but otherwise brownish. Lastly, the Water is to be evaporated with a very gentle Heat in a shallow Vessel, the Salt, as it dries, being frequently stirred, that the Humidity may the sooner be discharged. The Salt must be kept in a close Vessel, that it may not run by the Moisture of the Air.

The Salt ought to be very white, and should dissolve wholly, either in Water, or Spirit of Wine, without leaving any Faeces; if the Salt, tho' ever so white, leave in the Spirit any Faeces, after it is dissolved in this Spirit, it is to be filtred thro' Paper, and dried again. *L.*

We are told, that the Success of this Operation depends upon three Circumstances; completing the Saturation, duly calcining afterwards, and drying it at last, without too much Heat. For the First, it is necessary to make the finishing Trial when the Liquor is almost evaporated away. The Degree of Calcination may be judged of, by dropping a little into Water, and observing, when it begins to part with its Blackness very
readily;

readily; and this Point muſt be carefully watched; for the Solution of the Salt will be coloured, if the Salt is too much calcined, as well as when too little. In the laſt Drying, Care ſhould be taken not to melt it; for then it will loſe, in ſome Degree, its Whiteneſs; and will, upon Solution, again depoſite Dregs; tho' if it is not melted, it will not have that foliated Appearance, from which this Salt has obtained a Name, viz. *Terra foliata Tartari*, the foliated Earth of Tartar. But when it is prepared, ſo as to diſſolve intire, it is more agreeable to the Stomach, and a greater Doſe can be given of it, than when it does not diſſolve ſo compleatly.

In all theſe Preparations of regenerated Tartar, the Evaporation of the Moiſture, and Formation of a Salt, ſhould ſeem abſolutely ſuperfluous; becauſe the Vinegar ſaturated with the alcaline Salt, muſt be in all reſpects as good, and in many a better Medicine, than the Salt, when made with all this Trouble.

Tartarus Vitriolatus.

Vitriolated Tartar.

Take three Ounces of pure Oil of Vitriol; dilute it with thrice the Quantity of warm Water in a tall capacious glaſs Body, with a narrow Neck: Add to it, Drop by Drop, a Quantity of Oil of Tartar *per Deliquium*, till the Point of Saturation is perfectly obtain'd; otherwiſe a pernicious Acrimony, either acid or alcaline, remains. In this Operation a violent Efferveſcence will ariſe, and a white Salt begin to appear at the Bottom, long before the Saturation is completed. After this Point is found, ſhake the Veſſel for a conſiderable time, and taſte the Liquor; if it taſtes neither acid nor alcaline, take a little thereof, and heat it: Divide it into two Parts,

and to one add a Drop of Oil of Vitriol, and to the other a Drop of Oil of Tartar *per Deliquium*; and, if no Efferveſcence appears in either, the Point of Saturation, here ſo requiſite for medicinal Uſe, is exactly hit. If any Efferveſcence ariſe, upon the Addition of the Acid, the Alcali prevails; and, if the Alcali cauſes any Efferveſcence, the Acid prevails; but when the Equilibrium is obtain'd, let the Liquor be intirely diſſolved by the Addition of hot Water, ſo that all the Salt may be taken up. Let the Liquor be ſtrain'd while it is hot, evaporated to a Pellicule, and cryſtalized. A white Salt will be obtained, of a neutral Taſte, that requires a large Proportion of Water to diſſolve it: What remains cannot be cryſtalized, as happens in the Caſe of Nitre, Sea-ſalt, and almoſt every other Salt.

The Virtue of this Salt is eſteem'd highly opening, if taken upon an empty Stomach, diluted with Broth or Whey, and aſſiſted with the Exerciſe of the Body; for thus, by attenuating, reſiſting Putrefaction, and ſtimulating, it opens the obſtructed Viſcera, ſo as to have acquired the Name of the *Univerſal Digeſtive*.

Some eminent Chymiſts, among whom we reckon *Tachenius*, imagine that the Oil of Vitriol, after having ſuffer'd ſo great a Fire, carries up with it ſome volatilized metallic Part, that gives a noxious Quality to this Salt, not to be eaſily deſtroyed: Hence they endeavoured to obtain this Acid, native and ſimple, without Fire, and join it with fix'd Alcali of Tartar. They, therefore, diſſolved Vitriol in Water, ſo as to make a dilute and pure Liquor; to which, when filter'd, they added Oil of Tartar *per Deliquium*, Drop by Drop; upon which the Liquor grows turbid,

turbid, and the Iron, in Form of yellow Oaker, falls to the Bottom: They carefully proceed thus, till no more Precipitate is obtained upon Addition of the Alcali. This Point they carefully obferve, and fet by the Mixture, till all the Metallic Fæces are precipitated; then filter the pure Liquor, infpiffate, and cryftalize as before. Thus a *Tartarum Vitriolatum* is obtained without Fire; and, as they feem to imagine, without any Sufpicion of a fharp corrofive Virtue. And if there be no blue or green Colour remaining in the Liquor, or the Salt prepared from it, the Preparation will be good; but, otherwife, it will retain fomething of Copper, and prove malignant.

When by the like Means, a Salt is prepared with any pure volatile Alcali and Oil of Vitriol, either alone, or diluted with Water, a like, but a femi-volatile and more penetrating Salt is obtained; whereas the former is wonderfully fixed. This Salt, in whatever Manner prepared, appears confiderably ponderous and folid; and yet, at the fame time, is mild and opening.

Practitioners feem to be deceived in nothing fo much as in the vitriolated Tartar, becaufe Medicines of very different, and even directly oppofite Virtues, are called by this Name. That ufually fold in the Shops by this Name, is fo ftrong an Acid, as even to excoriate the Lips and Tongue of thofe who take it; and I believe Chymifts feldom take the Trouble of making it, but fubftitute for it the *Refiduum* of the *Spiritus Nitri fortis Glauberi*; a very different Thing from the true vitriolated Tartar here intended, which is a perfectly neutral Salt, fomewhat bitterifh, and nothing lefs than Acid. If this is made exactly according to thefe Directions, it is a moft excellent Medicine in many Diftempers, where nothing will anfwer fo well.

Taken in the Quantity of a Dram, or more, it excellently purges the Stomach and Inteftines, and refolves the vifcid and tenacious Concretions contain'd therein, which are the Parents of many Diforders. If taken in fmaller Quantities, ten or fifteen Grains, for Example, and repeated frequently at due Intervals, it is excellent in *Rheumatifms*, inflammatory Diftempers, Fevers, and all Diforders attended with a Sizinefs of the Blood. And in acute Diftempers, it will raife a Sweat better than Alexipharmics, without exciting any Heat. It is alfo an admirable Diuretic. I have been the more particular with refpect to this Medicine, becaufe I find its Virtues are very little known or regarded; and becaufe I have very feldom been able to perfuade Apothecaries, that this vitriolated Tartar differs in Efficacy from the common Sort, fo far as to ufe it in my Prefcriptions, having generally found the latter ufed inftead of this.

In the *London* Difpenfatory it is thus directed, under the Title of

Tartarum Vitriolatum.

Vitriolated Tartar.

Take of green Vitriol, the Weight of eight Ounces; of Water, two Quarts. The Vitriol being diffolved in the Water boiling, throw in Salt of Tartar, or any other fix'd Alcali, till all Fermentation ceafes, which ufually happens after throwing in four Ounces, or fomething more, of the alcaline Salt; then ftrain thro' Paper, and evaporate duly, that the Salt may cryftallize. *L.*

The Liquor fhould be kept boiling a little while, every time the alcaline Salt is thrown in, that it may duly penetrate, and draw forth the acid Spirit from the Vitriol.

The Point of Saturation is moft exactly to be judged of, by dropping the he ſtrong Spirit or Oil of Vitriol into a Spoonful of the Liquor filter'd; or as long as no Beginnings of Effervescence hereby appear, the alcaline ſalt does not exceed. This Salt may otherwiſe be prepared with a fixed Alcali, and the ſtrong Spirit or Oil of Vitriol; but the preceding Method beſt ſecures againſt a Redundancy of Acidity in the Salt.

I have never known this Sort uſed; I can ſay nothing of it from Experience.

Tartarus Tartariſatus. Tartariſed Tartar, otherwiſe call'd

Tartarus Solubilis.

Soluble Tartar.

Reduce the pureſt white Tartar to fine Powder, and boil a ſufficient Quantity thereof, with ten times its Weight of Water, in a large Copper Veſſel, till the Tartar appears ſufficiently diſſolved: Let the Veſſel remain over the Fire, that the Water and the Tartar may continue conſtantly boiling. The Liquor, being now taſted, proves acid, and is almoſt tranſparent, and tolerably pure. Then let fall from an Height a Quantity of Oil of Tartar, Drop by Drop, into the boiling Liquor, which is ſtill to be kept boiling, whilſt the Oil of Tartar is dropt in. Upon the Falling of each Drop, there ariſes a great Ebullition in the Liquor, proceeding from the Meeting of the Acid and the Alcali; as appears from hence, that the Ebullition, ſoon after, ſpontaneouſly ceaſes, and is raiſed again by dropping in more of the alcaline Liquor; and, becauſe this is performed in a ſtrong boiling Heat, large ſpherical Bubbles are generated on the Surface of the boiling Liquor, that preſently crack, burſt, and appear again. The Operation is thus to be patiently continued, till at length no more Efferveſcence

ariſes upon dropping the alcaline Liquor into the boiling Lixivium. And now the Acidity of the Tartar will be ſo ſaturated with ſuch a Quantity of its own Alcali, as neither to appear acid nor alcaline, but a third new Salt. But this Point of Saturation muſt be exactly hit, otherwiſe the Salt will be acid, if too little Alcali were added; or Alcaline, if too much: Great Caution muſt, therefore, be uſed at the End. This Liquor is to be ſtrain'd hot and quick thro' Flannel, till it becomes clear. It will be of a blackiſh-brown Colour, of a particular bitteriſh, ſaline, unctuous Taſte, but ſcentleſs. If inſpiſſated by Heat till a Skin appears on its Surface, and then ſet for ſome time in a cold Place, it depoſites to the Bottom and Sides of the Veſſel certain ſaline Grains, which, when collected, are a Tartar eaſily ſoluble in Water, even in the Cold; whereas before, it could ſcarce be diſſolved therein without a boiling Heat: Whence this Preparation may properly be called *ſoluble Tartar.*

Tartar has a manifeſt Acidity; by the prevailing Force thereof it acts kindly upon the firſt Paſſages, and this Acidity is the Cauſe that it makes ſo ſtrong an Efferveſcence with its own fixed Alcali, which is ſo eaſily produced from it: For after this Acidity is overcome by the Alcali, the Tartar becomes eaſily ſoluble, and a new kind of Salt is form'd, which has a conſiderable Virtue in the Body, when taken upon an empty Stomach, diſſolved in Water: For thus it deterges, and gently purges, and helps to cure many inveterate Diſeaſes. Externally uſed, it cleanſes foul Ulcers, and diſpoſes them to heal. A Solution of this Salt in Water is one of the beſt Menſtruums hitherto known in Chymiſtry, as any

one

one may learn by boiling Gum-Lac, Myrrh, and the like, therein: Whence he will find it can fcarce fufficiently be commended; and hence it is plain, that, ufed as a Medicine, it will diffolve vifcous Concretions in the firft Paffages; and it is even fuppofed to diffolve the tartarous Matter of the human Stone, generated in the Receptacles and Paffages of the Bile and Urine, provided it be ufed plentifully every Day, the Dofe being gradually increafed. It is ufeful in the Stone, Jaundice, and hypochondriacal Diforders. Laftly, the Examination of this Procefs fhews how proper Cream of Tartar is in all thofe Diftempers, where the Bile in particular, and other Humours, putrify in the Inteftines, from a burning Fever, or other Caufes, and thus becomes alcaline; for this Difpofition is then corrected by the latent Acidity of the Tartar; and at the fame time converted, in the Body, into a mild aperitive and foluble Salt, which opens the Paffages, without greatly ftimulating them, and clears away Obftructions.

In the *Edinburgh* Difpenfatory this is directed under the Name of foluble Tartar, with this only Difference, that the Cryftals of Tartar are ufed inftead of the Tartar; but this makes no material Difference. This Medicine fhould feem to refemble *Seignette*'s Salt in Virtues.

In the *London* Difpenfatory the *Tartarum Solubile* is thus directed:

Take of alcaline fix'd Salt, a Pound; of Water, one Gallon: The Salt being diffolved in the Water boiling, throw in Cryftals of Tartar in Powder as long as any Fermentation is raifed, which ufually ceafes before thrice the Weight of the Alcali is thrown in. Then ftrain the Liquor thro' Paper, and, after due Evaporation, fet it by for the Salt to cryftallize; or elfe

evaporate the Liquor wholly away, that the Salt may be left dry. *L.*

Cryftalli Tartari.
Cryftals of Tartar.

Take any Quantity of white Tartar, reduced to Powder; diffolve it in twenty times its own Weight of Spring-water, and filtre the Solution, whilft it is yet hot, through Cap-paper, into a wooden Veffel: Then expofe it to the cold Air for a Night longer, that the Cryftals may fhoot to the Sides of the Veffel; after which pouring off the Water, let the Cryftals be taken out and dried. There is no Difference between this and that of the *Edinburgh*.

Cremor Tartari.
Cream of Tartar.

Take any Quantity of the foregoing filtred Solution of Tartar, and boil it over the Fire, till a thick Skin appear on the Surface, which is to be taken off with a perforated wooden Ladle; then boil it till a new Skin arifes, and take this off as the former; and continue to do this till all the Water is wafted in this Manner, and at length dry what was fo fkim'd off in the Sun. *E.*

Both thefe are very pretty cooling Purges; or may with very good Effect, be given in fmall Dofes as Alteratives. Their great Ufes are, in Cafes where there is a Tendency to an alcaline Putrefaction in the *Primæ Viæ*, or whole Habit. See the Remarks on the *Tartarus Tartarifatus. Cremor Tartari* is efteem'd a Specific in the dry Gripes excited by the Fumes of Lead; a Diftemper called the *Bellon*, by the Smelters of Lead It is to be taken frequently in this Cafe.

Sapo Tartareus.

Soap of Tartar.

te any Quantity of Salt of Tartar horoughly calcined, and whilst it et remains hot, reduce it to Power; put it into a wide glass Vessel, and immediately pour thereon wice its Weight of Oil of Turpentine, and let them stand together in a Cellar for some Weeks, ill the Oil shall have entered the alt; then by degrees add more Oil, till at length the Salt shall ave imbibed thrice its own Quanty thereof, and they both together incorporate into a Soap, which they will do in the Space f a Month or two, provided the Matter be kept daily stirring.

he Operation will be finished the ier, if the containing Vessel be n'd to the Sails of a Wind mill, any other Machine that has a t circular Motion. *E.*

Sapo Amygdalinus.

Almond Soap.

te any Quantity of fresh Oil of Almonds, and thrice its Measure f the Soap-leys: Digest them together for some time in such a Ieat, wherewith the Mixture shall nt just boil, and within a few Iours the Oil and Leys will be nited; after which the Liquor t Boiling, will soon become ropy, nd in a good degree transparent, nd will cool into the Consistence f a Jelly: Then throw in Sea-.lt, till the boiling Liquor has lost s Ropiness: Continue the Boil-.ig till Drops of the Liquor being :ceived upon a Tile, the Water is en to separate freely from the :oagulated Soap; then remove the ire, and the Soap will gradually se to the Top of the Liquor, which is to be taken out before it cold, and put into a wooden

Frame, which has a Cloth for its Bottom. In the last Place, being taken out, it is to be set by till it acquires its just Consistence.

After the same Manner may Soap be made with Olive Oil, in which the finest Oil ought to be employ'd, that the Soap may be as little ungrateful as possible, either to the Palate or Stomach. *L.*

See the Virtues of Soap in the *Materia Medica.*

Cauterium Potentiale.

The Potential Cautery.

Take one Part of Quicklime fresh prepared from Stone; and put it, whilst it remains perfectly dry, solid, and uncrack'd, into a clean iron Pot: Lay upon it two Parts of pure Pot-ash, so as every Way to cover the Lime. Cover the Pot with a Linnen Cloth, and leave it in this State till the Lime begins to split; then add four times their Weight of fair Water, and boil them together for an Hour or two. Strain the clear Lixivium through a close Linnen Bag, made of a conical Form, till it becomes as limpid as Water; then inspissate this Lixivium in a large iron Ladle, with Care to prevent Boiling over, till it becomes perfectly dry; making the Fire so strong, at last, as to ignite the Ladle and melt the Matter, after it ceases to fume. As soon as it runs, pour it out upon an hot Copper Plate; and, whilst it is yet soft, make it flat, and cut it into little Sticks fit for Surgeons Use: Put the Pieces immediately into a strong, heated, and dry Glass, which must be directly stopt with a sound and dry Cork, and then be carefully closed over, by having its upper End dipp'd in melted Pitch, to prevent any Moisture from insinuating; which with in-

F f f credible

credible Force, is attracted by the Alcali so prepared, even through Cork and Bladder; but by this Contrivance it may be kept perfect for Years. When any Part is taken out for Use, this should be done in a strong Heat, near the Fire, and in a dry Air, the Glass being again immediately closed as before.

The Salt acquires a very strong and quick corrosive Power on this Account, that the fiery fixed Alcali attracts the fiery Virtue of the Lime; for no such Power resides either in the Alcali or Lime alone. This Corrosiveness exceeds that of any other known Salt; for if a little Piece of it be applied to the Skin, contained in a small round Hole cut in a Plaister, first laid upon the Part, and then cover'd with another Plaister, it soon burns the Skin and the Fat; for which Reason Surgeons prefer it as their chiefest potential Cautery. While the fresh Lixivium is boiling over the Fire, it will immediately dissolve almost any Animal Substance thrown into it; as also many vegetable Bodies, and fossil Sulphurs. But a prudent Application of such a Lixivium is an incomparable Remedy for disposing deep gangrenated, and almost sphacelated Parts of the Body to Separation; tho' its Application requires the Caution of an experienced Surgeon. If the Lime were first flaked either in the Air or in Water, as almost all old Lime is, or be already reduced to fine Powder, it will not give this corrosive Salt with fixed Alcali.

This Salt acquires this particular Property, that it becomes extremely well disposed to unite with Oils, whether express'd or distill'd, Vegetable or Animal, and thus forms Soaps; being by the Preparation render'd so penetrating, as intimately to divide the Body of Oil, and unite therewith, which unassisted with the

Sharpness of the Lime, it could not well do; nor will fixed Alcali easily melt at the Fire without this Assistance.

These are *Boerhaave's* Directions for preparing Soap Leys, and the Potential Cautery. Those in the *London* Dispensatory are thus:

Lixivium Saponarium.

Soap Leys.

Take equal Weights of *Russia* Potash and Quicklime, and throw Water upon them by degrees, til the Lime is flaked; then throw on more Water, and stir all together, that the Salt of the Ashes may be dissolved: After some time pour the Liquor, filtred thro' Paper if needful into another Vessel. A true standard Wine Pint of this Liquor, measured with the greatest Exactness, ought to weigh just sixteen Ounces: If it is heavier, for every Dram it exceeds that Weight, an Ounce and a half of Water, in Measure, is to be added to each Pint of the Liquor; but if it is lighter, it must be boiled ti'l the like Quantity of Water is carried off, or else must be thrown upon fresh Lime and Ashes. *L.*

Our Makers of soft Soap prepare their Ley stronger than this: The Ley will be reduced to the Standard here proposed, by mixing it with something less than an equal Measure of Water.

Causticum commune fortius.

The stronger common Caustic.

Boil to a fourth Part any Quantity of the Soap Leys above described, then sprinkle in, while boiling, Lime that has been kept in a Vessel pretty close stopt for several Months. Continue to add the Lime, till all the Liquor is absorb'd, and the Whole reduced a Paſte, which is to be kept in a Veſſel well ſtopt. *L.*

The Deſign of thus keeping the ime before it is uſed is, that its crimony may be a little abated, his Cauſtic is preferable to that lled the *Lapis Infernalis*, as it will t liquify like that, by the Moi- re of the Part, on which it is ap- ied, and by this means keeps bet- r confined within the Limits in hich it is intended ro operate; for is Reaſon the *Lapis Infernalis* is lit- : uſed at preſent by our Surgeons.

Cauſticum commune mitius.

The common milder Cauſtic.

Take of ſoft Soap, and of freſh Quicklime, equal Parts, and mix them at the Time of uſing. *L.*

Here in the Soap the Acrimony of the Ley being, by the Mixture of Oil and Tallow, as it were, wholly retunded, the Lime ſhould be quite freſh, without any Abatement of its Corroſiveneſs; for thus the Cauſtic is a great deal milder than the former.

CHAP. II.

CHYMICAL PREPARATIONS of ANIMALS.

Spiritus, Sal, & Oleum Cornu Cervi.

Spirit, Salt, and Oil of Hartſhorn.

TAKE any Quantity of Hartſ- horn, broke into ſmall Pieces, and put it into an earthen or coated glaſs Retort, ſo as to fill the ſame up to the Neck: Fit a large Re- ceiver thereto, and diſtil with due Degrees of Heat in an open Fire. The *Phlegm* will firſt aſcend, then the *Spirit*. next the yellow *oily Salt*, and at laſt the duſky red Oil, together with the *volatile Salt*, a black *Earth* remaining at the Bottom; which being calcined in an open Fire till it becomes white; is called by the Name of calcined Hartſhorn. *E.*

The ſeveral Preparations, being ured out of the Receiver, are thus arated:

he Oil is ſeparated from the legm and Spirit by Filtration, the two latter paſſing thro', and leaving the Oil behind in the Paper.

The Phlegm is ſeparated from the Spirit by gentle Diſtillation in a tall Veſſel, the Spirit aſcending firſt, and leaving the Phlegm behind.

The Spirit may be reſolved into Salt and Phlegm, by diſtilling it in a very tall and narrow Cucurbit; for thus the dry Salt will fix itſelf to the Head, and leave the Phlegm at the Bottom.

The Salt is freed from the Oil by ſubliming it with ſix times its own Quantity of Chalk, or calcin'd Bones; for by this means the Oil is kept down whilſt the Salt ſublimes. *E.*

In the *London* Diſpenſatory we are told, that if the Oil be ſeparated, and the Spirit and Salt mixed toge- ther, be diſtilled again, with a very gentle Heat, they will both riſe more pure. If this is carefully repeated ſeveral times, the Salt will become

very

very white, and the Spirit as limpid as Water, with a grateful Smell.

If the Salt be separated from the Spirit and sublimed, first from an equal Weight of fine Chalk, and then again from a small Quantity of rectify'd Spirit of Wine, it will become sooner pure. Calcined Hartshorn is for the most part made by burning the Horns after they have passed thro' the preceding Operation. *L.*

A Spirit, Salt, and Water, may in the like Manner be distilled from all the solid Parts of Animals; as also from their Blood, provided it be first dried by a gentle Heat. The same may be done from Urine, evaporated to the Consistence of Honey, and putrified; or whilst it remains fresh, provided it be mixed with four times its own Quantity of Sand, or an equal Proportion of any fixed alcaline Salt. Urine, with the Addition of Quicklime, affords only an exceeding pungent Spirit. *E.*

In the *Pharmacopœia Reformata*, we are told, that of all the Preparations, which the Chymical Pharmacy supplies us with, there is no one in greater Esteem, or more universally prescribed, than the Spirit of Hartshorn; and yet perhaps there is no Medicine, whose Dose is more precarious and uncertain; for as the Spirit is nothing but the volatile Salt dissolved in Phlegm, so the Strength of the Spirit must be in Proportion to the Quantity of Salt contained in it, and this will vary according to the particular Circumstances of the Hartshorn, and as the Distillation, in rectifying it, is contained for a longer or shorter Time; and hence it is that we hardly ever meet with it twice of the same Strength in the Shops; but this Inconvenience might be avoided, and a certain Degree of Strength always kept to, by continuing the Rectification no longer

than till the Salt is almost dissolved and the Physician might, without Impeachment of his Judgment, insist upon this Caution being observed, which whether complied with or not, will easily appear upon Examination.

The Chymical Properties and Virtues of a pure, volatile, alcaline Salt, are principally these: It makes an Effervescence with all the known Acids, as strong and as durable as fixed alcaline Salt; closely joins the Acid with itself, and retains it so as to form a compound Salt according to the Nature of the Acid. And thus, when fully saturated, it increases 2/7 in its Weight. Whence we may understand the requisite Proportion for making the Balance betwixt an Acid and an Alcali, and how much of either may be again expected upon the Resolution of these compound Salts. But as soon as the Point of Saturation is exactly gain'd, the Action of the Salt, is produced, is neither to be esteemed from the Acid or the Alcali of its Composition, but from the new Nature the compound Salt has acquired. And hence the Error of those may be easily confuted, who conceive that the Virtues of compound Salts are such as they observe in the Parts produced by a Separation. 2. This Salt, actuated with the Heat of a healthy Body, presently inflames, burns, and causes a gangrenous Escar, and therefore perfectly destroys all the Parts of the human Body, to which it is so apply'd, as that its Action, arising from the Heat, may be driven in upon the Part. Thus, a Scruple of the pure volatile Salt of Hartshorn be laid upon the Skin and covered with an adhesive Plaster, it will in half a quarter of an Hour, raise a black Carbuncle, as a Piece of hot Iron had been applied; and the Colour, Pain, Heat, and Hardness of the Skin are such e fame as they would be in that fe; and it refolves the Humours to a thin, fanious Liquor. It is e moft moveable Body of any hierto known, as exceeding even lcobol in Volatility: For if Alcool, Water, and this Salt be put tother in a tall chymical Glafs fil l, with an Alembic-head, and a all Degree of Heat be applied, e Salt will rife by itfelf into the ead, long before the Alcohol; the cohol will next follow, and the ter at laft with Difficulty. And us this Salt flies off from every ated Point; and if laid upon warm Hand, it prefently flies ray without hurting the Hand, as this Cafe its Reaction is not great on the heating Body; wherein it atly differs from the fixed alcaline lt, which adheres by its Weight. t when thofe volatile alcaline Salts received into the Veffels of the dy, and there actuated by the vital wers, and the Force of the circulat Fluids, they act very powerfully by harp, ftimulating, and corroding rtue; efpecially upon the more fible fine Fibres of the nervous ftem, which they excite to greater tion; and at the fame Time nning the Humours, promote rfpiration, Sweat, Urine, and Sa a. They likewife frequently prove viceable, when their Exhalations receiv'd along with the Air, into Noftrils; for thus they irritate Membrana Pituitaria of the fe, Mouth, Jaws, Lungs; and, irritating thereof, diffolve the vi us Fhlegm, which may adhere reto, provided they be ufed with ution. Thefe Salts, therefore, are per, and have very good Effects, aqueous, acid, auftere Diftempers the Humours, as alfo in Torpi y of the nervous Syftem, and dif erly Motions of the Spirits, rufh irregularly and involuntarily into ticular Mufcles. And hence they

excellently cure hypochondriacal, hyfterical, epileptical, and fpafmo dical Diforders. Being diluted with Water, and received in the Form of Vapour into the *Vagina Uteri*, they are efteem'd one of the moft imme diate Remedies, when prudently ap plied, for promoting the Menfes, if required. But they prove poifonous in alcaline and putrid Diforders, where the Humours are diffolved, and the Body already too much agi tated. They may alfo be externally apply'd, by way of a Cauftic, for the making of Iffues, the extirpating of Warts, and taking off Styes upon the Eyelids. The Method of ufing this Salt in thefe Cafes, is by laying it upon a little Pellet of Lint, and applying it to the Part; then cover ing it with an adhefive Plaifter, and leaving it thus, till it may be thought to have performed its Office: Thus far *Boerhaave*.

The volatile Salt of Hartfhorn is by fome fo highly extoll'd, as al moft to be pronounced an univerfal Medicine in Epilepfies, Apoplexies, Lethargies, Vertigoes, and in a Word, all the Diforders incident to the Brain. The fame Virtues are afcribed to it in the Cure of hyfteric Fits, in opening Obftructions of the Vifcera, in removing all Fevers, Diforders of the Kidneys, and the Bladder, the Plague, and the fatal Effects of all Poifons. It is no lefs extoll'd in rendering the Body fo luble when coftive, and reducing it to a due State, when it runs into the oppofite Extreme; as alfo, in pro voking the Menfes, and at the fame Time, giving a feafonable Check to them, when they flow immoderately. According to *Ettmuller*, *Moebius* in forms us, that the volatile Salt of Hartfhorn, duly exhibited, not only excites a Diaphorefis, but alfo a Vo miting. It is given internally mixed with other Subftances, either in the Form of Powders, Pills, or Potions.

When put into a narrow-mouthed Glass, it is applied to the Nostrils for opening their Obstructions, created by a viscid Lymph. It is also used in the same Manner for recovering and animating apoplectic, epileptic, and hysteric Patients. If the Virtues of this Medicine are really so great as is pretended, and if it is indiscriminately proper in all the above-mention'd Disorders, there would scarcely be a Necessity for any other Medicine in the Shops, besides those of the refrigerating, emollient, and emplastic Kind, since the Effects produced by all the others might be expected from the volatile Salt of Hartshorn alone.

The rectify'd Spirit of Hartshorn, according to *Ettmuller*, is very much used in the Cure of Fevers, and acute malignant Disorders, in exciting a Diaphoresis; and removing Epilepsies. It penetrates the whole Body, corrects Malignity by its alexipharmic Quality, and expels it by a Diaphoresis. It corrects vicious Acids, and promotes the Eruptions of Pustules, Small-pox, and *Petechiæ*. Some account it an universal Medicine, and say that nothing is more proper in the Increase of malignant Disorders. *Ludovicus*, in his *Pharmacopœia*, calls it a highly penetrating Alexipharmic in most malignant Disorders, and an excellent Cephalic in those of the vertiginous and lethargic Kind, when apply'd to the Nostrils. *Sculzius*, in his *Prælectiones*, tells us, that it is exhibited internally from ten to thirty Drops; and that robust Country-men sometimes take a Dram of it in Brandy. It is of an aperient, antispasmodic, and sedative Quality. In Conjunction with a proper Regimen, it is highly diaphoretic; but when it has not the Advantage of this, it rather proves diuretic. In *Eph. Nat. Curios. Dec.* 3, a 1. 091. we are told, that, after the fruitless and ineffectual

Use of other Means, it happily cured a malignant epidemical Fever, which raged after a moderately warm and rainy Winter; for the Patients, after the Exhibition of it, were immediately freed from the Delirium, and convulsive Motions with which the Disorder was accompany'd. *Slessius* informs us, that it produced a surprising Effect upon a Woman, who, in consequence of an intemperate Method of Living, labour'd under Indigestion, Loathing of her Food, Restlessness, and Loss of Strength. At last, being seized with such a violent fainting Fit, that her Case was judged desperate, half a Dram of the Spirit of Hartshorn was exhibited to her, without her perceiving it; immediately after which, she rose up, vomited Worms, and was in a surprising Manner snatched from the Jaws of Death. *Hoffman*, in his *Acta Laboratorii Altdorfensis*, recommends its Use, by way of Topic, in the Cure of malignant, phagedenic, and cancerous Ulcers. He also orders a Mixture of it, with some proper Decoction, to be injected into Fistulas by means of a Syringe.

Sydenham recommends two, three, or four Drops of Spirit of Hartshorn, in a Spoonful or two of black Cherry Water, or of some proper Julap, five or six Times repeated, as an excellent Remedy against those feverish Disorders, to which Children are subject whilst breeding their Teeth. But to Adults it may be given in the Quantity of fourteen Drops, or more, if exhibited with a View of answering any Intention.

I shall say no more of the Virtues attributed to the Salt and Spirit of Hartshorn, which are by some celebrated with extravagant Encomiums, because their genuine Efficacy is specified in the preceding Quotation from *Boerhaave*. Mean time, I am abundantly sensible, that great Numbers of tender People do themselves ite. Prejudice by habituating themselves to take large Quantities Hartshorn Drops, and those frequently repeated, as this Custom ... the Way to Drams, excessive ...orders of the nervous Kind, and the End Death. And it may be ...arked, that it is no new Thing a Medicine of great Importance, ...en duly apply'd, to become deleterious, by an improper, or too frequent Use. But if the Salt or Spirit Hartshorn happens to be adulterated, which is generally the Case, ... Consequences of taking it may ...ppen to be much worse. *Quincy*, a pretty good Judge of Subjects relating to Pharmacy, observes, that these Preparations have hitherto ...od in the Front of nervous Medicines; but the wicked Sophistications of our Chymists have debased them into Disregard, and almost ex...l'd them out of Practice. To ...ve the Spirit an uncommon Pungency and Quickness of Smell, which all they want to recommend it to sale, a Way has been found to quicken it with Lime, and urinous Volatiles; and they have been so hardy therein, as to own it, and give it a place in their Catalogue, of *Spiritus cornu Cervi cum Calce*, Spirit of Hartshorn with Lime. And now the Fraud is so far improved, that they will make it without any Hartshorn at all, but with Bittern, that is, the Brine which they get from the Salters, Urine, and Lime, which will raise a strong scented Spirit; and this these very honest Men, give some Scent and Colour to, with a little of the fetid Oil of Hartshorn, and put off for what is genuine; or without that Oil, for Spirit of Sal Ammoniac. So that from eight and ten Shillings *per* Pound, which the genuine Medicine deserved, these Gentlemen, to oblige a good Customer, can afford it now for as many Pence. But a curious Person may

pretty easily discover this Cheat, by the rancid urinous Smell of the sophisticated Sort, and its whitening the Inside of a Glass in which it is long kept. The volatile Salt too, which is now sold in the Shops for that of Hartshorn, is a perfect Cheat, and more a Caustic than a Cordial, by the Quantity of Lime and urinous Salt that is thrown up with it; whereas that which is carefully to be collected in the Distillation of the Spirits, about the Top and Neck of the Receiver, is truly an Animal volatile Salt, soften'd with such a Portion of a highly subtilized Oil, as renders it an admirable and agreeable Medicine; but this is never to be met with, or made Use of, unless the Physician will be at the Trouble of attending the Laboratory, or find a Person honest enough to make it on purpose for him: For one Dram of this genuine Salt may be stretched out into a Pound of that used in the Shops.

Oleum Animalium.

Oil of Animals.

Take any Oil distilled from Animal Substances, that of human Blood, for Instance, that of Worms, Ivory, or Hartshorn; and, without the Addition of any Thing, let it be drawn off from a Glass Retort, and rectified to such a Degree, that no black and burnt Fæces may remain in the Bottom; which can scarce be obtained by twelve repeated Distillations.

This Oil, which was before thick, and of a disagreeable and fetid Smell, gradually assumes a more grateful one, and becomes more pungent to the Taste.

Twenty or more Drops of such an Oil taken on an empty Stomach, before the Access of an intermitting Fever, bring on a calm and gentle Sleep, and wonderfully carry off feverish Disorders. This is also an efficacious

efficacious Medicine for the Cure of Epilepsies of long Standing, and allaying convulsive Motions, especially when taken before the ordinary Time of the Access, and when such Medicines have been previously used, as are proper for evacuating the too great Quantity of Humours.

It produces its Effects by its gentle, safe, anodyne, and somniferous Qualities; for it produces a calm and pleasant Sleep, which often lasts for twenty Hours, and which is so far from being followed by Drowsiness, Torpor, and Weakness, that it rather exhilarates and enlivens the Body. Besides, it promotes a gentle Sweat, without increasing the Heat of the Blood. The Effects produced by this Medicine are owing to the prodigious Smallness of its sulphureous Parts, occasioned by its frequent and reiterated Rectifications; and since its sulphureous Particles, in consequence of their Subtilty, penetrate all the smallest Meanders of the Parts, and diffuse themselves thro' the whole Mass of Humours, the Tensity and Elasticity of the *Dura Mater*, and of the whole nervous and membranous System, the depraved and preternatural spasmodic Motion of which is the very Essence and Cause of intermitting Fevers, and epileptic Motions are by this Medicine so much changed and diminished, as afterwards to become unsusceptible of such spasmodic Motions.

By this Observation we are taught, that uncommon medicinal Virtues are treasured up in the minutest Particles of sulphureous and oily Substances; which Circumstance is owing to their reaching the inmost Recesses of the solid Parts, especially those of the Nerves and Membranes; upon the due Form and Motion of which, almost all the Functions and Motions of our Bodies depend.

This also proves, that the hottest Medicine, and such as when administer'd in a very small Dose, is sufficient to throw the whole Mass of Blood into a vastly quick Motion, may be render'd so mild and safe, that when exhibited in a larger Dose, it shall be so very far from increasing the Motion of the Blood, that it will rather quell it, and induce a moderate Calm; and we plainly find that this Circumstance is owing only to the Change produced in the Texture of the Medicine; that is, by rendering the tenacious viscid Oil as subtile as possible.

In fine, this explains and accounts for the anodyne and somniferous Qualities of Camphire, which is no more than a most subtile coagulated Oil when prudently used, and as Exigencies require. *Frederic Hoffman* gives this Character of the rectify'd Oil of Animals; and others affirm, that it is certainly possessed of many and considerable Virtues. Its Character is, that it is a most excellent Remedy against the Plague, or any pestilential Disorder: It cures the Pleurisy, it strongly fortifies Nature, it chears the Heart, and revives the Spirits; it causes a free Circulation of the Blood, and thoroughly cleanses the whole Mass, and clears the Skin from erisipelatous Scurfs and Scabs. It cures the Itch, Scald Heads, Tetters, Ringworms, &c. It is most powerful in the Cure of the Leprosy or Elephantiasis; it opens the Obstructions of the Liver and Spleen; it cures Disorders of the Head and Brain, as Lethargies, Apoplexies, Megrims, Vertigoes, Convulsions, Palsies, &c. It strengthens the Stomach, and helps Digestion; it surprisingly prevails in Faintings, Swoonings, and Palpitations of the Heart. A safer, speedier, better, or more effectual Medicine is not

be found in the whole Art of Phy-
[si]c. Its Dose is from twenty to
[th]irty Drops upon a Lump of Su-
[g]ar, drinking after it a Glass of
Wine.

Spiritus, Sal, & Oleum Fuliginis.

Spirit, Salt, and Oil of Soot.

[D]istil Wood Soot in the same Man-
ner as Hartshorn, but here more
Labour is required to render the
Spirit and Salt pure. *L.*

These are said to possess the same
[v]irtues as the Spirit, Salt, and Oil
[o]f Animals. The Spirit is at pre-
[se]nt much us'd in epileptic Cases, and
[D]isorders which affect the Nerves.

Sal Ammoniacum factitium.

Factitious Sal Ammoniacum.

[Ta]ke of human Urine, or that of
any Kind of labouring Cattle, three
Quarts; of Sea Salt, two Pounds;
of Wood Soot, one Pound, and
boil them together into a Mass;
put this into proper subliming
Pots, and urge it with a gradual
Fire to sublime the Salt; which
will become purer by repeated Solutions in Water, Filtration, and
Evaporation, continued till it remains dry; as also by repeated
Sublimation. But this is brought
from Abroad ready prepared to
our Hands. *E.*

Spiritus Salis Ammoniaci.

Spirit of Sal Ammoniac.

[T]ake of Sal Ammoniac, and Salt of
Tartar, each a like Quantity;
grind them separately, then mix
them together, and put them into
a Glass Retort, and pour thereon
as much Spring Water as wi'l serve
to dissolve the Salts; then distil
the whole in a Sand Heat, till the
Salt that is caked in the Receiver
Is dissolved by the rising Liquor.
If the Receiver be taken away
before any Moisture rises, you

will obtain the *Sal Ammoniacum
volatile,* or a volatile Sal Ammoniac. *E.*

In the *London* Dispensatory it is
thus directed:

Take of any fixed alcaline Salt, a
Pound and a half; of Sal Ammoniac, a Pound; of Water, two
Quarts. With a gentle Fire distil
off one Quart.

Sal volatilis Salis Ammoniaci.

Volatile Salt of Sal Ammoniac.

Take of the finest Chalk or Whiting,
two Pounds; of Sal Ammoniac,
one Pound. Sublime the volatile
Salt in a Retort with a strong Fire.
L.

The alcaline Spirit of Sal Ammoniac is a Water, impregnated with
as much pure alcaline Salt as it can
dissolve, and with this likewise all
the other alcaline volatile Spirits
may be compared; and indeed, no
other volatile alcaline Salts and Spirits are ever so pure and genuine as
these, but constantly infected by
some Oil, which occasions them to
act very differently. This Salt and
Spirit instantly make a violent Effervescence with all Acids. If the
Glass, containing either this Salt or
Spirit, stand open near another filled
with the strong acid Spirit of Nitre,
there immediately arises a considerable Effervescence in the Air, proceeding from the volatile Acid and
Alcali meeting therein. If this Salt
be applied to the warm Skin, and
kept close to it by a Plaister, to prevent its Exhaling, it presently burns
the Part with intolerable Pain, and
with a violent Inflammation turns it
to a black Gangrene, so that there is
scarce a more sudden Poison. Whence
it should seem imprudent to direct
the Use of those Salts or Spirits in
the Way of Smelling-Bottles, for
fear of corroding and inflaming
the

the Olfactory Nerves, the Membrane that lines the Nostrils, and the tender Vesicles of the Lungs. Both this Salt and Spirit are render'd still more fiery by subliming them afresh, from pure, dry, fixed Alcali.

Spiritus Salis Ammoniaci dulcis.

Dulcify'd Spirit of Sal Ammoniae.

Take of any fixt alcaline Salt, half a Pound; of Sal Ammoniac, four Ounces; of Proof Spirit, three Pints: Distil off with a gentle Fire, a Pint and a half. *L.*

This is used in making the *Spiritus Volatilis Aromaticus.*

Flos Salis Ammoniaci.

Flowers of Sal Ammoniac.

Take any Quantity of dry powder'd Sal Ammoniac, put it into an earthen Cucurbit, fit to it a blind Head, and sublime the Flowers, by gradually increasing the Fire. *E.*

Sal Ammoniac is half volatile; for tho' it will not ascend with the Heat of Boiling-water, yet it is not so fixed as Sea Salt. When thus purify'd, it loses the Transparency, which is in some Measure found in common Sal Ammoniac. This Salt does not grow alcaline by Sublimation; in which respect it differs from the Salt of Urine, as still remaining what it was, tho' more purified. It has this wonderful Property, that by thus rising dry in a close Vessel; it carries up with it almost all Animal, Vegetable, and Mineral Substances, and strangely subtilizes them in the Sublimation; whence it has been called, the Pestle of the Chymists; as those Bodies could scarce be so subtilized by any other Means. But if often sublimed with Sal Ammoniac, they are thus at length fixed therewith: And in this Method excellent Medicines are often prepar'd.

Butyrum Ceræ.

Butter of Wax.

Half fill a Glass Retort with fine Wax, cut into Pieces small enough to enter the wide Mouth thereof; then pour clean Sand upon it, so as to fill the Retort, which is now to be gently warmed till the Wax melts, and sufficiently imbibes and mixes among the Sand: Set the Retort in a Sand Furnace, apply a Receiver, and distil with a gradual Fire: There usually first comes over a little tartish Water, of a disagreeable fetid Odour, along with a little Spirit: When with a gentle Heat nothing more ascends, change the Receiver, and raise the Fire, by which means there will gradually arise a thin Oil of a whitish Colour, and concreted, like Butter, in the Receiver. When this ceases, apply a violent Fire of Suppression, upon which the whole Body of the Wax will soon come over into the Receiver, and there appear in a solid Form, like Butter, having lost the hard brittle Nature of Wax. So much Sand should be here mixed with the Wax, as to prevent its explosive Swelling, which would otherwise happen in the Boiling.

The Butter of Wax, thus prepared, affords an extremely soft anodyne Unguent, agreeable to the Nerves, highly emollient and relaxing: and, when rubbed upon the Parts, proves serviceable in Contractions of the Limbs, and successfully preserves the Skin from Roughness, Dryness, and Cracking in the Cold, or the Winter: It also proves excellent in the sharp Pains of the Piles.

See the Articles *Apes* in the *Materia Medica.*

Ol...

Oleum Ceræ.

Oil of Wax.

the Butter of Wax over a gen- Fire, to a liquid Oil, then pour thro' a Funnel, first well heated, to a Glass Retort, also well heat- beforehand, so as to half fill the Retort, with Care to prevent any the Butter from sticking to the Neck thereof, because in that Case the gross Matter would fall into the Receiver, which should here be avoided. Set the Retort in a Sand Furnace, lute on a clean Receiver, and distil cautiously, managing the Fire so, that one Drop may follow another at the Distance of six Seconds; when nothing more comes over with this Degree of Heat, raise the Fire, and distil as before, and continue in this Manner, increasing the Fire with the same Caution, so long as any Butter remains in the Retort; and, by this Means, all the Butter will come over, scarce leaving any Fæ- ces behind; and a thickish Oil, not much diminished in Quantity, will be found instead of Butter in the Receiver. If this Oil of Wax be again distilled in like Manner, it always becomes more limpid, soft, transparent, and thin, so as at last to resemble a subtile, lim- pid Oil : And the oftener the Di- stillation is repeated, the more mild and gentle, yet the more pe- netrating the Oil becomes.

This last Oil of Wax is an incom- parable Remedy for the Diseases of the nervous *Papillæ* on the external Skin; and has scarce its Equal in curing chapt Lips in the Winter, chapt Nipples in the Women who give Suck, and in the Cracking of the Skin of the Hands and Fingers, being sometimes gently anointed thereon. It is also serviceable in discussing cold Tumors arising on the Face or Fin- gers in the Winter; and curing con- tracted Tendons, and the Rigidity of the Limbs thence arising, being used along with Baths, Fomentations, and Motion; for it has a singular Virtue in thus restoring Flexibility to the Parts : Being frequently rub- bed upon the Abdomen, it prevents Costiveness; and is therefore excel- lent in effectually curing the Diseases of Children.

C H A P. III.

CHYMICAL PREPARATIONS *of* MINERALS.

Preparations *of* Salts.

Spiritus Salis.

Spirit of Salt.

TAKE of dried or decrepitated Sea Salt, a Pound; and three Pounds of Brick Dust. Mix them, and put them together into an earthen Retort, whereof they may fill but one half; place the Vessel in a reverberating Furnace, and fitting it with a capacious Receiver, keep a slow Fire at the first, in- crease the Heat, till all the Spirit shall, like Clouds, be driven into the Receiver; when the Vessels are cold, pour out the Liquor in- to a Glass Cucurbit, and rectify, that

that a pure Spirit may remain after the Phlegm is drawn off by a gentle Distillation. *E.*

Spiritus Salis Glauberi.

Glauber's Spirit of Sea Salt.

To three Parts of Sea Salt well depurated and cryſtalized, and put into a Glaſs Retort, pour one Part of the ſtrongeſt Oil of Vitriol ; at the Inſtant they mix, a volatile white Vapour riſes out, which is to be carefully avoided, as being ſuffocating, and capable, if but once drawn in with the Breath, to ſtop the Action of the Lungs irremediably. Directly apply a large and cold Glaſs Receiver, lute the Juncture, apply a very ſmall Quantity of Fire at firſt, for a Spirit will long continue to come over, ſo furiouſly, as to blow thro' the Luting, or break the Veſſel ; ſo that the Fire muſt be kept gentle for three or four Hours ; then increaſe it a little, and a leſs volatile Liquor will come over. After eight Hours have been employed upon the Operation, urge the Fire till the Iron Pot becomes ignited, and no more Liquor riſes ; then let all cool ; and when the Neck of the Retort is no longer hot, take off the Receiver, the Liquor will fume ; and beware of receiving it in with the Breath. Pour it into a Glaſs, well fitted with a Glaſs-ſtopper, and ſet it in a cold Place, otherwiſe the Glaſs often burſts, by means of the Motion of the Vapour. If thus kept for Years, a white ſuffocating Vapour immediately breaks out upon opening of the Veſſel ; but if the Spirit thus produced be carefully diſtill'd in a Glaſs-body, under a Chimney, into a Receiver, the volatile Spirit will come over, whilſt there remains at the Bottom a more fixed Liquor, of a Colour betwixt a yellow and a green. This Li-

quor remains quiet without exhaling ; but that which comes over into the Receiver, has a violent ſuffocating Volatility, and may be kept apart, as a pure volatile Spirit of Salt, in a cloſe Veſſel. Or,

To three Parts of purify'd and dry Sea Salt, put into a Retort, add two Parts of clean Rain Water, and one Part of the ſtrongeſt Oil of Vitriol. Let the Oil of Vitriol fall in by ſlow Drops, to prevent burſting the Veſſel, by the ſudden Heat that would riſe from mixing in the whole at once. The Mixture will grow hot ; place the Retort in a Sand Furnace, and apply a capacious Receiver ; diſtil gently for the firſt Hours, while the Water comes over ſlowly, otherwiſe, if made to riſe briſkly, it always cracks the Receiver. After this, increaſe the Fire gradually ; the Spirit of Sea Salt will come over, which is then known to riſe, when the Liquor runs in ſpiral Veins. Now raiſe the Fire, and gradually urge it, till at length the Pot grows of a red Heat, and no more Liquor comes over ; at which Time the Spirit will not fume. Then ſuffering all to cool, pour out the Spirit, which is now neither ſuffocating, nor ſmoking. If this be diſtilled again with a gentle Fire, in a Glaſs Body, there will come over a limpid, ungratefully acid Water, of excellent internal Uſe, being mixed with Juleps, in ſuch Diſtempers as require it ; an excellent oily Spirit will remain in the Bottom, of a Colour betwixt green and yellow.

In both Caſes there will be left behind a very white and fixed Salt, that can only be fuſed by a violent Fire.

Spirit of Salt is particularly grateful to the Stomach, excites the Appetite, attenuates mucous Humours,

reſiſts

ifts Putrefaction, corrects the
le, when either too acrimoni-
s, large in Quantity, or corrupted.
is of excellent Ufe in curing Gan-
enes of the Gums, Mouth, or
ongue ; it prevents the Generation
the Stone ; and, according to
lmont, helps to diffolve it : It is
viceable in the Strangury attending
l Age. If the ftrongeft Spirit of
lt be mixed with thrice its Weight
Alcohol, and the two be thorough-
united together, by two or three
iftillations, they make a volatile,
ly, acid, fragrant, and balfamic
irit of great Virtue.

Frederic Hoffman remarks, that the
ghly penetrating and fubtile Nature
this Acid is obvious from this, that
a gentle Heat, or even in Balneo
lariæ, it paffes over the Helm of
e Alembic ; and when plac'd in
en Glaffes, fo exhales as foon to
l the whole Room ; and that the
enetrating Nature of this acid Salt
urpaffes that of Nitre, I am induced
believe, becaufe the Acid of Salt
as a freer Accefs into the Pores of
old than that of Nitre, which dif-
lves all other Metals ; for with-
ut an Addition of common Salt, the
rm Compages of Gold cannot be dif-
lved. So great is the Subtilty of the A-
id of common Salt, that when taken
nternally, it diffufes its Operation and
fficacy to remote Parts, efpecially
hofe of the membranous Kind. But
t in a particular Manner exerts its
nfluence on the nervous and fenfible
Membranes of the Lungs, by ftimu-
ating and agitating which, it excites
gentle Cough ; for which Reafon,
he Acid of common Salt ought to
e very cautioufly ufed ; it alfo by
ts powerful Stimulus, penetrates to
he urinary Paffages ; for there is
ardly a more efficacious Medicine
or exciting a Difcharge of Urine,
han Spirit of common Salt. Thofe
who have Fontanels in their Bodies,

and frequently ufe Spirit of Salt, in
Broths prepared with Flefh, perceive
pungent Pains in their Fontanels.
The great Subtilty alfo of this Spirit,
is the Reafon, why by acting on the
nervous Coat of the Stomach, it excites the Appetite far better than
all other acid and mineral Spirits.
Strongly concentrated Spirit of
common Salt has this peculiar to it,
that it does not, like other corrofive
and highly concentrated Acids, fuch
as Oil of Vitriol, and fuming Spirit
of Nitre, by the Addition of a fufficient Quantity of highly rectified Spirit of Wine, lofe its acid Tafte, and
affume a fweet Tafte and Smell. The
ftrong Acid of common Salt remains
entire in the Bottom of the Cucurbit ;
for 'tis fufficiently known to Chymifts, that Oil of Vitriol, after the
Addition of a fufficient Quantity of
highly rectified Spirit of Wine, at
different times, may, by Diftillation,
be converted into a very penetrating
Spirit of a grateful Tafte and Smell.
Thus alfo the fuming Spirit, upon
an Admixture of twelve Parts of
highly rectified Spirit of Wine, becomes fweet, and affumes a graceful
Tafte and Smell ; becaufe by the oleous and fulphureous Parts of the Spirit of Wine, the Acid Spiculæ are fo
corrected and fheathed up, as to
affume a quite different Nature, Texture, and Efficacy. But this is not
found to happen in the Spirit of Salt,
which rejects this Union of the oleous and phlogiftic Spirit, for it retains
its Acidity entire, except that its
thinner fulphureous Part being united
with the inflammable Spirit, in fome
Meafure changes its Smell, and renders it more grateful.

'Tis alfo peculiar to Spirit of Salt
above that of Vitriol, and Nitre,
that it does not fo quickly diffolve
Filings of Steel, but leaves the Lapis
Hæmatitis and the moft fubtile Crocus Martis entirely untouched ;
whereas common Salt, or, which is
ftill

ftill better, *Sal Ammoniac* acts more quickly and powerfully on Chalybeate Minerals, the *Lapis Hæmatitis*, and Filings of Steel, and by diffolving them, converts them into a highly aftringent Vitriol; provided they are intimately mixed in a Crucible, and kept on the Fire for a confiderable Time, which neither happens with Vitriol nor Nitre.

No Acid fo foon extracts the Sulphur, with which Iron is richly impregnated, as the Acid of common Salt; for whether a Solution of Steel with Spirit of Salt, is infpiffated, or whether *Sal Ammoniac*, with Filings of Steel, is treated by a clofe Fire, a Vitriol is obtained of a yellowifh Colour, an aftringent Tafte, a grateful Smell, and which is not capable of Cryftallization, but melts away in the open Air; and if duly dephlegrated Spirit of Wine is poured upon it, the fulphureous Part of the Steel, and the thinner Portion of Salt immediately enters it, and by this Means is prepared a Tincture of Steel, which is of a yellow Colour, a fragrant Smell, a fubaftringent Tafte, and highly efficacious in reftoring the Tone of the Parts; for by this Means the fulphureous Subftance of Steel, which is of great Ufe in Medicine, may be moft commodioufly feparated. 'Tis, alfo, to be obferved, that highly concentrated Spirit of Salt, when mixed with Oil of Vitriol, produces a greater Effervefcence, than any other acid Spirit.

In the *London* Difpenfatory, the *Spiritus Salis Marini Glauberi* is thus directed:

Take Sea Salt, and the ftrong Spirit of Vitriol, of each two Pounds; of Water one Pint. The Oil and Water being firft mixed together add the Mixture gradually to the Salt under a Chimney, then diftil firft with a fmall, and afterwards with a ftronger Fire. *L.*

Spiritus Salis Dulcis.
Sweet Spirit of Salt.

Take one Part of Spirit of Salt, and three Parts of rectified Spirit of Wine; digeft them together for fome Days in a large Glafs Vial, then diftil according to Art in a Sand Heat, taking Care towards the End of the Operation, that the Retort break not with a too violent Fire.

See the Remarks on *Glauber*'s Spirit of Salt.

Spiritus Salis Marini coagulatus.
Spirit of Sea Salt coagulated.

Pour gradually upon the Spirit of Sea Salt the Lixivium of any fixt Alcali, till all Fermentation ceafes, and then evaporate to Drynefs. *L.*

In this Preparation the fix'd Alcali, of which the Spirit of Salt had been depriv'd, is again added, fo as to form a Salt exactly refembling common Sea Salt; and poffeffed of no other Virtues that I know of. It is properly called *Regenerated Sea Salt*.

Sal Catharticus Glauberi.
Glauber's Cathartic Salt.

Diffolve in Water the Cake, which remains after the Diftillation of *Glauber*'s Spirit of Sea Salt, purify the Solution thro' Paper, and then duly evaporate it that the Salt may cryftallize. *L.*

This is the Salt commonly known by the Name of *Sal Mirabile Glauberi*, or *Glauber*'s Salt.

Glauber, the Inventor of this Salt, called it by this Name of Wonderful, not only on account of its being new, but of the furprifing Effects it produces. Some Chymifts that are fond of Syftems pretend, that no more than a true *Tartarum Vitriolatum* is here produced, which was long known before the Time of *Glauber*.

Bu

ut *Tartarum Vitriolatum* has not the Properties which are found in his Salt, either with respect to Figure, Taste, Effects, or any thing else: For if this Salt be properly prepared, reduced to Powder, and mixed with thrice its Weight of Vinegar, Beer, Wine, or Water, and set apart, it freezes them. When melted in a Crucible, if a fourth Part of Antimony be thrown to it by a Piece at a time, it wonderfully dissolves it. In Surgery, this Salt is of excellent Use against Putrefaction and Gangrenes: It is, also, of Use, when internally taken, by gently stimulating, resolving, purging, and promoting of Urine. Perhaps there is not a better gentle Purge. But we very seldom or never meet with it in the Shops of Chymists; for the *Sal Catharticum* is generally sold instead of it. The common Dose is half an Ounce; but it may be exhibited in larger Quantities. And it may with good Effect be given in very small Doses, frequently repeated, as a Cooler, and Deobstruent; the Patient drinking copiously of some diluting Fluid.

The Refinement and Crystallization of Nitre.

Dissolve common Nitre in six times its Quantity of boiling Water; strain the hot Lixivium quick; put it into a clean cylindrical Vessel, and exhale it over a clear Fire, to a Pellicule; set it in a cool Place, with clean Sticks a-cross the Vessel; there will presently be formed long prismatic, hexagonal, transparent Crystals. Collect these, and put them into an earthen Colander, that the Liquor may drain from them; afterwards dry the Nitre in the open Air. Or Dissolve Nitre in eight times its Quantity of boiling Water; filter the Lixivium; then drop therein some pure Oil of Tartar; mix them well, then drop in more, and

continue to do this, till the Liquor appears no more disturbed. Boil the Lixivium for a single Minute; strain it hot to make it perfectly clear; exhale to a Pellicule; pour it out into a clean cylindrical Vessel, with little Sticks laid a-cross, and let it stand in a quiet Place. Prismatic Crystals, like the former, will thus be formed. No Experiment shews, that any Alcali here adheres to the Crystals of Nitre, which is thus made pure; nor does it appear, that any Method can afford it purer.

Let the Lixivium, that remains after this first Crystallization, be diluted with an equal Quantity of fair Water, then boiled for a Moment, filtered hot, inspissated to a Pellicule, and set in a cold Place, as before; it will thus shoot into Crystals of pure Nitre, which are to be dried as above. The remaining Lixivium being again treated in the same manner, and again set to crystallize, yields more of them. And now the remaining Liquor, which is fat and sharp, will afford no more Crystals, and dries with great Difficulty; and this happens, not only when Alcali has been used in the Refining; but also when nothing but pure Nitre was added.

By this means an excellent Nitre is procured for Medicinal Use; being very light, of a particular bitterish Taste; and, when taken into the Body, it easily dissolves therein, wonderfully cools and thins the Blood, giving a florid Colour thereto, and checking the Inclinations to Venery. It is changed in the Body, not being unalterable therein like Sea Salt, but turning into the human Salt. If the moist or solid Parts of Animals be salted with this Nitre, they are thereby kept extremely red, and free from Putrefaction; whence in all inflammatory Distempers, attended with

with an inflammatory Condensation of the Blood, this Salt proves excellently attenuating; and at the same time, no way offends by any violent Acrimony, nor proves prejudicial by its Weight. It does not occasion Thirst, and prevents the Salt of the Body from turning alcaline, and the Oil from putrefying: And on this Account, it may properly be called an antiphlogistic Salt.

Sal Prunellæ.
Salt Prunella.

Take of purified Nitre reduced to Powder two Pounds; fuse it in a Crucible, and gradually sprinkle thereon an Ounce of the Flowers of Sulphur; when the Deflagration is over, pour out the melted Salt upon a Copper Plate, first made clean, dry, and hot, so as that the Salt may be formed into thin Cakes. *E.*

Boerhaave says, that Nitre thus prepared, entirely agrees in Virtue and Use, with purified Nitre, which last he prefers, and with very good Reason; for it sometimes sits easy on the Stomach, when Sal Prunel will not.

This Preparation has obtained the Name of *Sal Prunellæ* from the *Germans*, who observing that a certain Kind of epidemica Camp-Fever, attended with a dangerous b'ack Quinsey, which they call, *Diebraune*, was happily cured by the Use of this Powder; they thence called it by that Name.

Sal Polychrestum.
Salt of many Virtues.

Take of powder'd Nitre, and of the Flowers of Sulphur, each a like Quantity, mix them well together, and, by degrees, throw them into an ignited Crucible. After the Deflagration ceases, keep the Crucible in the Fire for one Hour; then purify the Salt, by dissolving it in hot Water, filtring the Solution, and exhaling it till it becomes dry. *E.*

Physicians, especially those of *Paris,* having thoroughly experienced the Virtues of this Salt, called it *Polychrestus,* because of its various Effects, and proving successful in many different Diseases. If taken upon an empty Stomach, by a Person in Health, in the Quantity of two Drams, diluted with twenty times its Quantity of Water, the Person walking gently after it, and drinking four or six Ounces of new Whey, for three or four times, it sometimes proves gently vomiting, often purgative, but always diuretic and sudorific; so often as it is determined to operate that Way by Heat, Motion, and Sudorifics. It cuts cold viscous Phlegm, resolves Inflammations of the Blood, opens the Passages, corrects the Bile, when tending to Putrefaction, excites it, when languid, and stimulates it with Gentleness and Safety. Hence being prudently given in chronical and acute Distempers, it proves curative: It almost certainly cures inveterate Tertians, without any Danger of Relapse, or without obstructing the Viscera: It securely cures Quartans, by gradually resolving the sluggish Matter thereof; and therefore has deservedly obtained the Name of the *Salt of many Virtues.*

Spiritus Nitri.
Spirit of Nitre.

This is distilled from Nitre, in the same Manner as Spirit of Salt. *E.*

Spiritus Nitri Glauberi.
Glauber's Spirit of Nitre.

Take of Nitre three Pounds, of strong Spirit of Vitriol one Pound. Let them be mixed with Caution, and gradually under a Chimney, afterwards

afterwards let them be ꝺiſtilled firſt with a gentle Heat, and then with a ſtronger. *L.*

ꞇhe principal Uſe of Spirit of Niꞇis, to diſſolve Metals and Mineꞅ for Medicinal Uſes; and to ꞇke the *Spiritus Nitri Dulcis.*

Spiritus Nitri Dulcis.

Dulcified Spirit of Nitre.

ꞇke of rectified Spirit of Wine one Quart, of *Glauber*'s Spirit of Niꞇre half a Pound. Mix them by ꞁouring the Spirit of Wine on ꞇhe other, and diſtil the Mixture with a gentle Heat, as long as what comes off will not raiſe any Fermentation with a lixivial Salt. *L.*

ꞁ the *Pharmacopœia Reformata,* are told, that the Direction of ꞁtinuing the Diſtillation only till ꞇat comes over ferments with a ꞇꝺ alcaline Salt, is ſufficiently ꞇbleſome and unartful. If the ꞅrit of Wine be highly phlegmed, ꞁ ſix Parts, inſtead of four, be adand the Spirit of Nitre be pure ꞁ ſtrong, almoſt the whole Mixꞇe will riſe in the Heat of a Waterꞇh, be greatly odorous, and ſuffiꞇtly dulcified, ſo as not to give ꞅ, or but very little Marks of ꞁdity upon the Affuſion of an Alꞁi. The Spirit of Nitre ſhould be ꞅilled from equal Parts of ſtrong of Vitriol, and well-dried Nitre, ꞇh a gentle Fire: And the Spirit Wine ſhould be drawn over from ꞇhoroughly dried fixed alcaline ꞇ.

ꞅpon thus mixing together Alcaand Spiri of Nitre, there immeꞇely ariſes a fragrant Smell, like ꞇt of Southern-Wood; *Boerhaave* ꞅ, that there is obſerved a high ꞇgree of Efferveſcence betwixt this ꞇꞇile Acid and pure ſubtile Oil, ꞇhout the leaſt Interpoſition of an

Alcali: And yet the Efferveſcence is almoſt fiery; ſo that if a lighted Candle were applied to the Vapour, the Inſide of the Glaſs would appear on Flame, and the Whole inſtantly burſt in a dangerous Manner. The oftener theſe two Liquors are digeſted, and diſtilled together, the more exactly they unite, and thus afford a perfectly acid and oily Salt, which has an actual preſervative, balſamic, detergent, diſſolving Virtue, and prevents the Putrefaction of the Bile. Being properly diluted, and prudently uſed, it preſently gives a beautiful Whiteneſs to the Teeth; but if imprudently uſed, deſtroys them. It reſtores the Appetite, if depraved by a mucous Phlegm, or corrupt Bile, or if the Cauſe proceeds from a Weakneſs of the Stomach. It is a great Carminative; it is recommended as a Preſervative againſt the Stone; and even as a Solvent for it. It was the famous Lithontriptic of *Sylvius* held at a very dear Price. It promotes Sweat, provokes Urine, allays Thirſt, corrects a fetid Breath, and has particular Virtues in the Scurvy. It is conveniently taken upon an empty Stomach, to twenty or thirty Drops, or more, in Wine, Mead, or Beer.

Nitrum Vitriolatum.

Vitriolated Nitre.

Diſſolve the Cake left after the Diſtillation of *Glauber*'s Spirit of Niꞇtre, as deſcribed above, in hot Water, and after purifying thro' Paper, evaporate, that the Salt may ſhoot. *L.*

This is commonly called *Sal Enixus Paracelſi.* It is a Diuretic, and is commonly ſold in the Shops for vitriolated Tartar; a Fraud ſometimes of pernicious Conſequence.

    Alumen

Alumen uftum.

Burnt Alum.

Let Alum be put into an iron or earthen Pot, and calcined as long as it rifes up and fwells. *L.*

This is often ufed as an Efcharotic, to eat away proud Flefh.

Vitriolum Calcinatum.

Calcined Vitriol.

Put green Vitriol into an earthen Veffel, and calcine it with an open Fire as long as it exhales any Moifture; then take it out by breaking the Veffel, and fet it by for Ufe, well clofed from the Air. The Vitriol is moft perfectly calcined, if, at the Bottom and Sides of the containing Veffel, it is become red. *L.*

Aqua Fortis fimplex.

Single Aqua Fortis.

Take two Parts of Vitriol calcined till it becomes white, and one Part of powdered Nitre; mix them well together, and put them into an earthen Retort, whereof they may fill two thirds; then fitting a very large Receiver thereto, diftil as was ordered of Spirit of Salt. *E.*

Aqua Fortis duplex.

Double Aqua Fortis.

Take of green Vitriol calcined to Whitenefs, of powdered Nitre, as alfo of Clay dried and reduced to Powder, each a like Quantity. Mix them well together, put them into an earthen Retort, whereof they may fill two thirds, and diftil as in making fingle *Aqua Fortis.* *E.*

In the *London* Difpenfatory, *Aqua Fortis* is thus directed:

Take Nitre, green Vitriol not calcined, of each three Pounds; of the fame Vitriol calcined, one Pound and half; mix all together, and diftil with a very ftrong Fire as long as red Fumes arife. *L.*

Aqua Fortis compofita.

Compound Aqua Fortis.

Take of Aqua Fortis fixteen Ounces in Weight, of Sea Salt one Dram. Diftil to Drynefs. *L.*

We are told, that our Chemifts in Practice find a Difficulty in preparing, with their common *Aqua Fortis,* what is ufually called Red Precipitate, but is here named *Mercurius corrofivus Ruber;* infomuch, that fome few, who make it with us, employ another compound Spirit: but the Succefs of the Procefs may be very well fecured by diftilling the *Aqua Fortis* firft from a fmall Quantity of Salt; and for this Purpofe fuch a Preparation is here inferted under the Title of *Aqua Fortis compofita.*

Aqua Regia.

Take an Ounce of Sal Ammoniac reduced to Powder, put it into a large Cucurbit; by Degrees mix therewith four Ounces of the Spirit of Nitre, or double *Aqua Fortis,* and let them ftand together in a Sand Furnace till the Salt is totally diffolved. *E.*

This is intended for the Solution of Gold, a Thing of very little Confequence in Medicine.

Spiritus & Oleum Vitrioli.

Spirit and Oil of Vitriol.

Take any Quantity of green Vitriol calcined till it becomes white, and afterwards reduced to Powder; put it into an earthen Retort fo as

to fill one half, and place the Veſſel in a reverberatory Furnace;
then having fitted the Retort with
a very capacious Receiver, and
luted the Junctures, diſtil with a
Heat gradually increas'd to the
extreme Degree, which continue
as long as any Vapours ariſe. The
Phlegm, Spirit, and Oil are to be
ſeparated by a Retort in a Sand
Heat. The Phlegm comes over
with a gentle Heat; the Spirit
with a ſtronger, and the Oil remains. What remains in the
Retort after the firſt Diſtillation is
called by the Name of *Colcothar.*
E.

n the *London* Diſpenſatory; the Oil
Vitriol is called *Spiritus Vitrioli
tis.*

Spiritus Vitrioli dulcis.

Dilcify'd Spirit of Vitriol.

ake of ſtrong Spirit of Vitriol,
called the Oil, one Pound; of
rectify'd Spirit of Wine, one Pint;
mix them cautiouſly and by Degrees,
and diſtil them with a gentle Heat,
till a black Froth begins to riſe;
then remove all from the Fire, that
this Froth may not ſwell over into
the Receiver, and fruſtrate the O-
peration. *L.*

n the *Edinburgh* Diſpenſatory this
edicine is thus directed:

ake of rectify'd Spirit of Wine,
four Pints; drop gradually and
cautiouſly into it of Oil of Vitriol, ſix Ounces. Digeſt for three
Days, and diſtil according to Art.
loth theſe ſeem intended to imitate
e following Preparation.

quor Mineralis Anodynus Hoffmanni.

ederic *Hoffman*'s Anodyne Mineral
Liquor.

ake of the beſt Oil of Vitriol, and
Indian Nitre, each four Ounces:

Diſtil the Spirit from a Retort by
a Fire, gradually raiſed to a great
Briſkneſs, about the End of the
Proceſs: Pour two Ounces of this
Spirit cautiouſly and ſucceſſively,
into fifteen Ounces of highly rectify'd Spirit of Wine; then by a
careful Diſtillation, we obtain an
highly fragrant and aromatic Spirit.
But in this Proceſs, great Care is
to be taken, that we neither fall
ſhort, nor exceed, in extracting
the ſulphureous Spirit, but endeavour to obtain the whole of it as
pure and genuine as we poſſibly
can; for as ſoon as the Phlegm
is about to riſe, with the crude
acid Spirit, the Receiver is to be
changed with all Expedition. But,
as this ſulphureous Spirit is not
yielded entirely pure, and free
from a Mixture of the crude and
acid Spirit, it is to be rectify'd
with an equal Quantity of Water,
and duly ſhaken, by which means,
the acid Principle will ſubſide in
the Water, and the ſulphureous
Spirit be diſtill'd pure and un-adul-
terated. When all the Spirit is
obtained, and the Phlegm juſt ready to come over, the former is to
be immediately removed, and
kept in a Veſſel carefully cloſed.
The mild and ſoporiferous Virtue
of this Spirit may be ſtill heightened, if before the Rectification
with Water, we add to it ſome
Quantity of the Oil of Cloves,
which is to be duly mixed with it,
by ſhaking both together in a Glaſs
Veſſel, cloſed with a Glaſs Stop-
per; for by this means, the Acrimony of the Oil of Cloves is deſtroyed; eſpecially if afterwards
both are mixed with Water, and
duly incorporated by ſhaking; for
thus the gentle, mild, and ethereal Quality is intimately united with
this Spirit. It is a Matter of no
Importance, whether this Compo-

ſition

sition is the genuine, anodyne, mineral Liquor of *Hoffman*, since the former is equally efficacious with the latter, in its gently stimulating, carminative, antiseptic, diaphoretic, and anodyne Virtues.

Gilla feu Sal Vitrioli.

Take any Quantity of white Vitriol, and dissolve it in a proper Proportion of hot Spring Water, filtre the Solution, and evaporate it till only one third remains behind; then set it in a cold Place for three Days, that the Crystals may shoot to the Sides of the Vessel, which are afterwards to be dried in the Sun. Exhale the remaining Liquor again till no more Crystals will shoot from it. *E.*

Quincy says, it works by Vomit, and is a gentle Puke enough for young Children, from three to eight Grains; and to grown People, from a Scruple to a Dram. It corrugates the Stomach into Contraction so soon, that it is fancied to come all up again, upon the first Ejectment; and therefore some give as many Doses of it as they would have the Patient vomit; giving each in a Porringer, or Bason of Posset-drink, or Carduus Tea.

In the *London* Dispensatory, the Salt of Vitriol is thus order'd:

Take of white Vitriol, a Pound; of the strong Spirit of Vitriol, one Ounce in Weight; of Water, as much as is sufficient. Dissolve the Vitriol by boiling, then strain the Decoction thro' Paper, and, after proper Exhalation, set it in a cold Place, that the Salt may shoot. *L.*

I don't apprehend, that this is in any Degree better than that order'd in the *Edinburgh* Dispensatory.

Ens Veneris.

Flowers of Copper.

Take Colcothar of blue Vitriol, first well edulcorated with Water, and dried; and of Sal Ammoniac, each a like Quantity; reduce them separately to Powder, then mix them together, and put them together into an earthen Cucurbit, whereof they may possess two thirds; place the Vessel with a blind Glass Head in a naked Fire, using only a moderate Heat at first, and increasing it by Degrees, as long as the Flowers rise of a yellow Colour inclined to red, which, when the Vessel is cooled, are to be carefully swept out with a Feather. *E.*

Boerhaave orders this Medicine to be prepared from the Colcothar of green Vitriol; and remarks, that when it is prepared with the Colcothar of blue Vitriol, it partakes of the Nature of Copper; but when green Vitriol is used, it is then more properly called *Ens Martis*, as being a Preparation of Iron.

Mr. *Boyle* promises great Effects from this Remedy, in Distempers proceeding from a Weakness of the Solids, as in the Rickets, or the like; and it is highly serviceable therein. *Helmont* also, in the Treatise he intitles *Butler*, greatly commends a like Preparation.

In the *London* Dispensatory this Medicine is thus directed, under the Title of,

Flores Martiales.

Martial Flowers.

Take of washed Colcothar of green Vitriol, or of Iron Filings, one Pound; of Sal Ammoniac, two Pounds. Mix and sublime them in a Retort, and mixing again the Bottom with the Flowers, renew the Sublimation, till the Flowers acquire a beautiful yellow Colour.

To the Residue may be added half a Pound of fresh Sal Ammoniac, and

Sublimation repeated, and the
e Procefs may be thus continued
as long as the Flowers rife duly
ured. *L.*

I apprehend Mr. *Boyle* has been
underftood, with refpect to the
paration of the *Ens Veneris*, I
l here tranfcribe what is faid upon
Subject, in the Narrative of the
nmittee; together with the Re-
rks of the Author of the *Phar-
opæia Reformata.*

he Committee have fubftituted an-
er Name for *Ens Veneris*, not on-
or the Sake of Propriety, but to
ıave the Occafion of the Miftake
ımitted in our prefent *Pharmaco-
a*, which has been followed by
ers, of directing the Preparation
h blue Vitriol; whereas it was
ginally made with a chalybeate
riol by Mr. *Boyle*, the Author of
as appears from his Account of
Colour of the Preparation, and
Property he afcribes to it, of turn-
a Tincture of Galls to an inky
cknefs, tho' from his not know-
the Qualities of the Vitriol he
d, he gave it the Name we
re changed, and afcribes its Ef-
ts to Copper. Vitriols are of va-
us Kinds; our Copperas fcarce
ıtains any Metal but Iron; the
e Vitriol, ufed by the Surgeons,
ıunds in Copper, tho' it is not
litute of Iron; in thofe of *Dant-
k* and *Goflar*, both which Mr.
yle recommends for this Purpofe.
ın is the principal Metal; tho'
y partake of Copper alfo, but in
fmall a Proportion, that when the
ıdicine is prepared with either of
fe two, it does not fenfibly differ from
it ufually made from our Copper s:
hereas in operating with blue Vi-
ol, the Appearances are wholly
ınged. This Vitriol does not
lcine red, which Mr. *Boyle* repre-
ıts to be the Cafe in his Prepara-

tion of the Medicine. The Salt alfo, in its firft Sublimation, rifes not
at all yellow, but of a greenifh Blue;
which in fubfequent Sublimations
becomes paler, and is changed by the
Iron contained in that Vitriol into
fuch a Hue, as a Mixture of the
firft Sublimation and *Flores Martiales* would compofe. Therefore, when
Mr. *Boyle* propofes the *Hungarian
Vitriol*, as the moft elegible for this
Preparation, he either did not mean,
what has been generally underftood
by it, the common blue Vitriol, or
muft never himfelf have made the
Preparation with it.

Thus far the Narrative of the Committee. The Author of the *Pharmacopæia Reformata* tells us, that,

Having feen this celebrated Medicine faithfully prepared of blue Vitriol, exactly according to the Directions of the *London Pharmacopæia*;
and finding the Sublimate to exactly
agree with the Author's Defcription,
not only in the yellow or reddifh
Colour, but likewife in turning an
Infufion of Galls black; and entertaining no fmall Opinion of its medicinal Virtues, from the Account
which Mr *Boyle* has given of it, he
was greatly furprifed at the Remarks
above, and therefore determined
thoroughly to inquire into them.
As to the Remark, that the Name
was originally impofed on it by Miftake, and that Mr. *Boyle* ufually
prepared it of Steel, I confulted the
Author's Works, and particularly
the Places quoted above. In his
Ufefulnefs of Natural Philofophy, he
tells us, that he and a Chymift endeavoured to imitate *Butler*'s Stone,
by a Preparation of calcined Vitriol;
and finding the Medicine upon Try-
al, tho' far fhort of what *Helmont*
afcribes to his, yet no ordinary one:
We did, fays he, for the Mineral's
Sake it was made of, call it *Ens
primum Veneris*. The Preparation

he

he gives us is this: Take good *Dantzick* Vitriol, if you cannot get *Hungarian* or *Goslarian*; this mixed with Sal Ammoniac, and sublimed, will give a yellow or reddish Sublimate. In another Place, he says, Take of the best *Hungarian*, or, if you cannot procure that, of *Dantzick*, or any other good venereal Vitriol. Again, we have always preferred such Vitriol as abounds with Copper, before our common *English* Vitriol, which abounds with Iron. The *Caput Mortuum*, he observes, will run *per Deliquium*, into a thick and high-coloured Liquor, very much impregnated with the somewhat opened Body of Copper. The celebrated Author, in his Treatise of the Origin and Production of Volatility, speaking of this Preparation, says thus, In which, that vitriolate Corpuscles of the Colcothar are really elevated, you may easily find by putting a Grain or two of that reddish Substance into a strong Infusion of Galls, which will thereby immediately acquire an inky Colour; Steel, also, will give the Sal Ammoniac a notable Colour, and an ironish Taste. From the above Quotations and Experiments, it plainly appears, that Mr. *Boyle* not only preferred such Vitriols as abounded with Copper, but likewise usually, if not always, prepared it of such as were strictly venereal, and consequently, that the Name was not originally imposed on it by Mistake, but given to it with Propriety, since it really was a Preparation from Copper.

The Committee are pleased to assert, that blue Vitriol does not calcine red; that the Salt also, in its first Sublimation, rises not at all yellow, but of a greenish Blue. I had some Years ago, says our Author, seen this Preparation made, and once made it myself; both the Processes succeeded

in such a Manner, as to occasion the preceding Remark. Since the Publication of the Committee's last Remarks, I carefully repeated the Experiment with common blue Vitriol, which I calcined at two different Times; both the Calces were of a dark red Colour. I then mixed one Part of the calcined Vitriol with two Parts of well dryed Sal Ammoniac, and ground them together in a Brass Mortar with a glass Pestle. When they were well mixed, I sublimed them with a smart Fire, some white Flowers arose at first, as *Boyle* himself has observed, which were soon succeeded with others manifestly yellow, without any Tinge of green or blue. To another Parcel of the Calx, I added two Parts of the Sal Ammoniac without drying it, and set the Mixture to sublime; before the Sublimation was finished, the Glass broke; this Sublimate appeared of a whitish Colour next to the Glass, and of a yellowish on its inner Surface. It was spotted in several Places of a bluish green Colour, which probably arose from some of the Copper liquefied and thrown up, by the aqueous Drops which had fallen from the upper Part of the subliming Glass, and which occasioned its being broke. Upon subliming some more of the Calx with dry'd Sal Ammoniac, a yellowish Sublimate arose, as in the three preceding Processes.

Lixivium Martis.

The Ley of Iron.

Set by the Residue after the Sublimation of the *Flores Martiales*, in a damp Place, that it may liquify by the Air. L.

Lapis Medicamentosus.

The Medicinal Stone.

Take Alum, Litharge, Bole Armenic

nic, or *French* Bole, of each half a Pound; of the Colcothar of green Vitriol, three Ounces; of Vinegar, a Quarter of a Pint; dry the whole Mixture together over a Fire, till it grows hard. *L.*

This is efteem'd a drying and aftrin-

gent Topic, and is recommended for faftening loofe Teeth; preferving the Gums; drying Ulcers, and Eyes abounding with Rheum; and is fometimes diffolv'd in a proper Water, and injected into the Urethra, to check a Running.

CHAP. IV.

PREPARATIONS *of* SULPHUR.

Flores Sulphuris.

Flowers of Sulphur.

LET Sulphur be fublimed in a fit Veffel, and any Part of the the Flowers which may have con-creted, are to be reduced to Pow-der by a wooden Mill, or in a Marble Mortar, with a wooden Peftle. *L.*

The Sulphur, by this Sublimation, is attenuated and purified; in other Refpects it is not changed; but thus it becomes very fit for internal Medicinal Ufe: For when thus divided, it exerts its Virtues to greater Advantage in the Body; and thus, alfo, it proves fit-ter for external Chirurgical Ufes, principally when it comes to be mix-ed with Balfams, Liniments, and Unguents. *Paracelfus* directs thefe Flowers to be fublimed from the red Calx of Vitriol, and recommends them for the Cure of exulcerated Lungs. *Boerhaave* fays, he made the Expe-riment, but without finding that thefe Flowers, which he fo much commends, had greater Virtues than the common Flowers of Brim-ftone.

Flores Sulphuris loti.

Flowers of Sulphur wafhed.

Pour Water on the Flowers, to the Height of three or four Fingers above them, and boil them for a Time; then pour off this Water, and with frefh cold Water, wafh the Remains of this away, then dry the Flowers for Ufe. *L.*

This Lotion is intended to take off a certain rough Acidity from the Flowers, to improve them for In-ternal Ufe, and prevent them from griping.

Spiritus Sulphuris per Campanam.

Spirit of Sulphur by the Bell.

Let Sulphur be fet on fire, under a Glafs Veffel fitted for that Pur-pofe, which is ufually called a Bell, and the acid Spirit will drop from it, which is to be received into a Difh placed underneath. *L.*

Sulphur when lighted, burns only on its Surface, contiguous to the Air; its blue Flame confifts of Fire, or the inflammable oily Part of the Sulphur, agitated by the Fire, and a mineral Acid, which is the other

con-

ent Part of the Sulphur now
l, attenuated, and made cau-
volatile by the Flame. Thus
ctuous combuftible Matter is
ed by the Fire, and the pon-
Acid diffipated, which foon
ondenfes by its own Weight,
t gets clear of the Flame that
it off. And hence this Va-
becomes mortal, becaufe the
ly cauftic Acid, thus ftrongly
d, comes in Contact with the
, which move the Mufcles,
in the Interftices of the carti-
us Rings of the Larynx, Bron-
and Veficulæ of the Lungs,
ntracts them fpafmodically, fo
imulate the Lungs into a pant-
deavour to cough, whilft they
tirely contracted, and not fuf-
to expand by the Weight of
r; altho' the Breaft be dilated
laborious, but fruitlefs En-
ur. The fame Vapour, fhut
th fermentable Liquors, ftops
ntation; and, if ftrongly re-
l, prevents Putrefaction in all
that otherwife eafily putrefy.
this Fume is a proper Prefer-
againft peftilential Poifon, and
ontagion that flies abroad, or
ns fixed in Goods, fo as to in-
hem. And hence we under-
why the Flame of Nitre and
ur together, but principally of
powder, afford a very healthy
in the Height of the Plague;
e explofive acid Vapour of Ni-
d Sulphur corrects the Air;
e fame Vapour, if received in
ll clofe pent up Place, kills In-
This Spirit of Sulphur, cal-
the Name of *Oleum Sulphuris*
mpanam, is no other than the
Vitriol, which was lodged in
riolic Pyrites; and afterwards
with the Oil of Coals, con-
Sulphur. This appears from
ds of Trials; only Oil of Vi-
s fufpected to contain fome
c Impreffion, which is want-

ing in the Spirit of Sulphur. The
great *Homberg* has, with much Labour and Subtlety, computed the
Quantity of this Acid contained in
Sulphur, and found it to be nearly a
tenth Part. This Spirit of Sulphur,
being purified, barely by ftanding,
then mixed with Juleps, gives them
an agreeable Acidity, and renders
them a wholfome Drink in all Inflammations, and hot Difeafes, attended with Thirft and Corruption.
Helmont fays, it is conducive to the
Prolongation of Life. Medicines
acidulated with this Spirit of Sulphur, are of good Effect in *Aphthæ.*

Aqua sulphurata.
Sulphurated Water.

Take of Water, a Quart; of Sulphur, half a Pound. Let fome
Portion of the Sulphur, fet on fire
in an Iron Ladle, be fufpended
over the Water in a clofe Veffel,
and let this be repeated, as often
as the Fumes from the laft Sulphur
fubfide, till the whole is burnt
away. *L.*

This was before called *Gas Sulphuris,* and is only Water impregnated
with the Acid of Sulphur.

Another Method of preparing the Gas Sulphuris.

Moiften fome Woollen Cloths in a
ftrong Solution of fix'd alkaline
Salt; hang thefe over the Fume
of burning Sulphur, till they grow
dry and ftiff: Steep them a-frefh
in the Ley, and repeat the Operation, till the Cloths are loaded
with Salt. On this Salt, placed
in a Retort, pour fome Water acidulated with Oil of Vitriol; diftil in Sand according to Art.

Hepar Sulphuris.
Liver of Sulphur.

Take of the Flowers of Sulphur, four
Ounces; and of Salt of Tartar, an
Ounce

Ounce and a half; grind the Salt, and mix the Flowers well therewith; then melt them together in a little earthen Difh, under a Chimney, continually ftirring the Mafs with a Spatula, till it becomes red, taking due Care to prevent its Firing. *E.*

this Liver of Sulphur is put whilft very hot and dry into a dry Glafs Veffel, and pure Spirit of Wine is poured upon it, fo as to be about five Fingers above it, a fine Gold-colour'd Tincture is immediately form'd, which by fhaking becomes richer; and if this is pour'd off, and more Spirit is added, it will afford more Tincture.

This Tincture of Sulphur affords a wonderful warming Medicine, that cures Eructation, refifts Acids, and cuts Phlegm; a few Drops of it being taken upon an empty Stomach, in Mead, *Spanifh* Wine, or any proper Syrup. But *Boerhaave* fays, that he could never difcover its antihifical Virtue, as a laft Refuge in ulcerated Lungs, tho' he diligently fought for it; notwithftanding the great Doctor *Willis* has wonderfully commended it in this Diftemper.

Lac Sulphuris.

Milk of Sulphur.

Take of the Liver of Sulphur powder'd, a fufficient Quantity; Spring Water, four times as much. Boil for three Hours, adding Water if it fhould be neceffary. Let the Liquor whilft hot be filter'd; and then drop into it a fufficient Quantity of Spirit of Vitriol, till the Effervefcence ceafes. Let the Powder precipitated be wafh'd with Water, and dry'd.

In making the Liver of Sulphur, the Body of the Sulphur is open'd by the fix'd Alcali, and render'd foluble in Water. And being thus precipitated, it fuits the delicate,

better than the crude Sulphur. But I don't know that it is a better Medicine.

Sulphur Præcipitatum.

Precipitated Sulphur.

Boil Flowers of Sulphur, with thrice their Weight of Quick Lime, till the Sulphur is diffolved, and filtre the Solution thro' Paper; then with weak Spirit of Vitriol make a Precipitation, which is to be often wafhed, till it becomes quite infipid. *L.*

This is another Way of preparing the *Lac Sulphuris*; but by no means preferable to the preceding.

Balfamum Sulphuris fimplex.

The fimple Balfam of Sulphur.

Boil Flowers of Sulphur in four times their Weight of Olive Oil, in a Pot lightly covered, till the Oil and Sulphur are joined into the Confiftence of a Balfam.

In the fame Manner is a Balfam of Sulphur alfo prepared with *Barbadoes* Tar. *L.*

This is the famous Balfam of Sulphur of *Helmont*, *Rulandus*, and *Boyle*, who very highly commend it for healing, mollifying, and refolving, when ufed externally; and internally, againft Putrefactions, and Suppurations of the Kidnies and Lungs efpecially, declaring they have thus found a fecret, but fufficient Remedy for Confumptions of the Lungs: But *Boerhaave* thinks, that by its acrimonious, indigeftible, and hot unctuous Part, it offends the weak Lungs, the Stomach and Vifcera of languid Perfons, fpoils the Appetite, increafes Thirft, and parches the Body, already too much dried by the Diftemper. And this, he fays, he fpeaks upon Experience and Confideration; and therefore advifes it to be fparingly and cautioufly tiously used, with a careful Observance of the Effect: Certainly, it is not without a burning Rancidness. It has been found, when externally used, successful in curing pale, cold, watery, mucous, sanious, running Ulcers: Perhaps, it was hence somewhat too hastily concluded to have the same Effects when used internally; for thus it raises and continues a Fever.

Balsamum Sulphuris Terebinthinatum.

Balsam of Sulphur, with Oil of Turpentine.

Take of the Flowers of Sulphur, two Ounces; of Oil of Turpentine, ten Ounces; and digest them together for some Hours in a circulating Vessel, placed in a Sand Heat, till the Oil appears of a red Colour, then suffering the Vessel to cool, separate the Balsam from the Sulphur that remains undissolved. *E.*

This Balsam is an extemporaneous anodyne Remedy in Pains of the Nerves, and an excellent Medicine in sanious, sinuous, weeping, watery, and fistulous Ulcers. Internally taken, it is heating, diuretic, and sudorific. It is recommended for cleansing and healing internal Ulcers; it is hence too highly commended for the Phthisic, Ulcers of the Kidnies, and for expelling and dissolving of the Stone: But the cautious Physician will recommend only the gentle Medicines, and be afraid of those that operate violently. It is certain, that the Urine is soon impregnated with a Violet Smell, upon taking a little of this Balsam. This is called the terebinthinated Balsam of Sulphur; and, as other distilled Oils may be thus mixed with Sulphur, the Balsams, so prepared, receive their Names from the distilled Oil employed, that gives them their prevailing Odour. Hence the *Balsa-*

mum Sulphuris Anisatum, Succinatum, Juniperinum, &c.

Sal volatile, Spiritus, & Oleum Succini.

Volatile Salt, Spirit, and Oil of Amber.

Take of bruised white Amber, one Part; of clean Sand, three Parts; mix and put them into a coated Glass Retort, whereof they may possess one half; then having fitted it with a large Receiver, distil in a Sand Heat by Degrees of Fire, with the first of which will come over a Spirit, and a little yellow Oil; with the second a yellow Oil and a little Salt, and with the third more Salt and a reddish Oil. Pour the Liquor out of the Receiver, and gather the Salt from the Sides of the Vessel; then press it between the Folds of Cap Paper, let it dry; afterwards by the Filtre separate the Oil from the filtrated Spirit, and rectify it by distilling it with muriatic Sea Salt. *E.*

Sal Succini rectificatum.

Rectify'd Salt of Amber.

Take any Quantity of the former distilled Salt of Amber, with twice its own Weight of decrepitated Sea Salt; powder and put them into a high large Glass Cucurbit, then having fitted it with a blind Head, sublime in *Balneo Arenæ*, but take Care the Oil does not ascend. When the Vessel grows cold, brush off the Salt with a Feather. *E.*

In the *London* Dispensatory we are directed to distil the Oil again, which will then part with a thinner Oil that will ascend, and a thicker Part will remain, called the Balsam of Amber, and we are told, that

The Salt is to be boiled either in the Spirit or Water, and set by to oot ; thus it will be freed from s Oil, and the oftener this Pro-ßs is repeated, the purer will ie Salt be. *L.*

ie Oils being purified by a re-ed Diftillation, have a fharp, amic, exciting, diaphoretic, diu-:, emmenagogic, and hyfteric rue ; and, when externally ufed, he Way of Liniment, are very

ferviceable in reftoring contracted, weak, paralytic, torpid Limbs : The volatile Salt is gratefully acid, bal-famic, unctuous, penetrating, pre-fervative, and ftimulating to the Nerves and Spirits, being a true vo-latile, acid, oily Salt ; and therefore a capital Antihyfteric and Diuretic, efpecially if purified by a fecond Diftillation.

CHAP. V.

PREPARATION *of* METALS.

Caufticum Lunare.
The Lunar Cauftic.

Iffolve pure Silver by a Sand Heat, in about twice its Weight of *Aqua fortis* ; then dry way the Humidity with a gentle Fire, afterwards melt it in a Cru-ible, that it may be poured into proper Moulds, carefully avoid-ing over much Heat, left the Mat-ter fhould grow too thick. *L.*

his is a moft powerful Caute-, and by a bare Touch inftant-burns the Parts of a live Body an Efchar, under which Na-e raifes an Inflammation that fe-rates the crude Efchar, and leaves Part pure ; fo that by repeated ouches with this Matter, all fuper-ial, foul, fungous Ulcers and Can-rs are excellently cured. Hence lful Surgeons highly extol the irtue of this Stone ; and Phyficians o learn the wonderful Power of an cid; when collected and fixed. If ven internally in this Form, it is immediate corrofive Poifon, and erefore is never to be ufed in this anner.

Calx Jovis.
Calx of Tin.

Take any Quantity of Tin, melt it in an unglazed earthen Veffel, and keep it continually ftirring with an Iron Spatula, till it turns to a Calx. *E.*

Stannum Pulveratum.
Powder'd Tin.

Let melted Tin be poured into a wooden Box chalked within, and while the Tin grows cold, let the Box be brifkly fhaken, and Part of the Tin will be reduced to Powder. The Remainder, by being treated in the fame Manner, may alfo be reduced to Powder. *L.*

Thefe Preparations of Tin are ef-teemed excellent for Worms and Acidities in the Inteftines, and Epi-lepfies, and Convulfions thence ari-fing.

Sal Jovis.
Salt of Tin.

Take any Quantity of the Calx of

of Tin, and as much *Aqua Regia* diluted with eight times its own Weight of Spring Water as will float some Inches above it; then make a slow Solution in a Sand-Heat; filtre the Liquor, and evaporate it to a Pellicle; then set it in a cold Place for three or four Days, till it shoots into Crystals, which are to be dried when the Liquor is poured away from them.

Separate the Calx remaining after the Solution; and by mixing it with the Liquor poured off from the Crystals, new Crystals will be thereby obtained. *E.*

This is esteemed an excellent Medicine against Epilepsies and Convulsions; and is very effectual in Case of Worms.

Amalgama Jovis.
Amalgama of Tin.

Take any Quantity of Tin, and melt it in a Crucible; and into another Crucible put an equal Weight of Quickfilver, and permit it to remain in the Fire till the Quickfilver begins to fume; then immediately pour it upon the melted Tin, and stir the Mass with an Iron Spatula till it grows cold. *E.*

Aurum Mosaicum.

Take of the Amalgama of Tin six Ounces, of Sal Ammoniac, and Flowers of Sulphur, each three Ounces; grind and mix them well together in a Marble Mortar, then put them into a Cucurbit, and leisurely raise your Fire thro' all the Degrees; at length breaking the Vessel, at the Bottom thereof you will find the *Aurum Mosaicum* free from the Scoria, which is sublimed. *E.*

In the *London* Dispensatory, the Proportion of the Ingredients is different. The Directions for making it stand thus under the Title of,

Aurum Musivum.
Mosaic Gold.

Take of Tin one Pound, of Flowers of Sulphur seven Ounces, Sal Ammoniac, purified Quickfilver, of each half a Pound. Add the Quickfilver to the Tin melted; when the Mixture is cold, reduce it to Powder; mix well with it the Sulphur and Sal Ammoniac, and sublime the Compound in a Mattras. The Mosaic Gold will be found under the Part sublimed, with a small Quantity of Foulness at the Bottom. *L.*

Its Operation is sudorific: It is said to be good in all chronical and nervous Cases, and particularly in Convulsions of young Children. And indeed it seems to be a very good Medicine, if duly prepared and exhibited.

Cerussa.
White Lead.

Take any Quantity of very thin Plates of Lead, and suspend them in an earthen Vessel, at the Bottom whereof is lodged a sufficient Quantity of Vinegar, so as the Fumes arising from the Liquor may surround the Plates; then digest in Horse-dung for three Weeks; during which, if the Plates be not entirely calcined, scrape off the white Powder, and again expose them to the Fumes of Vinegar, till they wholly turn into Powder. *E.*

The Ceruse, thus prepared, is compounded of the Acid of Vinegar, and the dissolved Body of the Lead. This Ceruse is of Use in watery, ulcerous, running Sores, or Diseases of the Skin, being sprinkled thereon. If this fine Powder be drawn along with

h the Breath into the Lungs, it
ıſes a violent, and almoſt incurable
mortal Aſthma. If received into
: Mouth, and ſwallowed along
h the Spittle, it occaſions invete-
e Diſtempers in the *Viſcera*, in-
erable Faintings, Weakneſſes,
ıns, Obſtructions, and, at laſt,
ath itſelf. Theſe terrible Effects
: daily ſeen among thoſe who do
ɣ Work in Lead, but principally
ıong the Makers of white Lead.
t all, therefore, beware of this Poi-
ı, which being both without Smell
d Taſte, proves the more pernici-
s, as it is the leſs diſcovered, and
es not ſhew itſelf till it has deſtroy-
the Body.

Minium.

Red Led.

ake any Quantity of Lead ; melt it
in an unglazed earthen Veſſel, and
keep it ſtirring with an Iron Spatula till it changes, firſt into a
blackiſh Powder, then into a yellow, and laſtly into an exceeding
red one, which is called *Red Lead* ;
but if it be urged with a ſtill
ſtronger Fire, it will vitrify. *E.*

The Medicinal Virtues of this are
ɔt different from thoſe of *Ceruſs.*

Saccharum Saturni.

Sugar of Lead.

'ake any Quantity, either of white
Lead, red Lead, or Litharge reduced to Powder ; put it into a Cucurbit, and pour thereon as much
diſtill'd Vinegar as will float four
Inches above it ; digeſt for ſome
Days in a Sand Heat, till the Vinegar becomes ſweet, which is then
to be ſeparated, or poured off clear,
after it is ſubſided, and new is to be
put on, till it ſhall be found to
have no Sweetneſs at all ; then let
all the Liquors firſt clarified by
Standing be evaporated in a glaſs

Veſſel to the Conſiſtence of Honey, ſo as that in a cold Place
they may ſhoot into Cryſtals,
which are to be dried in the
Shade. Exhale away the Remainder alſo to a Pellicle, and ſet
it in a cold Place that it may
ſhoot ; and repeat the Evaporation
· till no more Cryſtals appear. *E.*

It is aſtringent, ſtyptic, and preſently coagulates the Blood : Being
diſſolved in Water, it affords the
Vinegar of Litharge, good againſt
Inflammations, when externally uſed.
Internally, it is recommended for a
ſafe Remedy againſt Spitting of
Blood, Bleeding at the Noſe, making bloody Urine, the *Gonorrhæa,*
the *Fluor Albus,* and the like ; as
alſo for a mollifying Remedy againſt
the Acrimony of the Blood. *Boer-*
haave ſays, he never durſt make
Trial of it, becauſe he never ſaw it
ſucceſsfully uſed by others ; and becauſe there is ſcarce a more deceitful
and deſtructive Poiſon than this Lead,
which preſently returns to Ceruſs, as
ſoon as tne Acid is abſorbed from it,
by any thing it may meet with ;
whence it afterwards proves an exceeding dangerous, and almoſt incurable Poiſon to the Body.

Mars ſolubilis, ſeu Chalybs Tartariſatus.

Soluble Iron, or Tartarized Steel.

Take of the crude Filings of Iron,
and of the Cryſtals of Tartar, each
a like Quantity, and with a ſufficient Proportion of Rain-Water,
to bring them into a Maſs; make it
into Balls to be baked in an Oven ;
grind theſe Balls to Powder, and
again with a requiſite Quantity of
Water form it into Balls, and bake
them in an Oven as, before, and
repeat the Operation till the Powder become impalpable. *E.*

Mars

Mars Sulphuratus.

Iron prepared with Sulphur.

Take any Quantity of crude Filings of Steel, and twice their Weight of Sulphur reduced to Powder, and with a sufficient Quantity of Spring-Water make them into a Paste, and suffer it to ferment for six Hours; then put it into a Crucible, and deflagrate it, keeping it continually stirring with an Iron Spatula, that it may become a very black Powder; if farther urged with the Fire, it grows red, and is then called

Crocus Martis aperiens.

Opening Saffron of Iron;

Which does not at all differ from *Chalybs præparatus,* gently calcined in a Crucible till it appears of a red Colour. *E.*

Crocus Martis astringens.

Astringent Saffron of Iron.

This is made of *Crocus Martis aperiens,* reverberated a long time in a very vehement Fire. *E.*

Chalybs cum Sulphure præparatus.

Steel prepared with Sulphur.

Touch the Steel heated to a white Heat with a Roll of Brimstone, that the Steel may melt, and drop into Water placed under it; then let it be separated from the Sulphur, which has dropt along with it into the Water, and be reduced into the finest Powder. *L.*

The Virtues of these Preparations may be learn'd from those of the Filings of Iron, from which they differ but very little. The Filings, however, are as good.

Sal Martis.

Salt of Iron.

Take of the strong Spirit or Oil of Vitriol, the Weight of eight Ounces, of Filings of Iron four Ounces, of Water a Quart; mix them, and when the Ebullition has ceased, set the Mixture some time upon a Sand-Heat; then filtre the Liquor thro' Paper, and evaporate it, that the Salt may crystallize. *L.*

If the Salt of Iron be diluted with a hundred times its Quantity of Water, and drank in the Dose of twelve Ounces, upon an empty Stomach, walking gently after it, it opens and relaxes the Body, purges, proves diuretic, kills and expels Worms, tinges the Excrements black, or forms them to a Matter like Clay, strengthens the Fibres, and thus cures many different Distempers. The like Taste, Odour and Colour, and the like Blackness of the Excrements, have occasioned many to imagine, that the Chalybeate Waters were thus produced by Nature; especially, because these Liquors, when exposed to the Air, deposite a copious yellow Sediment or Oaker: But Dr. *Hoffman* has prudently corrected this Error, by Means of Experiments, in his noble Work of Mineral Water. However we must observe, that this Salt of Iron, meeting with alkalescent and putrid Matters, and thus having its acid Solvent drank up thereby, is turned into an astringent, ponderous, sluggish, metallic Calx, that occasions inveterate Obstructions, and therefore proves hurtful in putrid Fevers. And we know, that when Iron Filings are taken in Female Disorders, where the Body is weak, languid, and abounds with Acidity, the Metal thus produces Eructations, as of Garlick and putrid Eggs, on Account of the Acid it meets with; and hence the Hez, before wanting in the Body, is excited, and the Excrements generally turn black; and in this Case, the Powder of Iron-filings proves much

more

re serviceable, than when ever so
riously prepared by Chemistry.
ence Iron is known to prove use-
if Acids abound in the Body,
hurtful where the Body is bili-
, or hot.

Flores Martis.

Flowers of Iron.

te of the crude Filings of Iron,
f Sal Ammoniac reduced to Power, each a like Quantity; grind
nd mix them well together for
ome Time; set them in a moist
Place, and afterwards sublime them
n an earthen Cucurbit, with a glass
Head; the Spirit of the Sal Ammoniac will rise first, and is to be
aught in a Receiver; then white
Flowers will ascend, which are
o be thrown away as useless; and
t length the red Flowers inclining
o Yellow, which are to be swept
vith a Feather out of the Head.

e *Tinctura Martis*, or Tincture
f Iron, may be prepared from the
Caput Mortuum, as also from the
Flowers. *E.*

e the Remarks on the *Ens Vene-*
or *Flores Martiales* above.

hese Flowers have the same Virtues as Mr. *Boyle* commnds in the
Ens Veneris; for they are wonderfully restorative, warming, and
opening, containing the open Body of the metallic Sulphur. They
have, also, an Anodyne Virtue, and
are often somewhat soporiferous. The
dry Flowers, being digested with *Alcohol*, afford a copious golden Tincture, both metallic and sulphureous;
and the remaining *Caput Mortuum*,
after the Sublimation, affords the
same with Alcohol.

Chalybis Rubigo præparata.

The Rust of Steel prepared.

Expose Filings of Steel to the Air,
and moisten them sometimes with
Water or Vinegar, till they are
turned into Rust; then rub them
in a Mortar; and by pouring on
Water, wash off the finest Powder; the Residue, which by moderate Rubbing was not brought
to a Powder fine enough to be
washed off, is again to be exposed
moist to the Air; and, when farther rusted, is to be treated as before. The Powder thus washed
off, is to be dried and kept for
Use. *L.*

CHAP. VI.

PREPARATIONS of METALLINE MINERALS.

Argenti Vivi Purificatio.

The Purification of Quicksilver.

Istil the Quicksilver in a Retort, and then wash it well
with Water and Salt, or Vinegar.
L.

Mercurii Solutio.

Solution of Quicksilver.

ke of clean Quicksilver, and double *Aqua Fortis*, each a like Quantity, and digest them in a Phial
placed in a Sand-Heat, so that
there may be made a limpid Solution of the Quicksilver. *E.*

This Solution is violently caustic, so
that it can scarce be touched, as burning all Parts of the Body with violent
Pain and Heat: Whence it becomes
effectual in extirpating Warts. If a
small

small Part of a Drop touches the Skin, it presently turns it purple.

Mercurii Calx.

Calx of Quickfilver.

Take any Quantity of the Solution of Quickfilver, and with a gentle Fire evaporate it to a white and dry Mass. *E.*

Mercurius calcinatus.

Calcined Quickfilver.

Set Quickfilver purified, in a Sand Heat, for several Months in a Glass Vessel with a broad Bottom, and opening to the Air by a small Hole, till it is reduced to a red Powder. *L.*

Thus a red Powder is made, commonly called *Mercurius Praecipitatus per se.* It is much recommended in Venereal Disorders; cutaneous Eruptions of the chronical Kind; Rheumatisms, and many chronical Distempers. The Dose is one or two Grains. But a double Dose of this, with a double Dose of Opium, is said to be the celebrated Pill of *Mifaubin.* But I have Reason to think the following Preparation of much greater Effect.

Mercurius animatus solaris.

Animated Solar Mercury.

Take of the genuine Martial Regulus of Antimony, one Part; of pure Silver, two Parts; melt them together, and with a sufficient Quantity of Quickfilver, make an Amalgama, adding a sufficient Quantity of Salt of Tartar and Sal Ammoniac; triturate this Amalgama strongly in a Glass Mortar; pouring upon it, at due Intervals, a sufficient Quantity of Rain Water, which by this means becomes black; continue the Trituration, with frequent Affusions of Rain Water, till all is so effectually washed off, that nothing but the pure Amalgama is left. After this, the Amalgama is to be put into a Glass Retort, and the Mercury abstracted by a Sand Heat. By this means the pure Silver is left in the Bottom of the Retort; and this Silver, when again mixed with the Regulus of Antimony, is again to be amalgamated by the Addition of the Salts, afterwards depurated by the like Trituration, and last of all distilled. When these Measures are repeated for at least seven or nine times, a much more pure and subtle Mercury is afforded, which not only acts more powerfully upon other Metals, but, also, produces more conspicuous and salutary Effects on the human Body. The Mercury must be exalted in this Manner, in order to render it fit for the Preparation of this celebrated and efficacious Medicine. The Mercury produced by this laborious Preparation is to be afterwards added to pure Gold; to one Part of which, three or four, or, according to others, only two Parts of Mercury, are to be united and joined by the common Method of Amalgamation. After this, the Amalgama is to be put into a Glass Phial, with a flat Bottom, that the Heat may act on a larger Surface. Then the Phial, when the grosser Air is exhausted, left being expanded by the Heat, it should burst the Vessel, is to be hermetically sealed; and in that Species of Furnace called an *Athanor,* exposed to a proper Digestion, for seven, or even nine solar Months successively, gradually proceeding from a fainter to a stronger Degree of Fire. As in this Digestion the whole of the Affair consists, so if it is duly made, the Amalgama will be gradually converted into a reddish Powder; which, during the first Months of the Digestion, is not so corrected, but that it will excite Fluxes or Salivations, especially in tender Constitutions. But by a protracted Digestion it is so perfected,

fected

ed, and divefted of all its draftic
lities, that the fixed Powder pro-
ed by it, may be fafely exhibited
the Quantity of two, three, or
r Grains for a Dofe, and thus
fifted in for fome Days ; fo that
fe of the moft delicate Conftitu-
s have no Reafon to be afraid of
ing a Salivation, or any Commo-
s produced by the other Prepa-
ions of crude Mercury, excited
it.

The Character which *Frederic*
ffman gives of this Medicine is,
t it has, with uncommon Succefs,
n prefcribed for various obftinate
feafes, which would not yield to
Efficacy of other Medicines. It
s frequently ufed by *Crelles*, an
inent and fuccefsful Practitioner.
e Efficacy, alfo, of this folar ani-
ted Mercury was at *Hall* often
ppily experienc'd by the celebrated
ymift *Hochgraff*; efpecially in fub-
ing thofe Reproaches of Medicine,
artan Fevers, and the Gout : So
t fome who laboured long under
e former, and one afflicted with it
r four Years fucceffively, were, by
few Dofes of this Medicine, re-
red to perfect Health and Eafe.
t among the gouty Patients, who
re by this Medicine quickly cured,
e may juftly reckon a certain Man,
ho, being miferably racked with
ed arthritic Pains, and Contrac-
ns of his Limbs, was perfectly re-
red to his former Health, with-
t ever having had a Relapfe. The
uccefs of *Cnoeffelius*, in curing the
out with Mercury thus fixed, may
e feen in *Append. ad Mifcel. Nat.*
riof. and confirmed by unexcep-
onable Witneffes, that is, the Per-
ns cured. Thefe Inftances fuffici-
tly prove, that the Encomiums
eftowed on this Medicine are not
roundlefs and overdone, but fup-
rted by Experience : So that there
no manner of Doubt, but that,
ithout any Dread of Danger, this

Medicine is capable of producing
fuch falutary Effects in obftinate Diforders, if really curable, as can neither be obtained by any other Remedies of the Animal or Vegetable
Kingdom hitherto known, nor by a
mercurial Salivation, which is not only
harfh, and attended with violent and
often dangerous Commotions, but is
alfo frequently highly tedious The
Ufe of the folar animated Mercury
is preferable to a Salivation, becaufe
it may be gratefully exhibited to the
moft delicate Conftitutions in a due
Manner; and fmall Dofes, provided
it is once or twice a Day taken, and
its Ufe perfifted in, according to the
Circumftances of the Patient ; which
may be done in a fufficiently grateful Manner; if the Dofe is mixed
with Conferve of Rofes, or any o-
ther agreeable Conferve, without the
Ufe of any other Medicines. But,
before the Exhibition of this Preparation, the *Primæ Viæ* muft be freed
from thofe *Sordes*, which might prevent the Efficacy of the Medicine,
by Abftergents, whofe Efficacy is
heightened by a gently ftimulating
refinous Purgative ; fince draftic Purgatives, as they are rarely proper,
fo they are always prejudicial in the
Beginning of a Cure. The *Primæ*
Viæ may alfo, according to the Situation of the Patient, be freed from
the Sordes contained in them, by a
Vomit ; which, however, is not to
be exhibited without the previous
Ufe of faline and inciding Medicines.
When this Medicine is taken, after
fuch a previous Preparation of the
Body, it is proper to drink after it
fome warm aqueous Liquor ; fuch
as Tea, Coffee, an Infufion of *Paul*'s
Betony, or a Decoction of Sarfaparilla and China, heightened by Saffafras Bark. Thefe diluting Liquors
make the Medicine exert its proper
Efficacy, render the Body perfpirable, and receive the faline Sordes,
difengaged by the Force and Energy

H h h   of

of the Medicine, and which, being dispersed in them, may be without any Violence afterwards eliminated from the Body thro' proper Emunctories, especially thro' the Pores of the Skin, provided they are kept sufficiently open by a due Regimen, in which, by proper Cloths, the external Cold is excluded, without inducing an intolerable and troublesome Heat, and the whole Body is preserved in a gentle and moist Warmth ; for profuse Sweats are so far from being necessary, or productive of happy Effects, in the Cure of almost all chronical Diseases, that they rather exhaust the Strength, already too much impaired in the Course of a slow Disorder. But if such Sweats are forced, and as it were extorted, as they often are, the greatest Misfortunes, easily productive of Infarctions of the Viscera, are to be dreaded. Let all violent and sudden Commotions, therefore, be avoided, as much as possible ; and, as this Medicine is not productive of such Effects, the viscid and peccant Matter will not, by one or two Doses of it, which Quacks affirm of their Medicines, be subdued and eliminated, but must be conquered by the continual and un-interrupted, tho' mild and gentle Action of it. Thus, tho' *Lucas Torzi*, Physician to Pope *Innocent* XII, in his *Praxis Medica*, asserts, that by Mercury thus fixed, exhibited only seven times, he totally removed a *Lues Venerea*, and a Quartan Fever, without being so arrogant as to call his Veracity into Question, I must only say, that I can hardly believe, that in cold Climates, such as are more Northerly, and where, in chronical Disorders, there is such a Viscidity and Redundance of the peccant Humours, the like Effects can be so speedily, and in so few Days produced by this Medicine. Such an happy and salutary Effect will, how-

ever, without any Violence to the Patient, be much accelerated, if, after the repeated Use of the Medicine for some Days, we interpose balsamic and saline sulphureous Medicines, the most considerable and efficacious of which are the *Elixir Balsamicum*, or the *Spiritus volatilis Oleosus*, and accommodated to the Situation of the Patients : And certainly a moderate Dose of these, daily taken between Meals, and duly persisted in, calmly accelerates the Cure of chronical Disorders; an Effect not to be produced by more violent Means : For, as the languid Digestion is by this means excited, the Chyle, before not sufficiently subdued, and by its Viscidity contaminating the Humours, is corrected, and, as it were, sheathed up in these balsamic Substances. The vital Energy and Turgescence of the Humours before suppressed, and, as it were, suffocated, by their preternatural Lentor, is so animated with fresh Vigour, that the Fumes of the obstinate Disorder are thereby seasonably destroyed, especially if the Efficacy of the Medicine is promoted by a proper Regimen.

Mercurius Præcipitatus albus.

White Precipitate of Mercury.

Take any Quantity of the Solution of Quicksilver, and gradually pour upon it exceeding strong Brine, till all the Quicksilver be precipitated into a very white Powder, which is to be washed with hot Water in the Filtre, till it communicates no more Sharpness thereto ; afterwards the Powder is to be dried between folded Paper with a very gentle Heat. £.

Boerhaave says, that the Powder thus prepared, is perhaps the best Remedy hitherto afforded by Mercury, for internal Use. It operates effectually, and with considerable

Safe

Safety. If ground with thrice its Weight of Loaf Sugar, it makes, what may more properly be called a mercurial *Panacea*; than perhaps other laborious Preparations of Mercury; for however Mercury may be treated, its medicinal Virtue principally depends upon a certain Quantity of Acid adhering to its metallic Part. This acid Virtue, if it abound and appear externally in the Mercury, acts with more Violence, but with less Safety : If sparingly added, and more united to the Mercury, it acts more slowly, more mildly, and safely ; and this is the Case with our present Precipitate. If the Saccharine Powder above mentioned, be given in the Quantity of nine Grains to a Person fasting, it purges, vomits, gently kills Worms, opens, and cleanses the Vessels concerned in preparing the Chyle, resolves Phlegm, and thus cures many Distempers such as the Gonorrhœa, Itch, Venereal Ulcers, &c. If this Dose be several times repeated daily, it raises a kind of Salivation. If a Dram of this white Precipitate be well mixed with an Ounce of Pomatum, or the Ointment of Roses, it makes an excellent and safe Unguent in cutaneous Disorders, and proper for curing the Itch, Breakings out in the Face, and inveterate Ulcers. If this Powder be put into a Glass, set over the Fire, and kept constantly stirring with a Glass Rod, and thus be long and gently calcined; it becomes so mild, as scarce to purge, vomit, or salivate, and therefore acts very gently when taken internally ; and in this Form the Chymists commend it as a Diaphoretic, and Corrective : But thus treated, it is so mild, as to have little curative Virtue.

In the *London* Dispensatory, another Method of making the *Præcipitatus albus* is directed thus:

Take of Sal Ammoniac, and of corrosive Sublimate, equal Weights ; dissolve them together in Water, filtre the Solution thro' Paper, and with a Solution of some alcaline fixt Salt, make a Precipitation, then wash off all Acrimony from the precipitated Powder. **L.**

Mercurius Præcipitatus dulcis.

Dulcify'd Precipitate of Mercury.

Take of corrosive Mercury sublimate, any Quantity ; dissolve it in a sufficient Quantity of Spring Water, and drop into the Solution Spirit of Sal Ammoniac so long as any white Powder will precipitate ; then wash the Powder in a Filtre, with repeated Affusions of warm Water. **E.**

Mercurius Præcipitatus fuscus, vulgo Wurtzii.

Brown Precipitate of Mercury.

Take any Quantity of the Solution of Quicksilver, and gradually drop into it a due Proportion of Oil of Tartar *per Deliquium* ; that is, so much as will put a Stop to the Effervescence, and cause the Powder to fall to the Bottom, and this is also to be edulcorated with Water, like the white Precipitate. **E.**

Mercurius calcinatus, vulgo Præcipitatus ruber.

Red Precipitate of Mercury.

Take any Quantity of the Calx of Quicksilver, gradually reverberate it in a Crucible, and it will first change from white to brown, then to a yellow, and at length upon increasing the Fire become an exceeding red Powder. **E.**

This Precipitate, which goes by the Name of *Vigo*'s Precipitate, is sharp and corrosive, occasioning Pain, and producing an Eschar, when externally

nally applied; and hence afterwards it always occafions a thick, white Pus; and thus cleanfes the Lips and Bottoms of putrid Ulcers, and difpofes them to heal. It is dangerous to give internally, as inflaming the Vifcera by its cauftic Virtue, and occafioning Anxiety, Pain, Vomiting, Purging, Griping, and operating alfo by Urine and Sweat. If given in too large a Dofe, which fhould never exceed three Grains, or if too often repeated, it occafions a Salivation, with all its Symptoms; and thus cures many Diftempers, that are not eafily curable any other Way. It is more violent and dangerous than the white Precipitate. *Paracelfus* and *Helmont* fhew how to mitigate it, by feveral times diftilling *Alcohol* from it; and thus indeed it becomes milder, by lofing much of its Acid: But, at the fame Time, it requires to be given in a larger Dofe. They alfo correfted it with the fame Succefs, by diftilling from it the Water of the Whites of Eggs. Others diffolve it in ftrong diftilled Vinegar by boiling, then ftrain and purify; and, by feveral times diftilling the Vinegar off, render the Powder more mild: But there feems to be little gained by all this; white Precipitate being already the Thing here required. In fhort, the acrimonious Acid adhering to the Mercury, caufes it to operate in a very fmall Dofe; and the more this Acid is in it, and the more external to the Mercury, the more violently it afts, and *vice verfa*. If this Precipitate be put into a thin hollow Glafs Difh, fet over the Fire, and continually ftirred with a Tobacco Pipe, it will change of a deeper Colour; and if long continued thus, it becomes fo much the milder, fo as at length fcarce to aft at all. The Chymifts frequently mix red Lead with this Precipitate, in order to increafe their Profit.

In the *London* Difpenfatory this Precipitate is fomewhat differently directed, under the Title of

Mercurius corrofivus ruber.

The Mercurial red Corrofive.

Take of Quickfilver purified, and of the Compound *Aqua fortis,* equal Weights; fet them together in a Glafs with a flat Bottom, upon a Sand Heat, till a Humidity is exhaled, and the dry Mafs has acquired a red Colour. *L.*

Mercurius Corallinus.

Coralline Mercury.

Pour upon the mercurial red Corrofive, thrice its Weight of rectify'd Spirit of Wine, and digeft them together two or three Days in a gentle Heat, often fhaking the Veffel; then fet fire to the Spirit, ftirring the Powder continually, till the Spirit is quite burnt away. *L.*

See the Remarks on the *Mercurius Calcinatus.* This is generally known by the Name of *Arcanum Corallinum.*

Mercurius Præcipitatus viridis.

Green Precipitate of Mercury.

Take of corrofive Mercury fublimate powder'd, four Ounces; hot Spring Water, a Quart; in which diffolve the Sublimate. Take alfo, of Filings of Copper, an Ounce and half; of Spirit of Sal Ammoniac, eight Ounces; digeft in a Mattras, till a high green Tincture is extracted, which, when filter'd, gradually drop into the mercurial Solution; when the Precipitation is finifh'd, evaporate in a Sand Heat to Drynefs.

Some efteem this much in the Cure of a *Gonorrhæa,* but I dont know that it excels the other Precipitates.

Mer-

Mercurius Emeticus flavus, vel *Turpethum Minerale*.

The yellow Mercurial Emetic, or Turpeth Mineral.

ur upon purify'd Quicksilver in a Glafs Veffel, double its Weight of the ftrong Spirit of Vitriol. Let the Liquor heat gradually, and then boil, till in the Bottom of the Glafs there remains a white Mafs, whioh is to be perfectly dried with a ftrong Heat; this upon the Affufion of warm Water will turn yellow, and fall into Powder. Rub this Powder and warm Water diligently together in a glafs Mortar; when the Powder is fubfided, pour off this Water, and wafh the Powder often with frefh Water, till it becomes perfectiy free of all Acrimony. *L*.

his Medicine is generally known the Name of Turpeth Mineral, the yellow Precipitate of Mercu-
It is certainly a Medicine of y great Confequence in Practice; which Reafon I fhall give Remarks of *Boerhaave* thereon. his feems, fays he, to be the Pow-, with which, when rightly pre-ed, *Paracelfus* performed Won-s; as appears from his little Hofl Surgeon : And this is fufficient-ttefted by *Operinus*, who declares has frequently been employed in king it. It may be rendered mild-y burning Spirit of Wine upon after the Manner of the ancient ymifts, who by this Means took y from their metalline Calces Salts, that externally adhering eto, render'd them too fharp, fo only the Salts intimatefy united, ht remain behind. The prudent *nham*, who is a cautious and ing Commender of the Chymifts, efully acknowledges, that by ns of this Medicine, Difeafes, rwife incurable, might be cured.
Boyle relates, that by a fmall e hereof, ufed as a Sternutatory,

the whole Body has been changed, and even Cataracts cured. A Woman at *Paris* is alfo faid to have herewith cured Perfons given over. Hence it feems an extraordinary Medicine in ftubborn and obftinate Cafes; but it requires a fkilful Phyfician, and fhould not be ufed when milder Remedies may fuffice. It is ferviceable in the Dropfy, as well as in the venereal Difeafe; and alfo in the moft obftinate Difeafes of the Glands. *Helmont* fays, that Oil of Vitriol is here converted into Alum, barely by the Contact of Mercury; but this is either fpeaking improperly, or not juftly : But when that excellent Author directs the *Fire of the Vitriol of Copper* to be poured upon *Vigo*'s Powder, and thence diftilled, for preparing the fecret Cathartic of *Paracelfus*, if I underftand him right, fays *Boerhaave*, it makes this Medicine. For if the *Fire of the Vitriol of Copper* be the ftrongeft Oil of Vitriol, as foon as this is poured upon red Precipitate, it immediately renders the Spirit of Nitre volatile, caufes it to fly off from the fixed Mercury, and foon after, fupplying its Place, produces the Calx of Mercury as above. If the Water of White of Eggs be feveral times diftilled from it, this takes away the Acid externally adhering thereto, and renders the Powder milder; tho' it will ftill operate fufficiently. Metals alone have little Effect upon the Body, except by their Bulk, Figure, and Weight; but by the Addition of Salts, efpecially the acid Kind, they acquire new Properties, often ftrange ones, and very different, according as the Acids are more fixed therein, or adhere more externally. In the Form of Vitriol they act very violently; but if calcined in this Form, the Calx grows gradually milder, and by a long continued ftrong Calcination, which drives out the Acids, they become mild, tho' before ex-

ceeding'r

ceedingly fharp, as we fee happens in Turbith: And thus their Operation becomes milder, and, at the fame Time, proportionably lefs effectual. Thofe Chymifts and Phyficians therefore are miftaken, who, having found that this Turbith performed extraordinary Things, but operated violently, endeavoured to mitigate its Virulence; which indeed, may be eafily done, but not fo as to have the fame Effects when mitigated, as before. The Ways of mitigating the Acrimony, are by taking away the Acid by wafhing the Preparation with Water; by frequently diftilling pure Water upon it to Drynefs; by pouring Alcohol upon it; by diftilling feveral Parcels of *Alcohol* upon it to Drynefs; by grinding it along with more metallic Matter; by the Addition of alcaline Salts, which abforb the Acid; by grinding the Matter with Chalk, Crabs-eyes, teftaceous Powders, or the like Abforbers of Acids; by a long continued Calcination; and, laftly, by Fixation with a Fire gradually increafed, from a moderate Heat, to the higheft the Glafs will bear.

Mercurius Sublimatus corrofivus.

Corrofive Mercury Sublimate.

Take of the Calx of Quickfilver, and of decrepitated Sea Salt, each a like Quantity; reduce them to Powder, mix them, and put them into a Phial, whereof they may poffefs near a Half; and in a Sand Furnace, firft with a gentle Fire, then gradually increafing it, a white cryftalline Mafs will fublime to the Top Part of the Glaf, and every where adhere thereto, which is afterwards to be feparated from the red *Scoriæ*, and to be purified, if there be Occafion, by repeated Sublimation. *E.*

There are many other Methods of making this Preparation. In the *London* Difpenfatory it is thus directed, under the Title of

Mercurius corrofivus Sublimatus vel Albus.

Corrofive Mercury Sublimate, or white corrofive Mercury.

Take of purified Quickfilver forty Ounces; of Sea Salt, thirty-three Ounces; of Nitre, twenty-eight Ounces; of calcined green Vitriol forty fix Ounces: Rub the Quickfilver firft with about an Ounce or more of corrofive Sublimate in a wooden or ftone Veffel, till it breaks into fmall Grains; then mix it with the Nitre, afterwards with the Sea Salt, till the Quickfilver quite difappe·rs: Laftly, add the calcined Vitriol, but don't rub the Mixture too long with it, left the Quickfilver fhould begin to part again. Sublime the Mixture in a Mattras, to which may be fitted an Alembic Head, that a Spirit, which will afcend in a fmall Quantity, may be faved. *L.*

I am inform'd, that the Sublimate generally us'd is imported from *Holland*; and I believe it is certain that a great deal of Arfenic is mix'd with the *Dutch* Sublimate. Hence the Calomel made from it will be very different from that made with genuine Sublimate. The Apothecary, who trufts the Preparation of this to another, is guilty of an inexcufable Neglect. This Preparation is a *Lapis infernalis* of Mercury, and a moft violent Corrofive, prefently converting all the Parts of the Body it touches, into an Efchar, that foon falls off; whence it confumes obftinate Callofities in Ulcers, as alfo Warts, and indurated Glands. That eminent Surgeon *Johannes a Vigo* was acquainted herewith, and hence compofed his Troches of *Minium*, which are an incomparable Remedy for confuming fcrophulous Tumours nd eradicating them by Suppura-on. The Taste of this Vitriol is bominably austere. A Grain of it issolved in an Ounce of Water, af-ords an excellent Cosmetic, if cau-iously used. It proves poisonous to all cutaneous Insects by bare Lotion. If a Dram of this Solution be soft-ned with Syrup of Violets, and drank twice or thrice a Day, it performs Wonders in many reputed incurable Diseases; but it requires to be cau-tiously used, by a prudent Physician, and should not be ventured upon, unless the Method of managing it is well known.

Mercurius Sublimatus dulcis.

Sweet Mercury Sublimate.

Take of corrosive Mercury Subli-mate, ground in a glass Mortar, four Ounces; and of clean Quick-silver three Ounces; mix them well in the Mortar, till the Globules of Quicksilver disappear, then put the Powder into an oblong Phial, whereof it may possess only one Third, and bury it half Way in a Sand Heat; then with successive Degrees of Fire, nearly the whole Quantity of Mercury will sublime, and stick all around to the upper Part of the Glass, which being broke, and the red Powder about the Bottom, and the White about the Neck cleared away, the white Mercury is again to be three or four Times sublimed.

If the Operation be seven Times repeated, the Preparation is called *Calomel*, or *Aquila alba*. *E.*

In the *London* Dispensatory it is thus directed:

Take of corrosive Sublimate one Pound; of purified Quicksilver nine Ounces. Add the Quicksil-ver to the Sublimate reduced to Powder, and in a glass Mattrass digest them together, in a gentle Sand Heat, often shaking the Glass, till they are united. Then augmenting the Heat, sublime the Mixture: After the acrid Part on the Top of the Sublimation is scraped off, and if any Globules of Quicksilver chance to appear, they likewise being separated, the Mass sublimed is to be reduced to Powder, and sublimed again; the Sublimation is to be six Times re-peated. *L.*

The College have here drop'd the Distinction betwixt *Mercurius dulcis*, and *Calomel*, as of very little Conse-quence; because the Chymists have long neglected this Distinction, and sold the same Preparation for both. But if Apothecaries would be at the Trouble of making it themselves, and take proper Care, it would be well to have it thus distinguish'd; for the *Calomel* will operate more mildly than the *Mercurius dulcis*, as I have experienc'd when the Preparations have been began and finish'd under my own Inspection. Sir *Theodore Mayerne* is said to have been the In-troducer of this into Practice. The usual Dose is fifteen Grains for Adults, and in Proportion for Children. It is an admirable Remedy for the Worms; but for this Purpose and all others, except raising a Salivation, it must be either mix'd with cathar-tic Ingredients, or Purges must be given at a short Interval after it. And even with this Precaution, it will be very subject to affect the Mouth, if the Patient takes the least Cold. For the farther Virtues of *Mercurius dulcis*, see the Article of *Mercury* in the *Materia Medica*.

Panacæa Mercurii.

Panacæa of Mercury.

Take any Quantity of levigated Ca-lomel, and digest it in a Sand Heat for twenty Days with four Times its own Weight of Spirit of Wine, observing frequently to

shake

hake the containing Veel; then pour off the Spirit, and dry the Powder. *E.*

I don't know that this Treatment renders the Calomel in any Degree a better Medicine.

Æthiops Mineralis.
Æthiops Mineral.

Take equal Parts of Quickilver purified, and of Flowers of Sulphur unwahed; rub them together in a Mortar of Glafs or Marble, till the Quickilver perfectly diappears, and the Union is perfected. *L.*

Great Controverfies have arofe among Practitioners with Refpect to the medicinal Virtues of this Preparation. Some affert that it enters into the Blood, and penetrates fo far as to be found adhering to Plaifters laid upon old Ulcers; and that it is an excellent Alterative. But *Boerhaave* fays that it is an infipid Powder, not at all harp, nor eafy to be thoroughly mixed with any Thing; and that when given internally, it cannot enter the abforbent Veels, the Lacteals, or Lymphatics, but paes directly thro' the inteftinal Tube; where it may happen to defroy Worms. They are therefore deceived, fays he, who expect any other Effects from it; at leaft, *Boerkaave* himfelf, as he fays, could never find them. He is afraid it is too unwarily given in fuch large Quantities to Children, and Perfons of tender Conftitutions, as being a foil Mafs foreign to the Body, and unconquerable by the Nature thereof; and hould be the more fufpected as it there continues long fluggih and unactive. And affirms that it does not raife a Salivation, becaufe it cannot come into the Blood. When any great Man ftarts a Notion in Phyfic, with however little Foundation, the whole Tribe of Imitators who can-

not think for themfelves, immediately affent, and treat it as a certain Fact. In the prefent Cafe, it is difficult to conceive how two fuch penetrating Subftances as Quickilver and Sulphur, can by their Union form fo inert a Mafs as is reprefented above. And, indeed, Experience informs us, that it is of fuch good Service in fome chronical Diftempers, that without getting into the Blood it could not perform. I muft confefs, however, that it is the moft infignificant of all the Mercurials; and perhaps fometimes if taken for a long Time, without the due Interpofition of Cathartics, it may lodge in the inteftinal Tube, and caufe fome Inconveniences. There is fcarcely a better Remedy for Worms. But for this Purpofe Cathartics muft be given with it, or interpos'd in the Intervals of taking it.

Æthiops Antimonialis.
Antimonial Æthiops.

Firft flux equal Parts of Antimony and Sea Salt in a Crucible for an Hour; then let the Matter cool; break the Crucible, and knock off off the Scoriæ; then rub equal Parts of the Regulus made in this Manner, and Mercury, together, till they are incorporated,

It will cure moft chronical Diforders of the Skin, and is admirable in all Sorts of Obftructions. Hence it becomes ferviceable in the King's-Evil, and the moft obftinate glandular Difeafes, and many chronical Diftempers, that are out of the Reach of other Medicines. I have feen better Effects from it in cancerous Tumors, than from any other Remedy. In veneral Diforders of a long Standing, I have often been a Witnefs of fuch Effects as I have not feen from any other mercurial Medicine whatever. This, like all Antimonials, will contract an emetic Quality

by being expofed to the Air,
:h is probably owing to the Acid
nbibes. It may be given in the
ntity of a Scruple, or more in
: Conftitutions, but at firft it
ld be taken in much fmaller
ntities gradually increafing the
=, becaufe otherwife it will in
: Conftitutions excite a *Naufea*.

Mercurius Saccharatus.

Sugar'd Mercury.

:e of pure Quickfilver, and brown
agar-Candy, each half an Ounce;
aymical Oil of Juniper, fixteen
rops. Rub them in a glafs Mor-
ar, till all the Mercurial Globules
xtirely difappear. *E.*

Mercurius Alcalifatus.

Alcalis'd Mercury.

:e pure Quickfilver, three Drams;
repar'd Crabs Eyes, five Drams,
:ub them in a glafs Mortar as in
ae preceding Preparation. *E.*

aefe are very good Methods of
paring Mercurial Alteratives, but
hink not the beft. The Patient
t be purg'd at Intervals, other-
: they will falivate.

Cinnabaris Factitia.

Artificial Cinnabar.

:e of purified Quickfilver twenty-
ive Ounces; of Sulphur feven
Ounces; ftir the Quickfilver with
he Sulphur melted, and if the
Mixture takes fire, it is to be ex-
inguifhed by covering the Veffel;
hen let the Matter be reduced to
Powder, and fublimed. *L.*

he firft Part of the Procefs makes
Æthiops, without the tedious La-
ar of Trituration, which is as
ad as that made without Fire, as
cted above. *Boerhaave* fays, this
inabar is a Mixture of Mercury
l Sulphur united by the Fire, in the
rm of a fimple Foffil; which is
nd natural in many Mines, and is

like the factitious, without much
Difference. It has nearly the fame
Virtue in the Body, as Æthiops.
Crato called it the Magnet of the
Epilepfy; but *Boerhaave* fays, he
never faw it produce any great Effects. If it be mixed with Purgatives, then, like Æthiops, it is driven
quicker thro' the Inteftines, with the
Succefs of Æthiops. It is mixed
with red Cofmetics in the Form of
Pomatum. It is ufed in Fumigations,
againft venereal Ulcers in the Nofe,
Mouth, and Throat, with little, and
often with bad Succefs. The Mercury may be revived very pure from
the Cinnabar, by grinding it with
twice its Weight of Iron-filings, and
diftilling it in a Retort, with the
ftrongeft Heat of a Sand Furnace,
into Water.

Crocus Antimonii, vel Metallorum.

Crocus of Antimony.

Take of Antimony and Nitre equal
Weights, being feparately reduced
to Powder; let them be well mixed, and then gradually thrown into a hot Crucible to melt; the
Matter being poured out, is to be
feparated from its Scoriæ. It will
not always appear of the fame
Colour; it is the more yellow the
longer it has been melted. *L.*

This has hitherto been call'd *Crocus
Metallorum.* Sulphur and Nitre
make a Kind of Gunpowder with
black Antimony, and therefore flafh
off in the fame Manner. The metallic Part calcines to a Glafs and a
Scoria, both of them violently emetic, and communicating that Virtue
to Wine by Infufion; whereas native Antimony is not emetic. It is
of little other Ufe in Medicine, but
in making the emetic Wine.

Crocus Antimonii lotus.

Wafhed Crocus of Antimony.

Boil the Crocus of Antimony reduced

to a very fine Powder in Water, and this Water being poured away, wafh the Powder often with hot Water, till the Water comes off infipid. *L.*

This is ufed in making emetic Tartar.

What is ufually call'd Liver of Antimony, is made of the fame Ingredients, mix'd in the fame Proportion. But inftead of throwing them gradually into a hot Crucible, they are put into a Mortar, and fir'd, by throwing in a Piece of lighted Charcoal, or hot Iron. This, or the *Crocus Antimonii*, which is nearly the fame, are much recommended as a Prefervative, or Cure for the Murrain in Cattle; and nothing is fo likely to fucceed. A late anonymous Author recommends five Drams for an Ox; three for a Cow; and one for a Calf, or Sheep, once in ten Days, as a Prefervative. By way of Cure, the Dofe, and its Repetitions, muft be fuited to the Circumftances.

Crocus Metallorum mitior.
The milder Crocus of Metals.

This is prepar'd with one Part of Nitre to two of Antimony, in the fame Manner as the *Crocus* of Antimony.

When Antimony is mixed with half its Weight of Nitre, and thrown into a Crucible red-hot, it deflagrates; and if the Fire be raifed high enough, the Mixture melts, and *Scoriæ* feparate, as in the other *Crocus*; but if the Heat be not fo ftrong, it does not melt, nor is this Separation made. We are informed in the Narrative of the Committee of the College, that the Gentleman, who propofed this Medicine to the Committee, prepares it with this lefter Degree of Fire. I am well informed, that a Dofe of a few Grains, eight for Example, has an admirable Effect in Fevers, the

Small Pox, and many chronical Diftempers, by way of Emetic.

Antimonium Diaphoreticum Nitratum.
Diaphoretic Antimony with Nitre.

Take of Antimony half a Pound, of Nitre a Pound and a half; pulverize them feparately; then mix them together, and throw them, by a Spoonful at a time, into an ignited Crucible: After the Detonation, let the white Mafs be detained for half an Hour in the Fire, and let the Powder be kept in a glafs Veffel ftopt clofe. *E.*

Boerhaave fays, that this being taken in the Quantity of half a Dram, has fcarcely any fenfible Effect, except that it moderately opens on account of the fixing Nitre adhering thereto; whence it may prove ferviceable in acute Cafes. In this State, the Chymifts call it diaphoretic; and judge, that the arfenical Poifon of the Antimony is fixed by a large Proportion of Nitre; but there was nothing emetic in the Antimony before, tho' taken in the Quantity of feveral Drams crude, or without any Nitre; whereas an equal Proportion of Nitre excites this emetic Virtue. *Bafil Valentine*, therefore, and other Chymifts, need not to have been fo anxious to free this diaphoretic Antimony from its fixing Nitre; for it caufes no Anxiety, Naufea, or Vomiting, and only ftimulates mildly.

Antimonium Diaphoreticum dulce.
Sweet-Diaphoretic Antimony.

Take any Quantity of nitrated diaphoretic Antimony; powder it; then pour on as much Spring Water as will rife above it fome Inches; digeft for a Night, afterwards pour off the Water, and add frefh, and thus repeat the Ablution five or fix times. All the Wafhings being mixed together, filtrated, and

and evaporated over a gentle Fire to a Pellicle, afford the *Nitrum Stibiatum,* or Stibiated Nitre. *E.* This is the common diaphoretic Antimony, now called in the *London* dispensatory *Calx Antimonii,* or Calx of Antimony. It is a very great reproach to Physic, that the Virtues of a Medicine so long in Use, and so much in Practice as this, should be so little ascertain'd, that at this time it is asserted, that it is possessed of none at all, by very considerable authors; whilst others are of a different Opinion. *Boerhaave,* to whose Opinion I pay the utmost Regard, affirms, that it is an indolent, noxious Calx, without any Activity discoverable by Observation; and loses all the Virtue it had before it was washed. And that it only acts sensibly, when mixed in a double Proportion with Purgatives; the Virtues whereof it actually excites, as appears by the *Pulvis Cornacchini*. After this Declaration from so great an Author, it is not surprizing, that all those who never think for themselves should assent without farther Inquiry; and that this Medicine should fall into Disgrace. I can't from Experience say much with Respect to its Virtues; but I have sometimes known a profuse Sweat arise upon taking it, which has been attended with more happy Consequences than those excited by the warmer Diaphoretics. *Helvetius* recommends it as excellent in the Small Pox.

Regulus Antimonii.

Regulus of Antimony.

Take of Antimony, Nitre, and crude Tartar, each a like Quantity; reduce them to Powder separately; mix them together, and grind them again; at several times put the Whole into an ignited Crucible: when the Detonation is over, build up a large Fire, so as to make the

Matter flow like Water; then pour it out into a melting Cone first heated, and greased with Tallow, and keep it shaking, that the Regulus may separate and fall to the Bottom: When all is cold, free the Regulus from the *Scoriae* at the Top. *E.*

This renders Wine, in which it has been infus'd, Emetic.

Regulus Antimonii Martialis.

Regulus of Antimony with Iron.

Take of Antimony, Nitre, and crude Tartar, each a Pound; of Pieces of Iron half a Pound; make the Iron red-hot in a Crucible, and gradually add the other Ingredients to it, having first ground and mixed them together, and proceed entirely after the same Manner as in making the Regulus of Antimony.

If the Regulus of Antimony with Iron, be thus several times fused with Nitre and Tartar, it will at length become the *Regulus Antimonii Stellatus,* or Starry Regulus of Antimony. *E.*

Regulus Antimonii Medicinalis.

The Medicinal Regulus of Antimony.

Take five Parts of pure Antimony, four Parts of common Salt, and one Part of Salt of Tartar. Some alter the Proportion of the Ingredients, and take eight Parts of Antimony, seven of common Salt, and one of Salt of Tartar; but the first Proportions are most generally adhered to. These Ingredients, when beat and mixed together, are to be successively put into a red-hot Crucible: Let the Action of the Fire be raised to such a Height, that the Matter may be sufficiently and thoroughly fused. Then, after the Matter is sufficiently fused, which

which generally happens in a Quarter of an Hour, let it be poured into a Veffel of a conical Form, befmeared with Tallow, or fmoaked with a Candle. This Veffel is to be fhaken, that, by this Means, the Regulus may be fufficiently feparated from the Scoriæ, and carried to the Bottom of the Veffel. Some reckon this Circumftance of fhaking fo much the more neceffary, becaufe as this Regulus is lighter than any others prepared from Antimony, it muft of Confequence be feparated from the Scoriæ, and fall to the Bottom with more Difficulty. Thus if fuch a Concuffion, or Shaking, fhould be neglected, and the Mixture poured when boiling, as it were, from the red-hot Crucible into a cold conical Veffel, it frequently happens, that during the Continuation of the Ebullition, a a Portion of the Scoriæ is intermixed with the Regulus ; and, *vice verfa*, a Portion of the Regulus remains in the Scoriæ ; fo that by the Overfight, we do not obtain it fo pure or uncontaminated, or at leaft fo beautiful and fhining, as it would otherwife be. The Regulus, when feparated from the Scoriæ, refembles polifhed Steel or Iron ; but if either in a Mortar, or upon a Marble, with, or without the Addition of Water, it is reduced to a Powder fo fine, that the fhining Particles entirely difappear, it affumes a reddifh, or rather a purple Colour.

The Efficacy of this *Regulus* is highly extolled in chronical Diforders, and fuch as arife from long-continued Obftructions of the Vifcera : Hence it is much recommended in Dropfies, Epilepfies, Scurvies, and Fevers ; for as thefe Diforders are of a ftubborn and obftinate Nature, they require Medicines which do not, like Vegetable Subftances, too quickly produce

their Effects, but remain for a confiderable Time in the Body ; and by often impelling the tenacious Matter, at laft entirely break and fubdue it. Hence we may eafily conceive why this Regulus muft be a Medicine of fingular Efficacy in furmounting the Obftinacy of chronical Diforders. There are alfo not a few who highly extol its Efficacy againft Fevers. *Maetfius* fays, that it is a fpecific Diaphoretic in Fevers of all forts. The fame Author commends it *in all Diforders, where*, to ufe his own Words, *Sweats are wanted, becaufe it does not, like vegetable Subftances, inflame the Blood. Frederic Hoffman* afferts, that he was informed, by People who were acquainted with this Author when alive, that he made daily Ufe of this Regulus ; and his own *Praxis Chymiatrica* is a concurring and additional Proof, that he did fo ; for in that Work he maintains, that it is of uncommon Efficacy in all Difeafes where the Motion of the Lymph, and infenfible Tranfpiration, are to be promoted. Thus he commends it in the Gout, the Apoplexy, *&c* but more particularly in Fevers. This he has alfo done in *Act. Curiof. Lugd.* where he orders it to be ufed with a diaphoretic Regimen. *Barkhyifen* agrees with *Maetfius*, and highly extols its fudorific Virtues in Fevers, and cutaneous Diforders. *Koenig* declares himfelf of the fame Sentiments in his *Regnum Minerale.* This Medicine is alfo commended by fome in Cafes where the State of the Lymph is bad, in Dropfies, Anafarcas, *&c.* but particularly with Regard to its Ufe in an Anafarca. *Hoffman* fays, that the learned and judicious *Hennike* mixed it with *Mercurius Dulcis*, and ufed it under that Form with uncommon Succefs. *Frederic Hoffman* orders it to be prefcribed in fmall Dofes, with the Bezoardic Powders, in the firft Stages of malignant Fevers, Small

Pox,

x, and Dyfenteries. Becaufe, fays
, by its Means a gentle Diaphorefis'
brought on, and the Mucus of the
imæ Viæ being attenuated, the
eavinefs and Uneafinefs of the Præ-
rdia are removed. And he adds,
at when malignant Fevers raged
etty much in his own Country,
at excellent Chymift *Rollwagius*
ten ufed this Regulus with the
eateft Succefs ; of it, together
ith fome earthy Abforbents, he
mpofed an alexipharmic Powder,
hich is in conftant Ufe at this very
ime. He farther fays, that the
egulus was ufed by the above-
entioned Dr. *Hennike* in thefe Difders. *Maetfius* commends the Lixi-
ium of its Scoriæ apply'd externally
a proper Medicine for the Itch ;
id *Hoffman* fays, that, by his Fa-
er's Advice, not only himfelf, but
great many others, labouring un-
r this Diforder, ufed this Medicine
ith incredible Succefs ; and that he
members to have feen the Regulus
felf, mixt with earthy Subftances,
fed in the Itch ; and has known it
that Form, and in Conjunction
ith a fudorific Regimen, to remove
edematous Swellings, efpecially of
le Feet. Hence we may plainly
erceive the Efficacy of this Regu-
is, in augmenting the Motions of
le Humours.

Its Dofe is from fix Grains to one
cruple, and upwards, as the State
f the Patient fhall require. But be-
re this Regulus is ufed, it muft be
thoroughly triturated, and, upon
Marble, reduced to a Powder fo fine,
at none of the fhining Particles may
the leaft appear : For this Re-
uction of it to fo fine a Powder is
bfolutely requifite, both to its eafy
olution, and its fpeedy Operation ;
nd if this Caution fhould not be ob-
rved, it remains too long in the
nteftines, and may poffibly give
life to troublefome Symptoms.

Vitrum Antimonii.
Glafs of Antimony.

Put two Pounds of powdered Antimony into a large and unglazed
earthen Difh, with a flat Bottom ;
fet it over a Fire in the Air, fo
that the Powder may fume, but not
melt ; in which Management the
whole Art confifts. Keep the
Powder conftantly ftirring with an
Iron Rod ; there flies off a thick
white fetid Fume, pernicious to
the Lungs, and therefore to be
avoided by the Operator, ftanding with his Back to the Wind.
Continue the Calcination uniformly, till the Matter ceafes to fume ;
then increafe the Fire a little, and
if the Matter again begins to fume,
continue ftirring it till it leaves off.
Again increafe the Fire, till at
length the Difh begins to grow
red, whilft the Matter emits no
more Fume : The Calx will be of
a greyifh Colour ; but if the Calcination be longer continued with
a ftronger Fire, fo as to ignite the
Matter, the Calx will be yellow,
and better purified from its volatile
Parts. If the Fire fhould be ftrong
at the firft, fo as to melt the Antimony, and make it lumpy, the
Lumps are directly to be broke to
Powder, and the Fire to be diminifhed. Put this Calx into a Crucible, and apply Fire round it,
firft at fome Diftance, gradually
approaching it nearer, and at
length bringing it quite clofe, fo
that the Crucible being exactly
covered to prevent the Coals and
Afhes from falling in, may be thus
uniformly heated and ignited. Increafe the Fire till the Calx melts ;
keep it fufed for half a Quarter of
an Hour ; then pour it out upon
a dry and hot Marble. It will be
a dufky, yellowifh, brittle, fomewhat tranfparent, and livid Cake,
called

called the Glaſs of Antimony: It will appear the more tranſparent, the longer it was fuſed in the Fire.

This Glaſs of Antimony is almoſt mortally emetic; and when infuſed in Wine, that is not conſiderably acid, it renders the Liquor alſo emetic, without any great Loſs of its Subſtance; tho' this Virtue is ſoon exhauſted, by often repeating the Infuſion.

Vitrum Antimonii Ceratum.

Take Glaſs of Antimony in Powder one Ounce; Bees Wax one Dram: Melt the Wax in an Iron Ladle, then add the Powder; ſet them on a ſlow Fire without Flame for the Space of half an Hour, continually ſtirring them with a Spatula; then take it from the Fire; pour it upon a Piece of clean white Paper, powder it, and keep it for Uſe. E.

The *Edinburgh* Medical Eſſays have the Honour of having publiſhed this Preparation; a Remedy of ſo much Conſequence in obſtinate Diarrhœas and Dyſenteries, that I think it exceeds all other Medicines in Efficacy for thoſe Diſtempers. I ſhall therefore give the Directions with Reſpect to its Uſes, as I find them particulariſed by the Publiſher in the above-quoted Eſſays.

The ordinary Doſe for an Adult, is ten or twelve Grains; but for the greater Safety, I commonly began, ſays he, with ſix; to a ſtrong Man I have given a Scruple, which ſometimes worked ſo mildly, that I have thought it too weak. To weakly Conſtitutions I give five or ſix Grains, increaſing the Doſe afterwards, according to the Operation. To a Boy of ten Years of Age, give three or four Grains. To a Child of three or four Years, two or three. This

Medicine has been practiſed with Succeſs for the Dyſentery, and the Preparation was kept a Secret for many Years. When firſt it was communicated to me, ſays he, I thought it ſo harſh and dangerous a Medicine, that I had no Courage to try it for ſome Years; and even then began the Doſe with one Grain, and increaſed it gradually to twenty, which was the largeſt Doſe I ever gave. As ſoon as I was convinced by a Number of Experiments, that it was both mild and efficacious in curing the Dyſentery, I publiſhed the Receipt in our *Edinburgh* News-Papers, being under no Promiſe of Secreſy with Regard to this. I do not, ſays he, expect that any Phyſician will incline to give a full Doſe at firſt, without better Authority than I can give to Strangers; but the Cautious may give as ſmall a Doſe as they pleaſe, and make Trials almoſt in any Diſeaſe, where Purgatives will do no Harm; and increaſe it gradually as they find it operate. He farther tells us, he gave it in Dyſenteries, with or without a Fever, whether epidemic or not. He tried it often where Bleeding and Vomiting had been premiſed, and where they had not, with very good Succeſs. He never choſe to give Opiates in the Beginning, eſpecially where there was a great Sickneſs; becauſe altho' Opiates give great Relief to ſome, yet at other times he thought both the Sickneſs and Purging thereby increaſed the following Day. He never began with a larger Doſe than ten Grains, becauſe it frequently operates as violently at firſt, as twenty Grains at laſt, even upon the ſame Patient. In its Operation, it ſometimes makes the Patient ſick, and vomit; it purges almoſt every Perſon; but he has known it cure without any ſenſible Evacuation or Sickneſs; and in violent Dyſenteries, they purge ſeldomer with it than without it. If it purge ſufficiently,

tly, or fatigue the Patient any ay, then intermit a Day or two betwixt each Dose, as with other Purtives. As some have been cured ith one Dose, to others he has been obliged to give five or six, especially hen the first Doses have been too ild; and has often thought, a weak ose did no good in chronic Cases. fter the second or third Dose, the tools are seldom bloody, the Gripes d Sickness are much abated, and e mucous Stools are less viscid. ive it on an empty Stomach; for en it operates most mildly. Forid Drinking any thing after it for hree Hours, unless the Patient is ery sick, or disposed to vomit; in hich Case, give warm Water, as other Vomits. Beware of giving : for a Diarrhæa in the End of a Consumption. Some Diarrhæas have een cured of long Standing, with arge Doses of it; but it has failed ftener here than in Dysenteries. e forbids the Use of all fermented Liquors; and recommends a Milk-Diet, with Rice, or Bread, Chicken-roth, or Water-gruel. Nothing old should be given, unless it be a Tea Spoonful of Jelly of Hartshorn, s often as the Patients please; and ometimes indulge them with a little Jelly of Currans to refresh their Tongue. It may be given safely to Women with Child; and to Children on the Breast you may give half a Grain.

Experience has abundantly confirmed to me the Virtues of this Remedy, as represented in the preceding Remarks. And I am inform'd, that crude Antimony mix'd with melted Wax, instead of the Glass of Antimony, will have very good Effects in curing a Diarrhæa and Dysentery. The last I have only once experienced, and then not till after the cerated Glass had been taken; but I had Reason to think it attended with very salutary Consequences.

Sulphur Auratum Antimonii.
Golden Sulphur of Antimony.

Take any Quantity of the Scoriæ of Regulus of Antimony; grind them to Powder whilst they are hot, and boil them for a considerable Time in thrice their Weight of Spring Water; filter the Solution (which appears of a Colour between a Yellow and a Red) thro' Cap-paper, then by dropping into it a due Proportion of Spirit of Vitriol, the Powder will precipitate, which is to be washed with Water, so as to edulcorate and free it from its ill Scent. E.

In the *London* Dispensatory this Medicine is called *Sulphur Antimonii præcipitatum*; and the Precipitation is directed to be made with Spirit of Sea-Salt. It is Carthartic and Emetic; and the Dose is said to be from one to eight Grains.

Æthiops Medicinalis Plummerii.
Plummer's Medicinal Æthiops.

Take of Calomel, and the Golden Sulphur of Antimony, each two Drams; reduce the Calomel to a gross Powder, and then levigate it upon a Marble, adding gradually the Sulphur of Antimony; and by long Trituration rub the Whole into a fine Powder.

This has been found by Experience to be an excellent Remedy in all cutaneous Distempers, the Leprosy not excepted; in venereal Disorders, and many glandular and obstinate Distempers. The Dose is seven or eight Grains twice a-day. An Æthiops of not inferior Virtues may be made, by rubbing crude Mercury with the Sulphur of Antimony, till the Mercurial Globules disappear.

Butyrum Antimonii.
Butter of Antimony.

Grind two Pounds of corrosive Mercury

cury sublimate to fine Powder, in a warm and dry Glass Mortar, with a Glass Pestle; grind also separately a Pound of the best Antimony perfectly fine; mix the two together in the Glass Mortar; they will thus grow warm; and let the Vapour be carefully avoided; have at Hand a dry Glass Retort, capable of holding three or four times this Quantity of Matter, with its Neck cut off, so as to leave a wide Mouth. Put the Powder, whilst thoroughly dry, into this heated and dry Retort, so that no Blackness may stick internally to the short Neck; put the Retort into a Sand-Furnace fit for the Purpose, so as almost to touch the Bottom of the Iron Pot, the Neck of the Retort inclining a little downwards; apply a Glass Receiver, with the Neck cut off, so as exactly to receive the Retort. Cover the Retort with Sand, and let the Operation be performed under a Chimney that entirely carries up the Fumes. The Retort being now warmed by a very gentle Fire, and luted on with a Mixture of Lime and Clay, raise the Fire cautiously by Degrees; the Retort will first appear cloudy, and a little Liquor come into the Receiver: Keep up this Degree till no more Liquor comes over; then increase the Fire gradually, and carefully, till an unctuous Matter rises into the Neck of the Retort, distils into the Receiver, and coagulates in falling. Continue this Degree of Fire, and a white icy Matter will concrete, and remain in the Neck of the Retort; on both Sides of which place live Coals at a Distance, and approach them nearer by Degrees, that the Neck of the Retort may become as hot as the Belly; the Matter will thus be melted, and run down into the Receiver. Continue carefully with this Degree of Fire, and afterwards increase it a little, till no more Butter rises, and all of it be melted down into the Receiver, which is now to be removed with great Care, to prevent any of the Vapour coming to the Lungs. Immediately stop the Receiver, and set it by; apply another, fitted in the same Manner for the Purpose; lute it on, increase the Fire, and a yellow, red, blackish, variously coloured Mass will arise; then increase the Fire to the utmost, at last raising a Fire of Suppression, till the Sand almost grows red-hot; and leave it thus for two Hours. Let all cool; take off the Receiver, wherein some Quantity of of running Mercury will be found, and an impure Butter from the sulphureous Fumes of the Sulphur of the Antimony. In the Neck of the Retort will also appear a Matter of various Colours, consisting of the Mercury, Sulphur, and Butter, compounded together; and at the Bottom of the Retort, when broke, appear Antimonial *Fæces*: In the Beginning of the Neck is a compact, hard, opake, highly ponderous Mass, which shines on the Surface contiguous to the Glass, but is rough on the other: This being ground to Powder is the true Cinnabar of Antimony, and a thing of Value. Great Patience and Care are required in this Process; because if the Vessels or Luting crack, or the Fumes any other way escape, and are received into the Lungs, they are poisonous, on Account of their caustic Property.

The Butter of Antimony is to be rectify'd in a Glass Retort, till it appears of a very white Colour; taking great Care to avoid the Fumes, which may prove fatal. This Butter of Antimony

ry is a most immediate Caustic,
ng an Eschar the quickest of any
; known, and which generally
rates the same Day it was formed.
se to give this Preparation from
baave, as being more circum-
ial than it is delivered either in
Edinburgh or London Dispensato-
; a Circumstance which ought to
egarded in a Procefs attended
much Danger.

Cinnabaris Antimonii.

Cinnabar of Antimony.

e of crude Mercury fifteen Oun-
s, of common Sulphur five Oun-
s, Antimony crude one Ounce
d an half; mix them well toge-
er, and sublime them in a luted
olt-head in a naked Fire: Let
e Fire be strong enough to make
e Bolt-head red-hot.

the Procefs for making Butter of
imony, another Method of mak-
Cinnabar of Antimony is taken
ice of. And the London Dispen-
y orders what remains after the
illation of Butter of Antimony,
e sublim'd in a coated Retort, in
r to make this Cinnabar. Much
ame Virtues are ascribed to this
the native Cinnabar. The usual
e is a Scruple, but it may be gi-
in larger Quantities.

Mercurius Vitæ.

a Glafs of fair Water let fall
Drop of the rectified Oil of An-
mony; the Moment it falls it
comes white, turns to Powder,
d sinks to the Bottom of the
essel. Continue to drop in more,
l a fourth Part of the Oil be
ed in Respect to the Water; it
stantly sinks to the Bottom, in
orm of an exceeding white pon-
erous Powder. Stir all with a
lafs Rod; let them rest; a lim-
d acid Liquor will float above,
hich is gently to be decanted;
rfectly edulcorate the Powder,

by washing it in several fresh Waters, till it is entirely insipid: Dry
it with a gentle Fire, and thus there
will be obtained a white, insipid,
ponderous Powder, called Mercu-
curius Vitæ.

This Powder, being given in the
Quantity of two or three Grains, is
violently emetic. If it be for a long
Time exposed upon Glass to a gentle Fire, and kept constantly stirred, it
loses of its Violence, and becomes
less active. This Powder contains
not the least Mercury, but is a pure
Regulus of Antimony.

Bezoardicum Minerale.

Bezoar Mineral.

Take any Quantity of newly rectified
Butter of Antimony, and gradually
pour to it a due Proportion of Spirit
of Nitre, that is so much as will stop
the Effervescence; then draw off
the floating Liquor from a Glass
Veffel placed in a Sand-heat, till
the Powder is left dry; upon which
again pour a little Spirit of Nitre,
and dry it a second time. Repeat
the Operation a third time; then
put the Powder into a Crucible,
and commit it to the naked Fire,
till it becomes almost red-hot; in
which State let it be detained for
half an Hour. E.

Its Operation is by Sweat; tho'
it will also sometimes purge. It will
eradicate even Leprofies, as Quincy
informs us, and the most obstinate
Cafes of that Kind, if rightly managed. Some count it a Refifter of
Poifons, and commend it in Pestilential Diftempers. Its Dofe is from
ten Grains to half a Dram, according to the above-quoted Author.

Bezoardicum Joviale.

Bezoar of Tin.

Take Regulus of Antimony three
Ounces; melt it in a Crucible,
and add to it two Ounces of very

pure Tin, so as to make a new Regulus thereof; which being levigated, mix therewith five Ounces of corrosive Mercury sublimate; distil it in a Retort, and fix the Butter thence distilled, by three repeated Distillations, with thrice its Weight of Spirit of Nitre; afterwards calcine it, and whilst ignited, quench it in a sufficient Quantity of Spirit of Wine, and lastly dry the Powder. *E.*

This much resembles Bezoar Mineral.

Antihecticum Poterii.
Poterius's Antihectic.

Take of the Regulus of Antimony, made with Iron, six Ounces; of the best Tin, three Ounces; melt these together in a Crucible, and pour them into a Mortar first heated and greased with Tallow; and when the Mass is cold, reduce it to Powder; then add thereto thrice its Weight of very pure Nitre, and throw the whole into an ignited Crucible, by a Spoonful at a time, where it will make a Detonation, and calcine for an Hour; then grind the Mass again to a very fine Powder, and pour thereto a due Proportion of hot Spring-Water, and stir them about with a Pestle till the Water grows milky, which being thus saturated with the fine Powder is to be poured off; and fresh hot Water again added to the remaining Powder, and this to be repeated till nothing is left at the Bottom, but a dirty Matter that will not dissolve; then let all the milky Liquors stand at Rest together, that the fine Powder may be precipitated, which is afterwards to be several times washed in warm Water, and then dried. *E.*

The Character given of this Me-

dicine by *Quincy* is, that it is accounted a forcible, penetrating Medicine, insomuch as to make Way thro' the minute Passages, and search even the nervous Cells; whereupon in all Disorders from that Original, it is reckoned very effectual. In those Heavinesses of the Head, Giddinesses, and Dimness of Sight, whence proceed *Apoplexies* and *Epilepsies*, it does great Service. And in all Affections and Foulnesses of the *Viscera* of the lower Belly, it is reckon'd inferior to nothing, in cleansing away and discharging their Impurities. Thus it obtains in the *Jaundice, Dropsies,* and all Kinds of Cachexies. It is likewise esteem'd of great Service, even in obstinate venereal Cases; in clearing the Blood from all Impressions of Contagion; and cleansing the Glands from those corrosive Recrements which such Distempers frequently lodge upon them, and occasion Blotches and ulcerous Deformities. In short, there is hardly a Preparation in the *Chymical Pharmacy* of greater Efficacy in most obstinate Chronic Distempers; but is not often met with in Prescription, altho' constantly kept in the Shops. The Dose is from six Grains to a Scruple, in grown Persons; for it is seldom given to Children, their tender Vessels not well bearing the Force of such Medicines.

Tartarum Emeticum.
Emetic Tartar.

Take washed Crocus of Antimony, Crystals of Tartar, of each half a Pound; of Water three Pints; Boil them together for half an Hour, then filtre the Water thro' Paper, and after a due Evaporation set it by, that the Salt may crystallize. *L.*

This is a pretty brisk Emetic, in the Quantity of a few Grains. And I have Reasons to believe it much mor

e effectual than *Ipecacuanha,*
ch. is at present the fashionable
uit.

*rmes Mineralis, five Pulvis Car-
thusianorum.*

ermes's Mineral, or *Poudre des
Chartreux.*

e of Antimony four Pounds, So-
tion of fixed Nitre *per Deliquium*
ne Pound, Rain Water 3 Pounds,
d boil them for two Hours. Then
e boiling Decoction is to be passed
ro' Cap Paper ; set it in a quiet
lace for twenty-four Hours, till
yellowish, or saffron-coloured
owder sinks to the Bottom of the
essel, the Liquor remaining clear.
his Liquor being poured off by
nclination, the Powder is first
ashed by frequent Affusions of
arm Water, till it is deprived
f all its Salts, and then about
our Ounces of Spirit of Wine are
urnt upon it, and it is afterwards
ried, and kept for Use.

his Powder is looked upon almost
Panacea, or universal Remedy.
ometimes excites Vomiting, es-
ially when it meets with any Acid
the Stomach, and is sometimes
artic, diaphoretic, and sudori-
according as it is determined by
Disposition of the Patient to act
n any one Humour more than
ther. It is given from one to
r Grains, or sometimes when it
esigned only to attenuate and di-
e any Viscidities in the Fluids, in
Quantity of half a Grain, repeated
ry three, four, or six Hours. In
te Fevers, where there is a great
idity and Spissitude of the Hu-
ors, it is given in small Doses with
ress. It changes the crude and
ous Evacuations by Stool into a
re bilious Consistence, by attenu-
g the viscid Bile, and so disposing
pass off by Stool. It is often
a with Success in the Beginning

of the Small Pox and Measles, when
they are apprehended to be of a bad
Sort, at small Doses, mixed with
Bezoardic Powders, or Absorbents,
such as Crabs Eyes, red Coral,
Pearl, Egg-shells, Crabs-Claws, and
the like ; for thus it excites a Spitting and Diaphoresis, removes Anxieties, corrects the Lympha, and coagulated Serum, and raises such an
Effervescence in the Blood, as tends
to purify it. *Glauber* confirms these
Virtues by the Example of seven
Children in the Small Pox. *Frederic
Hoffman* commends the Use of this
Powder in stubborn autumnal Agues,
because it powerfully opens Obstructions, particularly of the Liver,
by which these Fevers are produced,
especially when taken in the Quantity
of a Grain, mixed with detergent
antifebrile Salts, such as the Salt of
Wormwood, the febrifugous Salt of
Sylvius, vitriolated Tartar, and the
like. *Schroder* order'd it in the
Quantity of half a Grain, or a Grain,
three or four times a-day in the intermitting Fevers of Children, and
commends it very much in correcting
the Acrimony of the Serum, and especially that of the Tears, which give
Pain in the Eyes, and produce very bad
Ophthalmias. The same Author
mentions a Woman labouring under
scorbutic Symptoms, and Defluxions
of so acid a Kind as to corrode her
Lungs, and bring on a Spitting of
Blood, who by using this Sulphur of
Antimony in very small Quantities,
corrected the Acrimony, and stopped
the Motion of this Serum, and thereby prevented the Growth of the
Disease, which must otherwise have
been of very fatal Consequence.
Hoffman says it is the most effectual
Remedy in such Chronical Diseases,
as arise from long Obstructions of the
Viscera. In a Dropsy, for Instance,
it is very properly mixed with Filings or *Crocus* of Steel and Nitre ;
in Epilepsies with all the *Cinnabars*

in the Scurvy with the *Arcanum Duplicatum*; in Dysenteries with the *Confectio de Hyacintho*; in a Dysury, or Complaints of the Stone, with white Nettle, or Pellitory Water; and even in Pleurisies and Peripneumonias, be frequently gives it in the Quantity of three or four Grains in a Glass of strong *Spanish* Wine, in *Carduus* Water, in an Infusion of red Poppies, or the Juice of Dendelion, or Borage. *Junker* observes, that this Powder has in many Patients suspended, in one Moment, the Effects of a suffocating Catarrh, sometimes by producing a gentle Vomiting, sometimes by Sweating, and sometimes without any sensible Evacuation; and he advises it to be mixed in these Cases with a certain digestive Salt. It may be given very advantageously to cachectic Girls, in the Quantity of a Grain mixed in ten Grains of *Crocus Martis aperiens*, and of the *Arcanum Duplicatum*, the Dose being repeated twice a-day; this Powder may be given either

..one, or mixed with a little S.. and diluted in Wine or Wat.. any other proper Liquor. It i.. wise sometimes given with O.. Sweet Almonds, or in Con.. of Violets, Borage, &c. in Fo.. a Bolus.

It is, however, to be careful.. served, that this Powder is so.. be given till the Quantity of I.. has been lessened, and all the F.. sufficiently diluted and attenu.. for as by the Use of it, the I.. is very suddenly rarified, and.. into a Kind of Effervescence, i.. Vessels are before full, they.. be still more distended, by the.. creased Heat and Motion of.. Blood, and other Fluids, and b.. ful Congestions may be forme.. the Viscera. It ought, ther.. never to be given till the Da.. from a Plethora are taken of.. till the Humours have become.. fluid by great Quantities of Dil.. often repeated.

F I N I S.

A
Copious INDEX
OF THE
ARTICLES ufed in PHYSICK, SURGERY, both in *Latin* and *English*, and of DISEASES, with numerous References to their Remedies.

TO avoid the Perplexity of fearching for any Particulars required, attending Three Indexes, and their referring to one another, we have thrown Our's into One only: And this directs to the Columns of the Page, diftinguifhed by i for the firft, and ii for the fecond.

The Difeafes and References to the Remedies are alfo more particularly pointed out, where requifite; as, for Inftance, in the Menfes, whether to promote, or reftrain them: So in Fevers, whether intermittent, putrid, &c. But where there is no fuch Diftinction, preceding the Figures directing to the Page, it is moftly to be underftood, that the Difeafe in general is intended.

It may not be improper always to view over the whole Column directed to, becaufe the fame Word many times occurs more than once therein.

It ought to be obferved, that the Words, more immediately preceding the Figures, often lead to the initial Words; as, for Inftance, Abortion, to promote, 213, ii.—to prevent, 439, ii.—are to be read, To promote, or to prevent Abortion: Again, Animals, poifonous, to keep at a Diftance, 257, ii.—is to be read, To keep at a Diftance poifonous Animals: And fo of the reft; after which Directions, it is prefumed, even the younger Pupils can make no Miftakes.

INDEX.

INDEX.

Dragon's-

INDEX.

Puge

INDEX.

INDEX.

INDEX.

INDEX.

Bb—

INDEX.

Z.

There having been some material Additions made, after the *Index* was committed to the Press, they have occasioned the following Alterations in the *Numbers*, which the Reader is desired to correct.

III. A Treatise on the Powers of Medicines, by the late learned Herman Boerhaave, Doctor of Philosophy and Physic, and Professor of Physic, Botany, and Chymistry in the University of Leyden. Translated from the most correct Latin Edition, by JOHN MARTYN Fellow of the Royal Society and Professor of Botany in the University. of Cambridge. Price bound in Calf 5 s.

IV. The Ladies Dispensatory; or, every Woman her own Physician: Treating of the Nature, Causes, and various Symptoms of all the Diseases, Infirmities, and Disorders, natural and contracted, that most peculiarly affect the Fair Sex, in all their different Situations of Life; as Maids, married Women, and Widows, &c. Price bound 2 s. 6 d.

V. Dr. SYDENHAM's compleat Method of curing all Diseases, and Description of all their Symptoms; to which are now added, five Discourses by the same Author, concerning the Pleurify, Gout, hysterical Passion, Dropsy, Rheumatism, &c. Price bound 1 s. 6 d.

VI. The whole Works of Dr. ARCHIBALD PITCAIRN, published by himself. Wherein are discover'd, the true Foundation and Principles of the Art of Phisic; with Cases and Observations upon most Distempers and Medicines. Done from the Latin Original by George Sewell, Mr. D. and J. T. Desaguliers, D. D. and F. R. S. To which is added an Account of the Author. Price bound in Calf 4 s.

VII. Nature Delineated: Being Philosophical Conversations; wherein the wonderful Works of Providence, in the Animal, Vegetable, and Mineral Creation are laid open; the Solar and Planetary System, and whatever is curious in the Mathematicks, explained. The Whole being a Compleat Course of Natural and Experimental Philosophy; calculated for the Instruction of Youth; in order to prepare them for an early Knowledge of Natural History, and create in their Minds an exalted Idea of the Wisdom of the GREAT CREATOR. Written by Way of Dialogue, to render the Conception more familiar and easy. Translated from the Original French, by JOHN KELLY, of the Inner Temple, Esq; D. BELLAMY of St. John's College, Oxford; and J. SPARROW, Surgeon and Mathematician. Neatly printed, on a new Letter, and Superfine Paper, in Four Volumes, 12mo. Price bound in Calf 12 s. The third Edition carefully revised and corrected, with large Additions, embellished with great Variety of Copper Plates, representing the principal Subjects treated of, with a Table of Contents, and a Compleat and Copious Index to each Volume.

These Volumes contain a curious Account of the Original and last State of all the various Productions of Nature, with the Uses they are applied to, and the Benefit Mankind receive therefrom, comprehending all Manner of Insects, Beasts, Birds, Fishes, Fruits, Flowers, Gardens, Orchards, Vineyards, Forests, Quarries, the several Sorts of Stones, as Diamonds, Rubies, &c. an Account of the Atmosphere, Sun, Moon, Eclipses, Painting, Engraving, Statuary, Dyalling, Geometry, &c. with whatever is curious and remarkable throughout the terrestrial Globe, being not only a useful Companion to those who are acquainted with the Subjects treated of, but also very necessary for instructing the Youth of both Sexes, having lately been introduced and well received in most of the great Schools throughout the Kingdoms of Great Britain and Ireland.

VIII. A Collection of scarce and valuable Treatises upon Metals, Mines, and Minerals: Being a Translation from the learned Albaro Alonso Barba, Director of the Mines at Potosi, in the Spanish West-Indies, and the Observations of several ingenious Persons of our own County, founded on many Years Experience. Price bound 3 s.

IX. The History of the Life and Reign of LEWIS XIV, King of France and Navarre. Containing an exact and comprehensive Relation of all the Battles, Sieges, Insurrections, Negotiations, Intrigues, and secret Designs; Literary and other Foundations. Inventions, and Improvements; Contests and Proceedings, Ecclesiastical and Civil; with whatever else is memorable in that long and active Reign. With Characters of the principal Persons concerned in them, and Reflections on the most remarkable Events. In 3 Vol.

X. The History of the Life and Reign of WILLIAM III. King of England, Prince of Orange, and Hereditary Statholder of the United Provinces: Containing a Series of memorable Efforts, Military and Political, for Maintaining the Liberties of Europe against the Encroachments of Popery and Arbitrary Power. Introduced with a brief Account of the History and Genealogy of his Family.

XI. A New History of the Life and Reign of the CZAR PETER the Great, Emperor of all Russia, and Father of his Country. Containing his Wars with the Swedes, Turks, Tartars, and Persians. His Travels, Studies, and Personal Fatigues. With a distinct Account of whatever is remarkable throughout his Reign; and a correct Geographical Description of that extensive Empire.

CPSIA information can be obtained at www.ICGtesting.com
Printed in the USA
LVOW131323040112

262375LV00013B/144/P